Caring for Our Children:

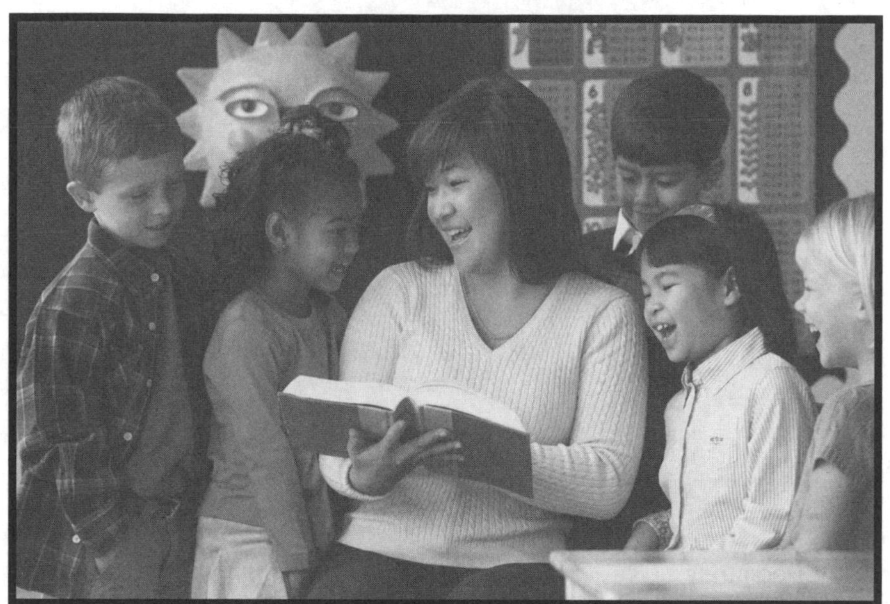

National Health and Safety Performance Standards; Guidelines for Early Care and Education Programs, Third Edition

A Joint Collaborative Project of

American Academy of Pediatrics
141 Northwest Point Boulevard
Elk Grove Village, IL 60007-1019

American Public Health Association
800 I Street, NW
Washington, DC 20001-3710

National Resource Center for Health and Safety in Child Care and Early Education
University of Colorado, College of Nursing
13120 E 19th Avenue
Aurora, CO 80045

Support for this project was provided by the
Maternal and Child Health Bureau,
Health Resources and Services Administration,
U.S. Department of Health and Human Services
(Cooperative Agreement #U46MC09810)

Second printing with minor corrections noted by asterisks, August 2011.
Go to http://nrckids.org for future changes/additions to this publication.

Suggested Citation:
American Academy of Pediatrics, American Public Health Association, National Resource Center for Health and Safety in Child Care and Early Education. 2011. *Caring for our children: National health and safety performance standards; Guidelines for early care and education programs*. 3rd Edition. Elk Grove Village, IL: American Academy of Pediatrics; Washington, DC: American Public Health Association. Also available at http://nrckids.org.

ISBN 978-1-58110-483-7 (American Academy of Pediatrics)
MA0552 (American Academy of Pediatrics)

Printed and bound in the United States of America
Design & Typesetting: Lorie Bircher, Betty Geer, Susan Paige Lehtola, Garrett T. Risley

2 3 4 5 6 7 8 9 10

Table of Contents

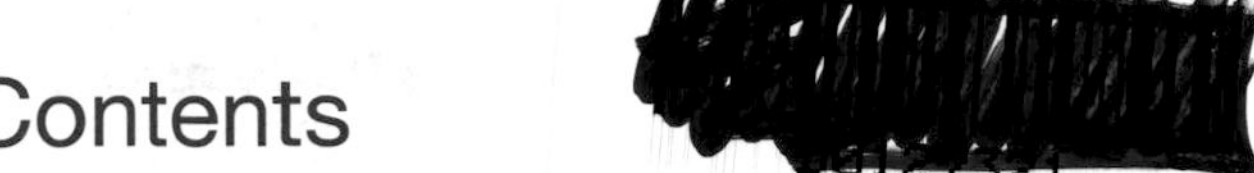

***Addition to Table of Contents in second printing, August 2011.

*Corrected page number in second printing, August 2011.

*Corrected page number in second printing, August 2011.

**Corrected to "Administration" from "Policies" in second printing, August 2011.

***Addition to Table of Contents in second printing, August 2011.

*Corrected page number in second printing, August 2011.

*Corrected page number in second printing, August 2011.
**Corrected to "Medical/Dental" from "Medical" in second printing, August 2011.
**Corrected to "Acronyms/Abbreviations" from "Acronyms" in second printing, August 2011

ACKNOWLEDGMENTS

The National Resource Center for Health and Safety in Child Care would like to acknowledge the outstanding contributions of all persons and organizations involved in the revision of *Caring for Our Children: National Health and Safety Performance Standards: Guidelines for Out-of-Home Child Care Programs, Third Edition*. The collaboration of the American Academy of Pediatrics, the American Public Health Association, and the Maternal and Child Health Bureau provided a wide scope of technical expertise from their constituents in the creation of this project. The subject-specific Technical Panels as listed provided the majority of the content and resources. Over 180 organizations and individuals were asked to review and validate the accuracy of the content and contribute additional expertise where applicable. The individuals representing these organizations are listed in *Stakeholder Reviewers/Additional Contributors* (see below). This broad collaboration and review from the best minds in the field has led to a more comprehensive and useful tool.

In a project of such scope, many individuals provide valuable input to the end product. We would like to acknowledge those individuals whose names may have been omitted.

Steering Committee

Danette Swanson Glassy, MD, FAAP
Co-Chair, American Academy of Pediatrics;
Mercer Island, WA

Jonathan B. Kotch, MD, MPH, FAAP
Co-Chair, American Public Health Association;
Chapel Hill, NC

Barbara U. Hamilton, MA
Project Officer, U.S. Department of Health and Human Services, Health Resources and Services Administration, Maternal and Child Health Bureau; Rockville, MD

Marilyn J. Krajicek, EdD, RN, FAAN
Director, National Resource Center for Health and Safety in Child Care and Early Education; Aurora, CO

Phyllis Stubbs-Wynn, MD, MPH
Former Project Officer, U.S. Department of Health and Human Services, Health Resources and Services Administration, Maternal and Child Health Bureau; Rockville, MD

The *Caring for Our Children,* 3rd Ed. Steering Committee would like to express special gratitude to the Co-Chairs of the First and/or Second Editions:
Dr. Susan Aronson, MD, FAAP;
Dr. Albert Chang, MD, MPH, FAAP; and
Dr. George Sterne, MD, FAAP.

Their leadership and dedication in setting the bar high for quality health and safety standards in early care and education ensured that children experienced healthier and safer lives and environments in child care and provided a valuable and nationally recognized resource for all in the field. We are pleased to build upon their foundational work in this Third Edition with new science and research.

Technical Panel Chairs and Members

Child Abuse

Anne B. Keith, DrPH, RN, C-PNP, Chair; New Gloucester, ME
Melissa Brodowski, MSW, MPH; Washington, DC
Gilbert Handal, MD, FAAP; El Paso, TX
Carole Jenny, MD, MBA, FAAP; Providence, RI
Salwa Khan, MD, MHS; Baltimore, MD
Ashley Lucas, MD, FAAP; Baton Rouge, LA
Hannah Pressler, MHS, PNP-BC; Portland, ME
Sara E. Schuh, MD, FAAP; Charleston, SC

Child Development

Angela Crowley, PhD, APRN, CS, PNP-BC, Chair; New Haven, CT
George J. Cohen, MD, FAAP; Rockville, MD
Christine Garvey, PhD, RN; Chicago, IL
Walter S. Gilliam, PhD; New Haven, CT
Peter A. Gorski, MD, MPA; Tampa, FL
Mary Louise Hemmeter, PhD; Nashville, TN
Michael Kaplan, MD; New Haven, CT
Cynthia Olson, MS; New Haven, CT
Deborah F. Perry, PhD; Baltimore, MD
June Solnit Sale, MSW; Los Angeles, CA

Children with Special Health Care Needs

Herbert J. Cohen, MD, FAAP, Chair; Bronx, NY
Elaine Donoghue, MD, FAAP; Neptune, NJ
Lillian Kornhaber, PT, MPH; Bronx, NY
Jack M. Levine, MD, FAAP; New Hyde Park, NY
Cordelia Robinson Rosenberg, PhD, RN; Aurora, CO
Sarah Schoen, PhD, OTR; Greenwood Village, CO
Nancy Tarshis, MA, CCC/SP; Bronx, NY
Melanie Tyner-Wilson, MS; Lexington, KY

Environmental Quality

Steven B. Eng, MPH, CIPHI(C), Chair; Port Moody, BC
Darlene Dinkins; Washington, DC
Hester Dooley, MS; Portland, OR
Bettina Fletcher; Washington, DC
C. Eve J. Kimball, MD, FAAP; West Reading, PA
Kathy Seikel, MBA; Washington, DC
Richard Snaman, REHS/RS; Arlington, VA
Brooke Stebbins, BSN; Concord, NH
Nsedu Obot Witherspoon, MPH; Washington, DC

General Health

CAPT. Timothy R. Shope, MD, MPH, FAAP, Chair; Portsmouth, VA
Abbey Alkon, RN, PNP, PhD; San Francisco, CA
Paul Casamassimo, DDS, MS; Columbus, OH
Sandra Cianciolo, MPH, RN; Chapel Hill, NC
Beth A. DelConte, MD, FAAP; Broomall, PA
Karen Leamer, MD, FAAP; Denver, CO
Judy Romano, MD, FAAP; Martins Ferry, OH

Linda Satkowiak, ND, RN, CNS; Denver, CO
Karen Sokal-Gutierrez, MD, MPH, FAAP; Berkeley, CA

Infectious Diseases

Larry Pickering, MD, FAAP, Chair; Atlanta, GA
Ralph L. Cordell, PhD; Atlanta, GA
Dennis L. Murray, MD; Augusta, GA
Thomas J. Sandora, MD, MPH; Boston, MA
Andi L. Shane, MD, MPH; Atlanta, GA

Injury Prevention

Seth Scholer, MD, MPH, Chair; Nashville, TN
Laura Aird, MS; Elk Grove Village, IL
Sally Fogerty, BSN, Med; Newton, MA
Paula Deaun Jackson, MSN, CRNP, LNC; Philadelphia, PA
Rhonda Laird; Nashville, TN
Sarah L. Myers, RN; Moorhead, MN
Susan H. Pollack, MD, FAAP; Lexington, KY
Ellen R. Schmidt, MS, OTR; Washington, DC
Alexander W. (Sandy) Sinclair; Washington, DC
Donna Thompson, PhD; Cedar Falls, IA

Nutrition

Catherine Cowell, PhD, Chair; New York, NY
Sara Benjamin Neelon, PhD, MPH, RD; Durham, NC
Donna Blum-Kemelor, MS, RD, LD; Alexandria, VA
Robin Brocato, MHS; Washington, DC
Kristen Copeland, MD, FAAP; Cincinnati, OH
Suzanne Haydu, MPH, RD; Sacramento, CA
Janet Hill, MS, RD, IBCLC; Sacramento, CA
Susan L. Johnson, PhD; Aurora, CO
Ruby Natale, PhD, PsyD; Miami, FL
Jeanette Panchula, BSW, RN, PHN, IBCLC
Shana Patterson, RD; Denver, CO
Barbara Polhamus, PhD, MPH, RD; Atlanta, GA
Susan Schlosser, MS, RD; Chappaqua, NY
Denise Sofka, MPH, RD; Rockville, MD
Jamie Stang, PhD, MPH, RD; Minneapolis, MN

Organization and Administration

Christopher A. Kus, MD, MPH, Chair; Albany, NY
Christine Ross–Baze; Topeka, KS
Janet Carter; Dover, DE
Sally Clausen, ARNP, BSN; Des Moines, IA
Judy Collins; Norman, OK
Pauline Koch; Newark, DE
Jackie Quirk; Raleigh, NC

Staff Health

Amy C. Cory, PhD, RN, CPNP, PCNS, BC, Chair; Valparaiso, IN
Patricia S. Cole; Indianapolis, IN
Susan Eckelt, CDA; Tulsa, OK
Bethany Geldmaker, PNP, PhD; Richmond, VA
Stephanie Olmore, MA; Washington, DC
Barbara Sawyer; Arvada, CO

Lead Organizations' Reviewers

American Academy of Pediatrics
Sandra G. Hassink, MD, MPH, FAAP
Jeanne VanOrsdal, MEd

American Public Health Association
Elizabeth L. M. Miller, BSN, RN, BC; Newtown Square, PA
Barbara Schwartz, PhD; New York, NY

U.S. Department of Health and Human Services, Health Resources and Services Administration, Maternal and Child Health Bureau
R. Lorraine Brown, RN, BS, CPHP; Rockville, MD
CAPT. Stephanie Bryn, MPH; Rockville, MD
Denise Sofka, MPH, RD; Rockville, MD

National Resource Center for Health and Safety in Child Care and Early Education Project Team
Marilyn J. Krajicek, EdD, RN, FAAN; Director
Jean M. Cimino, MPH; Professional Research Assistant
Betty Geer, MSN, RN, CPNP; Research Assistant
Barbara U. Hamilton, MA; Former Assistant Director
Susan Paige Lehtola, BBA, BS; Research Assistant
David Merten, BS; Former Research Assistant
Garrett T. Risley, MBA-HA; Research Assistant
Linda Satkowiak, ND, RN, CNS; Nurse Consultant
Gerri Steinke, PhD; Evaluator
Ginny Torrey, BA; Program Specialist

Stakeholder Reviewers/Additional Contributors

Kenneth C. Akwuole, PhD
U.S. Administration for Children and Families, Office of Child Care, DC

Duane Alexander, MD, FAAP
National Institute of Child Health and Human Development, MD

Abbey Alkon, RN, PNP, MPH, PhD
American Academy of Pediatrics, Section on Early Education and Child Care, IL
University of California San Francisco, California Childcare Health Program, CA

Krista Allison, RN, BSN
Parent, CO

Jamie Anderson, RNC, IBCLC
New Jersey Department of Health and Senior Services, Division of Family Health Services, NJ

Kristie Applegren, MD
American Academy of Pediatrics, Council on Communication and Media, IL

Lois D. W. Arnold, PhD, MPH
National Commission on Donor Milk Banking, American Breastfeeding Institute, MA

Susan Aronson, MD, FAAP
Healthy Child Care America Pennsylvania, Pennsylvania Chapter of the American Academy of Pediatrics, PA

Polly T. Barey, RN, MS
Connecticut Nurses Association, CT

Molly Bauer, ARNP, CPNP, RN
University of Iowa Health Care, IA

Kristen Becker
Parent, WA

Debbie Beirne
Virginia Department of Social Services and Division of Licensing, VA

Nancy P. Bernard, MPH
Washington State Department of Health, Indoor Air Quality/ School Environmental Health and Safety, WA

Wendy Bickford, MA
Buell Early Childhood Leadership Program, CO

Julia D. Block, MD, MPH, FAAP
American Academy of Pediatrics, NY

Kathie Boe
Knowledge Learning Corporation, OR

Kathie Boling
Zero to Three, DC

Suzanne Boulter, MD, FAAP
American Academy of Pediatrics, Section on Pediatric Dentistry and Oral Health, IL

Laurel Branen, PhD, RD, LD
University of Idaho, School of Family and Consumer Sciences, ID

Marsha R. Brookins
U.S. Administration for Children and Families, DC

Mary Jane Brown
Centers for Disease Control and Prevention, Environment Division, GA

Oscar Brown, MD, FAAP
American Academy of Pediatrics, Committee on Practice in Ambulatory Medicine and Immunizations, IL

Heather Brumberg, MD, MPH, FAAP
American Academy of Pediatrics, Committee on Environmental Health, IL

Barbara Cameron, MA, MSW
University of North Carolina, Carolina Breastfeeding Institute, NC

Charles Cappetta, MD, FAAP
American Academy of Pediatrics, Council on Sports Medicine and Fitness, IL

Anne Carmody, BS
Wisconsin Department of Children and Families, Bureau of Early Care Regulation, WI

Anna Carter
North Carolina Division of Child Development, NC

Susan Case
Oklahoma Department of Human Services, OK

Dimitri Christakis, MD, FAAP
American Academy of Pediatrics, Council on Communication and Media, IL

Tom Clark, MD, FAAP

Task Force of the Youth Futures Authority, GA

Sally Clausen, ARNP, BSN
Healthy Child Care America, IA

Abby J. Cohen, JD
National Child Care Information and Technical Assistance Center, CA

Herbert J. Cohen, MD, FAAP

Albert Einstein College of Medicine, Department of Pediatrics, NY

Teresa Cooper, RN
Washington Early Childhood Comprehensive Systems, State Department of Health, WA

Kristen A. Copeland, MD, FAAP
Cincinnati Children's Hospital Medical Center, OH

Ron Coté, PE
National Fire Protection Association, MA

William Cotton, MD, FAAP
American Academy of Pediatrics, Council on Community Pediatrics, IL

Melissa Courts
Ohio Early Childhood Comprehensive Systems, Healthy Child Care America, OH

Debby Cryer, PhD
University of North Carolina-Chapel Hill, FPG Child Development Institute, NC

Edward Curry, MD, FAAP
American Academy of Pediatrics, Committee on Practice in Ambulatory Medicine and Immunizations, IL

Nancy M. Curtis
Maryland Health and Human Services,
Montgomery County, MD

Cynthia Devore, MD, FAAP
American Academy of Pediatrics,
Council on School Health, IL

Ann Ditty, MA
National Association for Regulatory Administration, KY

Steven M. Donn, MD, FAAP
American Academy of Pediatrics, Committee on Medical Liability and Risk Management, IL

Elaine Donoghue, MD, FAAP
American Academy of Pediatrics, Committee on Early Childhood, Adoption, and Dependent Care, IL
American Academy of Pediatrics, Section on Early Education and Child Care, IL

Adrienne Dorf, MPH, RD, CD
Public Health - Seattle and King County, WA

Jacqueline Douge, MD, FAAP
American Academy of Pediatrics, Council on Communication and Media, IL

Benard Dreyer, MD, FAAP
American Academy of Pediatrics, Council on Communication and Media, IL

Jose Esquibel
Colorado Department of Public Health and Environment, CO

Karen Farley, RD, IBCLC
California WIC Association, CA

Rick Fiene, PhD
Penn State University, Capital Area Early Childhood Training Institute, PA

Margaret Fisher, MD, FAAP
American Academy of Pediatrics, Disaster Preparedness Advisory Council, IL
American Academy of Pediatrics, Section on Infectious Diseases, IL

Thomas Fleisher, MD, FAAP
American Academy of Pediatrics, Section on Allergy and Immunology, IL

Janice Fletcher, EdD
University of Idaho, School of Family and Consumer Sciences, ID

Carroll Forsch
South Dakota Department of Social Services, Division of Child Care Services, SD

Daniel Frattarelli, MD, FAAP
American Academy of Pediatrics, Section on Clinical Pharmacology and Therapeutics/Committee on Drugs, IL

Doris Fredericks, MEd, RD, FADA
Child Development, Inc., Choices for Children, CA

Gilbert Fuld, MD, FAAP
American Academy of Pediatrics, Council on Communication and Media, IL

Jill Fussell, MD, FAAP
American Academy of Pediatrics, Committee on Early Childhood, Adoption, and Dependent Care, Section on Developmental and Behavioral Pediatrics, IL

Carol Gage
U.S. Administration for Children and Families, Office of Child Care, DC

Robert Gilchick, MD, MPH
Los Angeles County Department of Public Health, Child and Adolescent Health Program and Policy, CA

Frances Page Glascoe, PhD
American Academy of Pediatrics, Section on Developmental and Behavioral Pediatrics, IL

Mary P. Glode, MD, FAAP
American Academy of Pediatrics, Committee on Infectious Diseases, IL

Eloisa Gonzalez, MD, MPH
Los Angeles County Department of Public Health, Physical Activity and Cardiovascular Health Program, CA

Rosario Gonzalez, MD, FAAP
American Academy of Pediatrics, Council on Communication and Media, IL

Joseph Hagan, MD, FAAP
American Academy of Pediatrics, Bright Futures, IL

Michelle Hahn, RN, PHN, BSN
Healthy Child Care Minnesota, MN

Cheryl Hall, RN, BSN, CCHC
Maryland State Department of Education, U.S. Administration for Children and Families, Office of Child Care, MD

Lawrence D. Hammer, MD, FAAP
American Academy of Pediatrics, Committee on Practice in Ambulatory Medicine and Immunizations, IL

Gil Handal, MD, FAAP
American Academy of Pediatrics, Council on Community Pediatrics, IL

Patty Hannah
KinderCare Learning Centers, OH

Jodi Hardin, MPH
Early Childhood Systems, CO

Thelma Harms, PhD
University of North Carolina-Chapel Hill, NC

Sandra Hassink, MD, FAAP
American Academy of Pediatrics, Obesity Initiatives, IL

James Henry
U.S. Administration for Children and Families, Office of Child Care, DC

Mary Ann Heryer, MA
University of Missouri at Kansas City, Institute of Human Development, MO

Karen Heying
National Infant and Toddler Child Care Initiative, Zero to Three, DC

Pam High, MD, MS, FAAP
American Academy of Pediatrics, Committee on Early Childhood Adoption and Dependent Care, IL

Chanda Nicole Holsey, DrPH, MPH, AE-C
San Diego State University, Graduate School of Public Health, CA

Sarah Hoover, MEd
University of Colorado School of Medicine,
JFK Partners, CO

Gail Houle, PhD
U.S. Department of Education, Early Childhood Programs Office of Special Education, DC

Bob Howard
Division of Child Day Care Licensing and Regulatory Services, SC

Julian Hsin-Cheng Wan, MD, FAAP
American Academy of Pediatrics, Section on Urology, IL

Moniquin Huggins
U.S. Administration for Children and Families, Office of Child Care, DC

Anne Hulick, RN, MS, JD
Connecticut Nurses Association, CT

Tammy Hurley
American Academy of Pediatrics, Section on Child Abuse and Neglect, IL

Mary Anne Jackson, MD, FAAP
American Academy of Pediatrics, Committee on Infectious Diseases, IL

Paula Deaun Jackson, MSN, CPNP, CCHC
Pediatric Nurse Practitioner and Child Care Health Consultant, PA

Paula James
Contra Costa Child Care Council, Child Health and Nutrition Program, CA

Laura Jana, MD, FAAP
American Academy of Pediatrics, Section on Early Education and Child Care, IL

Renee Jarrett, MPH
American Academy of Pediatrics, Section on Early Education and Child Care, IL

Paula Jaudes, MD, FAAP
American Academy of Pediatrics, Committee on Early Childhood, Adoption, and Dependent Care, IL

Lowest Jefferson, REHS/RS, MS, PHA
Department of Health, WA

Mark Jenkerson
Missouri Department of Health and Senior Services, MO

Lynn Jezyk
U.S. Administration for Children and Families, Office of Child Care Licensing, DC

Veronnie Faye Jones, MD, FAAP
American Academy of Pediatrics, Committee on Early Childhood, Adoption, and Dependent Care, IL

Mark Kastenbaum
Department of Early Learning, WA

Harry L. Keyserling, MD, FAAP
American Academy of Pediatrics, Committee on Infectious Diseases, IL

Matthew Edward Knight, MD, FAAP
American Academy of Pediatrics, Section on Clinical Pharmacology and Therapeutics/Committee on Drugs, IL

Pauline Koch
National Association for Regulatory Administration, DE

Bonnie Kozial
American Academy of Pediatrics, Section/Committee on Injury, Violence, and Poison Prevention, IL

Steven Krug, MD, FAAP
American Academy of Pediatrics, Disaster Preparedness Advisory Council, IL

Mae Kyono, MD, FAAP
American Academy of Pediatrics, Section on Early Education and Child Care, IL

Miriam Labbok, MD, MPH, FACPM, FABM, IBCLC
University of North Carolina, Carolina Breastfeeding Institute, NC

Mary LaCasse, MS, EdD
Department of Mental Health and Hygiene, MD

James Laughlin, MD, FAAP
American Academy of Pediatrics, Committee on Practice in Ambulatory Medicine and Immunizations, IL

Sharis LeMay
Alabama Department of Public Health, Healthy Child Care Alabama, AL

Vickie Leonard, RN, FNP, PhD
University of California San Francisco, California Childcare Health Program, CA

Herschel Lessin, MD, FAAP
American Academy of Pediatrics, Committee on Practice in Ambulatory Medicine and Immunizations, IL

Michael Leu, MD, MS, MHS, FAAP
American Academy of Pediatrics, Council on Communication and Media, IL

Katy Levenhagen, MS, RD
Snohomish Health District, WA

Linda L. Lindeke, PhD, RN, CNP
American Academy of Pediatrics,
Medical Home Initiatives, IL

Michelle Macias, MD, FAAP
American Academy of Pediatrics, Section on Developmental and Behavioral Pediatrics, IL

Karin A. Mack, PhD
Centers for Disease Control and Prevention, GA

Maxine M. Maloney
U.S. Administration for Children and Families, Office of Child Care, DC

Barry Marx, MD, FAAP
U.S. Office of Head Start, DC

Bryce McClamroch
Massachusetts Early Childhood Comprehensive Systems, State Department of Public Health, MA

Janet R. McGinnis
North Carolina Department of Public Instruction, Office of Early Learning, NC

Ellen McGuffey, CPNP
National Association of Pediatric Nurse Practitioners , NJ

Kandi Mell
Juvenile Products Manufacturers Association, NJ

Shelly Meyer, RN, BSN, PHN, CCHC
Missoula City-County Health Department, Child Care Resources, MT

Joan Younger Meek, MD, MS, RD, IBCLC
Orlando Health, Arnold Palmer Hospital for Children, Florida State University College of Medicine, FL

Angela Mickalide, PhD, CHES
Home Safety Council, DC

Jonathan D. Midgett, PhD
U.S. Consumer Product Safety Commission, MD

Mark Minier, MD, FAAP
American Academy of Pediatrics,
Council on School Health, IL

Mary Beth Miotto, MD, FAAP
American Academy of Pediatrics, Council on Communication and Media, IL

Antoinette Montgomery, BA
Parent, VA

Rachel Moon, MD, FAAP
American Academy of Pediatrics, Task Force on Infant Positioning and SIDS, IL

Len Morrissey
ASTM International, PA

Jane Morton, MD, FAAP
American Academy of Pediatrics,
Section on Breastfeeding, IL

Robert D. Murray, MD, FAAP
American Academy of Pediatrics,
Council on School Health, IL

Scott Needle, MD, FAAP
American Academy of Pediatrics, Disaster Preparedness Advisory Council, IL

Sara Benjamin Neelon, PhD, MPH, RD
Duke University Medical Center, Duke Global Health Institute, NC

Jeffrey Okamoto, MD, FAAP, FAACPDM
American Academy of Pediatrics,
Council on School Health, IL

Isaac Okehie
U.S. Administration for Children and Families, Office of Child Care, DC

Stephanie Olmore
National Association for the Education of Young Children, DC

John Pascoe, MD, MPH, FAAP
American Academy of Pediatrics, Committee on Psychosocial Aspects of Child and Family Health, IL

Shana Patterson, RD
Colorado Physical Activity and Nutrition Program, CO

Jerome A. Paulson, MD, FAAP
American Academy of Pediatrics, Committee on Environmental Health, IL

Kathy Penfold, MSN, RN
Department of Health and Human Services, MO

Leatha Perez-Chun, MS
U.S. Administration for Children and Families, Office of Child Care, DC

Christine Perreault, RN, MHA
The Children's Hospital, CO

Lauren Pfeiffer
Juvenile Products Manufacturers Association, NJ

Lisa Albers Prock, MD, MPH
American Academy of Pediatrics, Section on Adoption and Foster Care, IL

Susan K. Purcell, BS, MA
Grandparent, CO

Dawn Ramsburg, PhD
U.S. Administration for Children and Families, Office of Child Care, DC

Chadwick Rodgers, MD, FAAP
American Academy of Pediatrics, Committee on Practice in Ambulatory Medicine and Immunizations, IL

Judy Romano, MD, FAAP
American Academy of Pediatrics, Section on Early Education and Child Care, IL

Kate Roper, EdM
Massachusetts Early Childhood Comprehensive Systems, State Department of Public Health, MA

Bobbie Rose, RN
University of California San Francisco, California Childcare Health Program, CA

Lori Saltzman
U.S. Consumer Products Safety Commission, MD

Teresa Sakraida, PhD, MS, MSEd, BSN
University of Colorado, College of Nursing, CO

Kim Sandor, RN, MSN, FNP
Connecticut Nurses Association, CT

Karen Savoie, RDH, BS
Colorado Area Health Education Center System, Cavity Free at Three, CO

Barbara Sawyer
National Association for Family Child Care, CO

Beverly Schmalzried
National Association of Child Care Resource and Referral Agencies, VA

David J. Schonfeld, MD, FAAP
American Academy of Pediatrics, Disaster Preparedness Advisory Council, IL

Gordon E. Schutze, MD, FAAP
American Academy of Pediatrics, Committee on Infectious Diseases, IL

Lynne Shulster, PhD
Centers for Disease Control and Prevention, GA

Steve Shuman
Consultant, CA

Benjamin S. Siegel, MD, FAAP
American Academy of Pediatrics, Committee on Psychosocial Aspects of Child and Family Health, IL

Geoffrey Simon, MD, FAAP
American Academy of Pediatrics, Committee on Practice in Ambulatory Medicine and Immunizations, IL

Heather Smith
Parent, MO

Linda J. Smith, BSE, FACCE, IBCLC, FILCA
Bright Future Lactation Resource Centre, OH

Karen Sokal-Gutierrez, MD, MPH, FAAP
UCB-UCSF Joint Medical Program, CA

Robin Stanton, MA, RD, LD
Oregon Public Health Division,
Adolescent Health Section, OR

Brooke Stebbins
Healthy Child Care New Hampshire, Department of Public Health Services, NH

Kathleen M. Stiles, MA
Colorado Office of Professional Development, CO

Justine Strickland
Georgia Department of Early Care and Learning, Child Care Policy, GA

Jeanine Swenson, MD, FAAP
American Academy of Pediatrics, Council on Communication and Media, IL

Barbara Thompson
U.S. Department of Defense, Office of Family Policy/Children and Youth, VA

Lynne E. Torpy, RD
Colorado Department of Public Health and Environment, Colorado Child and Adult Care Food Program, CO

Michael Trautman, MD, FAAP
American Academy of Pediatrics, Section on Transport Medicine, IL

Patricia A. Treadwell, MD, FAAP
American Academy of Pediatrics, Section on Dermatology, IL

Mari Uehara, MD
University of Hawaii at Manoa, John A. Burns School of Medicine, Department of Pediatrics, HI

Taara Vedvik
Parent, CO

Darlene Watford
U.S. Environmental Protection Agency, Office of Pollution Prevention and Toxics, DC

Holly E. Wells
American Association of Poison Control Centers, VA

Lani Wheeler, MD, FAAP
American Academy of Pediatrics, Council on School Health, IL

Grace Whitney, PhD, MPA
Connecticut Head Start Collaboration Office, CT

Karen Cachevki Williams, PhD
University of Wyoming, Department of Family and Consumer Sciences, WY

David Willis, MD, FAAP
American Academy of Pediatrics, Section on Early Education and Child Care, IL

Cindy Young, MPH, RD, CLE
County of Los Angeles Department of Public Health, CA

INTRODUCTION

Every day millions of children attend early care and education programs. It is critical that they have the opportunity to grow and learn in healthy and safe environments with caring and professional caregivers/teachers. Following health and safety best practices is an important way to provide quality early care and education for young children. The American Academy of Pediatrics (AAP), the American Public Health Association (APHA), and the National Resource Center for Health and Safety in Child Care and Early Education (NRC) are pleased to release the 3rd edition of *Caring for Our Children: National Health and Safety Performance Standards; Guidelines for Early Care and Education Programs*. These national standards represent the best evidence, expertise, and experience in the country on quality health and safety practices and policies that should be followed in today's early care and education settings.

History

In 1992, the American Public Health Association (APHA) and the American Academy of Pediatrics (AAP) jointly published *Caring for Our Children: National Health and Safety Performance Standards; Guidelines for Out-of-Home Child Care Programs* (1). The publication was the product of a five year national project funded by the U.S. Department of Health and Human Services, Health Resources and Services Administration, Maternal and Child Health Bureau (MCHB). This comprehensive set of health and safety standards was a response to many years of effort by advocates for quality child care. In 1976, Aronson and Pizzo recommended development and use of national health and safety standards as part of a report to Congress in association with the *Federal Interagency Day Care Requirements* (FIDCR) *Appropriateness Study* (2). In the years that followed, experts repeatedly reaffirmed the need for these standards. For example, while the work to prepare *Caring for Our Children* was underway, the National Research Council's report, *Who Cares for America's Children? Child Care Policy for the 1990s*, called for uniform national child care standards (3). Subsequently a second edition of *Caring for Our Children* was published in 2002 addressing new knowledge generated by increasing research into health and safety in early care and education programs. The increased use of the standards both in practical onsite applications and in research documents the value of the standards and validates the importance of keeping the standards up-to-date (4). *Caring for Our Children* has been a yardstick for measuring what has been done and what still needs to be done, as well as a technical manual on how to do it.

Review Process

The Maternal and Child Health Bureau's continuing funding since 1995 of a National Resource Center for Health and Safety in Child Care and Early Education (NRC) at the University of Colorado, College of Nursing supported the work to coordinate the development of the second and third editions.

The revision of the standards for the third edition of *Caring for Our Children* was an extensive process. The third edition benefited from the contribution of eighty-six technical experts in the field of health and safety in early care and education. Reviews and recommendations were received from 184 stakeholder individuals - those representing consumers of the information and organizations representing major constituents of the early care and education community. Caregivers/teachers, parents/guardians, families, health care professionals, safety specialists, early childhood educators, early care and education advocates, regulators, and federal, military, and state agencies all brought their expertise and experience to the revision process. A complete listing of the Steering Committee, Lead Organizations' reviewers, Technical Panel members, and Stakeholder contributors appears on the Acknowledgment pages.

The process of revising the standards and the consensus building was organized in stages:

1) Technical panel chairs recruited members to their panels and reviewed the standards from the second edition. Using the best evidence available (peer reviewed scientific studies, published reports, and best practice information) they removed standards that were no longer applicable or out-of-date, identified those that were still applicable (in their original or in a revised form), and formulated many new standards that were deemed appropriate and necessary.

2) Telephone conference calls were convened among technical panel chairs to bring consensus on standards that bridge several technical areas.

3) A draft of these revised standards was sent to a national and state constituency of stakeholders for their comments and suggestions.

4) This feedback was subsequently reviewed and considered by the technical panels and a decision was made to further revise or not to revise a standard. It should be noted that the national review called attention to many important points of view and new information for additional discussion and debate.

5) The edited standards were then sent to review teams of the AAP, the APHA and the MCHB. Final copy was approved by the Steering Committee representing the four organizations (AAP, APHA, NRC and MCHB).

In projects of this scope and magnitude, the end product is only as good as the persons who participate in the effort. It is hard to enumerate in this introduction the countless hours of dedication and effort from contributors and reviewers. The project owes each of them a huge debt of gratitude. Their reward will come when high-quality early care and education services become available to all children and their families!

Overview of Content and Format Changes

Caring for Our Children, 3rd Edition contains ten chapters of 686 Standards and thirty-nine Appendices. We have made the following significant content and format changes in the third edition:

- Total of fifty-eight new standards and fifteen new appendices.
- Developed new and revised standards in all areas. Some key areas of change include:
  - o Use of early childhood mental health consultants and early education consultants;
  - o Monitoring children's development and obtaining consent for screening;
  - o Positive behavior management;
  - o Limiting screen time;
  - o Promoting physical activity;
  - o Swaddling;
  - o Healthy eating (including *MyPlate*, the United States Department of Agriculture (USDA) new primary food icon);
  - o Encouraging breastfeeding;
  - o Hand sanitizers;
  - o Sun safety and sunscreen;
  - o Integrated pest management;
  - o Influenza control; and
  - o Environmentally friendly settings and use of least toxic products.
- Updated and added new appendices including:
  - o Care plan for children with special health care needs;
  - o Helmet safety;
  - o Helping children in foster care make successful transitions;
  - o Medication administration forms;
  - o A poster on encouraging breastfeeding in early care and education settings;
  - o Authorization for emergency medical/dental care.
  - o Healthier eating as shown in the USDA *MyPlate*, which replaces *MyPyramid* to support healthier food choices.

For the list of new and significantly revised standards and appendices, see pages xxiv-xxix. See the Table of Contents for a list of all Appendices.

- Created new numbering system to differentiate third edition standards from the second edition. See Appendices LL and MM for conversion charts of the numbering system;
- Updated references for the rationale and comment sections and moved the references to be placed with the standard instead of at the back of the chapter;
- Added related standards at the bottom of each standard for easy referral.

Requirements of Other Organizations

We recognize that many organizations have requirements and recommendations that apply to out-of home early care and education. For example, the National Association for the Education of Young Children (NAEYC) publishes requirements for developmentally appropriate practice and accreditation of child care centers; Head Start follows Performance Standards; the AAP has many standards related to child health; the U.S. Department of Defense has standards for military child care; the Office of Child Care (OCC) produces health and safety standards for tribal child care; the National Fire Protection Association has standards for fire safety in child care settings. The Office of Child Care administers the Child Care and Development Fund (CCDF) which provides funds to states, territories, and tribes to assist low-income families, families receiving temporary public assistance, and those transitioning from public assistance in obtaining child care so that they can work or attend training/education. Caregivers/teachers serving children funded by CCDF must meet basic health and safety requirements set by states and tribes. All of these are valuable resources, as are many excellent state publications. By addressing health and safety as an integrated component of early care and education, contributors to *Caring for Our Children* have made every effort to ensure that these standards are consistent with and complement other child care requirements and recommendations.

Continuing Improvement

Standards are never static. Each year the knowledge base increases, and new scientific findings become available. New areas of concern and interest arise. These standards will assist individuals and organizations who are involved in the continuing work of standards improvement at every level: in early care and education practice, in regulatory administration, in research in early childhood systems building, in academic curricula, and in the professional performance of the relevant disciplines.

Each of these areas affects the others in the ongoing process of improving the way we meet the needs of children. Possibly the most important use of these standards will be to raise the level of understanding about what those needs are, and to contribute to a greater willingness to commit more resources to achieve quality early care and education where children can grow and develop in a healthy and safe environment.

***Caring for Our Children, 3rd Edition* Steering Committee**
Danette Swanson Glassy, MD, FAAP
Jonathan B. Kotch, MD, MPH, FAAP
Barbara U. Hamilton, MA
Marilyn Krajicek, EdD, RN, FAAN
Phyllis Stubbs-Wynn, MD, MPH

REFERENCES:

1. American Public Health Association, American Academy of Pediatrics. 1992. *Caring for our children. National health and safety performance standards: Guidelines for out-of-home child care programs.* Washington, DC: APHA.
2. USDHEW, Office of the Assistant Secretary for Planning and Evaluation. 1977. *Policy issues in day care: Summaries of 21 papers,* 109-15.
3. National Research Council, National Academy of Sciences. 1990. *Who Cares for America's Children? Child Care Policy in the 1990s.* Washington, DC: National Academy Press.
4. Crowley, A. A., J. Kulikowich. 2009. Impact of training on child care health consultant knowledge and practice. *Ped Nurs* 35:93-100.

GUIDING PRINCIPLES

The following are the guiding principles used in writing these standards:

1. The health and safety of all children in early care and education settings is essential. The child care setting offers many opportunities for incorporating health and safety education and life skills into everyday activities. Health education for children is an investment in a lifetime of good health practices and contributes to a healthier childhood and adult life. Modeling of good health habits, such as healthy eating and physical activity, by all staff in indoor and outdoor learning/play environments, is the most effective method of health education for young children.

2. Child care for infants, young children, and school-age children is anchored in a respect for the developmental needs, characteristics, and cultures of the children and their families; it recognizes the unique qualities of each individual and the importance of early brain development in young children and in particular children birth to three years of age.

3. To the extent possible, indoor and outdoor learning/play activities should be geared to the needs of all children.

4. The relationship between parent/guardian/family and child is of utmost importance for the child's current and future development and should be supported by caregivers/teachers. Those who care for children on a daily basis have abundant, rich observational information to share, as well as offer instruction and best practices to parents/guardians. Parents/guardians should share with caregivers/teachers the unique behavioral, medical and developmental aspects of their children. Ideally, parents/guardians can benefit from time spent in the child's caregiving environment and time for the child, parent/guardian and caregiver/teacher to be together should be encouraged. Daily communication, combined with at least yearly conferences between families and the principal caregiver/teacher, should occur. Communication with families should take place through a variety of means and ensure all families, regardless of language, literacy level, or special needs, receive all of the communication.

5. The nurturing of a child's development is based on knowledge of the child's general health, growth and development, learning style, and unique characteristics. This nurturing enhances the enjoyment of both child and parent/guardian as maturation and adaptation take place. As shown by studies of early brain development, trustworthy relationships with a small number of adults and an environment conducive to bonding and learning are essential to the healthy development of children. Staff selection, training, and support should be directed to the following goals:
   a) Promoting continuity of affective relationships;
   b) Encouraging staff capacity for identification with and empathy for the child;
   c) Emphasizing an attitude of involvement as an adult in the children's play without dominating the activity;
   d) Being sensitive to cultural differences; and
   e) Being sensitive to stressors in the home environment.

6. Children with special health care needs encompass those who have or are at increased risk for a chronic physical, developmental, behavioral, or emotional condition and who also require health and related services of a type or amount beyond that generally required by children. This includes children who have intermittent and continuous needs in all aspects of health. No child with special health care needs should be denied access to child care because of his/her disability(ies), unless one of the four reasons for denying care exists: level of care required; physical limitations of the site; limited resources in the community, or unavailability of specialized, trained staff. Whenever possible, children with special health care needs should be cared for and provided services in settings including children without special health care needs.

7. Developmental programs and care should be based on a child's functional status, and the child's needs should be described in behavioral or functional terms. Children with special needs should have a comprehensive interdisciplinary or multidisciplinary evaluation if determined necessary.

8. Written policies and procedures should identify facility requirements and persons and/or entities responsible for implementing such requirements including clear guidance as to when the policy does or does not apply.

9. Whenever possible, written information about facility policies and procedures should be provided in the native language of parents/guardians, in a form appropriate for parents/guardians who are visually impaired, and also in an appropriate literacy/readability level for parents/guardians who may have difficulty with reading. However, processes should never become more important than the care and education of children.

10. Confidentiality of records and shared verbal information must be maintained to protect the child, family, and staff. The information obtained at early care and education programs should be used to plan for a child's safe and appropriate participation. Parents/guardians must be assured of the vigilance of the staff in protecting such information. When sharing information, such as referrals to services that would benefit the child, attainment of parental consent to share information must be obtained in writing. It is also important to document key communication (verbal and written) between staff and parents/guardians.

11. The facility's nutrition activities complement and supplement those of home and community. Food provided in a child care setting should help to meet the child's daily nutritional needs while reflecting individual, cultural, religious, and philosophical differences and providing an opportunity for learning. Facilities can contribute to overall child development goals by helping the child and family understand the relationship of nutrition to health, the importance of positive child feeding practices, the factors that influence food practices, and the variety of ways to meet nutritional needs. All children should engage in daily physical activity in a safe environment that promotes developmentally appropriate movement skills and a healthy lifestyle.

12. The expression of, and exposure to, cultural and ethnic diversity enriches the experience of all children, families, and staff. Planning for cultural diversity through the provision of books, toys, activities and pictures and working with language differences should be encouraged.

13. Community resources should be identified and information about their services, eligibility requirements, and hours of operation should be available to the families and utilized as much as possible to provide consultation and related services as needed.

14. Programs should continuously strive for improvement in health and safety processes and policies for the improvement of the overall quality of care to children.

15. An emergency or disaster can happen at any time. Programs should be prepared for and equipped to respond to any type of emergency or disaster in order to ensure the safety and well-being of staff and children, and communicate effectively with parents/guardians.

16. Young children should receive optimal medical care in a family-centered medical home. Cooperation and collaboration between the medical home and caregivers/teachers lead to more successful outcomes.

17. Education is an ongoing, lifelong process and child care staff need continuous education about health and safety related subject matter. Staff members who are current on health related topics are better able to prevent, recognize, and correct health and safety problems. Subjects to be covered include the rationale for health promotion and information about physical and mental health problems in the children for whom the staff care. If staff turnover is high, training on health and safety related subjects should be repeated frequently.

18. Maintaining a healthy, toxic-free physical environment positively impacts the health and well-being of the children and staff served. Environmental responsibility is an important concept to teach and practice daily.

ADVICE TO THE USER

The intended users of the standards include all who care for young children in early care and education settings and who work toward the goal of ensuring that all children from day one have the opportunity to grow and develop appropriately, to thrive in healthy and safe environments, and to develop healthy and safe behaviors that will last a lifetime.

All of the standards are attainable. Some may have already been attained in individual settings; others can be implemented over time. For example, any organization that funds early care and education should, in our opinion, adopt these standards as funding requirements and should set a payment rate that covers the cost of meeting them.

Recommended Use

- **Caregivers/Teachers** can use the standards to develop and implement sound practices, policies, and staff training to ensure that their program is healthy, safe, age-appropriate for all children in their care.
- **Early Childhood Systems** can build integrated health and safety components into their systems that promote healthy lifestyles for all children.
- **Families** have sound information from the standards to select quality programs and/or evaluate their child's current early care and education program. They can work in partnership with caregivers/teachers in promoting healthy and safe behavior and practice for their child and family. Families may also want to incorporate many of these healthy and safe practices at home.
- **Health Care Professionals** can assist families and consult with caregivers/teachers by using the standards as guidance on what makes a healthy and safe and age appropriate environment that encourages children's development of healthy and safe habits. Consultants may use the standards to develop guidance materials to share with both caregivers/teachers and parents/guardians.
- **Licensing Professionals/Regulators** can use the evidence-based rationale to develop or improve regulations that require a healthy and safe learning environment at a critical time in a child's life and develop lifelong healthy behaviors in children.
- **National Private Organizations that will update standards** for accreditation or guidance purposes for a special discipline can draw on the new work and rationales of the third edition just as *Caring for Our Children's* expert contributors drew upon the expertise of these organizations in developing the new standards.
- **Policy-Makers** are equipped with sound science to meet emerging challenges to children's development of lifelong healthy behaviors and lifestyles.
- **State Departments of Education (DOEs) and local school administrations** can use the standards to guide the writing of standards for school operated child care and preschool facilities, and this guidance will help principals to implement good practice in early care and education programs.
- **States and localities who fund subsidized care and services for income-eligible families** can use the standards to determine the level and quality of service to be expected.
- **University/College Faculty** of early childhood education programs can instill healthy practices in their students to model and use with young children upon entering the early childhood workplace and transfer the latest research into their education.

Definitions

We have defined many terms in the Glossary found on page 541. Some of these are so important to the user that we are emphasizing them here as well.

Types of Requirements:

A **standard** is a statement that defines a goal of practice. It differs from a recommendation or a guideline in that it carries greater incentive for universal compliance. It differs from a regulation in that compliance is not necessarily required for legal operation. It usually is legitimized or validated based on scientific or epidemiological data, or when this evidence is lacking, it represents the widely agreed upon, state-of-the-art, high-quality level of practice.

The agency, program, or health practitioner that does not meet the standard may incur disapproval or sanction from within or without the organization. Thus, a standard is the strongest criterion for practice set by a health organization or association. For example, many manufacturers advertise that their products meet ASTM standards as evidence to the consumer of safety, while those products that cannot meet the standards are sold without such labeling to undiscerning purchasers.

A **guideline** is a statement of advice or instruction pertaining to practice. It originates in an organization with acknowledged professional standing. Although it may be unsolicited, a guideline often is developed in response to a stated request or perceived need for such advice or instruction. For example, the American Academy of Pediatrics (AAP) has a guideline for the elements necessary to make the diagnosis of Attention-Deficit/Hyperactivity Disorder.

A **regulation** takes a previous standard or guideline and makes it a requirement for legal operation. A regulation originates in an agency with either governmental or official authority and has the power of law. Such authority is usually accompanied by an enforcement activity. Examples of regulations are: State regulations pertaining to child:staff ratios in a licensed child care center, and immunizations required to enter an early care and education program. The components of the regulation will vary by topic addressed as well as by area of jurisdiction (e.g., municipality or state). Because a regulation prescribes a practice that every agency or program must comply with, it usually is the minimum or the floor below which no agency or program should operate.

Types of Facilities:

Child care offers developmentally appropriate care and education for young children who receive care in out-of-home settings (not their own home). Several types of facilities are covered by the general definition of child care and education. Although there are generally understood definitions for child care facilities, states vary greatly in their legal definitions, and some overlap and confusion of terms still exists in defining child care facilities. Although the needs of children do not differ from one setting to another, the declared intent of different types of facilities may differ. Facilities that operate part-day, in the evening, during the traditional work day and work week, or during a specific part of the year may call themselves by different names. These standards recognize that while children's needs do not differ in any of these settings, the way children's needs are met may differ by whether the facility is in a residence or a non-residence and whether the child is expected to have a longer or only a very short-term arrangement for care.

> A **Small family child care home** provides care and education of **one to six children**, including the caregiver's/teacher's own children in the home of the caregiver/teacher. Family members or other helpers may be involved in assisting the caregiver/teacher, but often, there is only one caregiver/teacher present at any one time.
>
> A **Large family child care home** provides care and education of **seven to twelve children**, including the caregiver's/teacher's own children in the home of the caregiver/teacher, with one or more qualified adult assistants to meet child: staff ratio requirements.
>
> A **Center** is a facility that provides care and education of **any number of children in a nonresidential setting**, or thirteen or more children in any setting if the facility is open on a regular basis.

For definitions of other special types of child care – drop-in, school-age, for the mildly ill – see Standard 10.4.1.1: Uniform Categories and Definitions.

The standards are to guide all the types of programs listed above.

Age Groups:

Although we recognize that designated age groups and developmental levels must be used flexibly to meet the needs of individual children, many of the standards are applicable to specific age and developmental categories. The following categories are used in *Caring for Our Children*.

	Age	**Functional Definition (By Developmental Level)**
Infant	Birth-12 months	Birth to ambulation
Toddler	13-35 months	Ambulation to accomplishment of self-care routines such as use of the toilet
Pre-schooler	36-59 months	From achievement of self-care routines to entry into regular school
School-Age Child	5-12 years	Entry into regular school, including kindergarten through 6th grade

Format and Language

Each standard unit has at least three components: the **Standard** itself, the **Rationale**, and the applicable **Type of Facility**. Most standards also have a **Comment** section, a **Related Standards** section and a **References** section. The reader will find the scientific reference and/or epidemiological evidence for the standard in the rationale section of each standard. The Rationale explains the intent of and the need for the standard. Where no scientific evidence for a standard is available, the standard is based on the best available professional consensus. If such a professional consensus has been published, that reference is cited. The Rationale both justifies the standard and serves as an educational tool. The Comments section includes other explanatory information relevant to the standard, such as applicability of the standard and, in some cases, suggested ways to measure compliance with the standard. Although this document reflects the best information available at the time of publication, as was the case with the first and second editions, this third edition will need updating from time to time to reflect changes in knowledge affecting early care and education.

Caring for Our Children is available at no cost online at http://nrckids.org. It is also available in print format for a fee from the American Academy of Pediatrics (AAP) and the American Public Health Association (APHA).

Standards have been written to be measurable and enforceable. Measurability is important for performance standards in a contractual relationship between a provider of service and a funding source. Concrete and specific language helps caregivers/teachers and facilities put the standards into practice. Where a standard is difficult to measure, we have provided guidance to make the requirement as specific as possible. Some standards required more technical terminology (e.g., certain infectious diseases, plumbing and heating terminology). We encourage readers to seek interpretation by appropriate specialists when needed. Where feasible, we have written the standards to be understood by readers from a wide variety of backgrounds.

The Steering Committee agreed to consistent use of the terms below to convey broader concepts instead of using a multitude of different terms.

- Caregiver/teacher – for the early care and education/ child care professional that provides care and learning opportunities to children—instead of child care provider, just caregiver or just teacher;
- Parents/guardians – for those adults legally responsible for a child's welfare;
- Primary care provider – for the licensed health professional, to name a few: pediatrician, pediatric nurse practitioner, family physician, who has responsibility for the health supervision of an individual child;
- Child abuse and neglect – for all forms of child maltreatment;
- Children with special health care needs – to encompass children with special needs, children with disabilities, children with chronic illnesses, etc.

Relationship of the Standards to Laws, Ordinances, and Regulations

The members of the technical panels could not annotate the standards to address local laws, ordinances, and regulations. Many of these legal requirements have a different intent from that addressed by the standards. Users of this document should check legal requirements that may apply to facilities in particular locales.

In general, child care is regulated by at least three different legal entities or jurisdictions. The first is the building code jurisdiction. Building inspectors enforce building codes to protect life and property in all buildings, not just child care facilities. Some of the standards should be written into state or local building codes, rather than into the licensing requirements.

The second major legal entity that regulates child care is the health system. A number of different codes are intended to prevent the spread of disease in restaurants, hospitals, and other institutions where hazards and risky practices might exist. Many of these health codes are not specific to child care; however, specific provisions for child care might be found in a health code. Some of the provisions in the standards might be appropriate for incorporation into a health code.

The third legal jurisdiction applied to child care is child care licensing. Usually, before a child care operator receives a license, the operator must obtain approvals from health and building safety authorities. Sometimes a standard is not included as a child care licensing requirement because it is covered in another code. Sometimes, however, it is not covered in any code. Since children need full protection, the issues addressed in this document should be addressed in some aspect of public policy, and consistently addressed within a community. In an effective regulatory system, different inspectors do not try to regulate the same thing. Advocates should decide which codes to review in making sure that these standards are addressed appropriately in their regulatory systems. Although the licensing requirements are most usually affected, it may be more appropriate to revise the health or building codes to include certain standards, and it may be necessary to negotiate conflicts among applicable codes.

The National Standards are for reference purposes only and should not be used as a substitute for medical or legal consultation, nor be used to authorize actions beyond a person's licensing, training, or ability.

NEW AND SIGNIFICANT CHANGES IN *Caring for Our Children* (*CFOC*) STANDARDS SINCE THE 2ND EDITION

Most of the 3rd Edition *CFOC* Standards have had some changes. Below are those standards and appendices that are new in the 3rd Edition or have had significant updates/changes to the content since the 2nd Edition.

CHAPTER 1 STAFFING

Standard 1.1.1.2: Ratios for Large Family Child Care. Lowered ratios for infants and toddlers to be more in line with small family child care.

Standard 1.1.2.1: Minimum Age to Enter Child Care – *NEW.* Recommends healthy full-term infants can be safely enrolled in child care settings beginning at three months of age. *Reader's Note:* This standard reflects a desirable goal when sufficient resources are available; it is understood that for some families, waiting until three months of age to enter their infant in child care may not be possible.

Standard 1.2.0.2: Background Screening. Changed terminology from background checks to background screening.

Standard 1.4.3.1: First Aid and CPR Training for Staff. Updated to be in compliance with the American Health Association's 2010 recommendations on CPR.

Standard 1.6.0.3: Early Childhood Mental Health Consultants – *NEW.* Recommends consultants engage with a minimum of quarterly visits, and outlines experience, knowledge base, and role of the mental health consultant.

Standard 1.6.0.4: Early Childhood Education Consultants – *NEW.* Recommends consultants engage with a minimum of semi-annual visits, and outlines the experience, knowledge base, and role of an education consultant.

CHAPTER 2 PROGRAM ACTIVITIES

Standard 2.1.1.3: Coordinated Child Care Health Program Model – *NEW.* Provides guidelines for coordinating care, including eight interactive components.

Standard 2.1.1.4: Monitoring Children's Development/Obtaining Consent for Screening – *NEW.* Defines the role of caregivers/teachers in monitoring a child's development, and includes policies on developmental screening, and sharing observation with parents/guardians.

Standard 2.1.1.6: Transitioning within Programs and Indoor and Outdoor Learning/Play Environments – *NEW.* Recommends ensuring positive transitions for children when entering a new program and beginning new routines or activities within existing program.

Standard 2.2.0.2: Limiting Infant/Toddler Time in Crib, High Chair, Car Seat, etc. – *NEW.* Guidelines to specific limit of time children should be confined in equipment.

Standard 2.2.0.3: Limiting Screen Time - Media, Computer Time – *NEW.* Provides specific limits outlined by age group and recommends what screen time is allowed be free of advertising. Also includes two exceptions.

Standard 2.2.0.4: Supervision Near Bodies of Water. Adds concept that supervising adult is within an arm's length, providing, "touch supervision."

Standard 2.2.0.6: Discipline Measures. Enhanced with information on positive behavior management and very limited use of time-out.

Standard 2.2.0.7: Handling Physical Aggression, Biting, and Hitting. Enhanced with more guidance on biting.

Standard 2.2.0.8: Preventing Expulsions, Suspensions, and Other Limitations in Services – *NEW.* Includes recommends procedures and policies for handling challenging behaviors to minimize expulsions.

Standard 2.2.0.10: Using Physical Restraint. Updates language on what a care plan should cover for the rare exception of a child with a special behavioral or mental health issue that may exhibit a behavior that endangers his/her safety and others.

Standard 2.4.1.2: Staff Modeling of Healthy and Safe Behavior and Health and Safety Education Activities. Enhanced with examples in the area of nutrition and physical activity.

CHAPTER 3 HEALTH PROMOTION AND PROTECTION

Standard 3.1.2.1: Routine Health Supervision and Growth Monitoring. Updated to include tracking BMI.

Standard 3.1.3.1: Active Opportunities for Physical Activity – *NEW.* Includes number, type, and frequency of physical activity by age group.

Standard 3.1.3.3: Protection from Air Pollution while Children are Outside – *NEW.* Recommends frequency of checking air quality index.

Standard 3.1.3.4: Caregivers'/Teachers' Encouragement of Physical Activity – *NEW.* Recommends staff promotion of children's active play throughout the day.

Standard 3.1.4.1: Safe Sleep Practices and SIDS/Suffocation Risk Reduction. Updated with new information on inappropriate infant sleeping equipment, pacifier use and swaddling.

Standard 3.1.4.2: Swaddling – *NEW.* Recommends that swaddling is not needed in child care settings.

Standard 3.1.4.3: Pacifier Use – *NEW.* Follows current American Academy of Pediatrics' recommendations and recommends written policy on use.

Standard 3.1.5.2: Toothbrushes and Toothpaste. Includes addition that toothbrushes should be replaced at least every three to four months.

Standard 3.2.1.5: Procedure for Changing Children's Soiled Underwear/Pull-Ups and Clothing – *NEW.* Outlines procedure consistent with and complimentary to the diaper changing procedure.

Standard 3.2.2.5: Hand Sanitizers – *NEW.* Describes appropriate use of hand sanitizers as alternative to traditional handwashing for children twenty-four months and older and staff. *Note to Reader:* This change is also reflected in several related standards.

Standard 3.2.3.1 - Procedures for Nasal Secretions and Use of Nasal Bulb Syringes. Provides guidance on the use of nasal bulb syringes.

Standard 3.2.3.2: Cough and Sneeze Etiquette – *NEW.* Describes appropriate etiquette to reduce the spread of respiratory pathogens.

Standard 3.3.0.1: Routine Cleaning, Sanitizing, and Disinfecting. Moved chart to Appendix K and updated definitions of sanitizer and disinfectant.

Standard 3.4.2.1: Animals that Might Have Contact with Children and Adults. Updated with more specificity to types of animals allowed and under what conditions.

Standard 3.4.2.2: Prohibited Animals. Updated with more specificity on types of animals that are prohibited and why.

Standard 3.4.2.3: Care for Animals. Updated with more specificity on caring for animals in child care settings.

Standard 3.4.4.3: Preventing and Identifying Shaken Baby Syndrome/Abusive Head Trauma – *NEW.*

Standard 3.4.4.5: Facility Layout to Reduce Risk of Child Abuse and Neglect. Removed recommending use of video surveillance due to privacy concerns.

Standard 3.4.5.1: Sun Safety Including Sunscreen – *NEW.* Explains procedures for protecting children from over exposure and the proper use and types of sunscreen.

Standard 3.4.5.2: Insect Repellent - Protection from Vector Borne Diseases – *NEW.* Outlines appropriate use and types of insect repellent; also instructions on protecting children and staff from ticks and proper removal of ticks.

Standard 3.5.0.1: Care Plan for Children with Special Health Care Needs. Describes for whom a care plan should be prepared and gives example in new Appendix O. Formerly, there was a separate standard on care plan for asthma.

Standard 3.6.1.1: Inclusion/Exclusion/Dismissal of Children. Provides updated information on those conditions for which children should or should not be temporarily excluded from child care.

Standard 3.6.1.2: Staff Exclusion for Illness. Provides updated information on those conditions for which staff should or should not be temporarily excluded from child care.

Standard 3.6.1.3: Thermometers for Taking Human Temperatures – *NEW.* Describes types of thermometers to use.

Standard 3.6.2.10: Inclusion and Exclusion of Children from Facilities that Serve Children Who are Ill. Provides updated information on those conditions for which children should or should not be temporarily excluded from child care.

Standard 3.6.3.1: Medication Administration. Reflects changes that no prescription or non-prescription medication (OTC) should be given without orders from a licensed health care provider and written permission from a parent/guardian. Exception: Non-prescription sunscreen and insect repellent must have parental consent but do not require instructions from each child's primary care provider.

Standard 3.6.3.2: Labeling, Storage, and Disposal of Medications. Recommends participating in community drug "take back" programs if available.

CHAPTER 4 NUTRITION

Overall: Strengthens the encouragement of **breastfeeding** throughout the document by incorporating supportive wording throughout the infant-related standards.

Standard 4.2.0.4: Categories of Foods. Overhauls detail information including limiting juice serving sizes, limiting fat content of milk, and avoiding concentrated sweets and limit salty food. *Note to Reader:* these changes are also reflected in several related standards.

Standard 4.2.0.5: Meal and Snack Pattern. Discusses breastfed infant feeding patterns in collaboration with families.

Standard 4.2.0.11: Ingestion of Substances that Do Not Provide Nutrition – *NEW.* Discusses monitoring of children to prevent ingestion of non-nutritive substances.

Standard 4.2.0.12: Vegetarian/Vegan Diets – *NEW.* Encourages accommodation of these diets in the child care setting.

Standard 4.3.1.2: Feeding Infants on Cue By a Consistent Caregiver/Teacher. Changes terminology and detail from "on demand" to "on cue".

Standard 4.3.1.3: Preparing, Feeding, and Storing Human Milk. Provides new guidelines on storage; use of glass or BPA-free plastic bottles; enhancement of preparing.

Standard 4.3.1.4: Feeding Human Milk to Another Mother's Child. Adds information about previous treatment related to potential HIV transmission, along with hepatitis B and C transmission issues.

Standard 4.3.1.5: Preparing, Feeding, and Storing Infant Formula. Adds more on safe handling and specifics on powdered formula.

Standard 4.3.1.6: Use of Soy-Based Formula and Soy Milk – *NEW.* Discusses allowing soy products with parent/guardian request. Encourages families and caregivers/teachers in securing community resources for soy-based formula.

Standard 4.3.1.8: Techniques of Bottle Feeding. Adds type of nipple to use and good example where breastfeeding is interlaced (i.e., bottle feeding should mimic approaches to breastfeeding).

Standard 4.3.1.9: Warming Bottles and Infant Foods. Recommends BPA free plastics.

Standard 4.3.1.11: Introduction of Age-Appropriate Solid Foods for Infants. Clarifies that solid foods should be introduced no sooner than four months and preferably at six months.

Standard 4.3.2.2: Serving Size for Toddlers and Preschoolers. Increases emphasis on age-appropriate portion size and eating from developmentally appropriate tableware and cups.

Standard 4.5.0.3: Activities that are Incompatible with Eating. Adds that watching TV and playing on a computer are incompatible with eating.

Standard 4.5.0.4: Socialization During Meals. Promotes using teachable moments on limiting portion size for those who need that.

Standard 4.5.0.8: Experience with Familiar and New Foods. Increases emphasis on introduction of a variety of "healthful" foods; food acceptance may take eight to fifteen times of offering food.

Standard 4.6.0.1: Selection and Preparation of Food Brought from Home. Adds that sweetened treats are highly discouraged. If provided, portion size should be small. Caregivers/teachers encouraged to inform families of healthy alternatives.

Standard 4.7.0.1: Nutrition Learning Experiences for Children. Strongly emphasizes teaching appropriate portion sizes.

Standard 4.7.0.2: Nutrition Education for Parents/Guardians. Emphasizes using teachable moments throughout year and importance of good nutrition and appropriate physical activity to prevent obesity.

Standard 4.9.0.8: Supply of Food and Water for Disasters. Increases allotment of food and water to seventy-two hour supply.

CHAPTER 5 FACILITIES

Overall: Standardizes height of fences to four to six feet (minimum four feet). Specifies use of nontoxic products if available and use of least toxic product for the job.

Standard 5.1.1.5: Environmental Audit of Site Location. Emphasizes comprehensive audit for environmental contaminants along with safety issues.

Standard 5.1.1.9: Unrelated Business in a Child Care Area. Adds elimination of residue in the air or on surfaces or materials/equipment that may be from activities performed in a child care area when children are not there.

Standard 5.1.2.1: Space Required by Child. Changes minimum space per child from thirty-five to forty-two square feet of useable floor space per child. Fifty square feet is preferred.

Standard 5.2.1.12: Fireplaces, Fireplace Inserts, and Wood/Corn Pellet Stoves. Adds that wood/corn pellet stoves should be inaccessible to children and should be certified that they along with fireplaces and fireplace inserts, meet air emission standards.

Standard 5.2.8.1: Integrated Pest Management. Expands guidance on adopting an integrated pest management program encouraging pest prevention and monitoring and then use of products that pose the least exposure hazard first.

Standard 5.2.9.5: Carbon Monoxide Detectors – *NEW.* Recommends installing in child care programs.

Standard 5.2.9.8: Use of Play Dough and Other Manipulative Art or Sensory Materials – *NEW.* Describes appropriate procedures when using manipulative art or sensory materials.

Standard 5.2.9.9: Plastic Containers and Toys – *NEW.* Recommends avoiding plastic materials used in child care that contain PVC, BPA, or phthalates.

Standard 5.2.9.12: Treatment of CCA Pressure-Treated Wood – *NEW.* Becomes a standalone standard on type of treatment for materials that have CCA treated surfaces; previously only covered for playground equipment.

Standard 5.2.9.15: Construction and Remodeling During Hours of Operation. Adds recommendation to use low volatile organic compound (VOC) paints.

Standard 5.3.1.2: Product Recall Monitoring – *NEW.* Recommends staff seek information regularly on recalls for juvenile products.

Standard 5.3.1.4: Surfaces of Equipment, Furniture, Toys, and Play Materials. Adds recommendation to choose materials with the least probability of containing materials that off-gas toxic elements.

Standard 5.3.1.5: Placement of Equipment and Furnishings. Adds that televisions must be anchored or mounted to prevent tipping over.

Standard 5.3.1.10: Restrictive Infant Equipment Requirements – *NEW.* Revises guidelines to specific limit of time children should be confined in equipment (max fifteen minutes, twice a day). Jumpers (attached to a door frame or ceiling) and infant walkers prohibited. Former 2nd Ed. *Baby walker* standard merged into this standard.

Standard 5.3.1.11: Exercise Equipment – *NEW*. Prohibits children from having access to adult exercise equipment.

Standard 5.4.5.1: Sleeping Equipment and Supplies. Adds that screens are not recommended to separate sleeping children. The ends of cribs do not suffice as screens. Also references new CPSC standards for toddler beds.

Standard 5.4.5.2: Cribs. Recommends programs follow current CPSC crib standards. Cribs with drop sides not permitted. Addition of information on evacuation cribs.

Standard 5.4.5.3: Stackable Cribs – *NEW.* Advises against use of stackable.

Standard 5.5.0.6: Inaccessibility to Matches, Candles, and Lighters. Adds candles as items to be inaccessible to children.

Standard 5.6.0.1: First Aid and Emergency Supplies. Adds items such as a flashlight, whistle, etc.; deletes syrup of ipecac.

Standard 5.6.0.4: Microfiber Cloths, Rags, Disposable Towels, and Mops Used for Cleaning. Adds microfiber cloths and mops as preferable for cleaning.

CHAPTER 6 PLAY AREAS/PLAYGROUNDS AND TRANSPORTATION

Overall: New Chapter. Moved selected standards from *Caring for Our Children, 2nd Ed.* Chapters 2 and 5. All playground requirements updated to conform to latest CPSC and ASTM requirements.

Standard 6.1.0.8: Enclosures for Outdoor Play Areas. Advises appropriate testing and treatment of fences and play structures for Chromated Copper Arsenate (CCA).

Standard 6.2.4.3: Sensory Table Materials – *NEW.* Requires using nontoxic materials and age-appropriate materials that do not cause choking. Children under eighteen months should not use sensory tables.

Standard 6.2.4.4: Trampolines – *NEW.* Prohibits trampolines in child care programs both onsite and during field trips.

Standard 6.2.4.5: Ball Pits – *NEW.* Prohibits children from playing in ball pits.

Standard 6.3.1.6: Pool Drain Covers. Updated in accordance with *Virginia Grame Baker Pool and Spa Safety Act.*

Standard 6.4.2.1: Riding Toys with Wheels and Wheeled Equipment. Updated to include requirements of riding toys and wheeled equipment including scooters and all riders should wear helmets.

Standard 6.4.2.2: Helmets. Updated on age requirements, use when riding any riding toy, bike, and meet CPSC standards.

Standard 6.5.2.2: Child Passenger Safety. Updated on current requirements for car safety seats, booster seats, seat belts, or harnesses.

Standard 6.5.3.1: Passenger Vans – NEW. Recommends to avoid use of fifteen-passenger vans and use vehicles meeting definition of a school bus.

CHAPTER 7 INFECTIOUS DISEASES

Overall: Updated standards on immunizations to the current Centers for Disease Control and Prevention's *Recommended immunization schedules for persons aged 0 through 18 years - United States, 2011.* **Users should always check for the current version at** www.cdc.gov/vaccines/. **Standards on immunizations moved from Chapter 3 to Chapter 7.** *Note: Infectious Diseases was formerly Chapter 6 in the 2nd Ed.*

Standard 7.2.0.3: Immunization of Caregivers/Teachers. Adds immunizations - Td/Tdap, HPV (ages eleven to twenty-six), seasonal influenza for all staff (no age restriction).

Standard 7.3.3.1: Influenza Immunizations for Children and Caregivers/Teachers – *NEW.* Recommends written documentation that a child six months of age and older has current annual vaccination against influenza unless there is a medical contraindication or philosophical or religious objection.

Standard 7.3.3.2: Influenza Control – *NEW.* Encourages parents/guardians to keep children with symptoms of acute respiratory tract illness with fever at home until their fever has subsided for at least twenty-four hours without use of fever reducing medication. Same for caregivers/teachers.

Standard 7.3.3.3: Influenza Prevention Education – *NEW.* Recommends refresher training for all staff and children on hand hygiene, cough and sneeze control, and influenza vaccine at beginning of influenza season.

Standard 7.3.4.1: Mumps – *NEW.* Recommends that children and staff with mumps should be excluded for five days following onset of parotid gland swelling.

Standard 7.3.8.1: Attendance of Children with Respiratory Syncytial Virus (RSV) Respiratory Tract Infection – *NEW.* Recommends that children may return to child care once symptoms have resolved and temperature has returned to normal.

Standard 7.3.10.1: Measures for Detection and Control of Tuberculosis. Updated that TB status of adolescents and caregivers/teachers present with children should be assessed with a tuberculin skin test (TST) or interferon-gamma release assay (IGRA) blood test before caregiving activities are initiated. Tests on those with negative results do not have to be repeated on a regular basis unless individual is at risk of acquiring new infection or state/local health department requires.

Standard 7.5.1.1: Conjunctivitis – *NEW.* Recommends that children with conjunctivitis should not be excluded unless meet certain criteria.

Standard 7.5.2.1: Enterovirus Infections – *NEW.* Recommends children with enterovirus infections should not be excluded unless meet certain criteria.

Standard 7.5.3.1: Human Papillomaviruses (HPV) (WARTS) – *NEW.* Recommends children with warts should not be excluded unless meet certain criteria.

Standard 7.5.4.1: Impetigo – *NEW.* Explains process for inclusion/exclusion of children or staff with impetigo.

Standard 7.5.5.1: Lymphadenitis – *NEW.* Outlines process for inclusion/exclusion of children or staff with lymphadenitis.

Standard 7.5.6.1: Immunization for Measles – *NEW.* Recommends all children have age appropriate immunizations, and those not immunized or not age appropriately immunized should be excluded immediately if there are documented cases.

Standard 7.5.7.1: Molluscum Contagiosum – *NEW.* Recommends not excluding children with molluscum contagiosum.

Standard 7.5.10.1: *Staphylococcus Aureus* Skin Infections Including MRSA – *NEW.* Recommends not excluding children and staff unless meet certain criteria. Lesions should be covered.

Standard 7.5.12.1: Thrush (Candidiasis) – *NEW.* Recommends not excluding children.

STANDARD 7.7.3.1: Roseola – *NEW.* Recommends not excluding children unless meet certain criteria.

CHAPTER 8 CHILDREN WITH SPECIAL HEALTH CARE NEEDS AND DISABILITIES

Overall: Improved consistency of language, referring to children with special health care needs. Note: Targeted information on *Children with Special Health Care Needs* was formerly Chapter 7 in the 2nd Ed.

CHAPTER 9 ADMINISTRATION

Overall: Encompasses policy and record changes reflecting major changes in process and procedures throughout document. Note: *Administration* was formerly Chapter 8 in the *CFOC,* 2nd Ed.

Standard 9.2.3.1: Policies and Practices that Promote Physical Activity – *NEW.* Outlines what policies should include: benefits, duration, setting, and clothing.

Standard 9.2.3.9: Written Policy on Use of Medications. Updated to include prohibition of administering OTC cough and cold, policies on prescriptions and OTC medications.

Standard 9.2.3.11: Food and Nutrition Service Policies and Plans. Adds to list of policies needed: Menu and meal planning, emergency preparedness for nutrition services, food brought from home, age-appropriate portion sizes, age-appropriate eating utensils and tableware, promotion of breastfeeding, and provision of community resources to support mothers.

Standard 9.2.3.14: Oral Health Policy – *NEW.* Outlines elements to be included in an oral health policy such as contact information for each child's dentist/dental home; provides resource list for children without a dentist/dental home; explains implementation of daily tooth brushing, restriction of sippy cup, etc.

Standard 9.2.4.1: Written Plan and Training for Handling Urgent Medical Care or Threatening Incidents. Expanded to cover mental health emergencies, emergencies involving parents/guardians/guests, and if/when threatening individual accesses the program.

Standard 9.2.4.3: Disaster Planning, Training and Communication. Outlines comprehensive approach on the details to be covered in an emergency/disaster plan, training requirements, and communication procedures with parents/guardians.

Standard 9.2.4.4: Written Plan for Seasonal and Pandemic Influenza – *NEW.* Recommends contents of a plan in the areas of planning and coordination, infection control policy and procedures, communications planning, and child learning and program operations.

Standard 9.2.4.5: Emergency and Evacuation Drills/Exercises Policy. Expands on types of events to have drills and exercises.

Standard 9.2.4.7: Sign-In/Sign-Out System – *NEW.* Recommends system to track who has entered and exited the facility as a means of security and of notification in case of situation requiring evacuation.

Standard 9.2.4.8: Authorized Persons to Pick Up Child. Expanded to include procedures for verifying persons who are not on the authorized list to pick up or to deny ability to pick up.

Standard 9.2.4.10: Documentation of Drop-Off, Pick-Up and Daily Attendance of Child, and Parent/Provider Communication. Expanded to include information on documenting whether or not a child is in attendance and communication procedures with parents/guardians.

Standard 9.2.5.1: Transportation Policy for Centers and Large Family Homes. Expanded to include policies such as procedures to ensure that no child is left in the vehicle at the end of the trip or left unsupervised outside or inside the vehicle during loading and unloading the vehicle, use of passenger vans, vehicle selection to safely transport children and others.

Standard 9.3.0.2: Written Human Resource Management for Small Family Child Care Homes – *NEW.* Addresses need for policies for caregivers/teachers in small family child care homes that address vacation leave, holidays, professional development leave, sick leave, and scheduled increases of small family child care home fees.

Standard 9.4.1.16: Evacuation and Shelter-In-Place Drill Record. Adds need for records of shelter-in-place drills.

CHAPTER 10 LICENSING AND COMMUNITY ACTION

Overall: Changed "Recommendations" to "Standards" for the first section of each standard. Chapter had major rearrangement. Most standards stayed but in different order. Note: *Licensing and Community Action* was formerly Chapter 9 in the *CFOC* 2nd Ed.

Standard 10.3.2.2: State Early Childhood Advisory Council: Changed terminology from old "Commission on Child Care" to reflect updated requirements from Head Start.

Standard 10.3.3.5: Licensing Agency Role in Communicating the Importance of Compliance with Americans with Disabilities Act – *NEW.* Explains that licensing agencies should inform child care programs on compliance with the ADA.

Standard 10.3.4.3: Support for Consultants to Provide Technical Assistance to Facilities. Expands types of consultants by adding early childhood education consultant, dental health consultant, and physical activity consultant.

Standard 10.4.1.1: Uniform Categories and Definitions. Updates definitions and completely revises the definition for drop-in care.

Standard 10.4.1.2: Quality Rating and Improvement Systems – *NEW.* Recommends that states develop QRIS systems.

Standard 10.4.2.1: Frequency of Inspections for Child Care Centers, Large Family Child Care Homes, and Small Family Child Care Homes. Increased inspections to two a year of which one should be unannounced.

APPENDICES

Appendix A: Signs and Symptoms Chart – *NEW.* Includes signs and symptoms of illness, whether to notify a child care health consultant, whether to notify parent/guardian, whether to exclude child and if excluded, when to readmit.

Appendix H: Recommended Adult Immunization Schedule – *NEW.*

Appendix J: Selecting an Appropriate Sanitizer and Disinfectant. Updated definitions on terms and expanded information.

Appendix K: Routine Schedule for Cleaning, Sanitizing and Disinfecting. Updated with new categories.

Appendix N: Protective Factors Regarding Child Abuse and Neglect – *NEW.* Includes early care and education program strategies to build protective factors.

Appendix O: Care Plan for Children with Special Health Care Needs – *NEW.*

Appendix Q: Getting Started with MyPlate – *NEW.* Displays new primary food icon for healthy eating.

Appendix R: Choose MyPlate: 10 Tips to a Great Plate – *NEW.* Shows food choices for a healthy lifestyle can be simple.

Appendix S: Physical Activity: How Much Is Needed? – *NEW.* A guide to age-appropriate physical activity.

Appendix T: Helping Children in Foster Care Make Successful Transitions Into Child Care – *NEW.* Includes advice for both foster parents and caregivers/teachers on how to make successful transitions for children into an early care and education program.

Appendix U: Recommended Safe Minimum Internal Cooking Temperatures – *NEW.*

Appendix AA: Medication Administration Packet – *NEW.* Includes authorization form to give medication, checklist on receiving medication, medication log, medication incident report form, and checklist for preparing to give medication.

Appendix DD: Injury Report Form for Indoor and Outdoor Injuries – *NEW.*

Appendix HH: Use Zones for Clearance Dimensions for Single- and Multi-Axis Swings – *NEW.*

Appendix II: Bicycle Helmets: Quick-Fit Check – *NEW.*

Appendix JJ: Our Child Care Center Supports Breastfeeding – *NEW.* Displays poster for programs to use to encourage breastfeeding at the program.

Appendix KK: Authorization for Emergency Medical/ Dental Care – *NEW.*

Chapter 1

1

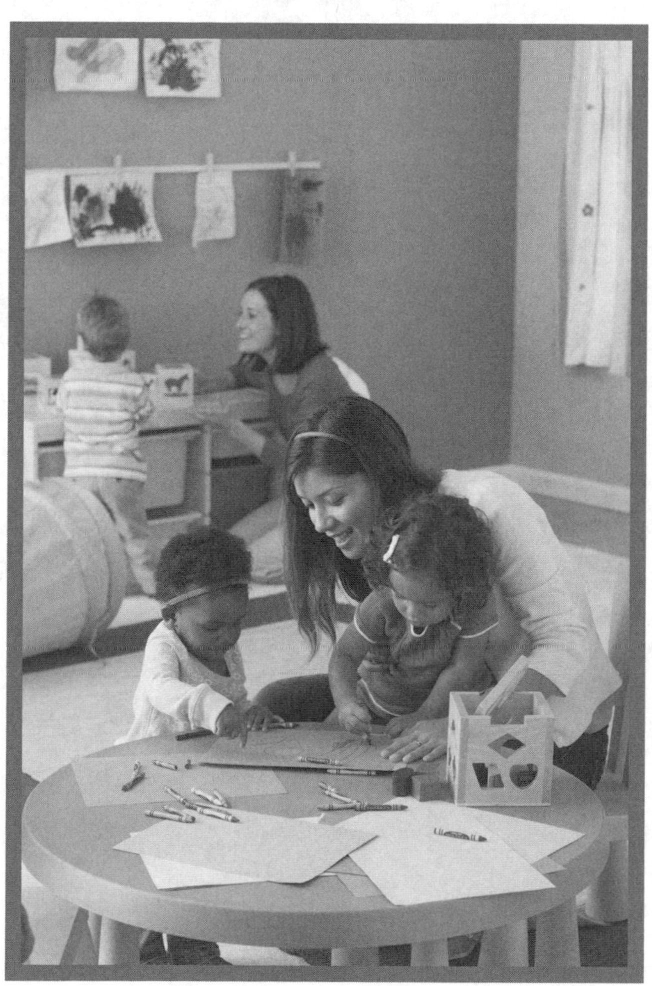

Staffing

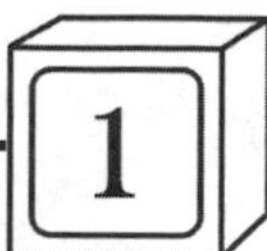

1.1 Child:Staff Ratio, Group Size, and Minimum Age

1.1.1 Child:Staff Ratio and Group Size

STANDARD 1.1.1.1: Ratios for Small Family Child Care Homes

The small family child care home caregiver/teacher child:staff ratios should conform to the following table:

If the small family child care home caregiver/teacher has no children under **two** years of age in care,	then the small family child care home caregiver/teacher may have one to six children over two years of age in care
If the small family child care home caregiver/teacher has one child under **two** years of age in care,	then the small family child care home caregiver/teacher may have one to three children over two years of age in care
If the small family child care home caregiver/teacher has **two** children under **two** years of age in care,	then the small family child care home caregiver/teacher may have no children over two years of age in care

The small family child care home caregiver's/teacher's own children as well as any other children in the home temporarily requiring supervision should be included in the child:staff ratio. During nap time, at least one adult should be physically present in the same room as the children.

RATIONALE: Low child:staff ratios are most critical for infants and toddlers (birth to thirty-six months) (1). Infant and child development and caregiving quality improves when group size and child:staff ratios are smaller (2). Improved verbal interactions are correlated with lower child:staff ratios (3). Small ratios are very important for young children's development (7). The recommended group size and child:staff ratio allow three- to five-year-old children to have continuing adult support and guidance while encouraging independent, self-initiated play and other activities (4).

The National Fire Protection Association (NFPA) requires in the *NFPA 101: Life Safety Code* that small family child care homes serve no more than two clients incapable of self-preservation (5).

Direct, warm social interaction between adults and children is more common and more likely with lower child:staff ratios. Caregivers/teachers must be recognized as performing a job for groups of children that parents/guardians of twins, triplets, or quadruplets would rarely be left to handle alone. In child care, these children do not come from the same family and must learn a set of common rules that may differ from expectations in their own homes (6,8).

COMMENTS: It is best practice for the caregiver/teacher to remain in the same room as the infants when they are sleeping to provide constant supervision. However in small family child care programs, this may be difficult in practice because the caregiver/teacher is typically alone, and all of the children most likely will not sleep at the same time. In order to provide constant supervision during sleep, caregivers/teachers could consider discontinuing the practice of placing infant(s) in a separate room for sleep, but instead placing the infant's crib in the area used by the other children so the caregiver/teacher is able to supervise the sleeping infant(s) while caring for the other children. Care must be taken so that placement of cribs in an area used by other children does not encroach upon the minimum usable floor space requirements. Infants do not require a dark and quiet place for sleep. Once they become accustomed, infants are able to sleep without problems in environments with light and noise. By placing infants (as well as all children in care) on the main (ground) level of the home for sleep and remaining on the same level as the children, the caregiver/teacher is more likely able to evacuate the children in less time; thus, increasing the odds of a successful evacuation in the event of a fire or another emergency. Caregivers/teachers must also continually monitor other children in this area so they are not climbing on or into the cribs. If the caregiver/teacher cannot remain in the same room as the infant(s) when the infant is sleeping, it is recommended that the caregiver/teacher should do visual checks every ten to fifteen minutes to make sure the infant's head is uncovered, and assess the infant's breathing, color, etc. Supervision is recommended for toddlers and preschoolers to ensure safety and prevent behaviors such as inappropriate touching or hurting other sleeping children from taking place. These behaviors may go undetected if a caregiver/teacher is not present. If caregiver/teacher is not able to remain in the same room as the children, frequent visual checks are also recommended for toddlers and preschoolers when they are sleeping.

Each state has its own set of regulations that specify child:staff ratios. To view a particular state's regulations, go to the National Resource Center for Health and Safety in Child Care and Early Education's (NRC) Website: http://nrckids.org. Some states are setting limits on the number of school-age children that are allowed to be cared for in small family child care homes, e.g., two school-age children in addition to the maximum number allowed for infants/preschool children. No data are available to support using a different ratio where school-age children are in family child care homes. Since school-age children require focused caregiver/teacher time and attention for supervision and adult-child interaction, this standard applies the same ratio to all children three-years-old and over. The family child care caregiver/teacher must be able to have a positive relationship and provide guidance for each child in care. This standard is consistent with ratio requirements for toddlers in centers as described in Standard 1.1.1.2.

Unscheduled inspections encourage compliance with this standard.

TYPE OF FACILITY: Small Family Child Care Home

RELATED STANDARDS:

Standard 1.1.2.1: Minimum Age to Enter Child Care

REFERENCES:
1. Zero to Three. 2007. *The infant-toddler set-aside of the Child Care and Development Block Grant: Improving quality child care for infants and toddlers.* Washington, DC: Zero to Three. http://main.zerotothree.org/site/DocServer/Jan_07_Child_Care_Fact_Sheet.pdf.
2. National Institute of Child Health and Human Development (NICHD). 2006. *The NICHD study of early child care and youth development: Findings for children up to age 4 1/2 years.* Rockville, MD: NICHD. http://www.nichd.nih.gov/publications/pubs/upload/seccyd_051206.pdf.
3. Goldstein, A., K. Hamm, R. Schumacher. *Supporting growth and development of babies in child care: What does the research say?* Washington, DC: Center for Law and Social Policy (CLASP); Zero to Three. http://main.zerotothree.org/site/DocServer/ChildCareResearchBrief.pdf.
4. De Schipper, E. J., J. M. Riksen-Walraven, S. A. E. Geurts. 2006. Effects of child-caregiver ratio on the interactions between caregivers and children in child-care centers: An experimental study. *Child Devel* 77:861-74.
5. National Fire Protection Association (NFPA). 2009. *NFPA 101: Life safety code.* 2009 ed. Quincy, MA: NFPA.
6. Fiene, R. 2002. *13 indicators of quality child care: Research update.* Washington, DC: U.S. Department of Health and Human Services, Office of the Assistant Secretary for Planning and Evaluation. http://aspe.hhs.gov/hsp/ccquality-ind02/.
7. Zigler, E., W. S. Gilliam, S. M. Jones. 2006. *A vision for universal preschool education*, 107-29. New York: Cambridge University Press.
8. Stebbins, H. 2007. *State policies to improve the odds for the healthy development and school readiness of infants and toddlers.* Washington, DC: Zero to Three. http://main.zerotothree.org/site/DocServer/NCCP_article_for_BM_final.pdf.

STANDARD 1.1.1.2: Ratios for Large Family Child Care Homes and Centers

Child:staff ratios in large family child care homes and centers should be maintained as follows during all hours of operation, including in vehicles during transport.

Large Family Child Care Homes

Age	Maximum Child:Staff Ratio	Maximum Group Size
≤ 12 months	2:1	6
13-23 months	2:1	8
24-35 months	3:1	12
3-year-olds	7:1	12
4- to 5-year-olds	8:1	12
6- to 8-year-olds	10:1	12
9- to 12-year-olds	12:1	12

During nap time for children birth through thirty months of age, the child:staff ratio must be maintained at all times regardless of how many infants are sleeping. They must also be maintained even during the adult's break time so that ratios are not relaxed.

Child Care Centers

Age	Maximum Child:Staff Ratio	Maximum Group Size
≤ 12 months	3:1	6
13-35 months	4:1	8
3-year-olds	7:1	14
4-year-olds	8:1	16
5-year-olds	8:1	16
6- to 8-year-olds	10:1	20
9- to 12-year-olds	12:1	24

During nap time for children ages thirty-one months and older, at least one adult should be physically present in the same room as the children and maximum group size must be maintained. Children over thirty-one months of age can usually be organized to nap on a schedule, but infants and toddlers as individuals are more likely to nap on different schedules. In the event even one child is not sleeping the child should be moved to another activity where appropriate supervision is provided.

If there is an emergency during nap time other adults should be on the same floor and should immediately assist the staff supervising sleeping children. The caregiver/teacher who is in the same room with the children should be able to summon these adults without leaving the children.

When there are mixed age groups in the same room, the child:staff ratio and group size should be consistent with the age of most of the children. When infants or toddlers are in the mixed age group, the child:staff ratio and group size for infants and toddlers should be maintained. In large family child care homes with two or more caregivers/teachers caring for no more than twelve children, no more than three children younger than two years of age should be in care.

Children with special health care needs or who require more attention due to certain disabilities may require additional staff on-site, depending on their special needs and the extent of their disabilities (1). See Standard 1.1.1.3.

At least one adult who has satisfactorily completed a course in pediatric first aid, including CPR skills within the past three years, should be part of the ratio at all times.

RATIONALE: These child:staff ratios are within the range of recommendations for each age group that the National Association for the Education of Young Children (NAEYC) uses in its accreditation program (5). The NAEYC recommends a range that assumes the director and staff members are highly trained and, by virtue of the accreditation process, have formed a staffing pattern that enables effective staff functioning. The standard for child:staff ratios in this

document uses a single desired ratio, rather than a range, for each age group. These ratios are more likely than less stringent ratios to support quality experiences for young children.

Low child:staff ratios for non-ambulatory children are essential for fire safety. The National Fire Protection Association (NFPA), in its *NFPA 101: Life Safety Code*, recommends that no more than three children younger than two years of age be cared for in large family child care homes where two staff members are caring for up to twelve children (6).

Children benefit from social interactions with peers. However, larger groups are generally associated with less positive interactions and developmental outcomes. Group size and ratio of children to adults are limited to allow for one to one interaction, intimate knowledge of individual children, and consistent caregiving (7).

Studies have found that children (particularly infants and toddlers) in groups that comply with the recommended ratio receive more sensitive and appropriate caregiving and score higher on developmental assessments, particularly vocabulary (1,9).

As is true in small family child care homes, Standard 1.1.1.1, child:staff ratios alone do not predict the quality of care. Direct, warm social interaction between adults and children is more common and more likely with lower child:staff ratios. Caregivers/teachers must be recognized as performing a job for groups of children that parents/guardians of twins, triplets, or quadruplets would rarely be left to handle alone. In child care, these children do not come from the same family and must learn a set of common rules that may differ from expectations in their own homes (10).

Similarly, low child:staff ratios are most critical for infants and young toddlers (birth to twenty-four months) (1). Infant development and caregiving quality improves when group size and child:staff ratios are smaller (2). Improved verbal interactions are correlated with lower ratios (3). For three- and four-year-old children, the size of the group is even more important than ratios. The recommended group size and child:staff ratio allow three- to five-year-old children to have continuing adult support and guidance while encouraging independent, self-initiated play and other activities (4).

In addition, the children's physical safety and sanitation routines require a staff that is not fragmented by excessive demands. Child:staff ratios in child care settings should be sufficiently low to keep staff stress below levels that might result in anger with children. Caring for too many young children, in particular, increases the possibility of stress to the caregiver/teacher, and may result in loss of the caregiver's/teacher's self-control (11).

Although observation of sleeping children does not require the physical presence of more than one caregiver/teacher for sleeping children thirty-one months and older, the staff needed for an emergency response or evacuation of the children must remain available on site for this purpose. Ratios are required to be maintained for children thirty months and younger during nap time due to the need for closer observation and the frequent need to interact with younger children during periods while they are resting. Close proximity of staff to these younger groups enables more rapid response to situations where young children require more assistance than older children, e.g., for evacuation. The requirement that a caregiver/teacher should remain in the sleeping area of children thirty-one months and older is not only to ensure safety, but also to prevent inappropriate behavior from taking place that may go undetected if a caregiver/teacher is not present. While nap time may be the best option for regular staff conferences, staff lunch breaks, and staff training, one staff person should stay in the nap room, and the above staff activities should take place in an area next to the nap room so other staff can assist if emergency evacuation becomes necessary. If a child with a potentially life-threatening special health care need is present, a staff member trained in CPR and pediatric first aid and one trained in administration of any potentially required medication should be available at all times.

COMMENTS: The child:staff ratio indicates the maximum number of children permitted per caregiver/teacher (8). These ratios assume that caregivers/teachers do not have time-consuming bookkeeping and housekeeping duties, so they are free to provide direct care for children. The ratios do not include other personnel (such as bus drivers) necessary for specialized functions (such as driving a vehicle).

Group size is the number of children assigned to a caregiver/teacher or team of caregivers/teachers occupying an individual classroom or well-defined space within a larger room (8). The "group" in child care represents the "home room" for school-age children. It is the psychological base with which the school-aged child identifies and from which the child gains continual guidance and support in various activities. This standard does not prohibit larger numbers of school-aged children from joining in occasional collective activities as long as child:staff ratios and the concept of "home room" are maintained.

Unscheduled inspections encourage compliance with this standard.

These standards are based on what children need for quality nurturing care. Those who question whether these ratios are affordable must consider that efforts to limit costs can result in overlooking the basic needs of children and creating a highly stressful work environment for caregivers/teachers. Community resources, in addition to parent/guardian fees and a greater public investment in child care, can make critical contributions to the achievement of the child:staff ratios and group sizes specified in this standard. Each state has its own set of regulations that specify child:staff ratios. To view a particular state's regulations, go to the National Resource Center for Health and Safety in Child Care and Early Education's (NRC) Website: http://nrckids.org.

TYPE OF FACILITY: Center; Large Family Child Care Home

RELATED STANDARDS:
Standards 1.1.1.3-1.1.1.5: Ratios and Supervision for Certain Scenarios

Standards 1.4.3.1-1.4.3.3: First Aid and CPR Training

REFERENCES:

1. Zero to Three. 2007. *The infant-toddler set-aside of the Child Care and Development Block Grant: Improving quality child care for infants and toddlers.* Washington, DC: Zero to Three. http://main.zerotothree.org/site/DocServer/Jan_07_Child_Care_Fact_Sheet.pdf.
2. National Institute of Child Health and Human Development (NICHD). 2006. *The NICHD study of early child care and youth development: Findings for children up to age 4 1/2 years.* Rockville, MD: NICHD. http://www.nichd.nih.gov/publications/pubs/upload/seccyd_051206.pdf.
3. Goldstein, A., K. Hamm, R. Schumacher. *Supporting growth and development of babies in child care: What does the research say?* Washington, DC: Center for Law and Social Policy (CLASP); Zero to Three. http://main.zerotothree.org/site/DocServer/ChildCareResearchBrief.pdf.
4. De Schipper, E. J., J. M. Riksen-Walraven, S. A. E. Geurts. 2006. Effects of child-caregiver ratio on the interactions between caregivers and children in child-care centers: An experimental study. *Child Devel* 77:861-74.
5. National Association for the Education of Young Children (NAEYC). 2007. *Early childhood program standards and accreditation criteria.* Washington, DC: NAEYC.
6. National Fire Protection Association (NFPA). 2009. *NFPA 101: Life safety code.* 2009 ed. Quincy, MA: NFPA.
7. Bradley, R. H., D. L. Vandell. 2007. Child care and the well-being of children. *Arch Ped Adolescent Med* 161:669-76.
8. Murph, J. R., S. D. Palmer, D. Glassy, eds. 2005. *Health in child care: A manual for health professionals.* 4th ed. Elk Grove Village, IL: American Academy of Pediatrics.
9. Vandell, D. L., B. Wolfe. 2000. *Child care quality: Does it matter and does it need to be improved?* Washington, DC: U.S. Department of Health and Human Services. http://aspe.hhs.gov/hsp/ccquality00/.
10. Fiene, R. 2002. *13 indicators of quality child care: Research update.* Washington, DC: U.S. Department of Health and Human Services, Office of the Assistant Secretary for Planning and Evaluation. http://aspe.hhs.gov/hsp/ccquality-ind02/.
11. Wrigley, J., J. Derby. 2005. Fatalities and the organization of child care in the United States. *Am Socio Rev* 70:729-57.

STANDARD 1.1.1.3: Ratios for Facilities Serving Children with Special Health Care Needs and Disabilities

Facilities enrolling children with special health care needs and disabilities should determine, by an individual assessment of each child's needs, whether the facility requires a lower child:staff ratio.

RATIONALE: The child:staff ratio must allow the needs of the children enrolled to be met. The facility should have sufficient direct care professional staff to provide the required programs and services. Integrated facilities with fewer resources may be able to serve children who need fewer services, and the staffing levels may vary accordingly. Adjustment of the ratio allows for the flexibility needed to meet each child's type and degree of special need and encourage each child to participate comfortably in program activities. Adjustment of the ratio produces flexibility without resulting in a need for care that is greater than the staff can provide without compromising the health and safety of other children. The facility should seek consultation with parents/guardians, a child care health consultant (CCHC), and other professionals, regarding the appropriate child:staff ratio. The facility may wish to increase the number of staff members if the child requires significant special assistance (1).

COMMENTS: These ratios do not include personnel who have other duties that might preclude their involvement in needed supervision while they are performing those duties, such as therapists, cooks, maintenance workers, or bus drivers.

TYPE OF FACILITY: Center; Large Family Child Care Home; Small Family Child Care Home

REFERENCES:

1. University of North Carolina at Chapel Hill, FPG Child Development Institute. The national early childhood technical assistance center. http://www.nectac.org.

STANDARD 1.1.1.4: Ratios and Supervision During Transportation

Child:staff ratios established for out-of-home child care should be maintained on all transportation the facility provides or arranges. Drivers should not be included in the ratio. No child of any age should be left unattended in or around a vehicle, when children are in a car, or when they are in a car seat. A face-to-name count of children should be conducted prior to leaving for a destination, when the destination is reached, before departing for return to the facility and upon return. Caregivers/teachers should also remember to take into account in this head count if any children were picked up or dropped off while being transported away from the facility.

RATIONALE: Children must receive direct supervision when they are being transported, in loading zones, and when they get in and out of vehicles. Drivers must be able to focus entirely on driving tasks, leaving the supervision of children to other adults. This is especially important with young children who will be sitting in close proximity to one another in the vehicle and may need care during the trip. In any vehicle making multiple stops to pick up or drop off children, this also permits one adult to get one child out and take that child to a home, while the other adult supervises the children remaining in the vehicle, who would otherwise be unattended for that time (1). Children require supervision at all times, even when buckled in seat restraints. A head count is essential to ensure that no child is inadvertently left behind in or out of the vehicle. Child deaths in child care have occurred when children were mistakenly left in vehicles, thinking the vehicle was empty.

TYPE OF FACILITY: Center; Large Family Child Care Home

RELATED STANDARDS:

Standard 5.6.0.1: First Aid and Emergency Supplies

REFERENCES:

1. Aird, L. D. 2007. Moving kids safely in child care: A refresher course. *Child Care Exchange* (January/February): 25-28. http://www.childcareexchange.com/library/5017325.pdf.

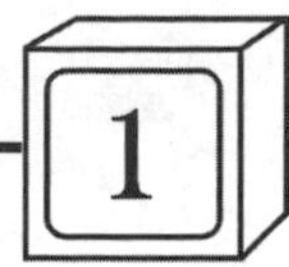

STANDARD 1.1.1.5: Ratios and Supervision for Swimming, Wading, and Water Play

The following child:staff ratios should apply while children are swimming, wading, or engaged in water play:

Developmental Levels	Child:Staff Ratio
Infants	1:1
Toddlers	1:1
Preschoolers	4:1
School-age Children	6:1

Constant and active supervision should be maintained when any child is in or around water (4). During any swimming/wading/water play activities where either an infant or a toddler is present, the ratio should always be one adult to one infant/toddler. The required ratio of adults to older children should be met without including the adults who are required for supervision of infants and/or toddlers. An adult should remain in direct physical contact with an infant at all times during swimming or water play (4). Whenever children thirteen months and up to five years of age are in or around water, the supervising adult should be within an arm's length providing "touch supervision" (6). The attention of an adult who is supervising children of any age should be focused on the child, and the adult should never be engaged in other distracting activities (4), such as talking on the telephone, socializing, or tending to chores.

A lifeguard should not be counted in the child:staff ratio.

RATIONALE: The circumstances surrounding drownings and water-related injuries of young children suggest that staffing requirements and environmental modifications may reduce the risk of this type of injury. Essential elements are close continuous supervision (1,4), four-sided fencing and self-locking gates around all swimming pools, hot tubs, and spas, and special safety covers on pools when they are not in use (2,7). Five-gallon buckets should not be used for water play (4). Water play using small (one quart) plastic pitchers and plastic containers for pouring water and plastic dish pans or bowls allow children to practice pouring skills. Between 2003 and 2005, a study of drowning deaths of children younger than five years of age attributed the highest percentage of drowning reports to an adult losing contact or knowledge of the whereabouts of the child (5). During the time of lost contact, the child managed to gain access to the pool (3).

COMMENTS: Water play includes wading. Touch supervision means keeping swimming children within arm's reach and in sight at all times. Drowning is a "silent killer" and children may slip into the water silently without any splashing or screaming.

Ratios for supervision of swimming, wading and water play do not include personnel who have other duties that might preclude their involvement in supervision during swimming/wading/water play activities while they are performing those duties. This ratio excludes cooks, maintenance workers, or lifeguards from being counted in the child:staff ratio if they are involved in specialized duties at the same time. Proper ratios during swimming activities with infants are important. Infant swimming programs have led to water intoxication and seizures because infants may swallow excessive water when they are engaged in any submersion activities (1).

TYPE OF FACILITY: Center; Large Family Child Care Home; Small Family Child Care Home

RELATED STANDARDS:

Standard 2.2.0.4: Supervision Near Bodies of Water
Standard 6.3.1.3: Sensors or Remote Monitors
Standard 6.3.1.4: Safety Covers for Swimming Pools
Standard 6.3.1.7: Pool Safety Rules
Standard 6.3.2.1: Lifesaving Equipment
Standard 6.3.2.2: Lifeline in Pool
Standard 6.3.5.2: Water in Containers
Standard 6.3.5.3: Portable Wading Pools

REFERENCES:

1. American Academy of Pediatrics, Committee on Injury, Violence, and Poison Prevention. 2010. Policy statement: Prevention of drowning. *Pediatrics* 126:178-85.
2. U.S. Consumer Product Safety Commission (CPSC). *Pool and spa safety: The Virginia Graeme Baker pool and spa safety act.* http://www.poolsafely.gov/wp-content/uploads/VGBA.pdf.
3. Gipson, K. 2008. *Pool and spa submersion: Estimated injuries and reported fatalities, 2008 report.* Bethesda, MD: U.S. Consumer Product Safety Commission. http://www.cpsc.gov/LIBRARY/poolsub2008.pdf.
4. U.S. Consumer Product Safety Commission (CPSC). 2009. CPSC warns of in-home drowning dangers with bathtubs, bath seats, buckets. Release #10-008. http://www.cpsc.gov/cpscpub/prerel/prhtml10/10008.html.
5. Gipson, K. 2008. *Submersions related to non-pool and non-spa products, 2008 report.* Washington, DC: U.S. Consumer Product Safety Commission. http://www.cpsc.gov/library/FOIA/FOIA09/OS/nonpoolsub2008.pdf.
6. American Academy of Pediatrics, Committee on Injury, Violence, and Poison Prevention, J. Weiss. 2010. Technical report: Prevention of drowning. *Pediatrics* 126: e253-62.
7. Consumer Product Safety Commission. Steps for safety around the pool: The pool and spa safety act. Pool Safely. http://www.poolsafely.gov/wp-content/uploads/360.pdf.

1.1.2 Minimum Age

STANDARD 1.1.2.1: Minimum Age to Enter Child Care

Reader's Note: This standard reflects a desirable goal when sufficient resources are available; it is understood that for some families, waiting until three months of age to enter their infant in child care may not be possible.

Healthy full-term infants can be enrolled in child care settings as early as three months of age. Premature infants or those with chronic health conditions should be evaluated by their primary care providers and developmental specialists to make an individual determination concerning the appropriate age for child care enrollment.

RATIONALE: Brain anatomy, chemistry, and physiology undergo rapid development over the first ten to twelve weeks of life (1-6). Concurrently, and as a direct consequence of these shifts in central nervous system structure and function, infants demonstrate significant growth, irregularity, and eventually, organization of their behavior, physiology, and social responsiveness (1-3,5). Arousal responses to stimulation mature before the ability to self-regulate and control such responses in the first six to eight weeks of life causing infants to demonstrate an expanding range and fluctuation of behavioral state changes from quiet to alert to irritable (1-3,6). Infant behavior is most disorganized, most difficult to read and most frustrating to support at the six to eight week period (2,3). At approximately eight to twelve weeks after birth, full term infants typically undergo changes in brain function and behavior that helps caregivers/teachers understand and respond effectively to infants' increasingly stable sleep-wake states, attention, self-calming efforts, feeding patterns and patterns of social engagement. Over the course of the third month, infants demonstrate an emerging capacity to sustain states of sleep and alert attention.

Infants, birth to three months of age, can become seriously ill very quickly without obvious signs (7). This increased risk to infants, birth to three months makes it important to minimize their exposure to children and adults outside their family, including exposures in child care (8). In addition, infants of mothers who return to work, particularly full-time, before twelve weeks of age, and are placed in group care may be at even greater risk for developing serious infectious diseases. These infants are less likely to receive recommended well-child care and immunizations and to be breastfed or are likely to have a shorter duration of breastfeeding (16,22).

Researchers report that breastfeeding duration was significantly higher in women with longer maternity leaves as compared to those with less than nine to twelve weeks leave (9,22). A leave of less than six weeks was associated with a much higher likelihood of stopping breastfeeding (10,22). Continuing breastfeeding after returning to work may be particularly difficult for lower income women who may have fewer support systems (11).

It takes women who have given birth about six weeks to return to the physical health they had prior to pregnancy (12). A significant portion of women reported child birth related symptoms five weeks after delivery (17). In contrast, women's general mental health, vitality, and role function were improved with maternity leaves at twelve weeks or longer (13).

Birth of a child or adoption of a newborn, especially the first, requires significant transition in the family. First time parents/guardians are learning a new role and even with subsequent children, integration of the new family member requires several weeks of adaptation. Families need time to adjust physically and emotionally to the intense needs of a newborn (14,15).

COMMENTS: In an analysis of twenty-one wealthy countries including Australia, New Zealand, Canada, United States, Japan, and several European countries, the U.S. ranked twentieth in terms of unpaid and paid parental leave available to two-parent families with the birth of their child (18,21). Although Switzerland ranked twenty-first with fourteen versus twenty-four weeks as compared to the U.S. for both parents/guardians, eleven weeks of leave are paid in Switzerland. In this study of twenty-one countries, only Australia and the U.S. do not provide for paid leave after the birth of a child (18).

Major social policies in the U.S. were established with the Social Security Act in 1935 at a time when the majority of women were not employed (19,20). The Family and Medical Leave Act (FMLA) of 1993, which allows twelve weeks of leave, established for the first time job protected maternity leave for qualifying employees (16,20). Despite the importance of FMLA, only about 60% of the women in the workforce are eligible for job protected maternity leave. FMLA does not provide paid leave, which may force many women to return to work sooner than preferred (18). FMLA is not transferable between parents/guardians. However, five U.S. states support five to six weeks of paid maternity leave and a few companies allow generous paid leaves for select employees (21).

In a nationally representative sample, 84% of women and 74% of men supported expansion of the FMLA; furthermore, 90% of women and 72% of men reported that employers and government should do more to support families (21).

Substantial evidence exists to strengthen social policies, specifically job protected paid leave for all families, for at least the first twelve weeks of life, in order to promote the health and development of children and families (22). Investing in families during an important life transition, the birth or adoption of a child, reflects a society's values and may in fact contribute to a healthier and more productive work force.

TYPE OF FACILITY: Center; Large Family Child Care Home; Small Family Child Care Home

RELATED STANDARDS:

Standard 2.1.1.5: Helping Families Cope with Separation

REFERENCES:

1. Staehelin, K., P. C. Bertea, E. Z. Stutz. 2007. Length of maternity leave and health of mother and child–a review. *Int J Public Health* 52:202-9.

2. Guendelman, S., J. L. Kosc, M. Pearl, S. Graham, J. Goodman, M. Kharrazi. 2009. Juggling work and breastfeeding: Effects of maternity leave and occupational characteristics. *Pediatrics* 123: e38-e46.

3. Kimbro, R. T. 2006. On-the-job moms: Work and breastfeeding initiation and duration for a sample of low-income women. *Maternal Child Health J* 10:19-26.

4. Cunningham, F. G., F. F. Gont, K. J. Leveno, L. C. Gilstrap, J. C. Hauth, K. D. Wenstrom. 2005. *Williams obstretrics.* 21st ed. New York: McGraw Hill.

5. McGovern P., B. Dowd, D. Gjerdingen, I. Moscovice, L. Kochevar, W. Lohman. 1997. Time off work and the postpartum health of employed women. *Medical Care* 35:507-21.

6. Carter, B., M. McGoldrick, eds. 2005. *The expanded family life cycle: Individual, family, and social perspectives.* 3rd ed. New York: Allyn and Bacon Classics.

7. Ishimine, P. 2006. Fever without source in children 0-36 months. Pediatric *Clinics North Am* 53:167.

8. Harper, M. 2004. Update on the management of the febrile infant. *Clin Pediatric Emerg Med* 5:5-12.

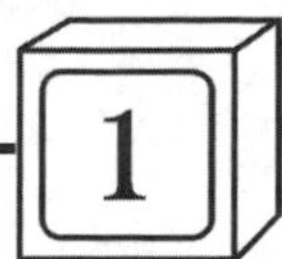

9. Carey, W. B., A. C. Crocker, E. R. Elias, H. M. Feldman, W. L. Coleman. 2009. *Developmental-behavioral pediatrics*. 4th ed. Philadelphia: W. B. Saunders.
10. Parmelee, A. H. Jr, W. Weiner, H. Schultz. 1964. Infant sleep patterns: From birth to 16 weeks of age. *J Pediatrics* 65:576-82.
11. Brazelton, T. B. 1962. Crying in infancy. *Pediatrics* 29:579-88.
12. Huttenlocher, P. R., C. de Courten. 1987. The development of synapses in striate cortex of man. *Human Neurobiology* 6:1-9.
13. Anders, T. F. 1992. Sleeping through the night: A developmental perspective. *Pediatrics* 90:554-60.
14. Edelstein, S., J. Sharlin, S. Edelstein. 2008. *Life cycle nutrition: An evidence-based approach*. Boston: Jones and Bartlett.
15. Robertson, S. S. 1987. Human cyclic motility: Fetal-newborn continuities and newborn state differences. *Devel Psychobiology* 20:425-42.
16. Berger, L. M., J. Hill, J. Waldfogel. 2005. Maternity leave, early maternal employment and child health and development in the US. *Economic J* 115: F29-F47.
17. McGovern, P., B. Dowd, D. Gjerdingen, C. R. Gross, S. Kenney, L. Ukestad, D. McCaffrey, U. Lundberg. 2006. Postpartum health of employed mothers 5 weeks after childbirth. *Annals Fam Med* 4:159-67.
18. Ray, R., J. C. Gornick, J. Schmitt. 2009. *Parental leave policies in 21 countries: Assessing generosity and gender equality.* Rev. ed. Washington, DC: Center for Economic and Policy Research.
19. Social Security Act. 1935. 42 USC 7.
20. Family and Medical Leave Act. 1993. 29 USC 2601.
21. Lovell, V., E. O'Neill, S. Olsen. 2007. Maternity leave in the United States: Paid parental leave is still not standard, even among the best U.S. employers. Washington, DC: Institute for Women's Policy Research. http://iwpr.org/pdf/parentalleaveA131.pdf.
22. Human Rights Watch. 2011. *Failing its families: Lack of paid leave and work-family supports in the U.S.* http://www.hrw.org/en/reports/2011/02/23/failing-its-families-0/.

1.2 Recruitment and Background Screening

STANDARD 1.2.0.1: Staff Recruitment

Staff recruitment should be based on a policy of non-discrimination with regard to gender, race, ethnicity, disability, or religion, as required by the Equal Employment Opportunity Act (EEOA). Centers should have a plan of action for recruiting and hiring a diverse staff that is representative of the children in the facility's care and people in the community with whom the child is likely to have contact as a part of life experience. Staff recruitment policies should adhere to requirements of the Americans with Disabilities Act (ADA) as it applies to employment. The job description for each position should be clearly written, and the suitability of an applicant should be measured with regard to the applicant's qualifications and abilities to perform the tasks required in the role.

RATIONALE: Child care businesses must adhere to federal law. In addition, child care businesses should model diversity and non-discrimination in their employment practices to enhance the quality of the program by supporting diversity and tolerance for individuals on the staff who are competent caregivers/teachers with different background and orientation in their private lives. Children need to see successful role models from their own ethnic and cultural groups and be able to develop the ability to relate to people who are different from themselves (1).

The goal of the ADA in employment is to reasonably accommodate applicants and employees with disabilities, to provide them equal employment opportunity and to integrate them into the program's staff to the extent feasible, given the individual's limitations. Under the ADA, employers are expected to make reasonable accommodations for persons with disabilities. Some disabilities may be accommodated, whereas others may not allow the person to do essential tasks. The fairest way to address this evaluation is to define the tasks and measure the abilities of applicants to perform them (2).

COMMENTS: In staff recruiting, the hiring pool should extend beyond the immediate neighborhood of the child's residence or location of the facility, to reflect the diversity of the people with whom the child can be expected to have contact as a part of life experience.

Reasons to deny employment include the following:

a) The applicant or employee is not qualified or is unable to perform the essential functions of the job with or without reasonable accommodations;
b) Accommodation is unreasonable or will result in undue hardship to the program;
c) The applicant's or employee's condition will pose a significant threat to the health or safety of that individual or of other staff members or children.

Accommodations and undue hardship are based on each individual situation.

The U.S. Equal Employment Opportunity Commission (EEOC) does not enforce the protections that prohibit discrimination and harassment based on sexual orientation, status as a parent, marital status, or political affiliation. However, other federal agencies and many states and municipalities do. For assistance in locating your state or local agency's rules go to http://www.eeoc.gov/field/ (3).

Caregivers/teachers can obtain copies of the EEOA and the ADA from their local public library. Facilities should consult with ADA experts through the U.S. Department of Education funded Disability and Business Technical Assistance Centers (DBTAC) throughout the country. These centers can be reached by calling 1-800-949-4232 (callers will be routed to the appropriate region), or by visiting http://www.adata.org/Static/Home.aspx.

TYPE OF FACILITY: Center; Large Family Child Care Home; Small Family Child Care Home

REFERENCES:

1. Chang, H. 2006. Developing a skilled, ethnically and linguistically diverse early childhood workforce. Adapted from *Getting ready for quality: The critical importance of developing and supporting a skilled, ethnically and linguistically diverse early childhood workforce.* http://www.buildinitiative.org/files/DiverseWorkforce.pdf.
2. U.S. Department of Justice, Civil Rights Division, Disability Rights Section. 1997. Commonly asked questions about child care centers and the Americans with Disabilities Act. http://www.ada.gov/childq&a.htm.

3. U.S. Equal Employment Opportunity Commission. Discrimination based on sexual orientation, status as a parent, marital status and political affiliation. http://www.eeoc.gov/federal/otherprotections.cfm.

STANDARD 1.2.0.2: Background Screening

Directors of centers and caregivers/teachers in large and small family child care homes should conduct a complete background screening before employing any staff member (including substitutes, cooks, clerical staff, transportation staff, bus drivers, or custodians who will be on the premises or in vehicles when children are present). The background screening should include:

a) Name and address verification;
b) Social Security number verification;
c) Education verification;
d) Employment history;
e) Alias search;
f) Driving history through state Department of Motor Vehicles records;
g) Background screening of:
   1) State and national criminal history records;
   2) Child abuse and neglect registries;
   3) Licensing history with any other state agencies (i.e., foster care, mental health, nursing homes, etc.);
   4) Fingerprints; and
   5) Sex offender registries;
h) Court records;
i) References.

All family members over age ten living in large and small family child care homes should also have background screenings.

Drug tests may also be incorporated into the background screening. Written permission to obtain the background screening (with or without a drug screen) should be obtained from the prospective employee. Consent to the background investigation should be required for employment consideration.

When checking references and when conducting employee or volunteer interviews, prospective employers should specifically ask about previous convictions and arrests, investigation findings, or court cases with child abuse/neglect or child sexual abuse. Failure of the prospective employee to disclose previous history of child abuse/neglect or child sexual abuse is grounds for immediate dismissal.

Persons should not be hired or allowed to work or volunteer in the child care facility if they acknowledge being sexually attracted to children or having physically or sexually abused children, or are known to have committed such acts.

Background screenings should be repeated periodically taking into consideration state laws and/or requirements. Screenings should be repeated more frequently if there are additional concerns.

RATIONALE: To ensure their safety and physical and mental health, children should be protected from any risk of abuse or neglect. Although few persons will acknowledge past child abuse or neglect to another person, the obvious attention directed to the question by the licensing agency or caregiver/teacher may discourage some potentially abusive individuals from seeking employment in child care. Performing diligent background screenings also protects the child care facility against future legal challenges (1). Having a state credentialing system can reduce the time required to ensure all those caring for children have had the required background screening review.

COMMENTS: Directors who are conducting screenings and caregivers/teachers who are asked to submit a background screening record should contact their state child care licensing agency for the appropriate documentation required. Fingerprinting can be secured at local law enforcement offices or the State Bureau of Investigation. Court records are public information and can be obtained from county court offices and some states have statewide online court records. When checking for prior arrests or previous court actions, the facility should check for misdemeanors as well as felonies. Driving records are available from the State Department of Motor Vehicles. A social security trace is a report, derived from credit bureau records that will return all current and reported addresses for the last seven to ten years on a specific individual based on his or her social security number. If there are alternate names (aliases) these are also reported. State child abuse registries can be accessed at http://www.hunter.cuny.edu/socwork/nrcfcpp/downloads/policy-issues/State_Child_Abuse_Registries.pdf. Sex offender registries can be accessed at http://www.prevent-abuse-now.com/register.htm. Companies also offer background check services. The National Association of Professional Background Screeners (http://www.napbs.com) provides a directory of their membership.

For more information on state licensing requirements regarding criminal background screenings, see the National Association for Regulatory Administration's (NARA) current Licensing Study at http://www.naralicensing.org.

TYPE OF FACILITY: Center; Large Family Child Care Home; Small Family Child Care Home

REFERENCES:

1. Privacy Rights Clearinghouse. 2011. Fact sheet 16: Employment background checks: A jobseeker's guide. http://www.privacyrights.org/fs/fs16-bck.htm.

1.3 Pre-service Qualifications

1.3.1 Director's Qualifications

STANDARD 1.3.1.1: General Qualifications of Directors

The director of a center enrolling fewer than sixty children should be at least twenty-one-years-old and should have all the following qualifications:

a) Have a minimum of a Baccalaureate degree with at least nine credit-bearing hours of specialized college-level course work in administration, leadership, or

management, and at least twenty-four credit-bearing hours of specialized college-level course work in early childhood education, child development, elementary education, or early childhood special education that addresses child development, learning from birth through kindergarten, health and safety, and collaboration with consultants OR documents meeting an appropriate combination of relevant education and work experiences (6);

b) A valid certificate of successful completion of pediatric first aid that includes CPR;
c) Knowledge of health and safety resources and access to education, health, and mental health consultants;
d) Knowledge of community resources available to children with special health care needs and the ability to use these resources to make referrals or achieve interagency coordination;
e) Administrative and management skills in facility operations;
f) Capability in curriculum design and implementation, ensuring that an effective curriculum is in place;
g) Oral and written communication skills;
h) Certificate of satisfactory completion of instruction in medication administration;
i) Demonstrated life experience skills in working with children in more than one setting;
j) Interpersonal skills;
k) Clean background screening.

Knowledge about parenting training/counseling and ability to communicate effectively with parents/guardians about developmental-behavioral issues, child progress, and in creating an intervention plan beginning with how the center will address challenges and how it will help if those efforts are not effective.

The director of a center enrolling more than sixty children should have the above and at least three years experience as a teacher of children in the age group(s) enrolled in the center where the individual will act as the director, plus at least six months experience in administration.

RATIONALE: The director of the facility is the team leader of a small business. Both administrative and child development skills are essential for this individual to manage the facility and set appropriate expectations. College-level coursework has been shown to have a measurable, positive effect on quality child care, whereas experience per se has not (1-3,5).

The director of a center plays a pivotal role in ensuring the day-to-day smooth functioning of the facility within the framework of appropriate child development principles and knowledge of family relationships (6).

The well-being of the children, the confidence of the parents/guardians of children in the facility's care, and the high morale and consistent professional growth of the staff depend largely upon the knowledge, skills, and dependable presence of a director who is able to respond to long-range and immediate needs and able to engage staff in decision-making that affects their day-to-day practice (5,6). Management skills are important and should be viewed primarily as a means of support for the key role of educational leadership that a director provides (6). A skilled director should know how to use early care and education consultants, such as health, education, mental health, and community resources and to identify specialized personnel to enrich the staff's understanding of health, development, behavior, and curriculum content. Past experience working in an early childhood setting is essential to running a facility.

Life experience may include experience rearing one's own children or previous personal experience acquired in any child care setting. Work as a hospital aide or at a camp for children with special health care needs would qualify, as would experience in school settings. This experience, however, must be supplemented by competency-based training to determine and provide whatever new skills are needed to care for children in child care settings.

COMMENTS: The profession of early childhood education is being informed by research on the association of developmental outcomes with specific practices. The exact combination of college coursework and supervised experience is still being developed. For example, the National Association for the Education of Young Children (NAEYC) has published the *Standards for Early Childhood Professional Preparation Programs* (4). The National Child Care Association (NCCA) has developed a curriculum based on administrator competencies; more information on the NCCA is available at http://www.nccanet.org.

TYPE OF FACILITY: Center

RELATED STANDARDS:
Standards 1.3.1.2-1.3.2.3: General Qualifications for all Caregivers/Teachers, Including Directors, of All Types of Facilities
Standards 1.4.2.1-1.4.2.3: Orientation Training
Standards 1.4.3.1-1.4.3.3: First Aid and CPR Training
Standards 1.4.4.1-1.4.6.2: Continuing Education/Professional Development

REFERENCES:

1. Roupp, R., J. Travers, F. M., Glantz, C. Coelen. 1979. *Children at the center: Summary findings and their implications.* Vol. 1 of *Final report of the National day care study*. Cambridge, MA: Abt Associates.
2. Howes, C. 1997. Children's experiences in center-based child care as a function of teacher background and adult:child ratio. *Merrill-Palmer Q* 43:404-24.
3. Helburn, S., ed. 1995. *Cost, quality and child outcomes in child care centers.* Denver, CO: University of Colorado at Denver.
4. National Association for the Education of Young Children (NAEYC). 2009. *Standards for early childhood professional preparation programs.* Washington, DC: NAEYC. http://www.naeyc.org/files/naeyc/file/positions/ProfPrepStandards09.pdf.
5. Fiene, R. 2002. *13 indicators of quality child care: Research update*. Washington, DC: U.S. Department of Health and Human Services, Office of the Assistant Secretary for Planning and Evaluation. http://aspe.hhs.gov/hsp/ccquality-ind02/.
6. National Association for the Education of Young Children (NAEYC). 2007. *NAEYC early childhood program standards and accreditation criteria: The mark of quality in early childhood education.* Washington, DC: NAEYC.

STANDARD 1.3.1.2: Mixed Director/Teacher Role

Centers enrolling thirty or more children should employ a non-teaching director. Centers with fewer than thirty children may employ a director who teaches as well.

RATIONALE: The duties of a director of a facility with more than thirty children do not allow the director to be involved in the classroom in a meaningful way.

COMMENTS: This standard does not prohibit the director from occasional substitute teaching, as long as the substitute teaching is not a regular and significant duty. Occasional substitute teaching may keep the director in touch with the caregivers'/teachers' issues.

TYPE OF FACILITY: Center

1.3.2 Caregiver's/Teacher's and Other Staff Qualifications

STANDARD 1.3.2.1: Differentiated Roles

Centers should employ a caregiving/teaching staff for direct work with children in a progression of roles, as listed in descending order of responsibility:

a) Program administrator or training/curriculum specialists;
b) Lead teachers;
c) Teachers;
d) Assistant teachers or teacher aides.

Each role with increased responsibility should require increased educational qualifications and experience, as well as increased salary.

RATIONALE: A progression of roles enables centers to offer career ladders rather than dead-end jobs. It promotes a mix of college-trained staff with other members of a child's own community who might have entered at the aide level and moved into higher roles through college or on-the-job training.

Professional education and pre-professional in-service training programs provide an opportunity for career progression and can lead to job and pay upgrades and fewer turnovers. Turnover rates in child care positions in 1997 averaged 30% (3).

COMMENTS: Early childhood professional knowledge must be required whether programs are in private centers, public schools, or other settings. The National Association for the Education of Young Children's (NAEYC) Academy of Early Childhood Programs recommends a multi-level training program that addresses pre-employment educational requirements and continuing education requirements for entry-level assistants, caregivers/teachers, and administrators. It also establishes a table of qualifications for accredited programs (1). The NAEYC requirements include development of an employee compensation plan to increase salaries and benefits to ensure recruitment and retention of qualified staff and continuity of relationships (2). The NAEYC's recommendations should be consulted in conjunction with the standards in this document.

TYPE OF FACILITY: Center

REFERENCES:

1. National Association for the Education of Young Children (NAEYC). 2005. *Accreditation criteria and procedures of the National Academy of Early Childhood Programs.* Washington, DC: NAEYC.
2. National Association for the Education of Young Children (NAEYC). 2009. *Standards for early childhood professional preparation programs.* Washington, DC: NAEYC. http://www.naeyc.org/files/naeyc/file/positions/ProfPrepStandards09.pdf.
3. Whitebook, M., C. Howes, D. Phillips. 1998. *Worthy work, unlivable wages: The national child care staffing study, 1988-1997.* Washington, DC: Center for the Child Care Workforce.

STANDARD 1.3.2.2: Qualifications of Lead Teachers and Teachers

Lead teachers and teachers should be at least twenty-one years of age and should have at least the following education, experience, and skills:

a) A Bachelor's degree in early childhood education, school-age care, child development, social work, nursing, or other child-related field, or an associate's degree in early childhood education and currently working towards a bachelor's degree;
b) A minimum of one year on-the-job training in providing a nurturing indoor and outdoor environment and meeting the child's out-of-home needs;
c) One or more years of experience, under qualified supervision, working as a teacher serving the ages and developmental abilities of the children in care;
d) A valid certificate in pediatric first aid, including CPR;
e) Thorough knowledge of normal child development and early childhood education, as well as knowledge of indicators that a child is not developing typically;
f) The ability to respond appropriately to children's needs;
g) The ability to recognize signs of illness and safety/injury hazards and respond with prevention interventions;
h) Oral and written communication skills;
i) Medication administration training (8).

Every center, regardless of setting, should have at least one licensed/certified lead teacher (or mentor teacher) who meets the above requirements working in the child care facility at all times when children are in care.

Additionally, facilities serving children with special health care needs associated with developmental delay should employ an individual who has had a minimum of eight hours of training in inclusion of children with special health care needs.

RATIONALE: Child care that promotes healthy development is based on the developmental needs of infants, toddlers, and preschool children. Caregivers/teachers are chosen for their knowledge of, and ability to respond appropriately to, the needs of children of this age generally, and the unique

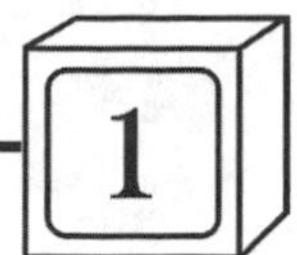

characteristics of individual children (1-4). Both early childhood and special educational experience are useful in a center. Caregivers/teachers that have received formal education from an accredited college or university have shown to have better quality of care and outcomes of programs. Those teachers with a four-year college degree exhibit optimal teacher behavior and positive effects on children (6).

Caregivers/teachers are more likely to administer medications than to perform CPR. Seven thousand children per year require emergency department visits for problems related to cough and cold medication (7).

COMMENTS: The profession of early childhood education is being informed by the research on early childhood brain development, child development practices related to child outcomes (5). For additional information on qualifications for child care staff, refer to the *Standards for Early Childhood Professional Preparation Programs* from the National Association for the Education of Young Children (NAEYC) (4). Additional information on the early childhood education profession is available from the Center for the Child Care Workforce (CCW).

TYPE OF FACILITY: Center

RELATED STANDARDS:
Standards 1.4.3.1-1.4.3.3: First Aid and CPR Training

REFERENCES:

1. National Institute of Child Health and Human Development (NICHD) Early Child Care Research Network. 1996. Characteristics of infant child care: Factors contributing to positive caregiving. *Early Child Res Q* 11:269-306.
2. Bredekamp, S., C. Copple, eds. 1997. *Developmentally appropriate practice in early childhood programs.* Rev ed. Washington, DC: National Association for the Education of Young Children.
3. U.S. Department of Justice. 2011. Americans with Disabilities Act. http://www.ada.gov.
4. National Association for the Education of Young Children (NAEYC). 2009. *Standards for early childhood professional preparation programs.* Washington, DC: NAEYC. http://www.naeyc.org/files/naeyc/file/positions/ProfPrepStandards09.pdf.
5. Committee on Integrating the Science of Early Childhood Development, Board on Children, Youth, and Families. 2000. *From neurons to neighborhoods.* Ed. J. P. Shonkoff, D. A. Phillips. Washington, DC: National Academy Press.
6. Kagan, S. L., K. Tarrent, K. Kauerz. 2008. *The early care and education teaching workforce at the fulcrum,* 44-47, 90-91. New York: Teachers College Press.
7. U.S. Department of Health and Human Services. 2008. CDC study estimates 7,000 pediatric emergency departments visits linked to cough and cold medication: Unsupervised ingestion accounts for 66 percent of incidents. Centers for Disease Control and Prevention (CDC). http://www.cdc.gov/media/pressrel/2008/r080128.htm.
8. American Academy of Pediatrics, Council on School Health. 2009. Policy statement: Guidance for the administration of medication in school. *Pediatrics* 124:1244-51.

STANDARD 1.3.2.3: Qualifications for Assistant Teachers, Teacher Aides, and Volunteers

Assistant teachers and teacher aides should be at least eighteen years of age, have a high school diploma or GED, and participate in on-the-job training, including a structured orientation to the developmental needs of young children and access to consultation, with periodic review, by a supervisory staff member. At least 50% of all assistant teachers and teacher aides must have or be working on either a Child Development Associate (CDA) credential or equivalent, or an associate's or higher degree in early childhood education/child development or equivalent (9).

Volunteers should be at least sixteen years of age and should participate in on-the-job training, including a structured orientation to the developmental needs of young children. Assistant teachers, teacher aides, and volunteers should work only under the continual supervision of lead teacher or teacher. Assistant teachers, teacher aides, and volunteers should never be left alone with children. Volunteers should not be counted in the child:staff ratio.

All assistant teachers, teacher aides, and volunteers should possess:

a) The ability to carry out assigned tasks competently under the supervision of another staff member;
b) An understanding of and the ability to respond appropriately to children's needs;
c) Sound judgment;
d) Emotional maturity; and
e) Clearly discernible affection for and commitment to the well-being of children.

RATIONALE: While volunteers and students can be as young as sixteen, age eighteen is the earliest age of legal consent. Mature leadership is clearly preferable. Age twenty-one allows for the maturity necessary to meet the responsibilities of managing a center or independently caring for a group of children who are not one's own.

Child care that promotes healthy development is based on the developmental needs of infants, toddlers, preschool, and school-age children. Caregivers/teachers should be chosen for their knowledge of, and ability to respond appropriately to, the general needs of children of this age and the unique characteristics of individual children (1,3-5).

Staff training in child development and/or early childhood education is related to positive outcomes for children. This training enables the staff to provide children with a variety of learning and social experiences appropriate to the age of the child. Everyone providing service to, or interacting with, children in a center contributes to the child's total experience (8).

Adequate compensation for skilled workers will not be given priority until the skills required are recognized and valued. Teaching and caregiving requires skills to promote development and learning by children whose needs and abilities change at a rapid rate.

COMMENTS: Experience and qualifications used by the Child Development Associate (CDA) program and the National Child Care Association (NCCA) credentialing program, and included in degree programs with field placement are valued (10). Early childhood professional knowledge must be required whether programs are in private homes, centers, public schools, or other settings. Go to http://www.cdacouncil.org/the-cda-credential/how-to-earn-a-cda/ to view appropriate training and qualification information on the CDA Credential.

The National Association for the Education of Young Children's (NAEYC) National Academy for Early Childhood Program Accreditation, the National Early Childhood Program Accreditation (NECPA) and the National Association of Family Child Care (NAFCC) have established criteria for staff qualifications (2,6,7).

Caregivers/teachers who lack educational qualifications may be employed as continuously supervised personnel while they acquire the necessary educational qualifications if they have personal characteristics, experience, and skills in working with parents, guardians and children, and the potential for development on the job or in a training program.

States may have different age requirements for volunteers.

TYPE OF FACILITY: Center; Large Family Child Care Home

RELATED STANDARDS:
Standard 6.5.1.2: Qualifications for Drivers

REFERENCES:

1. National Institute of Child Health and Human Development (NICHD) Early Child Care Research Network. 1996. Characteristics of infant child care: Factors contributing to positive caregiving. *Early Child Res Q* 11:269-306.
2. National Association for the Education of Young Children (NAEYC). 2005. *Accreditation and criteria procedures of the National Academy of Early Childhood Programs.* Washington, DC: NAEYC.
3. National Association for the Education of Young Children (NAEYC). 2009. *Developmentally appropriate practice in early childhood programs serving children from birth through age 8.* Washington, DC: NAEYC. http://www.naeyc.org/files/naeyc/file/positions/position statement Web.pdf.
4. U.S. Department of Justice. 2011. Americans with Disabilities Act. http://www.ada.gov.
5. National Association for the Education of Young Children (NAEYC). 2009. *Standards for Early Childhood professional preparation programs.* Washington, DC: NAEYC. http://www.naeyc.org/files/naeyc/file/positions/ProfPrepStandards09.pdf.
6. National Child Care Association (NCCA). NCCA official Website. http://www.nccanet.org.
7. National Association for Family Child Care (NAFCC). NAFCC official Website. http://nafcc.net.
8. Da Ros-Voseles, D., S. Fowler-Haughey. 2007. Why children's dispositions should matter to all teachers. *Young Children* (September): 1-7. http://www.naeyc.org/files/yc/file/200709/DaRos-Voseles.pdf.
9. National Association for the Education of Young Children (NAEYC). Candidacy requirements. http://www.naeyc.org/academy/pursuing/candreq/.
10. Council for Professional Recognition. 2011. How to obtaining a CDA. http://www.cdacouncil.org/the-cda-credential/how-to-earn-a-cda/.

STANDARD 1.3.2.4: Additional Qualifications for Caregivers/Teachers Serving Children Three to Thirty-Five Months of Age

Caregivers/teachers should be prepared to work with infants and toddlers and, when asked, should be knowledgeable and demonstrate competency in tasks associated with caring for infants and toddlers:

a) Diapering and toileting;
b) Bathing;
c) Feeding, including support for continuation of breastfeeding;
d) Holding;
e) Comforting;
f) Practicing safe sleep practices to reduce the risk of Sudden Infant Death Syndrome (SIDS) (3);
g) Providing warm, consistent, responsive caregiving and opportunities for child-initiated activities;
h) Stimulating communication and language development and pre-literacy skills through play, shared reading, song, rhyme, and lots of talking;
i) Promoting cognitive, physical, and social emotional development;
j) Preventing shaken baby syndrome/abusive head trauma;
k) Promoting infant mental health;
l) Promoting positive behaviors;
m) Setting age-appropriate limits with respect to safety, health, and mutual respect;
n) Using routines to teach children what to expect from caregivers/teachers and what caregivers/teachers expect from them.

Caregivers/teachers should demonstrate knowledge of development of infants and toddlers as well as knowledge of indicators that a child is not developing typically; knowledge of the importance of attachment for infants and toddlers, the importance of communication and language development, and the importance of nurturing consistent relationships on fostering positive self-efficacy development.

To help manage atypical or undesirable behaviors of children, caregivers/teachers, in collaboration with parents/guardians, should seek professional consultation from the child's primary care provider, an early childhood mental health professional, or an early childhood mental health consultant.

RATIONALE: The brain development of infants is particularly sensitive to the quality and consistency of interpersonal relationships. Much of the stimulation for brain development comes from the responsive interactions of caregivers/teachers and children during daily routines. Children need to be allowed to pursue their interests within safe limits and to be encouraged to reach for new skills (1-7).

COMMENTS: Since early childhood mental health professionals are not always available to help with the management of challenging behaviors in the early care and education setting early childhood mental health consultants may be able to help. The consultant should be viewed as an

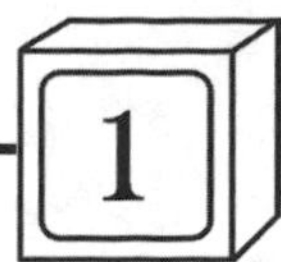

important part of the program's support staff and should collaborate with all regular classroom staff, consultants, and other staff. Qualified potential consultants may be identified by contacting mental health and behavioral providers in the local area, as well as accessing the National Mental Health Information Center (NMHIC) at http://store.samhsa.gov/mhlocator/ and Healthy Child Care America (HCCA) at http://www.healthychildcare.org/Contacts.html.

TYPE OF FACILITY: Center; Large Family Child Care Home; Small Family Child Care Home

RELATED STANDARDS:
Standards 1.3.1.1-1.3.2.3: General Qualifications for all Caregivers/Teachers, Including Directors, of All Types of Facilities
Standards 1.4.2.1-1.4.2.3: Orientation Training
Standards 1.4.3.1-1.4.3.3: First Aid and CPR Training
Standards 1.4.4.1-1.4.6.2: Continuing Education/Professional Development
Standard 1.6.0.3: Early Childhood Mental Health Consultants
Standard 3.1.4.1: Safe Sleep Practices and SIDS/Suffocation Risk Reduction
Standards 4.3.1.1-4.3.1.12: Nutrition for Infants

REFERENCES:

1. Shore, R. 1997. *Rethinking the brain: New insights into early development.* New York: Families and Work Inst.
2. National Forum on Early Childhood Policy and Programs, National Scientific Council on the Developing Child. 2007. *A science-based framework for early childhood policy: Using evidence to improve outcomes in learning, behavior, and health for vulnerable children.* http://developingchild.harvard.edu/index.php/library/reports_and_working_papers/policy_framework/.
3. Moon, R. Y., T. Calabrese, L. Aird. 2008. Reducing the risk of sudden infant death syndrome in child care and changing provider practices: Lessons learned from a demonstration project. *Pediatrics* 122:788-98.
4. Fiene, R. 2002. *13 indicators of quality child care: Research update.* Washington, DC: U.S. Department of Health and Human Services, Office of the Assistant Secretary for Planning and Evaluation. http://aspe.hhs.gov/hsp/ccquality-ind02/.
5. Centers for Disease Control and Prevention. Learn the signs. Act early. http://www.cdc.gov/ncbddd/actearly/.
6. Shonkoff, J. P., D. A. Phillips, eds. 2000. *From neurons to neighborhoods: The science of early childhood development.* Washington, DC: National Academy Press.
7. Cohen, J., N. Onunaku, S. Clothier, J. Poppe. 2005. *Helping young children succeed: Strategies to promote early childhood social and emotional development.* Washington, DC: National Conference of State Legislatures; Zero to Three. http://main.zerotothree.org/site/DocServer/help_yng_child_succeed.pdf.

STANDARD 1.3.2.5: Additional Qualifications for Caregivers/Teachers Serving Children Three to Five Years of Age

Caregivers/teachers should demonstrate the ability to apply their knowledge and understanding of the following to children three to five years of age within the program setting:

a) Typical and atypical development of three- to five-year-old children;
b) Social and emotional development of children, including children's development of independence, their ability to adapt to their environment and cope with stress, problem solve and engage in conflict resolution, and successfully establish friendships;
c) Cognitive, language, early literacy, scientific inquiry, and mathematics development of children;
d) Cultural backgrounds of the children in the facility's care;
e) Talking to parents/guardians about observations and concerns and referrals to parents/guardians;
f) Changing needs of populations served, e.g., culture, income, etc.

To help manage atypical or undesirable behaviors of children three to five years of age, caregivers/teachers serving this age group should seek professional consultation, in collaboration with parents/guardians, from the child's primary care provider, a mental health professional, a child care health consultant, or an early childhood mental health consultant.

RATIONALE: Three- and four-year-old children continue to depend on the affection, physical care, intellectual guidance, and emotional support of their caregivers/teachers (1,2).

A supportive, nurturing setting that supports a demonstration of feelings and accepts regression as part of development continues to be vital for preschool children. Preschool children need help building a positive self-image, a sense of self as a person of value from a family and a culture of which they are proud. Children should be enabled to view themselves as coping, problem-solving, competent, passionate, expressive, and socially connected to peers and staff (3).

TYPE OF FACILITY: Center; Large Family Child Care Home; Small Family Child Care Home

RELATED STANDARDS:
Standards 1.3.1.1-1.3.2.3: General Qualifications for all Caregivers/Teachers, Including Directors, of All Types of Facilities
Standards 1.4.2.1-1.4.2.3: Orientation Training
Standards 1.4.3.1-1.4.3.3: First Aid and CPR Training
Standards 1.4.4.1-1.4.6.2: Continuing Education/Professional Development

REFERENCES:

1. National Institute of Child Health and Human Development (NICHD) Early Child Care Research Network. 1999. Child outcomes when child center classes meet recommended standards for quality. *Am J Public Health* 89:1072-77.
2. Shore, R. 1997. *Rethinking the brain: New insights into early development.* New York: Families and Work Inst.
3. Fiene, R. 2002. *13 indicators of quality child care: Research update.* Washington, DC: U.S. Department of Health and Human Services, Office of the Assistant Secretary for Planning and Evaluation. http://aspe.hhs.gov/hsp/ccquality-ind02/.

STANDARD 1.3.2.6: Additional Qualifications for Caregivers/Teachers Serving School-Age Children

Caregivers/teachers should demonstrate knowledge about and competence with the social and emotional needs and developmental tasks of five- to twelve-year old children, be able to recognize and appropriately manage difficult behaviors, and know how to implement a socially and cognitively enriching program that has been developed with input from parents/guardians. Issues that are significant within school-age programs include having a sense of community, bullying, sexuality, electronic media, and social networking.

With this age group as well, caregivers/teachers, in collaboration with parents/guardians, should seek professional consultation from the child's primary care provider, a mental health professional, a child care health consultant, or an early childhood mental health consultant to help manage atypical or undesirable behaviors.

RATIONALE: A school-age child develops a strong, secure sense of identity through positive experiences with adults and peers (1,2). An informal, enriching environment that encourages self-paced cultivation of interests and relationships promotes the self-worth of school-age children (1). Balancing free exploration with organized activities including homework assistance and tutoring among a group of children also supports healthy emotional and social development (1,3).

When children display behaviors that are unusual or difficult to manage, caregivers/teachers should work with parents/guardians to seek a remedy that allows the child to succeed in the child care setting, if possible (4).

COMMENTS: The first resource for addressing behavior problems is the child's primary care provider. School personnel, including professional serving school-based health clinics may also be able to provide valuable insights. Support from a mental health professional may be needed. If the child's primary care provider cannot help or obtain help from a mental health professional, the caregiver/teacher and the family may need an early childhood mental health consultant to advise about appropriate management of the child. Local mental health agencies or pediatric departments of medical schools may offer help from child psychiatrists, psychologists, other mental health professionals skilled in the issues of early childhood, and pediatricians who have a subspecialty in developmental and behavioral pediatrics. Local or area education agencies serving children with special health or developmental needs may be useful. State Title V (Children with Special Health Care Needs) may be contacted. All state Maternal Child Health (MCH) programs are required to have a toll-free number to link consumers to appropriate programs for children with special health care needs. The toll-free number listing is located at https://perfdata.hrsa.gov/MCHB/MCHReports/search/program/prgsch16.asp. Dismissal from the program should be the last resort and only after consultation with the parent/guardian(s).

TYPE OF FACILITY: Center; Large Family Child Care Home; Small Family Child Care Home

RELATED STANDARDS:
Standards 1.3.1.1-1.3.2.3: General Qualifications for all Caregivers/Teachers, Including Directors, of All Types of Facilities
Standards 1.4.2.1-1.4.2.3: Orientation Training
Standards 1.4.3.1-1.4.3.3: First Aid and CPR Training
Standards 1.4.4.1-1.4.6.2: Continuing Education/Professional Development
Standard 2.2.0.8: Preventing Expulsions, Suspensions, and Other Limitations in Services

REFERENCES:
1. Deschenes, S. N., A. Arbreton, P. M. Little, C. Herrera, J. B. Grossman, H. B. Weiss, D. Lee. 2010. *Engaging older youth: Program and city-level strategies to support sustained participation in out-of-school time.* http://www.hfrp.org/out-of-school-time/publications-resources/engaging-older-youth-program-and-city-level-strategies-to-support-sustained-participation-in-out-of-school-time/.
2. New York State Department of Social Services, Cornell Cooperative Extension. 2004. A parent's guide to child care for school-age children. National Network for Child Care. http://www.nncc.org/choose.quality.care/parents.sac.html#anchor68421/. references
3. Fiene, R. 2002. *13 indicators of quality child care: Research update.* Washington, DC: U.S. Department of Health and Human Services, Office of the Assistant Secretary for Planning and Evaluation. http://aspe.hhs.gov/hsp/ccquality-ind02/.
4. Harvard Family Research Project. 2010. *Family engagement as a systemic, sustained, and integrated strategy to promote student achievement.* http://www.hfrp.org/publications-resources/browse-our-publications/family-engagement-as-a-systemic-sustained-and-integrated-strategy-to-promote-student-achievement/.

STANDARD 1.3.2.7: Qualifications and Responsibilities for Health Advocates

Each facility should designate at least one administrator or staff person as the health advocate to be responsible for policies and day-to-day issues related to health, development, and safety of individual children, children as a group, staff, and parents/guardians. In large centers it may be important to designate health advocates at both the center and classroom level. The health advocate should be the primary contact for parents/guardians when they have health concerns, including health-related parent/guardian/staff observations, health-related information, and the provision of resources. The health advocate ensures that health and safety is addressed, even when this person does not directly perform all necessary health and safety tasks.

The health advocate should also identify children who have no regular source of health care, health insurance, or positive screening tests with no referral documented in the child's health record. The health advocate should assist the child's parent/guardian in locating a Medical Home by referring them to a primary care provider who offers routine child health services.

For centers, the health advocate should be licensed/certified/credentialed as a director or lead teacher or should be a health professional, health educator, or social worker who works at the facility on a regular basis (at least weekly).

The health advocate should have documented training in the following:

a) Control of infectious diseases, including Standard Precautions, hand hygiene, cough and sneeze etiquette, and reporting requirements;
b) Childhood immunization requirements, record-keeping, and at least quarterly review and

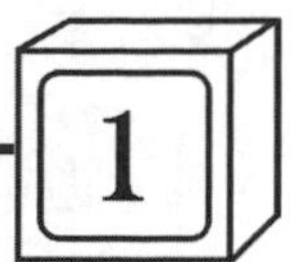

follow-up for children who need to have updated immunizations;

c) Child health assessment form review and follow-up of children who need further medical assessment or updating of their information;
d) How to plan for, recognize, and handle an emergency;
e) Poison awareness and poison safety;
f) Recognition of safety, hazards, and injury prevention interventions;
g) Safe sleep practices and the reduction of the risk of Sudden Infant Death Syndrome (SIDS);
h) How to help parents/guardians, caregivers/teachers, and children cope with death, severe injury, and natural or man-made catastrophes;
i) Recognition of child abuse, neglect/child maltreatment, shaken baby syndrome/abusive head trauma (for facilities caring for infants), and knowledge of when to report and to whom suspected abuse/neglect;
j) Facilitate collaboration with families, primary care providers, and other health service providers to create a health, developmental, or behavioral care plan;
k) Implementing care plans;
l) Recognition and handling of acute health related situations such as seizures, respiratory distress, allergic reactions, as well as other conditions as dictated by the special health care needs of children;
m) Medication administration;
n) Recognizing and understanding the needs of children with serious behavior and mental health problems;
o) Maintaining confidentiality;
p) Healthy nutritional choices;
q) The promotion of developmentally appropriate types and amounts of physical activity;
r) How to work collaboratively with parents/guardians and family members;
s) How to effectively seek, consult, utilize, and collaborate with child care health consultants, and in partnership with a child care health consultant, how to obtain information and support from other education, mental health, nutrition, physical activity, oral health, and social service consultants and resources;
t) Knowledge of community resources to refer children and families who need health services including access to State Children's Health Insurance (SCHIP), importance of a primary care provider and medical home, and provision of immunizations and Early Periodic Screening, Diagnosis, and Treatment (EPSDT).

RATIONALE: The effectiveness of an intentionally designated health advocate in improving the quality of performance in a facility has been demonstrated in all types of early childhood settings (1). A designated caregiver/teacher with health training is effective in developing an ongoing relationship with the parents/guardians and a personal interest in the child (2,3). Caregivers/teachers who are better trained are more able to prevent, recognize, and correct health and safety problems. An internal advocate for issues related to health and safety can help integrate these concerns with other factors involved in formulating facility plans.

Children may be current with required immunizations when they enroll, but they sometimes miss scheduled immunizations thereafter. Because the risk of vaccine-preventable disease increases in group settings, assuring appropriate immunizations is an essential responsibility in child care. Caregivers/teachers should contact their child care health consultant or the health department if they have a question regarding immunization updates/schedules. They can also provide information to share with parents/guardians about the importance of vaccines.

Child health records are intended to provide information that indicates that the child has received preventive health services to stay well, and to identify conditions that might interfere with learning or require special care. Review of the information on these records should be performed by someone who can use the information to plan for the care of the child, and recognize when updating of the information by the child's primary care provider is needed. Children must be healthy to be ready to learn. Those who need accommodation for health problems or are susceptible to vaccine-preventable diseases will suffer if the staff of the child care program is unable to use information provided in child health records to ensure that the child's needs are met (5,6).

COMMENTS: The director should assign the health advocate role to a staff member who seems to have an interest, aptitude, and training in this area. This person need not perform all the health and safety tasks in the facility but should serve as the person who raises health and safety concerns. This staff person has designated responsibility for seeing that plans are implemented to ensure a safe and healthful facility (1).

A health advocate is a regular member of the staff of a center or large or small family child care home, and is not the same as the child care health consultant recommended in Child Care Health Consultants, Standard 1.6.0.1. The health advocate works with a child care health consultant on health and safety issues that arise in daily interactions (4). For small family child care homes, the health advocate will usually be the caregiver/teacher. If the health advocate is not the child's caregiver/teacher, the health advocate should work with the child's caregiver/teacher. The person who is most familiar with the child and the child's family will recognize atypical behavior in the child and support effective communication with parents/guardians.

A plan for personal contact with parents/guardians should be developed, even though this contact will not be possible daily. A plan for personal contact and documentation of a designated caregiver/teacher as health advocate will ensure specific attempts to have the health advocate communicate directly with caregivers/teachers and families on health-related matters.

The immunization record/compliance review may be accomplished by manual review of child health records or by use of software programs that use algorithms with the currently recommended vaccine schedules and service intervals to test the dates when a child received recommended services and the child's date of birth to identify any gaps for which referrals should be made. On the Website of the Centers for Disease Control and Prevention (CDC), individual vaccine recommendations for children six years of age and younger can be checked at http://www.cdc.gov/vaccines/recs/scheduler/catchup.htm.

TYPE OF FACILITY: Center; Large Family Child Care Home; Small Family Child Care Home

RELATED STANDARDS:
Standards 1.3.1.1-1.3.2.3: General Qualifications for all Caregivers/Teachers, Including Directors, of All Types of Facilities
Standards 1.4.2.1-1.4.2.3: Orientation Training
Standards 1.4.3.1-1.4.3.3: First Aid and CPR Training
Standards 1.4.4.1-1.4.6.2: Continuing Education/Professional Development
Standard 1.6.0.1: Child Care Health Consultants
Standard 3.1.2.1: Routine Health Supervision and Growth Monitoring
Standards 3.1.3.1-3.1.3.4: Physical Activity and Limiting Screen Time
Standard 7.2.0.1: Immunization Documentation
Standard 7.2.0.2: Unimmunized Children
Standards 8.7.0.3: Review of Plan for Serving Children With Disabilities or Children With Special Health Care Needs
Appendices G and H: Immunization Schedules for Children and Adults

REFERENCES:
1. Uline, M. S. 1997. Health promotion and injury prevention in a child development center. *J Pediatr Nurs* 12:148-54.
2. Kendrick, A. S., R. Kaufmann, K. P. Messenger, eds. 1991. *Healthy young children: A manual for programs.* Washington, DC: National Association for the Education of Young Children.
3. Murph, J. R., S. D. Palmer, D. Glassy, eds. 2005. *Health in child care: A manual for health professionals*. 4th ed. Elk Grove Village, IL: American Academy of Pediatrics.
4. Alkon, A., J. Bernzweig, K. To, J. K. Mackie, M. Wolff, J. Elman. 2008. Child care health consultation programs in California: Models, services, and facilitators. *Public Health Nurs* 25:126-39.
5. Centers for Disease Control and Prevention (CDC). 2011. Immunization schedules. http://www.cdc.gov/vaccines/recs/schedules/.
6. Hagan, J. F., J. S. Shaw, P. M. Duncan, eds. 2008. *Bright futures: Guidelines for health supervision of infants, children, and adolescents.* 3rd ed. Elk Grove Village, IL: American Academy of Pediatrics.

1.3.3 Family Child Care Home Caregiver/Teacher Qualifications

STANDARD 1.3.3.1: General Qualifications of Family Child Care Caregivers/Teachers to Operate a Family Child Care Home

All caregivers/teachers in large and small family child care homes should be at least twenty-one years of age, hold an official credential as granted by the authorized state agency, meet the general requirements specified in Standard 1.3.2.4 through Standard 1.3.2.6, based on ages of the children served, and those in Section 1.3.3, and should have the following education, experience, and skills:

a) Current accreditation by the National Association for Family Child Care (NAFCC) (including entry-level qualifications and participation in required training) and a college certificate representing a minimum of three credit hours of early childhood education leadership or master caregiver/teacher training or hold an Associate's degree in early childhood education or child development;
b) A provider who has been in the field less than twelve months should be in the self-study phase of NAFCC accreditation;
c) A valid certificate in pediatric first aid, including CPR;
d) Pre-service training in health management in child care, including the ability to recognize signs of illness, knowledge of infectious disease prevention and safety injury hazards;
e) If caring for infants, knowledge on safe sleep practices including reducing the risk of sudden infant death syndrome (SIDS) and prevention of shaken baby syndrome/abusive head trauma (including how to cope with a crying infant);
f) Knowledge of normal child development, as well as knowledge of indicators that a child is not developing typically;
g) The ability to respond appropriately to children's needs;
h) Good oral and written communication skills;
i) Willingness to receive ongoing mentoring from other teachers;
j) Pre-service training in business practices;
k) Knowledge of the importance of nurturing adult-child relationships on self-efficacy development;
l) Medication administration training (6).

Additionally, large family child care home caregivers/teachers should have at least one year of experience serving the ages and developmental abilities of the children in their large family child care home.

Assistants, aides, and volunteers employed by a large family child care home should meet the qualifications specified in Standard 1.3.2.3.

RATIONALE: In both large and small family child care homes, staff members must have the education and experience to meet the needs of the children in care (7). Small family child care home caregivers/teachers often work alone and are solely responsible for the health and safety of small numbers of children in their care.

Most SIDS deaths in child care occur on the first day of care or within the first week; unaccustomed prone (tummy) sleeping increases the risk of SIDS eighteen times (3). Shaken baby syndrome/abusive head trauma is completely preventable. Pre-service training and frequent refresher training can prevent deaths (4).

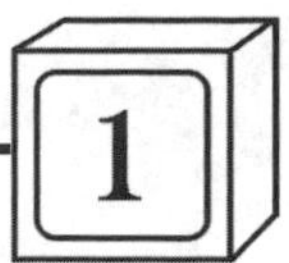

Caregivers/teachers are more likely to administer medications than to perform CPR. Seven thousand children per year require emergency department visits for problems related to cough and cold medications (5).

Age eighteen is the earliest age of legal consent. Mature leadership is clearly preferable. Age twenty-one is more likely to be associated with the level of maturity necessary to independently care for a group of children who are not one's own.

The NAFCC has established an accreditation process to enhance the level of quality and professionalism in small and large family child care (2).

COMMENTS: A large family child care home caregiver/teacher, caring for more than six children and employing one or more assistants, functions as the primary caregiver as well as the facility director. An operator of a large family-child-care home should be offered training relevant to the management of a small child care center, including training on providing a quality work environment for employees.

For more information on assessing the work environment of family child care employees, see *Creating Better Family Child Care Jobs: Model Work Standards,* a publication by the Center for the Child Care Workforce (CCW) (1).

TYPE OF FACILITY: Large Family Child Care Home; Small Family Child Care Home

RELATED STANDARDS:
Standards 1.3.1.1-1.3.2.6: Qualifications for all Caregivers/Teachers, Including Directors, of All Types of Facilities
Section 1.3.3: Family Child Care Home Caregiver/Teacher Qualifications
Standards 1.4.3.1-1.4.3.3: First Aid and CPR Training
Standard 3.1.4.1: Safe Sleep Practices and SIDS/Suffocation Risk Reduction

REFERENCES:

1. Center for Child Care Workforce. 1999. *Creating better family child care jobs: Model work standards.* Washington, DC: Center for Child Care Workforce.
2. National Association for Family Child Care. NAFCC official Website. http://nafcc.net.
3. Moon, R. Y., T. Calabrese, L. Aird. 2008. Reducing the risk of sudden infant death syndrome in child care and changing provider practices: Lessons learned from a demonstration project. *Pediatrics* 122:788-98.
4. Centers for Disease Control and Prevention. Learn the signs. Act early. http://www.cdc.gov/ncbddd/actearly/.
5. U.S. Department of Health and Human Services. 2008. CDC study estimates 7,000 pediatric emergency departments visits linked to cough and cold medication: Unsupervised ingestion accounts for 66 percent of incidents. Centers for Disease Control and Prevention (CDC). http://www.cdc.gov/media/pressrel/2008/r080128.htm.
6. American Academy of Pediatrics, Council on School Health. 2009. Policy statement: Guidance for the administration of medication in school. *Pediatrics* 124:1244-51.
7. National Association for Family Child Care (NAFCC). 2005. *Quality standards for NAFCC accreditation.* 4th ed. Salt Lake City, UT: NAFCC.

STANDARD 1.3.3.2: Support Networks for Family Child Care

Large and small family child care home caregivers/teachers should have active membership in a national, and/or state and local early care and education organization(s). National organizations addressing concerns of family child care home caregivers/teachers include the American Academy of Pediatrics (AAP), the National Association for Family Child Care (NAFCC), and the National Association for the Education of Young Children (NAEYC). In addition, belonging to a local network of family child care home caregivers/teachers that offers education, training and networking opportunities provides the opportunity to focus on local needs. Child care resource and referral agencies may provide additional support networks for caregivers/teachers that include professional development opportunities and information about electronic networking.

RATIONALE: Membership in peer professional organizations shows a commitment to quality child care and also provides a conduit for information to otherwise isolated caregivers/teachers. Membership in a family child care association and attendance at meetings indicate the desire to gain new knowledge about how to work with children (1).

COMMENTS: For more information about family child care associations, contact the NAFCC at http://nafcc.net and/or the NAEYC at http://www.naeyc.org. Also, caregivers/teachers should check to see if their state has specific accreditation standards.

TYPE OF FACILITY: Large Family Child Care Home; Small Family Child Care Home

RELATED STANDARDS:
Standards 1.3.1.1-1.3.2.3: General Qualifications for all Caregivers/Teachers, Including Directors, of All Types of Facilities
Standards 1.4.2.1-1.4.2.3: Orientation Training
Standards 1.4.3.1-1.4.3.3: First Aid and CPR Training
Standards 1.4.4.1-1.4.6.2: Continuing Education/Professional Development
Standard 10.6.2.1: Development of Child Care Provider Organizations and Networks

REFERENCES:

1. Fiene, R. 2002. *13 indicators of quality child care: Research update.* Washington, DC: U.S. Department of Health and Human Services, Office of the Assistant Secretary for Planning and Evaluation. http://aspe.hhs.gov/hsp/ccquality-ind02/.

1.4 Professional Development/Training

1.4.1 Pre-service Training

STANDARD 1.4.1.1: Pre-service Training

In addition to the credentials listed in Standard 1.3.1.1, upon employment, a director or administrator of a center or the lead caregiver/teacher in a family child care home should provide documentation of at least thirty clock-hours of pre-service training. This training should cover health,

psychosocial, and safety issues for out-of-home child care facilities. Small family child care home caregivers/teachers may have up to ninety days to secure training after opening except for training on basic health and safety procedures and regulatory requirements.

All directors or program administrators and caregivers/teachers should document receipt of pre-service training prior to working with children that includes the following content on basic program operations:

a) Typical and atypical child development and appropriate best practice for a range of developmental and mental health needs including knowledge about the developmental stages for the ages of children enrolled in the facility;
b) Positive ways to support language, cognitive, social, and emotional development including appropriate guidance and discipline;
c) Developing and maintaining relationships with families of children enrolled, including the resources to obtain supportive services for children's unique developmental needs;
d) Procedures for preventing the spread of infectious disease, including hand hygiene, cough and sneeze etiquette, cleaning and disinfection of toys and equipment, diaper changing, food handling, health department notification of reportable diseases, and health issues related to having animals in the facility;
e) Teaching child care staff and children about infection control and injury prevention through role modeling;
f) Safe sleep practices including reducing the risk of Sudden Infant Death Syndrome (SIDS) (infant sleep position and crib safety);
g) Shaken baby syndrome/abusive head trauma prevention and identification, including how to cope with a crying/fussy infant;
h) Poison prevention and poison safety;
i) Immunization requirements for children and staff;
j) Common childhood illnesses and their management, including child care exclusion policies and recognizing signs and symptoms of serious illness;
k) Reduction of injury and illness through environmental design and maintenance;
l) Knowledge of U.S. Consumer Product Safety Commission (CPSC) product recall reports;
m) Staff occupational health and safety practices, such as proper procedures, in accordance with Occupational Safety and Health Administration (OSHA) bloodborne pathogens regulations;
n) Emergency procedures and preparedness for disasters, emergencies, other threatening situations (including weather-related, natural disasters), and injury to infants and children in care;
o) Promotion of health and safety in the child care setting, including staff health and pregnant workers;
p) First aid including CPR for infants and children;
q) Recognition and reporting of child abuse and neglect in compliance with state laws and knowledge of protective factors to prevent child maltreatment;
r) Nutrition and age-appropriate child-feeding including food preparation, choking prevention, menu planning, and breastfeeding supportive practices;
s) Physical activity, including age-appropriate activities and limiting sedentary behaviors;
t) Prevention of childhood obesity and related chronic diseases;
u) Knowledge of environmental health issues for both children and staff;
v) Knowledge of medication administration policies and practices;
w) Caring for children with special health care needs, mental health needs, and developmental disabilities in compliance with the Americans with Disabilities Act (ADA);
x) Strategies for implementing care plans for children with special health care needs and inclusion of all children in activities;
y) Positive approaches to support diversity;
z) Positive ways to promote physical and intellectual development.

RATIONALE: The director or program administrator of a center or large family child care home or the small family child care home caregiver/teacher is the person accountable for all policies. Basic entry-level knowledge of health and safety and social and emotional needs is essential to administer the facility. Caregivers/teachers should be knowledgeable about infectious disease and immunizations because properly implemented health policies can reduce the spread of disease, not only among the children but also among staff members, family members, and in the greater community (1). Knowledge of injury prevention measures in child care is essential to control known risks. Pediatric first aid training that includes CPR is important because the director or small family child care home caregiver/teacher is fully responsible for all aspects of the health of the children in care. Medication administration and knowledge about caring for children with special health care needs is essential to maintaining the health and safety of children with special health care needs. Most SIDS deaths in child care occur on the first day of child care or within the first week due to unaccustomed prone (on the stomach) sleeping; the risk of SIDS increases eighteen times when an infant who sleeps supine (on the back) at home is placed in the prone position in child care (2). Shaken baby syndrome/abusive head trauma is completely preventable. It is crucial for caregivers/teachers to be knowledgeable of both syndromes and how to prevent them before they care for infants. Early childhood expertise is necessary to guide the curriculum and opportunities for children in programs (3). The minimum of a Child Development Associate credential with a system of required contact hours, specific content areas, and a set renewal cycle in addition to an assessment requirement would add significantly to the level of care and education for children.

The National Association for the Education of Young Children (NAEYC), a leading organization in child care and early childhood education, recommends annual training based on

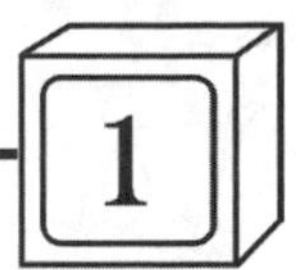

the needs of the program and the pre-service qualifications of staff (4). Training should address the following areas:

a) Health and safety (specifically reducing the risk of SIDS, infant safe sleep practices, shaken baby syndrome/abusive head trauma), and poison prevention and poison safety;
b) Child growth and development, including motor development and appropriate physical activity;
c) Nutrition and feeding of children;
d) Planning learning activities for all children;
e) Guidance and discipline techniques;
f) Linkages with community services;
g) Communication and relations with families;
h) Detection and reporting of child abuse and neglect;
i) Advocacy for early childhood programs;
j) Professional issues (5).

In the early childhood field there is often "crossover" regarding professional preparation (pre-service programs) and ongoing professional development (in-service programs). This field is one in which entry-level requirements differ across various sectors within the field (e.g., nursing, family support, and bookkeeping are also fields with varying entry-level requirements). In early childhood, the requirements differ across center, home, and school based settings. An individual could receive professional preparation (pre-service) to be a teaching staff member in a community-based organization and receive subsequent education and training as part of an ongoing professional development system (in-service). The same individual could also be pursuing a degree for a role as a teacher in a program for which licensure is required—this in-service program would be considered pre-service education for the certified teaching position. Therefore, the labels *pre-service* and *in-service* must be seen as related to a position in the field, and not based on the individual's professional development program (5).

COMMENTS: Training in infectious disease control and injury prevention may be obtained from a child care health consultant, pediatricians, or other qualified personnel of children's and community hospitals, managed care companies, health agencies, public health departments, EMS and fire professionals, pediatric emergency room physicians, or other health and safety professionals in the community.

For more information about training opportunities, contact the local Child Care Resource and Referral Agency (CCRRA), the local chapter of the American Academy of Pediatrics (AAP) (AAP provides online SIDS and medication administration training), the Healthy Child Care America Project, the National Resource Center for Health and Safety in Child Care and Early Education (NRC), or the National Training Institute for Child Care Health Consultants (NTI) at the University of North Carolina at Chapel Hill. California Childcare Health Program (CCHP) has free curricula for health and safety for caregivers/teachers to become child care health advocates. The curriculum (English and Spanish) is free to download on the Web at http://www.ucsfchildcarehealth.org/html/pandr/trainingcurrmain.htm, and is based on NTI's curriculum for child care health consultants. Online training for caregivers/teachers is also available through some state agencies.

For more information on social-emotional training, contact the Center on the Social and Emotional Foundations for Early Learning (CSEFEL) at http://csefel.vanderbilt.edu.

TYPE OF FACILITY: Center; Large Family Child Care Home; Small Family Child Care Home

RELATED STANDARDS:
Standard 1.3.1.1: General Qualifications of Directors
Standard 1.4.1.1: Pre-service Training
Standard 1.4.3.1: First Aid and CPR Training for Staff
Standard 1.7.0.1: Pre-Employment and Ongoing Adult Health Appraisals, Including Immunization
Chapter 3: Health Promotion and Protection
Standard 9.2.4.5: Emergency and Evacuation Drills/Exercises Policy
Standard 9.4.3.3: Training Record
Standards 10.6.1.1-10.6.1.2: Caregiver/Teacher Training

REFERENCES:

1. Hayney M. S., J. C. Bartell. 2005. An immunization education program for childcare providers. *J of School Health* 75:147-49.
2. Moon R. Y., R. P. Oden. 2003. Back to sleep: Can we influence child care providers? *Pediatrics* 112:878-82.
3. Fiene, R. 2002. *13 indicators of quality child care: Research update.* Washington, DC: U.S. Department of Health and Human Services, Office of the Assistant Secretary for Planning and Evaluation. http://aspe.hhs.gov/hsp/ccquality-ind02/.
4. Ritchie, S., B. Willer. 2008. *Teachers: A guide to the NAEYC early childhood program standard and related accreditation criteria.* Washington, DC: National Association for the Education of Young Children (NAEYC).
5. National Association for the Education of Young Children. 2010. *Definition of early childhood professional development*, 12. Eds. M. S. Donovan, J. D. Bransford, J. W. Pellegrino. Washington, DC: National Academy Press.

1.4.2 Orientation Training

STANDARD 1.4.2.1: Initial Orientation of All Staff

All new full-time staff, part-time staff and substitutes should be oriented to the policies listed in Standard 9.2.1.1 and any other aspects of their role. The topics covered and the dates of orientation training should be documented. Caregivers/teachers should also receive continuing education each year, as specified in Continuing Education, Standard 1.4.4.1 through Standard 1.4.6.2.

RATIONALE: Orientation ensures that all staff members receive specific and basic training for the work they will be doing and are informed about their new responsibilities. Because of frequent staff turnover, directors should institute orientation programs on a regular basis (3).

Orientation and ongoing training are especially important for aides and assistant teachers, for whom pre-service educational requirements are limited. Entry into the field at the level of aide or assistant teacher should be attractive and facilitated so that capable members of the families and cultural groups of the children in care can enter the field. Training ensures that staff members are challenged and stimulated, have access to current knowledge (2), and have access to education that will qualify them for new roles.

Use of videos and other passive methods of training should be supplemented by interactive training approaches that help verify content of training has been learned (4).

Health training for child care staff protects the children in care, staff, and the families of the children enrolled. Infectious disease control in child care helps prevent spread of infectious disease in the community. Outbreaks of infectious diseases and intestinal parasites in young children in child care have been shown to be associated with community outbreaks (1).

Child care health consultants can be an excellent resource for providing health and safety orientation or referrals to resources for such training.

COMMENTS: Many states have pre-service education and experience qualifications for caregivers/teachers by role and function. Offering a career ladder and utilizing employee incentives such as Teacher Education and Compensation Helps (TEACH) will attract individuals into the child care field, where labor is in short supply. Colleges, accrediting bodies, and state licensing agencies should examine teacher preparation guidelines and substantially increase the health content of early childhood professional preparation.

Child care staff members are important figures in the lives of the young children in their care and in the well-being of families and the community. Child care staff training should include new developments in children's health. For example; a new training program could discuss up-to-date information on the prevention of obesity and its impact on early onset of chronic diseases.

TYPE OF FACILITY: Center; Large Family Child Care Home; Small Family Child Care Home

RELATED STANDARDS:
Standards 1.4.4.1-1.4.6.2: Continuing Education/Professional Development
Standard 1.6.0.1: Child Care Health Consultants
Standard 9.2.1.1: Content of Policies
Standard 9.4.3.3: Training Record

REFERENCES:
1. Crowley, A. A. 1990. Health services in child care day care centers: A survey. *J Pediatr Health Care* 4:252-59.
2. Moon R. Y., R. P. Oden. 2003. Back to sleep: Can we influence child care providers? *Pediatrics* 112:878-82.
3. Fiene, R. 2002. *13 indicators of quality child care: Research update.* Washington, DC: U.S. Department of Health and Human Services, Office of the Assistant Secretary for Planning and Evaluation. http://aspe.hhs.gov/hsp/ccquality-ind02/.
4. National Association for the Education of Young Children (NAEYC). 2008. *Leadership and management: A guide to the NAEYC early childhood program standards and related accreditation criteria.* Washington, DC: NAEYC.

STANDARD 1.4.2.2: Orientation for Care of Children with Special Health Care Needs

When a child care facility enrolls a child with special health care needs, the facility should ensure that all staff members have been oriented in understanding that child's special health care needs and have the skills to work with that child in a group setting.

Caregivers/teachers in small family child care homes, who care for a child with special health care needs, should meet with the parents/guardians and meet or speak with the child's primary care provider (if the parent/guardian has provided prior, informed, written consent) or a child care health consultant to ensure that the child's special health care needs will be met in child care and to learn how these needs may affect his/her developmental progression or play with other children.

In addition to Orientation Training, Standard 1.4.2.1, the orientation provided to staff in child care facilities should be based on the special health care needs of children who will be assigned to their care. All staff oriented for care of children with special health needs should be knowledgeable about the care plans created by the child's primary care provider in their medical home as well as any care plans created by other health professionals and therapists involved in the child's care. A template for a care plan for children with special health care needs can be found in Appendix O. Child care health consultants can be an excellent resource for providing health and safety orientation or referrals to resources for such training. This training may include, but is not limited to, the following topics:

a) Positioning for feeding and handling, and risks for injury for children with physical/mental disabilities;
b) Toileting techniques;
c) Knowledge of special treatments or therapies (e.g., PT, OT, speech, nutrition/diet therapies, emotional support and behavioral therapies, medication administration, etc.) the child may need/receive in the child care setting;
d) Proper use and care of the individual child's adaptive equipment, including how to recognize defective equipment and to notify parents/guardians that repairs are needed;
e) How different disabilities affect the child's ability to participate in group activities;
f) Methods of helping the child with special health care needs or behavior problems to participate in the facility's programs, including physical activity programs;
g) Role modeling, peer socialization, and interaction;
h) Behavior modification techniques, positive behavioral supports for children, promotion of self-esteem, and other techniques for managing behavior;
i) Grouping of children by skill levels, taking into account the child's age and developmental level;
j) Health services or medical intervention for children with special health care problems;
k) Communication methods and needs of the child;

l) Dietary specifications for children who need to avoid specific foods or for children who have their diet modified to maintain their health, including support for continuation of breastfeeding;
m) Medication administration (for emergencies or on an ongoing basis);
n) Recognizing signs and symptoms of impending illness or change in health status;
o) Recognizing signs and symptoms of injury;
p) Understanding temperament and how individual behavioral differences affect a child's adaptive skills, motivation, and energy;
q) Potential hazards of which staff should be aware;
r) Collaborating with families and outside service providers to create a health, developmental, and behavioral care plan for children with special needs;
s) Awareness of when to ask for medical advice and recommendations for non-emergent issues that arise in school (e.g., head lice, worms, diarrhea);
t) Knowledge of professionals with skills in various conditions, e.g., total communication for children with deafness, beginning orientation and mobility training for children with blindness (including arranging the physical environment effectively for such children), language promotion for children with hearing-impairment and language delay/disorder, etc.;
u) How to work with parents/guardians and other professionals when assistive devices or medications are not consistently brought to the child care program or school;
v) How to safely transport a child with special health care needs.

RATIONALE: A basic understanding of developmental disabilities and special care requirements of any child in care is a fundamental part of any orientation for new employees. Training is an essential component to ensure that staff members develop and maintain the needed skills. A comprehensive curriculum is required to ensure quality services. However, lack of specialized training for staff does not constitute grounds for exclusion of children with disabilities (1).

Staff members need information about how to help children use and maintain adaptive equipment properly. Staff members need to understand how and why various items are used and how to check for malfunctions. If a problem occurs with adaptive equipment, the staff must recognize the problem and inform the parent/guardian so that the parent/guardian can notify the health care or equipment provider of the problem and request that it be remedied. While the parent/guardian is responsible for arranging for correction of equipment problems, child care staff must be able to observe and report the problem to the parent/guardian. Routine care of adaptive and treatment equipment, such as nebulizers, should be taught.

COMMENTS: These training topics are generally applicable to all personnel serving children with special health care needs and apply to child care facilities. The curriculum may vary depending on the type of facility, classifications of disabilities of the children in the facility, and ages of the children. The staff is assumed to have the training described in Orientation Training, Standard 1.4.2.1, including child growth and development. These additional topics will extend their basic knowledge and skills to help them work more effectively with children who have special health care needs and their families. The number of hours offered in any in-service training program should be determined by the staff's experience and professional background. Service plans in small family child care homes may require a modified implementation plan.

The parent/guardian is responsible for solving equipment problems. The parent/guardian can request that the child care facility remedy the problem directly if the caregiver/teacher has been trained on the maintenance and repair of the equipment and if the staff agrees to do it.

TYPE OF FACILITY: Center; Large Family Child Care Home; Small Family Child Care Home

RELATED STANDARDS:
Standard 1.4.2.1: Initial Orientation of All Staff
Standard 3.5.0.1: Care Plan for Children with Special Health Care Needs
Standard 9.4.3.3: Training Record
Appendix O: Care Plan for Children With Special Health Care Needs

REFERENCES:
1. U.S. Department of Justice. 2011. Americans with Disabilities Act. http://www.ada.gov.

STANDARD 1.4.2.3: Orientation Topics

During the first three months of employment, the director of a center or the caregiver/teacher in a large family home should document, for all full-time and part-time staff members, additional orientation in, and the employees' satisfactory knowledge of, the following topics:

a) Recognition of symptoms of illness and correct documentation procedures for recording symptoms of illness. This should include the ability to perform a daily health check of children to determine whether any children are ill or injured and, if so, whether a child who is ill should be excluded from the facility;
b) Exclusion and readmission procedures and policies;
c) Cleaning, sanitation, and disinfection procedures and policies;
d) Procedures for administering medication to children and for documenting medication administered to children;
e) Procedures for notifying parents/guardians of an infectious disease occurring in children or staff within the facility;
f) Procedures and policies for notifying public health officials about an outbreak of disease or the occurrence of a reportable disease;
g) Emergency procedures and policies related to unintentional injury, medical emergency, and natural disasters;
h) Procedure for accessing the child care health consultant for assistance;

i) Injury prevention strategies and hazard identification procedures specific to the facility, equipment, etc.;
j) Proper hand hygiene.

Before being assigned to tasks that involve identifying and responding to illness, staff members should receive orientation training on these topics. Small family child care home caregivers/teachers should not commence operation before receiving orientation on these topics in pre-service training (1).

RATIONALE: Children in child care are frequently ill (2). Staff members responsible for child care must be able to recognize illness and injury, carry out the measures required to prevent the spread of communicable diseases, handle ill and injured children appropriately, and appropriately administer required medications (4). Hand hygiene is one of the most important means of preventing spread of infectious disease (3).

RELATED STANDARDS:
Standard 3.1.1.1: Conduct of Daily Health Check
Standard 3.1.1.2: Documentation of the Daily Health Check
Standard 9.4.3.3: Training Record

TYPE OF FACILITY: Center; Large Family Child Care Home; Small Family Child Care Home

REFERENCES:

1. Fiene, R. 2002. *13 indicators of quality child care: Research update.* Washington, DC: U.S. Department of Health and Human Services, Office of the Assistant Secretary for Planning and Evaluation. http://aspe.hhs.gov/hsp/ccquality-ind02/.
2. Aronson, S. S., T. R. Shope, eds. 2009. *Managing infectious diseases in child care and schools: A quick reference guide.* 2nd ed. Elk Grove Village, IL: American Academy of Pediatrics.
3. Centers for Disease Control and Prevention (CDC). 2011. Handwashing: Clean hands save lives. http://www.cdc.gov/handwashing/.
4. American Academy of Pediatrics, Council on School Health. 2009. Policy statement: Guidance for the administration of medication in school. *Pediatrics* 124:1244-51.

1.4.3 First Aid and CPR Training

STANDARD 1.4.3.1: First Aid and CPR Training for Staff

The director of a center or a large family child care home and the caregiver/teacher in a small family child care home should ensure all staff members involved in providing direct care have documentation of satisfactory completion of training in pediatric first aid and pediatric CPR skills. Pediatric CPR skills should be taught by demonstration, practice, and return demonstration to ensure the technique can be performed in an emergency. These skills should be current according to the requirement specified for retraining by the organization that provided the training.

At least one staff person who has successfully completed training in pediatric first aid that includes CPR should be in attendance at all times with a child whose special care plan indicates an increased risk of needing respiratory or cardiac resuscitation.

Records of successful completion of training in pediatric first aid should be maintained in the personnel files of the facility.

RATIONALE: To ensure the health and safety of children in a child care setting, someone who is qualified to respond to life-threatening emergencies must be in attendance at all times (1). A staff trained in pediatric first aid, including pediatric CPR, coupled with a facility that has been designed or modified to ensure the safety of children, can mitigate the consequences of injury, and reduce the potential for death from life-threatening conditions. Knowledge of pediatric first aid, including pediatric CPR which addresses management of a blocked airway and rescue breathing, and the confidence to use these skills, are critically important to the outcome of an emergency situation.

Small family child care home caregivers/teachers often work alone. They must have the necessary skills to manage emergencies while caring for all the children in the group.

Children with special health care needs who have compromised airways may need to be accompanied to child care with nurses who are able to respond to airway problems (e.g., the child who has a tracheostomy and needs suctioning).

First aid skills are the most likely tools caregivers/teachers will need. Minor injuries are common. For emergency situations that require attention from a health professional, first aid procedures can be used to control the situation until a health professional can provide definitive care. However, management of a blocked airway (choking) is a life-threatening emergency that cannot wait for emergency medical personnel to arrive on the scene (2).

Documentation of current certification of satisfactory completion of pediatric first aid and demonstration of pediatric CPR skills in the facility assists in implementing and in monitoring for proof of compliance.

COMMENTS: The recommendations from the American Heart Association (AHA) changed in 2010 from "A-B-C" (Airway, Breathing, Chest compressions) to "C-A-B" (Chest compressions, Airway, Breathing) for adults and pediatric patients (children and infants, excluding newborns). Except for newborns, the ratio of chest compressions to ventilations in the 2010 guidelines is 30:2. CPR skills are lost without practice and ongoing education (3,5).

The most common renewal cycle required by organizations that offer pediatric first aid and pediatric CPR training is to require successful completion of training every three years (4), though the AHA requires successful completion of CPR class every two years.

Inexpensive self-learning kits that require only thirty minutes to review the skills of pediatric CPR with a video and an inflatable manikin are available from the AHA. See "Infant CPR Anytime" and "Family and Friends CPR Anytime" at http://www.heart.org/HEARTORG/.

Child care facilities should consider having an Automated External Defibrillators (AED) on the child care premises for

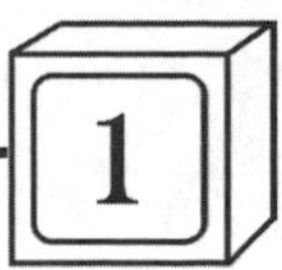

potential use with adults. The use of AEDs with children would be rare.

TYPE OF FACILITY: Center; Large Family Child Care Home; Small Family Child Care Home

RELATED STANDARDS:
Standard 1.4.3.2: Topics Covered in First Aid Training
Standard 1.4.3.3: CPR Training for Swimming and Water Play
Standard 9.4.3.3: Training Record
Standards 10.6.1.1-10.6.1.2: Caregiver/Teacher Training

REFERENCES:
1. Alkon, A., P. J. Kaiser, J. M. Tschann, W. T. Boyce, J. L. Genevro, M. Chesney. 1994. Injuries in child-care centers: Rates, severity, and etiology. *Pediatrics* 94:1043-46.
2. Stevens, P. B., K. A. Dunn. 1994. Use of cardiopulmonary resuscitation by North Carolina day care providers. *J School Health* 64:381-83.
3. American Heart Association (AHA). 2010 AHA guidelines for cardiopulmonary resuscitation and emergency cardiovascular care science. *Circulation* 122: S640-56.
4. Aronson, S. S., ed. 2007. *Pediatric first aid for caregivers and teachers.* Rev. 1st ed. Elk Grove Village, IL: American Academy of Pediatrics; Sudbury, MA: Jones and Bartlett.
5. American Heart Association (AHA). 2010. Hands-only CPR. http://handsonlycpr.org.

STANDARD 1.4.3.2: Topics Covered in First Aid Training

First aid training should present an overview of Emergency Medical Services (EMS), accessing EMS, poison center services, accessing the poison center, safety at the scene, and isolation of body substances. First aid instruction should include, but not be limited to, recognition and first response of pediatric emergency management in a child care setting of the following situations:

a) Management of a blocked airway and rescue breathing for infants and children with return demonstration by the learner (pediatric CPR);
b) Abrasions and lacerations;
c) Bleeding, including nosebleeds;
d) Burns;
e) Fainting;
f) Poisoning, including swallowed, skin or eye contact, and inhaled;
g) Puncture wounds, including splinters;
h) Injuries, including insect, animal, and human bites;
i) Poison control;
j) Shock;
k) Seizure care;
l) Musculoskeletal injury (such as sprains, fractures);
m) Dental and mouth injuries/trauma;
n) Head injuries, including shaken baby syndrome/abusive head trauma;
o) Allergic reactions, including information about when epinephrine might be required;
p) Asthmatic reactions, including information about when rescue inhalers must be used;
q) Eye injuries;
r) Loss of consciousness;
s) Electric shock;
t) Drowning;
u) Heat-related injuries, including heat exhaustion/heat stroke;
v) Cold related injuries, including frostbite;
w) Moving and positioning injured/ill persons;
x) Illness-related emergencies (such as stiff neck, inexplicable confusion, sudden onset of blood-red or purple rash, severe pain, temperature above 101°F [38.3°C] orally, above 102°F [38.9°C] rectally, or 100°F [37.8°C] or higher taken axillary [armpit] or measured by an equivalent method, and looking/acting severely ill);
y) Standard Precautions;
z) Organizing and implementing a plan to meet an emergency for any child with a special health care need;
aa) Addressing the needs of the other children in the group while managing emergencies in a child care setting;
ab) Applying first aid to children with special health care needs.

RATIONALE: First aid for children in the child care setting requires a more child-specific approach than standard adult-oriented first aid offers. To ensure the health and safety of children in a child care setting, someone who is qualified to respond to common injuries and life-threatening emergencies must be in attendance at all times. A staff trained in pediatric first aid, including pediatric CPR, coupled with a facility that has been designed or modified to ensure the safety of children, can reduce the potential for death and disability. Knowledge of pediatric first aid, including the ability to demonstrate pediatric CPR skills, and the confidence to use these skills, are critically important to the outcome of an emergency situation (1).

Small family child care home caregivers/teachers often work alone and are solely responsible for the health and safety of children in care. Such caregivers/teachers must have pediatric first aid competence.

COMMENTS: Other children will have to be supervised while the injury is managed. Parental notification and communication with emergency medical services must be carefully planned. First aid information can be obtained from the American Academy of Pediatrics (AAP) at http://www.aap.org and the American Heart Association (AHA) at http://www.heart.org/HEARTORG/.

TYPE OF FACILITY: Center; Large Family Child Care Home; Small Family Child Care Home

RELATED STANDARDS:
Standard 1.4.3.1: First Aid and CPR Training for Staff
Standard 9.4.3.3: Training Record

REFERENCES:
1. Aronson, S. S., ed. 2007. *Pediatric first aid for caregivers and teachers.* Rev. 1st ed. Elk Grove Village, IL: American Academy of Pediatrics; Sudbury, MA: Jones and Bartlett.

STANDARD 1.4.3.3: CPR Training for Swimming and Water Play

Facilities that have a swimming pool should require at least one staff member with current documentation of successful completion of training in infant and child (pediatric) CPR (Cardiopulmonary Resuscitation) be on duty at all times during business hours.

At least one of the caregivers/teachers, volunteers, or other adults who is counted in the child:staff ratio for swimming and water play should have documentation of successful completion of training in basic water safety, proper use of swimming pool rescue equipment, and infant and child CPR according to the criteria of the American Red Cross or the American Heart Association (AHA).

For small family child care homes, the person trained in water safety and CPR should be the caregiver/teacher. Written verification of successful completion of CPR and lifesaving training, water safety instructions, and emergency procedures should be kept on file.

RATIONALE: Drowning involves cessation of breathing and rarely requires cardiac resuscitation of victims. Nevertheless, because of the increased risk for cardiopulmonary arrest related to wading and swimming, the facility should have personnel trained to provide CPR and to deal promptly with a life-threatening drowning emergency. During drowning, cold exposure provides the possibility of protection of the brain from irreversible damage associated with respiratory and cardiac arrest. Children drown in as little as two inches of water. The difference between a life and death situation is the submersion time. Thirty seconds can make a difference. The timely administration of resuscitation efforts by a caregiver/teacher trained in water safety and CPR is critical. Studies have shown that prompt rescue and the presence of a trained resuscitator at the site can save about 30% of the victims without significant neurological consequences (1).

TYPE OF FACILITY: Center; Large Family Child Care Home; Small Family Child Care Home

RELATED STANDARDS:
Standard 1.1.1.5: Ratios and Supervision for Swimming, Wading, and Water Play
Standard 2.2.0.4: Supervision Near Bodies of Water
Standard 2.2.0.5: Behavior Around a Pool
Standard 6.3.1.7: Pool Safety Rules
Standard 6.4.1.1: Pool Toys
Standard 9.4.3.3: Training Record

REFERENCES:
1. Aronson, S. S., ed. 2007. *Pediatric first aid for caregivers and teachers.* Rev. 1st ed. Elk Grove Village, IL: American Academy of Pediatrics; Sudbury, MA: Jones and Bartlett.

1.4.4 Continuing Education/ Professional Development

STANDARD 1.4.4.1: Continuing Education for Directors and Caregivers/Teachers in Centers and Large Family Child Care Homes

All directors and caregivers/teachers of centers and large family child care homes should successfully complete at least thirty clock-hours per year of continuing education/ professional development in the first year of employment, sixteen clock-hours of which should be in child development programming and fourteen of which should be in child health, safety, and staff health. In the second and each of the following years of employment at a facility, all directors and caregivers/teachers should successfully complete at least twenty-four clock-hours of continuing education based on individual competency needs and any special needs of the children in their care, sixteen hours of which should be in child development programming and eight hours of which should be in child health, safety, and staff health.

Programs should conduct a needs assessment to identify areas of focus, trainer qualifications, adult learning strategies, and create an annual professional development plan for staff based on the needs assessment. The effectiveness of training should be evident by the change in performance as measured by accreditation standards or other quality assurance systems.

RATIONALE: Because of the nature of their caregiving/ teaching tasks, caregivers/teachers must attain multifaceted knowledge and skills. Child health and employee health are integral to any education/training curriculum and program management plan. Planning and evaluation of training should be based on performance of the staff member(s) involved. Too often, staff members make training choices based on what they like to learn about (their "wants") and not the areas in which their performance should be improved (their "needs"). Participation in training does not ensure that the participant will master the information and skills offered in the training experience. Therefore, caregiver/ teacher change in behavior or the continuation of appropriate practice resulting from the training, not just participation in training, should be assessed by supervisors and directors (4).

In addition to low child:staff ratio, group size, age mix of children, and stability of caregiver/teacher, the training/education of caregivers/teachers is a specific indicator of child care quality (2). Most skilled roles require training related to the functions and responsibilities the role requires. Staff members who are better trained are better able to prevent, recognize, and correct health and safety problems. The number of training hours recommended in this standard reflects the central focus of caregivers/teachers on child development, health, and safety.

Children may come to child care with identified special health care needs or special needs may be identified while attending child care, so staff should be trained in recogniz-

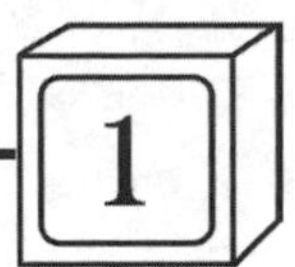

ing health problems as well as in implementing care plans for previously identified needs. Medications are often required either on an emergent or scheduled basis for a child to safely attend child care. Caregivers/teachers should be well trained on medication administration and appropriate policies should be in place.

The National Association for the Education of Young Children (NAEYC), a leading organization in child care and early childhood education, recommends annual training/professional development based on the needs of the program and the pre-service qualifications of staff (1). Training should address the following areas:

a) Promoting child growth and development correlated with developmentally appropriate activities;
b) Infant care;
c) Recognizing and managing minor illness and injury;
d) Managing the care of children who require the special procedures listed in Standard 3.5.0.2;
e) Medication administration;
f) Business aspects of the small family child care home;
g) Planning developmentally appropriate activities in mixed age groupings;
h) Nutrition for children in the context of preparing nutritious meals for the family;
i) Age-appropriate size servings of food and child feeding practices;
j) Acceptable methods of discipline/setting limits;
k) Organizing the home for child care;
l) Preventing unintentional injuries in the home (e.g., falls, poisoning, burns, drowning);
m) Available community services;
n) Detecting, preventing, and reporting child abuse and neglect;
o) Advocacy skills;
p) Pediatric first aid, including pediatric CPR;
q) Methods of effective communication with children and parents/guardians;
r) Socio-emotional and mental health (positive approaches with consistent and nurturing relationships);
s) Evacuation and shelter-in-place drill procedures;
t) Occupational health hazards;
u) Infant safe sleep environments and practices;
v) Standard Precautions;
w) Shaken baby syndrome/abusive head trauma;
x) Dental issues;
y) Age-appropriate nutrition and physical activity.

There are few illnesses for which children should be excluded from child care. Decisions about management of ill children are facilitated by skill in assessing the extent to which the behavior suggesting illness requires special management (3). Continuing education on managing infectious diseases helps prepare caregivers/teachers to make these decisions devoid of personal biases (5). Recommendations regarding responses to illnesses may change (e.g., H1N1), so caregivers/teachers need to know where they can find the most current information. All caregivers/teachers should be trained to prevent, assess, and treat injuries common in child care settings and to comfort an injured child and children witnessing an injury.

COMMENTS: Tools for assessment of training needs are part of the accreditation self-study tools available from the NAEYC, the National Association for Family Child Care (NAFCC), National Early Childhood Professional Accreditation (NECPA), Association for Christian Education International (ACEI), National AfterSchool Association (NAA), and the National Child Care Association (NCCA). Successful completion of training can be measured by a performance test at the end of training and by ongoing evaluation of performance on the job.

Resources for training on health and safety issues include:

a) State and local health departments (health education, environmental health and sanitation, nutrition, public health nursing departments, fire and EMS, etc.);
b) Networks of child care health consultants;
c) Graduates of the National Training Institute for Child Care Health Consultants (NTI);
d) Child care resource and referral agencies;
e) University Centers for Excellence on Disabilities;
f) Local children's hospitals;
g) State and local chapters of:
    1) American Academy of Pediatrics (AAP), including AAP Chapter Child Care Contacts;
    2) American Academy of Family Physicians (AAFP);
    3) American Nurses' Association (ANA);
    4) American Public Health Association (APHA);
    5) Visiting Nurse Association (VNA);
    6) National Association of Pediatric Nurse Practitioners (NAPNAP);
    7) National Association for the Education of Young Children (NAEYC);
    8) National Association for Family Child Care (NAFCC);
    9) National Association of School Nurses (NASN);
    10) National Training Institute for Child Care Health Consultants (NTI);
    11) Emergency Medical Services for Children (EMSC) National Resource Center;
    12) National Association for Sport and Physical Education (NASPE);
    13) American Dietetic Association (ADA);
    14) American Association of Poison Control Centers (AAPCC).

For nutrition training, facilities should check that the nutritionist/registered dietician (RD), who provides advice, has experience with, and knowledge of, child development, infant and early childhood nutrition, school-age child nutrition, prescribed nutrition therapies, food service and food safety issues in the child care setting. Most state Maternal and Child Health (MCH) programs, Child and Adult Care Food Programs (CACFP), and Special Supplemental Nutrition Programs for Women, Infants, and Children (WIC) have a nutrition specialist on staff or access to a local consultant. If this nutrition specialist has knowledge and experience in early childhood and child care, facilities might negotiate for this individual to serve or identify someone to serve as a consultant and trainer for the facility.

Many resources are available for nutritionists/RDs who provide training in food service and nutrition. Some resources to contact include:

a) Local, county, and state health departments to locate MCH, CACFP, or WIC programs;
b) State university and college nutrition departments;
c) Home economists at utility companies;
d) State affiliates of the American Dietetic Association;
e) State and regional affiliates of the American Public Health Association;
f) The American Association of Family and Consumer Services;
g) National Resource Center for Health and Safety in Child Care and Early Education;
h) Nutritionist/RD at a hospital;
i) High school home economics teachers;
j) The Dairy Council;
k) The local American Heart Association affiliate;
l) The local Cancer Society;
m) The Society for Nutrition Education;
n) The local Cooperative Extension office;
o) Local community colleges and trade schools.

Nutrition education resources may be obtained from the Food and Nutrition Information Center at http://fnic.nal.usda.gov. The staff's continuing education in nutrition may be supplemented by periodic newsletters and/or literature (frequently bilingual) or audiovisual materials prepared or recommended by the Nutrition Specialist.

Caregivers/teachers should have a basic knowledge of special health care needs, supplemented by specialized training for children with special health care needs. The type of special health care needs of the children in care should influence the selection of the training topics. The number of hours offered in any in-service training program should be determined by the experience and professional background of the staff, which is best achieved through a regular staff conference mechanism.

Financial support and accessibility to training programs requires attention to facilitate compliance with this standard. Many states are using federal funds from the Child Care and Development Block Grant to improve access, quality, and affordability of training for early care and education professionals. College courses, either online or face to face, and training workshops can be used to meet the training hours requirement. These training opportunities can also be conducted on site at the child care facility. Completion of training should be documented by a college transcript or a training certificate that includes title/content of training, contact hours, name and credentials of trainer or course instructor and date of training. Whenever possible the submission of documentation that shows how the learner implemented the concepts taught in the training in the child care program should be documented. Although on-site training can be costly, it may be a more effective approach than participation in training at a remote location.

Projects and Outreach: Early Childhood Research and Evaluation Projects, Midwest Child Care Research Consortium at http://ccfl.unl.edu/projects_outreach/projects/current/ecp/mwcrc.php, identifies the number of hours for education of staff and fourteen indicators of quality from a study conducted in four Midwestern states.

TYPE OF FACILITY: Center; Large Family Child Care Home

RELATED STANDARDS:

Standard 1.8.2.2: Annual Staff Competency Evaluation
Standard 3.5.0.2: Caring for Children Who Require Medical Procedures
Standard 3.6.3.1: Medication Administration
Standard 9.4.3.3: Training Record
Standard 10.3.3.4: Licensing Agency Provision of Child Abuse Prevention Materials
Standard 10.3.4.6: Compensation for Participation in Multidisciplinary Assessments for Children with Special Health Care or Education Needs
Standards 10.6.1.1-10.6.1.2: Caregiver/Teacher Training
Appendix C: Nutrition Specialist, Registered Dietician, Licensed Nutritionist, Consultant, and Food Service Staff Qualifications

REFERENCES:

1. National Association for the Education of Young Children (NAEYC). 2009. *Standards for early childhood professional preparation programs.* Washington, DC: NAEYC. http://www.naeyc.org/files/naeyc/file/positions/ProfPrepStandards09.pdf.
2. Whitebook, M., C. Howes, D. Phillips. 1998. *Worthy work, unlivable wages: The National child care staffing study, 1988-1997.* Washington, DC: Center for the Child Care Workforce.
3. Crowley, A. A. 1990. Health services in child care day care centers: A survey. *J Pediatr Health Care* 4:252-59.
4. Fiene, R. 2002. *13 indicators of quality child care: Research update.* Washington, DC: U.S. Department of Health and Human Services, Office of the Assistant Secretary for Planning and Evaluation. http://aspe.hhs.gov/hsp/ccquality-ind02/.
5. Aronson, S. S., T. R. Shope, eds. 2009. *Managing infectious diseases in child care and schools: A quick reference guide.* 2nd ed. Elk Grove Village, IL: American Academy of Pediatrics.

STANDARD 1.4.4.2: Continuing Education for Small Family Child Care Home Caregivers/Teachers

Small family child care home caregivers/teachers should have at least thirty clock-hours per year (2) of continuing education in areas determined by self-assessment and, where possible, by a performance review of a skilled mentor or peer reviewer.

RATIONALE: In addition to low child:staff ratio, group size, age mix of children, and continuity of caregiver/teacher, the training/education of caregivers/teachers is a specific indicator of child care quality (1). Most skilled roles require training related to the functions and responsibilities the role requires. Caregivers/teachers who engage in on-going training are more likely to decrease morbidity and mortality in their setting (3) and are better able to prevent, recognize, and correct health and safety problems.

Children may come to child care with identified special health care needs or may develop them while attending child care, so staff must be trained in recognizing health

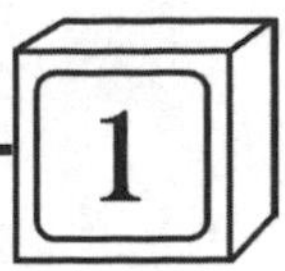

problems as well as in implementing care plans for previously identified needs.

Because of the nature of their caregiving/teaching tasks, caregivers/teachers must attain multifaceted knowledge and skills. Child health and employee health are integral to any education/training curriculum and program management plan. Planning and evaluation of training should be based on performance of the caregiver/teacher. Provision of workshops and courses on all facets of a small family child care business may be difficult to access and may lead to caregivers/teachers enrolling in training opportunities in curriculum related areas only. Too often, caregivers/teachers make training choices based on what they like to learn about (their "wants") and not the areas in which their performance should be improved (their "needs").

Small family child care home caregivers/teachers often work alone and are solely responsible for the health and safety of small numbers of children in care. Peer review is part of the process for accreditation of family child care and can be valuable in assisting the caregiver/teacher in the identification of areas of need for training. Self-evaluation may not identify training needs or focus on areas in which the caregiver/teacher is particularly interested and may be skilled already.

COMMENTS: The content of continuing education for small family child care home caregivers/teachers should include the following topics:

a) Promoting child growth and development correlated with developmentally appropriate activities;
b) Infant care;
c) Recognizing and managing minor illness and injury;
d) Managing the care of children who require the special procedures listed in Standard 3.5.0.2;
e) Medication administration;
f) Business aspects of the small family child care home;
g) Planning developmentally appropriate activities in mixed age groupings;
h) Nutrition for children in the context of preparing nutritious meals for the family;
i) Age-appropriate size servings of food and child feeding practices;
j) Acceptable methods of discipline/setting limits;
k) Organizing the home for child care;
l) Preventing unintentional injuries in the home (falls, poisoning, burns, drowning);
m) Available community services;
n) Detecting, preventing, and reporting child abuse and neglect;
o) Advocacy skills;
p) Pediatric first aid, including pediatric CPR;
q) Methods of effective communication with children and parents/guardians;
r) Socio-emotional and mental health (positive approaches with consistent and nurturing relationships);
s) Evacuation and shelter-in-place drill procedures;
t) Occupational health hazards;
u) Infant-safe sleep environments and practices;
v) Standard Precautions;
w) Shaken baby syndrome/abusive head trauma;
x) Dental issues;
y) Age-appropriate nutrition and physical activity.

Small family child care home caregivers/teachers should maintain current contact lists of community pediatric primary care providers, specialists for health issues of individual children in their care and child care health consultants who could provide training when needed.

In-home training alternatives to group training for small family child care home caregivers/teachers are available, such as distance courses on the Internet, listening to audiotapes or viewing media (e.g., DVDs) with self-checklists. These training alternatives provide more flexibility for caregivers/teachers who are remote from central training locations or have difficulty arranging coverage for their child care duties to attend training. Nevertheless, gathering family child care home caregivers/teachers for training when possible provides a break from the isolation of their work and promotes networking and support. Satellite training via down links at local extension service sites, high schools, and community colleges scheduled at convenient evening or weekend times is another way to mix quality training with local availability and some networking.

TYPE OF FACILITY: Small Family Child Care Home

RELATED STANDARDS:
Standard 1.4.4.1: Continuing Education for Directors and Caregivers/Teachers in Centers and Large Family Child Care Homes
Standard 1.7.0.4: Occupational Hazards
Standard 3.5.0.2: Caring for Children Who Require Medical Procedures
Standards 9.2.4.3-9.2.4.5: Emergency and Evacuation Plans, Training, and Communication
Standard 9.4.3.3: Training Record
Appendix B: Major Occupational Health Hazards

REFERENCES:
1. Whitebook, M., C. Howes, D. Phillips. 1998. *Worthy work, unlivable wages: The national child care staffing study, 1988-1997.* Washington, DC: Center for the Child Care Workforce.
2. The National Association of Family Child Care (NAFCC). 2005. *Quality standards for NAFCC accreditation.* 4th ed. Salt Lake City, UT: NAFCC. http://www.nafcc.org/documents/QualStd.pdf.
3. Fiene, R. 2002. *13 indicators of quality child care: Research update.* Washington, DC: U.S. Department of Health and Human Services, Office of the Assistant Secretary for Planning and Evaluation. http://aspe.hhs.gov/hsp/ccquality-ind02/.

1.4.5 Specialized Training/Education

STANDARD 1.4.5.1: Training of Staff Who Handle Food

All staff members with food handling responsibilities should obtain training in food service and safety. The director of a center or a large family child care home or the designated supervisor for food service should be a certified food protection manager or equivalent as demonstrated by completing an accredited food protection manager course. Small family child care personnel should secure training in food service and safety appropriate for their setting.

RATIONALE: Outbreaks of foodborne illness have occurred in many settings, including child care facilities. Some of these outbreaks have led to fatalities and severe disabilities. Young children are particularly susceptible to foodborne illness, due to their body size and immature immune systems. Because large centers serve more meals daily than many restaurants do, the supervisors of food handlers in these settings should have successfully completed food service certification, and the food handlers in these settings should have successfully completed courses on appropriate food handling (1).

COMMENTS: Sponsors of the Child and Adult Care Food Program (CACFP) provide this training for some small family child care home caregivers/teachers. For training in food handling, caregivers/teachers should contact the state or local health department, or the delegate agencies that handle nutrition and environmental health inspection programs for the child care facility. Training for food workers is mandatory in some jurisdictions. Other sources for food safety information are the Food and Drug Administration (FDA) *Food Code*, family child care associations, child care resource and referral agencies, licensing agencies, and state departments of education.

TYPE OF FACILITY: Center; Large Family Child Care Home; Small Family Child Care Home

RELATED STANDARDS:
Standard 9.4.3.3: Training Record

REFERENCES:
1. U.S. Department of Health and Human Services, Public Health Service, Food and Drug Administration (FDA). 2009. *Food code 2009.* College Park, MD: FDA. http://www.fda.gov/Food/FoodSafety/RetailFoodProtection/FoodCode/FoodCode2009/default.htm.

STANDARD 1.4.5.2: Child Abuse and Neglect Education

Caregivers/teachers should use child abuse and neglect prevention education to educate and establish child abuse and neglect prevention and recognition measures for the children, caregivers/teachers, and parents/guardians. The education should address physical, sexual, and psychological or emotional abuse and neglect. The dangers of shaking infants and toddlers and repeated exposure to domestic violence should be included in the education and prevention materials. Caregivers/teachers should also receive education on promoting protective factors to prevent child maltreatment. Caregivers/teachers should be able to identify signs of stress in families and assist families by providing support and linkages to resources when needed. Children with disabilities are at a higher risk of being abused. Special training in child abuse and neglect and children with disabilities should be provided (2).

Caregivers/teachers are mandatory reporters of child abuse or neglect. Caregivers/teachers should be trained in compliance with their state's child abuse reporting laws. Child abuse reporting requirements are known and available from the child care regulation department in each state.

RATIONALE: Education about the manifestations of child maltreatment can increase the likelihood of appropriate reports to child protection agencies and law enforcement agencies (1-3).

COMMENTS: Child abuse and neglect materials should be designed for non-medical audiences. Resources are available from the American Academy of Pediatrics (AAP) at http://www.aap.org, the Child Welfare Information Gateway at http://www.childwelfare.gov, and Prevent Child Abuse America at http://www.preventchildabuse.org.

TYPE OF FACILITY: Center; Large Family Child Care Home; Small Family Child Care Home

RELATED STANDARDS:
Standard 2.2.0.9: Prohibited Caregiver/Teacher Behaviors
Standards 3.4.4.1-3.4.4.5: Child Abuse and Neglect
Standard 9.4.3.3: Training Record

REFERENCES:
1. American Academy of Pediatrics. Children's health topics: Child abuse and neglect. http://www.aap.org/healthtopics/childabuse.cfm.
2. New York State Office of Children and Family Services. Child abuse and children with disabilities: A New York State perspective. http://childabuse.tc.columbia.edu.
3. Giardino, A. P., E. R. Giardino. 2002. *Recognition of child abuse for the mandated reporter.* 3rd ed. St. Louis, MO: G. W. Medical Publishing.

STANDARD 1.4.5.3: Training on Occupational Risk Related to Handling Body Fluids

All caregivers/teachers who are at risk of occupational exposure to blood or other blood-containing body fluids should be offered hepatitis B immunizations and should receive annual training in Standard Precautions and exposure control planning. Training should be consistent with applicable standards of the Occupational Safety and Health Administration (OSHA) Standard 29 CFR 1910.1030, "Occupational Exposure to Bloodborne Pathogens" and local occupational health requirements and should include, but not be limited to:

a) Modes of transmission of bloodborne pathogens;
b) Standard Precautions;
c) Hepatitis B vaccine use according to OSHA requirements;
d) Program policies and procedures regarding exposure to blood/body fluid;
e) Reporting procedures under the exposure control plan to ensure that all first-aid incidents involving exposure are reported to the employer before the end of the work shift during which the incident occurs (1).

RATIONALE: Providing first aid in situations where blood is present is an intrinsic part of a caregiver's/teacher's job. Split lips, scraped knees, and other minor injuries associated with bleeding are common in child care.

Caregivers/teachers who are designated as responsible for rendering first aid or medical assistance as part of their job duties are covered by the scope of this standard.

COMMENTS: OSHA has model exposure control plan materials for use by child care facilities. Using the model exposure control plan materials, caregivers/teachers can prepare a plan to comply with the OSHA requirements. The model plan materials are available from regional offices of OSHA.

TYPE OF FACILITY: Center; Large Family Child Care Home

RELATED STANDARDS:
Standard 9.4.3.3: Training Record

REFERENCES:

1. U.S. Department of Labor, Occupational Safety and Health Administration. 2008. *Toxic and hazardous substances: Bloodborne pathogens.* http://www.osha.gov/pls/oshaweb/owadisp.show_document?p_table=STANDARDS&p_id=10051.

STANDARD 1.4.5.4: Education of Center Staff

Centers should educate staff to support the cultural, language, and ethnic backgrounds of children enrolled in the program. In addition, all staff members should participate in diversity training that will ensure respectful service delivery to all families and a staff that works well together (2).

RATIONALE: Young children's identities cannot be separated from family, culture, and their home language. Children need both to see successful role models from their own ethnic and cultural groups and to develop the ability to relate to people who are different from themselves (1).

TYPE OF FACILITY: Center

RELATED STANDARDS:
Standard 9.4.3.3: Training Record

REFERENCES:

1. Chang, H. 2006. Developing a skilled, ethnically and linguistically diverse early childhood workforce. Adapted from *Getting ready for quality: The critical importance of developing and supporting a skilled, ethnically and linguistically diverse early childhood workforce.* http://www.buildinitiative.org/files/DiverseWorkforce.pdf.
2. National Association for the Education of Young Children (NAEYC). 2009. *Quality benchmark for cultural competence project.* Washington, DC: NAEYC. http://www.naeyc.org/files/naeyc/file/policy/state/QBCC_Tool.pdf.

1.4.6 Educational Leave/Compensation

STANDARD 1.4.6.1: Training Time and Professional Development Leave

A center, large family child care home or a support agency for a network of small family child care homes should make provisions for paid training time for staff to participate in required professional development (that includes training as well as education) during work hours, or reimburse staff for time spent attending professional development outside of regular work hours. Any hours worked in excess of forty hours in a week must be paid according to state and federal wage and hour regulations.

RATIONALE: Most caregivers/teachers work long hours and most are poorly paid (1). Using personal time for education required as a condition of employment is an unfair expectation until compensation for work done in child care is much more equitable. Many child care workers also employed in another vocation work at other jobs to make a living wage and would miss income from their other jobs or risk losing that employment. Additionally, the caregiver/teacher may incur stress in their family life when required to take time outside of child care hours to participate in work-related training.

COMMENTS: Professional development in child care often takes place when the participant is not released from other work-related duties, such as caring for children or answering phones. Providing substitutes and released time during work hours for such training is likely to enhance the effectiveness of training; and improve employee satisfaction/retention.

Large family child care homes employ staff in the same way as centers, except for size and location in a residence. For small family child care home caregivers/teachers, released time and compensation while engaged in training can be arranged only if the small family child care home caregiver/teacher is part of a support network that makes such arrangements. This standard does not apply to small family child care home caregivers/teachers independent of networks.

The Fair Labor Standard Act mandates payment of time and a half for all hours worked in excess of forty hours in a week.

TYPE OF FACILITY: Center; Large Family Child Care Homes; Small Family Child Care Homes

REFERENCES:

1. Center for the Child Care Workforce, American Federation of Teachers (AFT). 2009. *Wage data: Early childhood workforce hourly wage data.* 2009 ed. Washington, DC: AFT. http://www.ccw.org/storage/ccworkforce/documents/04-30-09 wwd fact sheet.pdf.

STANDARD 1.4.6.2: Payment for Continuing Education

Directors of centers and large family child care homes should arrange for continuing education that is paid for by the government, by charitable organizations, or by the facility, rather than by the employee. Small family child care home caregivers/teachers should avail themselves of training opportunities offered in their communities or online and claim their educational expenses as a business expense on tax forms.

RATIONALE: Caregivers/teachers often make low wages and may not be able to pay for mandated training. A majority of child care workers earnings are at or near minimum wage (1).

TYPE OF FACILITY: Center; Large Family Child Care Home; Small Family Child Care Home

REFERENCES:

1. Center for the Child Care Workforce, American Federation of Teachers. 2009. Wage data: Early childhood workforce hourly wage data. 2009 ed. Washington, DC: AFT. http://www.ccw.org/storage/ccworkforce/documents/04-30-09 wwd fact sheet.pdf.

1.5 Substitutes

STANDARD 1.5.0.1: Employment of Substitutes

Substitutes should be employed to ensure that child:staff ratios and requirements for direct supervision are maintained at all times. Substitutes and volunteers should be at least eighteen years of age and must meet the requirements specified throughout Standards 1.3.2.1-1.3.2.6. Those without licenses/certificates should work under direct supervision and should not be alone with a group of children.

A substitute should complete the same background screening processes as the caregiver/teacher. Obtaining substitutes to provide medical care for children with special health care needs is particularly challenging. A substitute nurse should be experienced in delivering the expected medical services. Decisions should be made on whether a parent/guardian will be allowed to provide needed on-site medical services. Substitutes should be aware of the care plans (including emergency procedures) for children with special health care needs.

RATIONALE: The risk to children from care by unqualified caregivers/teachers is the same whether the caregiver/teacher is a paid substitute or a volunteer (1).

COMMENTS: Substitutes are difficult to find, especially at the last minute. Planning for a competent substitute pool is essential for child care operation. Requiring substitutes for small family child care homes to obtain first aid and CPR certification forces small family child care home caregivers/teachers to close when they cannot be covered by a competent substitute. Since closing a child care home has a negative impact on the families and children they serve, systems should be developed to provide qualified alternative homes or substitutes for family child care home caregivers/teachers.

The lack of back-up for family child care home caregivers/teachers is an inherent liability in this type of care. Parents/guardians who use family child care must be sure they have suitable alternative care, such as family or friends, for situations in which the child's usual caregiver/teacher cannot provide the service.

Substitutes should have orientation and training on basic health and safety topics. Substitutes should not have an infectious disease when providing care.

TYPE OF FACILITY: Center; Large Family Child Care Home; Small Family Child Care Home

RELATED STANDARDS:
Standards 1.1.1.1-1.1.1.5: Child:Staff Ratio and Group Size
Standards 1.3.2.1-1.3.2.6: General Qualifications for All Caregivers/Teachers
Standard 1.3.3.1: General Qualifications of Family Child Care Caregivers/Teachers to Operate a Family Child Care Home
Standard 1.3.3.2: Support Networks for Family Child Care
Standard 1.5.0.2: Orientation of Substitutes
Standard 1.7.0.1: Pre-Employment and Ongoing Adult Health Appraisals, Including Immunization

REFERENCES:
1. National Association for Family Child Care (NAFCC). NAFCC official Website. http://nafcc.net.

STANDARD 1.5.0.2: Orientation of Substitutes

The director of any center or large family child care home and the small family child care home caregiver/teacher should provide orientation training to newly hired substitutes to include a review of ALL the program's policies and procedures (listed below is a sample). This training should include the opportunity for an evaluation and a repeat demonstration of the training lesson. In all child care settings the orientation should be documented. Substitutes should have background screenings.

All substitutes should be oriented to, and demonstrate competence in, the tasks for which they will be responsible. On the first day a substitute caregiver/teacher should be oriented on the following topics:

a) Safe infant sleep practices if an infant is enrolled in the program;
b) Any emergency medical procedure/medication needs of the children;
c) Any nutrition needs of the children.

All substitute caregivers/teachers, during the first week of employment, should be oriented to, and should demonstrate competence in at least the following items:

a) The names of the children for whom the caregiver/teacher will be responsible, and their specific developmental needs;
b) The planned program of activities at the facility;
c) Routines and transitions;
d) Acceptable methods of discipline;
e) Meal patterns and safe food handling policies of the facility (special attention should be given to life-threatening food allergies);
f) Emergency health and safety procedures;
g) General health policies and procedures as appropriate for the ages of the children cared for, including but not limited to the following:
    1) Hand hygiene techniques, including indications for hand hygiene;
    2) Diapering technique, if care is provided to children in diapers, including appropriate diaper disposal and diaper changing techniques, use and wearing of gloves;
    3) The practice of putting infants down to sleep positioned on their backs and on a firm surface along with all safe infant sleep practices to reduce the risk of Sudden Infant Death Syndrome (SIDS), as well as general nap time routines for all ages;
    4) Correct food preparation and storage techniques, if employee prepares food;
    5) Proper handling and storage of human milk when applicable and formula preparation if formula is handled;
    6) Bottle preparation including guidelines for human milk and formula if care is provided to children with bottles;

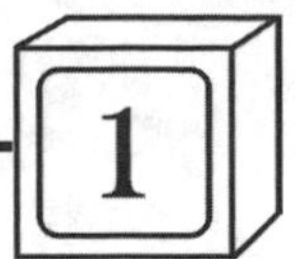

7) Proper use of gloves in compliance with Occupational Safety and Health Administration (OSHA) bloodborne pathogens regulations;
8) Injury prevention and safety including the role of mandatory child abuse reporter to report any suspected abuse/neglect.

h) Emergency plans and practices;
i) Access to list of authorized individuals for releasing children.

RATIONALE: Upon employment, substitutes should be able to carry out the duties assigned to them. Because facilities and the children enrolled in them vary, orientation programs for new substitutes can be most productive. Because of frequent staff turnover, child care programs must institute orientation programs as needed that protect the health and safety of children and new staff (1-3).

Most SIDS deaths in child care occur on the first day of care or within the first week due to unaccustomed prone (on stomach) sleeping. Unaccustomed prone sleeping increases the risk of SIDS eighteen times (4).

COMMENTS: Anyone who substitutes regularly should be up to date on all basic training as specified in this standard.

TYPE OF FACILITY: Center; Large Family Child Care Home; Small Family Child Care Home

RELATED STANDARDS:
Standard 1.2.0.2: Background Screening
Section 2.1: Program of Developmental Activities
Standards 2.2.0.6-2.2.0.9: Discipline
Standard 3.1.4.4: Scheduled Rest Periods and Sleep Arrangements
Standard 3.2.1.1: Type of Diapers Worn
Standards 3.2.2.1-3.2.2.5: Hand Hygiene
Standard 3.2.3.4: Prevention of Exposure to Blood and Bodily Fluids
Standards 3.4.3.1-3.4.3.3: Emergency Procedures
Chapter 4: Nutrition and Food Service
Standards 5.4.1.1-5.4.1.9: Sanitation, Disinfection, and Maintenance of Toilet Learning/Training Equipment, Toilets, and Bathrooms
Standards 5.4.5.1-5.4.5.5: Sleep and Rest Areas
Standard 9.2.2.3: Exchange of Information at Transitions
Standard 9.2.3.11: Food and Nutrition Service Policies and Plans
Standard 9.2.3.12: Infant Feeding Policy
Standard 9.2.4.1: Written Plan and Training for Handling Urgent Medical Care or Threatening Incidents
Standard 9.2.4.2: Review of Written Plan for Urgent Care
Standard 9.4.1.18: Records of Nutrition Service
Appendix D: Gloving

REFERENCES:

1. Gore, J. S. 1997. Does school-age child care staff training make a difference? *School-Age Connections,* vol. 6. http://www.canr.uconn.edu/ces/child/newsarticles/SAC643.html.
2. Crosland, K. A., G. Dunlap, W. Sager, et al. 2008. The effects of staff training on the types of interactions observed at two group homes for foster care children. *Research Soc Work* 18:410-20.
3. Cain, D. W., L. C. Rudd, T. F. Saxon. 2007. Effects of professional development training on joint attention engagement in low-quality childcare centers. *Early Child Devel Care* 177:159-85.
4. Moon, R. Y., T. Calabrese, L. Aird. 2008. Reducing the risk of sudden infant death syndrome in child care and changing provider practices: Lessons learned from a demonstration project. *Pediatrics* 122:788-98.

1.6 Consultants

STANDARD 1.6.0.1: Child Care Health Consultants

A facility should identify and engage/partner with a child care health consultant (CCHC) who is a licensed health professional with education and experience in child and community health and child care and preferably specialized training in child care health consultation.

CCHCs have knowledge of resources and regulations and are comfortable linking health resources with child care facilities.

The child care health consultant should be knowledgable in the following areas:

a) Consultation skills both as a child care health consultant as well as a member of an interdisciplinary team of consultants;
b) National health and safety standards for out-of-home child care;
c) Indicators of quality early care and education;
d) Day-to-day operations of child care facilities;
e) State child care licensing and public health requirements;
f) State health laws, Federal and State education laws (e.g., ADA, IDEA), and state professional practice acts for licensed professionals (e.g., State Nurse Practice Acts);
g) Infancy and early childhood development, social and emotional health, and developmentally appropriate practice;
h) Recognition and reporting requirements for infectious diseases;
i) American Academy of Pediatrics (AAP) and Early and Periodic Screening, Diagnosis, and Treatment (EPSDT) screening recommendations and immunizations schedules for children;
j) Importance of medical home and local and state resources to facilitate access to a medical home as well as child health insurance programs including Medicaid and State Children's Health Insurance Program (SCHIP);
k) Injury prevention for children;
l) Oral health for children;
m) Nutrition and age-appropriate physical activity recommendations for children including feeding of infants and children, the importance of breastfeeding and the prevention of obesity;
n) Inclusion of children with special health care needs, and developmental disabilities in child care;
o) Safe medication administration practices;
p) Health education of children;
q) Recognition and reporting requirements for child abuse and neglect/child maltreatment;
r) Safe sleep practices and policies (including reducing the risk of SIDS);

s) Development and implementation of health and safety policies and practices including poison awareness and poison prevention;
t) Staff health, including adult health screening, occupational health risks, and immunizations;
u) Disaster planning resources and collaborations within child care community;
v) Community health and mental health resources for child, parent and staff health;
w) Importance of serving as a healthy role model for children and staff.

The child care health consultant should be able to perform or arrange for performance of the following activities:

a) Assessing caregivers'/teachers' knowledge of health, development, and safety and offering training as indicated;
b) Assessing parents'/guardians' health, development, and safety knowledge, and offering training as indicated;
c) Assessing children's knowledge about health and safety and offering training as indicated;
d) Conducting a comprehensive indoor and outdoor health and safety assessment and on-going observations of the child care facility;
e) Consulting collaboratively on-site and/or by telephone or electronic media;
f) Providing community resources and referral for health, mental health and social needs, including accessing medical homes, children's health insurance programs (e.g., CHIP), and services for special health care needs;
g) Developing or updating policies and procedures for child care facilities (see comment section below);
h) Reviewing health records of children;
i) Reviewing health records of caregivers/teachers;
j) Assisting caregivers/teachers and parents/guardians in the management of children with behavioral, social and emotional problems and those with special health care needs;
k) Consulting a child's primary care provider about the child's individualized health care plan and coordinating services in collaboration with parents/guardians, the primary care provider, and other health care professionals (the CCHC shows commitment to communicating with and helping coordinate the child's care with the child's medical home, and may assist with the coordination of skilled nursing care services at the child care facility);
l) Consulting with a child's primary care provider about medications as needed, in collaboration with parents/guardians;
m) Teaching staff safe medication administration practices;
n) Monitoring safe medication administration practices;
o) Observing children's behavior, development and health status and making recommendations if needed to staff and parents/guardians for further assessment by a child's primary care provider;
p) Interpreting standards, regulations and accreditation requirements related to health and safety, as well as providing technical advice, separate and apart from an enforcement role of a regulation inspector or determining the status of the facility for recognition;
q) Understanding and observing confidentiality requirements;
r) Assisting in the development of disaster/emergency medical plans (especially for those children with special health care needs) in collaboration with community resources;
s) Developing an obesity prevention program in consultation with a nutritionist/registered dietitian (RD) and physical education specialist;
t) Working with other consultants such as nutritionists/RDs, kinesiologists (physical activity specialists), oral health consultants, social service workers, early childhood mental health consultants, and education consultants.

The role of the CCHC is to promote the health and development of children, families, and staff and to ensure a healthy and safe child care environment (11).

The CCHC is not acting as a primary care provider at the facility but offers critical services to the program and families by sharing health and developmental expertise, assessments of child, staff, and family health needs and community resources. The CCHC assists families in care coordination with the medical home and other health and developmental specialists. In addition, the CCHC should collaborate with an interdisciplinary team of early childhood consultants, such as, early childhood education, mental health, and nutrition consultants.

In order to provide effective consultation and support to programs, the CCHC should avoid conflict of interest related to other roles such as serving as a caregiver/teacher or regulator or a parent/guardian at the site to which child care health consultation is being provided.

The CCHC should have regular contact with the facility's administrative authority, the staff, and the parents/guardians in the facility. The administrative authority should review, and collaborate with the CCHC in implementing recommended changes in policies and practices. In the case of consulting about children with special health care needs, the CCHC should have contact with the child's medical home with permission from the child's parent/guardian.

Programs with a significant number of non-English-speaking families should seek a CCHC who is culturally sensitive and knowledgeable about community health resources for the parents'/guardians' native culture and languages.

RATIONALE: CCHCs provide consultation, training, information and referral, and technical assistance to caregivers/teachers (10). Growing evidence suggests that CCHCs support healthy and safe early care and education settings and protect and promote the healthy growth and development of children and their families (1-10). Setting health and safety policies in cooperation with the staff, parents/guardians, health professionals, and public health authorities will help ensure successful implementation of a quality program (3). The specific health and safety consultation needs for an individual facility depend on the characteristics of that facility (1-2). All facilities should have an overall child care health consultation plan (1,2,10).

The special circumstances of group care may not be part of the health care professional's usual education. Therefore, caregivers/teachers should seek child care health consultants who have the necessary specialized training or experience (10). Such training is available from instructors who are graduates of the National Training Institute for Child Care Health Consultants (NTI) and in some states from state-level mentoring of seasoned child care health consultants known to chapter child care contacts networked through the Healthy Child Care America (HCCA) initiatives of the AAP.

Some professionals may not have the full range of knowledge and expertise to serve as a child care health consultant but can provide valuable, specialized expertise. For example, a sanitarian may provide consultation on hygiene and infectious disease control and a Certified Playground Safety Inspector would be able to provide consultation about gross motor play hazards.

COMMENTS: The U.S. Department of Health and Human Services Maternal and Child Health Bureau (MCHB) has supported the development of state systems of child care health consultants through HCCA and State Early Childhood Comprehensive Systems grants and continues to support the NTI. Child care health consultants provide services to centers as well as family child care homes through on-site visits as well as phone or email consultation. Approximately twenty states are funding child care health consultant initiatives through a variety of funding sources, including Child Care Development Block Grants, TANF, and Title V. In some states a wide variety of health consultants, e.g., nutrition, kinesiology (physical activity), mental health, oral health, environmental health, may be available to programs and those consultants may operate through a team approach. Connecticut is an example of one state that has developed interdisciplinary training for early care and education consultants (health, education, mental health, social service, nutrition, and special education) in order to develop a multidisciplinary approach to consultation (8).

Certificates are provided for graduates of the NTI upon completion of the course and continuing education units are awarded. Some states offer CCHC training. Not all states implement CCHC training as modeled by the NTI. Some states offer continuing education units, college credit, and/or certificate of completion. Credentialing is an umbrella term referring to the various means employed to designate that individuals or organizations have met or exceeded established standards. These may include accreditation of *programs* or *organizations* and certification, registration, or licensure of *individuals.* Accreditation refers to a legitimate state or national organization verifying that an educational program or organization meets standards. Certification is the process by which a non-governmental agency or association grants recognition to an individual who has met predetermined qualifications specified by the agency or association. Certification is applied for by individuals on a voluntary basis and represents a professional status when achieved. Typical qualifications include 1) graduation from an accredited or approved program and 2) acceptable performance on a qualifying examination. While there is no national accreditation of CCHC training programs or individual CCHCs at this time, this is a future goal. Contact NTI at nti@unc.edu for additional information.

CCHC services may be provided through the public health system, resource and referral agency, private source, local community action program, health professional organizations, other non-profit organizations, and/or universities. Some professional organizations include child care health consultants in their special interest groups, such as the AAP's Section on Early Education and Child Care and the National Association of Pediatric Nurse Practitioners (NAPNAP).

CCHCs who are not employees of health, education, family service or child care agencies may be self-employed. Compensating them for their services via fee-for-service, an hourly rate, or a retainer fosters access and accountability.

Listed below is a sample of the policies and procedures child care health consultants should review and approve:

a) Admission and readmission after illness, including inclusion/exclusion criteria;
b) Health evaluation and observation procedures on intake, including physical assessment of the child and other criteria used to determine the appropriateness of a child's attendance;
c) Plans for care and management of children with communicable diseases;
d) Plans for prevention, surveillance and management of illnesses, injuries, and behavioral and emotional problems that arise in the care of children;
e) Plans for caregiver/teacher training and for communication with parents/guardians and primary care providers;
f) Policies regarding nutrition, nutrition education, age-appropriate infant and child feeding, oral health, and physical activity requirements;
g) Plans for the inclusion of children with special health or mental health care needs as well as oversight of their care and needs;
h) Emergency/disaster plans;
i) Safety assessment of facility playground and indoor play equipment;
j) Policies regarding staff health and safety;
k) Policy for safe sleep practices and reducing the risk of SIDS;
l) Policies for preventing shaken baby syndrome/abusive head trauma;
m) Policies for administration of medication;
n) Policies for safely transporting children;
o) Policies on environmental health – handwashing, sanitizing, pest management, lead, etc.

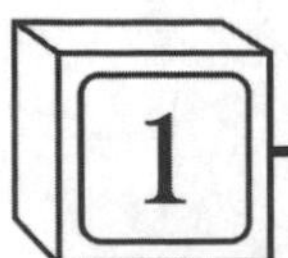

TYPE OF FACILITY: Center; Large Family Child Care Home; Small Family Child Care Home

RELATED STANDARDS:
Standard 1.6.0.3: Early Childhood Mental Health Consultants
Standard 1.6.0.4: Early Childhood Education Consultants

REFERENCES:

1. Alkon, A., J. Bernzweig, K. To, J. K. Mackie, M. Wolff, J. Elman. 2008. Child care health consultation programs in California: Models, services, and facilitators. *Public Health Nurs* 25:126-39.
2. Alkon, A., J. Farrer, J. Bernzweig. 2004. Roles and responsibilities of child care health consultants: Focus group findings. *Pediatric Nurs* 30:315-21.
3. Crowley, A. A. 2000. Child care health consultation: The Connecticut experience. *Maternal Child Health J* 4:67-75.
4. Gupta, R. S., S. Shuman, E. M. Taveras, M. Kulldorff, J. A. Finkelstein. 2005. Opportunities for health promotion education in child care. *Pediatrics* 116:499-505.
5. Farrer, J., A. Alkon, K. To. 2007. Child care health consultation programs: Barriers and opportunities. *Maternal Child Health J* 11:111-18.
6. Heath, J. M., et al. 2005. *Creating a statewide system of multi-disciplinary consultation system for early care and education in Connecticut.* Farmington, CT: Child Health and Development Institute of Connecticut. http://nitcci.nccic.acf.hhs.gov/resources/10262005_93815_901828.pdf.
7. Crowley, A. A., J. M Kulikowich. 2009. Impact of training on child care health consultant knowledge and practice. *Pediatric Nurs* 35:93-100.
8. Crowley, A. A., R. M. Sabatelli. 2008. Collaborative child care health consultation: A conceptual model. *J for Specialists in Pediatric Nurs* 13:74-88.
9. Dellert, J. C., D. Gasalberti, K. Sternas, P. Lucarelli, J. Hall. 2006. Outcomes of child care health consultation services for child care providers in New Jersey: A pilot study. *Pediatric Nurs* 32:530-37.
10. Alkon, A., J. Bernzweig, K. To, M. Wolff, J. F. Mackie. 2009. Child care health consultation improves health and safety policies and practices. *Academic Pediatrics* 9:366-70.
11. Crowley, A. A. 2001. Child care health consultation: An ecological model. *J Society Pediat Nurs* 6:170-81.

STANDARD 1.6.0.2: Frequency of Child Care Health Consultation Visits

The child care health consultant (CCHC) should visit each facility as needed to review and give advice on the facility's health component (1). Early childhood programs that serve any child younger than three years of age should be visited more frequently than child care programs that serve children three to five years of age. In both cases the frequency of visits should meet the needs of the composite group of children and be based on the needs of the program for training, support, and monitoring of child health and safety needs, including (but not limited to) infectious disease, injury prevention, safe sleep, nutrition, oral health, physical activity and outdoor learning, emergency preparation, medication administration, and the care of children with special health care needs. Written documentation of CCHC visits should be maintained at the facility.

RATIONALE: Almost everything that goes on in a facility and almost everything about the facility itself affects the health of the children, families, and staff it serves (1). Because infants are developing rapidly, environmental situations can quickly create harm. Their rapid changes in behavior make regular and frequent visits by the CCHC extremely important (2-4). In facilities where health and safety problems are present, staff require additional training and support to care for special health care needs or a high turnover rate of staff may occur, more frequent visits by the child care health consultant should be arranged (2).

COMMENTS: State child care regulations display a wide range of frequency and recommendations in states that require CCHC visits, from as frequently as once a week for programs serving children under three years of age to twice a year for programs serving children three to five years of age (2,5,6).

TYPE OF FACILITY: Center; Large Family Child Care Home; Small Family Child Care Home

RELATED STANDARDS:
Standard 1.1.1.3: Ratios for Facilities Serving Children with Special Health Care Needs and Disabilities
Standard 1.6.0.1: Child Care Health Consultants
Standard 1.6.0.5: Specialized Consultation for Facilities Serving Children with Disabilities
Standard 3.6.2.7: Child Care Health Consultants for Facilities That Care for Children Who Are Ill
Standard 4.4.0.1: Food Service Staff by Type of Facility and Food Service
Standard 4.4.0.2: Use of Nutritionist/Registered Dietitian
Standard 9.4.1.17: Documentation of Child Care Health Consultation/Training Visits
Standard 10.3.4.3: Support for Consultants to Provide Technical Assistance to Facilities
Standard 10.3.4.4: Development of List of Providers of Services to Facilities

REFERENCES:

1. Alkon, A., J. Bernzweig, K. To, J. K. Mackie, M. Wolff, J. Elman. 2008. Child care health consultation programs in California: Models, services, and facilitators. *Public Health Nurs* 25:126-39.
2. Crowley, A. A. 2000. Child care health consultation: The Connecticut experience. *Maternal Child Health J* 4:67-75.
3. Dellert, J. C., D. Gasalberti, K. Sternas, P. Lucarelli, J. Hall. 2006. Outcomes of child care health consultation services for child care providers in New Jersey: A pilot study. *Pediatric Nursing* 32:530-37.
4. Gupta, R. S., S. Shuman, E. M. Taveras, M. Kulldorff, J. A. Finkelstein. 2005. Opportunities for health promotion education in child care. *Pediatrics* 116:499-505.
5. Healthy Child Care Consultant Network Support Center, CHT Resource Group. 2006. *The influence of child care health consultants in promoting children's health and well-being: A report on selected resources.* http://hcccnsc.jsi.com/resources/publications/CC_lit_review_Screen_All.pdf.
6. National Resource Center for Health and Safety in Child Care and Early Education. 2010. Child care health consultant requirements and profiles by state. http://nrckids.org/RESOURCES/cchc by state.pdf.

STANDARD 1.6.0.3: Early Childhood Mental Health Consultants

A facility should engage a qualified early childhood mental health consultant who will assist the program with a range of early childhood social-emotional and behavioral issues and who will visit the program at minimum quarterly and more often as needed.

The knowledge base of an early childhood mental health consultant should include:

a) Training, expertise and/or professional credentials in mental health (e.g., psychiatry, psychology, clinical social work, nursing, developmental-behavioral medicine, etc.);
b) Early childhood development (typical and atypical) of infants, toddlers, and preschool age children;
c) Early care and education settings and practices;
d) Consultation skills and approaches to working as a team with early childhood consultants from other disciplines, especially health and education consultants, to effectively support directors and caregivers/teachers.

The role of the early childhood mental health consultant should be focused on building staff capacity and be both proactive in decreasing the incidence of challenging classroom behaviors and reactive in formulating appropriate responses to challenging classroom behaviors and should include:

a) Developing and implementing classroom curricula regarding conflict resolution, emotional regulation, and social skills development;
b) Developing and implementing appropriate screening and referral mechanisms for behavioral and mental health needs;
c) Forming relationships with mental health providers and special education systems in the community;
d) Providing mental health services, resources and/or referral systems for families and staff;
e) Helping staff facilitate and maintain mentally healthy environments within the classroom and overall system;
f) Helping address mental health needs and reduce job stress within the staff;
g) Improving management of children with challenging behaviors;
h) Preventing the development of problem behaviors;
i) Providing a classroom climate that promotes positive social-emotional development;
j) Recognizing and appropriately responding to the needs of children with internalizing behaviors, such as persistent sadness, anxiety, and social withdrawal;
k) Actively teaching developmentally appropriate social skills, conflict resolution, and emotional regulation;
l) Addressing the mental health needs and daily stresses of those who care for young children, such as families and caregivers/teachers;
m) Helping the staff to address and handle unforeseen crises or bereavements that may threaten the mental health of staff or children and families, such as the death of a caregiver/teacher or the serious illness of a child.

RATIONALE: As increasing numbers of children are spending longer hours in child care settings, there is an increasing need to build the capacity of caregivers/teachers to attend to the social-emotional and behavioral well-being of children as well as their health and learning needs. Early childhood mental health underlies much of what constitutes school readiness, including emotional and behavioral regulation, social skills (i.e., taking turns, postponing gratification), the ability to inhibit aggressive or anti-social impulses, and the skills to verbally express emotions, such as frustration, anger, anxiety, and sadness. Supporting children's health, mental health and learning requires a comprehensive approach. Child care programs need to have health, education, and mental health consultants who can help them implement universal, selected and targeted strategies to improve school readiness in young children in their care (1-5). Mental health consultants in collaboration with education and child care health consultants can reduce the risk for children being expelled, can reduce levels of problem behaviors, increase social skills and build staff efficacy and capacity (1-11).

COMMENTS: Access to an early childhood mental health consultant should be in the context of an ongoing relationship, with at least quarterly regular visits to the classroom to consult. However, even an on-call-only relationship is better than no relationship at all. Regardless of the frequency of contact, this relationship should be established before a crisis arises, so that the consultant can establish a useful proactive working relationship with the staff and be quickly mobilized when needs arise. This consultant should be viewed as an important part of the program's support staff and should collaborate with all regular classroom staff, administration, and other consultants such as child care health consultants and education consultants, and support staff. In most cases, there is no single place in which to look for early childhood mental health consultants. Qualified potential consultants may be identified by contacting mental health and behavioral providers (e.g., child clinical and school psychologists, licensed clinical social workers, child psychiatrists, developmental pediatricians, etc.), as well as training programs at local colleges and universities where these professionals are being trained. Colleges and universities may be a good place to find well-supervised consultants-in-training at a potentially reasonable cost, although consultant turnover may be higher.

TYPE OF FACILITY: Center; Large Family Child Care Home; Small Family Child Care Home

RELATED STANDARDS:

Standard 1.6.0.1: Child Care Health Consultants
Standard 1.6.0.4: Early Childhood Education Consultants

REFERENCES:

1. Brennan, E. M., J. Bradley, M. D. Allen, D. F. Perry. 2008. The evidence base for mental health consultation in early childhood settings: A research synthesis addressing staff and program outcomes. *Early Ed Devel* 19:982-1022.
2. National Scientific Council on the Developing Child. 2008. Mental health problems in early childhood can impair learning and behavior for life. Working Paper no. 6. http://developingchild.harvard.edu/library/reports_and_working_papers/working_papers/wp6/.
3. Perry, D. F., M. D. Allen, E. M. Brennan, J. R. Bradley. 2009. The evidence base for mental health consultation in early childhood

settings: A research synthesis addressing children's behavioral outcomes. *Early Ed Devel* 21:795-824.
4. Perry, D. F., R. Kaufmann, J. Knitzer. 2007. *Early childhood social and emotional health: Building bridges between services and systems.* Baltimore, MD: Paul Brookes Publishing.
5. Perry, D. F., M. C. Dunne, L. McFadden, D. Campbell. 2008. Reducing the risk for preschool expulsion: Mental health consultation for young children with challenging behaviors. *J Child Fam Studies* 17:44-54.
6. Committee on Integrating the Science of Early Childhood Development, Board on Children, Youth, and Families. 2000. *From neurons to neighborhoods.* Ed. J. P. Shonkoff, D. A. Phillips. Washington, DC: National Academy Press.
7. Gilliam, W. S. 2005. *Prekindergarteners left behind: Expulsion rates in state prekindergarten programs.* Foundation for Child Development (FCD). Policy Brief Series no. 3. New York: FCD. http://www.challengingbehavior.org/explore/policy_docs/prek_expulsion.pdf.
8. Gilliam, W. S., G. Shahar. 2006. Preschool and child care expulsion and suspension: Rates and predictors in one state. *Infants Young Children* 19:228-45.
9. Gilliam, W. S. 2007. *Early Childhood Consultation Partnership: Results of a random-controlled evaluation.* New Haven, CT: Yale Universty. http://www.chdi.org/admin/uploads/5468903394946c41768730.pdf.
10. American Academy of Pediatrics, Committee on School Health. 2003. Policy statement: Out-of-school suspension and expulsion. *Pediatrics* 122:1206-9.
11. Duran, F., K. Hepburn, M. Irvine, R. Kaufmann, B. Anthony, N. Horen, D. Perry. 2009. *What works?: A study of effective early childhood mental health consultation programs.* Washington, DC: Georgetown University Center for Child and Human Development. http://gucchdtacenter.georgetown.edu/publications/ECMHCStudy_Report.pdf.

STANDARD 1.6.0.4: Early Childhood Education Consultants

A facility should engage an early childhood education consultant who will visit the program at minimum semi-annually and more often as needed. The consultant must have a minimum of a Baccalaureate degree and preferably a Master's degree from an accredited institution in early childhood education, administration and supervision, and a minimum of three years in teaching and administration of an early care/education program. The facility should develop a written plan for this consultation which must be signed annually by the consultant. This plan should outline the responsibilities of the consultant and the services the consultant will provide to the program.

The knowledge base of an early childhood education consultant should include:

a) Working knowledge of theories of child development and learning for children from birth through eight years across domains, including socio-emotional development and family development;
b) Principles of health and wellness across the domains, including social and emotional wellness and approaches in the promotion of healthy development and resilience;
c) Current practices and materials available related to screening, assessment, curriculum, and measurement of child outcomes across the domains, including practices that aid in early identification and individualizing for a wide range of needs;
d) Resources that aid programs to support inclusion of children with diverse health and learning needs and families representing linguistic, cultural, and economic diversity of communities;
e) Methods of coaching, mentoring, and consulting that meet the unique learning styles of adults;
f) Familiarity with local, state, and national regulations, standards, and best practices related to early education and care;
g) Community resources and services to identify and serve families and children at risk, including those related to child abuse and neglect and parent education;
h) Consultation skills as well as approaches to working as a team with early childhood consultants from other disciplines, especially child care health consultants, to effectively support program directors and their staff.

The role of the early childhood education consultant should include:

a) Review of the curriculum and written policies, plans and procedures of the program;
b) Observations of the program and meetings with the director, caregivers/teachers, and parents/guardians;
c) Review of the professional needs of staff and program and provision of recommendations of current resources;
d) Reviewing and assisting directors in implementing and monitoring evidence based approaches to classroom management;
e) Maintaining confidences and following all Family Educational Rights and Privacy Act (FERPA) regulations regarding disclosures;
f) Keeping records of all meetings, consultations, recommendations and action plans and offering/providing summary reports to all parties involved;
g) Seeking and supporting a multidisciplinary approach to services for the program, children and families;
h) Following the National Association for the Education of Young Children (NAEYC) Code of Ethics;
i) Availability by telecommunication to advise regarding practices and problems;
j) Availability for on-site visit to consult to the program;
k) Familiarity with tools to evaluate program quality, such as the Early Childhood Environment Rating Scale–Revised (ECERS–R), Infant/Toddler Environment Rating Scale–Revised (ITERS–R), Family Child Care Environment Rating Scale–Revised (FCCERS–R), School-Age Care Environment Rating Scale (SACERS), Classroom Assessment Scoring System (CLASS), as well as tools used to support various curricular approaches.

RATIONALE: The early childhood education consultant provides an objective assessment of a program and essential knowledge about implementation of child development

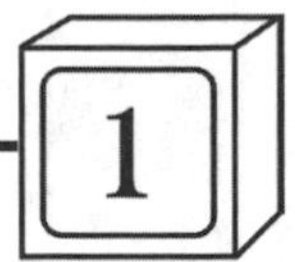

principles through curriculum which supports the social and emotional health and learning of infants, toddlers and preschool age children (1-5). Furthermore, utilization of an early childhood education consultant can reduce the need for mental health consultation when challenging behaviors are the result of developmentally inappropriate curriculum (6,7). Together with the child care health consultant, the early childhood education consultant offers core knowledge for addressing children's healthy development.

TYPE OF FACILITY: Center; Large Family Child Care Home; Small Family Child Care Home

RELATED STANDARDS:
Standard 1.6.0.1: Child Care Health Consultants
Standard 1.6.0.3: Early Childhood Mental Health Consultants

REFERENCES:

1. Dunn, L., K. Susan. 1997. What have we learned about developmentally appropriate practice? *Young Children* 52:4-13.
2. Wesley, P. W., V. Buysse. 2006. Ethics and evidence in consultation. *Topics Early Childhood Special Ed* 26:131-41.
3. Wesley, P. W., S. A. Palsha. 1998. Improving quality in early childhood environments through on-site consultation. *Topics Early Childhood Special Ed* 18:243-53.
4. Wesley, P. W., V. Buysee. 2005. *Consultation in early childhood settings.* Baltimore, MD: Brookes Publishing.
5. Bredekamp, S., C. Copple, eds. 2000. *Developmentally appropriate practice in early childhood programs serving children from birth through age 8.* Rev ed. National Association for the Education of Young Children (NAEYC). Publication no. 234. Washington, DC: NAEYC. http://www.naeyc.org/files/naeyc/file/positions/position statement Web.pdf.
6. The Connecticut Early Education Consultation Network. CEECN: Guidance, leadership, support. http://ctconsultationnetwork.org.
7. Connecticut Department of Public Health. Child day care licensing program. http://www.ct.gov/dph/cwp/view.asp?a=3141&Q=387158&dphNav_GID=1823/.

STANDARD 1.6.0.5: Specialized Consultation for Facilities Serving Children with Disabilities

When children at the facility include those with special health care needs, developmental delay or disabilities, and mental health or behavior problems, the staff or documented consultants should involve any of the following consultants in the child's care, with prior informed, written parental consent and as appropriate to each child's needs:

a) A registered nurse, nurse practitioner with pediatric experience, or child care health consultant;
b) A physician with pediatric experience, especially those with developmental-behavioral training;
c) A registered dietitian;
d) A psychologist;
e) A psychiatrist;
f) A physical therapist;
g) An adaptive equipment technician;
h) An occupational therapist;
i) A speech pathologist;
j) An audiologist for hearing screenings conducted on-site at child care;
k) A vision screener;
l) A respiratory therapist;
m) A social worker;
n) A parent/guardian of a child with special health care needs;
o) Part C representative/service coordinator;
p) A mental health consultant;
q) Special learning consultant/teacher (e.g., teacher specializing in work with visually impaired child or sign language interpreters);
r) A teacher with special education expertise;
s) The caregiver/teacher;
t) Individuals identified by the parent/guardian;
u) Certified child passenger safety technician with training in safe transportation of children with special needs.

RATIONALE: The range of professionals needed may vary with the facility, but the listed professionals should be available as consultants when needed. These professionals need not be on staff at the facility, but may simply be available when needed through a variety of arrangements, including contracts, agreements, and affiliations. The parent's participation and written consent in the native language of the parent, including Braille/sign language, is required to include outside consultants (1).

TYPE OF FACILITY: Center; Large Family Child Care Home; Small Family Child Care Home

REFERENCES:

1. Cohen, A. J. 2002. *Liability exposure and child care health consultation.* http://www.ucsfchildcarehealth.org/pdfs/forms/CCHCLiability.pdf.

1.7 Staff Health

STANDARD 1.7.0.1: Pre-Employment and Ongoing Adult Health Appraisals, Including Immunization

All paid and volunteer staff members should have a health appraisal before their first involvement in child care work. The appraisal should identify any accommodations required of the facility for the staff person to function in his or her assigned position.

Health appraisals for paid and volunteer staff members should include:

a) Physical exam;
b) Dental exam;
c) Vision and hearing screening;
d) The results and appropriate follow up of a tuberculosis (TB) screening, using the Tuberculin Skin Test (TST) or IGRA (interferon gamma release assay), once upon entering into the child care field with subsequent TB screening as determined by history of high risk for TB thereafter;
e) A review and certification of up-to-date immune status per the current Recommended Adult Immunization Schedule found in Appendix H, including annual influenza vaccination and up to date Tdap;

f) A review of occupational health concerns based on the performance of the essential functions of the job.

All adults who reside in a family child care home who are considered to be at high risk for TB, should have completed TB screening (1) as specified in Standard 7.3.10.1. Adults who are considered at high risk for TB include those who are foreign-born, have a history of homelessness, are HIV-infected, have contact with a prison population, or have contact with someone who has active TB.

Testing for TB of staff members with previously negative skin tests should not be repeated on a regular basis unless required by the local or state health department. A record of test results and appropriate follow-up evaluation should be on file in the facility.

RATIONALE: Caregivers/teachers need to be physically and emotionally healthy to perform the tasks of providing care to children. Performing their work while ill can spread infectious disease and illness to other staff and the children in their care (2). Under the Americans with Disabilities Act (ADA), employers are expected to make reasonable accommodations for persons with disabilities. Under ADA, accommodations are based on an individual case by case situation. Undue hardship is defined also on a case by case basis. Accommodation requires knowledge of conditions that must be accommodated to ensure competent function of staff and the well-being of children in care (3).

Since detection of tuberculosis using screening of healthy individuals has a low yield compared with screening of contacts of known cases of tuberculosis, public health authorities have determined that routine repeated screening of healthy individuals with previously negative skin tests is not a reasonable use of resources. Since local circumstances and risks of exposure may vary, this recommendation should be subject to modification by local or state health authorities.

COMMENTS: Child care facilities should provide the job description or list of activities that the staff person is expected to perform. Unless the job description defines the duties of the role specifically, under federal law the facility may be required to adjust the activities of that person. For example, child care facilities typically require the following activities of caregivers:

a) Moving quickly to supervise and assist young children;
b) Lifting children, equipment, and supplies;
c) Sitting on the floor and on child-sized furniture;
d) Washing hands frequently;
e) Responding quickly in case of an emergency;
f) Eating the same food as is served to the children (unless the staff member has dietary restrictions);
g) Hearing and seeing at a distance required for playground supervision or driving;
h) Being absent from work for illness no more often than the typical adult, to provide continuity of caregiving relationships for children in child care.

Healthy Young Children: A Manual for Programs, from the National Association for the Education of Young Children (NAEYC), provides a model form for an assessment by a health professional. See also *Model Child Care Health Policies*, from NAEYC and from the American Academy of Pediatrics (AAP).

Concern about the cost of health exams (particularly when many caregivers/teachers do not receive health benefits and earn minimum wage) is a barrier to meeting this standard. When staff members need hepatitis B immunization to meet Occupational Safety and Health Administration (OSHA) requirements (4), the cost of this immunization may or may not be covered under a managed care contract. If not, the cost of health supervision (such as immunizations, dental and health exams) must be covered as part of the employee's preparation for work in the child care setting by the prospective employee or the employer. Child care workers are among those for whom annual influenza vaccination is strongly recommended.

Facilities should consult with ADA experts through the U.S. Department of Education funded Disability and Business Technical Assistance Centers (DBTAC) throughout the country. These centers can be reached by calling 1-800-949-4232 (callers are routed to the appropriate region) or by accessing regional center's contacts directly at http://adata.org/Static/Home.aspx.

TYPE OF FACILITY: Center; Large Family Child Care Home; Small Family Child Care Home

RELATED STANDARDS:
Standard 1.7.0.1: Pre-Employment and Ongoing Adult Health Appraisals, Including Immunization
Standard 1.7.0.4: Occupational Hazards
Standards 7.2.0.1-7.2.0.3: Immunizations
Standard 7.3.10.1: Measures for Detection, Control, and Reporting of Tuberculosis
Standard 7.3.10.2: Attendance of Children with Latent Tuberculosis Infection or Active Tuberculosis Disease
Appendix B: Major Occupational Health Hazards
Appendix E: Child Care Staff Health Assessment
Appendix H: Recommended Adult Immunization Schedule

REFERENCES:

1. U.S. Department of Health and Human Services, Centers for Disease Control and Prevention. 2011. Recommended adult immunization schedule – United States, 2011. http://www.cdc.gov/vaccines/recs/schedules/.
2. Baldwin, D., S. Gaines, J. L. Wold, A. Williams. 2007. The health of female child care providers: Implications for quality of care. *J Comm Health Nurs* 24:1-7.
3. Keyes, C. R. 2008. Adults with disabilities in early childhood settings. *Child Care Info Exchange* 179:82-85.
4. Occupational Safety and Health Administration. 2008. *Bloodborne pathogens.* Title 29, pt. 1910.1030. http://www.osha.gov/pls/oshaweb/owadisp.show_document?p_table=standards&p_id=10051.

STANDARD 1.7.0.2: Daily Staff Health Check

On a daily basis, the administrator of the facility or caregiver/teacher should observe staff members, substitutes,

and volunteers for obvious signs of ill health. When ill, staff members, substitutes and volunteers may be directed to go home. Staff members, substitutes, and volunteers should be responsible for reporting immediately to their supervisor any injuries or illnesses they experience at the facility or elsewhere, especially those that might affect their health or the health and safety of the children. It is the responsibility of the administration, not the staff member who is ill or injured, to arrange for a substitute caregiver/teacher.

RATIONALE: Sometimes adults report to work when feeling ill or become ill during the day but believe it is their responsibility to stay. The administrator's or caregiver's/teacher's observation of illness followed by sending the staff member home may prevent the spread of illness. Arranging for a substitute caregiver/teacher ensures that the children receive competent care (1,2).

COMMENTS: Administrators and caregivers/teachers need guidelines to ensure proper application of this standard. For a demonstration of how to implement this standard, see the video series, *Caring for Our Children*, available from National Association for the Education of Young Children (NAEYC) and the American Academy of Pediatrics (AAP) (1).

TYPE OF FACILITY: Center; Large Family Child Care Home; Small Family Child Care Home

REFERENCES:

1. Baldwin D., S. Gaines, J. L. Wold, A. Williams. 2007. The health of female child care providers: Implications for quality of care. *J Comm Health Nurs* 24:1-7.

2. Murph, J. R., S. D. Palmer, D. Glassy, eds. 2005. *Health in child care: A manual for health professionals*. 4th ed. Elk Grove Village, IL: American Academy of Pediatrics.

STANDARD 1.7.0.3: Health Limitations of Staff

Staff and volunteers must have a primary care provider's release to return to work in the following situations:

a) When they have experienced conditions that may affect their ability to do their job or require an accommodation to prevent illness or injury in child care work related to their conditions (such as pregnancy, specific injuries, or infectious diseases);
b) After serious or prolonged illness;
c) When their condition or health could affect promotion or reassignment to another role;
d) Before return from a job-related injury;
e) If there are workers' compensation issues or if the facility is at risk of liability related to the employee's or volunteer's health problem.

If a staff member is found to be unable to perform the activities required for the job because of health limitations, the staff person's duties should be limited or modified until the health condition resolves or employment is terminated because the facility can prove that it would be an undue hardship to accommodate the staff member with the disability.

RATIONALE: Under the Americans with Disabilities Act (ADA), employers are expected to make reasonable accommodations for persons with disabilities. Under ADA, accommodations are based on an individual case by case situation (1). Undue hardship is defined also on a case by case basis (1).

COMMENTS: Facilities should consult with ADA experts through the U.S. Department of Education funded Disability and Business Technical Assistance Centers throughout the country. These centers can be reached by calling 1-800-949-4232 and callers are routed to the appropriate region or accessing contacts directly at http://adata.org/Static/Home.aspx.

TYPE OF FACILITY: Center; Large Family Child Care Home

RELATED STANDARDS:

Standard 7.6.1.4: Informing Public Health Authorities of HBV Cases
Standard 7.6.3.4: Ability of Caregivers/teachers with HIV Infection to Care for Children

REFERENCES:

1. ADA National Network. The Americans with Disabilities Act (ADA) from a civil rights perspective. http://adaanniversary.org/2010/ap03_ada_civilrights/03_ada_civilrights_09_natl.pdf.

STANDARD 1.7.0.4: Occupational Hazards

Written personnel policies of centers and large family child care homes should address the major occupational health hazards for workers in child care settings. Special health concerns of pregnant caregivers/teachers should be carefully evaluated, and up-to-date information regarding occupational hazards for pregnant caregivers/teachers should be made available to them and other workers. The occupational hazards including those regarding pregnant workers listed in Appendix B, Major Occupational Health Hazards, should be referenced and used in evaluations by caregivers/teachers and supervisors.

RATIONALE: Employees must be aware of the risks to which they are exposed so they can weigh those risks and take countermeasures (2). As a workforce composed primarily of women of childbearing age, pregnancy is common among caregivers/teachers in child care settings. In a study of child care personnel, one quarter of the study's sample reported becoming pregnant since beginning work in child care, with higher pregnancy rates for directors (33%) and family home caregivers/teachers (36%) than for center staff (15%) (1).

TYPE OF FACILITY: Center; Large Family Child Care Home

RELATED STANDARDS:

Appendix B: Major Occupational Health Hazards

REFERENCES:

1. The National Association of Family Child Care (NAFCC). 2005. *Quality standards for NAFCC accreditation*. 4th ed. Salt Lake City, UT: NAFCC. http://www.nafcc.org/documents/QualStd.pdf.

2. Aronson, S. S., T. R. Shope, eds. 2009. *Managing infectious diseases in child care and schools: A quick reference guide.* 2nd ed. Elk Grove Village, IL: American Academy of Pediatrics.

STANDARD 1.7.0.5: Stress

Caregivers/teachers should be able to:

a) Identify risks associated with stress;
b) Identify stressors specific to child caregiving;

   c) Identify specific ways to manage stress in the child care environment.

The following measures to lessen stress for the staff should be implemented to the maximum extent possible:

   a) Wages and benefits (including health care insurance) that fairly compensate the skills, knowledge, and performance required of caregivers/teachers, at the levels of wages and benefits paid for other jobs that require comparable skills, knowledge, and performance;
   b) Job security;
   c) Training to improve skills and hazard recognition;
   d) Stress management and reduction training;
   e) Written plan/policy in place for the situation in which a caregiver/teacher recognizes that s/he or a colleague is stressed and needs help immediately (the plan should allow for caregivers/teachers who feel they may lose control to have a short, but relatively immediate break away from the children at times of high stress);
   f) Regular work breaks and paid time-off;
   g) Appropriate child:staff ratios;
   h) Liability insurance for caregivers/teachers;
   i) Staff lounge separate from child care area with adult size furniture;
   j) The use of sound-absorbing materials in the workspace;
   k) Regular performance reviews which, in addition to addressing any areas requiring improvement, provide constructive feedback, individualized encouragement and appreciation for aspects of the job well performed;
   l) Stated provisions for back-up staff, for example, to allow caregivers/teachers to take necessary time off when ill without compromising the function of the center or incurring personal negative consequences from the employer (this back-up should also include a stated plan to be implemented in the event a staff member needs to have a short, but relatively immediate break away from the children);
   m) Adult size furniture in the classroom for the staff;
   n) Access to experts in child development and behavior to help problem solve child specific issues.

RATIONALE: One of the best indicators of quality child care is consistent staff with low turnover rates (5,6).

According to the Bureau of Labor Statistics' Website, "in 2007, hourly earnings of nonsupervisory workers in the child day care services industry averaged $10.53" (1). About 42% of all child care workers have a high school degree or less, reflecting the minimal training requirements for most jobs. Many child care workers leave the industry due to stressful working conditions and dissatisfaction with benefits and pay (1).

Stress reduction measures (particularly adequate wages and reasonable health care benefits) contribute to decreased staff turnover and thereby promote quality care (2). The health, welfare, and safety of adult workers in child care determine their ability to provide care for the children.

Serious physical abuse sometimes occurs when the caregiver/teacher is under high stress. Too much stress can not only affect the caregiver's/teacher's health, but also the quality of the care that the adult is able to give. A caregiver/teacher who is feeling too much stress may not be able to offer the praise, nurturing, and direction that children need for good development (3). Regular breaks with substitutes when the caregiver/teacher cannot continue to provide safe care can help ensure quality child care.

Sound-absorbing materials in the work area, break times, and a separate lounge allow for respite from noise and from non-auditory stress. Unwanted sound, or noise, can be damaging to hearing as well as to psychosocial well-being. The stress effects of noise will aggravate other stress factors present in the facility. Lack of adequate sound reduction measures in the facility can force the caregiver/teacher to speak at levels above those normally used for conversation, and thus may increase the risk of throat irritation. When caregivers/teachers raise their voices to be heard, the children tend to raise theirs, escalating the problem.

COMMENTS: Documentation of implementation of stress reduction measures should be on file in the facility.

Rest breaks of twenty minutes or less are customary in industry and are customarily paid for as working time. Meal periods (typically thirty minutes or more) generally need not be compensated as work time as long as the employee is completely relieved from duty for the entire meal period (4). For resources on respite or crisis care, contact the ARCH National Respite Network at http://archrespite.org.

Caregivers/teachers who use tobacco can experience stress related to nicotine withdrawals. For help dealing with stress from tobacco addiction, see the Tobacco Research and Intervention Program's *Forever Free* booklet on smoking, stress, and mood at http://www.smokefree.gov/pubs/FFree6.pdf. Or, for help quitting smoking, visit the Smoke Free Website at http://www.smokefree.gov.

TYPE OF FACILITY: Center; Large Family Child Care Home; Small Family Child Care Home

RELATED STANDARDS:
Standards 1.1.1.1-1.1.1.5: Child:Staff Ratio and Group Size

REFERENCES:
1. U.S. Department of Labor, Bureau of Labor Statistics. 2010. *Career guide to industries: Child day care services, 2010-11 Edition.* http://www.bls.gov/oco/cg/cgs032.htm.
2. U.S. Department of Labor, Bureau of Labor Statistics. 2010. *Occupational employment statistics: occupational employment and wages, May 2009.* http://www.bls.gov/oes/current/oes399011.htm.
3. Healthy Childcare Consultants (HCCI). *Stress management for child caregivers.* Pelham, AL: HCCI.
4. U.S. Department of Labor, Wage and Hour Division. 2009. *Fact sheet #46: Daycare centers and preschools under the Fair Labor Standards Act (FLSA).* Rev. ed. http://www.dol.gov/whd/regs/compliance/whdfs46.pdf.
5. Fiene, R. 2002. *13 indicators of quality child care: Research update.* Washington, DC: U.S. Department of Health and Human

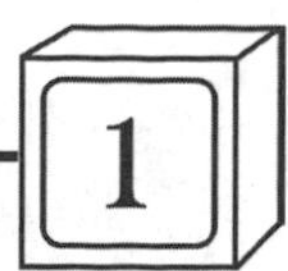

Services, Office of the Assistant Secretary for Planning and Evaluation. http://aspe.hhs.gov/hsp/ccquality-ind02/.
6. National Institute of Child Health and Human Development (NICHD). 2006. *The NICHD study of early child care and youth development: Findings for children up to age 4 1/2 years.* Rockville, MD: NICHD.

1.8 Human Resource Management

1.8.1 Benefits

STANDARD 1.8.1.1: Basic Benefits

The following basic benefits should be offered to staff:

a) Affordable health insurance;
b) Paid time-off (vacation, sick time, personal leave, holidays, family, parental and medical leave, etc.);
c) Social Security or other retirement plan;
d) Workers' compensation;
e) Educational benefits.

Centers and large family child care homes should have written policies that detail these benefits of employees at the facility.

RATIONALE: The quality and continuity of the child care workforce is the main determining factor of the quality of care. Nurturing the nurturers is essential to prevent burnout and promote retention. Fair labor practices should apply to child care as well as other work settings. Child care workers should be considered as worthy of benefits as workers in other careers.

Medical coverage should include the cost of the health appraisals and immunizations required of child care workers, and care for the increased incidence of communicable disease and stress-related conditions in this work setting.

The potential for acquiring injuries and infections when caring for young children is a health and safety hazard for child care workers. Information abounds about the risk of infectious disease for children in child care settings. Children are reservoirs for many infectious agents. Staff members come into close and frequent contact with children and their excretions and secretions and are vulnerable to these illnesses. In addition, many child care workers are women who are planning a pregnancy or who are pregnant, and they may be vulnerable to potentially serious effects of infection on the outcome of pregnancy (2).

Sick leave is important to minimize the spread of communicable diseases and maintain the health of staff members. Sick leave promotes recovery from illness and thereby decreases the further spread or recurrence of illness.

Workplace benefits contribute to higher morale and less staff turnover, and thus promote quality child care. Lack of benefits is a major reason reported for high turnover of child care staff (1).

COMMENTS: Staff benefits may be appropriately addressed in center personnel policies and in state and federal labor standards. Not all the material that has to be addressed in these policies is appropriate for state child care licensing requirements. Having facilities acknowledge which benefits they do provide will help enhance the general awareness of staff benefits among child care workers and other concerned parties. Currently, this standard is difficult for many facilities to achieve, but new federal programs and shared access to small business benefit packages will help. Many options are available for providing leave benefits and education reimbursements, ranging from partial to full employer contribution, based on time employed with the facility.

Caregivers/teachers should be encouraged to have health insurance. Health benefits can include full coverage, partial coverage (at least 75% employer paid), or merely access to group rates. Some local or state child care associations offer reduced group rates for health insurance for child care facilities and individual caregivers/teachers.

TYPE OF FACILITY: Center; Large Family Child Care Home; Small Family Child Care Home

RELATED STANDARDS:
Standard 1.4.6.1: Training Time and Professional Development Leave
Standard 1.4.6.2: Payment for continuing Education
Standard 9.3.0.1: Written Human Resource Management Policies for Centers and large Family Child Care Homes

REFERENCES:
1. Whitebook, M., C. Howes, D. Phillips. 1998. *Worthy work, unlivable wages: The National child care staffing study, 1988-1997.* Washington, DC: Center for the Child Care Workforce.
2. National Association for the Education of Young Children (NAEYC). 2008. *Leadership and management: A guide to the NAEYC early childhood program standards and related accreditation criteria.* Washington, DC: NAEYC.

1.8.2 Evaluation

STANDARD 1.8.2.1: Staff Familiarity with Facility Policies, Plans and Procedures

All caregivers/teachers should be familiar with the provisions of the facility's policies, plans, and procedures, as described in Chapter 9, Administration. The compliance with these policies, plans, and procedures should be used in staff performance evaluations and documented in the personnel file.

RATIONALE: Written policies, plans and procedures provide a means of staff orientation and evaluation essential to the operation of any organization (1).

TYPE OF FACILITY: Center; Large Family Child Care Home

RELATED STANDARDS:
Chapter 9: Administration

REFERENCES:
1. Boone, L. E., D. L. Kurtz. 2010. *Contemporary business.* Hoboken, NJ: John Wiley and Sons.

STANDARD 1.8.2.2: Annual Staff Competency Evaluation

For each employee, there should be a written annual self-evaluation, a performance review from the personnel supervisor, and a continuing education/professional development plan based on the needs assessment, described in Standard 1.4.4.1 through Standard 1.4.5.4.

RATIONALE: A system for evaluation of employees is a basic component of any personnel policy (1). Staff members who are well trained are better able to prevent, recognize, and correct health and safety problems (2).

COMMENTS: Formal evaluation is not a substitute for continuing feedback on day-to-day performance. Performance appraisals should include a customer satisfaction component and/or a peer review component. Compliance with this standard may be determined by licensing requirements set by the state and local regulatory processes, and by state and local funding requirements, or by accrediting bodies (1). In some states, a central Child Development Personnel Registry may track and certify the qualifications of staff.

TYPE OF FACILITY: Center; Large Family Child Care Home

RELATED STANDARDS:
Standards 1.4.4.1-1.4.6.2: Continuing Education/Professional Development
Standard 1.8.2.2: Annual Staff Competency Evaluation

REFERENCES:
1. National Association for the Education of Young Children (NAEYC). 2008. *Leadership and management: A guide to the NAEYC early childhood program standards and related accreditation criteria.* Washington, DC: NAEYC.
2. Owens, C. 1997. *Rights in the workplace: A guide for child care teachers.* Washington, DC: Worker Option Resource Center.

STANDARD 1.8.2.3: Staff Improvement Plan

When a staff member of a center or a large family child care home does not meet the minimum competency level, that employee should work with the employer to develop a plan to assist the person in achieving the necessary skills. The plan should include a timeline for completion and consequences if it is not achieved.

RATIONALE: Children must be protected from incompetent caregiving. A system for evaluation and a plan to promote continued development are essential to assist staff to meet performance requirements (1).

COMMENTS: Whether the caregiver/teacher meets the minimum competency level is related to the director's assessment of the caregiver's/teacher's performance.

TYPE OF FACILITY: Center; Large Family Child Care Home

RELATED STANDARDS:
Standard 1.4.1.1: Pre-service Training
Standards 1.4.2.1-1.4.2.3: Orientation Training
Standard 1.4.3.1: First Aid and CPR Training for Staff
Standards 1.4.4.1-1.4.6.2: Continuing Education/Professional Development
Standard 9.4.3.1: Maintenance and Content of Staff and Volunteer Records

REFERENCES:
1. University of California Berkeley Human Resources. Guide to managing human resources. Chapter 7: Performance management. http://hrweb.berkeley.edu/guides/managing-hr/managing-successfully/performance-management/introduction/.

STANDARD 1.8.2.4: Observation of Staff

Observation of staff by a designee of the program director should include an assessment of each member's adherence to the policies and procedures of the facility with respect to sanitation, hygiene, and management of infectious diseases. Routine, direct observation of employees is the best way to evaluate hygiene and safety practices. The observation should be followed by positive and constructive feedback to staff. Staff will be informed in their job description and/or employee handbook that observations will be made.

RATIONALE: Ongoing observation is an effective tool to evaluate consistency of staff adherence to program policies and procedures (1). It also serves to identify areas for additional orientation and training.

COMMENTS: Videotaping of these assessments may be a useful way to provide feedback to staff around their adherence to policies and procedures regarding hygiene and safety practices. If videotaping includes interactions with children, parent/guardian permission must be obtained before taping occurs. Desirable interactions can be encouraged and discussing methods of improvement can be facilitated through videotaping. Videotaped interactions can also prove useful to caregivers/teachers when informing, illustrating and discussing an issue with the parents/guardians. It gives the parents/guardians a chance to interpret the observations and begin a healthy, respectful dialogue with caregivers/teachers in developing a consistent approach to supporting their child's healthy development. Sharing videotaping must have participant approval to avoid privacy issues.

If the staff follows the National Association for the Education of Young Children (NAEYC) Code of Ethical Conduct, peers are expected to observe, support and guide peers. In addition within the role of the child care health consultant and the education consultant are guidelines for observation of staff within the classroom. It should be within the role of the director and assistant director guidelines for direct observation of staff for health, safety, developmentally appropriate practice, and curriculum. For more information on the NAEYC Code of Ethical Conduct, go to http://www.naeyc.org/files/naeyc/file/positions/PSETH05.pdf.

TYPE OF FACILITY: Center; Large Family Child Care Home

REFERENCES:
1. Nolan, Jr., J. F., L. A. Hoover. 2010. *Teacher supervision and evaluation.* Hoboken, NJ: John Wiley and Sons.

STANDARD 1.8.2.5: Handling Complaints About Caregivers/Teachers

When complaints are made to licensing or referral agencies about caregivers/teachers, the caregivers/teachers should receive formal notice of the complaint and the resulting

action, if any. Caregivers/teachers should maintain records of such complaints, post substantiated complaints with correction action, make them available to parents/guardians on request, and post a notice of how to contact the state agency responsible for maintaining complaint records.

RATIONALE: Parents/guardians seeking child care should know if previous complaints have been made, particularly if the complaint is substantiated. This information should be easily accessible to the parents/guardians. Parents/guardians can then evaluate whether or not the complaint is valid, and whether the complaint has been adequately addressed and necessary changes have been made.

COMMENTS: This policy requires program development by licensing agencies.

TYPE OF FACILITY: Center; Large Family Child Care Home; Small Family Child Care Home

Chapter 2

2

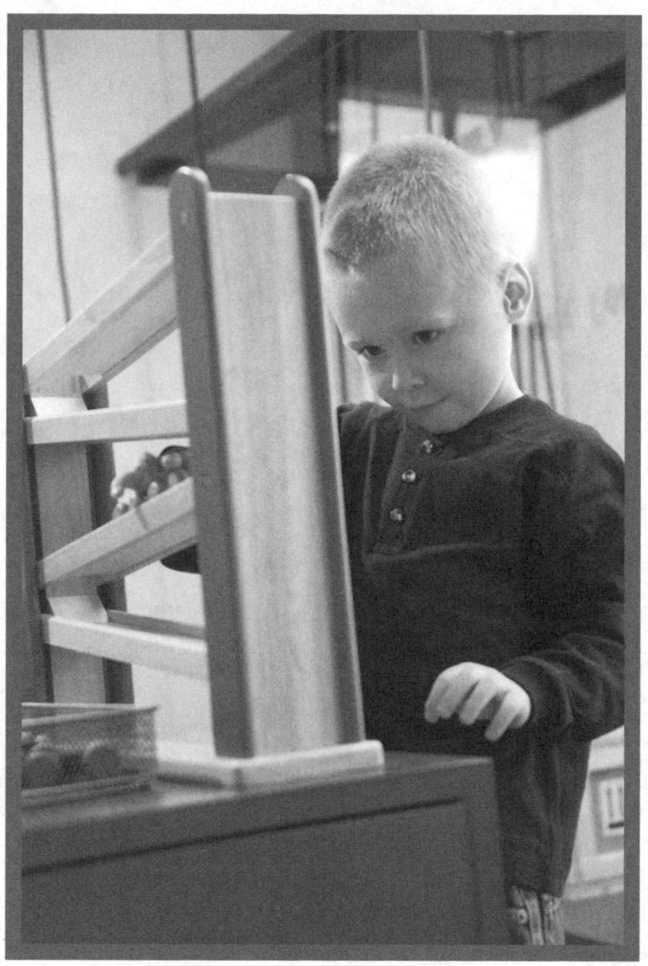

Program Activities for Healthy Development

2.1 Program of Developmental Activities

2.1.1 General Program Activities

STANDARD 2.1.1.1: Written Daily Activity Plan and Statement of Principles

Facilities should have a written comprehensive and coordinated planned program of daily activities based on a statement of principles for the facility and each child's individual development, as well as appropriate activities for groups of children at each stage of early childhood. The objective of the program of daily activities should be to foster incremental developmental progress in a healthy and safe environment and should be flexible to capture the interests of the children and the individual abilities of the children.

Centers, large and small family child care homes should develop a written statement of principles that set out the basic elements from which the daily indoor/outdoor program is to be built. These principles should include the following elements:

a) Overall child health and safety;
b) Physical development, which facilitates small and large motor skills;
c) Family development, which acknowledges the role of the family, including culture and language;
d) Social development, which leads to cooperative play with other children and the ability to make relationships with other children and adults and children of other backgrounds and ability levels;
e) Emotional development, which facilitates self awareness and self confidence;
f) Cognitive development, which includes an understanding of the world and environment in which they live and leads to understanding science, math, and literacy concepts, as well as increasing the use and understanding of language to express feelings and ideas.

The planned program should provide for the incorporation of specific health education topics on a daily basis throughout the year. Topics of health education should include health promotion and disease prevention topics, e.g., handwashing, oral health, nutrition, physical activity, etc.

Health and safety behaviors should be modeled by staff in order to insure that children and parents/guardians understand the need for a safe indoor and outdoor learning/play environment and feel comfortable.

Continuity and consistency by a caring staff is vital so that children and parents/guardians know what to expect. All of the principles should be developed with play being the foundation of the planned curriculum. Material such as blocks, clay, paints, books, puzzles, and/or other manipulatives should be available indoors and outdoors to the children to further the planned curriculum.

RATIONALE: Reviews of children's performance after attending out-of-home child care indicate that children attending facilities with well-developed curricula achieve appropriate levels of development (1,2).

Early childhood specialists agree on the:

a) Inseparability and interdependence of cognitive, physical, emotional, communication and social development. Social-emotional capacities do not develop or function separately;
b) Influence of the child's health and safety on all these areas;
c) Central importance of continuity and consistent relationships with affectionate care that is the formation of strong, nurturing relationships between caregivers/teachers and children;
d) Relevance of the phase or stage concept;
e) Importance of action (including play) as a mode of learning, and to express self (3).

Those who provide child care and early education must be able to articulate components of the curriculum they are implementing and the related values/principles on which the curriculum is based. In centers and large family child care homes, because more than two caregivers/teachers are involved in operating the facility, a written statement of principles helps achieve consensus about the basic elements from which all staff will plan the daily program (4).

A written description of the planned program of daily activities allows staff and parents/guardians to have a common understanding and gives them the ability to compare the program's actual performance to the stated intent. Child care is a "delivery of service" involving a contractual relationship between the caregiver/teacher and the consumer. A written plan helps to define the service and contributes to specific and responsible operations that are conducive to sound child development and safety practices and to positive consumer relations (4). For infants and toddlers who learn through healthy and ongoing relationships with primary caregivers/teachers, a relationship-based plan should be shared with parents/guardians that include opportunities for parents/guardians to be an integral partner and member of this relationship system. Professional development is often required to enable staff to develop proficiency in the development and implementation of a curriculum that they use to carry out daily activities appropriately (6).

Planning ensures that some thought goes into indoor and outdoor programming for children. The plans are tools for monitoring and accountability. Also, a written plan is a tool for staff orientation.

COMMENTS: The National Association for the Education of Young Children (NAEYC) Accreditation Criteria and Procedures, the National Association for Family Child Care (NAFCC) accreditation standards, and the National Child Care Association (NCCA) standards can serve as resources for planning program activities.

Parents/guardians and staff can experience mutual learning in an open, supportive setting. Suggestions for topics and methods of presentation are widely available. For example, the publication catalogs of the NAEYC and of the American Academy of Pediatrics (AAP) contain many materials for child, parent/guardian, and staff education on child development, the importance of attachment and temperament, and other health issues. A certified health education specialist (CHES) can also be a source of assistance. The American Association for Health Education (AAHE) at http://www.aahperd.org/AAHE/, and the National Commission for Health Education Credentialing (NCHEC) at http://www.nchec.org, provide information on this specialty.

TYPE OF FACILITY: Center; Large Family Child Care Home; Small Family Child Care Home

RELATED STANDARDS:
Standard 2.1.1.3: Coordinated Child Care Health Program Model
Standard 2.1.1.8: Diversity in Enrollment and Curriculum
Section 2.1.2: Program Activities for Infants and Toddlers from Three to Less Than Thirty-Six Months
Section 2.1.3: Program Activities for Three- to Five-Year-Olds
Section 2.1.4: Program Activities for School-Age Children
Section 2.4: Health Education

REFERENCES:
1. Colker L. J., A. L. Dombro, D. T. Dodge. 1996. Curriculum for infants and toddlers: Who needs it? *Child Care Info Exch* 112:74-78.
2. Smith A. B. 1996. Quality programs that care and educate. *Child Education* 72:330-36.
3. Dimidjian, V. J., ed. 1992. *Play's place in public education for young children*. National Education Association Early Childhood Education Series. Washington, DC: NEAECE.
4. The Family Child Care Accreditation Project, Wheelock College and The National Association for Family Child Care. 2005. *Quality standards for NAFCC accreditation*. 4th ed. http://www.nafcc.org/documents/QualStd.pdf.
5. National Child Care Information Center (NCCIC). NCCIC resources. U.S. Department of Health and Human Services, Administration for Children and Families. http://nccic.acf.hhs.gov/nccic-resources/.
6. Nell, M. 2009. Using the integrative research approach to facilitate early childhood teacher planning. *J Early Child Teach Edu* 30:79-88.

STANDARD 2.1.1.2: Health, Nutrition, Physical Activity, and Safety Awareness

Early care and education programs should have and implement written program plans addressing the health, nutrition, physical activity, and safety aspects of each formally structured activity documented in the written curriculum. These plans should include daily opportunities to learn health habits that prevent infection and significant injuries, and health habits that support healthful eating, nutrition education, and physical motor activity. Awareness of healthy and safe behaviors, including good nutrition and physical activity, should be an integral part of the overall program.

RATIONALE: Young children learn better through experiencing an activity and observing behavior than through didactic methods (1). There may be a reciprocal relationship between learning and play so that play experiences are closely related to learning (2,3). Children can live by rules about health and safety when their personal experience helps them to understand why these rules were created. National guidelines for children birth to age five encourage their engagement in daily physical activity that promotes movement, motor skills and the foundations of health-related fitness (4). Physical activity is important to overall health and to overweight and obesity prevention (5).

COMMENTS: Resources for activities can be found at:

- Fit Source – http://nccic.acf.hhs.gov/fitsource/;
- Go Out and Play – http://www.cdc.gov/ncbddd/actearly/pdf/ccp_pdfs/GOP_kit.pdf; and
- Center of Excellence for Training and Research Translation – http://www.center-trt.org.

TYPE OF FACILITY: Center; Large Family Child Care Home; Small Family Child Care Home

RELATED STANDARDS:
Standard 2.1.1.3: Coordinated Child Care Health Program Model
Standard 3.1.3.1: Active Opportunities for Physical Activity
Standard 4.5.0.4: Socialization During Meals
Standard 4.5.0.8: Experience with Familiar and New Foods
Standard 4.7.0.1: Nutrition Learning Experiences for Children
Appendix S: Physical Activity: How Much Is Needed?

REFERENCES:
1. Fleer, M., ed. 1996. *Play through profiles: Profiles through play*. Watson, Australia: Australian Early Childhood Association.
2. Evaldson, A., W. A. Corsaro. 1998. Play and games in the peer cultures of preschool and preadolescent children: An interpretative approach. *Childhood* 5:377-402.
3. Petersen, E. A. 1998. The amazing benefits of play. *Children and Families* 17:7-8, 10.
4. National Association for Sport and Physical Education (NASPE). 2009. *Active start: A statement of physical activity guidelines for children birth to five years*. 2nd ed. Reston, VA: NASPE.
5. U.S. Department of Health and Human Services, U.S. Department of Agriculture. 2010. *Dietary guidelines for Americans*. 7th ed. Washington, DC: Government Printing Office. http://www.cnpp.usda.gov/Publications/DietaryGuidelines/2010/PolicyDoc/PolicyDoc.pdf.

STANDARD 2.1.1.3: Coordinated Child Care Health Program Model

Caregivers/teachers should follow these guidelines for implementing coordinated health programs in all early care and education settings. These coordinated health programs should consist of health and safety education, physical activity and education, health services and child care health consultation, nutrition services, mental health services, healthy and safe indoor and outdoor learning environment, health and safety promotion for the staff, and family and community involvement. The guidelines consist of the following eight interactive components:

1. Health Education: A planned, sequential, curriculum that addresses the physical, mental, emotional, and social dimensions of health. The curriculum is designed to motivate and assist children in maintaining and improving their health, preventing disease and injury, and reducing health-related risk behaviors (1,2).

2. Physical Activity and Education: A planned, sequential curriculum that provides learning experiences in a variety of

activity areas such as basic movement skills, physical fitness, rhythms and dance, games, sports, tumbling, outdoor learning and gymnastics. Quality physical activity and education should promote, through a variety of planned physical activities indoors and outdoors, each child's optimum physical, mental, emotional, and social development, and should promote activities and sports that all children enjoy and can pursue throughout their lives (1,2,6).

3. Health Services and Child Care Health Consultants: Services provided for child care settings to assess, protect, and promote health. These services are designed to ensure access or referral to primary health care services or both, foster appropriate use of primary health care services, prevent and control communicable disease and other health problems, provide emergency care for illness or injury, promote and provide optimum sanitary conditions for a safe child care facility and child care environment, and provide educational opportunities for promoting and maintaining individual, family, and community health. Qualified professionals such as child care health consultants may provide these services (1,2,4,5).

4. Nutrition Services: Access to a variety of nutritious and appealing meals that accommodate the health and nutrition needs of all children. School nutrition programs reflect the U.S. Dietary Guidelines for Americans and other criteria to achieve nutrition integrity. The school nutrition services offer children a learning laboratory for nutrition and health education and serve as a resource for linkages with nutrition-related community services (1,2).

5. Mental Health Services: Services provided to improve children's mental, emotional, and social health. These services include individual and group assessments, interventions, and referrals. Organizational assessment and consultation skills of mental health professionals contribute not only to the health of students but also to the health of the staff and child care environment (1,2).

6. Healthy Child Care Environment: The physical and aesthetic surroundings and the psychosocial climate and culture of the child care setting. Factors that influence the physical environment include the building and the area surrounding it, natural spaces for outdoor learning, any biological or chemical agents that are detrimental to health, indoor and outdoor air quality, and physical conditions such as temperature, noise, and lighting. Unsafe physical environments include those such as where bookcases are not attached to walls and doors that could pinch children's fingers. The psychological environment includes the physical, emotional, and social conditions that affect the well-being of children and staff (1,2).

7. Health Promotion for the Staff: Opportunities for caregivers/teachers to improve their own health status through activities such as health assessments, health education, help in accessing immunizations, health-related fitness activities, and time for staff to be outdoors. These opportunities encourage caregivers/teachers to pursue a healthy lifestyle that contributes to their improved health status, improved morale, and a greater personal commitment to the child care's overall coordinated health program. This personal commitment often transfers into greater commitment to the health of children and creates positive role modeling. Health promotion activities have improved productivity, decreased absenteeism, and reduced health insurance costs (1,2).

8. Family and Community Involvement: An integrated child care, parent/guardian, and community approach for enhancing the health and safety, and well-being of children. Parent/guardian-teacher health advisory councils, coalitions, and broadly based constituencies for child care health can build support for child care health program efforts. Early care and education settings should actively solicit parent/guardian involvement and engage community resources and services to respond more effectively to the health-related needs of children (1,2).

RATIONALE: Early care and education settings provide a structure by which families, caregivers/teachers, administrators, primary care providers, and communities can promote optimal health and well-being of children (3,4). The coordinated child care health program model was adapted from the Center for Disease Control and Prevention (CDC) Division of Adolescent and School Health's (DASH) Coordinated School Health Program (CSHP) model (2).

TYPE OF FACILITY: Center; Large Family Child Care Home; Small Family Child Care Home

REFERENCES:

1. Centers for Disease Control and Prevention. 2008. Healthy youth! Coordinates school health programs. http://www.cdc.gov/healthyyouth/CSHP/.
2. Cory, A. C. 2007. The role of the child care health consultant in promoting health literacy for children, families, and educators in early care and education settings. Paper presented at the annual meeting of the American School Health Association.
3. Fiene, R. 2002. *13 indicators of quality child care: Research update*. Washington, DC: U.S. Department of Health and Human Services, Office of the Assistant Secretary for Planning and Evaluation. http://aspe.hhs.gov/hsp/ccquality-ind02/.
4. U.S. Department of health and Human Services, Office of Child Care. 2010. *Coordinating child care consultants: Combining multiple disciplines and improving quality in infant/toddler care settings.* http://nitcci.nccic.acf.hhs.gov/resources/consultation_brief.pdf.
5. Coordinated Health/Care. Maximize your benefits: FAQs about care coordination. https://www.cchcare.com/router.php?action=about.
6. Friedman, H. S., L. R. Martin, J. S. Tucker, M. H. Criqui, M. L. Kern, C. A. Reynolds. 2008. Stability of physical activity across the lifespan. *J Health Psychol* 13:1092-1104.

STANDARD 2.1.1.4: Monitoring Children's Development/Obtaining Consent for Screening

Child care settings provide daily indoor and outdoor opportunities for promoting and monitoring children's development. Caregivers/teachers should monitor the children's development, share observations with parents/guardians, and provide resource information as needed for screenings, evaluations, and early intervention and treatment. Caregivers/teachers should work in collaboration to monitor a child's development with parents/guardians and in conjunction with the child's primary care provider and health, education, mental health, and early intervention consultants. Caregivers/teachers should utilize the services of health and safety, education, mental health, and early intervention consultants to strengthen their observation skills, collaborate with families, and be knowledgeable of community resources.

Programs should have a formalized system of developmental screening with all children that can be used near the beginning of a child's placement in the program, at least yearly thereafter, and as developmental concerns become apparent to staff and/or parents/guardians. The use of authentic assessment and curricular-based assessments should be an ongoing part of the services provided to all children (5-9). The facility's formalized system should include a process for determining when a health or developmental screening or evaluation for a child is necessary. This process should include parental/guardian consent and participation.

Parents/guardians should be explicitly invited to:

a) Discuss reasons for a health or developmental assessment;
b) Participate in discussions of the results of their child's evaluations and the relationship of their child's needs to the caregivers'/teachers' ability to serve that child appropriately;
c) Give alternative perspectives;
d) Share their expectations and goals for their child and have these expectations and goals integrated with any plan for their child;
e) Explore community resources and supports that might assist in meeting any identified needs that child care centers and family child care homes can provide;
f) Give written permission to share health information with primary health care professionals (medical home), child care health consultants and other professionals as appropriate;

The facility should document parents'/guardians' presence at these meetings and invitations to attend.

If the parents/guardians do not attend the screening, the caregiver/teacher should inform the parents/guardians of the results, and offer an opportunity for discussion. Efforts should be made to provide notification of meetings in the primary language of the parents/guardians. Formal evaluations of a child's health or development should also be shared with the child's medical home with parent/guardian consent.

Programs are encouraged to utilize validated screening tools to monitor children's development, as well as various measures that may inform their work facilitating children's development and providing an enriching indoor and outdoor environment, such as authentic-based assessment, work sampling methods, observational assessments, and assessments intended to support curricular implementation (5,9). Programs should have clear policies for using reliable and valid methods of developmental screening with all children and for making referrals for diagnostic assessment and possible intervention for children who screen positive. All programs should use methods of ongoing developmental assessment that inform the curricular approaches used by the staff. Care must be taken in communicating the results. Screening is a way to identify a child *at risk* of a developmental delay or disorder. It is not a diagnosis.

If the screening or any observation of the child results in any concern about the child's development, after consultation with the parents/guardians, the child should be referred to his or her primary care provider (medical home), or to an appropriate specialist or clinic for further evaluation. In some situations, a direct referral to the Early Intervention System in the respective state may also be required.

RATIONALE: Seventy percent of children with developmental disabilities and mental health problems are not identified until school entry (10). Daily interaction with children and families in early care and education settings offers an important opportunity for promoting children's development as well as monitoring developmental milestones and early signs of delay (1-3). Caregivers/teachers play an essential role in the early identification and treatment of children with developmental concerns and disabilities (6-8) because of their knowledge in child development principles and milestones and relationship with families (4). Coordination of observation findings and services with children's primary care providers in collaboration with families will enhance children's outcomes (6).

COMMENTS: Parents/guardians need to be included in the process of considering, identifying and shaping decisions about their children, (e.g., adding, deleting, or changing a service). To provide services effectively, facilities must recognize parents'/guardians' observations and reports about the child and their expectations for the child, as well as the family's need of child care services. A marked discrepancy between professional and parent/guardian observations of, or expectations for, a child necessitates further discussion and development of a consensus on a plan of action.

Consideration should be given to utilizing parent/guardian-completed screening tools, such as the Ages and Stages Questionnaire (ASQ) (for a list of validated developmental screening tools, see the American Academy of Pediatric's [AAP] list of developmental screening tools at http://www.medicalhomeinfo.org/downloads/pdfs/DPIPscreeningtoolgrid.pdf). The caregiver/teacher should explain the results to parents/guardians honestly, with sensitivity, and without using technical jargon (11).

Resources for implementing a program that involves a formalized system of developmental screening are available at the Centers for Disease Control and Prevention (CDC) at http://www.cdc.gov/ncbddd/actearly/ and the AAP at http://www.healthychildcare.org.

Scheduling meetings at times convenient for parent/guardian participation is optimal. Those conducting an evaluation, and when subsequently discussing the findings with the family, should consider parents'/guardians' input. Parents/

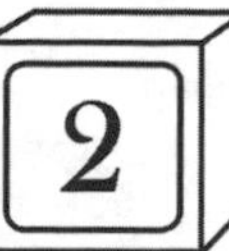

guardians have both the motive and the legal right to be included in decision-making and to seek other opinions.

A second, independent opinion could be provided by the program's child care health consultant or the child's primary care provider.

TYPE OF FACILITY: Center; Large Family Child Care Home; Small Family Child Care Home

RELATED STANDARDS:
Standard 1.3.2.5: Additional Qualifications for Caregivers/Teachers Serving Children Three to Five Years of Age
Standard 1.3.2.7: Qualifications and Responsibilities for Health Advocates
Standard 3.1.4.5: Conduct of Daily Health Check
Standard 9.4.1.3: Written Policy on Confidentiality of Records

REFERENCES:
1. Copple, C., S. Bredekamp. 2009. *Developmentally appropriate practice in early childhood programs serving children at birth through age 8*. 3rd ed. Washington, DC: National Association for the Education of Young Children.
2. Dworkin, P. H. 1989. British and American recommendations for developmental monitoring: The role of surveillance. *Pediatrics* 84:1000-1010.
3. Brothers, K. I., F. Glascoe, N. Robertshaw. 2008. PEDS: Developmental milestones - An accurate brief tool for surveillance and screening. *Clinical Pediatrics* 47:271-79.
4. Kostelnik, M. J., A. K. Soderman, A. P. Whiren. 2006. *Developmentally appropriate curriculum best practices in early childhood education.* Upper Saddle River, NJ: Prentice Hall.
5. Squires, J., D. Bricker. 2009. *Ages and stages questionnaires*. Baltimore: Brookes Publishing.
6. Centers for Disease Control and Prevention. Learn the signs. Act early. http://www.cdc.gov/ncbddd/actearly/.
7. American Academy of Pediatrics, Council on Children With Disabilities, Section on Developmental Behavioral Pediatrics, Bright Futures Steering Committee and Medical Home Initiatives for Children With Special Needs Project Advisory Committee. 2006. Identifying infants and young children with developmental disorders in the medical home: An alogorithm for developmental surveillance and screening. *Pediatrics* 118:405-20.
8. Hagan, J. F., J. S. Shaw, P. M. Duncan, eds. 2008. *Bright futures: Guidelines for health supervision of infants, children, and adolescents.* 3rd ed. Elk Grove Village, IL: American Academy of Pediatrics.
9. Gilliam, W. S., S. Meisels, L. Mayes. 2005. Screening and surveillance in early intervention systems. In *A developmental systems approach to early intervention: National and international perspectives,* ed. M. J. Guralnick, 73-98. Baltimore, MD: Brookes Publishing.
10. Glascoe, F. P. 2005. Screening for developmental and behavioral problems. *Mental Retardation Develop Disabilities* 11:173-79.
11. O'Connor, S., et al. 1996. *ASQ: Assessing school age child care quality*. Wellesly, MA: Center for Research on Women.

STANDARD 2.1.1.5: Helping Families Cope with Separation

The staff of the facility should engage strategies to help a child and parents/guardians cope with the experience of separation and reunion, such as death of family members, divorce, or placement in foster care.

For the child, this should be accomplished by:

a) Encouraging parents/guardians to spend time in the facility with the child and supporting the separation transition;
b) Providing a comfortable setting both indoors and outdoors for parents/guardians to be with their children to transition or to have conversation with staff;
c) Having established routines for drop-off and pick-up times to assist with transition;
d) Enabling the child to bring to child care tangible reminders of home/family (such as a favorite toy or a picture of self and parent/guardian);
e) Encouraging parents/guardians to reassure the child of their return and to calmly say "goodbye";
f) Helping the child play out themes of separation and reunion;
g) Frequently exchanging information between the child's parents/guardians and caregivers/teachers, including activities and routine care information particularly during greeting and departing;
h) Reassuring the child about the parent's/guardian's return;
i) Ensuring the caregivers/teachers are consistent both within the parts of a day and across days;
j) Requesting assistance from early childhood mental health consultants, mental health professionals, developmental-behavioral pediatricians, parent/guardian counselors, etc. when a child's adjustment continues to be problematic over time;
k) When a family is experiencing separation due to a military deployment, explore changes in children's behavior that may be related to feelings of anger, fear, sadness, or uncertainty related to changes in family structure as a result of deployment. Work with the parent/guardian at home to help the child adjust to these changes, including providing activities that help the child remain connected to the deployed parent/guardian and manage their emotions throughout the deployment cycle.

For the parents/guardians, this should be accomplished by:

a) Validating their feelings as a universal human experience;
b) Providing parents/guardians with information about the positive effects for children of high quality facilities with strong parent/guardian participation;
c) Encouraging parents/guardians to discuss their feelings;
d) Providing parents/guardians with evidence, such as photographs, that their child is being cared for and is enjoying the activities of the facility;
e) Ask parents/guardians to bring pictures from home that may be placed in the room or cubby and displayed throughout the indoor and outdoor learning/play environment at the child's eye level;
f) Where a family is experiencing separation due to a military deployment, collaborate with the parent/guardian at home to address changes in children's behavior that may be related to the deployment,

providing parents/guardians with information about activities in care and at home may help promote their child's positive adjustment throughout the deployment cycle (connect parents/guardians with services/resources in the community that can help to support them);

g) Requesting assistance from early childhood mental health consultants, mental health professionals, developmental-behavioral pediatricians, parent/guardian counselors, etc. when a child's adjustment continues to be problematic over time.

RATIONALE: In childhood, some separation experiences facilitate psychological growth by mobilizing new approaches for learning and adaptation. Other separations are painful and traumatic. The way in which influential adults provide support and understanding, or fail to do so, will shape the child's experience (1).

Many parents/guardians who prefer to care for their young children only at home may have no other option than to place their children in out-of-home child care before three months of age. Some parents/guardians prefer combining out-of-home child care with parental/guardian care to provide good experiences for their children and support for other family members to function most effectively. Whether parents/guardians view out-of-home child care as a necessary accommodation to undesired circumstances or a benefit for their family, parents/guardians and their children need help from the caregivers/teachers to accommodate the transitions between home and out-of-home settings (2).

Many parents/guardians experience distress at separation. For most parents/guardians, the younger their child and the less experience they have had with sharing the care of their children with others, the more intense their distress at separation (3).

Although children's responses to deployment separation will vary depending on age, personality, and support received, children will be aware of a parent's/guardian's long-term absence and may mourn. Children may feel uncertain, sad, afraid, or angry. These feelings can manifest as increased clinginess, aggression, withdrawal, changes in sleeping or eating patterns, regression or other behaviors. Young children don't often have the vocabulary to express their emotions, and may need support to express their feelings in healthy and safe ways (2). Additionally, the parent/guardian at home may be experiencing stress, anxiety, depression, or fear. These parents/guardians may benefit from additional outreach from caregivers/teachers, who are part of their community support system, and can help them with strategies to promote children's adjustment and connect them with resources in the community (3).

COMMENTS: Depending on the child's developmental stage, the impact of separation on the child and parent/guardian will vary. Child care facilities should understand and communicate this variation to parents/guardians and work with parents/guardians to plan developmentally appropriate coping strategies for use at home and in the child care setting. For example, a child at eighteen to twenty-four months of age is particularly vulnerable to separation issues and may show visible distress when experiencing separation from parents/guardians. Entry into child care at this age may trigger behavior problems, such as difficulty sleeping. Even for the child who has adapted well to a child care arrangement before this developmental stage, such difficulties can occur as the child continues in care and enters this developmental stage. For younger children, who are working on understanding object permanence (usually around nine to twelve months of age), parents/guardians who sneak out after bringing their children to the child care facility may create some level of anxiety in the child throughout the day. Sneaking away leaves the child unable to discern when someone the child trusts will leave without warning. Parents/guardians and caregivers/teachers reminding a child that the parent/guardian returned as promised reinforces truthfulness and trust. Parents/guardians of children of any age should be encouraged to visit the facility together before the child care officially begins. Parents/guardians of infants may benefit from feeling assured by the caregivers/teachers themselves. Depending on the child's temperament and prior care experience, several visits may be recommended before enrolling as well opportunities to practice the process and consistency of a separation experience in the first weeks of entering the child care. Using a phasing-in period can also be helpful (e.g., spend only a part of the day with parents/guardians on the first day, half-day on the second day, and parents/guardians leave earlier, etc.)

TYPE OF FACILITY: Center; Large Family Child Care Home; Small Family Child Care Home

RELATED STANDARDS:
Standard 1.1.2.1: Minimum Age to Enter Child Care
Standard 1.6.0.3: Early Childhood Mental Health Consultants

REFERENCES:
1. Blecher-Sass, H. 1997. Good-byes can build trust. *Young Child* 52:12-14.
2. Kim, A. M., J. Yeary. 2008. Making long-term separations easier for children and families. *Young Children* 63:32-37.
3. Gonzalez-Mena, J. 2007. Separation: Helping children and families. In *50 Early childhood strategies for working and communicating with diverse families,* 96-97. Upper Saddle River, NJ: Prentice Hall.

STANDARD 2.1.1.6: Transitioning within Programs and Indoor and Outdoor Learning/Play Environments

Caregivers/teachers should take into consideration the individual needs of children when transitioning them to a new indoor and outdoor learning/play environment. The transitioning child/children should be offered the opportunity to visit the new space with a familiar caregiver/teacher with enough time to allow them to display comfort in the new space. The program should allow time for communication with the families regarding the process and for each child to follow through a comfortable time line of adaptation to the new indoor and outdoor learning/play environment, caregiver/teachers, and peers.

Children need time to manipulate, explore and familiarize themselves with the new space and caregivers/teachers. This should be done before they are part of a new group to allow them time to explore to their personal satisfaction. Eating is a primary reinforcer and need. The opportunity to share food within the new space will help reassure a child and help adults assess how the transition is going. Toileting involves another level of trust. Diapering/toileting should be introduced in the new space with a familiar teacher.

New routines should be introduced by the new staff with a familiar caregiver/teacher present to support the child/children. Transitions to the indoor and outdoor learning/play environment, especially if the space is different than the one from which they are familiar, should follow similar procedures as moving to another indoor space. Parents/guardians should be part of the transition as they too are in the process of learning to trust a new indoor and outdoor learning/play environment for their child. Primary needs need to be met to support a smooth transition.

Transitions should be planned in advance, based on the child's readiness. A written plan should be developed and shared with parents/guardians, describing how and when the transition will occur. Children should not be moved to a new indoor and outdoor learning/play environment for the sole purpose of maintaining child: staff ratios.

RATIONALE: Supporting the achievement of developmental tasks for young children is essential for their social and emotional health. Establishing trust with caregivers/teachers and successful adaptation to a new indoor and outdoor learning/play environment is a critical component of quality care. Young children need predictability and routine. They need to feel secure and to understand the expectations of their environment. By taking time to allow them to familiarize themselves with their new caregivers/teachers and environment, they are better able to handle the emotional, cognitive, and social requirements of their new space (1-5).

TYPE OF FACILITY: Center; Large Family Child Care Home; Small Family Child Care Home

RELATED STANDARDS:
Standard 2.1.2.5: Toilet Learning/Training

REFERENCES:

1. Erikson, E. H. 1950. *Childhood and society*. New York: W.W. Norton and Co.
2. Gorski, P. A., S. P. Berger. 2005. Emotional health in child care. In *Health in child care: A manual for health professionals*, ed. J. R. Murph, S. D. Palmer, D. Glassy, 173-86. Elk Grove Village, IL: American Academy of Pediatrics.
3. Lally, R. L., L. Y. Torres, P. C. Phelps. 1994. Caring for infants and toddlers in groups: Necessary considerations for emotional, social, and cognitive development. *Zero to Three* 14:1-8.
4. Mahler, M., F. Pine, A. Bergman. 1975. *The Psychological birth of the human infant*. New York: Basic Books.
5. Maslow, A. 1943. A theory of human motivation. *Psychological Review* 50:370-96

STANDARD 2.1.1.7: Communication in Native Language Other Than English

At least one member of the staff should be able to communicate with the parents/guardians and children in the family's native language (sign or spoken), or the facility should work with parents/guardians to arrange for a translator to communicate with parents/guardians and children. Efforts should be made to support a child's and family's native language while providing resources and opportunities for learning English (2). Children should not be used as translators. They are not developmentally able to understand the meaning of all words as used by adults, nor should they participate in all conversations that may be regarding the child.

RATIONALE: The future development of the child depends on his/her command of language (1). Richness of language increases as a result of experiences as well as through the child's verbal interaction with adults and peers. Basic communication with parents/guardians and children requires an ability to speak their language. Learning English while maintaining a family's native language enriches child development and strengthens family cultural traditions.

COMMENTS: For resources on bilingual and dual language learning, see the American Academy of Pediatrics Section on Developmental and Behavioral Pediatrics (SODBP) at http://www.aap.org/sections/dbpeds/.

TYPE OF FACILITY: Center; Large Family Child Care Home; Small Family Child Care Home

REFERENCES:

1. Moerk, E. L. 2000. The guided acquisition of first language skills. *Advances Applied Dev Psychol* 20:248.
2. Olsen, L. 2006. Ensuring academic success of English learners. 2006. *U.C. Linguistic Minority Research Institute* 15:1-7.

STANDARD 2.1.1.8: Diversity in Enrollment and Curriculum

Programs should work to increase understanding of cultural, ethnic, and other similarities and differences by enrolling children who reflect the cultural and ethnic diversity of the community. Programs should provide cultural curricula that engage children and families and teach multicultural learning activities. Indoor and outdoor learning/play environments should have an array of toys, materials, posters, etc. that reflect diverse cultures and ethnicities. Stereotyping of any culture must be avoided.

RATIONALE: Children who participate in programs that reflect and show respect for the cultural diversity of their communities learn to understand and value cultural diversity. This learning in early childhood enables their healthy participation in a democratic pluralistic society (peaceful coexistence of different interests, convictions, and lifestyles) throughout life (1-3,11,12). By facilitating the expression of cultural development or ethnic identity and by encouraging familiarity with different groups and practices through ordinary interaction and activities integrated into a developmentally appropriate curriculum, a facility can foster children's

ability to relate to people who are different from themselves, their sense of possibility, and their ability to succeed in a diverse society, while also promoting feelings of belonging and identification with a tradition.

COMMENTS: Sharing information about the child on a daily basis with the children's families shows respect for the children's cultures by creating an opportunity to learn more about the families' background, beliefs, and traditions (5-9). Materials, displays, and learning activities must represent the cultural heritage of the children and the staff to instill a sense of pride and positive feelings of identification in all children and staff members (4). In order to enroll a diverse group, the facility should market its services in a culturally sensitive way and should make sincere efforts to employ staff members that represent the culture of the children and their families (10). Children need to see members of their own community in positions of influence in the services they use. Scholarships and tuition assistance can be used to increase the diversity among enrolled children.

TYPE OF FACILITY: Center; Large Family Child Care Home; Small Family Child Care Home

REFERENCES:

1. Wardle, F. 1998. Meeting the needs of multicultural and multiethnic children in early childhood settings. *Early Child Education J* 26:7-11.
2. Ramsey, P. G. 1998. *Teaching and learning in a diverse world: Multicultural education for young children*. 2nd ed. New York: Teachers College Press.
3. Ramsey, P. G. 1995. Growing up with the contradictions of race and class. *Young Child* 50:18-22.
4. Maschinot, B. 2008. *The changing face of the United States: The influence of culture on early child development*. Washington, DC: Zero to Three. http://www.zerotothree.org/site/DocServer/Culture_book.pdf?docID=6921.
5. Williams, K. C., M. H. Cooney. 2006. Young children and social justice. *Young Children* 61:75-82.
6. Gonzalex-Mena, J. 2008. *Diversity in early care and education: Honoring differences*. 5th ed. Boston: McGraw-Hill.
7. Gonzalez-Mena, J. 2007. *50 early childhood strategies for working and communicating with diverse families*. Upper Saddle River, NJ: Pearson Merrill Prentice Hall.
8. Bradely, J., P. Kibera. 2006. Closing the gap: Culture and promotion of inclusion in child care. *Young Children* 61:34-40.
9. Romero, M. 2008. Promoting tolerance and respect for diversity in early childhood: Toward a research and practice agenda. Report of the Promoting Tolerance and Respect for Diversity in Early Childhood Meeting, Brooklyn, NY, June 25, 2007. http://www.nccp.org/publications/pdf/text_812.pdf.
10. Matthews, H. 2008. Supporting a diverse and culturally competent workforce: Charting progress for babies in child care. Charting Progress for Babies in Child Care: A CLASP Child Care and Early Education Project, Washington, DC. http://www.clasp.org/babiesinchildcare/recommendations?id=0005.
11. Parent Services Project (PSP). Making room in the circle. Training Curriculum, PSP, San Rafael, CA.
12. Fox, R. K. 2007. One of the hidden diversities in schools: Families with parents who are Lesbian or Gay. *Childhood Education* 83:277-81.

STANDARD 2.1.1.9: Verbal Interaction

The child care facility should assure that a rich environment of spoken language by caregivers/teachers surrounds and includes all children with opportunities to expand their language communication skills. Each child should have at least one speaking adult person who engages the child in frequent verbal exchanges linked to daily events and experiences. To encourage the development of language, the caregiver/teacher should demonstrate skillful verbal communication and interaction with the child.

a) For infants, these interactions should include responses to, and encouragement of, soft infant sounds, as well as identifying objects, feelings, and desires by the caregiver/teacher.
b) For toddlers, the interactions should include naming of objects, feelings, listening to the child and responding, along with actions and supporting, but not forcing, the child to do the same.
c) For preschool and school-age children, interactions should include respectful listening and responses to what the child has to say, amplifying and clarifying the child's intent, and not reinforcing mispronunciations (e.g., Wambulance instead of Ambulance).
d) Frequent interchange of questions, comments, and responses to children, including extending children's utterances with a longer statement, by teaching staff.
e) For children with special needs, alternative methods of communication should be available, including but not limited to: sign language, assistive technology, picture boards, picture exchange communication systems (PECS), FM systems for hearing aids, etc. Communication through methods other than verbal communication can result in the same desired outcomes.
f) Profanity should not be used at any time.

RATIONALE: Conversation with adults is one of the main channels through which children learn about themselves, others, and the world in which they live. While adults speaking to children teaches the children facts and relays information, the social and emotional communications and the atmosphere of the exchange are equally important. Reciprocity of expression, response, and the initiation and enrichment of dialogue are hallmarks of the social function and significance of the conversations (1-4).

The future development of the child depends on his/her command of language (5). Research suggests that language experiences in a child's early years have a profound influence on that child's language and vocabulary development, which in turn has an impact on future school success (6). Richness of the child's language increases as it is nurtured by verbal interactions and learning experiences with adults and peers. Basic communication with parents/guardians and children requires an ability to speak their language. Discussing the impact of actions on feelings for the child and others helps to develop empathy.

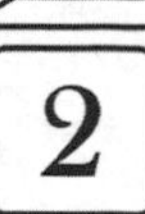

TYPE OF FACILITY: Center; Large Family Child Care Home; Small Family Child Care Home

REFERENCES:

1. Mayr, T., M. Ulich. 1999. Children's well-being in day care centers: An exploratory empirical study. *Int J Early Years Education* 7:229-39.
2. Baron, N., L. W. Schrank. 1997. *Children learning language: How adults can help*. Lake Zurich, IL: Learning Seed.
3. Szanton, E. S., ed. 1997. *Creating child-centered programs for infants and toddlers, birth to 3 year olds, step by step: A Program for children and families*. New York: Children's Resources International, Inc.
4. Kontos, S., A. Wilcox-Herzog. 1997. Teachers' interactions with children: Why are they so Important? *Young Child* 52:4-12.
5. Moerk, E. L. 2000. The guided acquisition of first language skills. *Advances in Applied Dev Psychol* 20:248.
6. Pikulski, J. J., Templeton, S. 2004. *Teaching and developing vocabulary: Key to long-term reading success.* Geneva, IL: Houghton Mifflin Company. http://www.eduplace.com/state/author/pik_temp.pdf.

2.1.2 Program Activities for Infants and Toddlers from Three Months to Less Than Thirty-Six Months

STANDARD 2.1.2.1: Personal Caregiver/Teacher Relationships for Infants and Toddlers

The facility should practice a relationship-based philosophy that promotes consistency and continuity of caregivers/teachers for infants and toddlers. The facility should limit the number of caregivers/teachers who interact with any one infant (1,2) to no more than five caregivers/teachers across the period that the child is an infant in child care. The caregiver/teacher should:

a) Hold and comfort children who are upset;
b) Engage in frequent, multiple, and rich social interchanges such as smiling, talking, touching, singing, and eating;
c) Be play partners as well as protectors;
d) Be attuned to children's feelings and reflect them back;
e) Communicate consistently with parents/guardians;
f) Interact with children and develop a relationship in the context of everyday routines (diapering, feeding, etc.)

Opportunities should be provided for each child to develop a personal and affectionate relationship with, and attachment to, that child's parents/guardians and one or a small number of caregivers/teachers whose care for and responsiveness to the child ensure relief of distress, experiences of comfort and stimulation, and satisfaction of the need for a personal relationship.

RATIONALE: Trustworthy adults who give of themselves as they provide care and learning experiences play a key role in a child's development as an active, self-knowing, self-respecting, thinking, feeling, and loving person (3,6). Limiting the number of adults with whom an infant interacts fosters reciprocal understanding of communication cues that are unique to each child. This leads to a sense of trust of the adult by the infant that the infant's needs will be understood and met promptly (5). Studies of infant behavior show that infants have difficulty forming trusting relationships in settings where many adults interact with a child, e.g., in hospitalization of infants when shifts of adults provide care (4,6). This difficulty occurs even if each of the many adults is very caring in their interaction with the child (7). There should be breaks at least every four hours and in accordance with U.S. Department of Labor laws.

COMMENTS: Hugging, holding, and cuddling infants and children are expressions of wholesome love that should be encouraged. Caregivers/teachers should be advised that it is alright to demonstrate affection for children of both sexes. At all times, caregivers/teachers should respect the wishes of children, regardless of their ages, with regard to physical contact and their comfort or discomfort with it. Caregivers/teachers should avoid even "friendly contact" (such as touching the shoulder or arm) with a child if the child is uncomfortable with it.

TYPE OF FACILITY: Center; Large Family Child Care Home; Small Family Child Care Home

REFERENCES:

1. Creyer, D., S. Hurwitz, M. Wolery. 2003. Continuity of caregiver for infants and toddlers. ERIC Clearinghouse on Elementary and Early Care Education. http://www.ericdigests.org/2004-3/infants.html.
2. Theilheimer, R. 2006. Molding to the children: Primary caregiving and continuity of care. *Zero to Three* 26:50-54.
3. Baron, N., L. W. Schrank. 1997. *Children learning language: How adults can help*. Lake Zurich, IL: Learning Seed.
4. Botkin, D., et al. 1991. Children's affectionate behavior: Gender differences. *Early Education Dev* 2:270-86.
5. Cassidy J., Shaver, P., eds. 1999. *Handbook of attachment: Theory, research and clinical applications*, 671-87. 2nd ed. New York: Guilford Press.
6. Raikes, H. 1996. A secure base for babies: Applying attachment concepts to the infant care setting. *Young Children* 51:59-67.
7. Lally, R. J. 2000. Infants have their own curriculum: A responsive approach to curriculum planning for infants and toddlers. U.S. Department of Health and Human Services, Administration for Children and Families, Early Childhood Learning and Knowledge Center. http://eclkc.ohs.acf.hhs.gov/hslc/tta-system/teaching/eecd/Curriculum/Definition and Requirements/edudev_art_00032_071005.html.

STANDARD 2.1.2.2: Interactions with Infants and Toddlers

Caregivers/teachers should provide consistent, continuous and inviting opportunities to talk, listen to, and otherwise interact with young infants throughout the day (indoors and outdoors) including feeding, changing, playing with, and cuddling them.

RATIONALE: Richness of language increases by nurturing it through verbal interactions between the child and adults and peers. Adults' speech is one of the main channels through which children learn about themselves, others, and the world in which they live. While adults speaking to children teach the children facts, the social and emotional communications and the atmosphere of the exchange are equally important. Reciprocity of expression, response, the initiation and enrichment of dialogue are hallmarks of the social function and significance of the conversations (2-5). Infants and toddlers learn through meaningful relationships and interaction with consistent adults and peers.

The future development of the child depends on his/her command of language (1). Richness of language increases as it is nurtured by verbal interactions of the child with adults and peers. Basic communication with parents/guardians and children requires an ability to speak their language. A language-rich environment and warm, responsive interactions between staff and children are among the elements that produce positive impacts (6).

COMMENTS: Live, real-time interaction with caregivers/teachers is preferred. For example, caregivers/teachers naming objects in the indoor and outdoor learning/play environment or singing rhymes to all children supports language development. Children's stories and poems presented on recordings with a fixed speed for sing-along can actually interfere with a child's ability to participate in the singing or recitation. With fixed-speed activities, the pace may be too fast for some children, and the activity may have to be repeated for some children or the caregiver/teacher will need to try a different method for learning.

TYPE OF FACILITY: Center; Large Family Child Care Home; Small Family Child Care Home

RELATED STANDARDS:
Standard 2.2.0.3: Limiting Screen Time – Media, Computer Time

REFERENCES:
1. Moerk, E. L. 2000. The guided acquisition of first language skills. *Advances Applied Dev Psychol* 20:248.
2. Baron, N., L. W. Schrank. 1997. *Children learning language: How adults can help*. Lake Zurich, Ill: Learning Seed.
3. Szanton, E. S., ed. 1997. *Creating child-centered programs for infants and toddlers, birth to 3 year olds, step by step: A Program for children and families*. New York: Children's Resources International.
4. Kontos, S., A. Wilcox-Herzog. 1997. Teachers' interactions with children: Why are they so important? *Young Child* 52:4-12.
5. Snow, C. E., M. S. Burns, P. Griffin. 1999. Language and literacy environments in preschools. *ERIC Digest* (January).
6. National Forum on Early Childhood Program Evaluation, National Scientific Council on the Developing Child. 2007. *A science-based framework for early childhood policy: Using evidence to improve outcomes in learning, behavior, and health for vulnerable children*. Cambridge, MA: Center on the Developing Child, Harvard University. http://developingchild.harvard.edu/index.php/library/reports_and_working_papers/policy_framework/.

STANDARD 2.1.2.3: Space and Activity to Support Learning of Infants and Toddlers

The facility should provide a safe and clean learning environment, both indoors and outdoors, colorful materials and equipment arranged to support learning. The indoor and outdoor learning/play environment should encourage and be comfortable with staff on the floor level when interacting with active infant crawlers and toddlers. The indoor and outdoor play and learning settings should provide opportunities for the child to act upon the environment by experiencing age-appropriate obstacles, frustrations, and risks in order to learn to negotiate environmental challenges. The facility should provide opportunities for play that:

a) Lessen the child's anxiety and help the child adapt to reality and resolve conflicts;
b) Enable the child to explore and experience the natural world;
c) Help the child practice resolving conflicts;
d) Use symbols (words, numbers, etc.);
e) Manipulate objects;
f) Exercise physical skills;
g) Encourage language development;
h) Foster self-expression;
i) Strengthen the child's identity as a member of a family and a cultural community;
j) Promote sensory exploration.

For infants and toddlers the curriculum should be based on the child's development at the time and connected to a sound understanding as to where they are in their developmental course.

RATIONALE: Opportunities to be an active learner are vitally important for the development of motor competence and awareness of one's own body and person, the development of sensory motor skills, the ability to demonstrate initiative through active outdoor and indoor play, and feelings of mastery and successful coping. Coping involves original, imaginative, and innovative behavior as well as previously learned strategies.

Learning to resolve conflicts constructively in childhood is essential in preventing violence later in life (1,2). A physical and social environment that offers opportunities for active mastery and coping enhances the child's adaptive abilities (3,4,9). The importance of play for developing cognitive skills, for maintaining an affective and intellectual equilibrium, and for creating and testing new capacities is well recognized (8). Play involves a balance of action and symbolization, and of feeling and thinking (5-7). Children need access to age-appropriate toys and safe household objects.

COMMENTS: For more information regarding appropriate play materials for young children, see "Which Toy for Which Child: A Consumer's Guide for Selecting Suitable Toys" from the U.S. Consumer Product Safety Commission (CPSC) and "The Right Stuff for Children Birth to 8: Selecting Play Materials to Support Development" from the National Association for the Education of Young Children (NAEYC). For information regarding appropriate materials for outdoor play, see POEMS: Preschool Outdoor Environment Measurement Scale (10).

TYPE OF FACILITY: Center; Large Family Child Care Home; Small Family Child Care Home

RELATED STANDARDS:
Standard 3.1.3.1: Active Opportunities for Physical Activity
Standard 5.1.2.1: Space Required Per Child
Standard 5.2.9.14: Shoes in Infant Play Areas
Standard 5.3.1.1: Safety of Equipment, Materials, and Furnishings

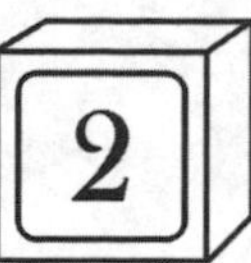

Standard 5.3.1.5: Placement of Equipment and Furnishings
Chapter 6: Play Areas/Playgrounds and Transportation

REFERENCES:

1. Massey, M. S. 1998. Early childhood violence prevention. *ERIC Digest* (October).
2. Levin, D. E. 1994. *Teaching young children in violent times: Building a peaceable classroom, A preschool-grade 3 violence prevention and conflict resolution guide*. Cambridge, MA: Educators for Social Responsibility.
3. Mayr, T., M. Ulich. 1999. Children's well-being in day care centers: An exploratory empirical study. *Int J Early Years Education* 7:229-39.
4. Cartwright, S. 1998. Group trips: An invitation to cooperative learning. *Child Care Infor Exch* 124:95-97.
5. Evaldson, A., W. A. Corsaro. 1998. Play and games in the peer cultures of preschool and preadolescent children: An interpretative approach. *Childhood* 5:377-402.
6. Petersen, E. A. 1998. The amazing benefits of play. *Child Family* 17:7-8.
7. Pica, R. 1997. Beyond physical development: Why young children need to move. *Young Child* 52:4-11.
8. Tepperman, J., ed. 2007. *Play in the early years: Key to school success, a policy brief*. El Cerrito, CA: Early Childhood Funders. http://www.4children.org/images/pdf/play07.pdf.
9. Torelli, L., C. Durrett. 1996. Landscape for learning: The impact of classroom design on infants and toddlers. *Early Childhood News* 8 (March-April): 12-17. http://www.spacesforchildren.com/landc1.pdf.
10. DeBord, K., L. Hestenes, R. Moore, N. Cosco, J. McGinnis. 2005. *Preschool outdoor environment measurement scale*. Lewisville, NC: Kaplan Early Learning Co.

STANDARD 2.1.2.4: Separation of Infants and Toddlers from Older Children

Infants and toddlers younger than three years of age should be cared for in a closed room(s) that separates them from older children, except in small family child care homes with closed groups of mixed aged children.

In facilities caring for three or more children younger than three years of age, activities that bring children younger than three years of age in contact with older children should be prohibited, unless the younger children already have regular contact with the older children as part of a group.

Pooling, as a practice in larger settings where the infants/toddlers are not part of the group all day – as in home care – should be avoided for the following reasons:

a) Unfamiliarity with caregivers/teachers if not the primary one during the day;
b) Concerns of noise levels, space ratios, social-emotional well-being, etc.;
c) Occurs at times when children are least able to handle transitions;
d) Increases the number of transitions for children,
e) Increases the number of adults caring for infants and toddlers, a practice to be avoided if possible.

Caregivers/teachers of infants should not be responsible for the care of older children who are not a part of the infants' closed child care group.

Groups of younger infants should receive care in closed room(s) that separates them from other groups of toddlers and older children.

When partitions are used, they must control interaction between groups, provide separated ventilation of the spaces and control sound transmission. The acoustic controls should limit significant transmission of sound from one group's activity into other group environments.

RATIONALE: Infants need quiet, calm environments, away from the stimulation of older children. Younger infants should be cared for in rooms separate from the more boisterous toddlers. In addition to these developmental needs of infants, separation is important for reasons of disease prevention. Rates of hospitalization for all forms of acute infectious respiratory tract diseases are highest during the first year of life, indicating that respiratory tract illness becomes less severe as the child gets older (1). Therefore, infants should be a focus for interventions to reduce the incidence of respiratory tract diseases. Handwashing and sanitizing practices are key.

Depending on the temperament of the child, an increase in transitions can increase anxiety in young children by reducing the opportunity for routine and predictability (2), and it increases basic health and safety concerns of cross contamination with older children who have more contact with the environment.

COMMENTS: This separation of younger children from older children ideally should be implemented in all facilities, but may be less feasible in small or large family child care homes.

Separation of groups of children by low partitions that divide a single common space is not acceptable. Without sound attenuation, limitation of shared air pollutants including airborne infectious disease agents, or control of interactions among the caregivers/teachers who are working with different groups, the separate smaller groups are essentially one large group.

TYPE OF FACILITY: Center

RELATED STANDARDS:

Standard 3.2.2.2: Handwashing Procedure
Chapter 7: Infectious Disease
Appendix J: Selecting an Appropriate Sanitizer or Disinfectant
Appendix K: Routine Schedule for Cleaning, Sanitizing, and Disinfecting

REFERENCES:

1. Izurieta, H. S., W. W. Thompson, P. Kramarz, et al. 2000. Influenza and the rates of hospitalization for respiratory disease among infants and young children. *New England J Med* 342:232-39.
2. Poole, C. 1998. Routine matters. *Scholastic Parent Child* (August/September).

STANDARD 2.1.2.5: Toilet Learning/Training

The facility should develop and implement a plan that teaches each child how and when to use the toilet. Toilet learning/training, when initiated, should follow a prescribed, sequential plan that is developed and coordinated with the parent's/guardian's plan for implementation in the home environment. Toilet learning/training should be based on the child's developmental level rather than chronological age.

To help children achieve bowel and bladder control, caregivers/teachers should enable children to take an active role in using the toilet when they are physically able to do so and when parents/guardians support their children's learning to use the toilet.

Diapering/toilet training should not be used as rationale for not spending time outdoors. Practices and policies should be offered to address diapering/toileting needs outdoors such as providing staff who can address children's needs, or provide outdoor diapering and toileting that meets all sanitation requirements.

Caregivers/teachers should take into account the preferences and customs of the child's family.

For children who have not yet learned to use the toilet, the facility should defer toilet learning/training until the child's family is ready to support this learning and the child demonstrates:

a) An understanding of the concept of cause and effect;
b) An ability to communicate, including sign language;
c) The physical ability to remain dry for up to two hours;
d) An ability to sit on the toilet, to feel/understand the sense of elimination;
e) A demonstrated interest in autonomous behavior.

For preschool and school-age children, an emphasis should be placed on appropriate handwashing after using the toilet and they should be provided frequent and unrestricted opportunities to use the toilet.

Children with special health care needs may require specific instructions, training techniques, adapted toilets, and/or supports or precautions. Some children will need to be taught special techniques like catheterization or care of ostomies. This can be provided by trained staff or older children can sometimes learn self-care techniques. Any special techniques should be documented in a written care plan. The child care health consultant can provide training or coordinate resources necessary to accommodate special toileting techniques while in child care.

Cultural expectations of toilet learning/training need to be recognized and respected.

RATIONALE: A child's achievements of motor and cognitive or developmental skills assist in determining when s/he is ready for toilet learning/training (1). Physical ability/neurological function also includes the ability to sit on the toilet and to feel/understand the sense of elimination.

Toilet learning/training is achieved more rapidly once expectations from adults across environments are consistent (3). The family may not be prepared, at the time, to extend this learning/training into the home environment (2).

School-age and preschool children may not respond when their bodies signal a need to use the toilet because they are involved in activities or embarrassed about needing to use the toilet. Holding back stool or urine can lead to constipation and urinary tract problems (4). Also, unless reminded, many children forget to correctly wash their hands after toileting.

COMMENTS: The area of toilet learning/training for children with special health care needs is difficult because there are no age-related, disability-specific rules to follow. As a result, support and counseling for parents/guardians and caregivers/teachers are required to help them deal with this issue. Some children with multiple disabilities do not demonstrate any requisite skills other than being dry for a few hours. Establishing a toilet routine may be the first step toward learning to use the toilet, and at the same time, improving hygiene and skin care. The child care health consultant should be considered a resource to assist is supporting special health care needs.

Sometimes children need to increase their fluid intake to help a medical condition and this can lead to increased urination. Other conditions can lead to loose stools. Children should be given unrestricted access to toileting facilities, especially in these situations. Children who are recovering from gastrointestinal illness might temporarily lose continence, especially if they are recently toilet trained, and may need to revert to diapers or training pants for a short period of time. Children who are experiencing stress (e.g., a new infant in the family) may regress and also return to using diapers for a period of time.

For more information on toilet learning/training, see "Toilet Training: Guidelines for Parents," available from the American Academy of Pediatrics (AAP) at http://www.aap.org and the AAP Section on Developmental and Behavioral Pediatrics at http://www.aap.org/sections/dbpeds/.

TYPE OF FACILITY: Center; Large Family Child Care Home; Small Family Child Care Home

RELATED STANDARDS:

Standard 3.2.1.5: Procedure for Changing Children's Soiled Underwear/Pull-Ups and Clothing
Standards 5.4.1.1-5.4.1.7: Toilets and Toilet Learning/Training Equipment
Standards 5.4.1.8-5.4.1.9: Sanitation, Disinfection, and Maintenance of Toilet Learning/Training Equipment, Toilets, and Bathrooms

REFERENCES:

1. Mayo Clinic. 2009. Potty training: How to get the job done. http://www.mayoclinic.com/health/potty-training/CC00060/.
2. American Academy of Pediatrics. 2009. When is the right time to start toilet training? http://www.aap.org/publiced/BR_ToiletTrain.htm.
3. Anthony-Pillai, R. 2007. What's potty about early toilet training? *British Med J* 334:1166.
4. Schmitt, B. D. 2004. Toilet training problems: Underachievers, refusers, and stool holders. *Contemporary Pediatrics* 21:71-77.

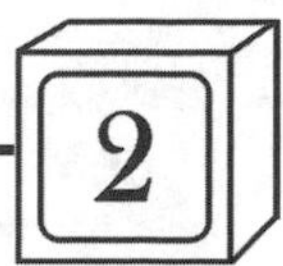

2.1.3 Program Activities for Three- to Five-Year-Olds

STANDARD 2.1.3.1: Personal Caregiver/Teacher Relationships for Three- to Five-Year-Olds

Facilities should provide opportunities for each child to build long-term, trusting relationships with a few caring caregivers/teachers by limiting the number of adults the facility permits to care for any one child in child care to a maximum of eight adults in a given year and no more than three primary caregivers/teachers in a day. Children with special health care needs may require additional specialists to promote health and safety and to support learning; however, relationships with primary caregivers/teachers should be supported.

RATIONALE: Children learn best from adults who know and respect them; who act as guides, facilitators, and supporters within a rich learning environment; and with whom they have established a trusting relationship (1,2). When the facility allows too many adults to be involved in the child's care, the child does not develop a reciprocal, sustained, responsive, and trusting relationship with any of them.

Children should have continuous friendly and trusting relationships with several caregivers/teachers who are reasonably consistent within the child care facility. Young children can extract from these relationships a sense of themselves with a capacity for forming trusting relationships and self-esteem. Relationships are fragmented by rapid staff turnover, staffing reassignment, or if the child is frequently moved from one room to another or one child care facility to another.

COMMENTS: Compliance should be measured by staff and parent/guardian interviews. Turnover of staff lowers the quality of the facility. High quality facilities maintain low turnover through their wage policies, training and support for staff (3).

TYPE OF FACILITY: Center; Large Family Child Care Home; Small Family Child Care Home

REFERENCES:

1. Rodd, J. 1996. *Understanding young children's behavior: A guide for early childhood professionals*. New York: Teacher's College Press.

2. Greenberg, P. 1991. *Character development: Encouraging self-esteem and self-discipline in infants, toddlers, and two-year-olds*. Washington, DC: National Association for the Education of Young Children.

3. Whitebook, M., D. Bellm. 1998. *Taking on turnover: An action guide for child care center teachers and directors*. Washington, DC: Center for the Child Care Workforce.

STANDARD 2.1.3.2: Opportunities for Learning for Three- to Five-Year-Olds

Programs should provide children a balance of guided and self-initiated play and learning indoors and outdoors. These should include opportunities to observe, explore, order and reorder, to make mistakes and find solutions, and to move from the concrete to the abstract in learning.

RATIONALE: The most meaningful learning has its source in the child's self-initiated activities. The learning environment that supports individual differences, learning styles, abilities, and cultural values fosters confidence and curiosity in learners (1,2).

TYPE OF FACILITY: Center; Large Family Child Care Home; Small Family Child Care Home

REFERENCES:

1. Rodd, J. 1996. *Understanding young children's behavior: A guide for early childhood professionals*. New York: Teacher's College Press.

2. Ritchie, S., B. Willer. 2008. *Teaching: A guide to the NAEYC early childhood standard and related accreditation criteria*. Washington, DC: National Association for the Education of Young Children.

STANDARD 2.1.3.3: Selection of Equipment for Three- to Five-Year-Olds

The program should select, for both indoor and outdoor play and learning, developmentally appropriate equipment and materials, for safety, for its ability to provide large and small motor experiences, and for its adaptability to serve many different ideas, functions, and forms of creative expression.

RATIONALE: An aesthetic, orderly, appropriately stimulating, child-oriented indoor and outdoor learning/play environment contributes to the preschooler's sense of well-being and control (1,2,4,5).

COMMENTS: "Play and learning settings that motivate children to be physically active include pathways, trails, lawns, loose parts, anchored playground equipment, and layouts that stimulate all forms of active play" (3). If traditional playground equipment is used, caregivers/teachers may want to consult with an early childhood specialist or a certified playground inspector for recommendations on developmentally appropriate play equipment. For more information on play equipment also contact the National Program for Playground Safety (http://www.uni.edu/playground/).

TYPE OF FACILITY: Center; Large Family Child Care Home; Small Family Child Care Home

RELATED STANDARDS:

Standard 5.2.9.9: Plastic Containers and Toys
Standard 5.2.9.12: Treatment of CCA Pressure-Treated Wood
Chapter 6: Play Areas/Playgrounds and Transportation

REFERENCES:

1. Torelli, L., C. Durrett. 1996. Landscape for learning: The impact of classroom design on infants and toddlers. *Early Child News* 8:12-17.

2. Center for Environmental Health. The safe playgrounds project. http://www.safe2play.org.

3. DeBord, K., L. Hestenes, R. Moore, N. Cosco, J. McGinnis. 2005. *Preschool outdoor environment measurement scale*. Lewisville, NC: Kaplan Early Learning Co.

4. Banning, W., G. Sullivan. 2009. *Lens on outdoor learning*. St. Paul, MN: Red Leaf Press.

5. Keeler, R. 2008. *Natural playscapes: Creating outdoor play environments for the soul*. Redmond, WA: Exchange Press.

STANDARD 2.1.3.4: Expressive Activities for Three- to Five-Year-Olds

Caregivers/teachers should encourage and enhance expressive activities that include play, painting, drawing, storytelling, sensory play, music, singing, dancing, and dramatic play.

RATIONALE: Expressive activities are vehicles for socialization, conflict resolution, and language development. They are vital energizers and organizers for cognitive development (2). Stifling the preschooler's need to play damages a natural integration of thinking and feeling (1).

TYPE OF FACILITY: Center; Large Family Child Care Home; Small Family Child Care Home

REFERENCES:

1. Cooney, M., L. Hutchinson, V. Costigan. 1996. From hitting to tattling to communication and negotiation: The young child's stages of socialization. *Early Child Education J* 24:23-27.
2. Tepperman, J., ed. 2007. *Play in the early years: Key to school success, a policy brief*. El Cerrito, CA: Early Childhood Funders. http://www.4children.org/images/pdf/play07.pdf.

STANDARD 2.1.3.5: Fostering Cooperation of Three- to Five-Year-Olds

Programs should foster a cooperative rather than a competitive indoor and outdoor learning/play environment.

RATIONALE: As three-, four-, and five-year-olds play and work together, they shift from almost total dependence on the adult to seeking social opportunities with peers that still require adult monitoring and guidance. The rules and responsibilities of a well-functioning group help children of this age to internalize impulse control and to become increasingly responsible for managing their behavior. A dynamic curriculum designed to include the ideas and values of a broad socioeconomic group of children will promote socialization. The inevitable clashes and disagreements are more easily resolved when there is a positive influence of the group on each child (1).

COMMENTS: Encouraging communication skills and attentiveness to the needs of individuals and the group as a whole supports a cooperative atmosphere. Adults need to model cooperation.

TYPE OF FACILITY: Center; Large Family Child Care Home; Small Family Child Care Home

REFERENCES:

1. Pica, R. 1997. Beyond physical development: Why young children need to move. *Young Child* 52:4-11.

STANDARD 2.1.3.6: Fostering Language Development of Three- to Five-Year-Olds

The indoor and outdoor learning/play environment should be rich in first-hand experiences that offer opportunities for language development. They should also have an abundance of books of fantasy, fiction, and nonfiction, and provide chances for the children to relate stories. Caregivers/teachers should foster language development by:

a) Speaking with children rather than at them;
b) Encouraging children to talk with each other by helping them to listen and respond;
c) Giving children models of verbal expression;
d) Reading books about the child's culture and history, which would serve to help the child develop a sense of self;
e) Reading to children and re-reading their favorite books;
f) Listening respectfully when children speak;
g) Encouraging interactive storytelling;
h) Using open-ended questions;
i) Provide opportunities during indoor and outdoor learning/play to use writing supplies and printed materials;
j) Provide and read books relevant to their natural environment outdoors (for example, books about the current season, local wildlife, etc.);
k) Provide settings that encourage children to observe nature, such as a butterfly garden, bird watching station, etc.;
l) Providing opportunities to explore writing, such as through a writing area or individual journals.

RATIONALE: Language reflects and shapes thinking. A curriculum created to match preschoolers' needs and interests enhances language skills. First-hand experiences encourage children to talk with each other and with adults, to seek, develop, and use increasingly more complex vocabulary, and to use language to express thinking, feeling, and curiosity (1-3).

COMMENTS: Compliance with development should be measured by structured observation. Examples of verbal encouragement of verbal expression are: "ask Johnny if you may play with him"; "tell him you don't like being hit"; "tell Sara what you saw downtown yesterday;" "can you tell Mommy about what you and Johnny played this morning?" These encouraging statements should be followed by respectful listening, without pressuring the child to speak.

TYPE OF FACILITY: Center; Large Family Child Care Home; Small Family Child Care Home

RELATED STANDARDS:

Standard 2.3.2.3: Support Services for Parents/Guardians

REFERENCES:

1. Szanton, E. S., ed. 1997. *Creating child-centered programs for infants and toddlers, birth to 3 year olds, step by step: A Program for children and families*. New York: Children's Resources International.
2. Snow, C. E., M. S. Burns, P. Griffin. 1999. Language and literacy environments in preschools. *ERIC Digest* (January).
3. Maschinot, B. 2008. *The changing face of the United States: The influence of culture on early child development*. Washington, DC: Zero to Three. http://www.zerotothree.org/site/DocServer/Culture_book.pdf?docID=6921.

STANDARD 2.1.3.7: Body Mastery for Three- to Five-Year-Olds

The caregivers/teachers should offer children opportunities, indoors and outdoors, to learn about their bodies and how their bodies function in the context of socializing with others. Caregivers/teachers should support the children in their curiosity and body mastery, consistent with parental/guardian expectations and cultural preferences. Body mastery includes feeding oneself, learning how to use the toilet, running, skipping, climbing, balancing, playing with peers, displaying affection, and using and manipulating objects.

RATIONALE: Achieving the pleasure and gratification of feeling physically competent on a voluntary basis is a basic component of developing self-esteem and the ability to socialize with adults and other children inside and outside the family (1-5).

COMMENTS: Self-stimulatory behaviors, such as thumb sucking or masturbation, should be ignored. If the masturbation is excessive, interferes with other activities, or is noticed by other children, the caregiver/teacher should make a brief non-judgmental comment that touching of private body parts is normal, but is usually done in a private place (7,8). After making such a comment, the caregiver/teacher should offer friendly assistance in going on to other activities. These behaviors may be signs of stress in the child's life, or simply a habit. If the child's sexual play is more explicit or forceful toward other children or the child witnessed or was exposed to adult sexuality, the caregiver/teacher may need to consider that abuse is possible (6).

TYPE OF FACILITY: Center; Large Family Child Care Home; Small Family Child Care Home

REFERENCES:

1. Botkin, D., et al. 1991. Children's affectionate behavior: Gender differences. *Early Education Dev* 2:270-86.
2. Mayr, T., M. Ulich. 1999. Children's well-being in day care centers: An exploratory empirical study. *Int J Early Years Education* 7:229-39.
3. Cartwright, S. 1998. Group trips: An invitation to cooperative learning. *Child Care Infor Exch* 124:95-97.
4. Rodd, J. 1996. *Understanding young children's behavior: A guide for early childhood professionals*. New York: Teacher's College Press.
5. Cooney, M., L. Hutchinson, V. Costigan. 1996. From hitting to tattling to communication and negotiation: The young child's stages of socialization. *Early Child Education J* 24:23-27.
6. Kellogg, N., American Academy of Pediatrics Committee on Child Abuse and Neglect. 2005. Clinical report: The evaluation of sexual abuse in children. *Pediatrics* 116:506-12.
7. Johnson, T. C. 2007. *Understanding children's sexual behaviors: What's natural and healthy*. San Diego: Institute on Violence, Abuse and Trauma.
8. Friedrich, W. N., J. Fisher, D. Broughton, M. Houston, C. R. Shafran. 1998. Normative sexual behavior in children: A contemporary sample. *Pediatrics* 101: e9.

2.1.4 Program Activities for School-Age Children

STANDARD 2.1.4.1: Supervised School-Age Activities

The facility should have a program of supervised activities designed especially for school-age children, to include:

a) Free choice of play;
b) Opportunities, both indoors and outdoors, for vigorous physical activity which engages each child daily for at least sixty minutes and are not limited to opportunities to develop physical fitness through a program of focused activity that only engages some of the children in the group;
c) Opportunities for concentration, alone or in a group, indoors and/or outdoors;
d) Time to read or do homework, indoors and/or outdoors;
e) Opportunities to be creative, to explore the arts, sciences, and social studies, and to solve problems, indoors and/or outdoors;
f) Opportunities for community service experience (museums, library, leadership development, elderly citizen homes, etc.);
g) Opportunities for adult-supervised skill-building and self-development groups, such as scouts, team sports, and club activities (as transportation, distance, and parental permission allow);
h) Opportunities to rest;
i) Opportunities to seek comfort, consolation, and understanding from adult caregivers/teachers;
j) Opportunities for exercise and exploration out of doors.

RATIONALE: Programs organized for older children after school or during vacation time should provide indoor and outdoor learning/play environments that meet the needs of these children for physical activity, recreation, responsible completion of school work, expanding their interests, learning cultural sensitivity, exploring community resources, and practicing pro-social skills (1,2).

COMMENTS: For more information on school-age standards, see [*The NAA Standards for Quality School-Age Care,*] available from the National AfterSchool Association (NAA).

TYPE OF FACILITY: Center; Large Family Child Care Home; Small Family Child Care Home

RELATED STANDARDS:

Standard 3.1.3.1: Active Opportunities for Physical Activity

REFERENCES:

1. Coltin, L. 1999. Enriching children's out-of-school time. *ERIC Digest* (May).
2. Fashola, O. S. 1999. Implementing effective after-school programs. *Here's How* 17:1-4

STANDARD 2.1.4.2: Space for School-Age Activity

The facility should provide a space for indoor and outdoor activities for children in school-age child care.

RATIONALE: A safe and secure environment that fosters the growing independence of school-age children is essential for their development (1,2). Active connection with nature promotes children's sensitivity, confidence, exploration, and self-regulation.

TYPE OF FACILITY: Center; Large Family Child Care Home; Small Family Child Care Home

RELATED STANDARDS:
Chapter 6: Playgrounds/Play Areas and Transportation

REFERENCES:
1. Greenspan, S. L. 1997. Building children's minds: Early childhood development for a better future. *Our Child* 23:6-10.
2. Maxwell, L. E. 1996. Designing early childhood education environments: A partnership between architect and educator. *Education Facility Planner* 33:15-17.

STANDARD 2.1.4.3: Developing Relationships for School-Age Children

The facility should offer opportunities to school-age children for developing trusting, supportive relationships with the staff and with peers.

RATIONALE: Although school-age children need more independent experiences, they continue to need the guidance and support of adults. Peer relationships take on increasing importance for this age group. Community service opportunities can be valuable for this age group.

TYPE OF FACILITY: Center; Large Family Child Care Home; Small Family Child Care Home

STANDARD 2.1.4.4: Planning Activities for School-Age Children

The facility should offer a program based on the needs and interests of the age group, as well as of the individuals within it. Children should participate in planning the program activities. Parents/guardians should be engaged and their work commitments should be honored when planning program activities.

RATIONALE: A child care facility for school-age children should provide an enriching contrast to the formal school program, but also offer time for children to complete homework assignments. Programs that offer a wide range of activities (such as team sports, cooking, dramatics, art, music, crafts, games, open time, quiet time, outdoor play and learning, and use of community resources) allow children to explore new interests and relationships.

TYPE OF FACILITY: Center; Large Family Child Care Home; Small Family Child Care Home

STANDARD 2.1.4.5: Community Outreach for School-Age Children

The facility should provide opportunities for school-age children to participate in community outreach and involvement, such as field trips and community improvement projects.

RATIONALE: As the world of the school-age child encompasses the larger community, facility activities should reflect this stage of development. Field trips and other opportunities to explore the community should enrich the child's experience (1).

TYPE OF FACILITY: Center; Large Family Child Care Home; Small Family Child Care Home

REFERENCES:
1. Taras, H. L. 2005. School-aged child care. In *Health in child care: A manual for health professionals,* ed. J. R. Murph, S. D. Palmer, D. Glassy, 411-21. 4th ed. Elk Grove Village, IL: American Academy of Pediatrics.

STANDARD 2.1.4.6: Communication Between Child Care and School

Facilities that accept school-age children directly from school should arrange a system of communication with the child's school teacher. Families should be included in this communication loop.

RATIONALE: Activities and experiences that occurred during the school day may be important in anticipating and understanding children's after-school behavior (1). The connection between children's learning at school experience and their out-of-school activities is important (1).

COMMENTS: This communication may be facilitated by phone or email between the child's teacher and the school-age child care facility. School-age child care programs should include parent/guardian permissions which allow school teachers to communicate relevant information to caregivers/teachers. Parents/guardians should also be notified of any significant event so that a system of communication is established between and among family, school, and caregivers/teachers. The child's school teacher and a staff member from the facility should meet at least once to exchange telephone numbers and to offer a contact in the event relevant information needs to be shared.

TYPE OF FACILITY: Center; Large Family Child Care Home; Small Family Child Care Home

RELATED STANDARDS:
Standard 9.4.1.3: Written Policy on Confidentiality of Records

REFERENCES:
1. National Association of Elementary School Principals, National AfterSchool Association. *Leading a new day for learning.* http://www.naaweb.org/downloads/Principal Documents/leading_joint_statement-r3_.pdf.

2.2 Supervision and Discipline

STANDARD 2.2.0.1: Methods of Supervision of Children

Caregivers/teachers should directly supervise infants, toddlers, and preschoolers by sight and hearing at all times, even when the children are going to sleep, napping or sleeping, are beginning to wake up, or are indoors or outdoors. School-age children should be within sight or hearing at all times. Caregivers/teachers should not be on one floor level of the building, while children are on another floor or room. Ratios should remain the same whether inside or outside.

School-age children should be permitted to participate in activities off the premises with appropriate adult supervision and with written approval by a parent/guardian and by the caregiver. If parents/guardians give written permission for the school-age child to participate in off-premises activities,

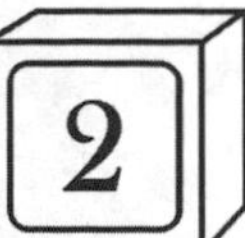

the facility would no longer be responsible for the child during the off-premises activity and not need to provide staff for the off-premises activity.

Caregivers/teachers should regularly count children (name to face on a scheduled basis, at every transition, and whenever leaving one area and arriving at another), going indoors or outdoors, to confirm the safe whereabouts of every child at all times. Additionally, they must be able to state how many children are in their care at all times.

Developmentally appropriate child:staff ratios should be met during all hours of operation, including indoor and outdoor play and field trips, and safety precautions for specific areas and equipment should be followed. No center-based facility or large family child care home should operate with fewer than two staff members if more than six children are in care, even if the group otherwise meets the child:staff ratio. Although centers often downsize the number of staff for the early arrival and late departure times, another adult must be present to help in the event of an emergency. The supervision policies of centers and large family child care homes should be written policies.

RATIONALE: Supervision is basic to safety and the prevention of injury and maintaining quality child care. Parents/guardians have a contract with caregivers/teachers to supervise their children. To be available for supervision or rescue in an emergency, an adult must be able to hear and see the children. In case of fire, a supervising adult should not need to climb stairs or use a ramp or an elevator to reach the children. Stairs, ramps, and elevators may become unstable because they can be pathways for fire and smoke.

Children who are presumed to be sleeping might be awake and in need of adult attention. A child's risk-taking behavior must be detected and illness, fear, or other stressful behaviors must be noticed and managed.

The importance of supervision is not only to protect children from physical injury, but from harm that can occur from topics discussed by children or by teasing/bullying/inappropriate behavior. It is the responsibility of caregivers/teachers to monitor what children are talking about and intervene when necessary.

Children like to test their skills and abilities. This is particularly noticeable around playground equipment. Even if the highest safety standards for playground layout, design and surfacing are met, serious injuries can happen if children are left unsupervised. Adults who are involved, aware, and appreciative of young childrens' behaviors are in the best position to safeguard their well-being. Active and positive supervision involves:

a) Knowing each child's abilities;
b) Establishing clear and simple safety rules;
c) Being aware of and scanning for potential safety hazards;
d) Standing in a strategic position;
e) Scanning play activities and circulating around the area;
f) Focusing on the positive rather than the negative to teach a child what is safe for the child and other children;
g) Teaching children the appropriate and safe use of each piece of equipment (e.g., using a slide correctly – feet first only – and teaching why climbing up a slide can cause injury, possibly a head injury).

Children are going to be more active in the outdoor learning/play environment and need more supervision rather than less outside. Playground supervisors need to be designated and trained to supervise children in play areas (1). Supervision of the playground is a strategy of watching all the children within a specific territory and not engaging in prolonged dialog with any one child or group of children (or other staff). Other adults not designated to supervise may facilitate outdoor learning/play activities and engage in conversations with children about their exploration and discoveries. Facilitated play is where the adult is engaged in helping children learn a skill or achieve specific outcome of an activity. Facilitated play is not supervision (2).

Children need spaces, indoors and out, in which they can withdraw for alone-time or quiet play in small groups. However, program spaces should be designed with visibility that allows constant unobtrusive adult supervision. To protect children from maltreatment, including sexual abuse, the environment layout should limit situations in which an adult or older child is left alone with a child without another adult present (3,4).

Many instances have been reported where a child has hidden when the group was moving to another location, or where the child wandered off when a door was opened for another purpose. Regular counting of children (name to face) will alert the staff to begin a search before the child gets too far, into trouble, or slips into an unobserved location.

Caregivers/teachers should record the count on an attendance sheet or on a pocket card, along with notations of any children joining or leaving the group. Caregivers/teachers should do the counts before the group leaves an area and when the group enters a new area. The facility should assign and reassign counting responsibility as needed to maintain a counting routine. Facilities might consider counting systems such as using a reminder tone on a watch or musical clock that sounds at timed intervals (about every fifteen minutes) to help the staff remember to count.

Caregivers/teachers should be ready to provide help and guidance when children are ready to use the toilet correctly and independently. Caregivers/teachers should make sure children correctly wash their hands after every use of the toilet, as well as monitor the bathroom to make sure that the toilet is flushed, the toilet seat and floor are free from stool or urine, and supplies (toilet paper, soap, and paper towels) are available.

Older preschool children and school-age children may use toilet facilities without direct visual observation but must remain within hearing range in case children need assis-

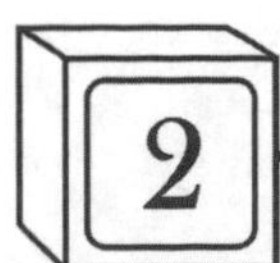

tance and to prevent inappropriate behavior. If toilets are not on the same floor as the child care area or within sight or hearing of a caregiver/teacher, an adult should accompany children younger than five years of age to and from the toilet area. Younger children who request privacy and have shown capability to use toilet facilities properly should be given permission to use separate and private toilet facilities.

Planning must include advance assignments, monitoring, and contingency plans to maintain appropriate staffing. During times when children are typically being dropped off and picked up, the number of children present can vary. There should be a plan in place to monitor and address unanticipated changes, allowing for caregivers/teachers to receive additional help when needed. Sufficient staff must be maintained to evacuate the children safely in case of emergency. Compliance with proper child:staff ratios should be measured by structured observation, by counting caregivers/teachers and children in each group at varied times of the day, and by reviewing written policies.

TYPE OF FACILITY: Center; Large Family Child Care Home; Small Family Child Care Home

RELATED STANDARDS:

Standards 1.1.1.1-1.1.1.5: Child:Staff Ratios
Standard 3.4.4.5: Facility Layout to Reduce Risk of Child Abuse and Neglect
Standard 5.4.1.2: Location of Toilets and Privacy Issues

REFERENCES:

1. National Program for Playground Safety. 2006. Playground supervision training for childcare providers. University of Northern Iowa. http://www.playgroundsafety.org/training/online/childcare/course_supervision.htm.
2. National Program for Playground Safety. 2006. NPPS Website. http://www.playgroundsafety.org.
3. National Association for the Education of Young Children. 1996. Position Statement. Prevention of child abuse in early childhood programs and the responsibilities of early childhood professionals to prevent child abuse.
4. Fiene, R. 2002. *13 indicators of quality child care: Research update*. Washington, DC: U.S. Department of Health and Human Services, Office of the Assistant Secretary for Planning and Evaluation. http://aspe.hhs.gov/hsp/ccquality-ind02/.

ADDITIONAL READINGS:

Harms, T., R. M. Clifford, D. Cryer. 2005. Early childhood environment rating scale, revised ed. Frank Porter Graham Child Development Institute, University of North Carolina. http://ers.fpg.unc.edu/node/82/.
Harms, T., D. Cryer, R. M. Clifford. 2005. Infant/toddler environment rating scale, revised ed. Frank Porter Graham Child Development Institute, University of North Carolina. http://ers.fpg.unc.edu/node/84/.
Chen, X., M. Beran, R. Altkorn, S. Milkovich, K. Gruaz, G. Rider, A. Kanti, J. Ochsenhirt. 2006. Frequency of caregiver supervision of young children during play. *Intl J Injury Control and Safety Promotion* 14:122-24.
Schwebel, D. C., A. L. Summerlin, M. L. Bounds, B. A. Morrongiello. 2006. The stamp-in-safety program: A behavioral intervention to reduce behaviors that can lead to unintentional playground injury in a preschool setting. *J Pediatric Psychology* 31:152-62.
U.S. Consumer Product Safety Commission (CPSC). 2010. Public playground safety handbook. http://www.cpsc.gov/cpscpub/pubs/325.pdf.

STANDARD 2.2.0.2: Limiting Infant/Toddler Time in Crib, High Chair, Car Seat, Etc.

A child should not sit in a high chair or other equipment that constrains his/her movement (1,2) indoors or outdoors for longer than fifteen minutes, other than at meals or snack time. Children should never be left out of the view and attention of adult caregivers/teachers while in these types of equipment/furniture. A least restrictive environment should be encouraged at all times. Children should not be left to sleep in equipment, such as car seats, swings, or infant seats that does not meet ASTM International (ASTM) product safety standards for sleep equipment.

RATIONALE: Children are continually developing their physical skills. They need opportunities to use and build on their physical abilities. This is especially true for infants and toddlers who are eagerly using their bodies to explore their environment. Extended periods of time in the crib, high chair, car seat, or other confined space limits their physical growth and also affects their social interactions. Injuries and Sudden Infant Death Syndrome (SIDS) have occurred when children have been left to sleep in car seats or infant seats when the straps have entrapped body parts, or the children have turned the seats over while in them. Sleeping in a seated position can restrict breathing and cause oxygen desaturation in young infants (3). Sleeping should occur in equipment manufactured for this activity. When children are awake, restricting them to a seat may limit social interactions. These social interactions are essential for children to gain language skills, develop self-esteem, and build relationships (4).

TYPE OF FACILITY: Center; Large Family Child Care Home; Small Family Child Care Home

RELATED STANDARDS:

Standard 3.1.3.1: Active Opportunities for Physical Activity
Standard 3.1.4.1: Safe Sleep Practices and SIDS/Suffocation Risk Reduction
Standard 5.3.1.10: Restrictive Infant Equipment Requirements
Standard 5.4.5.1: Sleeping Equipment and Supplies
Standard 5.4.5.2: Cribs

REFERENCES:

1. Kornhauser Cerar, L., C.V. Scirica, I. Stucin Gantar, D. Osredkar, D. Neubauer, T.B. Kinane. 2009. A comparison of respiratory patterns in healthy term infants placed in care safety seats and beds. *Pediatrics* 124:e396-e402.
2. Benjamin, S.E., S.L. Rifas-Shiman, E.M. Taveras, J. Haines, J. Finkelstein, K. Kleinman, M.W. Gillman. 2009. Early child care and adiposity at ages 1 and 3 years. *Pediatrics* 124:555-62.
3. Bass, J. L., M. Bull. 2008. Oxygen desaturation in term infants in car safety seats. *Pediatrics* 110:401-2.
4. New York State Office of Children and Family Services. Website. http://www.ocfs.state.ny.us/main/.

STANDARD 2.2.0.3: Limiting Screen Time – Media, Computer Time

In early care and education settings, media (television [TV], video, and DVD) viewing and computer use should not be permitted for children younger than two years. For children two years and older in early care and early education settings, total media time should be limited to not more than thirty minutes once a week, and for educational or physical activity use only. During meal or snack time, TV, video, or DVD viewing should not be allowed (1). Computer use should be limited to no more than fifteen-minute increments except for school-age children completing homework assignments (2) and children with special health care needs who require and consistently use assistive and adaptive computer technology.

Parents/guardians should be informed if screen media are used in the early care and education program. Any screen media used should be free of advertising and brand placement. TV programs, DVD, and computer games should be reviewed and evaluated before participation of the children to ensure that advertising and brand placement are not present.

RATIONALE: In the first two years of life, children's brains and bodies are going through critical periods of growth and development. It is important for infants and young children to have positive interactions with people and not sit in front of a screen that takes time away from social interaction with parents/guardians and caregivers/teachers. Before age three, television viewing can have modest negative effects on cognitive development of children (3). For that reason, the American Academy of Pediatrics (AAP) recommends television viewing be discouraged for children younger than two years of age (4). Interactive activities that promote brain development can be encouraged, such as talking, playing, singing, and reading together.

For children two years and older, the AAP recommends limiting children's total (early care and education, and home) media time (with entertainment media) to no more than one to two hours of quality programming per twenty-four hour period (3). Because children may watch television before and after attending early care and education settings, limiting media time during their time in early care and education settings will help meet the AAP recommendation. When TV watching is intended to be interactive, with the adult interacting with children about what they are watching, caregivers/teachers can sing along and comment on what children are watching. Caregivers/teachers should always consider whether children could learn the skill better in another way through hands-on experiences.

Studies have shown a relationship between TV viewing and overweight in young children. For example, watching more than eight hours of television per week has been associated with an increased risk of obesity in young children and exposure to two or more hours of television per day increased the risk of overweight for three- to five-year-olds (5,6). Among four-year-olds, research has shown that as body mass index increases, average hours of TV viewing increases (7). Also, young children who watch TV have been shown to have poor diet quality. For each one-hour increment of TV viewing per day, three-year-olds were found to have higher intakes of sugar-sweetened beverage and lower fruit and vegetable intakes (8). Children are exposed to extensive advertising for high-calorie and low-nutrient dense foods and drinks and very limited advertising of healthful foods and drinks during their television viewing. Television advertising influences the food consumption of children two-to eleven-years-old (9).

About two-thirds (66%) of children ages six months to six years watch television every day. About a quarter (24%) watch videos or DVDs every day, and nearly two-thirds (65%) watch them several times a week or more. Additionally, young children engage in other forms of screen activity several times a week or more including using a computer (27%), playing console video games (13%), and playing handheld video games (8%) (10). Survey data show that by three months of age, about 40% of infants regularly watch television, DVDs, or videos. By twenty-four months, this rose to 90% (1).

Caregivers/teachers cannot determine which child does and does not watch TV at home. It is important for early care and education programs to limit TV viewing so that the AAP goal of less than two hours a day, accompanied by more physical activity and increased interaction with reading, can be achieved. A study of TV viewing in early care and education settings reported that, on average, preschool-aged children watched more than four times as much television while at home-based programs than at center-based programs (1.39 hours per day vs. 0.36 hours per day); with significant differences between groups in the type of television content viewed, and in the proportions of programs in which no television viewing occurred at all. The proportion of programs where preschool-aged children watched no television during the early care and education day was 65% in center-based programs and 11% in home-based programs (11).

COMMENTS: It is important for caregivers/teachers to be a role model for children in early care and education settings by not watching TV during the care day. In addition, when adults watch television (including the news) in the presence of children, children may be exposed to inappropriate language or frightening images. The USDA has tips on limiting media time – "How Much Inactive Time Is Too Much" at http://www.choosemyplate.gov/foodgroups/physicalactivity_why.html.

The AAP provides a description of the TV programming rating scale and tips for parents/guardians at http://www.healthychildren.org/English/family-life/Media/Pages/TV-Ratings-A-Guide-for-Parents.aspx. Caregivers/teachers are discouraged from having a TV in a room where children are present.

Caregivers/teachers should begin reading to children when they are six months of age and facilities should have age-appropriate books available for each cognitive stage of development. See "Reach Out and Read" at http://www.reachoutandread.org for more information.

TYPE OF FACILITY: Center; Large Family Child Care Home; Small Family Child Care Home

RELATED STANDARDS:

Standard 3.1.3.1: Active Opportunities for Physical Activity
Appendix S: Physical Activity: How Much Is Needed?

REFERENCES:

1. Zimmerman, F. J., D. A. Christakis, A. N. Meltzoff. 2007. Television and DVD/video viewing in children younger than 2 years. *Arch Pediatric Adolescent Med* 161:473-79.
2. Harms, T., R. M. Clifford, D. Cryer. 2005. Early childhood environment rating scale, revised ed. Frank Porter Graham Child Development Institute, University of North Carolina. http://ers.fpg.unc.edu/node/82/.
3. Zimmerman, F. J., D. A. Christakis. 2005. Children's television viewing and cognitive outcomes. *Arch Pediatric Adolescent Med* 159:619-25.
4. American Academy of Pediatrics, Council on Communications and Media. 2009. Policy statement: Media violence. *Pediatrics* 124:1495-1503.
5. Reilly, J. J., J. Armstrong, A. R. Dorosty. 2005. Early life risk factors for obesity in childhood: Cohort study. *British Medical J* 330:1357.
6. Lumeng, J. C., S. Rahnama, D. Appugliese, N. Kaciroti, R. H. Bradley. 2006. Television exposure and overweight risk in preschoolers. *Arch Pediatric Adolescent Med* 160:417-22.
7. Levin, S., M. W. Martin, W. F. Riner. 2004. TV viewing habits and Body Mass Index among South Carolina Head Start children. *Ethnicity and Disease* 14:336-39.
8. Miller, S. A., E. M. Taveras, S. L. Rifas-Shiman, M. W. Gillman. 2008. Association between television viewing and poor diet quality in young children. *Int J Pediatric Obesity* 3:168-76.
9. Committee on Food Marketing and the Diets of Children and Youth. 2006. *Food marketing to children and youth: Threat or opportunity*. Ed. J. M. McGinnis, J. A. Gootman, V. I. Kraak. Washington, DC: National Academies Press.
10. Taveras, E. M., T. J. Sandora, M. C. Shih, D. Ross-Degnan, D. A. Goldmann, M. W. Gillman. 2006. The association of television and video viewing with fast food intake by preschool-age children. *Obesity* 14:2034-41.
11. Christakis, D. A., M. M. Garrison, F. J. Zimmerman. 2006. Television viewing in child care programs: A national survey. *Communication Reports* 19:111-20.

ADDITIONAL READINGS:

Dennison, B. A., T. A. Erb, P. L. Jenkins. 2002. Television viewing and television in bedroom associated with overweight risk among low-income preschool children. *Pediatrics* 109:1028-35.

Funk, J. B., J. Brouwer, K. Curtiss, E. McBroom. 2009. Parents of preschoolers: Expert media recommendations and ratings knowledge, media-effects beliefs, and monitoring practices. *Pediatrics* 123:981-88.

National Association for the Education of Young Children. 1994. Media violence in children's lives. Position Statement. http://www.naeyc.org/files/naeyc/file/positions/PSMEVI98.PDF.

Martinez-Gomez, D., J. Tucker, K. A. Heelan, G. J. Welk, J. C. Eisenmann. 2009. Associations between sedentary behavior and blood pressure in young children. *Arch Pediatr Adolesc Med* 163:724-30.

Nixon, G. M., J. M. D. Thompson, D. Y. Han, et al. 2009. Falling asleep: The determinants of sleep latency. *Arch Dis Child* 94:686-89.

McMurray, R. G., S. I. Bangdiwala, J. S. Harrell, L. D. Amorim. 2008. Adolescents with metabolic syndrome have a history of low aerobic fitness and physical activity levels. *Dynamic Med* 7:5.

McDonough, P. 2009. TV viewing among kids at an eight-year high. Nielsen Wire (October 26). http://blog.nielsen.com/nielsenwire/media_entertainment/tv-viewing-among-kids-at-an-eight-year-high/.

Tandon, P. S., C. Zhou, P. Lozano, D. A. Christakis. 2010. Preschoolers' total daily screen time at home and by type of child care. *J Pediatr* 158:297-300.

STANDARD 2.2.0.4: Supervision Near Bodies of Water

Constant and active supervision should be maintained when any child is in or around water (1). During any swimming/wading/water play activities where either an infant or a toddler is present, the ratio should always be one adult to one infant/toddler. Children ages thirteen months to five years of age should not be permitted to play in areas where there is any body of water, including swimming pools, ponds and irrigation ditches, built-in wading pools, tubs, pails, sinks, or toilets unless the supervising adult is within an arm's length providing "touch supervision".

Caregivers/teachers should ensure that all pools meet the Virginia Graeme Baker Pool and Spa Safety Act, requiring the retrofitting of safe suction-type devices for pools and spas to prevent underwater entrapment of children in such locations with strong suction devices that have led to deaths of children of varying ages (2).

RATIONALE: Small children can drown within thirty seconds, in as little as two inches of liquid (3).

In a comprehensive study of drowning and submersion incidents involving children under five years of age in Arizona, California, and Florida, the U.S. Consumer Product Safety Commission (CPSC) found that:

a) Submersion incidents involving children usually happen in familiar surroundings;
b) Pool submersions involving children happen quickly, 77% of the victims had been missing from sight for five minutes or less;
c) Child drowning is a silent death, and splashing may not occur to alert someone that the child is in trouble (4).

Drowning is the second leading cause of unintentional injury-related death for children ages one to fourteen (5).

In 2006, approximately 1,100 children under the age of twenty in the U.S died from drowning (11). A national study that examined where drowning most commonly takes place concluded that infants are most likely to drown in bathtubs, toddlers are most likely to drown in swimming pools and older children and adolescents are most likely to drown in freshwater (rivers, lakes, ponds) (11).

While swimming pools pose the greatest risk for toddlers, about one-quarter of drowning among toddlers are in freshwater sites, such as ponds or lakes.

The American Academy of Pediatrics (AAP) recommends:

a) Swimming lessons for children based on the child's frequency of exposure to water, emotional maturity, physical limitations, and health concerns related to swimming pools;
b) "Touch supervision" of infants and young children through age four when they are in the bathtub or around other bodies of water;

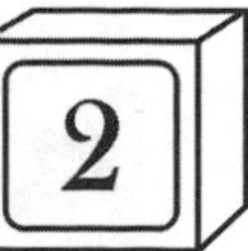

c) Installation of four-sided fencing that completely separates homes from residential pools;
d) Use of approved personal flotation devices (PFDs) when riding on a boat or playing near a river, lake, pond, or ocean;
e) Teaching children never to swim alone or without adult supervision;
f) Stressing the need for parents/guardians and teens to learn first aid and cardiopulmonary resuscitation (CPR) (3).

Deaths and nonfatal injuries have been associated with infant bathtub "supporting ring" devices that are supposed to keep an infant safe in the tub. These rings usually contain three or four legs with suction cups that attach to the bottom of the tub. The suction cups, however, may release suddenly, allowing the bath ring and infant to tip over. An infant also may slip between the legs of the bath ring and become trapped under it. Caregivers/teachers must not rely on these devices to keep an infant safe in the bath and must never leave an infant alone in these bath support rings (1,6,7).

Thirty children under five years of age died from drowning in buckets, pails, and containers from 2003-2005 (10). Of all buckets, the five-gallon size presents the greatest hazard to young children because of its tall straight sides and its weight with even just a small amount of liquid. It is nearly impossible for top-heavy (their heads) infants and toddlers to free themselves when they fall into a five-gallon bucket head first (8).

The Centers for Disease Control (CDC) National Center for Injury Prevention and Control recommends that whenever young children are swimming, playing, or bathing in water, an adult should be watching them constantly. The supervising adult should not read, play cards, talk on the telephone, mow the lawn, or do any other distracting activity while watching children (1,9).

COMMENTS: "Touch supervision" means keeping swimming children within arm's reach and in sight at all times. Flotation devices should never be used as a substitute for supervision. Knowing how to swim does not make a child drown-proof.

The need for constant supervision is of particular concern in dealing with very young children and children with significant motor dysfunction or developmental delays. Supervising adults should be CPR-trained and should have a telephone accessible to the pool and water area at all times should emergency services be required.

TYPE OF FACILITY: Center; Large Family Child Care Home; Small Family Child Care Home

RELATED STANDARDS:

Standard 1.1.1.5: Ratios and Supervision for Swimming, Wading, and Water Play
Standard 1.4.3.3: CPR Training for Swimming and Water Play
Standard 6.3.1.1: Enclosure of Bodies of Water
Standard 6.3.1.7: Pool Safety Rules

REFERENCES:

1. U.S. Consumer Product Safety Commission. 2009. *CPSC warns of in-home drowning dangers with bathtubs, bath seats, buckets.* Release #10-008. Washington, DC: CPSC. http://www.cpsc.gov/cpscpub/prerel/prhtml10/10008.html.
2. U.S. Congress. 2007. *Virginia Graeme Baker Pool and Spa Safety Act*. 15 USC 8001. http://www.cpsc.gov/businfo/vgb/pssa.pdf.
3. American Academy of Pediatrics, Committee on Injury, Violence, and Poison Prevention. 2010. Policy statement-prevention of drowning. *Pediatrics* 126: 178-85.
4. U.S. Consumer Product Safety Commission. 2002. *How to plan for the unexpected: Preventing child drownings*. Publication #359. Washington, DC: CPSC. http://www.cpsc.gov/CPSCPUB/PUBS/359.pdf.
5. Centers for Disease Control and Prevention (CDC). 2010. Unintentional drowning: Fact sheet. http://www.cdc.gov/HomeandRecreationalSafety/Water-Safety/waterinjuries-factsheet.html.
6. U.S. Consumer Product Safety Commission. 1994. *Drowning hazard with baby "supporting ring" devices.* Document #5084. Washington, DC: CPSC. http://www.cpsc.gov/cpscpub/pubs/5084.html.
7. Rauchschwalbe, R., R. A. Brenner, S. Gordon. 1997. The role of bathtub seats and rings in infant drowning deaths. *Pediatrics* 100:e1.
8. U.S. Consumer Product Safety Commission. 1994. *Infants and toddlers can drown in 5-gallon buckets: A hidden hazard in the home*. Document #5006. Washington, DC: CPSC. http://www.cpsc.gov/cpscpub/pubs/5006.html.
9. U.S. Consumer Product Safety Commission. 1997. *CPSC reminds pool owners that barriers, supervision prevent drowning*. Release #97-152. Washington, DC: CPSC. http://www.cpsc.gov/CPSCPUB/PREREL/PRHTML97/97152.html.
10. Gipson, K. 2008. *Submersions related to non-pool and non-spa products, 2008 report.* Washington, DC: U.S. Consumer Product Safety Commission. http://www.cpsc.gov/library/FOIA/FOIA09/OS/nonpoolsub2008.pdf.
11. American Academy of Pediatrics Committee on Injury, Violence, and Poison Prevention, J. Weiss. 2010. Technical report: Prevention of drowning. *Pediatrics* 126: e253-62.

STANDARD 2.2.0.5: Behavior Around a Pool

When children are in or around a pool, caregivers/teachers should teach age-appropriate behavior and safety skills including not pushing each other, holding each other under water, or running at the poolside. Children should be shown the depth of the water at different part of the pool. They should be taught that when going into a body of water, they should go in feet first the first time to check the depth. Children should be instructed what an emergency would be and to only call for help only in a real/genuine emergency. They should be taught to never dive in shallow water.

RATIONALE: Caregivers/teachers should take the opportunities to explain how certain behaviors could injure other children. Also such behavior can distract caregivers/teachers from supervising other children, thereby placing the other children at risk (1).

TYPE OF FACILITY: Center; Large Family Child Care Home; Small Family Child Care Home

REFERENCES:

1. U.S. Department of Health and Human Services, Maternal and Child Health Bureau. 1999. *Basic emergency lifesaving skills (BELS): A framework for teaching emergency lifesaving skills to children and adolescents*. Newton, MA: Children's Safety Network, Education

Development Center. http://bolivia.hrsa.gov/emsc/Downloads/BELS/BELS.htm.

STANDARD 2.2.0.6: Discipline Measures

Reader's Note: The word discipline means to teach and guide. Discipline is not punishment. The discipline standard therefore reflects an approach that focuses on preventing behavior problems by supporting children in learning appropriate social skills and emotional responses.

Caregivers/teachers should guide children to develop self-control and appropriate behaviors in the context of relationships with peers and adults. Caregivers/teachers should care for children without ever resorting to physical punishment or abusive language. When a child needs assistance to resolve a conflict, manage a transition, engage in a challenging situation, or express feelings, needs, and wants, the adult should help the child learn strategies for dealing with the situation. Discipline should be an ongoing process to help children learn to manage their own behavior in a socially acceptable manner, and should not just occur in response to a problem behavior. Rather, the adult's guidance helps children respond to difficult situations using socially appropriate strategies. To develop self-control, children should receive adult support that is individual to the child and adapts as the child develops internal controls. This process should include:

a) Forming a positive relationship with the child. When children have a positive relationship with the adult, they are more likely to follow that person's directions. This positive relationship occurs when the adult spends time talking to the child, listening to the child, following the child's lead, playing with the child, and responding to the child's needs;
b) Basing expectations on children's developmental level;
c) Establishing simple rules children can understand (e.g., you can't hurt others, our things, or yourself) and being proactive in teaching and supporting children in learning the rules;
d) Adapting the physical indoor and outdoor learning/play environment or family child care home to encourage positive behavior and self regulation by providing engaging materials based on children's interests and ensuring that the learning environment promotes active participation of each child. Well-designed child care environments are ones that are supportive of appropriate behavior in children, and are designed to help children learn about what to expect in that environment and to promote positive interactions and engagement with others;
e) Modifying the learning/play environment (e.g., schedule, routine, activities, transitions) to support the child's appropriate behavior;
f) Creating a predictable daily routine and schedule. When a routine is predictable, children are more likely to know what to do and what is expected of them. This may decrease anxiety in the child. When there is less anxiety, there may be less acting out. Reminders need to be given to the children so they can anticipate and prepare themselves for transitions within the schedule. Reminders should be individualized such that each child understands and anticipates the transition;
g) Using encouragement and descriptive praise. When clear encouragement and descriptive praise are used to give attention to appropriate behaviors, those behaviors are likely to be repeated. Encouragement and praise should be stated positively and descriptively. Encouragement and praise should provide information that the behavior the child engaged in was appropriate. Examples: "I can tell you are ready for circle time because you are sitting on your name and looking at me." "Your friend looked so happy when you helped him clean up his toys." "You must be so proud of yourself for putting on your coat all by yourself." Encouragement and praise should label the behaviors, not the child (e.g., good listening, good eating, instead of good boy);
h) Using clear, direct, and simple commands. When clear commands are used with children, they are more likely to follow them. The caregiver/teacher should tell the child what to do rather than what NOT to do. The caregiver/teacher should limit the number of commands. The caregiver/teacher should use if/then and when/then statements with logical and natural consequences. These practices help children understand they can make choices and that choices have consequences;
i) Showing children positive alternatives rather than just telling children "no";
j) Modeling desired behavior;
k) Using planned ignoring and redirection. Certain behaviors can be ignored while at the same time the adult is able to redirect the children to another activity. If the behavior cannot be ignored, the adult should prompt the child to use a more appropriate behavior and provide positive feedback when the child engages in the behavior;
l) Individualizing discipline based on the individual needs of children. For example, if a child has a hard time transitioning, the caregiver/teacher can identify strategies to help the child with the transition (individualized warning, job during transition, individual schedule, peer buddy to help, etc.) If a child has a difficult time during a large group activity, the child might be taught to ask for a break;
m) Using time-out for behaviors that are persistent and unacceptable. Time-out should only be used in combination with instructional approaches that teach children what to do in place of the behavior problem. (See guidance for time-outs below.)

Expectations for children's behavior and the facility's policies regarding their response to behaviors should be written and shared with families and children of appropriate age. Further, the policies should address proactive as well as reactive strategies. Programs should work with families to support their children's appropriate behaviors before it becomes a problem.

RATIONALE: Common usage of the word "discipline" has corrupted the word so that many consider discipline as synonymous with punishment, most particularly corporal punishment (2,3). Discipline is most effective when it is consistent, reinforces desired behaviors, and offers natural and logical consequences for negative behaviors. Research studies find that corporal punishment has limited effectiveness and potentially harmful side effects (4-9). Children have to be taught expectations for their behavior if they are to develop internal control of their actions. The goal is to help children learn to control their own behavior.

COMMENTS: Children respond well when they receive descriptive praise/attention for behaviors that the caregiver/teacher wants to see again. It is best if caregivers/teachers are sincere and enthusiastic when using descriptive praise. On the contrary, children should not receive praise for undesirable behaviors, but instead be praised for honest efforts towards the behaviors the caregivers/teachers want to see repeated (1). Discipline is best received when it includes positive guidance, redirection, and setting clear-cut limits that foster the child's ability to become self-disciplined. In order to respond effectively when children display challenging behavior, it is beneficial for caregivers/teachers to understand typical social and emotional development and behaviors. Discipline is an ongoing process to help children develop inner control so they can manage their own behavior in a socially approved manner. A comprehensive behavior plan is often based first on a positive, affectionate relationship between the child and the caregiver/teacher. Measures that prevent behavior problems often include developmentally appropriate environments, supervision, routines, and transitions. Children can benefit from receiving guidance and repeated instructions for navigating the various social interactions that take place in the child care setting such as friendship development, problem-solving, and conflict-resolution.

Time-out (also known as temporary separation) is one strategy to help children change their behavior and should be used in the context of a positive behavioral support approach which works to understand undesired behaviors and teach new skills to replace the behavior. Listed below are guidelines when using time-out (8):

a) Time-outs should be used for behaviors that are persistent and unacceptable, used infrequently and used only for children who are at least two years of age. Time-outs can be considered an extended ignore or a time-out from positive enforcement;
b) The caregiver/teacher should explain how time-out works to the child BEFORE s/he uses it the first time. The adult should be clear about the behavior that will lead to time-out;
c) When placing the child in time-out, the caregiver/teacher should stay calm;
d) While the child is in time-out, the caregiver/teacher should not talk to or look at the child (as an extended ignore). However, the adult should keep the child in sight. The child could 1) remain sitting quietly in a chair or on a pillow within the room or 2) participate in some activity that requires solitary pursuit (painting, coloring, puzzle, etc.) If the child cannot remain in the room, s/he will spend time in an alternate space, with supervision;
e) Time-outs do not need to be long. The caregiver/teacher should use the one minute of time-out for each year of the child's age (e.g., three-years-old = three minutes of time-out);
f) The caregiver/teacher should end the time-out on a positive note and allow the child to feel good again. Discussions with the child to "explain WHY you were in time-out" are not usually effective;
g) If the child is unable to be distracted or consoled, parents/guardians should be contacted.

How to respond to failure to cooperate during time-out:

Caregivers/teachers should expect resistance from children who are new to the time-out procedure. If a child has never experienced time-out, s/he may respond by becoming very emotional. Time-out should not turn into a power struggle with the child. If the child is refusing to stay on time-out, the caregiver/teacher should give the child an if/then statement. For example, "if you cannot take your time-out, then you cannot join story time." If the child continues to refuse the time-out, then the child cannot join story time. Note that children should not be restrained to keep them in time-out.

More resources for caregivers/teachers on discipline can be found at the following organizations' Websites: a) Center on the Social and Emotional Foundations for Early Learning (CSEFEL) at http://csefel.vanderbilt.edu and b) Technical Assistance Center on Social Emotional Intervention (TACSIE) at http://www.challengingbehavior.org.

TYPE OF FACILITY: Center; Large Family Child Care Home; Small Family Child Care Home

RELATED STANDARDS:

Standard 2.1.1.6: Transitioning Within Programs and Indoor and Outdoor Learning/Play Environments
Standard 2.2.0.7: Handling Physical Aggression, Biting, and Hitting
Standard 2.2.0.8: Preventing Expulsions, Suspensions, and Other Limitations in Services
Standards 3.4.4.1-3.4.4.5: Child Abuse and Neglect
Standard 9.2.1.1: Content of Policies
Standard 9.2.1.3: Enrollment Information to Parents/Guardians and Caregivers/Teachers
Standard 9.2.1.6: Written Discipline Policies
Standard 9.4.1.6: Availability of Documents to Parents/Guardians

REFERENCES:

1. Henderlong, J., M. Lepper. 2002 The effects of praise on children's intrinsic motivation: A review and synthesis. *Psychological Bulletin* 128:774-95.
2. Hodgkin, R. 1997. Why the "gentle smack" should go: Policy review. *Child Soc* 11:201-4.
3. Fraiberg, S. H. 1959. *The Magic Years*. New York: Charles Scribner's Sons.
4. Straus, M. A., et al. 1997. Spanking by parents and subsequent antisocial behavior of children. *Arch Pediatric Adolescent Medicine* 151:761-67.

5. Deater-Deckard, K., et al. 1996. Physical discipline among African American and European American mothers: Links to children's externalizing behaviors. *Dev Psychol* 32:1065-72.
6. Weiss, B., et al. 1992. Some consequences of early harsh discipline: Child aggression and a maladaptive social information processing style. *Child Dev* 63:1321-35.
7. American Academy of Pediatrics, Committee on School Health. 2006. Policy statement: Corporal punishment in schools. *Pediatrics* 118:1266.
8. Dunlap, S., L. Fox, M. L. Hemmeter, P. Strain. 2004. *The role of time-out in a comprehensive approach for addressing challenging behaviors of preschool children*. CSEFEL What Works Series. http://csefel.vanderbilt.edu/briefs/wwb14.pdf.
9. Fiene, R. 2002. *13 indicators of quality child care: Research update*. Washington, DC: U.S. Department of Health and Human Services, Office of the Assistant Secretary for Planning and Evaluation. http://aspe.hhs.gov/hsp/ccquality-ind02/.

ADDITIONAL READINGS:
Gross, D., C. Garvey, W. Julion, L. Fogg, S. Tucker, H. Mokos. 2009. Efficacy of the Chicago Parent Program with low-income multi-ethnic parents of young children. *Preventions Science* 10:54-65.
Breitenstein, S., D. Gross, I. Ordaz, W. Julion, C. Garvey, A. Ridge. 2007. Promoting mental health in early childhood programs serving families from low income neighborhoods. *J Am Psychiatric Nurses Assoc* 13:313-20.
Gross, D., C. Garvey, W. Julion, L. Fogg. 2007. Preventive parent training with low-income ethnic minority parents of preschoolers. In *Handbook of parent training: Helping parents prevent and solve problem behaviors*. Ed. J. M. Briesmeister, C. E. Schaefer. 3rd ed. Hoboken, NJ: Wiley.
Gartrell, D. 2007. He did it on purpose! *Young Children* 62:62-64.
Gartrell, D. 2004. *The power of guidance: Teaching social-emotional skills in early childhood classrooms*. Clifton Park, NY: Thomson Delmar Learning; Washington, DC: NAEYC.
Gartrell, D., K. Sonsteng. 2008. Promoting physical activity: It's proactive guidance. *Young Children* 63:51-53.
Shiller, V. M., J. C. O'Flynn. 2008. Using rewards in the early childhood classroom: A reexamination of the issues. *Young Children* 63:88, 90-93.
Reineke, J., K. Sonsteng, D. Gartrell. 2008. Nurturing mastery motivation: No need for rewards. *Young Children* 63:89, 93-97.
Ryan, R. M., E. L. Deci. 2000. When rewards compete with nature: The undermining of intrinsic motivation and self-regulation. In *Intrinsic and extrinsic motivation: The search for optimal motivation and performance*, ed. C. Sanstone, J. M. Harackiewicz, 13-54. San Diego, CA: Academic Press.

STANDARD 2.2.0.7: Handling Physical Aggression, Biting, and Hitting

Caregivers/teachers should intervene immediately when a child's behavior is aggressive and endangers the safety of others. It is important that the child be clearly told verbally, "no hitting" or "no biting." The caregiver/teacher should use age–appropriate interventions. For example, a toddler can be picked up and moved to another location in the room if s/he bites other children or adults. A preschool child can be invited to walk with you first but, if not compliant, taken by the hand and walked to another location in the room. The caregiver/teacher should remain calm and make eye contact with the child telling him/her the behavior is unacceptable. If the behavior persists, parents/guardians, caregivers/teachers, the child care health consultant and the early childhood mental health consultant should be involved to create a plan targeting this behavior. For example, a plan may be developed to recognize non-aggressive behavior. Children who might not have the social skills or language to communicate appropriately may use physical aggression to express themselves and the reason for and antecedents of the behavior must be considered when developing a plan for addressing the behavior.

RATIONALE: Caregiver/teacher intervention protects children and encourages children to exhibit more acceptable behavior (1).

COMMENTS: Biting is a phase. Here are some specific steps to deal with biting:

Step 1: If a child bites another child, the caregiver/teacher should comfort the child who was bitten and remind the biter that biting hurts and we do not bite. Children should be given some space from each other for an appropriate amount of time.

Step 2: The caregiver/teacher should follow first aid instructions (available from the American Academy of Pediatrics [AAP] and the American Red Cross) and use the Center for Disease Control and Prevention's (CDC's) Standard Precautions to handle potential exposure to blood.

Step 3: The caregiver/teacher should allow for "dignity of risk," and let the children back in the same space with increased supervision. Interactions should be structured between children such that the child learns to use more appropriate social skills or language rather than biting. If there is another incident, caregivers/teachers should repeat step one. The biter can play with children they have not bitten.

Step 4: The adult needs to shadow the biter to ensure safety of the other children. This can be challenging but imperative for the biter.

Step 5: For all transitions when the biter would be in close contact, the caregiver/teacher should hold him/her on her/his hip or if possible hold hands, keep a close watch, and keep the biter from close proximity with peers.

Step 6: The child (biter) should play with one or two other children whom they have not bitten with a favored adult in a section separate from the other children. Sometimes, until a phase (biting is a phase) passes, the caregiver/teacher needs to extinguish the behavior by not allowing it to happen and thereby reducing the attention given to the behavior.

Step 7: Parents/guardians of both children of the incident should be informed.

Step 8: The caregiver/teacher should determine whether the incident necessitates documentation (see Standard 9.4.1.9). If so, s/he should complete a report form.

Caregivers/teachers need to consider why the child is biting and teach the child a more appropriate way to communicate the same need. Possible reasons why a child would bite include:

a) Lack of words (desire to stop the behavior of another child);
b) Teething;
c) Tired (is nap time too late?);
d) Hungry (is lunch time too late?);
e) Lack of toys – consider buying duplicates of popular items;
f) Lack of supervision – more staff should be added, staff are near children during transitions, and room is set up to ensure visibility;
g) Child is bored – too much sitting, activities are too frustrating;
h) Child has oral motor needs – teethers are offered;
i) Child is avoiding something, and biting gets him/her out of it;
j) Lack of attention – child receives attention when biting.

Other important strategies to consider:

a) The caregiver/teacher should point out the effect of the child's biting on the victim: "Emma is crying. Biting hurts. Look at her face. See how sad she is?" Label feelings and give victims the words to respond. "Emma, you can say 'No biting!' to Josh";
b) The child should help the victim feel better. He can get a wet paper towel, a blankie or favorite toy for the victim and sit near them until the other child is feeling better. This encourages children to take responsibility for their actions, briefly removes the child from other activities and also lets the child experience success as a helper.

Discussing aggressive behavior in group time with the children can be an effective way to gain and share understanding among the children about how it feels when aggressive behavior occurs. Although bullying has not been studied in the preschool population, it is a form of aggression (2). Here are some helpful Websites: http://stopbullying.gov and http://www.eyesonbullying.org/preschool.html.

For more helpful strategies for handling aggression, see Center on the Social and Emotional Foundations for Early Learning Website at http://csefel.vanderbilt.edu. In addition, a child care health consultant or child care mental health consultant can help when the biting behavior continues.

TYPE OF FACILITY: Center; Large Family Child Care Home; Small Family Child Care Home

RELATED STANDARDS:

Standard 2.2.0.6: Discipline Measures
Standard 2.2.0.8: Preventing Expulsions, Suspensions, and Other Limitations in Services
Standard 2.3.1.1: Mutual Responsibility of Parents/Guardians and Staff
Standard 3.2.3.3: Cuts and Scrapes
Standard 3.2.3.4: Prevention of Exposure to Blood and Body Fluids
Standard 9.4.1.9: Records of Injury

REFERENCES:

1. Rush, K. L. 1999. Caregiver-child interactions and early literacy development of preschool children from low-income environments. *Topics Early Child Special Education* 19:3-14.
2. Ross, Scott W., Horner, Robert H. 2009. Bully prevention in positive behavior support. *J Applied Behavior Analysis* 42:747-59.

STANDARD 2.2.0.8: Preventing Expulsions, Suspensions, and Other Limitations in Services

Child care programs should not expel, suspend, or otherwise limit the amount of services (including denying outdoor time, withholding food, or using food as a reward/punishment) provided to a child or family on the basis of challenging behaviors or a health/safety condition or situation unless the condition or situation meets one of the two exceptions listed in this standard.

Expulsion refers to terminating the enrollment of a child or family in the regular group setting because of a challenging behavior or a health condition. Suspension and other limitations in services include all other reductions in the amount of time a child may be in attendance of the regular group setting, either by requiring the child to cease attendance for a particular period of time or reducing the number of days or amount of time that a child may attend. Requiring a child to attend the program in a special place away from the other children in the regular group setting is included in this definition.

Child care programs should have a comprehensive discipline policy that includes an explicit description of alternatives to expulsion for children exhibiting extreme levels of challenging behaviors, and should include the program's protocol for preventing challenging behaviors. These policies should be in writing and clearly articulated and communicated to parents/guardians, staff and others. These policies should also explicitly state how the program plans to use any available internal mental health and other support staff during behavioral crises to eliminate to the degree possible any need for external supports (e.g., local police departments) during crises.

Staff should have access to in-service training on both a proactive and as-needed basis on how to reduce the likelihood of problem behaviors escalating to the level of risk for expulsion and how to more effectively manage behaviors throughout the entire class/group. Staff should also have access to in-service training, resources, and child care health consultation to manage children's health conditions in collaboration with parents/guardians and the child's primary care provider. Programs should attempt to obtain access to behavioral or mental health consultation to help establish and maintain environments that will support children's mental well-being and social-emotional health, and have access to such a consultant when more targeted child-specific interventions are needed. Mental health consultation may be obtained from a variety of sources, as described in Standard 1.6.0.3.

When children exhibit or engage in challenging behaviors that cannot be resolved easily, as above, staff should:

a) Assess the health of the child and the adequacy of the curriculum in meeting the developmental and educational needs of the child;
b) Immediately engage the parents/guardians/family in a spirit of collaboration regarding how the

child's behaviors may be best handled, including appropriate solutions that have worked at home or in other settings;

c) Access an early childhood mental health consultant to assist in developing an effective plan to address the child's challenging behaviors and to assist the child in developing age-appropriate, pro-social skills;
d) Facilitate, with the family's assistance, a referral for an evaluation for either Part C (early intervention) or Part B (preschool special education), as well as any other appropriate community-based services (e.g., child mental health clinic);
e) Facilitate with the family communication with the child's primary care provider (e.g., pediatrician, family medicine provider, etc.), so that the primary care provider can assess for any related health concerns and help facilitate appropriate referrals.

The only possible reasons for considering expelling, suspending or otherwise limiting services to a child on the basis of challenging behaviors are:

a) Continued placement in the class and/or program clearly jeopardizes the physical safety of the child and/or his/her classmates as assessed by a qualified early childhood mental health consultant AND all possible interventions and supports recommended by a qualified early childhood mental health consultant aimed at providing a physically safe environment have been exhausted; or
b) The family is unwilling to participate in mental health consultation that has been provided through the child care program or independently obtain and participate in child mental health assistance available in the community; or
c) Continued placement in this class and/or program clearly fails to meet the mental health and/or social-emotional needs of the child as agreed by both the staff and the family AND a different program that is better able to meet these needs has been identified and can immediately provide services to the child.

In either of the above three cases, a qualified early childhood mental health consultant, qualified special education staff, and/or qualified community-based mental health care provider should be consulted, referrals for special education services and other community-based services should be facilitated, and a detailed transition plan from this program to a more appropriate setting should be developed with the family and followed. This transition could include a different private or public-funded child care or early education program in the community that is better equipped to address the behavioral concerns (e.g., therapeutic preschool programs, Head Start or Early Head Start, prekindergarten programs in the public schools that have access to additional support staff, etc.), or public-funded special education services for infants and toddlers (i.e., Part C early intervention) or preschoolers (i.e., Part B preschool special education).

To the degree that safety can be maintained, the child should be transitioned directly to the receiving program. The program should assist parents/guardians in securing the more appropriate placement, perhaps using the services of a local child care resource and referral agency. With parent/guardian permission, the child's primary care provider should be consulted and a referral for a comprehensive assessment by qualified mental health provider and the appropriate special education system should be initiated. If abuse or neglect is suspected, then appropriate child protection services should be informed. Finally, no child should ever be expelled or suspended from care without first conducting an assessment of the safety of alternative arrangements (e.g., Who will care for the child? Will the child be adequately and safely supervised at all times?) (1).

RATIONALE: The rate of expulsion in child care programs has been estimated to be as high as one in every thirty-six children enrolled, with 39% of all child care classes per year expelling at least one child. In state-funded prekindergarten programs, the rate has been estimated as one in every 149 children enrolled, with 10% of prekindergarten classes per year expelling at least one child. These expulsions prevent children from receiving potentially beneficial mental health services and deny the child the benefit of continuity of quality early education and child care services. Mental health consultation has been shown in rigorous research to help reduce the likelihood of behaviors leading to expulsion decisions. Also, research suggests that expulsion decisions may be related to teacher job stress and depression, large group sizes, and high child:staff ratios (1-6).

Mental health services should be available to staff to help address challenging behaviors in the program, to help improve the mental health climate of indoor and outdoor learning/play environments and child care systems, to better provide mental health services to families, and to address job stress and mental health needs of staff.

TYPE OF FACILITY: Center; Large Family Child Care Home; Small Family Child Care Home

RELATED STANDARDS:

Standard 1.6.0.1: Child Care Health Consultants
Standard 1.6.0.3: Early Childhood Mental Health Consultants
Standard 1.6.0.5: Early Childhood Education Consultants
Standard 2.2.0.6: Discipline Measures
Standard 2.2.0.7: Handling Physical Aggression, Biting, and Hitting
Standard 2.2.0.9: Prohibited Caregiver/Teacher Behaviors
Standard 2.2.0.10: Using Physical Restraint
Standards 3.4.4.1-3.4.4.5: Child Abuse and Neglect
Standard 4.5.0.11: Prohibited Uses of Food
Standard 9.2.1.6: Written Discipline Policies

REFERENCES:

1. American Academy of Pediatrics, Committee on School Health. 2008. Policy statement: Out-of-school suspension and expulsion. *Pediatrics* 122:450.
2. Gilliam, W. S. 2005. Prekindergarteners left behind: Expulsion rates in state prekindergarten programs. Foundation for Child Development, Policy Brief Series no. 3. http://medicine.yale.edu/childstudy/zigler/Images/National Prek Study_expulsion brief _tcm350-34775.pdf.
3. Gilliam, W. S., G. Shahar. 2006. Preschool and child care expulsion and suspension: Rates and predictors in one state. *Infants Young Children* 19:228-45.

4. Gilliam, W. S. 2008. Implementing policies to reduce the likelihood of preschool expulsion. Foundation for Child Development, Policy Brief Series no. 7. http://medicine.yale.edu/childstudy/zigler/Images/PreKExpulsionBrief2_tcm350-34772.pdf.
5. National Scientific Council on the Developing Child. 2008. Mental health problems in early childhood can impair learning and behavior for life. Working paper #6. http://developingchild.harvard.edu/library/reports_and_working_papers/working_papers/wp6/.
6. Perry, D. F., M. C. Dunne, L. McFadden, D. Campbell. 2008. Reducing the risk for preschool expulsion: Mental health consultation for young children with challenging behaviors. *J Child Family Studies* 17:44-54.

STANDARD 2.2.0.9: Prohibited Caregiver/ Teacher Behaviors

The following behaviors should be prohibited in all child care settings and by all caregivers/teachers:

a) The use of corporal punishment. Corporal punishment means punishment inflicted directly on the body including, but not limited to:
   1) Hitting, spanking (refers to striking a child with an open hand on the buttocks or extremities with the intention of modifying behavior without causing physical injury), shaking, slapping, twisting, pulling, squeezing, or biting;
   2) Demanding excessive physical exercise, excessive rest, or strenuous or bizarre postures;
   3) Compelling a child to eat or have in his/her mouth soap, food, spices, or foreign substances;
   4) Exposing a child to extremes of temperature.

b) Isolating a child in an adjacent room, hallway, closet, darkened area, play area, or any other area where a child cannot be seen or supervised;

c) Binding or tying to restrict movement, such as in a car seat (except when travelling) or taping the mouth;

d) Using or withholding food as a punishment or reward;

e) Toilet learning/training methods that punish, demean, or humiliate a child;

f) Any form of emotional abuse, including rejecting, terrorizing, extended ignoring, isolating, or corrupting a child;

g) Any abuse or maltreatment of a child, either as an incident of discipline or otherwise. Any child care program must not tolerate, or in any manner condone, an act of abuse or neglect of a child by an older child, employee, volunteer, or any person employed by the facility or child's family;

h) Abusive, profane, or sarcastic language or verbal abuse, threats, or derogatory remarks about the child or child's family;

i) Any form of public or private humiliation, including threats of physical punishment (1);

j) Physical activity/outdoor time should not be taken away as punishment.

RATIONALE: Corporal punishment may be physical abuse or may easily become abusive. Corporal punishment is clearly prohibited in family child care homes and centers in the majority of states (2-4). Research links corporal punishment with negative effects such as later aggression (5) behavior problems in school (6,7), antisocial and criminal behavior, and impairment of learning (8-12).

Factors supporting prohibition of certain methods of discipline include current child development theory and practice, legal aspects (namely, that a caregiver/teacher does not foster a relationship with the child in place of the parents/guardians), and increasing liability suits. The American Academy of Pediatrics (AAP) is opposed to the use of corporal punishment (12). Physicians, educators, and caregivers/teachers should neither inflict nor sanction corporal punishment (11).

COMMENTS: Appropriate alternatives to corporal punishment vary as children grow and develop. As infants become more mobile, the caregiver/teacher must create a safe space and impose limitations by encouraging activities that distract them from harmful situations. Brief verbal expressions of disapproval help prepare infants and toddlers for later use of reasoning. However, the caregiver/teacher cannot expect infants and toddlers to be controlled by verbal reprimands. Preschoolers have begun to develop an understanding of rules and can be expected to understand "time-out" (out-of-group activity) under adult supervision as a consequence for undesirable behavior. School-age children begin to develop a sense of personal responsibility and self-control and will recognize the removal of privileges (12). This standard covers any behaviors that threaten the safety and security of children. This would include behaviors that occur among or between staff. Children should not see hitting, ridicule, etc. among staff members. Even though adults may state that the behaviors are "playful," children cannot distinguish this.

"In the wake of well-publicized allegations of child abuse in out-of-home settings and increased concerns regarding liability, some programs have instituted no-touch policies, either explicitly or implicitly. No-touch policies are misguided efforts that fail to recognize the importance of touch to children's healthy development. Touch is especially important for infants and toddlers. Warm, responsive touches convey regard and concern for children of any age. Adults should be sensitive to ensuring that their touches (such as pats on the back, hugs, or ruffling the child's hair) are welcomed by the children and appropriate to their individual characteristics and cultural experience. Careful, open communication between the program and families about the value of touch in children's development can help to achieve consensus as to acceptable ways for adults to show their respect and support for children in the program" (13).

TYPE OF FACILITY: Center; Large Family Child Care Home; Small Family Child Care Home

RELATED STANDARDS:
Standard 2.2.0.5: Discipline Measures
Standard 2.2.0.7: Handling Physical Aggression, Biting, and Hitting
Standard 2.2.0.10: Using Physical Restraint
Standards 3.4.4.1-3.4.4.5: Child Abuse and Neglect
Standard 4.5.0.11: Prohibited Uses of Food
Standard 9.2.1.6: Written Discipline Policies

REFERENCES:

1. New York State Office of Children and Family Services. Child care forms, licensed/ registered provider. http://www.ocfs.state.ny.us/main/forms/day_care/.
2. The Children's Foundation. *Family child care licensing study*. 2000. Washington, DC: The Children's Foundation.
3. Azer, S., D. Eldred. 1998. *Training requirements in child care licensing regulations*. Boston, MA: Center for Career Development in Early Care and Education, Wheelock College.
4. Meadows, A., ed. 1991. *Caring for America's Children*. Washington, DC: National Academy of Sciences and National Research Council.
5. Gershoff, E. T. 2002. Corporal punishment by parents and associated child behaviors and experiences: A meta-analytic and theoretical review. *Psychological Bulletin* 128:539-79.
6. Slade, E. P., L. S. Wissow. 2004. Spanking in early childhood and later behavior problems: A prospective study of infants and young toddlers. *Pediatrics* 113:1321-30.
7. Grogan-Kaylor, A. 2005. Corporal punishment and the growth trajectory of children's antisocial behavior. *Child Maltreatment* 10:283-92.
8. Straus, M. A., et al. 1997. Spanking by parents and subsequent antisocial behavior of children. *Arch Pediatric Adolescent Medicine* 151:761-67.
9. Deater-Deckard, K., et al. 1996. Physical discipline among African American and European American mothers: Links to children's externalizing behaviors. *Dev Psychology* 32:1065-72.
10. Weiss, B., et al. 1992. Some consequences of early harsh discipline: Child aggression and a maladaptive social information processing style. *Child Dev* 63:1321-35.
11. American Academy of Pediatrics, Committee on School Health. 2006. Policy statement: Corporal punishment in schools. *Pediatrics* 188:1266.
12. American Academy of Pediatrics, Committee on Psychological Aspects of Child and Family Health. 2004. Policy statement: Guidance for effective discipline. *Pediatrics* 114:1126.
13. National Association for the Education of Young Children. 1996. Position Statement. Prevention of child abuse in early childhood programs and the responsibilities of early childhood professionals to prevent child abuse.

STANDARD 2.2.0.10: Using Physical Restraint

Reader's Note: It should never be necessary to physically restrain a typically developing child unless his/her safety and/or that of others are at risk.

When a child with special behavioral or mental health issues is enrolled who may frequently need the cautious use of restraint in the event of behavior that endangers his or her safety or the safety of others, a behavioral care plan should be developed with input from the child's primary care provider, mental health provider, parents/guardians, center director/family child care home caregiver/teacher, child care health consultant, and possibly early childhood mental health consultant in order to address underlying issues and reduce the need for physical restraint.

That behavioral care plan should include:

a) An indication and documentation of the use of other behavioral strategies before the use of restraint and a precise definition of when the child could be restrained;
b) That the restraint be limited to holding the child as gently as possible to accomplish the restraint;
c) That such child restraint techniques do not violate the state's mental health code;
d) That the amount of time the child is physically restrained should be the minimum necessary to control the situation and be age-appropriate; reevaluation and change of strategy should be used every few minutes;
e) That no bonds, ties, blankets, straps, car seats, heavy weights (such as adult body sitting on child), or abusive words should be used;
f) That a designated and trained staff person, who should be on the premises whenever this specific child is present, would be the only person to carry out the restraint.

RATIONALE: A child could be harmed if not restrained properly (1). Therefore, staff who are doing the restraining must be trained. A clear behavioral care plan needs to be in place. And, clear documentation with parent/guardian notification needs to be done after a restraining incident occurs in order to conform with the mental health code.

COMMENTS: If all strategies described in Standard 2.2.0.6 are followed and a child continues to behave in an unsafe manner, staff need to physically remove the child from the situation to a less stimulating environment. Physical removal of a child is defined according the development of the child. If the child is able to walk, staff should hold the child's hand and walk him/her away from the situation. If the child is not ambulatory, staff should pick the child up and remove him/her to a quiet place where s/he cannot hurt themselves or others. Staff need to remain calm and use a calm voice when directing the child. Certain procedures described in Standard 2.2.0.6 can be used at this time, including not giving a lot of attention to the behavior, distracting the child and/or giving a time-out to the child. If the behavior persists, a plan needs to be made with parental/guardian involvement. This plan could include rewards or a sticker chart and/or praise and attention for appropriate behavior. Or, loss of privileges for inappropriate behavior can be implemented, if age-appropriate. Staff should request or agree to step out of the situation if they sense a loss of their own self-control and concern for the child.

The use of safe physical restraint should occur rarely and only for brief periods to protect the child and others. Staff should be alert to repeated instances of restraint for individual children or within a indoor and outdoor learning/play environment and seek consultation from health and mental health consultants in collaboration with families to develop more appropriate strategies.

TYPE OF FACILITY: Center; Large Family Child Care Home; Small Family Child Care Home

RELATED STANDARDS:
Standard 2.2.0.6: Discipline Measures

REFERENCES:

1. Safe and Responsive Schools. 2003. Effective responses: Physical restraint. http://www.unl.edu/srs/pdfs/physrest.pdf.

2.3 Parent/Guardian Relationships

2.3.1 General

STANDARD 2.3.1.1: Mutual Responsibility of Parents/Guardians and Staff

The quality of the relationship between parents/guardians and caregivers/teachers has an influence on the child. There should be a reciprocal responsibility of the family and caregivers/teachers to observe, participate, and be trained in the care that each child requires, and they should be encouraged to work together as partners in providing care.

During the enrollment process, caregivers/teachers should clarify who is/are the legal guardian(s) of the child. All relevant legal documents, court orders, etc., should also be collected and filed during the enrollment process (1). Caregivers/teachers should comply with court orders and written consent from the parent/guardian with legal authority, and not try to make the determination themselves regarding the best interests of the child.

All aspects of child care programs should be designed to facilitate parent/guardian input and involvement. Non-custodial parents should have access to the same developmental and behavioral information given to the custodial parent/guardian, if they have joint legal custody, permission by court order, or written consent from the custodial parent/guardian.

Caregivers/teachers should also clarify with whom the child spends significant time and with whom the child has primary relationships as they will be key informants for the caregivers/teachers about the child and his/her needs.

Parent/guardian involvement is needed at all levels of the program, including program planning for indoors and outdoors, provision of quality care, screening for children who are ill, and support for other parents/guardians. Communication between the administrator, caregiver/teacher and parent/guardian are essential to facilitate the involvement and commitment of parents/guardians. Parents/guardians should be invited to participate on the program board or planning meetings for the program. Parents/guardians should meet with their child's caregiver/teacher or the director annually to discuss how their child is doing in the program. On a daily basis, parents/guardians and caregivers/teachers should share information about the child's health, changes in drop-off or pick-up times, and changes in family routines or family events. Caregivers/teachers should communicate regularly with parents/guardians by providing injury report forms if their child sustains an injury, posting notices of exposures to infectious diseases, and greeting the parent/guardian at drop-off each day. Parents/guardians should receive a copy of the child care programs' written policies, including health and safety policies.

Caregivers/teachers should informally share with parents/guardians daily information about their child's needs and activities.

Transition reports on any symptoms that the child developed, differences in patterns of appetite or urinating, and activity level should be exchanged to keep parents/guardians informed.

RATIONALE: This plan will help achieve the important goal of carryover of facility components from the child care setting to the child's home environment. The child's learning of new skills is a continuous process occurring both at home and in child care.

Research, practice, and accumulated wisdom attest to the crucially important influence of children's relationships with those closest to them. Children's experience in child care will be most beneficial when parents/guardians and caregivers/teachers develop feelings of mutual respect and trust. In such a situation, children feel a continuity of affection and concern, which facilitates their adjustment to separation and use of the facility. Especially for infants and toddlers, attention to consistency across settings will help minimize stress that can result from notable differences in routines across caregivers/teachers and settings.

Another ongoing source of stress for an infant or a young child is the separation from those they love and depend upon. Of the various programmatic elements in the facility that can help to alleviate that stress, by far the most important is the comfort in knowing that parents/guardians and caregivers/teachers know the children and their needs and wishes, are in close contact with each other, and can respond in ways that enable children to deal with separation.

The encouragement and involvement of parents/guardians in the social and cognitive leaps of the child provides parents/guardians with the confidence vital to their sense of competence. Caregivers/teachers should be able to direct parents/guardians to sources of information and activities that support child's development and learning and be able to assist them to obtain appropriate screening and assessment when there are concerns. Communication should be sensitive to ethnic and cultural practices. The parent/guardian/caregiver/teacher partnership models positive adult behavior for school-age children and demonstrates a mutual concern for the child's well-being (2-16).

In families where the parents/guardians are separated, it is usually in the child's best interest for both parents/guardians to be involved in the child's care, and informed about the child's progress and problems in care. However, it is up to the courts to decide who has legal custody of the child.

TYPE OF FACILITY: Center; Large Family Child Care Home; Small Family Child Care Home

RELATED STANDARDS:
Standard 2.1.1.7: Communication in Native Language Other than English
Standard 2.1.1.8: Diversity in Enrollment and Curriculum
Standard 2.1.1.9: Verbal Interaction

REFERENCES:
1. Public Counsel Law Center in California. Guidelines for Releasing Children and Custody Issues. http://www.publiccounsel.org/publications/release.pdf.

2. Mayr, T., M. Ulich. 1999. Children's well-being in day care centers: An exploratory empirical study. *Int J Early Years Educ* 7:229-39.
3. Marshall, N. L. 1991. *Empowering low-income parents: The role of child care*. Boston, MA: EDRS.
4. Greenman, J. 1998. Parent partnerships: What they don't teach you can hurt. *Child Care Infor Exch* 124:78-82.
5. Shores, E. J. 1998. *A call to action: Family involvement as a critical component of teacher education programs*. Tallahassee, FL: Southeastern Regional Vision for Education.
6. Massachusetts State Office for Children. *Establishing a successful family daycare home: A resource guide for providers*. 1990. Boston: MA State Office for Children.
7. Tijus, C. A., et al. 1997. The impact of parental involvement on the quality of day care centers. *Int J Early Years Educ* 5:7-20.
8. Jones, R. 1996. Producing a school newsletter parents will read. *Child Care Infor Exch* 107:91-3.
9. O'Connor, S., et al. 1996. *ASQ: Assessing school age child care quality*. Wellesly, MA: Center for Research on Women.
10. Powell, D. R. 1998. Reweaving parents back into the fabric of early childhood programs: Research in review. *Young Child* 53:60-67.
11. Miller, S. H., et al. 1995. Family support in early education and child care settings: Making a case for both principles and practices. *Child Today* 23:26-29.
12. Dombro, A. L. 1995. Sharing the care: What every provider and parent needs to know. *Child Today* 23:22-5.
13. Larner, M. 1995. *Linking family support and early childhood programs: Issues, experiences, opportunities: Best practices project*, 1-40. Chicago, IL: Family Resource Coalition.
14. Endsley, R. C., et al. 1993. Parent involvement and quality day care in proprietary centers. *J Res Child Educ* 7:53-61.
15. Fagan, J. 1994. Mother and father involvement in day care centers serving infants and young toddlers. *Early Child Dev Care* 103:95-101.
16. Seibel, N. L., L. G. Gillespie, and T. Temple. 2008. The role of child care providers in child abuse prevention. *Zero to Three* 28:33-40.

STANDARD 2.3.1.2: Parent/Guardian Visits

Parents/guardians are welcome any time their child is in attendance.

Caregivers/teachers should inform all parents/guardians that they may visit the site at any time when their child is there, and that, under normal circumstances, they will be admitted without delay. This open-door policy should be part of the "admission agreement" or other contract between the parent/guardian and the facility/caregiver/teacher. Parents/guardians should be welcomed and encouraged to speak freely to staff about concerns and suggestions. Parents/guardians must be informed what appropriate and inappropriate parental/guardian behavior is and the consequences for inappropriate behavior.

Authorized family members and parents/guardians should check in with the facility staff every visit to ensure safety of the children in the facility.

RATIONALE: Requiring unrestricted access of parents/guardians to their children is essential to preventing the abuse and neglect of children in child care (1,2). When access is restricted, areas observable by the parents/guardians may not reflect the care the children actually receive.

COMMENTS: Caregivers/teachers should not release a child to a parent/guardian who appears impaired (see Standard 9.2.4.1). Caregivers/teachers should not attempt on their own to handle an unstable (e.g., intoxicated) parent/guardian who wants to be admitted but whose behavior poses a risk to the children. Caregivers/teachers should consult local police or the local child protection agency about their recommendations for how staff can obtain support from law enforcement authorities.

Parents/guardians can be interviewed to see if the open-door policy is consistently implemented.

TYPE OF FACILITY: Center; Large Family Child Care Home; Small Family Child Care Home

RELATED STANDARDS:
Standard 2.1.1.7: Communication in Native Language Other than English
Standards 2.3.2.1-2.3.3.1: Parent/Guardian Involvement
Standard 9.2.1.1: Content of Policies
Standard 9.2.1.3: Enrollment Information to Parents/Guardians and Caregivers/Teachers
Standard 9.2.4.1: Written Plan and Training for Handling Urgent Medical Care or Threatening Incidents

REFERENCES:

1. Koralek, D., U.S. Department of Health and Human Services. 1992. *Caregivers of young children: Preventing and responding to child maltreatment*. Rev ed. The user manual series. McLean, VA: Circle, Inc.
2. Baglin, C. A., M. Bender, eds. 1994. *Handbook on quality child care for young children: Settings standards and resources*. San Diego, CA: Singular Publishing Group.

2.3.2 Regular Communication

STANDARD 2.3.2.1: Parent/Guardian Conferences

Along with short informal daily conversations between parents/guardians and caregivers/teachers, and as a supplement to the collaborative relationships caregivers/teachers and parents/guardians form specifically to support infants and toddlers, periodic and regular planned communication (e.g., parent/guardian conferences) should be scheduled with at least one parent/guardian of every child in care:

a) To review the child's adjustment to care and development over time;
b) To reach agreement on appropriate disciplinary measures;
c) To discuss the child's strengths, specific health issues, special needs, and concerns;
d) To stay informed of family issues that may affect the child's behavior in care;
e) To identify goals for the child;
f) To discuss resources that parents/guardians can access;
g) To discuss the results of developmental screening.

At these planned conferences a caregiver/teacher should review with the parent/guardian the child's health report, and the health record and assessments of development and learning that the program may do to identify medical and developmental issues that require follow-up or adjustment by the facility.

Each review should be documented in the child's health record with the signature of the parent/guardian and the staff reviewer. These planned conferences should occur:

a) As part of the intake process;
b) At each health update interval;
c) On a calendar basis, scheduled according to the child's age:
    1) Every six months for children under six years of age and for children with special health care needs;
    2) Every year for children six years of age and older;
d) Whenever new information is added to the child's facility health record.

Additional conferences should be scheduled if the parent/guardian or caregiver/teacher has a concern at any time about a particular child. Any concern about a child's health or development should not be delayed until a scheduled conference date.

Notes about these planned communications should be maintained in each child's record at the facility and should be available for review.

RATIONALE: Parents/guardians and caregivers/teachers alike should be aware of, and should have arrived at, an agreement concerning each other's beliefs and knowledge about how to care for children. Reviewing the health record with parents/guardians ensures correct information and can be a valuable teaching and motivational tool (1). It can also be a staff learning experience, through insight gained from parents/guardians on a child's special circumstances.

Studies have shown that parent–child interactions characterized as structured and responsive to the child's needs and emotions were positively related to school readiness, social skills, and receptive communication skills development (2).

A health history is the basis for meeting the child's health, mental, safety, and social needs in the child care setting (1). Review of the health record can be a valuable educational tool for parents/guardians, through better understanding of the health report and immunization requirements (1). A goal of out-of-home care of infants and children is to identify parents/guardians who are in need of instruction so they can provide preventive health/nutrition/physical activity care at a critical time during the child's growth and development. It is in the child's best interest that the staff communicates with parents/guardians about the child's needs and progress. Parent/guardian support groups and parent/guardian involvement at every level of facility planning and delivery are usually beneficial to the children, parents/guardians, and staff. Communication among parents/guardians whose children attend the same facility helps the parents/guardians to share useful information and to be mutually supportive.

COMMENTS: The need for follow-up on needed intervention increases when an understanding of the need and motivation for the intervention has been achieved through personal contact. A health history ensures that all information needed to care for the child is available to the appropriate staff member. Special instructions, such as diet, can be copied for everyday use. Compliance can be assessed by reviewing the records of these planned communications.

Parents/guardians who use child care services should be regarded as active participants and partners in facilities that meet their needs as well as their children's. Especially for infants and toddlers, authentic relationships are crucial to the optimal development of the child. Compliance can be measured by interviewing parents/guardians and staff.

TYPE OF FACILITY: Center; Large Family Child Care Home; Small Family Child Care Home

RELATED STANDARDS:
Standard 1.3.2.7: Qualifications and Responsibilities for Health Advocates
Standard 4.2.0.2: Assessment and Planning of Nutrition for Individual Children
Standards 9.2.3.4-9.2.3.8: Plan for Child Health Services
Standards 9.4.2.1-9.4.2.8: Health Reports/Records

REFERENCES:
1. Aronson, S. 2002. *Model Child Care Health Policies*. 4th ed. Bryn Mawr, PA: American Academy of Pediatrics, Pennsylvania Chapter.
2. Connell, C. M., R. J. Prinz. 2002. The impact of childcare and parent–child interactions on school readiness and social skills development for low-income African American children. *J of School Psychology* 40:177-93.

STANDARD 2.3.2.2: Seeking Parent/Guardian Input

At least twice a year, each caregiver/teacher should seek the views of parents/guardians about the strengths and needs of the indoor and outdoor learning/play environment and their satisfaction with the services offered. Caregivers/teachers should honor parents'/guardians' requests for more frequent reviews. Anonymous surveys can be offered as a way to receive parent/guardian input without parents/guardians feeling concerned if they have negative comments or concerns about the facility or practices within a facility.

RATIONALE: Parents/guardians and caregiver/teacher alike recognize that parents/guardians have essential rights in helping to shape the kind of child care service their children receive (1).

COMMENTS: Asking parents/guardians about their concerns and observations is essential so they can share issues and engage with staff in collaborative problem-solving. Small and large family child care homes should have group meetings of all parents/guardians once or twice a year. This standard avoids mention of procedures that are inappropriate to small family child care, as it does not require any explicit mechanism (such as a parent/guardian advisory council) for obtaining or offering parental/guardian input. Individual or group meetings with parents/guardians would suffice to meet this standard. Seeking consumer input is a cornerstone of facility planning and evaluation. Centers can offer parents/guardians the chance to respond in writing.

Accreditation organizations such as the National Association for the Education of Young Children (NAEYC) or the National Association for Family Child Care (NAFCC) have guidance on conducting parent/guardian surveys.

TYPE OF FACILITY: Center; Large Family Child Care Home; Small Family Child Care Home

REFERENCES:

1. National Association of Child Care Resource and Referral Agencies. It's a win-win situation: When parents and providers work together. Child Care Aware. http://ccaapps.childcareaware.org/en/subscriptions/dailyparent/volume.php?id=29.

STANDARD 2.3.2.3: Support Services for Parents/Guardians

Caregivers/teachers should establish parent/guardian groups and parent/guardian support services. Caregivers/teachers should have a regularly established means of communicating to parents/guardians the existence of these groups and support services. Caregivers/teachers should document these services and should include intra-agency activities or other community support group offerings. The caregiver/teacher should record parental/guardian participation in these on-site activities in the facility record.

One strategy for supporting parents/guardians is to facilitate communication among parents/guardians. The facility should give consenting parents/guardians a list of names and phone numbers of other consenting parents/guardians whose children attend the same facility. The list should include an annotation encouraging parents/guardians whose children attend the same facility to communicate with one another about the service. The facility should update the list at least annually.

RATIONALE: Parental/guardian involvement at every level of program planning and delivery and parent/guardian support groups are elements that are usually beneficial to the children, parents/guardians, and staff of the facility (1). The parent/guardian association group facilitates mutual understanding between the program and parents/guardians. Parental/guardian involvement also helps to broaden parents'/guardians' knowledge of administration of the facility and develops and enhances advocacy efforts (1).

Encouraging parents'/guardians' communication is simple, inexpensive, and beneficial. Such communication may include the exchange of positive aspects of the facility and positive knowledge about children's peers. If parents/guardians communicate with each other, they can share concerns about the behavior of a specific caregiver/teacher and can identify patterns of action suggestive of abuse/neglect. Parents/guardians can encourage each other to report all concerns to the director or owner of the program.

COMMENTS: Parent/guardian meetings within a facility are useful means of communication that supplement mailings and indirect contacts.

TYPE OF FACILITY: Center; Large Family Child Care Home; Small Family Child Care Home

REFERENCES:

1. National Association of Child Care Resource and Referral Agencies. It's a win-win situation: When parents and providers work together. Child Care Aware. http://ccaapps.childcareaware.org/en/subscriptions/dailyparent/volume.php?id=29.

STANDARD 2.3.2.4: Parent/Guardian Complaint Procedures

Facilities should have in place complaint resolution procedures to jointly resolve with parents/guardians any problems that may arise. Arrangements for hearing (or receiving) the complaint and the actions (or discussion) resulting in resolution should be documented along with dates and people involved. Facilities should develop mechanisms for holding formal and informal meetings between staff and groups of parents/guardians. Substantiated complaints and their resolution(s) should be posted in a prominent location. Facilities should post the complaint and resolution procedure where parents/guardians can easily see (or view) them.

RATIONALE: Coordination between the facility and the parents/guardians is essential to promote their respective child care roles and to avoid confusion or conflicts surrounding values. In addition to routine meetings, special meetings can deal with crises and unique problems. Complaint and resolution documentation records can help program directors assess problem areas of the facility, staff, and services.

COMMENTS: Special meetings could identify facility needs, assist in developing resources, and recommend facility and policy changes to the governing body. It is most helpful to document the proceedings of these meetings to facilitate future communications and to ensure continuity of service delivery. Facility-sponsored activities could take place outside facility hours and at other venues.

TYPE OF FACILITY: Center; Large Family Child Care Home; Small Family Child Care Home

RELATED STANDARDS:

Standard 1.8.2.5: Handling Complaints About Caregivers/Teachers
Standard 9.1.0.1: Governing Body of the Facility
Standard 9.1.0.2: Written Delegation of Administrative Authority
Standard 9.4.1.4: Access to Facility Records
Standard 10.4.3.1: Procedure for Receiving Complaints

2.3.3 Health Information Sharing

STANDARD 2.3.3.1: Parents'/Guardians' Provision of Information on Their Child's Health and Behavior

The facility should ask parents/guardians for information regarding the child's health, nutrition, level of physical activity, and behavioral status upon registration or when there has been an extended gap in the child's attendance at the facility. The child's health record should be updated if s/he have had any changes in their health or immunization status. Parents/guardians should be encouraged to sign a release of information/agreement so that child care workers can communicate directly with the child's medical home/primary care provider.

RATIONALE: Admission of children without this information will leave the center unprepared to deal with daily and emergent health needs of the child, other children, and staff if there is a question of communicability of disease.

COMMENTS: It would be helpful to also have updated information about the health status of parents/guardians and siblings, noting any special conditions, circumstances, or stress that may be affecting the child in care. Some parents/guardians may resist providing this information. If so, the caregiver/teacher should invite them to view this exchange of information as an opportunity to express their own concerns about the facility (1).

TYPE OF FACILITY: Center; Large Family Child Care Home; Small Family Child Care Home

RELATED STANDARDS:
Standards 3.6.1.1-3.6.1.2: Inclusion/Exclusion Due to Illness
Standard 9.2.1.3: Enrollment Information to Parents/Guardians and Caregivers/Teachers
Standard 9.4.2.1: Contents of Child's Records

REFERENCES:
1. Crowley, A. A., G. C. Whitney. 2005. Connecticut's new comprehensive and universal early childhood health assessment form. *J School Health* 75:281-85.

STANDARD 2.3.3.2: Communication from Specialists

Health and safety, education, and other specialists/professionals who come into the facility to furnish special services to a child should communicate at each visit with the caregiver/teacher at the facility. The specialist/professional must also be certain that all communication shared with caregivers/teachers is shared directly with the parent/guardian. These specialists may include, but are not limited to, physicians, registered nurses, child care health consultants, behavioral consultants (e.g., psychologists, counselors, clinical social workers), occupational therapists, physical therapists, speech therapists, educational therapists, registered dietitians, and play facilitator. The discussions should be documented in the child's Care Plan.

Specialists should use the facility's sign in/sign out system for accurate tracking of their interactions with or on behalf of the child.

RATIONALE: Therapeutic services must be coordinated with the child's general education program and with the parents/guardians and caregivers/teachers so everyone understands the child's needs. To be most useful, the service providers must share the therapeutic techniques with the caregivers/teachers and parents/guardians and integrate them into the child's daily routines, not just at therapy sessions. Parent/guardian consent to share information may be necessary. A child care health consultant can be helpful in coordinating these techniques and treatments.

TYPE OF FACILITY: Center; Large Family Child Care Home; Small Family Child Care Home

RELATED STANDARDS:
Standard 9.2.4.7: Sign-In/Sign-Out System
Standards 9.4.2.1-9.4.2.8: Child Records

2.4 Health Education

2.4.1 Health Education for Children

STANDARD 2.4.1.1: Health and Safety Education Topics for Children

Health and safety education for children should include physical, oral, mental, emotional, nutritional, and social health and should be integrated daily into the program of activities, to include such topics as:

a) Body awareness and use of appropriate terms for body parts;
b) Families (including information that all families are different and have unique beliefs and cultural heritage);
c) Personal social skills such as sharing, being kind, helping others, and communicating appropriately;
d) Expression and identification of feelings;
e) Self-esteem;
f) Nutrition, healthy eating (preventing obesity);
g) Outdoor learning/play;
h) Fitness and age-appropriate physical activity;
i) Personal and dental hygiene including wiping, flushing, handwashing, cough and sneezing etiquette and toothbrushing;
j) Safety (such as home, vehicular car seats and safety belts, playground, bicycle, fire, and firearms, water safety, personal safety, what to do in an emergency, getting help and/or dialing 9-1-1 for emergencies);
k) Conflict management, violence prevention, and bullying prevention;
l) Age-appropriate first aid concepts;
m) Healthy and safe behaviors;
n) Poisoning prevention and poison safety;
o) Awareness of routine preventive and special health care needs;
p) Importance of rest and sleep;
q) Health risks of secondhand smoke;
r) Taking medications;
s) Handling food safely; and
t) Preventing choking and falls.

RATIONALE: For young children, health and safety education are inseparable from one another. Children learn about health and safety by experiencing risk taking and risk control, fostered by adults who are involved with them. Whenever opportunities for learning arise; caregivers/teachers should integrate education to promote healthy and safe behaviors (1). Health and safety education does not have to be seen as a structured curriculum, but as a daily component of the planned program that is part of child development. Health and safety education supports and reinforces a healthy and safe lifestyle (1,2).

COMMENTS: Teaching children the appropriate names for their body parts is a good way to increase self esteem and personal safety. Learning about routine health maintenance practices such as receiving vaccines, having vision screening, blood pressure screening, oral health examinations,

and blood tests helps children understand these activities and appreciate their value rather than fearing them. Similarly, learning about the importance of fitness choices helps children make responsible healthful decisions when facing abundant temptation to do otherwise.

Certified health education specialists (CHES) are good resources for this instruction. The American Association for Health Education (AAHE), the National Commission for Health Education Credentialing. (NCHEC), and the State and Territorial Injury Prevention Directors' Association (STIPDA) provide information on this specialty.

TYPE OF FACILITY: Center; Large Family Child Care Home; Small Family Child Care Home

REFERENCES:

1. Gupta, R. S., S. Shuman, E. M. Taveras, M. Kulldorff, J. A. Finkelstein. 2005. Opportunities for health promotion education in child care. *Pediatrics* 116: e499-e505.
2. Hemmeter, M. L., L. Fox, S. Jack, L. Broyles. 2007. A program-wide model of positive behavior support in early childhood settings. *J Early Intervention* 29:337-55.

STANDARD 2.4.1.2: Staff Modeling of Healthy and Safe Behavior and Health and Safety Education Activities

The program should strongly encourage all staff members to model healthy and safe behaviors and attitudes in their contact with children in the indoor and outdoor learning/play environment, including, eating nutritious foods, drinking water or nutritious beverages when with the children, sitting with children during mealtime, and eating some of the same foods as the children. Caregivers/teachers should engage in daily movement and physical activity, limiting sedentary behaviors when in the outdoor learning/play environment (e.g., not sitting in structured chairs), not watching TV, and should comply with tobacco and drug use policies and handwashing protocols.

Caregivers/teachers should talk about and model healthy and safe behaviors while they carry out routine daily activities. Activities should be accompanied by words of encouragement and praise for achievement.

Facilities should encourage and support staff who wish to breastfeed their own infants and those who engage in gardening to enhance interest in healthy food, science, inquiries and learning. Staff are consistently a model for children and should be cognizant of the environmental information and print messages they bring into the indoor and outdoor learning/play environment. The labels and print messages that are present in the indoor and outdoor learning/play environment or family child care home should be in line with the healthy and safe behaviors and attitudes they wish to impart to the children.

Facilities should use developmentally appropriate health and safety education materials in the children's activities and should also share these with the families whenever possible. All health and safety education activities should be geared to the child's developmental age and should take into account individual personalities and interests.

RATIONALE: Modeling is an effective way of confirming that a behavior is one to be imitated. Young children are particularly dependent on adults for their nutritional needs in both the home (1) and child care environment (2). Thus, modeling healthy and safe behaviors is an important way to demonstrate and reinforce healthy and safe behaviors of caregivers/teachers and children. Young children learn better through experiencing an activity and observing behavior than through didactic training (3,4). Learning and play have a reciprocal relationship; play experiences are closely related to learning (5).

Caregivers/teachers impact the nutrition habits of the children under their care, not only by making choices regarding the types of foods that are available but by influencing children's attitudes and beliefs about that food as well as social interactions at mealtime. This provides a unique opportunity for programs to guide children's choices by assigning parents/guardians and caregivers/teachers to the role of nutritional gatekeepers for the young children in their care. Such intervention is consistent with the USDA and U.S. Department of Health and Human Services (DHHS) recent release of 2010 Dietary Guidelines for Americans. The Dietary Guidelines focus on increased healthy eating and physical activity to reduce the current rate of overweight or obesity in American children (one in three in the nation) (6).

The effectiveness of health and safety education is enhanced when shared between the caregiver/teacher and the parents/guardians (7).

COMMENTS: Caregivers/teachers are important in the lives of the young children in their care. They should be educated and supported to be able to interact optimally with the children in their care. Compliance should be documented by observation. Consultation can be sought from a child care health consultant or certified health education specialist. The American Association for Health Education (AAHE) and the National Commission for Health Education Credentialing (NCHEC) provide information on this specialty.

An extensive education program to make such experiential learning possible indoors and outdoors should be supported by strong community resources in the form of both consultation and materials from sources such as the health department, nutrition councils, and so forth. Suggestions for topics and methods of presentation are widely available (8). Examples include, but are not limited to, routine preventive care by health professionals, nutrition education and physical activity to prevent obesity, crossing streets safely, how to develop and use outdoor learning/play environments, car restraint safety, poison safety, latch key programs, health risks from secondhand smoke, personal hygiene, and oral health, including limiting sweets, rinsing the mouth with water after sweets, and regular tooth brushing. It can be helpful to place visual cues in the indoor and outdoor learning/play environments to serve as reminders (e.g., posters). "Risk Watch" is a prepared curriculum from the National

Fire Protection Association (NFPA) offering comprehensive injury prevention strategies for children in preschool through eighth grade (9).

TYPE OF FACILITY: Center; Large Family Child Care Home; Small Family Child Care Home

RELATED STANDARDS:
Standard 2.2.0.3: Limiting Screen Time – Media, Computer Time
Standard 2.4.1.1: Health and Safety Education Topics for Children
Standard 2.4.1.2: Staff Modeling of Healthy and Safe Behavior and Health and Safety Education Activities
Standard 3.1.3.1: Active Opportunities for Physical Activity
Standard 3.1.3.2: Playing Outdoors
Standard 3.1.3.4: Caregivers'/Teachers' Encouragement of Physical Activity
Standard 3.2.2.1: Situations that Require Handwashing
Standard 3.2.2.2: Handwashing Procedure
Standard 3.4.1.1: Use of Tobacco, Alcohol, and Illegal Drugs
Standard 4.2.0.1: Written Nutrition Plan
Standard 4.2.0.6: Availability of Drinking Water
Standard 4.3.1.1: General Plan for Feeding Infants
Standard 4.3.1.3: Preparing, Feeding, and Storing Human Milk
Standard 4.3.2.2: Serving Size for Toddlers and Preschoolers
Standard 4.3.3.1: Meal and Snack Patterns for School-Age Children
Standard 4.5.0.4: Socialization During Meals
Standard 4.5.0.7: Participation of Older Children and Staff in Mealtime Activities
Standard 4.6.0.2: Nutritional Quality of Food Brought from Home
Standard 4.7.0.1: Nutrition Learning Experiences for Children

REFERENCES:
1. Lindsay, A. C., K. M. Sussner, J. Kim, S. Gortmaker. 2006. The role of parents in preventing childhood obesity. *Future Child* 16:169-86.
2. McBean, L. D., G. D. Miller. 1999. Enhancing the nutrition of America's youth. *J Am College of Nutrition* 18:563-71.
3. Evaldson, A., W. A. Corsaro. 1998. Play and games in the peer cultures of preschool and preadolescent children: An interpretative approach. *Childhood* 5:377-402.
4. Hemmeter, M. L., L. Fox, S. Jack, L. Broyles. 2007. A program-wide model of positive behavior support in early childhood settings. *J Early Intervention* 29:337-55.
5. Petersen, E. A. 1998. The amazing benefits of play. *Child Fam* 17:7-8.
6. U.S. Department of Agriculture, "USDA and HHS Announce New Dietary Guidelines to Help Americans Make Healthier Food Choices and Confront Obesity Epidemic," press release June 2, 2011.
7. Holmes, M., et al. 1996. *Promising partnerships: How to develop successful partnerships in your community*. Alexandria, VA: National Head Start Association.
8. Gupta, R. S., S. Shuman, E. M. Taveras, M. Kulldorff, J. A. Finkelstein. 2005. Opportunities for health promotion education in child care. *Pediatrics* 116: e499-505.
9. Kendrick, D., L. Groom, J. Stewart, M. Watson, C. Mulvaney, R. Casterton. 2007. Risk Watch: Cluster randomized controlled trial evaluating an injury prevention program. *Injury Prevention* 13:93-99.

STANDARD 2.4.1.3: Gender and Body Awareness

The facility should prepare caregivers/teachers to appropriately discuss with the children anatomical facts related to gender identity and sex differences. When talking with parents/guardians, caregivers/teachers should take a general approach, while respecting cultural differences, acknowledging that all children engage in fantasy play, dressing up and trying out different roles (1). Caregivers/teachers should give children messages that contrast with stereotypes, such as men and women in non-traditional roles (2). Facilities should strive for developing common language and understanding among all the partners.

RATIONALE: Open discussions among adults concerning childhood sexuality increase their comfort with the subject. The adults' comfort may reduce children's anxiety about sexuality (3,4).

COMMENTS: Discussing sexuality and gender identity topics with young children is not always easy because the views of facility administrators, caregivers/teachers, parents/guardians, and community leaders on these topics may differ.

TYPE OF FACILITY: Center; Large Family Child Care Home; Small Family Child Care Home

REFERENCES:
1. Stein, M., K. Zuckert, S. Dixon. 2001. Sammy: Gender identity concerns in a six year old boy. *Pediatrics* 107:850-854.
2. National Association for the Education of Young Children (NAEYC). 1997. *Teaching young children to resist bias*. Early Years are Learning Years Series. Washington, DC: NAEYC.
3. Couchenour, D., K. Chrisman. 2002. *Healthy sexuality development: A guide for early childhood educators and families*. Washington, DC: National Association for the Education of Young Children.
4. Brill, S. A., R. Pepper. 2008. *The transgender child: A handbook for families and professionals*. San Francisco: Cleis.

2.4.2 Health Education for Staff

STANDARD 2.4.2.1: Health and Safety Education Topics for Staff

Health and safety education for staff should include physical, oral, mental, emotional, nutritional, physical activity, and social health of children. In addition to the health and safety topics for children in Standard 2.4.1.1, health education topics for staff should include:

a) Promoting healthy mind and brain development through child care;
b) Healthy indoor and outdoor learning/play environments;
c) Behavior/discipline;
d) Managing emergency situations;
e) Monitoring developmental abilities, including indicators of potential delays;
f) Nutrition (i.e., healthy eating to prevent obesity);
g) Food safety;
h) Water safety;
i) Safety/injury prevention;
j) Safe use, storage, and clean-up of chemicals;
k) Hearing, vision, and language problems;
l) Physical activity and outdoor play and learning;
m) Appropriate antibiotic use;
n) Immunizations;
o) Gaining access to community resources;
p) Maternal or parental/guardian depression;

q) Exclusion policies;
r) Tobacco use/smoking;
s) Safe sleep environments and SIDS prevention;
t) Breastfeeding support (1);
u) Environmental health and reducing exposures to environmental toxins;
v) Children with special needs;
w) Shaken baby syndrome and abusive head trauma;
x) Safe use, storage of firearms;
y) Safe medication administration.

RATIONALE: When child care staff are knowledgeable in health and safety practices, programs are more likely to be healthy and safe (2). Compliance with twenty hours per year of staff continuing education in the areas of health, safety, child development, and abuse identification was the most significant predictor for compliance with state child care health and safety regulations (3). Child care staff often receive their health and safety education from a child care health consultant. Data support the relationship between child care health consultation and the increased health and safety of a center (4,5).

COMMENTS: Community resources can provide written health- and safety-related materials. Consultation or training can be sought from a child care health consultant (CCHC) or certified health education specialist (CHES).

Child care programs should consider offering "credit" for health education classes or encourage staff members to attend accredited education programs that can give education credits.

The American Association for Health Education (AAHE), the National Commission for Health Education Credentialing (NCHEC), and the National Training Institute for Child Care Health Consultants (NTI) provide information on certified health education specialists.

TYPE OF FACILITY: Center; Large Family Child Care Home; Small Family Child Care Home

RELATED STANDARDS:
Standards 1.4.2.1-1.4.6.2: Professional Training, Education, and Compensation
Standard 2.4.1.1: Health Education Topics for Children

REFERENCES:

1. Gupta, R. S., S. Shuman, E. M. Taveras, M. Kulldorff, J. A. Finkelstein. 2005. Opportunities for health promotion education in child care. *Pediatrics* 116: e499-e505.
2. Alkon, A., J. Bernzweig, K. To, M. Wolff, J. F. Mackie. 2009. Child care health consultation improves health and safety policies and practices. *Academic Pediatrics* 9:366–70.
3. Crowley, A. A., M. S. Rosenthal. 2009. Ensuring the health and safety of Connecticut's early care and education programs. Farmington, CT: The Child Health and Development Institute of Connecticut. http://www.chdi.org/admin/uploads/3074013304b154ef428c1a.pdf.
4. Snohomish Health District: Child Care Health Program. Child care health consultation: Evidence based effectiveness. http://www.napnap.org/docs/CCS_SIG_Evidence_ Based_ CCHP.pdf.
5. Rosenthal, M. S., A. A. Crowley, L. Curry. 2009. Promoting child development and behavioral health: Family child care providers' perspectives. *J Pediatric Health Care* 23:289-97.

2.4.3 Health Education for Parents/Guardians

STANDARD 2.4.3.1: Opportunities for Communication and Modeling of Health and Safety Education for Parents/Guardians

Parents/guardians should be given opportunities to observe staff members modeling healthy and safe behavior and facilitating child development, both indoors and outdoors. Parents/guardians should also have opportunities to ask questions and to describe how effective the modeling has been. For parents/guardians who may not have the opportunity to visit their child or observe during the day, there should be alternate forms of communication between the staff and the parents/guardians. This can be handouts, written journals that would go between facility and home, newsletters, electronic communication, or events.

RATIONALE: Modeling and communication about healthy and safe behaviors that promote positive development can be an effective educational tool (1,2).

TYPE OF FACILITY: Center; Large Family Child Care Home; Small Family Child Care Home

REFERENCES:

1. Lehman, G. R., E. S. Geller. 1990. Participative education for children: An effective approach to increase safety belt use. *J Appl Behav Anal* 23:219-25.
2. Lindsay, A. C., K. M. Sussner, J. Kim, S. Gortmaker. 2006. The role of parents in preventing childhood obesity. *Future Child* 16:169-86.

STANDARD 2.4.3.2: Parent/Guardian Education Plan

The content of a parent/guardian education plan should be individualized to meet each family's needs and should be sensitive to cultural values and beliefs. Written material, at a minimum, should address the most important health and safety issues for all age groups served, should be in a language understood by families, and may include the topics listed in Standard 2.4.1.1, with special emphasis on the following:

a) Safety (such as home, community, playground, firearm, seat belts, safe medication administration procedures, poison awareness, vehicular, or bicycle, and awareness of environmental toxins and healthy choices to reduce exposure);
b) Value of developing healthy and safe lifestyle choices early in life and parental/guardian health (such as exercise and routine physical activity, nutrition, weight control, breastfeeding, avoidance of substance abuse and tobacco use, stress management, maternal depression, HIV/AIDS prevention);
c) Importance of outdoor play and learning;
d) Importance of role modeling;
e) Importance of well-child care (such as immunizations, hearing/vision screening, monitoring growth and development);

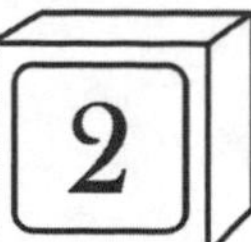

f) Child development and behavior including bonding and attachment;
g) Domestic and relational violence;
h) Conflict management and violence prevention;
i) Oral health promotion and disease prevention;
j) Effective toothbrushing, handwashing, diapering, and sanitation;
k) Positive discipline, effective communication, and behavior management;
l) Handling emergencies/first aid;
m) Child advocacy skills;
n) Special health care needs;
o) Information on how to access services such as the supplemental food and nutrition program (i.e., The Women, Infants and Children [WIC] Supplemental Food Program), Food Stamps (SNAP), food pantries, as well as access to medical/health care and services for developmental disabilities for children;
p) Handling loss, deployment, and divorce;
q) The importance of routines and traditions (including reading and early literacy) with a child.

Health and safety education for parents/guardians should utilize principles of adult learning to maximize the potential for parents/guardians to learn about key concepts. Facilities should utilize opportunities for learning, such as the case of an illness present in the facility, to inform parents/guardians about illness and prevention strategies.

The staff should introduce seasonal topics when they are relevant to the health and safety of parents/guardians and children.

RATIONALE: Adults learn best when they are motivated, comfortable, and respected; when they can immediately apply what they have learned; and when multiple learning strategies are used. Individualized content and approaches are needed for successful intervention. Parent/guardian attitudes, beliefs, fears, and educational and socioeconomic levels all should be given consideration in planning and conducting parent/guardian education (1,2). Parental/guardian behavior can be modified by education. Parents/guardians should be involved closely with the facility and be actively involved in planning parent/guardian education activities. If done well, adult learning activities can be effective for educating parents/guardians. If not done well, there is a danger of demeaning parents/guardians and making them feel less, rather than more, capable (1,2).

The concept of parent/guardian control and empowerment is key to successful parent/guardian education in the child care setting. Support and education for parents/guardians lead to better parenting skills and abilities.

Knowing the family will help the staff such as the health and safety advocate determine content of the parent/guardian education plan and method for delivery. Specific attention should be paid to the parents'/guardians' need for support and consultation and help locating resources for their problems. If the facility suggests a referral or resource, this should be documented in the child's record. Specifics of what the parent/guardian shared need not be recorded.

COMMENTS: Community resources can provide written health- and safety-related materials. School-age child care facilities may incorporate child health education into their programs as they can be integrated into their regular activities, (e.g., handwashing before snack, making healthful snack choices, pointing out why screen time limits are in place to promote physical activity, safe playground behaviors, and where possible, making an attempt to coordinate with formal health education enrollees receive in school).

TYPE OF FACILITY: Center; Large Family Child Care Home; Small Family Child Care Home

RELATED STANDARDS:

Standard 1.3.2.7: Qualifications and Responsibilities for Health Advocates
Standard 2.4.1.1: Health Education Topics for Children

REFERENCES:

1. Gonzalez-Mena, J. 1996. When values collide: Exploring a cross cultural issue. *Child Care Infor Exch* 108:30-32.
2. Hendricks, C., M. Russell, C. J. Smith. 1997. Staying healthy: Strategies for helping parents ensure their children's health and well being. *Child Fam* 16:10-17.

Chapter 3

3

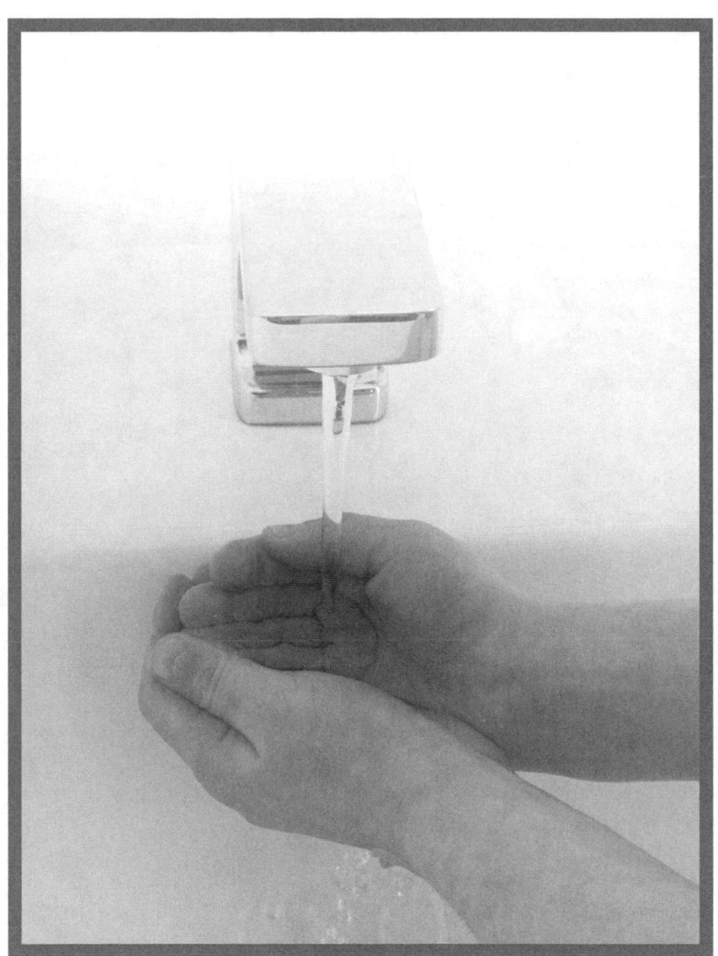

Health Promotion and Protection

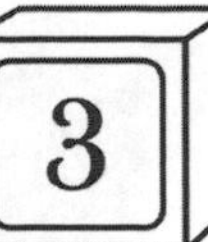

3.1 Health Promotion in Child Care

3.1.1 Daily Health Check

STANDARD 3.1.1.1: Conduct of Daily Health Check

Every day, a trained staff member should conduct a health check of each child. This health check should be conducted as soon as possible after the child enters the child care facility and whenever a change in the child's behavior or appearance is noted while that child is in care. The health check should address:

a) Reported or observed illness or injury affecting the child or family members since the last date of attendance;
b) Reported or observed changes in behavior of the child (such as lethargy or irritability) or in the appearance (e.g., sad) of the child from the previous day at home or the previous day's attendance at child care;
c) Skin rashes, impetigo, itching or scratching of the skin, itching or scratching of the scalp, or the presence of one or more live crawling lice;
d) A temperature check if the child appears ill (a daily screening temperature check is not recommended);
e) Other signs or symptoms of illness and injury (such as drainage from eyes, vomiting, diarrhea, cuts/lacerations, pain, or feeling ill).

The caregiver/teacher should gain information necessary to complete the daily health check by direct observation of the child, by querying the parent/guardian, and, where applicable, by conversation with the child.

RATIONALE: Daily health checks seek to identify potential concerns about a child's health including recent illness or injury in the child and the family. Health checks may serve to reduce the transmission of infectious diseases in child care settings by identifying children who should be excluded, and enable the caregivers/teachers to plan for necessary care while the child is in care at the facility.

COMMENTS: The daily health check should be performed in a relaxed and comfortable manner that respects the family's culture as well as the child's body and feelings. The child care health consultant should train the caregiver/teacher(s) in conducting a health check. The items in the standard can serve as a checklist to guide learning the procedure until it becomes routine.

The obtaining of information from the parent/guardian should take place at the time of transfer of care from the parent/guardian to the staff of the child care facility. If this exchange of information happens outside the facility (e.g., when the child is put on a bus), the facility should use an alternative means to accurately convey important information. Handwritten notes, electronic communications, health checklists, and/or daily logs are examples of how parents/guardians and staff can exchange information when face-to-face is not possible.

TYPE OF FACILITY: Center; Large Family Child Care Home; Small Family Child Care Home

RELATED STANDARDS:
Standard 1.6.0.1: Child Care Health Consultants
Standard 3.6.1.1: Inclusion/Exclusion/Dismissal of Children
Appendix A: Signs and Symptoms Chart
Appendix F: Enrollment/Attendance/Symptom Record
Appendix G: Recommended Immunization Schedules for Persons Aged 0 Through 18 Years–United States, 2011

STANDARD 3.1.1.2: Documentation of the Daily Health Check

The caregiver/teacher should conduct and document a daily health check of each child upon arrival. The daily health check documentation should be kept for one month.

RATIONALE: The vast majority of infectious diseases of concern in child care have incubation periods of less than twenty-one days (1). This information may be helpful to public health authorities investigating occasional outbreaks.

COMMENTS: The documentation should note that the daily health check was done and any deviation from the usual status of the child and family.

TYPE OF FACILITY: Center; Large Family Child Care Home; Small Family Child Care Home

RELATED STANDARDS:
Standards 9.4.1.9-9.4.1.11: Incidence Logs of Illness, Injury, and Other Problems
Standards 9.4.2.1-9.4.2.8: Child Records

REFERENCES:
1. California Childcare Health Program. CCHP health and safety checklist. Rev. ed. http://www.ucsfchildcarehealth.org/html/pandr/formsmain.htm#hscr/.

3.1.2 Routine Health Supervision

STANDARD 3.1.2.1: Routine Health Supervision and Growth Monitoring

The facility should require that each child has routine health supervision by the child's primary care provider, according to the standards of the American Academy of Pediatrics (AAP) (3). For all children, health supervision includes routine screening tests, immunizations, and chronic or acute illness monitoring. For children younger than twenty-four months of age, health supervision includes documentation and plotting of sex-specific charts on child growth standards from the World Health Organization (WHO), available at http://www.who.int/childgrowth/standards/en/, and assessing diet and activity. For children twenty-four months of age and older, sex-specific height and weight graphs should be plotted by the primary care provider in addition to body mass index (BMI), according to the Centers for Disease Control and Prevention (CDC). BMI is classified as underweight (BMI less than 5%), healthy weight (BMI 5%-84%), overweight (BMI 85%-94%), and obese (BMI equal to or greater than 95%).

Follow-up visits with the child's primary care provider that include a full assessment and laboratory evaluations should be scheduled for children with weight for length greater than 95% and BMI greater than 85% (5).

School health services can meet this standard for school-age children in care if they meet the AAP's standards for school-age children and if the results of each child's examinations are shared with the caregiver/teacher as well as with the school health system. With parental/guardian consent, pertinent health information should be exchanged among the child's routine source of health care and all participants in the child's care, including any school health program involved in the care of the child.

RATIONALE: Provision of routine preventive health services for children ensures healthy growth and development and helps detect disease when it is most treatable. Immunization prevents or reduces diseases for which effective vaccines are available. When children are receiving care that involves the school health system, such care should be coordinated by the exchange of information, with parental/guardian permission, among the school health system, the child's medical home, and the caregiver/teacher. Such exchange will ensure that all participants in the child's care are aware of the child's health status and follow a common care plan.

The plotting of height and weight measurements and plotting and classification of BMI by the primary care provider or school health personnel, on a reference growth chart, will show how children are growing over time and how they compare with other children of the same chronological age and sex (1,3,4). Growth charts are based on data from national probability samples, representative of children in the general population. Their use by the primary care provider may facilitate early recognition of growth concerns, leading to further evaluation, diagnosis, and the development of a plan of care. Such a plan of care, if communicated to the caregiver/teacher, can direct the caregiver's/teacher's attention to disease, poor nutrition, or inadequate physical activity that requires modification of feeding or other health practices in the early care and education setting (2).

COMMENTS: Periodic and accurate height and weight measurements that are obtained, plotted, and interpreted by a person who is competent in performing these tasks provide an important indicator of health status. If such measurements are made in the early care and education facility, the data from the measurements should be shared by the facility, subject to parental/guardian consent, with everyone involved in the child's care, including parents/guardians, caregivers/teachers, and the child's primary care provider. The child care health consultant can provide staff training on growth assessment. It is important to maintain strong linkage among the early care and education facility, school, parent/guardian, and the child's primary care provider. Screening results (physical and behavioral) and laboratory assessments are only useful if a plan for care can be developed to initiate and maintain lifestyle changes that incorporate the child's activities during their time at the early care and education program.

The Special Supplemental Nutrition Program for Women, Infants, and Children (WIC) can also be a source for the BMI data with parental/guardian consent, as WIC tracks growth and development if the child is enrolled.

For BMI charts by sex and age, see http://www.cdc.gov/growthcharts/clinical_charts.htm.

TYPE OF FACILITY: Center; Large Family Child Care Home; Small Family Child Care Home

RELATED STANDARDS:
Standard 4.2.0.2: Assessment and Planning of Nutrition for Individual Children

REFERENCES:
1. Paige, D. M. 1988. *Clinical nutrition.* 2nd ed. St. Louis: Mosby.
2. Kleinman, R. E. 2009. *Pediatric nutrition handbook.* 6th ed. Elk Grove Village, IL: American Academy of Pediatrics.
3. Hagan, J. F., J. S. Shaw, P. M. Duncan, eds. 2008. *Bright futures: Guidelines for health supervision of infants, children, and adolescents.* 3rd ed. Elk Grove Village, IL: American Academy of Pediatrics.
4. Story, M., K. Holt, D. Sofka, eds. 2002. *Bright futures in practice: Nutrition.* 2nd ed. Arlington, VA: National Center for Education in Maternal and Child Health.
5. Centers for Disease Control and Prevention. 2011. About BMI for children and teens. http://www.cdc.gov/healthyweight/assessing/bmi/childrens_bmi/about_childrens_bmi.html.

3.1.3 Physical Activity and Limiting Screen Time

STANDARD 3.1.3.1: Active Opportunities for Physical Activity

The facility should promote children's active play every day. Children should have ample opportunity to do moderate to vigorous activities such as running, climbing, dancing, skipping, and jumping. All children, birth to six years, should participate daily in:

a) Two to three occasions of active play outdoors, weather permitting (see Standard 3.1.3.2: Playing Outdoors for appropriate weather conditions);
b) Two or more structured or caregiver/teacher/adult-led activities or games that promote movement over the course of the day—indoor or outdoor;
c) Continuous opportunities to develop and practice age-appropriate gross motor and movement skills.

The total time allotted for outdoor play and moderate to vigorous indoor or outdoor physical activity can be adjusted for the age group and weather conditions.

a) Outdoor play:
    1) Infants (birth to twelve months of age) should be taken outside two to three times per day, as tolerated. There is no recommended duration of infants' outdoor play;
    2) Toddlers (twelve months to three years) and preschoolers (three to six years) should be allowed sixty to ninety total minutes of outdoor play. These outdoor times can be curtailed somewhat during adverse weather conditions in which children may

still play safely outdoors for shorter periods, but should increase the time of indoor activity, so the total amount of exercise should remain the same;

b) Total time allotted for moderate to vigorous activities:
   1) Toddlers should be allowed sixty to ninety minutes per eight-hour day for moderate to vigorous physical activity, including running;
   2) Preschoolers should be allowed ninety to one hundred and twenty minutes per eight-hour day (4).

Infants should have supervised tummy time every day when they are awake. Beginning on the first day at the early care and education program, caregivers/teachers should interact with an awake infant on their tummy for short periods of time (three to five minutes), increasing the amount of time as the infant shows s/he enjoys the activity (27).

Time spent outdoors has been found to be a strong, consistent predictor of children's physical activity (1-3). Children can accumulate opportunities for activity over the course of several shorter segments of at least ten minutes each. Because structured activities have been shown to produce higher levels of physical activity in young children, it is recommended that caregivers/teachers incorporate two or more short structured activities (five to ten minutes) or games daily that promote physical activity.

Opportunities to be actively enjoying physical activity should be incorporated into part-time programs by prorating these recommendations accordingly, i.e., twenty minutes of outdoor play for every three hours in the facility.

Active play should never be withheld from children who misbehave (e.g., child is kept indoors to help another caregiver/teacher while the rest of the children go outside) (5). However, children with out-of-control behavior may need five minutes or less to calm themselves or settle down before resuming cooperative play or activities.

Infants should not be seated for more than fifteen minutes at a time, except during meals or naps. Infant equipment such as swings, stationary activity centers (ex. exersaucers), infant seats (ex. bouncers), molded seats, etc. if used should only be used for short periods of time. A least restrictive environment should be encouraged at all times (5,6,26).

Children should have adequate space for both inside and outside play.

RATIONALE: Free play, active play and outdoor play are essential components of young children's development (2). Children learn through play, developing gross motor, socio-emotional, and cognitive skills. In outdoor play, children learn about their environment, science, and nature.

Infants' and young children's participation in physical activity is critical to their overall health, development of motor skills, social skills, and maintenance of healthy weight (7). Daily physical activity promotes young children's gross motor development and provides numerous health benefits including improved fitness and cardiovascular health, healthy bone development, improved sleep, and improved mood and sense of well-being. Tummy time prepares infants for the time when they will be able to slide on their bellies and crawl. As infants grow older and stronger they will need more time on their tummies to build their own strength (27).

Daily physical activity is an important part of preventing excessive weight gain and childhood obesity. Some evidence also suggests that children may be able to learn better during or immediately after bursts of physical activity, due to improved attention and focus (8,9).

Numerous reports suggest that children are not meeting daily recommendations for physical activity, and that children spend 70% (10) to 87% (11) of their time in early care and education being sedentary, (i.e., sitting or lying down). Excluding nap time, children are sedentary 83% of the time (11). Children may only spend about 2% to 3% of time being moderately or vigorously active (11).

Very young children are entirely dependent on their caregivers/teachers for opportunities to be active (12-15). Especially for children in full-time care and for children who live in unsafe neighborhoods, the early care and education facility may provide the child's only daily opportunity for active play. Evidence suggests that physical activity habits learned early in life may track into adolescence and adulthood supporting the importance for children to learn lifelong healthy physical activity habits while in the early care and education program (13,16-25).

COMMENTS: There are many ways to promote tummy time with infants:

a) Place yourself or a toy just out of the infant's reach during playtime to get him to reach for you or the toy;
b) Place toys in a circle around the infant. Reaching to different points in the circle will allow him/her to develop the appropriate muscles to roll over, scoot on his/her belly, and crawl;
c) Lie on your back and place the infant on your chest. The infant will lift his/her head and use his/her arms to try to see your face (27).

There are a multitude of short, structured activities that are appropriate for toddlers and preschoolers. Structured activities could include popular children's games such as Simon Says, Mother May I, Red Rover, Get the Wiggles Out, Musical Chairs, or a simple walk through the neighborhood. For training materials and more ideas of effective and age-appropriate games for young children, consider the following resources:

a) "Nutrition and Physical Activity Self Assessment for Child Care - NAP SACC Program" – http://www.napsacc.org;
b) "Color Me Healthy Preschoolers Moving and Eating" – http://www.colormehealthy.com;
c) "Let's Move, Learn, and Have Fun" physical activity curriculum from Kansas State University;
d) "I am Moving I am Learning: Intervention in Head Start" – http://eclkc.ohs.acf.hhs.gov/hslc/tta-system/health/Health/Nutrition/Nutrition Program Staff/IamMovingIam.htm;

e) "Moving and Learning: The Physical Activity Specialists for Birth through Age 8" – http://www.movingandlearning.com;
f) "How to Lower Your Risk for Type 2 Diabetes: National Diabetes Education Program" – http://ndep.nih.gov/media/kids-tips-lower-risk.pdf;
g) "Motion Moments" – http://nrckids.org/Motion_Moments/.

Experts disagree about the appropriate amount of physical activity for toddlers and preschoolers, what proportion of children's physical activity should be structured, and to what extent structured activities are effective in producing children's physical activity. Researchers do agree that toddlers and preschoolers generally accumulate moderate to vigorous physical activity over the course of the day in very short bursts (fifteen to thirty seconds) (23). For additional recommendations by other national groups and experts, see:

a) The National Association for Sport and Physical Education's *Active Start: A Statement of Physical Activity Guidelines for Children From Birth to Age 5, 2nd Edition* at http://www.aahperd.org/naspe/standards/nationalGuidelines/ActiveStart.cfm and *Physical Activity for Children: A Statement of Guidelines for Children 5 - 12, 2nd Edition* at http://www.aahperd.org/naspe/standards/nationalGuidelines/PA-Children-5-12.cfm;
b) U.S. Department of Health and Human Services' *2008 Physical Activity Guidelines for Americans* at http://www.health.gov/PAGuidelines/Report/pdf/CommitteeReport.pdf;
c) U.S. Department of Health and Human Services and the U.S. Department of Agriculture's *Dietary Guidelines for Americans, 2010* at http://www.cnpp.usda.gov/DGAs2010-DGACReport.htm.

TYPE OF FACILITY: Center; Large Family Child Care Home; Small Family Child Care Home

RELATED STANDARDS:

Standard 2.1.1.2: Health, Nutrition, Physical Activity, and Safety Awareness
Standard 3.1.3.2: Playing Outdoors
Standard 3.1.3.4: Caregivers'/Teachers' Encouragement of Physical Activity
Standard 5.3.1.10: Restrictive Infant Equipment Requirements
Standard 9.2.3.1: Policies and Practices that Promote Physical Activity
Appendix S: Physical Activity: How Much Is Needed?

REFERENCES:

1. Brown, W. H., K. A. Pfeiffer, K. L. McIver, M. Dowda, C. L. Addy, R. R. Pate. 2009. Social and environmental factors associated with preschoolers' nonsedentary physical activity. *Child Devel* 80:45-58.
2. Burdette, H. L., R. C. Whitaker. 2005. Resurrecting free play in young children: Looking beyond fitness and fatness to attention, affiliation, and affect. Arch Pediatr Adolesc *Med* 159:46-50.
3. Burdette, H. L., R. C. Whitaker, S. R. Daniels. 2004. Parental report of outdoor playtime as a measure of physical activity in preschool-aged children. *Arch Pediatr Adolesc Med* 158:353-57.
4. Bower, J. K., D. P. Hales, D. F. Tate, D. A. Rubin, S. E. Benjamin, D. S. Ward. 2008. The childcare environment and children's physical activity. *Am J Prev Med* 34:23-29.
5. Benjamin, S. E., A. Ammerman, J. Sommers, J. Dodds, B. Neelon, D. S. Ward. 2007. *The nutrition and physical activity self-assessment for child care (NAP SACC).* Rev ed. Raleigh and Chapel Hill, NC: UNC Center for Health Promotion and Disease Prevention, Center of Excellence for Training and Research Translation. http://www.center-trt.org/downloads/obesity_prevention/interventions/napsacc/NAPSACC_Template.pdf.
6. National Association for Sport and Physical Education (NASPE). 2002. *Active start: A statement of physical activity guidelines for children birth to five years.* Washington, DC: NASPE.
7. Patrick, K., B. Spear, K. Holt, D. Sofka, eds. 2001. *Bright futures in practice: Physical activity.* Arlington, VA: National Center for Education in Maternal and Child Health. http://www.brightfutures.org/physicalactivity/pdf/index.html.
8. Pellegrini, A., C. Bohn. 2005. The role of recess in children's cognitive performance and school adjustment. *Educ Res* 34:13-19.
9. Mahar, M. T., S. K. Murphy, D. A. Rowe, J. Golden, A. T. Shields, T. D. Raedeke. 2006. Effects of a classroom-based program on physical activity and on-task behavior. *Med Sci Sports Exerc* 38:2086-94.
10. Pate, R. R., K. A. Pfeiffer, S. G. Trost, P. Ziegler, M. Dowda. 2004. Physical activity among children attending preschools. *Pediatrics* 114:1258-63.
11. Pate, R. R., K. McIver, M. Dowda, W. H. Brown, A. Cheryl. 2008. Directly observed physical activity levels in preschool children. *J Sch Health* 78:438-44.
12. McKenzie, T. L., J. F. Sallis, J. P. Elder, C. C. Berry, P. L. Hoy, P. R. Nader, M. M. Zive, S. L. Broyles. 1997. Physical activity levels and prompts in young children at recess: A two-year study of a bi-ethnic sample. *Res Q Exerc Sport* 68:195-202.
13. McKenzie, T. L., J. F. Sallis, P. R. Nader, S. L. Broyles, J. A. Nelson. 1992. Anglo- and Mexican-American preschoolers at home and at recess: Activity patterns and environmental influences. *J Dev Behav Pediatr* 13:173-80.
14. Sallis, J. F., T. L. McKenzie, J. P. Elder, S. L. Broyles, P. R. Nader. 1997. Factors parents use in selecting play spaces for young children. *Arch Pediatr Adolesc Med* 151:414-17.
15. Sallis, J. F., P. R. Nader, S. L. Broyles, J. P. Elder, T. L. McKenzie, J. A. Nelson. 1993. Correlates of physical activity at home in Mexican-American and Anglo-American preschool children. *Health Psychol* 12:390-98.
16. Davis, K., K. K. Christoffel. 1994. Obesity in preschool and school-age children: Treatment early and often may be best. *Arch Pediatr Adolesc Med* 148:1257-61.
17. Sallis, J. F., C. C. Berry, S. L. Broyles, T. L. McKenzie, P. R. Nader. 1995. Variability and tracking of physical activity over 2 yr in young children. *Med Sci Sports Exerc* 27:1042-49.
18. Pate, R. R., T. Baranowski, S. G. Trost. 1996. Tracking of physical activity in young children. *Med Sci Sports Exerc* 28:92-96.
19. Birch, L. L., J. O. Fisher. 1998. Development of eating behaviors among children and adolescents. *Pediatrics* 101:539-49.
20. Sallis, J. F., J. J. Prochaska, W. C. Taylor. 2000. A review of correlates of physical activity of children and adolescents. *Med Sci Sports Exerc* 32:963-75.
21. Skinner, J. D., B. R. Carruth, W. Bounds, P. Ziegler, K. Reidy. 2002. Do food-related experiences in the first 2 years of life predict dietary variety in school-aged children? *J Nutr Educ Behav* 34:310-15.
22. Skinner, J. D., B. R. Carruth, B. Wendy, P. J. Ziegler. 2002. Children's food: A longitudinal analysis. *J Am Diet Assoc* 102:1638-47.
23. Oliver, M., G. M. Schofield, G. S. Kolt. 2007. Physical activity in preschoolers: Understanding prevalence and measurement issues. *Sports Med* 37:1045-70.

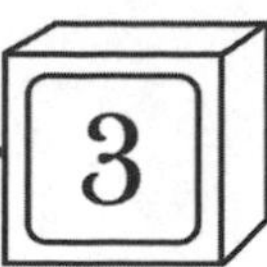

24. American Academy of Pediatrics, Council on Sports Medicine and Fitness, and Council on School Health. 2006. Active healthy living: Prevention of childhood obesity through increased physical activity. *Pediatrics* 117:1834-42.
25. Physical Activity Guidelines Advisory Committee. 2008. *Physical activity guidelines advisory committee report, 2008.* Washington, DC: U.S. Department of Health and Human Services. http://www.health.gov/PAGuidelines/Report/pdf/CommitteeReport.pdf.
26. American Physical Therapy Association. 2008. *Lack of time on tummy shown to hinder achievement of developmental milestones, say physical therapists. News Release.*
27. American Academy of Pediatrics (AAP). 2008. *Back to sleep, tummy to play.* Elk Grove Village, IL: AAP. http://www.healthychildcare.org/pdf/SIDStummytime.pdf.

STANDARD 3.1.3.2: Playing Outdoors

Children should play outdoors when the conditions do not pose a safety risk, individual child health risk, or significant health risk of frostbite or of heat related illness. Caregivers/teachers must protect children from harm caused by adverse weather, ensuring that children wear appropriate clothing and/or appropriate shelter is provided for the weather conditions. Outdoor play for infants may include riding in a carriage or stroller; however, infants should be offered opportunities for gross motor play outdoors, as well.

Weather that poses a significant health risk should include wind chill factor at or below minus 15°F and heat index at or above 90°F, as identified by the National Weather Service (NWS).

Sunny weather:

a) Children should be protected from the sun by using shade, sun-protective clothing, and sunscreen with UVB-ray and UVA-ray protection of SPF 15 or higher, with permission from parents/guardians;
b) Children should wear sun-protective clothing, such as hats, when playing outdoors between the hours of 10 AM and 2 PM.

Warm weather:

a) Children should be well hydrated before engaging in prolonged periods of physical activity and encouraged to drink water during periods of prolonged physical activity;
b) Caregivers/teachers should encourage parents/guardians to have children dress in clothing that is light-colored, lightweight, and limited to one layer of absorbent material that will maximize the evaporation of sweat;
c) On hot days, infants receiving human milk in a bottle can be given additional human milk in a bottle but should not be given water, especially in the first six months of life. Infants receiving formula and water can be given additional formula in a bottle.

Cold weather:

a) Children should wear layers of loose-fitting, lightweight clothing. Outer garments such as coats should be tightly woven, and be at least water repellent when precipitation is present, such as rain or snow;
b) Children should wear a hat, coat, and gloves/mittens kept snug at the wrist;
c) Caregivers/teachers should check children's extremities for maintenance of normal color and warmth at least every fifteen minutes.

Caregivers/teachers should also be aware of environmental hazards such as contaminated water, loud noises, and lead in soil when selecting an area to play outdoors. Children should be observed closely when playing in dirt/soil, so that no soil is ingested. Play areas should be secure and away from heavy traffic areas.

RATIONALE: Outdoor play is not only an opportunity for learning in a different environment; it also provides many health benefits. Outdoor play allows for physical activity that supports maintenance of a healthy weight (2). Short exposure of the skin to sunlight promotes the production of vitamin D that growing children require.

Open spaces in outdoor areas, even those confined to screened rooftops in urban play spaces, encourage children to develop gross motor skills and fine motor play in ways that are difficult to duplicate indoors. Nevertheless, some weather conditions make outdoor play hazardous.

Children need protection from adverse weather and its effects. Wind chill conditions that pose a risk of frostbite as well as heat and humidity that pose a significant risk of heat-related illness are defined by the NWS and are announced routinely.

Heat-induced illness and cold injury are preventable. Children have greater surface area-to-body mass ratio than adults. Therefore, children do not adapt to extremes of temperature as effectively as adults when exposed to a high climatic heat stress or to cold. Children produce more metabolic heat per mass unit than adults when walking or running. They also have a lower sweating capacity and cannot dissipate body heat by evaporation as effectively (1).

Generally, infectious disease organisms are less concentrated in outdoor air than indoor air.

COMMENTS: Wind chill temperature is the temperature it "feels like" outside and is based on the rate of heat loss from exposed skin caused by the effects of wind and cold. As the wind increases, the body is cooled at a faster rate causing the skin temperature to drop. Many layers of clothing traps air between the layers and provides better insulation than one thick layer of clothing.

The NWS provides up to date weather information and warnings. The NWS Website will inform the public when wind chill conditions reach critical thresholds. A Wind Chill Warning is issued when wind chill temperatures are life threatening. A Wind Chill Advisory is issued when wind chill temperatures are potentially hazardous.

The NWS provides convenient color-coded guides for caregivers/teachers to use to determine which weather conditions are comfortable for outdoor play, which require caution, and which are dangerous. These guides are available on the NWS Website at http://www.nws.noaa.gov/om/

windchill/index.shtml for wind chill and http://www.nws.noaa.gov/om/heat/index.shtml for heat index.

The National Oceanic and Atmospheric Administration (NOAA) Weather Radio All Hazards (NWR) broadcasts continuous weather information twenty-four hours a day, seven days a week, directly from the nearest NWR office. NWR is an "All Hazards" radio network, making it a single source for comprehensive weather and emergency information. In conjunction with Federal, State, and Local Emergency Managers and other public officials, NWR also broadcasts warning and post-event information for all types of hazards – including natural (such as earthquakes or avalanches), environmental (such as chemical releases or oil spills), and public safety (such as AMBER alerts or 9-1-1 telephone outages). NWR requires a special radio receiver or scanner capable of picking up the signal. NWR radios/receivers can usually be found in most electronic store chains across the country or you can also purchase NOAA weather radios online at http://www.noaaweatherradios.com.

Email and Text Message Weather Alerts: These weather alert services send out weather warnings, watches, and hurricane information. Alerts are sent to subscribers in the warned areas via text messages and email. Select a service that sends warnings based on county, state, or national advisories. Some alerts may be delayed or missed because of problems on the Internet or the cell-phone network. Thus, do not rely solely on this system. Weather radio or local news affiliates should also be monitored for weather warnings.

Some flexibility is needed depending on the location of the program. For example, in some climates where children do not have warm winter clothing even 20°F could be too cold. In some southern climates it is always above 90°F, but older children are acclimated and can play in shaded areas.

To access the latest local weather information and warnings, contact the National Weather Service at http://www.weather.gov.

Frostbite is an injury to the body caused by freezing body tissue. The most susceptible parts of the body are the extremities such as fingers, toes, ear lobes, or the tip of the nose. Symptoms include a loss of feeling in the extremity and a white or pale appearance. Medical attention is needed immediately for frostbite. The affected area should be SLOWLY re-warmed by immersing frozen areas in warm water (around 100° Fahrenheit) or apply warm compresses for thirty minutes. If warm water is not available, wrap gently in warm blankets (4).

Hypothermia is a medical emergency that occurs when the body loses heat faster than it can produce heat, causing a dangerously low body temperature. An infant with hypothermia may have bright red, cold skin and very low energy. A child's symptoms may include shivering, clumsiness, slurred speech, stumbling, confusion, poor decision making, drowsiness or low energy, apathy, weak pulse, or shallow breathing (3). Call 9-1-1 if a child has these symptoms.

Winter can be problematic for children with asthma for two reasons. Indoor allergens such as dust and dust mites are common triggers for asthma symptoms and levels of these allergens can become elevated during the winter, when doors and windows are kept shut to keep out cold air. Cold temperatures also may, in some cases, serve as a trigger to asthma symptoms for children with asthma. Children for whom cold weather is an asthma trigger may be helped by wearing a scarf during periods of cold weather. All children with asthma can safely play outdoors as long as their asthma is well controlled, and the parents/guardians of children with asthma should be encouraged to work with their child's primary care provider to develop a plan the child can self-manage that incorporates opportunities for outdoor play.

The thought is often expressed that children are more likely to become sick if exposed to cold air, however upper respiratory infections and flu are caused by viruses, not exposure to cold air. These viruses spread easily during the winter when children are kept indoors in close proximity. The best protection against the spread of illness is regular and proper hand hygiene for children and caregivers/teachers, as well as proper sanitation procedures during mealtimes, and when there is any contact with bodily fluids.

TYPE OF FACILITY: Center; Large Family Child Care Home; Small Family Child Care Home

RELATED STANDARDS:

Standard 3.1.3.1: Active Opportunities for Physical Activity
Standard 3.1.3.4: Caregivers'/Teachers' Encouragement of Physical Activity
Standard 3.4.5.1: Sun Safety Including Sunscreen
Standard 8.2.0.1: Inclusion in All Activities
Appendix S: Physical Activity: How Much Is Needed?

REFERENCES:

1. American Academy of Pediatrics, Committee on Sports Medicine and Fitness. 2007. Policy statement: Climatic heat stress and the exercising child and adolescent. *Pediatrics* 120:683-84.
2. Hagan, J. F., J. S. Shaw, P. M. Duncan, eds. 2008. Promoting physical activity. In *Bright futures: Guidelines for health supervision of infants, children, and adolescents,* 147-54. 3rd ed. Elk Grove Village, IL: American Academy of Pediatrics.
3. Mayo Clinic. 2009. Hypothermia: Symptoms. http://www.mayoclinic.com/health/hypothermia/DS00333/.
4. Kids Health. 2008. Frostbite. Nemours. http://kidshealth.org/parent/firstaid_safe/emergencies/frostbite.html.

STANDARD 3.1.3.3: Protection from Air Pollution While Children Are Outside

Supervising adults should check the air quality index (AQI) each day and use the information to determine whether all or only certain children should be allowed to play outdoors.

RATIONALE: Children need protection from air pollution. Air pollution can contribute to acute asthma attacks in sensitive children and, over multiple years of exposure, can contribute to permanent decreased lung size and function (1,2).

COMMENTS: The federal Clean Air Act requires that the Environmental Protection Agency (EPA) establish ambient air quality health standards. Most local health departments monitor weather and air quality in their jurisdiction and make

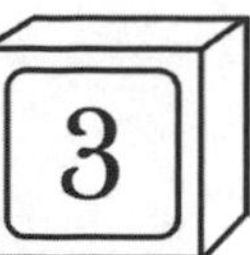

appropriate announcements. AQI is usually reported with local weather reports on media outlets or individuals can sign up for email or text message alerts at http://www.enviroflash.info.

The AQI (available at http://www.airnow.gov) is a cumulative indicator of potential health hazards associated with local or regional air pollution. The AQI is divided into six categories; each category corresponds to a different level of health concern. The six levels of health concern and what they mean are:

a) "Good" AQI is 0 - 50. Air quality is considered satisfactory, and air pollution poses little or no risk.
b) "Moderate" AQI is 51 - 100. Air quality is acceptable, however, for some pollutants there may be a moderate health concern for a very small number of people. For example, people who are unusually sensitive to ozone may experience respiratory symptoms.
c) "Unhealthy for Sensitive Groups" AQI is 101 - 150. Although general public is not likely to be affected at this AQI range, people with heart and lung disease, older adults, and children are at a greater risk from exposure to ozone and the presence of particles in the air.
d) "Unhealthy" AQI is 151 - 200. Everyone may begin to experience some adverse health effects, and members of the sensitive groups may experience more serious effects.
e) "Very Unhealthy" AQI is 201 - 300. This would trigger a health alert signifying that everyone may experience more serious health effects.
f) "Hazardous" AQI greater than 300. This would trigger a health warning of emergency conditions. The entire population is more likely to be affected.

TYPE OF FACILITY: Center; Large Family Child Care Home; Small Family Child Care Home

RELATED STANDARDS:
Standard 3.1.3.2: Playing Outdoors
Standard 5.2.1.1: Fresh Air

REFERENCES:
1. Gauderman, W. J., E. Avol, F. Gilliland, et al. 2004. The effect of air pollution on lung development from 10 to 18 years of age. *N Engl J Med* 351:1057-67.
2. Hao, M., S. Comier, M. Wang, J. J. Lee, A. Nel. 2003. Diesel exhaust particles exert acute effects on airway inflammation and function in murine allergen provocation models. *J Allergy Clin Immunol* 112:905-14.

STANDARD 3.1.3.4: Caregivers'/Teachers' Encouragement of Physical Activity

Caregivers/teachers should promote children's active play, and participate in children's active games at times when they can safely do so. Caregivers/teachers should:

a) Lead structured activities to promote children's activities two or more times per day;
b) Wear clothing and footwear that permits easy and safe movement (2);
c) Not sit during active play;
d) Provide prompts for children to be active (3,4), e.g., "good throw";
e) Encourage children's physical activities that are appropriate and safe in the setting, e.g., do not prohibit running on the playground when it is safe to run;
f) Have orientation and annual training opportunities to learn about age-appropriate gross motor activities and games that promote children's physical activity (1,3);
g) Limit screen time (TV, DVD, computer, etc.), except for 1) school-age children completing homework assignments and 2) children with special health care needs who require and consistently use assistive and adaptive computer technology.

RATIONALE: Children learn from the modeling of healthy and safe behavior.

Chairs for adults on playgrounds inhibit the promotion of children's physical activity. They may also pose a safety hazard if caregivers/teachers sitting in them cannot see all parts of the playground.

COMMENTS: Caregivers/teachers may not feel comfortable promoting active play, perhaps due to inhibitions about their own physical activity skills, or due to lack of training. Caregivers/teachers may feel that their sole role on the playground is to supervise and keep children safe, rather than to promote physical activity. Continuing education activities are useful in disseminating knowledge about effective games to promote physical activity in early care and education while keeping children safe (1). Caregivers/teachers should consider incorporating structured activities into the curriculum indoors, or after children have been on playground for ten to fifteen minutes, as children tend to be less active after the first ten to fifteen minutes on the playground. Caregivers/teachers, if they are facilitating physical activity with a small group, must ensure that there is adequate supervision of all children on the playground.

Caregivers/teachers should be aware that there is often a high level of TV and computer exposure in the home. Early care and education settings offer caregivers/teachers the opportunity to model the limitation of media and computer time and to educate parents/guardians about alternative activities that families can do with their children (3).

TYPE OF FACILITY: Center; Large Family Child Care Home; Small Family Child Care Home

RELATED STANDARDS:
Standard 2.2.0.3: Limiting Screen Time – Media, Computer, Etc.
Standard 3.1.3.1: Active Opportunities for Physical Activity
Standard 3.1.3.2: Playing Outdoors
Standard 9.2.3.1: Policies and Practices that Promote Physical Activity
Appendix S: Physical Activity: How Much Is Needed?

REFERENCES:
1. Ward, D. S., A. Vaughn, C. McWilliams, D. Hales. 2010. Interventions for increasing physical activity at child care. *Med Sci Sports Exercise* 42:526-34.

2. Copeland, K. A., S. N. Sherman, C. A. Kendeigh, B. E. Saelens, H. J. Kalkwarf. 2009. Flip-flops, dress clothes and no coat: Clothing barriers to children's physical activity in child-care centers. *Int J Behav Nutr Activ* 74(6).
3. Trost, S. G., D. S. Ward, M. Senso. 2010. Effects of child care policy and environment on physical activity. *Med Sci Sports Exercise* 42:520-25.
4. Brown, W. H., K. A. Pfeiffer, K. L. McIver, M. Dowda, C. L. Addy, R. R. Pate. 2009. Social and environmental factors associated with preschoolers' nonsedentary physical activity. *Child Devel* 80:45-58.

3.1.4 Safe Sleep

STANDARD 3.1.4.1: Safe Sleep Practices and SIDS/Suffocation Risk Reduction

Facilities should develop a written policy that describes the practices to be used to promote safe sleep when infants are napping or sleeping. The policy should explain that these practices aim to reduce the risk of sudden infant death syndrome (SIDS) or suffocation death and other infant deaths that could occur when an infant is in a crib or asleep.

All staff, parents/guardians, volunteers and others approved to enter rooms where infants are cared for should receive a copy of the Safe Sleep Policy and additional educational information and training on the importance of consistent use of safe sleep policies and practices before they are allowed to care for infants (i.e., first day of employment/volunteering/subbing). Documentation that training has occurred and that these individuals have received and reviewed the written policy should be kept on file.

All staff, parents/guardians, volunteers and others who care for infants in the child care setting should follow these required safe sleep practices as recommended by the American Academy of Pediatrics (AAP) (1):

a) Infants up to twelve months of age should be placed for sleep in a supine position (wholly on their back) for every nap or sleep time unless the infant's primary care provider has completed a signed waiver indicating that the child requires an alternate sleep position;
b) Infants should be placed for sleep in safe sleep environments; which includes: a firm crib mattress covered by a tight-fitting sheet in a safety-approved crib (the crib should meet the standards and guidelines reviewed/approved by the U.S. Consumer Product Safety Commission [CPSC] and ASTM International [ASTM]), no monitors or positioning devices should be used unless required by the child's primary care provider, and no other items should be in a crib occupied by an infant except for a pacifier;
c) Infants should not nap or sleep in a car safety seat, bean bag chair, bouncy seat, infant seat, swing, jumping chair, play pen or play yard, highchair, chair, futon, or any other type of furniture/equipment that is not a safety-approved crib (that is in compliance with the CPSC and ASTM safety standards) (4);
d) If an infant arrives at the facility asleep in a car safety seat, the parent/guardian or caregiver/teacher should immediately remove the sleeping infant from this seat and place them in the supine position in a safe sleep environment (i.e., the infant's assigned crib);
e) If an infant falls asleep in any place that is not a safe sleep environment, staff should immediately move the infant and place them in the supine position in their crib;
f) Only one infant should be placed in each crib (stackable cribs are not recommended);
g) Soft or loose bedding should be kept away from sleeping infants and out of safe sleep environments. These include, but are not limited to: bumper pads, pillows, quilts, comforters, sleep positioning devices, sheepskins, blankets, flat sheets, cloth diapers, bibs, etc. Also, blankets/items should not be hung on the sides of cribs. Swaddling infants when they are in a crib is not necessary or recommended, but rather one-piece sleepers should be used (see Standard 3.1.4.2 for more detail information on swaddling);
h) Toys, including mobiles and other types of play equipment that are designed to be attached to any part of the crib should be kept away from sleeping infants and out of safe sleep environments;
i) When caregivers/teachers place infants in their crib for sleep, they should check to ensure that the temperature in the room is comfortable for a lightly clothed adult, check the infants to ensure that they are comfortably clothed (not overheated or sweaty), and that bibs, necklaces, and garments with ties or hoods are removed (clothing sacks or other clothing designed for sleep can be used in lieu of blankets);
j) Infants should be directly observed by sight and sound at all times, including when they are going to sleep, are sleeping, or are in the process of waking up;
k) Bedding should be changed between children, and if mats are used, they should be cleaned between uses.

The lighting in the room must allow the caregiver/teacher to see each infant's face, to view the color of the infant's skin, and to check on the infant's breathing and placement of the pacifier (if used).

A caregiver/teacher trained in safe sleep practices and approved to care for infants should be present in each room at all times where there is an infant. This caregiver/teacher should remain alert and should actively supervise sleeping infants in an ongoing manner. Also, the caregiver/teacher should check to ensure that the infant's head remains uncovered and re-adjust clothing as needed.

The construction and use of sleeping rooms for infants separate from the infant group room is not recommended due to the need for direct supervision. In situations where there are existing facilities with separate sleeping rooms, facilities should develop a plan to modify room assignments and/or practices to eliminate placing infants to sleep in separate rooms.

Facilities should be aware of the current recommendation of the AAP about pacifier use (1). If pacifiers are allowed, facilities should have a written policy that describes relevant procedures and guidelines. Pacifier use outside of a crib in rooms and programs where there are mobile infants or toddlers is not recommended.

RATIONALE: Despite the decrease in deaths attributed to SIDS and the decreased frequency of prone (tummy) infant sleep positioning over the past two decades, many caregivers/teachers continue to place infants to sleep in positions or environments that are not safe. Deaths in child care facilities attributable to SIDS continue to occur at an alarming rate, with a majority occurring in the first day or first week that an infant starts attending a child care program (2,3). Many of these deaths appear to be associated with prone positioning, especially when the infant is unaccustomed to being placed in that position (2,4).

Infants who are cared for by adults other than their parent/guardian or primary caregiver/teacher are at increased risk for dying from SIDS. Recent research and demonstration projects (2) have revealed that:

a) Caregivers/teachers are unaware of the dangers or risks associated with prone or side infant sleep positioning, and many believe that they are using the safest practices possible, even when they are not;
b) Although training programs are effective in improving the knowledge of caregivers/teachers, these programs alone do not always lead to changes in caregiver/teacher practices, beliefs, or attitudes;
c) Caregivers/teachers report the following major barriers to implementing safe sleep practices:
   1) They have been misinformed about methods shown to reduce the risk of SIDS;
   2) Facilities do not have or use written "safe sleep" policies or guidelines;
   3) State child care regulations do not mandate the use of supine (wholly on their back) sleep position for infants in child care and/or training for infant caregivers/teachers;
   4) Other caregivers/teachers or parents/guardians have objections to use of safe sleep practices, either because of their concern for choking or aspiration, and/or their concern that some infants do not sleep well in the supine position;
   5) Parents/guardians model their practices after what happens in the hospital or what others recommend. Infants who were placed to sleep in other positions in the hospital or home environments may have difficulty transitioning to supine positioning at home and later in child care.

Training that includes observations and addresses barriers to changing caregiver/teacher practices would be most effective. Use of safe sleep policies, continued education of parents/guardians, expanded training efforts for child care professionals, statewide regulations and mandates, and increased monitoring and observation are critical to reduce the risk of SIDS and other infant deaths in child care (3).

Loose or ill-fitting sheets have caused infants to be strangled or suffocated (8).

COMMENTS: Background: Deaths of infants who are asleep in child care (whether attributable to SIDS, suffocation, or other causes) may be under-reported because of the lack of consistency in training and regulating death scene investigations and determining and reporting cause of death. Not all states require documentation that clarifies that an infant died while being cared for by someone other than their parents/guardians.

Although the cause of SIDS is not known, researchers believe that some infants develop in a manner that makes it challenging for them to be aroused or to breathe when they experience a life-threatening challenge during sleep. Although some state regulations require that caregivers/teachers "check on" sleeping infants every ten, fifteen, or thirty minutes, an infant can suffocate or die in only a few minutes. It is for this reason that the standards above discourage toys or mobiles in cribs and recommend direct, active, and ongoing supervision when infants are falling to sleep, are sleeping, or are becoming awake. This is also why *Caring for Our Children* describes a safe sleep environment as one that includes a safety-approve crib, firm mattress, firmly fitted sheet, and the infant placed on their back at all times, in comfortable, safe garments, but nothing else – not even a blanket.

When infants are being dropped off, staff may be busy. Requiring parents/guardians to remove the infant from the car seat and re-position them in the supine position in their crib (if they are sleeping), will reinforce safe sleep practices and reassure parents/guardians that their child is in a safe position before they leave the facility.

Challenges: National recommendations for reducing the risk of SIDS or suffocation and other infant deaths are provided for use in the general population. Most research reviewed to guide the development of these recommendations was not conducted on children in child care. Because infants are at increased risk for dying from SIDS in child care (5) and because caregivers/teachers are liable for their actions, they must err on the side of caution and must provide the safest sleep environment for the infants in their care for liability and other reasons.

When hospital staff or parents/guardians of infants who may attend child care place the infant in a position other than supine for sleep, the infant becomes accustomed to this and can have a more difficult time adjusting to child care, especially when they are placed for sleep in a new unfamiliar position.

Parents/guardians and caregivers/teachers want infants to transition to child care facilities in a comfortable and easy manner. It can be challenging for infants to fall asleep in a new environment because there are different people, equipment, lighting, noises, etc. When infants sleep well in child care, adults feel better. Placing personal items in cribs with infants and covering or wrapping infants with blankets may help the adults to believe that the child is more comfort-

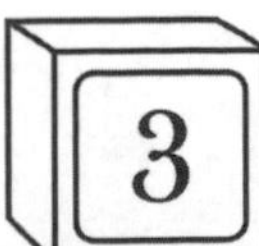

able or feels comforted. However, this may or may not be true. These practices are not the safest practices for infants in child care, and they should not be allowed. Efforts to educate the public about reducing the risk of SIDS and suffocation and promoting the use of consistent safe sleep practices need to continue.

Special Care Plans: Some facilities require staff to place infants in a supine position for sleep unless there is documentation in a child's special care plan indicating a medical need for a different position. This can provide the caregiver/teacher with more confidence in implementing the safe sleep policy and refusing parental demands that are not consistent with safe sleep practices. It is likely that an infant will be unaccustomed to sleeping supine if his or her parents/guardians object to the supine position (and are therefore placing the infant prone to sleep at home). By providing educational information on the importance of consistent use of safe sleep policies and practices to expectant parents, facilities will help raise awareness of these issues, promote infant safety, and increase support for proper implementation of safe sleep policies and practices in the future.

Use of Blankets: AAP recommendations state that blankets may be hazardous, and use of blankets is not advisable. Parents/guardians and caregivers/teachers sometimes experience difficulty in placing infants to sleep without a blanket. If blankets are used, the "Feet to Foot Rule" should be followed. This involves placing the child's feet to the foot of the crib, and tucking a light blanket along the sides and the foot of the mattress. The blanket is placed only up to the infant's chest with their arms outside of the blanket. The infant's head must remain uncovered, so if a blanket is used, frequent visual checks are required to make sure the infant has not pulled the blanket over his/her head.

Use of Pacifiers: Caregivers/teachers should be aware of the current recommendation of the AAP about pacifier use to reduce the risk of SIDS. While using pacifiers to reduce the risk of SIDS seems prudent (especially if the infant is already sleeping with a pacifier at home), pacifier use has also been shown to be associated with an increased risk of ear infections. Keeping pacifiers clean and limiting their use to sleep time is best. Using pacifiers in a sanitary and safe fashion in group care settings requires special diligence.

Pacifiers should be inspected for tears before use. Pacifiers should not be clipped to an infant's clothing or tied around an infant's neck.

For children in the general population, the AAP recommends:

a) Consider offering a pacifier when placing the infant down for nap and sleep time;
b) If the infant refuses the pacifier, s/he should not be forced to take it;
c) If the infant falls asleep and the pacifier falls out of the infant's mouth, it should be removed from the crib and does not need to be reinserted. A pacifier has been shown to reduce the risk of SIDS, even if the pacifier falls out during sleep (1);
d) Pacifiers should not be coated in any sweet solution, and they should be cleaned and replaced regularly;
e) For breastfed infants, delay pacifier introduction until fifteen days of age to ensure that breastfeeding is well-established (7);
f) Written permission from the child's parent/guardian is required for pacifier use in the facility.

Swaddling: Hospital personnel or physicians, particularly those who work in neonatal intensive care units or infant nurseries in hospitals may recommend that newborns be swaddled in the hospital setting. Although parents/guardians may choose to continue this practice at home, swaddling infants when they are being placed to sleep or are sleeping in a child care facility is not necessary or recommended. See Standard 3.1.4.2 for more detailed information.

Concern about Plagiocephaly: If parents/guardians or caregivers/teachers are concerned about positional plagiocephaly (flat head or flat spot on head), they can continue to use safe sleep practices but also do the following:

a) Offer infants opportunities to be held upright and participate in supervised "tummy time" when they are awake;
b) Alter the position of the infant, and thereby alter the supine position of the infant's head and face. This can easily be accomplished by alternating the placement of the infant in the crib – place the infant to sleep with their head facing to one side for a week and then turning the infant so that their head and face are placed the other way. Infants typically turn their head to one side toward the room or door, so if they are placed with their head toward one side of the bed for one sleep time and then placed with their head toward the other side of the bed the next time, this changes the area of the head that is in contact with the mattress.

A common question among caregivers/teachers and parents/guardians is whether they should return the infant to the supine position if they roll onto their side or their tummies. Infants up to twelve months of age should be placed wholly supine for sleep every time. In fact, all children should be placed (or encouraged to lie down) on their backs to sleep. When infants are developmentally capable of rolling comfortably from their backs to their fronts and back again, there is no evidence to suggest that they should be re-positioned into the supine position.

The California Childcare Health Program has available a Safe Sleep Policy for infants in child care programs at http://ucsfchildcarehealth.org/pdfs/forms/SafeSleep_policy1108.pdf (6). AAP provides a free online course on safe sleep practices at http://www.healthychildcare.org/sids.html.

TYPE OF FACILITY: Center; Large Family Child Care Home; Small Family Child Care Home

RELATED STANDARDS:
Standard 3.1.4.2: Swaddling
Standard 3.1.4.3: Pacifier Use
Standard 3.1.4.4: Scheduled Rest Periods and Sleep Arrangements

Standard 3.6.4.5: Death
Standard 4.3.1.1: General Plan for Feeding Infants
Standard 4.5.0.3: Activities That are Incompatible With Eating
Standard 5.4.5.1: Sleeping Equipment and Supplies
Standard 5.4.5.2: Cribs
Standard 6.4.1.3: Crib Toys

REFERENCES:

1. American Academy of Pediatrics, Task Force on Sudden Infant Death Syndrome. 2009. Policy statement: The changing concept of SIDS: Diagnostic coding shifts, controversies regarding the sleeping environment, and new variables to consider in reducing risk. *Pediatrics* 123:188.
2. Moon R. Y., T. Calabrese, L. Aird. 2008. Reducing the risk of sudden infant death syndrome in child care and changing provider practices: Lessons learned from a demonstration project. *Pediatrics* 122:788-79.
3. American Academy of Pediatrics, Back to Sleep, Healthy Child Care America, First Candle. 2008. *Reducing the risk of SIDS in child care*. http://www.healthychildcare.org/pdf/SIDSfinal.pdf.
4. ECELS, Healthy Child Care Pennsylvania. 2007. Car seats and swings are not safe for sleeping. *Health Link Online* 18:1-2. http://www.ecels-healthychildcarepa.org/content/3-27-07 April-May 2007 HL Online.pdf.
5. Leonard, V. 2009. *Health and safety notes: Reducing the risk of SIDS for infants in our care*. Berkeley, CA: California Childcare Health Program. http://www.ucsfchildcarehealth.org/pdfs/healthandsafety/SIDS_en1009.pdf.
6. California Childcare Health Program (CCHP). 2008. *Safe sleep policy for infants in child care*. Berkeley, CA: CCHP. http://ucsfchildcarehealth.org/pdfs/forms/SafeSleep_policy1108.pdf.
7. Jenik, A. G., N. E. Vain, A. N. Gorestein, N. E. Jacobi, Pacifier and Breastfeeding Trial Group. 2009. Does the recommendation to use a pacifier influence the prevalence of breastfeeding? *J Pediatrics* 155:350-54.
8. National MCH Center for Child Death Review. Sudden infant death syndrome (SIDS)/Sudden unexplained infant death (SUID): Fact sheet. http://www.childdeathreview.org/causesSI.htm.

STANDARD 3.1.4.2: Swaddling

In child care settings, swaddling is not necessary or recommended.

RATIONALE: There is evidence that swaddling can increase the risk of serious health outcomes, especially in certain situations. The risk of sudden infant death is increased if an infant is swaddled and placed on his/her stomach to sleep (4) or if the infant can roll over from back to stomach. Loose blankets around the head can be a risk factor for sudden infant death syndrome (SIDS) (3). With swaddling, there is an increased risk of developmental dysplasia of the hip, a hip condition that can result in long-term disability (1,5). Hip dysplasia is felt to be more common with swaddling because infants' legs can be forcibly extended. With excessive swaddling, infants may overheat (i.e., hyperthermia) (2).

COMMENTS: Most infants in child care centers are at least six-weeks-old. Even with newborns, research does not provide conclusive data about whether swaddling should or should not be used. Benefits of swaddling may include decreased crying, increased sleep periods, and improved temperature control. However, temperature can be maintained with appropriate infant clothing and/or an infant sleeping bag. Although swaddling may decrease crying, there are other, more serious health concerns to consider, including SIDS and hip disease. If swaddling is used, it should be used less and less over the course of the first few weeks and months of an infant's life.

TYPE OF FACILITY: Center; Large Family Child Care Home; Small Family Child Care Home

RELATED STANDARDS:
Standard 3.1.4.1: Safe Sleep Practices and SIDS/Suffocation Risk Reduction

REFERENCES:

1. Van Sleuwen, B. E., A. C. Engelberts, M. M. Boere-Boonekamp, W. Kuis, T. W. J. Schulpen, M. P. L'Hoir. 2007. Swaddling: A systematic review. *Pediatrics* 120:e1097-e1106.
2. Franco, P., N. Seret, J. N. Van Hees, S. Scaillet, J. Groswasser, A. Kahn. 2005. Influence of swaddling on sleep and arousal characteristics of healthy infants. *Pediatrics* 115:1307-11.
3. Contemporary Pediatrics. 2004. *Guide for parents: Swaddling 101*. http://www.aap.org/sections/scan/practicingsafety/Toolkit_Resources/Module1/swadling.pdf.
4. Richardson, H. L., A. M. Walker, R. S. Horne. 2010. Influence of swaddling experience on spontaneous arousal patterns and autonomic control in sleeping infants. *J Pediatrics* 157:85-91.
5. Mahan, S. T., Kasser J. R. 2008. Does Swaddling Influence Developmental Dysplasia of the Hip? *Pediatrics* 121:177-78.

STANDARD 3.1.4.3: Pacifier Use

Facilities should be informed and follow current recommendations of the American Academy of Pediatrics (AAP) about pacifier use (1-3).

If pacifiers are allowed, facilities should have a written policy that indicates:

a) Rationale and protocols for use of pacifiers;
b) Written permission and any instructions or preferences from the child's parent/guardian;
c) If desired, parent/guardian should provide at least two new pacifiers (labeled with their child's name using a waterproof label or non-toxic permanent marker) on a regular basis for their child to use. The extra pacifier should be available in case a replacement is needed;
d) Staff should inspect each pacifier for tears or cracks (and to see if there is unknown fluid in the nipple) before each use;
e) Staff should clean each pacifier with soap and water before each use;
f) Pacifiers with attachments should not be allowed; pacifiers should not be clipped, pinned, or tied to an infant's clothing, and they should not be tied around an infant's neck, wrist, or other body part;
g) If an infant refuses the pacifier, s/he should not be forced to take it;
h) If the pacifier falls out of the infant's mouth, it does not need to be reinserted;
i) Pacifiers should not be coated in any sweet solution;
j) Pacifiers should be cleaned and stored open to air; separate from the diapering area, diapering items, or other children's personal items.

Infants should be directly observed by sight and sound at all times, including when they are going to sleep, are sleeping, or are in the process of waking up. The lighting in the room must allow the caregiver/teacher to see each infant's face, to view the color of the infant's skin, and to check on the infant's breathing and placement of the pacifier.

Pacifier use outside of a crib in rooms and programs where there are mobile infants or toddlers is not recommended.

Caregivers/teachers should work with parents/guardians to wean infants from pacifiers as the suck reflex diminishes between three and twelve months of age. Objects which provide comfort should be substituted for pacifiers (6).

RATIONALE: Mobile infants or toddlers may try to remove a pacifier from an infant's mouth, put it in their own mouth, or try to reinsert it in another child's mouth. These behaviors can increase risks for choking and/or transmission of infectious diseases.

Cleaning pacifiers before and after each use is recommended to ensure that each pacifier is clean before it is inserted into an infant's mouth (5). This protects against unknown contamination or sharing. Cleaning a pacifier before each use allows the caregiver/teacher to worry less about whether the pacifier was cleaned by another adult who may have cared for the infant before they did. This may be of concern when there are staffing changes or when parents/guardians take the pacifiers home with them and bring them back to the facility.

If a caregiver/teacher observes or suspects that a pacifier has been shared, the pacifier should be cleaned. Caregivers/teachers should make sure the nipple is free of fluid after cleaning to ensure the infant does not ingest it. For this reason, submerging a pacifier is not recommended. If the pacifier nipple contains any unknown fluid, or if a caregiver/teacher questions the safety or ownership, the pacifier should be discarded (4).

While using pacifiers to reduce the risk of sudden infant death syndrome (SIDS) seems prudent (especially if the infant is already sleeping with a pacifier at home), pacifier use has been associated with an increased risk of ear infections and oral health issues (7).

COMMENTS: To keep current with the AAP's recommendations on the use of pacifiers, go to http://www.aap.org.

TYPE OF FACILITY: Center; Large Family Child Care Home; Small Family Child Care Home

REFERENCES:

1. American Academy of Pediatrics, Task Force on Sudden Infant Death Syndrome. 2009. Policy statement: The changing concept of SIDS: Diagnostic coding shifts, controversies regarding the sleeping environment, and new variables to consider in reducing risk. *Pediatrics* 123:188.
2. Hauck, F. R. 2006. Pacifiers and sudden infant death syndrome: What should we recommend? *Pediatrics* 117:1811-12.
3. Mitchell, E. A., P. S. Blair, M. P. L'Hoir. 2006. Should pacifiers be recommended to prevent sudden infant death syndrome? *Pediatrics* 117:1755-58.
4. Reeves, D. L. 2006. Pacifier use in childcare settings. *Healthy Child* Care 9:12-13.
5. Cornelius, A. N., J. P. D'Auria, L. M. Wise. 2008. Pacifier use: A systematic review of selected parenting web sites. *J Pediatric Health Care* 22:159-65.
6. American Academy of Pediatrics, Back to Sleep, Healthy Child Care America, First Candle. 2008. *Reducing the risk of SIDS in child care.* http://www.healthychildcare.org/pdf/SIDSfinal.pdf.
7. Mayo Clinic. 2009. Infant and toddler health. Pacifiers: Are they good for your baby? http://www.mayoclinic.com/health/pacifiers/PR00067/.

STANDARD 3.1.4.4: Scheduled Rest Periods and Sleep Arrangements

The facility should provide an opportunity for, but should not require, sleep and rest. The facility should make available a regular rest period for preschool and school-aged children, if the child desires. For children who are unable to sleep, the facility should provide time and space for quiet play.

Facilities that offer infant care should use a written Safe Sleep Policy that describes the practices to be used to reduce the risk of sudden infant death syndrome (SIDS) and other infant deaths.

RATIONALE: Conditions conducive to sleep and rest for younger children include a consistent caregiver, a routine quiet place, regular times for rest (1), and use of similar routines and safe practices. Most preschool children in all-day care benefit from scheduled periods of rest. This rest may take the form of actual napping, a quiet time, or a change of pace between activities. The times of naps will affect behavior at home (1).

Studies suggest that sleep is essential for optimal health and growth for young children. There are studies that show the amount of time young children sleep in a twenty-four-hour period is related to obesity later in life (2). Preschool children who sleep less than other children are at higher risk of being obese adults. In a meta-analysis of the association between sleep duration and childhood obesity, children with shorter sleep durations had a 58% higher risk of developing obesity compared to children with longer sleep durations (3). Children with ten hours or less of sleep ages six to seven years of age are more likely to be obese adults than children who sleep more than ten hours.

In a nationally representative sample, three-year-olds slept an average of ten and one-half hours and five-year-olds slept an average of ten hours on weekdays (2). Daytime naps supplement the nighttime sleep period to meet the total sleep requirement. Daily sleep duration of less than twelve hours during infancy also appears to be a risk factor for overweight and adiposity in preschool-aged children (4).

COMMENTS: In the young infant, favorable conditions for sleep and rest include being dry, well-fed, and comfortable. Infants may need one or two (or sometimes more naps during the time they are in child care). As infants age, they typically transition to one nap per day, and having one nap per day is consistent with the schedule that most facilities follow. A facility that includes preschool and school-age children should make available books, board games and other forms of quiet play. Different practices such as rock-

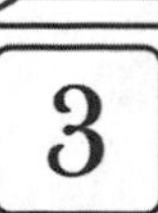

ing, holding a child while swaying, singing, reading, patting an arm or back, etc. could be included. Lighting does not need to be turned off during nap time.

TYPE OF FACILITY: Center; Large Family Child Care Home; Small Family Child Care Home

RELATED STANDARDS:
Standard 3.1.4.1: Safe Sleep Practices and SIDS/Suffocation Risk Reduction
Standard 5.2.2.1: Levels of Illumination
Standard 5.4.5.1: Sleeping Equipment and Supplies
Standard 5.4.5.2: Cribs

REFERENCES:

1. Murph, J. R., S. D. Palmer, D. Glassy, eds. 2005. *Health in child care: A manual for health professionals.* Elk Grove Village, IL: American Academy of Pediatrics.
2. Snell, E. K., E. K. Adam, G. J. Duncan. 2007. Sleep and body mass index and overweight status of children and adolescents. *Child Development.* 78:309-23.
3. Chen, Z., M. A. Beydoun, Y. Wang. 2008. Is sleep duration associated with childhood obesity? A systematic review and meta-analysis. *Obesity.* 16:265-74.
4. Taveras, E. M., S. L. Rifas-Shiman, E. Oken, E. P. Gunderson, M. W. Gillman. 2008. Short sleep duration in infancy and risk of childhood overweight. *Arch Pediatr Adolesc Med* 162:305-11.

STANDARD 3.1.4.5: Unscheduled Access to Rest Areas

All children should have access to rest or nap areas whenever the child desires to rest. These rest or nap areas should be set up to reduce distraction or disturbance from other activities. All facilities should provide rest areas for children, including children who become ill, at least until the child leaves the facility for care elsewhere. Children need to be within sight and hearing of caregivers/teachers when resting.

RATIONALE: Any child, especially children who are ill (1), may need more opportunity for rest or quiet activities.

TYPE OF FACILITY: Center; Large Family Child Care Home; Small Family Child Care Home

RELATED STANDARDS:
Standard 3.1.4.1: Safe Sleep Practices and SIDS/Suffocation Risk Reduction
Standard 3.1.4.4: Scheduled Rest Periods and Sleep Arrangements
Standards 3.6.2.2-3.6.2.10: Caring for Children Who Are Ill
Standard 5.4.5.1: Sleeping Equipment and Supplies
Standard 5.4.6.1: Space for Children Who Are Ill

REFERENCES:

1. Pickering, L. K., C. J. Baker, D. W. Kimberlin, S. S. Long, eds. 2009. *Red book: 2009 report of the Committee on Infectious Diseases,* 153. 28th ed. Elk Grove Village, IL: American Academy of Pediatrics.

3.1.5 Oral Health

STANDARD 3.1.5.1: Routine Oral Hygiene Activities

Caregivers/teachers should promote the habit of regular tooth brushing. All children with teeth should brush or have their teeth brushed at least once during the hours the child is in child care. Children under two years of age should have only a smear of toothpaste (rice grain) on the brush when brushing. Those over two years of age should use a pea-sized amount of fluoride toothpaste. An ideal time to brush is after eating. The caregiver/teacher should either brush the child's teeth or supervise as the child brushes his/her own teeth. Disposable gloves should be worn by the caregiver/teacher if contact with a child's oral fluids is anticipated. The younger the child, the more the caregiver/teacher needs to be involved. The caregiver/teacher should be able to evaluate each child's motor activity and to teach the child the correct method of tooth brushing when the child is capable of doing this activity. The caregiver/teacher should monitor the tooth brushing activity and thoroughly brush the child's teeth after the child has finished brushing, preferably for a total of two minutes. Children whose teeth are brushed at home twice a day may be exempted since additional brushing has little additive benefit and may expose a child to excess fluoride toothpaste.

The cavity-causing effect of frequent exposure to food or juice should be reduced by offering the children rinsing water after snacks and meals when tooth brushing is not possible. Local dental health professionals can facilitate compliance with these activities by offering education and training for the child care staff and providing oral health presentations for the children and parents/guardians.

RATIONALE: Regular tooth brushing with fluoride toothpaste is encouraged to reinforce oral health habits and prevent gingivitis and tooth decay. There is currently no (strong) evidence that shows any benefit to wiping the gums of a baby who has no teeth. Good oral hygiene is as important for a six-month-old child with one tooth as it is for a six-year-old with many teeth (2). Tooth brushing at least once a day reduces build-up of decay-causing plaque (2,3). The development of tooth decay-producing plaque begins when an infant's first tooth appears in his/her mouth (1). Tooth decay cannot develop without this plaque which contains the acid-producing bacteria in a child's mouth. The ability to do a good job brushing the teeth is a learned skill, improved by practice and age. There is general consensus that children do not have the necessary hand eye coordination for independent brushing until around age six so either caregiver/teacher brushing or close supervision is necessary in the preschool child. Tooth brushing and activities at home may not suffice to develop this skill or accomplish the necessary plaque removal, especially when children eat most of their meals and snacks during a full day in child care.

COMMENTS: The caregiver/teacher should use a small amount of fluoride toothpaste (a smear about the size of a rice grain spread across the width of the toothbrush for children under two years of age and a pea-sized amount for children two years of age and over). Children should attempt to spit out excess toothpaste after brushing. Fluoride is the single most effective way to prevent tooth decay. Brushing of teeth with fluoridated toothpaste is the most efficient way to apply fluoride to the teeth. Young children may occasionally swallow a small amount of toothpaste and this is not a health risk. However, if children swallow more than recommended amounts of fluoride toothpaste on a consistent basis, they are at risk for fluorosis, a condition caused by ingesting excessive levels of fluoride (6). Other products such as fluoride rinses can pose a poisoning hazard if ingested (7).

The children can also rinse with water and spit out after a snack or a meal if their teeth have already been brushed earlier. Rinsing with water helps to remove food particles from teeth, diluting sugars and may help prevent cavities.

A sink is not necessary to accomplish tooth brushing in child care. Each child can use a cup of water for tooth brushing. The child should wet the brush in the cup, brush and then spit excess toothpaste into the cup.

Caregivers/teachers should encourage replacement of toothbrushes when the bristles become worn or frayed or approximately every three to four months (4,5).

Caregivers/teachers should encourage parents/guardians to establish a dental home for their child within six months after the first tooth erupts or by one year of age, whichever is earlier (1). The dental home is the ongoing relationship between the dentist and the patient, inclusive of all aspects of oral health care delivered in a comprehensive, continuously accessible, coordinated and family-centered way. Currently there are insufficient numbers of dentists who are able to incorporate infants and toddlers into their practices so primary care providers may provide oral health screening during well child care in this population while promoting the establishment of a dental home (2).

Fluoride varnish applied at primary care visits reduce decay rates by one-third, and lead to significant cost savings in restorative dental care and associated hospital costs. Coupled with parent/guardian and caregiver/teacher education, fluoride varnish is an important tool to improve children's health (8,9).

TYPE OF FACILITY: Center; Large Family Child Care Home; Small Family Child Care Home

RELATED STANDARDS:
Standard 3.1.5.2: Toothbrushes and Toothpaste
Standard 3.1.5.3: Oral Health Education
Standards 9.4.2.1-9.4.2.8: Child Records

REFERENCES:
1. American Academy of Pediatrics, Section on Pediatric Dentistry. 2009. Policy statement: Oral health risk assessment timing and establishment of the dental home. *Pediatrics* 124:845.
2. American Academy of Pediatrics, Section on Pediatric Dentistry. 2008. Preventive oral health intervention for pediatricians. *Pediatrics* 122:1387-94.
3. American Academy of Pediatric Dentistry, Clinical Affairs Committee, Council on Clinical Affairs. 2008-2009. Guideline on periodicity of examination, preventive dental services, anticipatory guidance/counseling, and oral treatment for infants, children, and adolescents. *Pediatric Dentistry* 30:112-18.
4. American Academy of Pediatric Dentistry. Early childhood caries. Chicago: AAPD. http://www.aapd.org/media/ECCstats.pdf.
5. American Dental Association. ADA positions and statements. ADA statement on toothbrush care: Cleaning, storage, and replacement. Chicago: ADA. http://www.ada.org/1887.aspx.
6. Centers for Disease Control and Prevention, Fluoride Recommendations Work Group. 2001. Recommendations for using fluoride to prevent and control dental caries in the United States. *MMWR* 50(RR14): 1-42.
7. Centers for Disease Control and Prevention. 2009. Community water fluoridation. Other fluoride products. http://www.cdc.gov/fluoridation/other.htm.
8. Marinho, V. C., et al. 2002. Fluoride varnishes for preventing dental caries in children and adolescents. *Cochrane Database System Rev* 3, no. CD002279. http://www2.cochrane.org/reviews/en/ab002279.html.
9. American Academy of Pediatric Dentistry. 2006. Talking points: AAPD perspective on physicians or other non-dental providers applying fluoride varnish. Dental Home Resource Center. http://www.aapd.org/dentalhome/1225.pdf.

STANDARD 3.1.5.2: Toothbrushes and Toothpaste

In facilities where tooth brushing is an activity, each child should have a personally labeled, age-appropriate toothbrush. No sharing or borrowing should be allowed. After use, toothbrushes should be stored on a clean surface with the bristle end of the toothbrush up to air dry in such a way that the toothbrushes cannot contact or drip on each other and the bristles are not in contact with any surface (6). Racks and devices used to hold toothbrushes for storage should be labeled and disinfected as needed. The toothbrushes should be replaced at least every three to four months, or sooner if the bristles become frayed (2-4,6). When a toothbrush becomes contaminated through contact with another brush or use by more than one child, it should be discarded and replaced with a new one.

If toothpaste is used, each child should have his/her own labeled toothpaste tube. If toothpaste from a single tube is shared among the children, it should be dispensed onto a clean piece of paper or paper cup for each child rather than directly on the toothbrush (1,6). A pea-sized amount should be used for each brushing. Toothpaste should be stored out of children's reach.

When children require assistance with brushing, caregivers/teachers should wash their hands thoroughly between brushings for each child. If children have bleeding gums, caregivers/teachers should wear gloves when assisting such children with brushing their teeth.

RATIONALE: Toothbrushes and oral fluids that collect in the mouth during tooth brushing are contaminated with infectious agents and must not be allowed to serve as a conduit of infection from one individual to another (6). Individually labeling the toothbrushes will prevent different children from sharing the same toothbrush. As an alternative to racks, children can have individualized, labeled cups and their brush can be stored bristle-up in their cup. Some bleeding may occur during tooth brushing in children who have inflammation of the gums. In child care, saliva is considered an infectious vehicle if it contains blood, so caregivers/teachers should protect themselves from exposure to blood in such situations, as required by standard precautions.

The Occupational Safety and Health Administration (OSHA) regulations apply where there is potential exposure to blood.

COMMENTS: Children can use an individually labeled or disposable cup of water to brush their teeth (6).

Toothpaste is not necessary if removal of food and plaque is the primary objective of tooth brushing. However, no anti-caries benefit is achieved from brushing without fluoride toothpaste.

Some risk of infection is involved when numerous children brush their teeth into sinks that are not sanitized between uses.

Toothbrushing ability varies by age. Preschool children most likely will require assistance. Adults helping children brush their teeth not only help them learn how to brush, but also improve the removal of plaque and food debris from all teeth (5).

TYPE OF FACILITY: Center; Large Family Child Care Home; Small Family Child Care Home

RELATED STANDARDS:
Standard 3.6.1.5: Sharing of Personal Articles Prohibited
Standard 5.5.0.1: Storage and Labeling of Personal Articles

REFERENCES:
1. Davies, R. M., G. M. Davies, R. P. Ellwood, E. J. Kay. 2003. Prevention. Part 4: Toothbrushing: What advice should be given to patients? *Brit Dent Jour* 195:135-41.
2. American Dental Association, Council on Scientific Affairs. 2005. ADA statement on toothbrush care: Cleaning, storage, and replacement. http://www.ada.org/1887.aspx.
3. American Academy of Pediatric Dentistry. 2004. *Early childhood caries (ECC).* http://www.aapd.org/media/ECCstats.pdf.
4. American Dental Hygienists' Association. *Proper brushing.* http://www.adha.org/oralhealth/brushing.htm.
5. 12345 First Smiles. 2006. Oral health considerations for children with special health care needs (CSHCN). http://www.first5oralhealth.org/page.asp?page_id=432.
6. Centers for Disease Control and Prevention. 2005. Infection control in dental settings: The use and handling of toothbrushes. http://www.cdc.gov/OralHealth/InfectionControl/factsheets/toothbrushes.htm.

STANDARD 3.1.5.3: Oral Health Education

All children with teeth should have oral hygiene education as a part of their daily activity.

Children three years of age and older should have developmentally appropriate oral health education that includes:

a) Information on what plaque is;
b) The process of dental decay;
c) Diet influences on teeth, including the contribution of sugar-sweetened beverages and foods to cavity development; and
d) The importance of good oral hygiene behaviors.

School-age children should receive **additional** information including:

a) The preventive use of fluoride;
b) Dental sealants;
c) Mouth guards for protection when playing sports;
d) The importance of healthy eating behaviors; and
e) Regularly scheduled dental visits.

Adolescent children should be informed about the effect of tobacco products on their oral health and additional reasons to avoid tobacco.

Caregivers/teachers and parents/guardians should be taught to not place a child's pacifier in the adult's mouth to clean or moisten it or share a toothbrush with a child due to the risk of promoting early colonization of the infant oral cavity with *Streptococcus mutans* (5).

Caregivers/teachers should limit juice consumption to no more than four to six ounces per day for children one through six years of age.

RATIONALE: Studies have reported that the oral health of participants improved as a result of educational programs (1).

COMMENTS: Caregivers/teachers are encouraged to advise parents/guardians on the following recommendations for preventive and early intervention dental services and education:

a) Dental or primary care provider visits to evaluate the need for supplemental fluoride therapy (prescription pills or drops if tap water does not contain fluoride) starting at six months of age, and professionally applied topical fluoride treatments for high risk children (4);
b) First dental visit within six months after the first tooth erupts or by one year of age, whichever is earlier and whenever there is a question of an oral health problem;
c) Dental sealants generally at six or seven years of age for first permanent molars, and for primary molars if deep pits and grooves or other high risk factors are present (2,3).

Caregivers/teachers should provide education for parents/guardians on good oral hygiene practices and avoidance of behaviors that increase the risk of early childhood caries, such as inappropriate use of a bottle, frequent consumption of carbohydrate-rich foods, and sweetened beverages such as juices with added sweeteners, soda, sports drinks, fruit nectars, and flavored teas.

For more resources on oral health education, see:

Parent's Checklist for Good Dental Health Practices in Child Care, a parent handout in English and Spanish, developed by the National Resource Center for Health and Safety in Child Care and Early Education at http://nrckids.org/dentalchecklist.pdf;

Bright Futures for Oral Health at http://brightfutures.aap.org/practice_guides_and_other_resources.html;

California Childcare Health Program *Health and Safety in the Child Care Setting: Promoting Children's Oral Health A Curriculum for Health Professionals and Child Care Providers* (in English and Spanish) at http://www.ucsfchildcarehealth.org and its *12345 first smiles* program at http://first5oralhealth.org; and

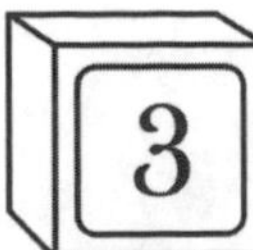

National Training Institute for Child Care Health Consultant's *Healthy Smiles Through Child Care Health Consultation* course at http://nti.unc.edu/healthy_smiles/.

TYPE OF FACILITY: Center

RELATED STANDARDS:
Section 2.4: Health Education
Standard 3.1.4.3: Pacifier Use
Standard 3.1.5.1: Routine Oral Hygiene Activities
Standard 3.1.5.2: Toothbrushes and Toothpaste
Standard 4.2.0.7: 100% Juice
Standard 9.2.3.14: Oral Health Policy

REFERENCES:

1. Dye, B. A., J. D. Shenkin, C. L. Ogden, T. A. Marshould, S. M. Levy, M. J. Kanellis. 2004. The relationship between healthful eating practices and dental caries in children aged 2-5 years in the United States. *J Am Dent Assoc* 135:55-66.
2. American Academy of Pediatrics, Section on Pediatric Dentistry. 2009. Policy statement: Oral health risk assessment timing and establishment of the dental home. *Pediatrics* 124:845.
3. American Academy of Pediatrics, Section on Pediatric Dentistry.2008. Preventive oral health intervention for pediatricians. *Pediatrics* 122:1387-94.
4. American Academy of Pediatric Dentistry, Clinical Affairs Committee, Council on Clinical Affairs. 2008-2009. Guideline on periodicity of examination, preventive dental services, anticipatory guidance/counseling, and oral treatment for infants, children, and adolescents. *Pediatric Dentistry* 30:112-18.
5. American Academy of Pediatrics, Oral Health Initiative. Protecting all children's teeth (PACT): A pediatric oral health training program. Factors in development: Bacteria. http://www.aap.org/oralhealth/pact/ch4_sect2.cfm.

3.2 Hygiene

3.2.1 Diapering and Changing Soiled Clothing

STANDARD 3.2.1.1: Type of Diapers Worn

Diapers worn by children should be able to contain urine and stool and minimize fecal contamination of children, caregivers/teachers, environmental surfaces, and objects in the child care setting. Only disposable diapers with absorbent material (e.g., polymers) may be used unless the child has a medical reason that does not permit the use of disposable diapers (such as allergic reactions). When children cannot use disposable diapers for a medical reason, the reason should be documented by the child's primary care provider. Children of all ages who are incontinent of urine or stool should wear a barrier method to prevent contamination of their environment.

If cloth diapers are used, the diaper should have an absorbent inner lining completely contained within an outer covering made of waterproof material that prevents the escape of feces and urine. An alternative is the use of cloth diapers that contain a waterproof cover that is adherent to the cloth material. If a cloth diaper with a separate lining is used, the outer covering and inner lining should be changed together at the same time as a unit and should not be reused in the child care facility. No rinsing or dumping of the contents of cloth diapers should be performed at the child care facility. Soiled cloth diapers should be completely wrapped in a non-permeable material, stored in a location inaccessible to children, and given directly to the parent/ guardian upon discharge of the child.

RATIONALE: Gastrointestinal tract disease caused by bacteria, viruses, parasites, and hepatitis A virus infection of the liver are spread from infected persons through fecal contamination of objects in the environment and hands of caregivers/teachers and children. Procedures that reduce fecal contamination, such as minimal handling of soiled diapers and clothing, thorough hand hygiene, and containment of fecal matter and articles containing fecal matter control the spread of these diseases. Diapering practices that require significant manipulation of the diaper and waterproof covering, particularly reuse of the covering before it is cleaned and disinfected, present increased opportunities for fecal contamination of the caregivers/teachers' hands, the child, and consequently, objects and surfaces in the environment. Environmental contamination has been associated with increased diarrheal rates in child care facilities (1). Fecal contamination in the center environment may be less when single-use, disposable diapers are used than when cloth diapers worn with pull-on waterproof pants are used (3). When clothes are worn over either disposable or cloth diapers with pull-on waterproof pants, there is a reduction in contamination of the environment (1,3).

Diaper dermatitis occurs frequently in diapered children. Diapering practices that reduce the frequency and severity of diaper dermatitis will require less application of skin creams and ointments, thereby decreasing the likelihood for fecal contamination of caregivers/teachers' hands. Most common diaper dermatitis represents an irritant contact dermatitis; the source of irritation is prolonged contact of the skin with urine, feces, or both (1). The action of fecal digestive enzymes on urinary urea and the resulting production of ammonia make the diapered area more alkaline, which has been shown to damage skin (1,2). Damaged skin is more susceptible to other biological, chemical, and physical insults that can cause or aggravate diaper dermatitis (1). Frequency and severity of diaper dermatitis are lower when diapers are changed more often, regardless of the diaper used (1). The use of modern disposable diapers with absorbent material has been associated with less frequent and less severe diaper dermatitis in some children than with the use of cloth diapers and pull-on pants made of a waterproof material (3).

COMMENTS: Several types of diapers or diapering systems are currently available: disposable paper diapers, reusable cloth diapers worn with pull-on waterproof pants, reusable cloth diapers worn with a modern front closure waterproof cover, and single unit reusable diaper systems with an inner cotton lining attached to an outer waterproof covering. Two types of diapers meet the physical requirements of the standard: modern disposable paper diapers with absorbent material, and single unit reusable diaper systems with an inner cotton lining attached to an outer waterproof covering. A

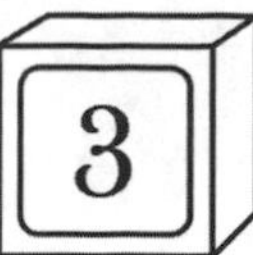

third type, reusable cloth diapers worn with a modern front closure waterproof cover, meets the standard only:

a) If the cloth diaper and cover are removed simultaneously as a unit and are not removed as two separate pieces; and
b) If the cloth diaper and outer cover are not reused until both are cleaned and disinfected.

Caregivers/teachers should follow this recommendation unless they have a care plan noting a different procedure from the child's primary care provider.

Reusable cloth diapers worn either without a covering or with pull-on pants made of waterproof material do not meet the physical requirements of the standard and should not be permitted in facilities. Whichever diapering system is used in the facility, clothes should be worn over diapers while the child is in the facility. Rigorous protocols should be implemented for diaper handling and changing, personal hygiene, and environmental decontamination. While single unit reusable diaper systems, with an inner cloth lining attached to an outer waterproof covering, and reusable cloth diapers, worn with a modern front closure waterproof cover, meet the physical criteria of this standard (if used as described), they have not been evaluated for their ability to reduce fecal contamination, or for their association with diaper dermatitis. Moreover, it has not been demonstrated that the waterproof covering materials remain waterproof with repeated cleaning and disinfecting. Therefore, single-use disposable diapers should be encouraged for use in child care facilities.

TYPE OF FACILITY: Center; Large Family Child Care Home; Small Family Child Care Home

RELATED STANDARDS:
Standard 3.2.1.2: Handling Cloth Diapers
Standard 3.2.1.4: Diaper Changing Procedure
Standards 3.2.2.1-3.2.2.5: Hand Hygiene
Standard 5.2.7.4: Containment of Soiled Diapers
Standard 5.4.1.10: Handwashing Sinks

REFERENCES:

1. Van, R., A. L. Morrow, R. R. Reves, L. K. Pickering. 1991. Environmental contamination in child day care centers. *Am J Epidemiol* 133:460-70.
2. Gorski, P. A. 1999. Toilet training guidelines: Day care providers-the role of the day care provider in toilet training. *Pediatrics* 103:1367-68.
3. Kubiak, M., B. Kressner, W. Raynor, J. Davis, R. E. Syverson. 1993. Comparison of stool containment in cloth and single-use diapers using a simulated infant feces. *Pediatrics* 91:632-36.

STANDARD 3.2.1.2: Handling Cloth Diapers

If cloth diapers are used, soiled cloth diapers and/or soiled training pants should never be rinsed or carried through the child care area to place the fecal contents in a toilet. Reusable diapers should be laundered by a commercial diaper service. Soiled cloth diapers should be stored in a labeled container with a tight-fitting lid provided by an accredited commercial diaper service, or in a sealed plastic bag for removal from the facility by an individual child's family. The sealed plastic bag should be sent home with the child at the end of the day. The containers or sealed diaper bags of soiled cloth diapers should not be accessible to any child (1).

RATIONALE: Containing and minimizing the handling of soiled diapers so they do not contaminate other surfaces is essential to prevent the spread of infectious disease. Putting stool into a toilet in the child care facility increases the likelihood that other surfaces will be contaminated during the disposal (2). There is no reason to use the toilet for stool if disposable diapers are being used. Commercial diaper laundries use a procedure that separates solid components from the diapers and does not require prior dumping of feces into the toilet.

TYPE OF FACILITY: Center; Large Family Child Care Home; Small Family Child Care Home

RELATED STANDARDS:
Standard 3.2.1.1: Type of Diapers Worn

REFERENCES:

1. Healthy Child Care. Diapering. 2006. http://www.globalhealthychildcare.org/default.aspx?page=poi&content_id=4&language=content.
2. Pickering, L. K., C. J. Baker, D. W. Kimberlin, S. S. Long, eds. 2009. *Red book: 2009 report of the Committee on Infectious Diseases.* 28th ed. Elk Grove Village, IL: American Academy of Pediatrics.

STANDARD 3.2.1.3: Checking For the Need to Change Diapers

Diapers should be checked for wetness and feces at least hourly, visually inspected at least every two hours, and whenever the child indicates discomfort or exhibits behavior that suggests a soiled or wet diaper. Diapers should be changed when they are found to be wet or soiled.

RATIONALE: Frequency and severity of diaper dermatitis is lower when diapers are changed more often, regardless of the type of diaper used (1). Diaper dermatitis occurs frequently in diapered children. Most common diaper dermatitis represents an irritant contact dermatitis; the source of irritation is prolonged contact of the skin with urine, feces, or both (2). The action of fecal digestive enzymes on urinary urea and the resulting production of ammonia make the diapered area more alkaline, which has been shown to damage skin (1,2). Damaged skin is more susceptible to other biological, chemical, and physical insults that can cause or aggravate diaper dermatitis (2).

Modern disposable diapers can be checked for wetness by feeling the diaper through the clothing and fecal contents can be assessed by odor. Nonetheless, since these methods of checking may be inaccurate, the diaper should be opened and checked visually at least every two hours. Even though modern disposable diapers can continue to absorb moisture for an extended period of time when they are wet, they should be changed after two hours of wearing if they are found to be wet. This prevents rubbing of wet surfaces against the skin, a major cause of diaper dermatitis.

TYPE OF FACILITY: Center; Large Family Child Care Home; Small Family Child Care Home

REFERENCES:

1. Healthy Children. 2010. Ages and stages: When diaper rash strikes. http://www.healthychildren.org/English/ages-stages/baby/diapers-clothing/Pages/When-Diaper-Rash-Strikes.aspx.
2. Shelov, S. P., T. R. Altmann, eds. 2009. *Caring for your baby and young child: Birth to age 5.* 5th ed. Elk Grove Village, IL: American Academy of Pediatrics.

STANDARD 3.2.1.4: Diaper Changing Procedure

The following diaper changing procedure should be posted in the changing area, should be followed for all diaper changes, and should be used as part of staff evaluation of caregivers/teachers who diaper. The signage should be simple and should be in multiple languages if caregivers/teachers who speak multiple languages are involved in diapering. All employees who will diaper should undergo training and periodic assessment of diapering practices. Caregivers/teachers should never leave a child unattended on a table or countertop, even for an instant. A safety strap or harness should not be used on the diaper changing table. If an emergency arises, caregivers/teachers should bring any child on an elevated surface to the floor or take the child with them.

An EPA-registered disinfectant suitable for the surface material that is being disinfected should be used. If an EPA-registered product is not available, then household bleach diluted with water is a practical alternative. All cleaning and disinfecting solutions should be stored to be accessible to the caregiver/teacher but out of reach of any child. Please refer to Appendix J, Selecting an Appropriate Sanitizer or Disinfectant.

Step 1: Get organized. Before bringing the child to the diaper changing area, perform hand hygiene, gather and bring supplies to the diaper changing area:

a) Non-absorbent paper liner large enough to cover the changing surface from the child's shoulders to beyond the child's feet;
b) Unused diaper, clean clothes (if you need them);
c) Wipes for cleaning the child's genitalia and buttocks removed from the container or dispensed so the container will not be touched during diaper changing;
d) A wet cloth or paper towel;
e) A plastic bag for any soiled clothes or cloth diapers;
f) Disposable gloves, if you plan to use them (put gloves on before handling soiled clothing or diapers) and remove them before handling clean diapers and clothing;
g) A thick application of any diaper cream (e.g., zinc oxide ointment), when appropriate, removed from the container to a piece of disposable material such as facial or toilet tissue.

Step 2: Carry the child to the changing table, keeping soiled clothing away from you and any surfaces you cannot easily clean and sanitize after the change.

a) Always keep a hand on the child;
b) If the child's feet cannot be kept out of the diaper or from contact with soiled skin during the changing process, remove the child's shoes and socks so the child does not contaminate these surfaces with stool or urine during the diaper changing.

Step 3: Clean the child's diaper area.

a) Place the child on the diaper change surface and unfasten the diaper, but leave the soiled diaper under the child;
b) If safety pins are used, close each pin immediately once it is removed and keep pins out of the child's reach (never hold pins in your mouth);
c) Lift the child's legs as needed to use disposable wipes to clean the skin on the child's genitalia and buttocks and prevent recontamination from a soiled diaper. If there is a need to clean between the labia of an infant girl, use only a wet cloth or paper towel. Remove stool and urine from front to back and use a fresh wipe each time you swipe. Put the soiled wipes into the soiled diaper or directly into a plastic-lined, hands-free covered can.

Step 4: Remove the soiled diaper and clothing without contaminating any surface not already in contact with stool or urine.

a) Fold the soiled surface of the diaper inward;
b) Put soiled disposable diapers in a covered, plastic-lined, hands-free covered can. If reusable cloth diapers are used, put the soiled cloth diaper and its contents (without emptying or rinsing) in a plastic bag or into a plastic-lined, hands-free covered can to give to parents/guardians or laundry service;
c) Put soiled clothes in a plastic-lined, hands-free plastic bag;
d) If gloves were used, remove them using the proper technique (see Appendix D) and put them into a plastic-lined, hands-free covered can;
e) Whether or not gloves were used, use a disposable antibacterial wipe or alcohol-based hand sanitizer to clean the surfaces of the caregiver/teacher's hands and an application to clean the child's hands, and put the wipes, if used, into the plastic-lined, hands-free covered can. Allow sanitized hands to dry completely before proceeding;
f) Check for spills under the child. If there are any, use the paper that extends under the child's feet to fold over the soiled area so a fresh, unsoiled paper surface is now under the child's buttocks.

Step 5: Put on a clean diaper and dress the child.

a) Slide a fresh diaper under the child;
b) Use a facial or toilet tissue or wear clean disposable glove to apply any necessary diaper creams, discarding the tissue or glove in a covered, plastic-lined, hands-free covered can;
c) Note and plan to report any skin problems such as redness, skin cracks, or bleeding;
d) Fasten the diaper; if pins are used, place your hand between the child and the diaper when inserting the pin.

Step 6: Wash the child's hands and return the child to a supervised area.

a) Use soap and warm water, between 60°F and 120°F, at a sink to wash the child's hands, if you can.

Step 7: Clean and disinfect the diaper-changing surface.

a) Dispose of the disposable paper liner used on the diaper changing surface in a plastic-lined, hands-free covered can;
b) If clothing was soiled, securely tie the plastic bag used to store the clothing and send home;
c) Remove any visible soil from the changing surface with a water saturated disposable paper towel or wipe;
d) Wet the entire changing surface with a disinfectant that is appropriate for the surface material you are treating. Follow the manufacturer's instructions for use;
e) Put away the disinfectant. Some types of disinfectants may require rinsing the change table surface with fresh water afterwards.

Step 8: Perform hand hygiene according to the procedure in Standard 3.2.2.2 and record the diaper change in the child's daily log.

a) In the daily log, record what was in the diaper and any problems (such as a loose stool, an unusual odor, blood in the stool, or any skin irritation), and report as necessary (2).

RATIONALE: The procedure for diaper changing is designed to reduce the contamination of surfaces that will later come in contact with uncontaminated surfaces such as hands, furnishings, and floors (1,3). Posting the multi-step procedure may help caregivers/teachers maintain the routine.

Assembling all necessary supplies before bringing the child to the changing area will ensure the child's safety, make the change more efficient, and reduce opportunities for contamination. Taking the supplies out of their containers and leaving the containers in their storage places reduces the likelihood that the storage containers will become contaminated during diaper changing.

Commonly, caregivers/teachers do not use disposable paper that is large enough to cover the area likely to be contaminated during diaper changing. If the paper is large enough, there will be less need to remove visible soil from surfaces later and there will be enough paper to fold up so the soiled surface is not in contact with clean surfaces while dressing the child.

If the child's foot coverings are not removed during diaper changing, and the child kicks during the diaper changing procedure, the foot coverings can become contaminated and subsequently spread contamination throughout the child care area.

If the child's clean buttocks are put down on a soiled surface, the child's skin can be resoiled.

Children's hands often stray into the diaper area (the area of the child's body covered by diaper) during the diapering process and can then transfer fecal organisms to the environment. Washing the child's hands will reduce the number of organisms carried into the environment in this way. Infectious organisms are present on the skin and diaper even though they are not seen. To reduce the contamination of clean surfaces, caregivers/teachers should use an antibacterial wipe or alcohol-based hand sanitizer to wipe their hands after removing the gloves, or, if no gloves were used, before proceeding to handle the clean diaper and the clothing.

Some states and credentialing organizations may recommend wearing gloves for diaper changing. Although gloves may not be required, they may provide a barrier against surface contamination of a caregiver/teacher's hands. This may reduce the presence of enteric pathogens under the fingernails and on hand surfaces. Even if gloves are used, caregivers/teachers must perform hand hygiene after each child's diaper changing to prevent the spread of disease-causing agents. To achieve maximum benefit from use of gloves, the caregiver/teacher must remove the gloves properly after cleaning the child's genitalia and buttocks and removing the soiled diaper. Otherwise, retained contaminated gloves could transfer organisms to clean surfaces. Note that sensitivity to latex is a growing problem. If caregivers/teachers or children who are sensitive to latex are present in the facility, non-latex gloves should be used. See Appendix D, for proper technique for removing gloves.

A safety strap cannot be relied upon to restrain the child and could become contaminated during diaper changing. Cleaning and disinfecting a strap would be required after every diaper change. Therefore safety straps on diaper changing surfaces are not recommended.

Prior to disinfecting the changing table, clean any visible soil from the surface with a detergent and rinse well with water. Always follow the manufacturer's instructions for use, application and storage. If the disinfectant is applied using a spray bottle, always assume that the outside of the spray bottle could be contaminated. Therefore, the spray bottle should be put away before hand hygiene is performed, (the last and essential part of every diaper change) (4).

Diaper-changing areas should never be located in food preparation areas and should never be used for temporary placement of food, drinks, or eating utensils.

If parents use the diaper changing area, they should be required to follow the same diaper changing procedure to minimize contamination of the diaper changing area and child care.

TYPE OF FACILITY: Center; Large Family Child Care Home; Small Family Child Care Home

RELATED STANDARDS:

Standard 3.2.1.1: Type of Diapers Worn
Standard 3.2.1.2: Handling Cloth Diapers
Standard 3.2.1.3: Checking for the Need to Change Diapers
Standard 3.2.2.1: Situations that Require Hand Hygiene
Standard 3.2.2.2: Handwashing Procedure
Standard 3.3.0.1: Routine Cleaning, Sanitizing, and Disinfecting

Standard 5.2.7.4: Containment of Soiled Diapers
Appendix D: Gloving

REFERENCES:

1. Pickering, L. K., C. J. Baker, D. W. Kimberlin, S. S. Long, eds. 2009. *Red book 2009: Report of the Committee on Infectious Diseases.* 28th ed. Elk Grove Village, IL: American Academy of Pediatrics.
2. National Association for the Education of Young Children. 2007. *Keeping healthy: Parents, teachers, and children.* Rev ed. Washington, DC: NAEYC.
3. Fiene, R. 2002. *13 indicators of quality child care: Research update*. Washington, DC: U.S. Department of Health and Human Services, Office of the Assistant Secretary for Planning and Evaluation. http://aspe.hhs.gov/hsp/ccquality-ind02/.
4. North Carolina Child Care Health and Safety Resource Center. Diapering procedure poster. http://www.healthychildcarenc.org/PDFs/diaper_procedure_english.pdf.

STANDARD 3.2.1.5: Procedure for Changing Children's Soiled Underwear/Pull-Ups and Clothing

The following changing procedure for soiled pull-ups or underwear and clothing should be posted in the changing area, should be followed for all changes, and should be used as part of staff evaluation of caregivers/teachers who change pull-ups or underwear and clothing. The signage should be simple and should be in multiple languages if caregivers/teachers who speak multiple languages are involved in changing pull-ups or underwear. All employees who will change pull-ups or underwear and clothing should undergo training and periodic assessment of these practices.

Changing a child from the floor level or on a chair puts the adult in an awkward position and increases the risk of contamination of the environment. Using a toddler changing table helps establish a well-organized changing area for both the child and the caregiver/teacher. Changing tables with steps that allow the child to climb with the caregiver/teacher's help and supervision are a good idea. This would help reduce the risk of back injury for the adults that may occur from lifting the child onto the table (1).

Caregivers/teachers should never leave a child unattended on a table or countertop, even for an instant. A safety strap or harness should not be used on the changing surface. If an emergency arises, caregivers/teachers should bring any child on an elevated surface to the floor or take the child with them.

An EPA-registered disinfectant suitable for the surface material that is being disinfected should be used. If an EPA-registered product is not available, then household bleach diluted with water is a practical alternative. All cleaning and disinfecting solutions should be stored to be accessible to the caregiver/teacher but out of reach of any child. Please refer to Appendix J, Selecting an Appropriate Sanitizer or Disinfectant.

Step 1: Get organized. Before bringing the child to the changing area, perform hand hygiene, gather and bring supplies to the changing area.

a) Non-absorbent paper liner large enough to cover the changing surface from the child's shoulders to beyond the child's feet;
b) Unused pull-up or underwear, clean clothes (if you need them);
c) Wipes for cleaning the child's genitalia and buttocks removed from the container or dispensed so the container will not be touched during changing;
d) A wet cloth or paper towel;
e) A plastic bag for any soiled clothes, including underwear, or pull-ups;
f) Disposable gloves, if you plan to use them (put gloves on before handling soiled clothing or pull-ups) and remove them before handling clean pull-ups or underwear and clothing.

Step 2: Avoid contact with soiled items.

a) Consider whether to change the child lying down or standing up;
b) If the child is standing, it may cause the clothing, shoes and socks to become soiled. The caregiver/teacher must remove these items before the change begins;
c) To avoid contaminating the child's clothes, have the child hold their shirt, sweater, etc. up above their waist during the change. This keeps the child's hands busy and the caregiver/teacher knows where the child's hands are during the changing process. Caregivers/teachers can also use plastic clothes pins that can be washed and sanitized to keep the clothing out of the way;
d) If disposable pull-ups were used, pull the sides apart, rather than sliding the garment down the child's legs. If underwear is being changed, remove the soiled underwear and any soiled clothing, doing your best to avoid contamination of surfaces;
e) To avoid contamination of the environment and/or the increased risk of spreading germs to the other children in the room, do not rinse the soiled clothing in the toilet or elsewhere. Place all soiled garments in a plastic-lined, hands-free plastic bag to be cleaned at the child's home;
f) If the child's shoes are soiled, the caregiver/teacher must wash and sanitize them before putting them back on the child. It is a good idea for the child care facility to request a few extra pair of socks and shoes from the parent/caregiver to be kept at the facility in case these items become soiled (1);
g) Check for spills under the child. If there are any, use the paper that extends under the child's feet to fold over the soiled area so a fresh, unsoiled paper surface is now under the child's buttocks.

Step 3: Clean the child's skin.

a) Lift the child's legs as needed to use disposable wipes to clean the skin on the child's genitalia and buttocks. If there is a need to clean between the labia of a toddler girl, use only a wet cloth or paper towel. Remove stool and urine from front to back and use a fresh wipe each time you swipe. Put the soiled wipes

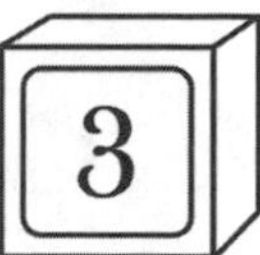

into the soiled pull-up or directly into a plastic-lined, hands-free covered can;

b) If gloves were used, remove them using the proper technique (see Appendix D) and put them into a plastic-lined, hands-free covered can;

c) Whether or not gloves were used, use a disposable antibacterial wipe or alcohol-based hand sanitizer to clean the surfaces of the caregiver/teacher's hands and an application to clean the child's hands, and put the wipes, if used, into the plastic-lined, hands-free covered can. Allow sanitized hands to dry completely before proceeding.

Step 4: Put on a clean pull-up or underwear and clothing, if necessary.

a) Assist the child, as needed, in putting on a clean disposable pull-up or underwear, then in re-dressing (1);

b) Note and plan to report any skin problems such as redness, skin cracks, or bleeding;

c) Put the child's socks and shoes back on if they were removed during the changing procedure (1).

Step 5: Wash the child's hands and return the child to a supervised area.

a) Use soap and warm water, between 60°F and 120°F, at a sink to wash the child's hands, if you can.

Step 6: Clean and disinfect the changing surface.

a) Dispose of the disposable paper liner used on the changing surface in a plastic-lined, hands-free covered can;

b) If clothing was soiled, securely tie the plastic bag used to store the clothing and send home;

c) Remove any visible soil from the changing surface with a water saturated disposable paper towel or wipe;

d) Wet the entire changing surface with a disinfectant that is appropriate for the surface material you are treating. Follow the manufacturer's instructions for use;

e) Put away the disinfectant. Some types of disinfectants may require rinsing the change table surface with fresh water afterwards.

Step 7: Perform hand hygiene according to the procedure in Standard 3.2.2.2 and record the change in the child's daily log.

a) In the daily log, record what was in the pull-up or underwear and any problems (such as a loose stool, an unusual odor, blood in the stool, or any skin irritation), and report as necessary (3).

RATIONALE: Children who are learning to use the toilet may still wet/soil their pull-ups or underwear and clothing. Changing these undergarments can lead to risk for spreading infection due to the contamination of surfaces from urine or feces (1). The procedure for changing a child's soiled undergarment and clothing is designed to reduce the contamination of surfaces that will later come in contact with uncontaminated surfaces such as hands, furnishings, and floors (2,4). Posting the multi-step procedure may help caregivers/teachers maintain the routine.

Assembling all necessary supplies before bringing the child to the changing area will ensure the child's safety, make the change more efficient, and reduce opportunities for contamination. Taking the supplies out of their containers and leaving the containers in their storage places reduces the likelihood that the storage containers will become contaminated during changing.

Commonly, caregivers/teachers do not use disposable paper that is large enough to cover the area likely to be contaminated during changing. If the paper is large enough, there will be less need to remove visible soil from surfaces later and there will be enough paper to fold up so the soiled surface is not in contact with clean surfaces while dressing the child.

If the child's foot coverings are not removed during changing, and the child kicks during the changing procedure, the foot coverings can become contaminated and subsequently spread contamination throughout the child care area.

If the child's clean buttocks are put down on a soiled surface, the child's skin can be resoiled.

Children's hands often stray into the changing area (the area of the child's body covered by the soiled pull-ups or underwear) during the changing process and can then transfer fecal organisms to the environment. Washing the child's hands will reduce the number or organisms carried into the environment in this way. Infectious organisms are present on the skin and pull-ups or underwear even though they are not seen. To reduce the contamination of clean surfaces, caregivers/teachers should use an antibacterial wipe or alcohol-based hand sanitizer to wipe their hands after removing the gloves or, if no gloves were used, before proceeding to handle the clean pull-up or underwear and the clothing.

Some states and credentialing organizations may recommend wearing gloves for changing. Although gloves may not be required, they may provide a barrier against surface contamination of a caregiver/teacher's hands. This may reduce the presence of enteric pathogens under the fingernails and on hand surfaces. Even if gloves are used, caregivers/teachers must perform hand hygiene after each child's changing to prevent the spread of disease-causing agents. To achieve maximum benefit from use of gloves, the caregiver/teacher must remove the gloves properly after cleaning the child's genitalia and buttocks and removing the soiled pull-up or underwear. Otherwise, retained contaminated gloves could transfer organisms to clean surfaces. Note that sensitivity to latex is a growing problem. If caregivers/teachers or children who are sensitive to latex are present in the facility, non-latex gloves should be used. See Appendix D for proper technique for removing gloves.

A safety strap cannot be relied upon to restrain the child and could become contaminated during changing. Cleaning and disinfecting a strap would be required after every change. Therefore safety straps on changing surfaces are not recommended.

Prior to disinfecting the changing table, clean any visible soil from the surface with a detergent and rinse well with water. Always follow the manufacturer's instructions for use, application and storage. If the disinfectant is applied using a spray bottle, always assume that the outside of the spray bottle could be contaminated. Therefore, the spray bottle should be put away before hand hygiene is performed (the last and essential part of every change) (5).

Changing areas should never be located in food preparation areas and should never be used for temporary placement of food, drinks, or eating utensils.

COMMENTS: Children with disabilities may require diapering and the method of diapering will vary according to their abilities. However, principles of hygiene should be consistent regardless of method. Toddlers and preschool age children without physical disabilities frequently have toileting issues as well. These soiling/wetting episodes can be due to rapid onset gastroenteritis, distraction due to the intensity of their play, and emotional disruption secondary to new transition. These include new siblings, stress in the family, or anxiety about changing classrooms or programs, all of which are based on their inability to recognize and articulate their stress and to manage a variety of impulses.

Development is not a straight trajectory, but rather a cycle of forward and backward steps as children gain mastery over their bodies in a wide variety of situations. It is normal and developmentally appropriate for children to revert to immature behaviors as they gain developmental milestones while simultaneously dealing with immediate struggles which they are internalizing. Even for preschool and kindergarten aged children, these accidents happen and these incidents are called 'accidents' because of the frequency of these episodes among normally developing children. It is important for caregivers/teachers to recognize that the need to assist young children with toileting is a critical part of their work and that their attitude regarding the incident and their support of children as they work toward self regulation of their bodies is a component of teaching young children.

TYPE OF FACILITY: Center; Large Family Child Care Home; Small Family Child Care Home

RELATED STANDARDS:
Standard 3.2.1.3: Checking for the Need to Change Diapers
Standard 3.2.2.1: Situations that Require Hand Hygiene
Standard 3.2.2.2: Handwashing Procedure
Standard 3.3.0.1: Routine Cleaning, Sanitizing, and Disinfecting
Standard 5.2.7.4: Containment of Soiled Diapers
Appendix D: Gloving
Appendix J: Selecting an Appropriate Sanitizer or Disinfectant

REFERENCES:
1. ECELS-Healthy Child Care Pennsylvania. Changing soiled underwear for toddlers. http://www.ecels-healthychildcarepa.org/content/2-11-10 v2ChangingSoiledUnderwear.pdf.
2. Pickering, L. K., C. J. Baker, D. W. Kimberlin, S. S. Long, eds. 2009. *Red book 2009: Report of the Committee on Infectious Diseases.* 28th ed. Elk Grove Village, IL: American Academy of Pediatrics.
3. National Association for the Education of Young Children. 2007. *Keeping healthy: Parents, teachers, and children.* Rev ed. Washington, DC: NAEYC.
4. Fiene, R. 2002. *13 indicators of quality child care: Research update.* Washington, DC: U.S. Department of Health and Human Services, Office of the Assistant Secretary for Planning and Evaluation. http://aspe.hhs.gov/hsp/ccquality-ind02/.
5. North Carolina Child Care Health and Safety Resource Center. Diapering procedure poster. http://www.healthychildcarenc.org/PDFs/diaper_procedure_english.pdf.

3.2.2 Hand Hygiene

STANDARD 3.2.2.1: Situations that Require Hand Hygiene

All staff, volunteers, and children should follow the procedure in Standard 3.2.2.2 for hand hygiene at the following times:

a) Upon arrival for the day, after breaks, or when moving from one child care group to another;
b) Before and after:
   1) Preparing food or beverages;
   2) Eating, handling food, or feeding a child;
   3) Giving medication or applying a medical ointment or cream in which a break in the skin (e.g., sores, cuts, or scrapes) may be encountered;
   4) Playing in water (including swimming) that is used by more than one person;
   5) Diapering;
c) After:
   1) Using the toilet or helping a child use a toilet;
   2) Handling bodily fluid (mucus, blood, vomit), from sneezing, wiping and blowing noses, from mouths, or from sores;
   3) Handling animals or cleaning up animal waste;
   4) Playing in sand, on wooden play sets, and outdoors;
   5) Cleaning or handling the garbage.

Situations or times that children and staff should perform hand hygiene should be posted in all food preparation, hand hygiene, diapering, and toileting areas.

RATIONALE: Hand hygiene is the most important way to reduce the spread of infection. Many studies have shown that improperly cleansed hands are the primary carriers of infections. Deficiencies in hand hygiene have contributed to many outbreaks of diarrhea among children and caregivers/teachers in child care centers (1).

In child care centers that have implemented hand hygiene training program, the incidence of diarrheal illness has decreased by 50% (2). Several studies demonstrate a reduction in upper respiratory symptoms (colds) when frequent and proper hand hygiene practices were incorporated into a child care center's curriculum (2-4).

Hand hygiene after exposure to soil and sand will reduce opportunities for the ingestion of zoonotic parasites that could be present in contaminated sand and soil (6,7).

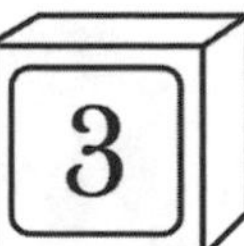

Thorough handwashing with soap for at least twenty seconds using comfortably warm, running water (between 60°F and 120°F) removes organisms from the skin and allows them to be rinsed away (5). Hand hygiene is effective in preventing transmission of disease. Hand hygiene with an alcohol-based sanitizer is an alternative to traditional handwashing with soap and water when visible soiling is not present.

Infectious organisms may be spread in a variety of ways:

a) In human waste (urine, stool);
b) In body fluids (saliva, nasal discharge, secretions from open injuries; eye discharge, blood);
c) Cuts or skin sores;
d) By direct skin-to-skin contact;
e) By touching an object that has live organisms on it;
f) In droplets of body fluids, such as those produced by sneezing and coughing, that travel through the air.

Since many infected people carry infectious organisms without symptoms and many are contagious before they experience a symptom, caregivers/teachers routine hand hygiene is the safest practice (4).

If caregivers/teachers smoke off premises before starting work, they should wash their hands before caring for children to prevent children from receiving third-hand smoke exposure (8).

TYPE OF FACILITY: Center; Large Family Child Care Home; Small Family Child Care Home

RELATED STANDARDS:
Standard 3.2.2.2: Handwashing Procedure
Standard 3.2.2.3: Assisting Children with Hand Hygiene
Standard 3.2.2.4: Training and Monitoring for Hand Hygiene
Standard 3.2.2.5: Hand Sanitizers
Standard 3.4.1.1: Use of Tobacco, Alcohol, and Illegal Drugs

REFERENCES:

1. Hawks, D., J. Ascheim, G. S. Giebink, S. Graville, A. J. Solnit. 1994. Science, prevention, and practice VII: Improving child day care, a concurrent summary of the American Public Health Association/American Academy of Pediatrics National health and safety guidelines for child-care programs; featured standards and implementation. *Pediatrics* 94:1110-12.
2. Soto. J. C., M. Guy, L. Belanger. 1994. Science, prevention and practice II: Preventing infectious diseases, abstracts on handwashing and infection control in day-care centers. *Pediatrics* 94:1030.
3. Roberts, L., E. Mapp, W. Smith, L. Jorm, M. Pate, R. M. Douglas, C. McGilchrist. 2000. Effect of infection control measures on the frequency of upper respiratory infection in child care: A randomized, controlled trial. *Pediatrics* 105:738-42.
4. Niffenegger, J. P. 1997. Proper handwashing promotes wellness in child care. *J Pediatr Health Care* 11:26-31.
5. Donowitz, L. G., ed. 1996. *Infection control in the child care center and preschool*, 18, 19, 68. 2nd ed. Baltimore, MD: Williams and Wilkins.
6. Palmer, S. R., L. Soulsby, D. I. H. Simpson, eds. 1998. *Zoonoses: Biology, clinical practice, and public health control*. New York: Oxford University Press.
7. Weinberg, A. N. and D. J. Weber, eds. 1991. Respiratory infections transmitted from animals. *Infect Dis Clin North Am* 5:649-61.
8. Mayo Clinic. 2010. Secondhand smoke: Avoid dangers in the air. http://www.mayoclinic.com/health/secondhand-smoke/CC00023/.

STANDARD 3.2.2.2: Handwashing Procedure

Children and staff members should wash their hands using the following method:

a) Check to be sure a clean, disposable paper (or single-use cloth) towel is available;
b) Turn on warm water, between 60°F and 120°F, to a comfortable temperature;
c) Moisten hands with water and apply soap (not antibacterial) to hands;
d) Rub hands together vigorously until a soapy lather appears, hands are out of the water stream, and continue for at least twenty seconds (sing Happy Birthday silently twice) (2). Rub areas between fingers, around nailbeds, under fingernails, jewelry, and back of hands. Nails should be kept short; acrylic nails should not worn (3);
e) Rinse hands under running water, between 60°F and 120°F, until they are free of soap and dirt. Leave the water running while drying hands;
f) Dry hands with the clean, disposable paper or single use cloth towel;
g) If taps do not shut off automatically, turn taps off with a disposable paper or single use cloth towel;
h) Throw the disposable paper towel into a lined trash container; or place single-use cloth towels in the laundry hamper; or hang individually labeled cloth towels to dry. Use hand lotion to prevent chapping of hands, if desired.

The use of alcohol based hand sanitizers is an alternative to traditional handwashing with soap and water by children over twenty-four months of age and adults on hands that are not visibly soiled. A single pump of an alcohol-based sanitizer should be dispensed. Hands should be rubbed together, distributing sanitizer to all hand and finger surfaces and hands should be permitted to air dry.

Situations/times that children and staff should wash their hands should be posted in all handwashing areas.

Use of antimicrobial soap is not recommended in child care settings. There are no data to support use of antibacterial soaps over other liquid soaps.

Children and staff who need to open a door to leave a bathroom or diaper changing area should open the door with a disposable towel to avoid possibly re-contaminating clean hands. If a child can not open the door or turn off the faucet, they should be assisted by an adult.

RATIONALE: Running water over the hands removes visible soil. Wetting the hands before applying soap helps to create a lather that can loosen soil. The soap lather loosens soil and brings it into solution on the surface of the skin. Rinsing the lather off into a sink removes the soil from the hands that the soap brought into solution. Warm water, between 60°F and 120°F, is more comfortable than cold water; using warm water also promotes adequate rinsing during handwashing (1).

Acceptable forms of soap include liquid and powder.

COMMENTS: Pre-moistened cleansing towlettes do not effectively clean hands and should not be used as a substitute for washing hands with soap and running water. When running water is unavailable or impractical, the use of alcohol-based hand sanitizer (Standard 3.2.2.5) is a suitable alternative.

Outbreaks of disease have been linked to shared wash water and wash basins (4). Water basins should not be used as an alternative to running water. Camp sinks and portable commercial sinks with foot or hand pumps dispense water as for a plumbed sink and are satisfactory if filled with fresh water daily. The staff should clean and disinfect the water reservoir container and water catch basin daily.

Single-use towels should be used unless an automatic electric hand-dryer is available.

The use of cloth roller towels is not recommended for the following reasons:

a) Children often use cloth roll dispensers improperly, resulting in more than one child using the same section of towel; and
b) Incidents of unintentional strangulation have been reported (U.S. Consumer Product Safety Commission Data Office, pers. comm.)

TYPE OF FACILITY: Center; Large Family Child Care Home; Small Family Child Care Home

RELATED STANDARDS:
Standard 3.2.2.1: Situations that Require Hand Hygiene
Standard 3.2.2.3: Assisting Children with Hand Hygiene
Standard 3.2.2.5: Hand Sanitizers
Appendix K: Routine Schedule for Cleaning, Sanitizing, and Disinfecting

REFERENCES:
1. Donowitz, L. G., ed. 1996. *Infection control in the child care center and preschool.* 2nd ed. Baltimore, MD: Williams and Wilkins.
2. Centers for Disease Control and Prevention. 2011. Handwashing: Clean hands save lives. http://www.cdc.gov/handwashing/.
3. McNeil, S. A., C. L. Foster, S. A. Hedderwick, C. A. Kauffman. 2001. Effect of hand clensing with antimicrobial soap or alcohol-based gel on microbial colonization of artificial fingernails worn by health care workers. *Clin Infect Dis* 32:367-72.
4. Ogunsola, F. T., Y. O. Adesiji. 2008. Comparison of four methods of hand washing in situations of inadequate water supply. *West Afr J Med* 27:24-28.

STANDARD 3.2.2.3: Assisting Children with Hand Hygiene

Caregivers/teachers should provide assistance with handwashing at a sink for infants who can be safely cradled in one arm and for children who can stand but not wash their hands independently. A child who can stand should either use a child-height sink or stand on a safety step at a height at which the child's hands can hang freely under the running water. After assisting the child with handwashing, the staff member should wash his or her own hands. Hand hygiene with an alcohol-based sanitizer is an alternative to handwashing with soap and water by children over twenty-four months of age and adults when there is no visible soiling of hands (1).

RATIONALE: Encouraging and teaching children good hand hygiene practices must be done in a safe manner. A "how to" poster that is developmentally appropriate should be placed wherever children wash their hands.

For examples of handwashing posters, see:

California Childcare Health Program at http://www.ucsfchildcarehealth.org;

North Carolina Child Care Health and Safety Resource Center at http://www.healthychildcarenc.org/training_materials.htm.

TYPE OF FACILITY: Center; Large Family Child Care Home; Small Family Child Care Home

RELATED STANDARDS:
Standard 3.2.2.1: Situations that Require Hand Hygiene
Standard 3.2.2.2: Handwashing Procedure
Standard 3.2.2.5: Hand Sanitizers

REFERENCES:
1. Centers for Disease Control and Prevention. 2009. Preventing the spread of influenza (the flu) in child care settings: Guidance for administrators, caregivers/teachers, and other staff. http://www.cdc.gov/flu/professionals/infectioncontrol/childcaresettings.htm.

STANDARD 3.2.2.4: Training and Monitoring for Hand Hygiene

The program should ensure that staff members and children who are developmentally able to learn personal hygiene are instructed in, and monitored on performing hand hygiene as specified in Standard 3.2.2.2.

RATIONALE: Education of the staff and children regarding hand hygiene and other cleaning procedures can reduce the occurrence of illness in the group of children in care (1,2).

Staff training and monitoring of hand hygiene has been shown to reduce transmission of organisms that cause disease (3-6). Periodic training and monitoring is needed to result in sustainable changes in practice (7).

COMMENTS: Training programs may utilize some type of verbal cue such as singing the alphabet song, twinkle, twinkle little star or the birthday song during handwashing.

TYPE OF FACILITY: Center; Large Family Child Care Home; Small Family Child Care Home

RELATED STANDARDS:
Standard 3.2.2.1: Situations that Require Hand Hygiene
Standard 3.2.2.2: Handwashing Procedure

REFERENCES:
1. Hawks, D., J. Ascheim, G. S. Giebink, S. Graville, A. J. Solnit. 1994. Science, prevention, and practice VII: Improving child day care, a concurrent summary of the American Public Health Association/American Academy of Pediatrics national health and safety guidelines for child-care programs; featured standards and implementation. *Pediatrics* 95:1110-12.
2. Roberts, L., E. Mapp, W. Smith, L. Jorm, M. Pate, R. M. Douglas, C. McGilchrist. 2000. Effect of infection control measures on the

frequency of upper respiratory infection in child care: A randomized, controlled trial. *Pediatrics* 105:738-42.
3. Black, R. E., A. C. Dykes, K. E. Anderson. 1981. Handwashing to prevent diarrhea in day care centers. *Am J Epidemiol* 113:445-51.
4. Roberts, L., L. Jorm, M. Patel, W. Smith, R. M. Douglas, C. McGilchrist. 2000. Effect of infection control measures on the frequency of diarrheal episodes in child care: A randomized, controlled trial. *Pediatrics* 105:743-46.
5. Carabin, H., T. W. Gyorkos, J. C. Soto, L. Joseph, P. Payment, J. P. Collet. 1999. Effectiveness of a training program in reducing infections in toddlers attending daycare centers. *Epidemiol* 10:219-27.
6. Bartlett, A. V., B. A. Jarvis, V. Ross, T. M. Katz, M. A. Dalia, S. J. Englender, L. J. Anderson. 1988. Diarrheal illness among infants and toddlers in day care centers: Effects of active surveillance and staff training without subsequent monitoring. *Am J Epidemiol* 127:808-17.
7. Alkon, A., J. Bernzweig, K. To, M. Wolff, J. F. Mackie. 2009. Child care health consultation improves health and safety policies and practices. *Academic Pediatrics* 9:366-70.

STANDARD 3.2.2.5: Hand Sanitizers

The use of hand sanitizers by children over twenty-four months of age and adults in child care programs is an appropriate alternative to the use of traditional handwashing with soap and water. For visibly dirty hands, rinsing under running water or wiping with a water-saturated towel should be used to remove as much dirt as possible before using a hand sanitizer.

Hand sanitizers using an alcohol-based active ingredient must contain 60% to 95% alcohol in order to be effective to kill germs, including multi-drug resistant pathogens. Child care programs should follow the manufacturer's instructions for use, check instructions to determine how long the hand sanitizer needs to remain on the skin surface to be effective.

Supervision of children is required to monitor effective use and to avoid potential ingestion or inadvertent contact of hand sanitizers with eyes and mucous membranes.

When alcohol based hand sanitizers are offered in a child care facility, the facility should encourage parents/guardians to teach their children about their use at home.

Where alcohol-based hand sanitizer dispensers are used:

a) The maximum individual dispenser fluid capacity should be as follows:
b) 0.32 gal (1.2 L) for dispensers in rooms, corridors, and areas open to corridors;
c) 0.53 gal (2.0 L) for dispensers in suites of rooms;
d) Where aerosol containers are used, the maximum capacity of the aerosol dispenser should be 18 oz. (0.51 kg) and should be limited to Level 1 aerosols as defined in NFPA 30B: Code for the Manufacture and Storage of Aerosol Products;
e) Wall mounted dispensers should be separated from each other by horizontal spacing of not less than 48 in. (1,220 mm);
f) Wall mounted dispensers should not be installed above or adjacent to ignition sources such as electrical outlets;
g) Wall mounted dispensers installed directly over carpeted floors should be permitted only in child care facilities protected by automatic sprinklers (1).

RATIONALE: Studies have demonstrated that using an alcohol-based hand sanitizer after washing hands with soap and water is effective in reducing illness transmission in the home, in child care centers and in health care settings (2-5). Hand sanitizer products may be dangerous or toxic if ingested in amounts greater than the residue left on hands after cleaning. It is important for caregivers/teachers to monitor children's use of hand sanitizers to ensure the product is being used appropriately.

Alcohol-based hand sanitizers have the potential to be toxic due to the alcohol content if ingested in a significant amount. As with any hand hygiene product, supervision of children is required to monitor effective use and to avoid potential ingestion or inadvertent contact with eyes and mucous membranes.

COMMENTS: Even in health care settings, the Centers for Disease Control and Prevention (CDC) guidelines recommend washing hands that are visibly soiled or contaminated with organic material with soap and water as an adjunct to the use of alcohol-based sanitizers (6).

Some hand sanitizing products contain non-alcohol and "natural" ingredients. The efficacy of non-alcohol containing hand sanitizers is variable and therefore a non-alcohol-based product is not recommended for use.

TYPE OF FACILITY: Center; Large Family Child Care Home; Small Family Child Care Home

RELATED STANDARDS:

Standard 3.2.2.1: Situations that Require Hand Hygiene
Standard 3.2.2.2: Handwashing Procedure
Standard 5.5.0.5: Storage of Flammable Materials***

REFERENCES:

1. National Fire Protection Association (NFPA). 2009. *NFPA 101: Life safety code.* 2009 ed. Quincy, MA: NFPA.
2. Boyce, J. M., D. Pittet, Healthcare Infection Control Practices Advisory Committee, HICPAC/SHEA/APIC/IDSA Hand Hygiene Task Force. 2002. Guideline for hand hygiene in health-care settings. *MMWR* 25:1-45.
3. Lennell, A., S. Kuhlmann-Berenzon, P. Geli, K. Hedin, C. Petersson, O. Cars, et al. 2008. Alcohol-based hand-disinfection reduced children's absence from Swedish day care centers. *Acta Paediatrica* 97:1672-80.
4. Sandora, T. J., E. M. Taveras, M. C. Shih, E. A. Resnick, G. M. Lee, D. Ross-Degnan, et al. 2005. Hand sanitizer reduces illness transmission in the home. *Pediatrics* 116:587-94.
5. Vessey, J. A., J. J. Sherwood, D. Warner, D. Clark. 2007. Comparing hand washing to hand sanitizers in reducing elementary school students' absenteeism. *Pediatric Nurs* 33:368-72.
6. U.S. Department of Health and Human Services, Centers for Disease Control and Prevention. 2011. Handwashing: Clean hands save lives! http://www.cdc.gov/handwashing/.

***Addition to Related Standards in second printing, August 2011

3.2.3 Exposure to Body Fluids

STANDARD 3.2.3.1: Procedure for Nasal Secretions and Use of Nasal Bulb Syringes

Staff members and children should blow or wipe their noses with disposable, single use tissues and then discard them in a plastic-lined, covered, hands-free trash container. After blowing the nose, they should practice hand hygiene, as specified in Standards 3.2.2.1 and 3.2.2.2.

Use of nasal bulb syringes is permitted. Nasal bulb syringes should be provided by the parents/guardians for individual use and should be labeled with the child's name.

If nasal bulb syringes are used, facilities should have a written policy that indicates:

a) Rationale and protocols for use of nasal bulb syringes;
b) Written permission and any instructions or preferences from the child's parent/guardian;
c) Staff should inspect each nasal bulb syringe for tears or cracks (and to see if there is unknown fluid in the nasal bulb syringe) before each use;
d) Nasal bulb syringes should be cleaned with warm soapy water and stored open to air.

RATIONALE: Hand hygiene is the most effective way to reduce the spread of infection (1).

TYPE OF FACILITY: Center; Large Family Child Care Home; Small Family Child Care Home

RELATED STANDARDS:
Standard 3.2.2.2: Handwashing Procedure
Standard 3.2.2.3: Assisting Children with Hand Hygiene

REFERENCES:
1. Pickering, L. K., C. J. Baker, D. W. Kimberlin, S. S. Long, eds. 2009. *Red book: 2009 report of the Committee on Infectious Diseases*. 28th ed. Elk Grove Village, IL: American Academy of Pediatrics.

STANDARD 3.2.3.2: Cough and Sneeze Etiquette

Staff members and children should be taught to cover their mouths and noses with a tissue when they cough or sneeze. Staff members and children should also be taught to cough or sneeze into their inner elbow/upper sleeve and to avoid covering the nose or mouth with bare hands. Hand hygiene, as specified in Standards 3.2.2.1 and 3.2.2.2, should follow a cough or sneeze that could result in the spread of respiratory droplets to the skin.

RATIONALE: Proper respiratory etiquette can prevent transmission of respiratory pathogens (1).

COMMENTS: Multi-lingual videos, posters, and handouts should be part of an active educational effort of caregivers/teachers and children to reinforce this practice. For free downloadable posters and flyers in multiple languages, go to http://www.cdc.gov/flu/protect/covercough.htm.

TYPE OF FACILITY: Center; Large Family Child Care Home; Small Family Child Care Home

RELATED STANDARDS:
Standard 3.2.2.1: Situations that Require Hand Hygiene
Standard 3.2.2.2: Handwashing Procedure
Standard 3.2.2.3: Assisting Children with Hand Hygiene
Standard 3.2.2.5: Hand Sanitizers

REFERENCES:
1. Centers for Disease Control and Prevention. 2010. Seasonal flu: Cover your cough. http://www.cdc.gov/flu/protect/covercough.htm.

STANDARD 3.2.3.3: Cuts and Scrapes

Cuts or sores that are actively dripping, oozing, or draining body fluids should be covered with a dressing to avoid contamination of surfaces in child care. The caregiver/teacher should wear gloves if there is contact with any wound (cut or scrape) that has material that could be transmitted to another surface.

A child or caregiver/teacher with a cut or sore that is leaking a body fluid that cannot be contained or cannot be covered with a dressing, should be excluded from the facility until the cut or sore is scabbed over or healed.

RATIONALE: Touching a contaminated object or surface may spread infectious organisms. Body fluids may contain infectious organisms (1).

Gloves can provide a protective barrier against infectious organisms that may be present in body fluids.

COMMENTS: Covering sores on lips and on eyes is difficult. Children or caregivers/teachers who are unable to prevent contact with these exposed lesions should be excluded until lesions do not present a risk of transmission of a pathogen.

TYPE OF FACILITY: Center; Large Family Child Care Home; Small Family Child Care Home

RELATED STANDARDS:
Standard 3.6.1.1: Inclusion/Exclusion/Dismissal of Children

REFERENCES:
1. Pickering, L. K., C. J. Baker, D. W. Kimberlin, S. S. Long, eds. 2009. *Red book: 2009 report of the Committee on Infectious Diseases*. 28th ed. Elk Grove Village, IL: American Academy of Pediatrics.

STANDARD 3.2.3.4: Prevention of Exposure to Blood and Body Fluids

Child care facilities should adopt the use of Standard Precautions developed for use in hospitals by The Centers for Disease Control and Prevention (CDC). Standard Precautions should be used to handle potential exposure to blood, including blood-containing body fluids and tissue discharges, and to handle other potentially infectious fluids.

In child care settings:

a) Use of disposable gloves is optional unless blood or blood containing body fluids may contact hands. Gloves are not required for feeding human milk, cleaning up of spills of human milk, or for diapering;
b) Gowns and masks are not required;

c) Barriers to prevent contact with body fluids include moisture-resistant disposable diaper table paper, disposable gloves, and eye protection.

Caregivers/teachers are required to be educated regarding Standard Precautions to prevent transmission of bloodborne pathogens before beginning to work in the facility and at least annually thereafter. Training must comply with requirements of the Occupational Safety and Health Administration (OSHA).

Procedures for Standard Precautions should include:

a) Surfaces that may come in contact with potentially infectious body fluids must be disposable or of a material that can be disinfected. Use of materials that can be sterilized is not required.
b) The staff should use barriers and techniques that:
    1) Minimize potential contact of mucous membranes or openings in skin to blood or other potentially infectious body fluids and tissue discharges; and
    2) Reduce the spread of infectious material within the child care facility. Such techniques include avoiding touching surfaces with potentially contaminated materials unless those surfaces are disinfected before further contact occurs with them by other objects or individuals.
c) When spills of body fluids, urine, feces, blood, saliva, nasal discharge, eye discharge, injury or tissue discharges occur, these spills should be cleaned up immediately, and further managed as follows:
    1) For spills of vomit, urine, and feces, all floors, walls, bathrooms, tabletops, toys, furnishings and play equipment, kitchen counter tops, and diaper-changing tables in contact should be cleaned and disinfected as for the procedure for diaper changing tables in Standard 3.2.1.4, Step 7;
    2) For spills of blood or other potentially infectious body fluids, including injury and tissue discharges, the area should be cleaned and disinfected. Care should be taken and eye protection used to avoid splashing any contaminated materials onto any mucus membrane (eyes, nose, mouth);
    3) Blood-contaminated material and diapers should be disposed of in a plastic bag with a secure tie;
    4) Floors, rugs, and carpeting that have been contaminated by body fluids should be cleaned by blotting to remove the fluid as quickly as possible, then disinfected by spot-cleaning with a detergent-disinfectant. Additional cleaning by shampooing or steam cleaning the contaminated surface may be necessary. Caregivers/teachers should consult with local health departments for additional guidance on cleaning contaminated floors, rugs, and carpeting.

Prior to using a disinfectant, clean the surface with a detergent and rinse well with water. Facilities should follow the manufacturer's instruction for preparation and use of disinfectant (3,4). For guidance on disinfectants, refer to Appendix J, Selecting an Appropriate Sanitizer or Disinfectant.

If blood or bodily fluids enter a mucous membrane (eyes, nose, mouth) the following procedure should occur. Flush the exposed area thoroughly with water. The goal of washing or flushing is to reduce the amount of the pathogen to which an exposed individual has contact. The optimal length of time for washing or flushing an exposed area is not known. Standard practice for managing mucous membrane(s) exposures to toxic substances is to flush the affected area for at least fifteen to twenty minutes. In the absence of data to support the effectiveness of shorter periods of flushing it seems prudent to use the same fifteen to twenty minute standard following exposure to bloodborne pathogens (5).

RATIONALE: Some children and adults may unknowingly be infected with HIV or other infectious agents, such as hepatitis B virus, as these agents may be present in blood or body fluids. Thus, the staff in all facilities should adopt Standard Precautions for all blood spills. Bacteria and viruses carried in the blood, such as hepatitis B, pose a small but specific risk in the child care setting (3). Blood and body fluids containing blood (such as watery discharges from injuries) pose a potential risk, because bloody body fluids contain the highest concentration of viruses. In addition, hepatitis B virus can survive in a dried state in the environment for at least a week and perhaps even longer. Some other body fluids such as saliva contaminated with blood or blood-associated fluids may contain live virus (such as hepatitis B virus) but at lower concentrations than are found in blood itself. Other body fluids, including urine and feces, do not pose a risk for bloodborne infections unless they are visibly contaminated with blood, although these fluids may pose a risk for transmission of other infectious diseases.

Touching a contaminated object or surface may spread illnesses. Many types of infectious germs may be contained in human waste (urine, feces) and body fluids (saliva, nasal discharge, tissue and injury discharges, eye discharges, blood, and vomit). Because many infected people carry infectious diseases without having symptoms, and many are contagious before they experience a symptom, staff members need to protect themselves and the children they serve by adhering to Standard Precautions for all activities.

Gloves have proven to be effective in preventing transmission of many infectious diseases to health care workers. Gloves are used mainly when people knowingly contact or suspect they may contact blood or blood-containing body fluids, including blood-containing tissue or injury discharges. These fluids may contain the viruses that transmit HIV, hepatitis B, and hepatitis C. While human milk can be contaminated with blood from a cracked nipple, the risk of transmission of infection to caregivers/teachers who are feeding expressed human milk is almost negligible and this represents a theoretical risk. Wearing of gloves to feed or clean up spills of expressed human milk is unnecessary, but caregivers/teachers should avoid getting expressed human milk on their hands, if they have any open skin or sores on their hands. If caregivers/teachers have open wounds they should be protected by waterproof bandages or disposable gloves.

Cleaning and disinfecting rugs and carpeting that have been contaminated by body fluids is challenging. Extracting as much of the contaminating material as possible before it penetrates the surface to lower layers helps to minimize this challenge. Cleaning and disinfecting the surface without damaging it requires use of special cleaning agents designed for use on rugs, or steam cleaning (3). Therefore, alternatives to the use of carpeting and rugs are favored in the child care environment.

COMMENTS: The sanctions for failing to comply with OSHA requirements can be costly, both in fines and in health consequences. Regional offices of OSHA are listed at http://www.epa.gov/aboutepa/index.html#regional/ and in the telephone directory with other federal offices.

Either single-use disposable gloves or utility gloves should be used when disinfecting. Single-use disposable gloves should be used only once and then discarded immediately without being handled. If utility gloves are used, they should be cleaned after every use with soap and water and then dipped in disinfectant solution up to the wrist. The gloves should then be allowed to air dry. The wearing of gloves does not prevent contamination of hands or of surfaces touched with contaminated gloved hands. Hand hygiene and sanitizing of contaminated surfaces is required when gloves are used.

Ongoing exposures to latex may result in allergic reactions in both the individual wearing the latex glove and the individual who contacts the latex glove. Reports of such reactions have increased (1).

Caregivers/teachers should take the following steps to protect themselves, children, volunteers, and visitors from latex exposure and allergy in the workplace (6):

a) Use non-latex gloves for activities that are not likely to involve contact with infectious materials (food preparation, diapering, routine housekeeping, general maintenance, etc.);
b) Use appropriate barrier protection when handling infectious materials. Avoid using latex gloves BUT if latex gloves are chosen, use powder-free gloves with reduced protein content;
    1) Such gloves reduce exposures to latex protein and thus reduce the risk of latex allergy;
    2) Hypoallergenic latex gloves do not reduce the risk of latex allergy. However, they may reduce reactions to chemical additives in the latex (allergic contact dermatitis);
c) Use appropriate work practices to reduce the chance of reactions to latex;
d) When wearing latex gloves, do not use oil-based hand creams or lotions (which can cause glove deterioration);
e) After removing latex gloves, wash hands with a mild soap and dry thoroughly;
f) Practice good housekeeping, frequently clean areas and equipment contaminated with latex-containing dust;
g) Attend all latex allergy training provided by the facility and become familiar with procedures for preventing latex allergy;
h) Learn to recognize the symptoms of latex allergy: skin rash; hives; flushing; itching; nasal, eye, or sinus symptoms; asthma; and (rarely) shock.

Natural fingernails that are long or wearing artificial fingernails or extenders is not recommended. Child care facilities should develop an organizational policy on the wearing of non-natural nails by staff (2).

For more information on safety with blood and body fluids, consult Healthy Child Care Pennsylvania's "Keeping Safe When Touching Blood or Other Body Fluids" at http://www.ecels-healthychildcarepa.org/content/Keeping Safe 07-27-10.pdf.

TYPE OF FACILITY: Center; Large Family Child Care Home; Small Family Child Care Home

RELATED STANDARDS:
Standard 3.2.1.4: Diaper Changing Procedure
Appendix D: Gloving
Appendix J: Selecting an Appropriate Sanitizer or Disinfectant

REFERENCES:
1. De Queiroz, M., S. Combet, J. Berard, A. Pouyau, H. Genest, P. Mouriquand, D. Chassard. 2009. Latex allergy in children: Modalities and prevention. *Pediatric Anesthesia* 19:313-19.
2. Siegel, J. D., E. Rhinehart, M. Jackson, L. Chiarello, Healthcare Infection Control Practices Advisory Committee. 2007. *2007* Guideline for isolation precautions: Preventing transmission of infectious agents in healthcare settings. http://www.cdc.gov/ncidod/dhqp/pdf/guidelines/Isolation2007.pdf.
3. Kotch, J. B., P. Isbell, D. J. Weber, et al. 2007. Hand-washing and diapering equipment reduces disease among children in out-of-home child care centers. *Pediatrics* 120: e29-e36.
4. Rutala, W. A., D. J. Weber, HICPAC. 2008. Guideline for disinfection and sterilization in healthcare facilities. Center for Disease Control and Prevention. http://www.cdc.gov/ncidod/dhqp/pdf/guidelines/Disinfection_Nov_2008.pdf.
5. Email communication from Amy V. Kindrick, MD, MPH, Senior Consultant, National Clinicians' Post-Exposure Prophylaxis Hotline (PEPline), UCSF School of Medicine at San Francisco General Hospital to Elisabeth L.M. Miller, BSN, RN, BC, PA Chapter American Academy of Pediatrics, Early Childhood Education Linkage System – Healthy Child Care Pennsylvania. November 11, 2009.
6. American Association of Nurse Anesthetists. 2003. Creating a latex-safe school for latex-sensitive children. http://www.anesthesiapatientsafety.com/patients/latex/school.asp.

3.3 Cleaning, Sanitizing, and Disinfecting

STANDARD 3.3.0.1: Routine Cleaning, Sanitizing, and Disinfecting

Keeping objects and surfaces in a child care setting as clean and free of pathogens as possible requires a combination of:

a) Frequent cleaning; and

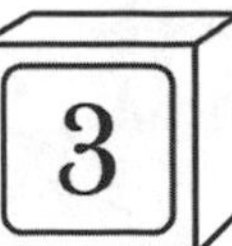

b) When necessary, an application of a sanitizer or disinfectant.

Facilities should follow a routine schedule of cleaning, sanitizing, and disinfecting as outlined in Appendix K, Routine Schedule for Cleaning, Sanitizing, and Disinfecting.

Cleaning, sanitizing and disinfecting products should not be used in close proximity to children, and adequate ventilation should be maintained during any cleaning, sanitizing or disinfecting procedure to prevent children and caregivers/teachers from inhaling potentially toxic fumes.

RATIONALE: Young children sneeze, cough, drool, use diapers and are just learning to use the toilet. They hug, kiss, and touch everything and put objects in their mouths (1). Illnesses may be spread in a variety of ways, such as by coughing, sneezing, direct skin-to-skin contact, or touching a contaminated object or surface. Respiratory tract secretions that can contain viruses (including respiratory syncytial virus and rhinovirus) contaminate environmental surfaces and may present an opportunity for infection by contact (2-4).

COMMENTS: The terms cleaning, sanitizing and disinfecting are sometimes used interchangeably which can lead to confusion and result in cleaning procedures that are not effective (3).

For example, a spray bottle containing a mixture of bleach and water might be incorrectly used as the "first step" to clean a soiled diaper change table or a table surface after a meal. The solution in the spray bottle cannot be used as a "first step" because the purpose of the bleach and water solution is to sanitize (it is not designed to clean and is not effective as a disinfectant on dirty surfaces). In this example, cleaning with detergent and water, and then rinsing the surface with water, should occur before spraying the surface with the bleach and water solution (5).

Each term has a specific purpose and there are many methods that may be used to achieve such purpose.

Task	Purpose
Clean	To physically remove all dirt and contamination. The friction of cleaning removes most germs and exposes any remaining germs to the effects of a sanitizer or disinfectant used later.
Sanitize	To reduce germs on inanimate surfaces to levels considered safe by public health codes or regulations.
Disinfect	To destroy or inactivate most germs on any inanimate object, but not bacterial spores.

Note: The term "germs" refers to bacteria, viruses, fungi and molds that may cause infectious disease. Bacterial spores are dormant bacteria that have formed a protective shell, enabling them to survive extreme conditions for years. The spores reactivate after entry into a host (such as a person), where conditions are favorable for them to live and reproduce (6).

Only U.S. Environmental Protection Agency (EPA)-registered products that have an EPA registration number on the label can make public health claims that can be relied on for reducing or destroying germs. The EPA registration label will also describe the product as a cleaner, sanitizer, or disinfectant. It is important to use the least toxic cleaner, sanitizer and disinfectant for the particular job. Products that are labeled as "green" sanitizers and disinfectants should be EPA-registered. Products must be used according to manufacturer's instructions.

Employers should provide staff with hazard information, including access to and review of the Material Safety Data Sheets (MSDS) as required by the Occupational Safety and Health Administration (OSHA), about the presence of toxic substances such as, cleaning, sanitizing and disinfecting supplies in use in the facility. The MSDS explain the risk of exposure to products so that appropriate precautions may be taken.

TYPE OF FACILITY: Center; Large Family Child Care Home; Small Family Child Care Home

RELATED STANDARDS:
Standard 3.3.0.2: Cleaning and Sanitizing Toys
Standard 3.3.0.3: Cleaning and Sanitizing Objects Intended for the Mouth
Standard 5.2.1.6: Ventilation to Control Odors
Appendix K: Routine Schedule for Cleaning, Sanitizing, and Disinfecting

REFERENCES:

1. California Childcare Health Program. 2009. Sanitize safely and effectively: Bleach and alternatives in child care programs. *Health and Safety Notes* (July). http://www.ucsfchildcarehealth.org/pdfs/healthandsafety/SanitizeSafely_En0709.pdf.
2. Thompson, S. C. 1994. Infectious diarrhoea in children: Controlling transmission in the child care setting. *J Paediatric Child Health* 30:210-19.
3. Butz, A. M., P. Fosarelli, D. Dick, et al. 1993. Prevalence of rotavirus on high-risk fomites in day-care facilities. *Pediatrics* 92:202-5.
4. Grenier, D., D. Leduc, eds. 2008. *Well beings: A guide to health in child care.* 3rd ed. Ottawa, Ontario: Canadian Paediatric Society.
5. North Carolina Child Care Health and Safety Resource Center. Diapering procedure poster. http://www.healthychildcarenc.org/training_materials.htm.
6. Microbiology Procedure. Sporulation in bacteria. http://www.microbiologyprocedure.com/microorganisms/sporulation-in-bacteria.htm.

STANDARD 3.3.0.2: Cleaning and Sanitizing Toys

Toys that cannot be cleaned and sanitized should not be used. Toys that children have placed in their mouths or that are otherwise contaminated by body secretion or excretion should be set aside until they are cleaned by hand with water and detergent, rinsed, sanitized, and air-dried or in a mechanical dishwasher that meets the requirements of Standard 4.9.0.11 through Standard 4.9.0.13. Play with plastic or play foods, play dishes and utensils, should be closely supervised to prevent shared mouthing of these toys.

Machine washable cloth toys should be used by one individual at a time. These toys should be laundered before being used by another child.

Indoor toys should not be shared between groups of infants or toddlers unless they are washed and sanitized before being moved from one group to the other.

RATIONALE: Contamination of hands, toys and other objects in child care areas has played a role in the transmission of diseases in child care settings (1). All toys can spread disease when children put the toys in their mouths, touch the toys after putting their hands in their mouths during play or eating, or after toileting with inadequate hand hygiene. Using a mechanical dishwasher is an acceptable labor-saving approach for sanitizing plastic toys as long as the dishwasher can wash and sanitize the surfaces and dishes and cutlery are not washed at the same time (1).

COMMENTS: Small toys with hard surfaces can be set aside for cleaning by putting them into a dish pan labeled "soiled toys." This dish pan can contain soapy water to begin removal of soil, or it can be a dry container used to bring the soiled toys to a toy cleaning area later in the day. Having enough toys to rotate through cleaning makes this method of preferred cleaning possible.

TYPE OF FACILITY: Center; Large Family Child Care Home; Small Family Child Care Home

RELATED STANDARDS:
Standard 3.3.0.1: Routine Cleaning, Sanitizing, and Disinfecting
Standards 4.9.0.11-4.9.0.13: Dishwashing
Appendix J: Selecting an Appropriate Sanitizer or Disinfectant
Appendix K: Routine Schedule for Cleaning, Sanitizing, and Disinfecting

REFERENCES:
1. Grenier, D., D. Leduc, eds. 2008. Preventing infections. In *Well beings.* 3rd ed. Ottawa, Ontario: Canadian Paediatric Society.

STANDARD 3.3.0.3: Cleaning and Sanitizing Objects Intended for the Mouth

Thermometers, pacifiers, teething toys, and similar objects should be cleaned, and reusable parts should be sanitized between uses. Pacifiers should not be shared.

RATIONALE: Contamination of hands, toys and other objects in child care areas has played a role in the transmission of diseases in child care settings (1).

TYPE OF FACILITY: Center; Large Family Child Care Home; Small Family Child Care Home

RELATED STANDARDS:
Standard 3.1.4.3: Pacifier Use
Standard 3.3.0.1: Routine Cleaning, Sanitizing, and Disinfecting
Standard 3.6.1.3: Thermometers for Taking Human Temperatures
Appendix K: Routine Schedule for Cleaning, Sanitizing, and Disinfecting

REFERENCES:
1. Grenier, D., D. Leduc, eds. 2008. Preventing infections. In *Well beings*. 3rd ed. Ottawa, Ontario: Canadian Paediatric Society.

STANDARD 3.3.0.4: Cleaning Individual Bedding

Bedding (sheets, pillows, blankets, sleeping bags) should be of a type that can be washed. Each child's bedding should be kept separate from other children's bedding, on the bed or stored in individually labeled bins, cubbies, or bags. Bedding that touches a child's skin should be cleaned weekly or before use by another child.

RATIONALE: Toddlers often nap or sleep on mats or cots and the mats or cots are taken out of storage during nap time, and then placed back in storage. Providing bedding for each child and storing each set in individually labeled bins, cubbies, or bags in a manner that separates the personal articles of one individual from those of another are appropriate hygienic practices (1).

TYPE OF FACILITY: Center; Large Family Child Care Home; Small Family Child Care Home

RELATED STANDARDS:
Standard 5.4.5.1: Sleeping Equipment and Supplies

REFERENCES:
1. Pickering, L. K., C. J. Baker, D. W. Kimberlin, S. S. Long, eds. 2009. *Red book: 2009 report of the Committee on Infectious Diseases,* 153. 28th ed. Elk Grove Village, IL: American Academy of Pediatrics.

STANDARD 3.3.0.5: Cleaning Crib Surfaces

Cribs and crib mattresses should have a nonporous, easy-to-wipe surface. All surfaces should be cleaned as recommended in Appendix K, Routine Schedule for Cleaning, Sanitizing, and Disinfecting.

RATIONALE: Contamination of hands, toys and other objects in child care areas has played a role in the transmission of diseases in child care settings (1).

TYPE OF FACILITY: Center; Large Family Child Care Home; Small Family Child Care Home

RELATED STANDARDS:
Standard 5.4.5.1: Sleeping Equipment and Supplies
Standard 5.4.5.2: Cribs

REFERENCES:
1. Grenier, D., D. Leduc, eds. 2008. Preventing infections. In *Well beings*. 3rd ed. Ottawa, Ontario: Canadian Paediatric Society.

3.4 Health Protection in Child Care

3.4.1 Tobacco and Drug Use

STANDARD 3.4.1.1: Use of Tobacco, Alcohol, and Illegal Drugs

Tobacco use, alcohol, and illegal drugs should be prohibited on the premises of the program (both indoor and outdoor environments) and in any vehicles used by the program at all times. Caregivers/teachers should not use tobacco, alcohol, or illegal drugs off the premises during the child care program's paid time including break time.

RATIONALE: Scientific evidence has linked respiratory health risks to secondhand smoke. No children, especially those with respiratory problems, should be exposed to additional risk from the air they breathe. Infants and young children exposed to secondhand smoke are at risk of developing bronchitis, pneumonia, and middle ear infections when they experience common respiratory infections (1-5). Separation of smokers and nonsmokers within the same air space does not eliminate or minimize exposure of nonsmokers to secondhand smoke. Tobacco smoke contamination lingers after a cigarette is extinguished and children come in contact with the toxins (6). Thirdhand smoke exposure also presents hazards. Thirdhand smoke refers to gases and particles clinging to smokers' hair and clothing, cushions and carpeting, and outdoor equipment, after tobacco smoke has dissipated (1). The residue includes heavy metals, carcinogens and radioactive materials that young children can get on their hands and ingest, especially if they're crawling or playing on the floor. Residual toxins from smoking at times when the children are not using the space can trigger asthma and allergies when the children do use the space (1,2).

Cigarettes used by adults are the leading cause of ignition of fatal house fires (7-9).

Adults under the influence of alcohol and other drugs cannot take care of young children and keep them safe. Alcohol use, illegal drug use and misuse of prescription or over the counter (OTC) drugs prevent caregivers/teachers from providing appropriate care to infants and children by impairing motor coordination, judgment, and response time. Safe child care necessitates alert, unimpaired caregivers/teachers.

The use of alcoholic beverages in family child care homes after children are not in care is not prohibited.

COMMENTS: The age, defenselessness, and dependence upon the judgment of caregivers/teachers of the children under care make this prohibition an absolute requirement.

TYPE OF FACILITY: Center; Large Family Child Care Home; Small Family Child Care Home

RELATED STANDARDS:

Standard 9.2.3.15: Policy on Prohibiting Tobacco, Alcohol, Illegal Drugs, and Toxic Substances

REFERENCES:

1. U.S. Department of Health and Human Services. 2007. *Children and secondhand smoke exposure*. Excerpts from the health consequences of involuntary exposure to tobacco smoke: A report of the Surgeon General. Atlanta, GA: U.S. Department of Health and Human Services, Centers for Disease Control and Prevention, Coordinating Center for Health Promotion, National Center for Chronic Disease Prevention and Health Promotion, Office on Smoking and Health.
2. Schwartz, J., K. L. Timonen, J. Pekkanen. 2000. Respiratory effects of environmental tobacco smoke in a panel study of asthmatic and symptomatic children. *Am J Resp Crit Care Med* 161:802-6.
3. Stenstrom, R., P. A. Bernard, H. Ben-Simhon. 1993. Exposure to environmental tobacco smoke as a risk factor for recurrent acute otitis media in children under the age of five years. *Inter J Pediatr Otorhinolaryngol* 27:127-36.
4. Pershagen, G. 1999. Accumulating evidence on health hazards of passive smoking. *Acta Paediatr* 88:490-92.
5. Gergen, P. J., J. A. Fowler, K. R. Maurer, et al. 1998. The burden of environmental tobacco smoke exposure on the respiratory health of children 2 months through 5 years of age in the United States: Third national health and nutritional examination survey, 1988 to 1994. *Pediatrics* 101: e8.
6. Winickoff, J. P., J. Friebely, S. E. Tanski, C. Sherrod, G. E. Matt, M. F. Hovell, R. C. McMillen. 2009. Beliefs about the health effects of "thirdhand" smoke and home smoking bans. *Pediatrics* 123: e74-e79.
7. Runyan, C. W., S. I. Bangdiwala, M. A. Linzer, et al. 1992. Risk factors for fatal residential fires. *N Eng J Med* 327:856-63.
8. Brigham, P. A., A. McGuire 1995. Progress towards a fire-safe cigarette. *J Public Health Policy* 16:433-39.
9. Ballard, J. E., T. D. Koepsell, F. Rivara. 1992. Association of smoking and alcohol drinking with residential fire injuries. *Am J Epidemiol* 135:26-34.

3.4.2 Animals

STANDARD 3.4.2.1: Animals that Might Have Contact with Children and Adults

The following domestic animals may have contact with children and adults if they meet the criteria specified in this standard:

a) Dog;
b) Cat;
c) Ungulate (e.g., cow, sheep, goat, pig, horse);
d) Rabbit;
e) Rodent (e.g., mice, rats, hamsters, gerbils, guinea pigs, chinchillas).

Fish are permissible but must be inaccessible to children.

Any animal present at the facility, indoors or outdoors, should be trained/adapted to be with young children, in good health, show no evidence of carrying any disease, fleas or ticks, be fully immunized, and be maintained on an intestinal parasite control program. A current (time-specified) certificate from each animal's attending veterinarian should be on file in the facility, stating that all animals on the facility premises meet these conditions and meet local and state requirements.

Only animals that do not pose a health or safety risk will be allowed on the premises of the facility.

The caregiver/teacher should instruct children on the humane and safe procedures to follow when in close proximity to animals (for example, not to provoke or startle animals or touch them when they are near food).

All contact between animals and children should be supervised by a caregiver/teacher who is close enough to remove the child immediately if the animal shows signs of distress (e.g., growling, baring teeth, tail down, ears back) or the child shows signs of treating the animal inappropriately.

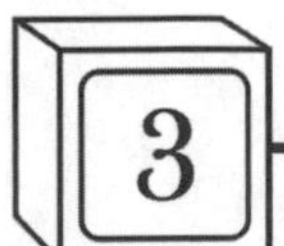

Children should not be allowed to feed animals directly from their hands.

No food and beverages should be allowed in animal areas. In addition, adults and children should not carry toys, use pacifiers, cups, and infant bottles in animal areas.

The animals should be housed within some "barrier" that protects them from competition by other animals while being fed which would also provide protection for the children yet they could still observe the animals eating. Animal food dishes should not be placed in areas accessible to children during hours when children are present.

Children should be discouraged from "kissing" animals or having them in close contact with their faces.

All children and caregivers/teachers who handle animals or animal-related equipment (e.g., leashes, dishes, toys, etc.) should be instructed to use hand hygiene immediately after handling.

Immunocompromised children, such as children with organ transplants, human immunodeficiency virus (HIV), acquired immunodeficiency syndrome (AIDS), or currently receiving cancer chemotherapy or radiation therapy, and/or children with allergies, should have an individualized health care plan in place that specifies if there are precautionary measures to be taken before the child has direct or indirect contact with animals or equipment.

Uncaged animals, such as dogs and cats, should wear a proper collar, harness, and/or leash when on the facility premises and the owner or responsible adult should stay with the animal at all times. Animals should not be permitted in food preparation or service areas at any time.

RATIONALE: The risk of injury, infection, and aggravation of allergy from contact between children and animals is significant. The staff must plan carefully when having an animal in the facility and when visiting a zoo or local pet store (5,9,10). Children should be brought into direct contact only with animals known to be friendly and comfortable in the company of children.

Dog bites to children under four years of age usually occur at home, and the most common injury sites are the head, face, and neck (1-4). Many human illnesses can be acquired from animals (5,7,8,11). Many allergic children have symptoms when they are around animals.

Special precautions may be needed to minimize the risk of disease transmission to immunocompromised children (13).

When animals are taken out of their natural environment and are in situations unusual to them, the stress that the animals experience may cause them to act aggressively or attempt to escape (the "flight or fight" phenomenon). Appropriate restraint devices will allow the holder to react quickly, prevent harm to children and/or the escape of the animal (9).

Pregnant women need to be aware of a potential risk associated with contact with cats' feces (stool). Toxoplasmosis is an infection caused by a parasite called *Toxoplasma gondii*. This parasite is carried by cats and is passed in their feces. Toxoplasmosis can cause problems with pregnancy, including abortion (8). The CDC advises pregnant women to avoid pet rodents because of the risk of lymphocytic choriomeningitis virus (6,12).

COMMENTS: Bringing animals and children together has both risks and benefits. Animals teach children about how to be gentle and responsible, about life and death, and about unconditional love (9). Nevertheless, animals can pose serious health and safety risks.

Special accommodations for children with allergies may be necessary. Cleaning air filters more often if animals are in childcare areas may be helpful in reducing animal dander.

Some dogs complete training and are certified as part of "dog-assisted therapy programs." Certification requires that dogs meet specific criteria, complete screening/training, and be a member of Therapy Dogs International for liability purposes. Although these programs are typically based in hospitals, certified therapy animals also help with disaster relief and other efforts. Facilities that want to offer educational information to staff or hands-on learning opportunities for children may find it helpful to contact their local hospital to identify a trainer for dog-assisted therapy programs. For more information on this program and resources, contact Therapy Dogs International at http://www.tdi-dog.org.

TYPE OF FACILITY: Center; Large Family Child Care Home; Small Family Child Care Home

RELATED STANDARDS:
Standards 3.2.2.1-3.2.2.5: Hand Hygiene
Standard 3.4.2.2: Prohibited Animals
Standard 3.4.2.3: Care for Animals

REFERENCES:

1. Gilchrist, J., J. J. Sacks, D. White, M. J. Kresnow. 2008. Dog bites: Still a problem? *Injury Prevention* 14:296-301.
2. Reisner, I. R., F. S. Shofer. 2008. Effects of gender and parental status on knowledge and attitudes of dog owners regarding dog aggression toward children. *J Am Vet Med Assoc* 233:1412-19.
3. Information from Your Family Doctor. 2004. Dog bites: Teaching your child to be safe. *Am Family Physician* 69:2653.
4. Bernardo, L. M., M. J. Gardner, R. L. Rosenfield, B. Cohen, R. Pitetti. 2002. A comparison of dog bite injuries in younger and older children treated in a pediatric emergency department. *Pediatric Emergency Care* 18:247-49.
5. National Association of State Public Health Veterinarians. 2007. Compendium of measures to prevent disease associated with animals in public settings. *MMWR* 56:1-13. 6. U.S. Department of Health and Human Services, Centers for Disease Control and Prevention. 2009. Appendix D: Guidelines for animals in school and child-care settings. *MMWR* 58:20-21.
7. U.S. Department of Health and Human Services, Centers for Disease Control and Prevention. 2000. Compendium of measures to control Chlamydia psittaci infection among humans (psittacosis) and pet birds (avian chlamydiosis). *MMWR* 49:3-17.
8. U.S. Department of Health and Human Services, Centers for Disease Control and Prevention. *Pregnant women and Toxoplasmosis.* http://www.cdc.gov/healthypets/pregnant.htm.
9. Hansen, G. R. 2004. *Animals in Kansas schools: Guidelines for visiting and resident pets.* Topeka, KS: Kansas Department of Health and Environment. http://www.kdheks.gov/pdf/hef/ab1007.pdf.

10. Massachusetts Department of Public Health Division of Epidemiology and Immunization. 2001. Recommendations for petting zoos, petting farms, animal fairs, and other events and exhibits where contact between animals and people is permitted. http://www.mass.gov/Eeohhs2/docs/dph/cdc/rabies/reduce_zoos_risk.pdf.
11. Pickering, L. K., N. Marano, J. A. Bocchini, F. J. Angulo. 2008. Exposure to nontraditional pets at home and to animals in public settings: risks to children. *Pediatrics* 122:876-86.
12. Centers for Disease Control and Prevention. 2010. Lymphocytic choriomeningitis (LCMV). http://www.cdc.gov/ncidod/dvrd/spb/mnpages/dispages/lcmv.htm.
13. Hemsworth, S., B. Pizer. 2006. Pet ownership in immunocompromised children – A review of the literature and survey of existing guidelines. *Eur J Oncol Nurs* 10:117-27.

STANDARD 3.4.2.2: Prohibited Animals

The following animals should not be kept at or brought onto the grounds of the child care facility (4,6,7):

a) Bats;
b) Hermit crabs;
c) Poisonous animals - Inclusive of spiders, venomous insects, venomous reptiles (including snakes), and venomous amphibians;
d) Wolf-dog hybrids - These animals are crosses between a wolf and a domestic dog and have shown a propensity for aggression, especially toward young children;
e) Stray animals - Stray animals should never be present at a child care facility because the health and vaccination status of these animals is unknown;
f) Chickens and ducks - These animals excrete E. coli O157:H7, *Salmonella*, *Campylobacter*, *S. paratyphoid*;
g) Aggressive animals - Animals which are bred or trained to demonstrate aggression towards humans or other animals, or animals which have demonstrated such aggressive behavior in the past, should not be permitted on the grounds of the child care facility. Exceptions may be sentry or canine corps dogs for a demonstration. These dogs must be under the control of trained military or law enforcement officials;
h) Reptiles and amphibians - Inclusive of non-venomous snakes, lizards, and iguanas, turtles, tortoises, terrapins, crocodiles, alligators, frogs, tadpoles, salamanders, and newts;
i) Psittacine birds unless tested for *psittacosis* - Inclusive of parrots, parakeets, budgies, and cockatiels. Psittacine birds can carry diseases that can be transferred to humans;
j) Ferrets - Ferrets have a propensity to bite when startled;
k) Animals in estrus - Female dogs and cats should be determined not to be in estrus (heat) when at the child care facility;
l) Animals less than one year of age - Incorporating young animals (animal that are less than one year of age) into child care programs is not permitted because of issues regarding unpredictable behavior and elimination control. Additionally, the immune systems of very young puppies and kittens are not completely developed, thereby placing the health of these animals at risk.

RATIONALE: Animals, including pets, are a source of illness for people, and people may be a source of illness for animals (1-2,4-5). Reptiles usually carry salmonella and pose a risk to children who are likely to put unwashed hands in their mouths (3,5).

TYPE OF FACILITY: Center; Large Family Child Care Home; Small Family Child Care Home

RELATED STANDARDS:
Standard 3.4.2.1: Animals That Might Have Contact with Children and Adults
Standard 3.4.2.3: Care for Animals

REFERENCES:

1. Weinberg, A. N., D. J. Weber, eds. 1991. Respiratory infections transmitted from animals. *Infect Dis Clin North Am* 5:649-61.
2. National Association of State Public Health Veterinarians. 2007. Compendium of measures to prevent disease associated with animals in public settings. *MMWR* 56:1-13.
3. Hansen, G. R. 2004. Animals in Kansas schools: Guidelines for visiting and resident pets. Topeka, KS: Kansas Department of Health and Environment. http://www.kdheks.gov/pdf/hef/ab1007.pdf.
4. U.S. Department of Health and Human Services, Centers for Disease Control and Prevention. 2009. Appendix D: Guidelines for animals in school and child-care settings. *MMWR* 58:20-21.
5. Pickering, L. K., N. Marano, J. A. Bocchini, F. J. Angulo. 2008. Exposure to nontraditional pets at home and to animals in public settings: risks to children. *Pediatrics* 122:876-86.
6. PETCO Animal Supplies. 2006. Hermit crab: Care sheet. http://www.petco.com/caresheets/invertebrates/HermitCrab.pdf.
7. Kahn, C. M., S. Line, eds. 2010. *The Merck veterinary manual.* 10th ed. Whitehouse Station, NJ: Merck.

STANDARD 3.4.2.3: Care for Animals

The facility should care for all animals as recommended by the health department and in consultation with licensed veterinarian. When animals are kept on the premises, the facility should write and adhere to procedures for their humane care and maintenance. When animals are kept in the child care facility, the following conditions should be met:

Humane Care: An environment will be maintained in which animals experience:

a) Good health;
b) Are able to effectively cope with their environment;
c) Are able to express a diversity of species specific behaviors.

Health Care: Proof of appropriate current veterinary certificate meeting local and state health requirement is kept on file at the facility for each animal kept on the premises or visiting the child care facility.

Animal care: Specific areas should be designated for animal contact.

Live animals should be prohibited from:

a) Food preparation, food storage, and dining areas;
b) The vicinity of sinks where children wash their hands;

c) Clean supply rooms;
d) Areas where children routinely play or congregate (e.g., sandboxes, child care facility playgrounds).

The living quarters of animals should be enclosed and kept clean of waste to reduce the risk of human contact with this waste.

Animal food supplies should be kept out of reach of children.

Animal litter boxes should not be located in areas accessible to children. Children and food handlers should not handle or clean up any form of animal waste (feces, urine, blood, etc).

All animal waste and litter should be removed immediately from children's areas and will be disposed of in a way where children cannot come in contact with the material, such as in a plastic bag or container with a well-fitted lid or via the sewage waste system for feces.

Used fish tank water should be disposed of in sinks that are not used for food preparation or used for obtaining water for human consumption.

Disposable gloves should be used when cleaning aquariums and hands should be washed immediately after cleaning is finished. Eye and oral contamination by splashing of contaminated water during the cleaning process should be prevented. Children should not be involved in the cleaning of aquariums.

Areas where feeders, water containers, and cages are cleaned should be disinfected after cleaning activity is finished.

Pregnant persons should not handle cat waste or litter. Cat litter boxes should be cleaned daily.

All persons who have contact with animals, animal products, or animal environments should wash their hands immediately after the contact.

RATIONALE: Animals, including pets, are a source of illness for people; likewise, people may be a source of illness for animals (1). All contact with animals, and animal wastes should occur in a fashion that minimizes staff and children's risk of injury, infection and aggravation of allergy (2,4,5). Hand hygiene is the most important way to reduce the spread of infection. Unwashed or improperly washed hands are primary carriers of germs which may lead to infections.

Just as food intended for human consumption may become contaminated, an animal's food can become contaminated by standing at room temperature, or by being exposed to animals, insects, or people.

Pregnant woman can acquire toxoplasmosis from infected cat waste. The infection can be transmitted to her unborn child. Congenital toxoplasmosis infection can lead to miscarriage or an array of malformations of the developing child prior to birth. Cat litter boxes should be cleaned daily since it takes one to five days for feces containing toxoplasma oocysts to become infectious with toxoplasmosis (3).

COMMENTS: Ensuring animal welfare is a human responsibility that includes consideration for all aspects of animal well-being, inclusive of secure housing, suitable temperature, adequate exercise and proper diet, disease prevention and treatment, humane handling, and, when necessary, humane euthanasia (6). Animal well-being also includes continued care of animals during the days that child care is not in session and in the event of an emergency evacuation.

TYPE OF FACILITY: Center; Large Family Child Care Home; Small Family Child Care Home

RELATED STANDARDS:
Standards 3.2.2.1-3.2.2.5: Hand Hygiene
Standard 3.4.2.1: Animals That Might Have Contact with Children and Adults
Standard 3.4.2.2: Prohibited Animals

REFERENCES:
1. Weinberg, A. N., D. J. Weber, eds. 1991. Respiratory infections transmitted from animals. *Infect Dis Clin North Am* 5:649-61.
2. National Association of State Public Health Veterinarians. 2007. Compendium of measures to prevent disease associated with animals in public settings. *MMWR* 56:1-13.
3. Centers for Disease Control and Prevention (CDC). Pregnant women and toxoplasmosis. http://www.cdc.gov/healthypets/pregnant.htm.
4. Hansen, G. R. 2004. *Animals in Kansas schools: Guidelines for visiting and resident pets.* Topeka, KS: Kansas Department of Health and Environment. http://www.kdheks.gov/pdf/hef/ab1007.pdf.
5. U.S. Department of Health and Human Services, Centers for Disease Control and Prevention. 2009. Appendix D: Guidelines for animals in school and child-care settings. *MMWR* 58:20-21.
6. American Veterinary Medical Association. Animal welfare principles. http://www.avma.org/issues/animal_welfare/default.asp.

3.4.3 Emergency Procedures

STANDARD 3.4.3.1: Emergency Procedures

When an immediate emergency medical response is required, the following emergency procedures should be utilized:

a) First aid should be employed and an emergency medical response team should be called such as 9-1-1 and/or the poison center if a poison emergency (1-800-222-1222);
b) The program should implement a plan for emergency transportation to a local emergency medical facility;
c) The parent/guardian or parent/guardian's emergency contact person should be called as soon as practical;
d) A staff member should accompany the child to the hospital and will stay with the child until the parent/guardian or emergency contact person arrives. Child to staff ratio must be maintained, so staff may need to be called in to maintain the required ratio.

Programs should develop contingency plans for emergencies or disaster situations when it may not be possible or feasible to follow standard or previously agreed upon emergency procedures (see also Standard 9.2.4.3, Disaster Planning, Training, and Communication). Children with known medical conditions that might involve emergent care require a Care Plan created by the child's primary care provider.

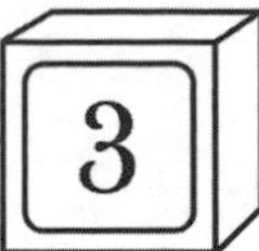

All staff need to be trained to manage an emergency until emergency medical care becomes available.

RATIONALE: The staff must know how to carry out the written disaster and emergency plans as described in Standard 9.2.4.3 to help prevent or minimize severe injury to children and other staff. The staff should review and practice the emergency plan regularly (1).

COMMENTS: First aid instructions are available from the American Academy of Pediatrics (AAP) and the American Red Cross.

TYPE OF FACILITY: Center; Large Family Child Care Home; Small Family Child Care Home

RELATED STANDARDS:
Standard 9.2.4.3: Disaster Planning, Training, and Communication

REFERENCES:
1. Aronson, S. 2005. *Pediatric first aid for caregivers and teachers.* Sudbury, MA: Jones and Bartlett; Elk Grove Village, IL: American Academy of Pediatrics.

STANDARD 3.4.3.2: Use of Fire Extinguishers

The staff should demonstrate the ability to locate and operate the fire extinguishers. Facilities should develop a plan for responding in the event of a fire in or near the facility that includes staff responsibilities and protocols regarding evacuation, notifying emergency personnel, and using fire extinguishers. The staff should demonstrate the ability to recognize a fire that is larger than incipient stage and should not be fought with a portable fire extinguisher.

RATIONALE: A fire extinguisher may be used to put out a small fire or to clear an escape path (1). Developing a plan that includes staff use of fire extinguishers and conducting fire drills/exercises can increase preparedness and help staff better understand what to do to respond to a fire. It is just as important that staff know when not to try to fight a fire with portable fire extinguishers.

COMMENTS: Staff should be trained that the first priority is to remove the children from the facility safely and quickly. Putting out the fire is secondary to the safe exit of the children and staff. However, depending upon the situation at hand and the number of available staff, the facility's plan could identify which caregivers/teachers evacuate the children, where they will all meet outside, who should call emergency personnel, and who should locate/use the fire extinguishers. These efforts can take place simultaneously.

TYPE OF FACILITY: Center; Large Family Child Care Home; Small Family Child Care Home

RELATED STANDARDS:
Standard 9.2.4.3: Disaster Planning, Training, and Communication

REFERENCES:
1. American Academy of Pediatrics, Committee on Injury and Poison Prevention. 2000. Reducing the number of deaths and injuries from residential fires. *Pediatrics* 105:1355-57.

STANDARD 3.4.3.3: Response to Fire and Burns

Children who are developmentally able to understand, should be instructed to STOP, DROP, and ROLL when garments catch fire. Children should be instructed to crawl on the floor under the smoke if necessary when they evacuate the building. This instruction is part of ongoing health and safety education and fire drills/exercise.

Cool water should be applied to burns immediately. The injury should be covered with a loose bandage or clean, dry cloth. Medical assessment/care should be immediate.

RATIONALE: Running when garments have been ignited will fan the fire. Removing heat from the affected area will prevent continued burning and aggravation of tissue damage. Asphyxiation causes more deaths in house fires than does thermal injury (1).

COMMENTS: For resources for children: see *Stop, Drop, and Roll – A Jessica Worries Book: Fire Safety*.

TYPE OF FACILITY: Center; Large Family Child Care Home; Small Family Child Care Home

REFERENCES:
1. American Academy of Pediatrics, Committee on Injury and Poison Prevention. 2000. Reducing the number of deaths and injuries from residential fires. *Pediatrics* 105:1355-57.

3.4.4 Child Abuse and Neglect

STANDARD 3.4.4.1: Recognizing and Reporting Suspected Child Abuse, Neglect, and Exploitation

Each facility should have a written policy for reporting child abuse and neglect. Caregivers/teachers are mandated reporters of child abuse and neglect. The facility should report to the child abuse reporting hotline, department of social services, child protective services, or police as required by state and local laws, in any instance where there is reasonable cause to believe that child abuse and neglect has occurred. Every staff person should be oriented to what and how to report. Phone numbers and reporting system as required by state or local agencies should be clearly posted by every phone.

Caregivers/teachers should receive initial and ongoing training to assist them in preventing child abuse and neglect and in recognizing signs of child abuse and neglect. Programs are encouraged to partner with primary care providers, child care health consultants and/or child protection advocates to provide training and to be available for consultation.

Employees and volunteers in centers and large family child care homes should receive an instruction sheet about child abuse and neglect reporting that contains a summary of the state child abuse reporting statute and a statement that they will not be discharged/disciplined solely because they have made a child abuse and neglect report. Some states have specific forms that are required to be completed when abuse and neglect is reported. Some states have forms that

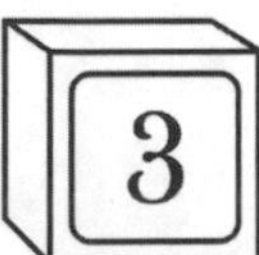

are not required but assist mandated reporters in documenting accurate and thorough reports. In those states, facilities should have such forms on hand and all staff should be trained in the appropriate use of those forms.

Parents/guardians should be notified upon enrollment of the facility's child abuse and neglect reporting requirement and procedures.

RATIONALE: While caregivers/teachers are not expected to diagnose or investigate child abuse and neglect, it is important that they be aware of common physical and emotional signs and symptoms of child maltreatment (see Appendix M, Clues to Child Abuse and Neglect) (1,2,4).

All states in the U.S. have laws mandating the reporting of child abuse and neglect to child protection agencies and/or police. Laws about when and to whom to report vary by state (3). Failure to report abuse and neglect is a crime in all states and may lead to legal penalties.

COMMENTS: Child abuse includes physical, sexual, psychological, and emotional abuse. Other components of abuse include shaken baby syndrome/acute head trauma and repeated exposure to violence including domestic violence. Neglect occurs when the parent/guardian does not meet the child's basic needs and includes physical, medical, educational, and emotional neglect (5). Caregivers/teachers and health professionals may contact individual state hotlines where available. While almost all states have hotlines, they may not operate twenty-four-hours a day, and some toll free numbers may only be accessible within that particular state. ChildHelp USA provides a national hotline: 1-800-4-A-CHILD or 1-800-422-4453.

Many health departments will be willing to provide contact for experts in child abuse and neglect prevention and recognition. The American Academy of Pediatrics (AAP), http://www.aap.org, can also assist in recruiting and identifying physicians who are skilled in this work.

The caregiver/teacher is still liable for reporting even when their supervisor indicates they don't need to or says that someone else will report it. Caregivers/teachers who report in good faith may do so confidentially and are protected by law.

For more information on Mandated Reporting, go to the Child Welfare Information Gateway, Mandated Reporting at http://www.childwelfare.gov/responding/mandated.cfm. Information regarding specific state laws is accessible via the Child Welfare Information Gateway at http://www.childwelfare.gov/systemwide/laws_policies/state/.

TYPE OF FACILITY: Center; Large Family Child Care Home; Small Family Child Care Home

RELATED STANDARDS:
Standard 1.6.0.1: Child Care Health Consultants
Standard 1.7.0.5: Stress
Standard 3.4.4.2: Immunity for Reporters of Child Abuse and Neglect
Standard 3.4.4.3: Preventing and Identifying Shaken Baby Syndrome/Abusive Head Trauma
Standard 3.4.4.4: Care for Children Who Have Been Abused/Neglected
Standard 9.4.1.9: Records of Injury
Appendix M: Clues to Child Abuse and Neglect
Appendix N: Protective Factors Regarding Child Abuse and Neglect

REFERENCES:
1. Hussey, J. M., J. J. Chang, J. B. Kotch. 2006. Child maltreatment in the United States: Prevalence, risk factors, and adolescent health consequences. *Pediatrics* 118:933-42.
2. Jenny, C. 2007. Recognizing and responding to medical neglect. *Pediatrics* 120:1385-89.
3. U.S. Department of Health and Human Services, Administration for Children and Families, Administration on Children, Youth, and Families, and Children's Bureau. Child welfare information gateway: State statutes. http://www.childwelfare.gov/systemwide/laws_policies/state/.
4. Fiene, R. 2002. *13 indicators of quality child care: Research update.* Washington, DC: U.S. Department of Health and Human Services, Office of the Assistant Secretary for Planning and Evaluation. http://aspe.hhs.gov/hsp/ccquality-ind02/.
5. U.S. Department of Health and Human Services, Administration for Children and Families, Administration on Children, Youth, and Families, and Children's Bureau. What is child abuse and neglect? Child Welfare Information Gateway. http://www.childwelfare.gov/pubs/factsheets/whatiscan.cfm.

STANDARD 3.4.4.2: Immunity for Reporters of Child Abuse and Neglect

Caregivers/teachers who report suspected abuse and neglect in the settings where they work should be immune from discharge, retaliation, or other disciplinary action for that reason alone, unless it is proven that the report was malicious.

RATIONALE: Cases which are reported suggest that sometimes workers are intimidated by superiors in the centers where they work, and for that reason, fail to report abuse and neglect (1). In some cases the abuser may be a staff member or superior.

TYPE OF FACILITY: Center; Large Family Child Care Home; Small Family Child Care Home

RELATED STANDARDS:
Standard 3.4.4.1: Recognizing and Reporting Suspected Child Abuse, Neglect, and Exploitation
Standard 3.4.4.3: Preventing and Identifying Shaken Baby Syndrome/Abusive Head Trauma
Standard 3.4.4.4: Care for Children Who Have Been Abused/Neglected
Standard 3.7.0.5: Stress
Standard 9.4.1.9: Records of Injury
Appendix M: Clues to Child Abuse and Neglect
Appendix N: Protective Factors Regarding Child Abuse and Neglect

REFERENCES:
1. Goldman, R. 1990. An educational perspective on abuse. In *Children at risk: An interdisciplinary approach to child abuse and neglect.* Ed. R. Goldman, R. Gargiulo. Austin, TX: Pro-Ed.

STANDARD 3.4.4.3: Preventing and Identifying Shaken Baby Syndrome/Abusive Head Trauma

All child care facilities should have a policy and procedure to identify and prevent shaken baby syndrome/abusive head trauma. All caregivers/teachers who are in direct contact with children including substitute caregivers/teachers and volunteers, should receive training on preventing shaken baby syndrome/abusive head trauma, recognition of potential signs and symptoms of shaken baby syndrome/abusive head trauma, strategies for coping with a crying, fussing or distraught child, and the development and vulnerabilities of the brain in infancy and early childhood.

RATIONALE: Over the past several years there has been increasing recognition of shaken baby syndrome/abusive head trauma which is the occurrence of brain injury in young children under three years of age due to shaking a child. Even mild shaking can result in serious, permanent brain damage or death. The brain of the young child may bounce inside of the skull resulting in brain damage, hemorrhaging, blindness, or other serious injuries or death. There have been several reported incidents occurring in child care (1). Caregivers/teachers experience young children who may be fussy or constantly crying. It is important for caregivers/teachers to be educated about the risks of shaking and provided with strategies to cope if they are frustrated (3). Many states have passed legislation requiring education and training for caregivers/teachers. Caregivers/teachers should check their individual state's specific requirements (2). Staff can also recognize the signs and symptoms of shaken baby syndrome/abusive head trauma in children in their care.

COMMENTS: For more information and resources on shaken baby syndrome/abusive head trauma, contact the National Center on Shaken Baby Syndrome at http://www.dontshake.org.

TYPE OF FACILITY: Center; Large Family child Care Home; Small Family child Care Home

RELATED STANDARDS:

Standard 3.4.4.1: Recognizing and Reporting Suspected Child Abuse, Neglect, and Exploitation

REFERENCES:

1. American Academy of Pediatrics, Committee on Child Abuse and Neglect. 2009. Abusive head trauma in infants and children. *Pediatrics* 123:1409-11.
2. National Resource Center for Health and Safety in Child Care and Early Education. State licensing database. http://nrckids.org/STATES/states.htm.
3. Calm a Crying Baby. Shaken baby syndrome prevention. http://www.calmacryingbaby.com.

STANDARD 3.4.4.4: Care for Children Who Have Been Abused/Neglected

Caregivers/teachers should have access to specialized training and expert advice for children with behavioral abnormalities related to abuse or neglect are enrolled.

RATIONALE: All children who have been abused or neglected have had their physical and emotional boundaries violated and crossed. With this violation often comes a breach of the child's sense of security and trust. Abused and neglected children may come to believe that the world is not a safe place and that adults are not trustworthy. Abused and neglected children may have more emotional needs and may require more individual staff time and attention than children who are not maltreated. Children who are victims of abuse or neglect, in addition to having more developmental problems, also have behavior problems such as emotional lability, depression, and aggressive behaviors (3). These problems may persist long after the maltreatment occurred and may have significant psychiatric and medical consequences into adulthood. In particular, children who have suffered abuse or neglect or been exposed to violence, including domestic violence, often have excessive responses to environmental stress. Their responses are often misinterpreted by caregivers/teachers and responded to inappropriately which, in turn, reinforces their hyper-vigilance and maladaptive behavior in a counter-productive feedback cycle (1,2). Child care staff may need to work closely with the child's primary care provider, therapist, social worker, and parents/guardians to formulate a more personalized behavior management plan.

COMMENTS: Centers serving children with a history of maltreatment related behavior problems may require professionally trained staff. Resources on caring for a child who has been abused or neglected are available from the National Children's Advocacy Center at http://www.nationalcac.org/professionals/.

TYPE OF FACILITY: Center

RELATED STANDARDS:

Standard 1.6.0.1: Child Care Health Consultants

REFERENCES:

1. American Academy of Pediatrics. 2008. Understanding the behavioral and emotional consequences of child abuse. *Pediatrics* 122:667-73.
2. Felitti, V. J., R. F. Anda, P. Nordenber, D. F. Williamson, A. M. Spitz, V. Edwards, M. P. Koss, J. S. Marks. 1998. Relationship of childhood abuse and household dysfunction to many of the leading causes of death in adults. The Adverse Childhood Experiences (ACE) Study. *Am J Prev Med* 14:245-58.
3. Child Welfare Information Gateway. 2008. *Parenting a child who has been sexually abused: A guide for foster and adoptive parents – factsheet for families.* Washington, DC: U.S. Department of Health and Human Services. http://www.childwelfare.gov/pubs/f_abused/.

STANDARD 3.4.4.5: Facility Layout to Reduce Risk of Child Abuse and Neglect

The physical layout of facilities should be arranged so that there is a high level of visibility in the inside and outside areas as well as diaper changing areas and toileting areas used by children. All areas should be viewed by at least one other adult in addition to the caregiver/teacher at all times when children are in care. For center-based programs, rooms should be designed so that there are windows to the hallways to keep classroom activities from being too private. Ideally each area of the facility should have two adults at all times. Such an arrangement reduces the risk of child

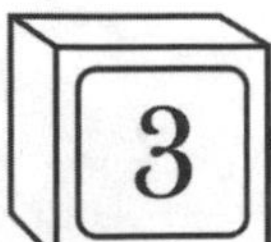

abuse and neglect and the likelihood of extended periods of time in isolation for individual caregivers/teachers with children, especially in areas where children may be partially undressed or in the nude.

Caregivers/teachers should have increased awareness regarding risk of abuse and neglect when a caregiver/teacher is alone with a child. Other caregivers/teachers should periodically walk into a room with one caregiver/teacher to ensure there is no abuse and neglect.

RATIONALE: The presence of multiple caretakers greatly reduces the risk of serious abusive injury. Maltreatment tends to occur in privacy and isolation, and especially in toileting areas (1). A significant number of cases of abuse have been found involving young children being diapered in diaper changing areas (1).

COMMENTS: This standard does not mean to disallow privacy for children who are developmentally able to toilet independently and who may need privacy (2).

TYPE OF FACILITY: Center; Large Family child Care Home; Small Family child Care Home

RELATED STANDARDS:
Standard 2.1.2.5: Toilet Learning/Training
Standards 5.4.1.1-5.4.1.9: Toilets and Toilet Learning/Training Equipment

REFERENCES:

1. Goldman, R. 1990. An educational perspective on abuse. In *Children at risk: An interdisciplinary approach to child abuse and neglect.* R. Goldman, R. Gargiulo, eds. Austin, TX: Pro-Ed.
2. Child Development Institute. 2010. Child development. http://childdevelopmentinfo.com/development/.

3.4.5 Sun Safety and Insect Repellent

STANDARD 3.4.5.1: Sun Safety Including Sunscreen

Caregivers/teachers should implement the following procedures to ensure sun safety for themselves and the children under their supervision:

a) Keep infants younger than six months out of direct sunlight. Find shade under a tree, umbrella, or the stroller canopy;
b) Wear a hat or cap with a brim that faces forward to shield the face;
c) Limit sun exposure between 10 AM and 2 PM, when UV rays are strongest;
d) Wear child safe shatter resistant sunglasses with at least 99% UV protection;
e) Apply sunscreen (1).

Over-the-counter ointments and creams, such as sunscreen that are used for preventive purposes do not require a written authorization from a primary care provider with prescriptive authority. However, parent/guardian written permission is required, and all label instructions must be followed. If the skin is broken or an allergic reaction is observed, caregivers/teachers should discontinue use and notify the parent/guardian.

If parents/guardians give permission, sunscreen should be applied on all exposed areas, especially the face (avoiding the eye area), nose, ears, feet, and hands and rubbed in well especially from May through September. Sunscreen is needed on cloudy days and in the winter at high altitudes. Sun reflects off water, snow, sand, and concrete. "Broad spectrum" sunscreen will screen out both UVB and UVA rays. Use sunscreen with an SPF of 15 or higher, the higher the SPF the more UVB protection offered. UVA protection is designated by a star rating system, with four stars the highest allowed in an over-the-counter product.

Sunscreen should be applied thirty minutes before going outdoors as it needs time to absorb into the skin. If the children will be out for more than one hour, sunscreen will need to be reapplied every two hours as it can wear off. If children are playing in water, reapplication will be needed more frequently. Children should also be protected from the sun by using shade and sun protective clothing. Sun exposure should be limited between the hours of 10 AM and 2 PM when the sun's rays are the strongest.

Sunscreen should be applied to the child at least once by the parents/guardians and the child observed for a reaction to the sunscreen prior to its use in child care.

RATIONALE: Sun exposure from ultraviolet rays (UVA and UVB) causes visible and invisible damage to skin cells. Visible damage consists of freckles early in life. Invisible damage to skin cells adds up over time creating age spots, wrinkles, and even skin cancer (2,4).

Exposure to UV light is highest near the equator, at high altitudes, during midday (10 AM to 4 PM), and where light is reflected off water or snow (5).

COMMENTS: Protective clothing must be worn for infants younger than six months. For infants older than six months, apply sunscreen to all exposed areas of the body, but be careful to keep away from the eyes (3). If an infant rubs sunscreen into her/his eyes, wipe the eyes and hands clean with a damp cloth. Unscented sunblocks or sunscreen with titanium dioxide or zinc oxide are generally safer for children and less likely to cause irritation problems (6). If a rash develops, have parents/guardians talk with the child's primary care provider (1).

Sunscreen needs to be applied every two hours because it wears off after swimming, sweating, or just from absorbing into the skin (1).

There is a theoretical concern that daily sunscreen use will lower vitamin D levels. UV radiation from sun exposure causes the important first step in converting vitamin D in the skin into a usable form for the body. Current medical research on this topic is not definitive, but there does not appear to be a link between daily normal sunscreen use and lower vitamin D levels (7). This is probably because the vitamin D conversion can still occur with sunscreen use at lower levels of UV exposure, before the skin becomes pink or tan. However, vitamin D levels can be influenced significantly by amount of sun exposure, time of the day, amount of protective clothing, skin color and geographic location (8). These

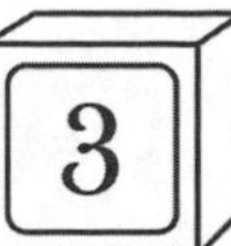

factors make it difficult to apply a safe sunscreen policy for all settings. A health consultant may assist the program develop a local sunscreen policy that may differ from above if there is a significant public health concern regarding low vitamin D levels.

EPA provides specific UV Index information by City Name, Zip Code or by State, to view go to http://www.epa.gov/sunwise/uvindex.html.

A good resource for reading materials for young children and parents/guardians can be found at Healthy Child Care Pennsylvania's Self Learning Module "Sun Safety" at http://www.ecels-healthychildcarepa.org/content/Sun Safey SLM 6-23-10 v5%20.pdf.

TYPE OF FACILITY: Center; Large Family Child Care Home; Small Family Child Care Home

RELATED STANDARDS:
Standard 3.4.5.2: Insect Repellent and Protection from Vector-Borne Diseases
Standard 3.6.3.1: Medication Administration
Standard 6.1.0.7: Shading of Play Area

REFERENCES:

1. American Academy of Pediatrics. 2008. Sun safety. http://www.healthychildren.org/english/safety-prevention/at-play/pages/Sun-Safety.aspx.
2. American Academy of Dermatology. 2010. Skin, hair and nail care: Protecting skin from the sun. Kids Skin Health. http://www.kidsskinhealth.org/grownups/skin_habits_sun.html.
3. Kenfield, S., A. Geller, E. Richter, S. Shuman, D. O'Riordan, H. Koh, G. Colditz. 2005. Sun protection policies and practices at child care centers in Massachusetts. *J Comm Health* 30:491-503.
4. Maguire-Eisen, M., K, Rothman, M. F. Demierre. 2005. The ABCs of sun protection for children. *Dermatology Nurs* 17:419-22,431-33.
5. Weinberg, N., M. Weinberg, S. Maloney. Traveling safely with infants and children. Medic8. http://www.medic8.com/travel/child-safety.htm.
6. Yan, X. S., G. Riccardi, M. Meola, A. Tashjian, J. SaNogueira, T. Schultz. 2008. A tear-free, SPF50 sunscreen product. Cutan Ocul Toxicol 27:231-39.
7. Norval, M., H. C. Wulf. 2009. Does chronic sunscreen use reduce vitamin D production to insufficient levels? British J Dermatology 161:732-36.
8. Misra, M., D. Pacaud, A. Petryk, P. F. Collett-Solberg, M. Kappy. 2008. Vitamin D deficiency in children and its management: Review of current knowledge and recommendations. Pediatrics 122:398-417.

STANDARD 3.4.5.2: Insect Repellent and Protection from Vector-Borne Diseases

Insect repellents offer varying levels of protection from insect bites. Most insects do not carry human disease and most bites only cause mild irritation. Insect repellents may be used with children in child care in areas of the country due to specific disease outbreaks and alerts. Parents/guardians and caregivers/teachers should decide about the use of repellents depending upon the likelihood that local insects are carrying diseases (e.g., local cases of meningitis from mosquito bites). Caregivers/teachers should consult with a child care health consultant, the primary care provider, or the local health department about the appropriateness of use.

Insect repellent used for preventive purposes does not require a written authorization from a primary care provider. Parent/guardian written permission is required, and all label instructions must be followed. If the skin is broken or an allergic reaction is observed, discontinue use and notify the parent/guardian.

Repellents with 10%-30% DEET offer the broadest protection against mosquitoes, ticks, flies, chiggers, and fleas. The concentration of DEET that is used should be dependent upon how much time the child will be exposed. Products with 10% DEET are effective for approximately two hours whereas products with 24% DEET offers protection for approximately five hours. Caregivers/teachers should read the product label and confirm that the product is safe for children and contains a concentration of 30% DEET or less. Some repellents may contain up to 100% DEET and could be very dangerous if applied to a child. DEET is not approved for infants less than two months of age.

Application of this product for children older than two months is acceptable using the following guidelines:

a) Apply insect repellent to the caregiver/teacher's hands first and then put it on the child;
b) Use just enough repellent to cover exposed skin;
c) Do not apply under clothing;
d) Do not use DEET on the hands of young children;
e) Avoid applying to areas around the eyes and mouth;
f) Do not use over cuts or irritated skin;
g) Do not use near food;
h) Do not use products that combine insect repellent and sunscreen. If sunscreen is used, apply sunscreen first;
i) Do not apply a second application to the skin (1);
j) DEET concentration should not exceed 30% for use with children (1);
k) After returning indoors, wash treated skin immediately with soap and water;
l) If the child gets a rash or other bad reaction from an insect repellent, stop using the repellent, wash the repellent off with mild soap and water, and call a local poison center (1-800-222-1222) for further guidance. (1,3,4)

Oil of lemon and eucalyptus products should NOT be used on CHILDREN UNDER THREE YEARS OF AGE (1). Most product labels for registrations containing DEET recommend consultation with a physician if applying to a child less than six months of age.

Picaridin and IR3535 are other products registered at the Environmental Protection Agency (EPA) identified as providing repellent activity sufficient to help people avoid the bites of disease carrying mosquitoes (3).

Caregivers/teachers should practice hand hygiene after applying insect repellent to the children in the group.

Written parent/guardian permission is required before applying any insect repellent to children.

In places where ticks are likely to be found, caregivers/teachers should take the following steps to protect children in their care from ticks:

a) Wear light colored clothing, long sleeves and pants, tuck pants into socks;
b) Conduct tick checks when returning indoors (2).
c) Caregivers/teachers should also take the following protective measures against ticks and mosquitoes with children's play areas:
d) Remove stagnant water sources to prevent breeding grounds for mosquito larvae;
e) Remove leaf litter and clear tall grasses and brush around homes and buildings and at the edges of lawns;
f) Place wood chips or gravel between lawns and wooded areas to restrict tick migration to recreational areas;
g) Mow the lawn and clear brush and leaf litter frequently;
h) Keep playground equipment, decks, and patios away from yard edges and trees.

RATIONALE: Ticks and mosquitoes can carry pathogens that may cause life threatening diseases (i.e., vector-borne diseases such as Lyme Disease) (2).

COMMENTS: Repellent does not have to contain DEET but must be approved for use in the child's age range. If not approved, the parent/guardian must obtain a prescription from the child's primary care provider.

Aerosol sprays are not recommended. Pump sprays are a better choice. Regardless of the type of spray used, caregivers/teachers should spray the insect repellent into her/his hand and then apply to the child. It is not recommended to directly spray the child with the insect repellent to prevent unintentional injury to eyes and mouth. Preschool children, toddlers, and infants should not apply insect repellent to themselves. School age children can apply insect repellent to themselves if they are supervised to make sure that they are applying it correctly.

Parents/guardians should be notified when insect repellent is applied to their child since it is recommended that treated skin is washed with soap and water.

If a product gets in the eyes, flush with water and consult the poison center at 1-800-222-1222.

How to Remove a Tick:

It is important to remove the tick as soon as possible. Use the following steps:

a) If possible, clean the area with an antiseptic solution or soap and water. Take care not to scrub the tick too hard. Just clean the skin around it;
b) Use blunt, fine tipped tweezers or gloved fingers to grasp the tick as close to the skin as possible;
c) Pull slowly and steadily upwards to allow the tick to release;
d) If the tick's head breaks off in the skin, use tweezers to remove it like you would a splinter;
e) Wash the area around the bite with soap;
f) Following the removal of the tick, wash your hands, the tweezers, and the area thoroughly with soap and warm water.

Take care not to do the following:

a) Do not use sharp tweezers.
b) Do not crush, puncture, or squeeze the tick's body.
c) Do not use a twisting or jerking motion to remove the tick.
d) Do not handle the tick with bare hands.
e) Do not try to make the tick let go by holding a hot match or cigarette close to it.
f) Do not try to smother the tick by covering it with petroleum jelly or nail polish.

Several resources are available on reducing exposure to ticks and mosquitoes based on habits, protective attire, and insect repellent use. The following Websites offer detailed information on preventing exposure to ticks and mosquitoes which may cause disease: "Integrated Pest Management (IPM) of Mosquitoes in Early Childhood Education (ECE) Settings" by the California Childcare Health Program at http://www.ucsfchildcarehealth.org/pdfs/healthandsafety/Mosquitoes_en_0709.pdf, and Protect Yourself from Tick Bites by the Centers for Disease Control and Prevention at http://www.cdc.gov/ncidod/dvbid/lyme/Prevention/ld_Prevention_Avoid.htm.

Additional resources:

- http://www.cdc.gov/ncidod/diseases/list_mosquitoborne.htm;
- http://www.epa.gov/pesticides/health/mosquitoes/ai_insectrp.htm; and
- http://www.lymediseaseassociation.org/index.php?option=com_content&view=category&id=29&Itemid=180.

TYPE OF FACILITY: Center; Large Family Child Care Home; Small Family Child Care Home

RELATED STANDARDS:

Standard 3.2.2.1: Situations that Require Hand Hygiene
Standard 3.4.5.1: Sun Safety Including Sunscreen
Standard 5.2.8.1: Integrated Pest Management

REFERENCES:

1. American Academy of Pediatrics, Committee on Environmental Health. 2003. Follow safety precautions when using DEET on children. *AAP News* 22. http://aapnews.aappublications.org/cgi/content/full/e200399v1/.
2. Centers for Disease Control and Prevention, Division of Vector-Borne Infectious Diseases. 2010. Lyme disease: Protect yourself from tick bites. http://www.cdc.gov/ncidod/dvbid/lyme/Prevention/ld_Prevention_Avoid.htm.
3. Centers for Disease Control and Prevention, Division of Vector-Borne Infectious Diseases. 2009. West nile virus: Updated information regarding insect repellents. http://www.cdc.gov/ncidod/dvbid/westnile/RepellentUpdates.htm.
4. Roberts J. R., Weil W. B., Shannon, M. W. 2005. DEET alternatives considered to be effective mosquito repellents. *AAP News.* http://aap.org/family/wnv-jun05.htm.

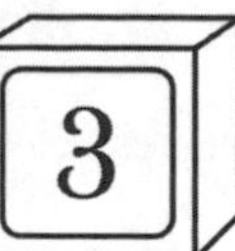

3.4.6 Strangulation

STANDARD 3.4.6.1: Strangulation Hazards

Strings and cords (such as those that are parts of toys and those found on window coverings) long enough to encircle a child's neck should not be accessible to children in child care. Miniblinds and venetian blinds should not have looped cords. Vertical blinds, continuous looped blinds, and drapery cords should have tension or tie-down devices to hold the cords tight. Inner cord stops should be installed. Shoulder straps on guitars and chin straps on hats should be removed (1).

Straps/handles on purses/bags used for dramatic play should be removed or shortened. Ties, scarves, necklaces, and boas used for dramatic play should not be used for children under three years. If used by children three years and over, children should be supervised.

Pacifiers attached to strings or ribbons should not be placed around infants' necks or attached to infants' clothing.

Hood and neck strings from all children's outerwear, including jackets and sweatshirts, should be removed. Drawstrings on the waist or bottom of garments should not extend more than three inches outside the garment when it is fully expanded. These strings should have no knots or toggles on the free ends. The drawstring should be sewn to the garment at its midpoint so the string cannot be pulled out through one side.

RATIONALE: Window covering cords are associated with strangulation of young children under (2,4). Infants can become entangled in cords from window coverings near their cribs. Since 1990, more than 200 infants and young children have died from unintentional strangulation in window cords (5).

Cords and ribbons tied to pacifiers can become tightly twisted, or can catch on crib cornerposts or other protrusions, causing strangulation.

Clothing strings on children's clothing, necklaces and scarves can catch on playground equipment and strangle children. The U.S. Consumer Product Safety Commission (CPSC) has reported deaths and injuries involving the entanglement of children's clothing drawstrings (3).

COMMENTS: Children's outerwear that has alternative closures (e.g., snaps, buttons, hook and loop, and elastic) are recommended (3).

It is advisable that caregivers avoid wearing necklaces or clothing with drawstrings that could cause entanglement.

For additional information regarding the prevention of strangulation from strings on toys, window coverings, clothing, contact the CPSC. See http://www.windowcoverings.org for the latest blind cord safety information.

RELATED STANDARDS:
Standard 5.3.1.1: Safety of Equipment, Materials, and Furnishings

TYPE OF FACILITY: Center; Large Family Child Care Home; Small Family Child Care Home

REFERENCES:
1. U.S. Consumer Product Safety Commission. Strings and straps on toys can strangle young children. http://www.cpsc.gov/CPSCPUB/PUBS/5100.html.
2. Window Covering Safety Council. Basic cord safety. http://www.windowcoverings.org/basic_cord_safety.html.
3. U.S. Consumer Product Safety Commission (CPSC). 1999. *Guidelines for drawstrings on children's outerwear.* Bethesda, MD: CPSC. http://www.cpsc.gov/cpscpub/pubs/208.pdf.
4. U.S. Consumer Product Safety Commission (CPSC). *Are your window coverings safe?* Washington, DC: CPSC.
5. Window Covering Safety Council. 2011. New study released on window covering safety awareness. http://www.windowcoverings.org/nr_2011-3.html.

3.5 Care Plans and Adaptations

STANDARD 3.5.0.1: Care Plan for Children with Special Health Care Needs

Reader's Note: Children with special health care needs are defined as "...those who have or are at increased risk for a chronic physical, developmental, behavioral, or emotional condition and who also require health and related services of a type or amount beyond that required by children generally" (1).

Any child who meets these criteria should have a Routine and Emergent Care Plan completed by their primary care provider in their medical home. In addition to the information specified in Standard 9.4.2.4 for the Health Report, there should be:

a) A list of the child's diagnosis/diagnoses;
b) Contact information for the primary care provider and any relevant sub-specialists (i.e., endocrinologists, oncologists, etc.);
c) Medications to be administered on a scheduled basis;
d) Medications to be administered on an emergent basis with clearly stated parameters, signs, and symptoms that warrant giving the medication written in lay language;
e) Procedures to be performed;
f) Allergies;
g) Dietary modifications required for the health of the child;
h) Activity modifications;
i) Environmental modifications;
j) Stimulus that initiates or precipitates a reaction or series of reactions (triggers) to avoid;
k) Symptoms for caregiver/teachers to observe;
l) Behavioral modifications;
m) Emergency response plans – both if the child has a medical emergency and special factors to consider in programmatic emergency, like a fire;
n) Suggested special skills training and education for staff.

A template for a Care Plan for children with special health care needs is provided in Appendix O.

The Care Plan should be updated after every hospitalization or significant change in health status of the child. The Care Plan is completed by the primary care provider in the medical home with input from parents/guardians, and it is implemented in the child care setting. The child care health consultant should be involved to assure adequate information, training, and monitoring is available for child care staff.

RATIONALE: Children with special health care needs could have a variety of different problems ranging from asthma, diabetes, cerebral palsy, bleeding disorders, metabolic problems, cystic fibrosis, sickle cell disease, seizure disorder, sensory disorders, autism, severe allergy, immune deficiencies, or many other conditions (2). Some of these conditions require daily treatments and some only require observation for signs of impending illness and ability to respond in a timely manner (3).

COMMENTS: A collaborative approach in which the primary care provider and the parent/guardian complete the Care Plan and the parent/guardian works with the child care staff to implement the plan is helpful. Although it is usually the primary care provider in the medical home completing the Care Plan, sometimes management is shared by specialists, nurse practitioners, and case managers, especially with conditions such as diabetes or sickle cell disease.

Child care health consultants are very helpful in assisting in implementing Care Plans and in providing or finding training resources. The child care health consultant may help in creating the care plan, through developing a draft and/or facilitate the primary care provider to provide specific directives to follow within the child care environment. The child care health consultant should write out directives into a "user friendly" language document for caregivers/teachers and/or staff to implement with ease.

Communication between parents/guardians, the child care program and the primary care provider (medical home) requires the free exchange of protected medical information (4). Confidentiality should be maintained at each step in compliance with any laws or regulations that are pertinent to all parties such as the Family Educational Rights and Privacy Act (commonly known as FERPA) and/or the Health Insurance Portability and Accountability Act (commonly known as HIPAA) (4).

For additional information on care plans and approaches for the most prevalent chronic diseases in child care see the following resources:

Asthma: How Asthma-Friendly Is Your Child-Care Setting? at http://www.nhlbi.nih.gov/health/public/lung/asthma/chc_chk.htm;

Autism: Learn the Signs/ACT Early at http://www.cdc.gov/ncbddd/autism/actearly/;

Food Allergies: Guides for School, Childcare, and Camp at http://www.foodallergy.org/section/guidelines1/;

Diabetes: "Diabetes Care in the School and Day Care Setting" at http://care.diabetesjournals.org/content/29/suppl_1/s49.full;

Seizures: Seizure Disorders in the ECE Setting at http://www.ucsfchildcarehealth.org/pdfs/healthandsafety/SeizuresEN032707_adr.pdf.

TYPE OF FACILITY: Center; Large Family Child Care Home; Small Family Child Care Home

RELATED STANDARDS:
Standard 3.6.3.1: Medication Administration
Standard 4.2.0.10: Care for Children with Food Allergies
Chapter 8: Children with Special Health Care Needs and Disabilities
Standard 9.4.2.4: Contents of Child's Primary Care Provider's Assessment

REFERENCES:

1. McPherson, M., P. Arango, H. Fox, C. Lauver, M. McManus, P. Newacheck, J. Perrin, J. Shonkoff, B. Strickland. 1998. A new definition of children with special health care needs. *Pediatrics* 102:137-40.
2. U.S. Department of Health and Human Services, Health Resources and Services Administration. The national survey of children with special health care needs: Chartbook 2005-2006. http://mchb.hrsa.gov/cshcn05/.
3. American Association of Nurse Anesthetists. 2003. Creating a latex-safe school for latex-sensitive children. http://www.anesthesiapatientsafety.com/patients/latex/school.asp.
4. Donoghue, E. A., C. A. Kraft, eds. 2010. *Managing chronic health needs in child care and schools: A quick reference guide.* Elk Grove Village, IL: American Academy of Pediatrics.

STANDARD 3.5.0.2: Caring for Children Who Require Medical Procedures

A facility that enrolls children who require the following medical procedures: tube feedings, endotracheal suctioning, supplemental oxygen, postural drainage, or catheterization daily (unless the child requiring catheterization can perform this function on his/her own), checking blood sugars or any other special medical procedures performed routinely, or who might require special procedures on an urgent basis, should receive a written plan of care from the primary care provider who prescribed the special treatment (such as a urologist for catheterization). Often, the child's primary care provider may be able to provide this information. This plan of care should address any special preparation to perform routine and/or urgent procedures (other than those that might be required in an emergency for any typical child, such as cardiopulmonary resuscitation [CPR]). This plan of care should include instructions for how to receive training in performing the procedure, performing the procedure, a description of common and uncommon complications of the procedure, and what to do and who to notify if complications occur. Specific/relevant training for the child care staff should be provided by a qualified health care professional in accordance with state practice acts. Facilities should follow state laws where such laws require RN's or LPN's under RN supervision to perform certain medical procedures. Updated, written medical orders are required for nursing procedures.

RATIONALE: The specialized skills required to implement these procedures are not traditionally taught to early childhood caregivers/teachers, or educational assistants as part

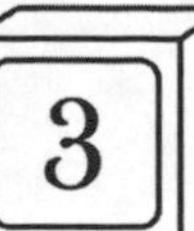

of their academic or practical experience. Skilled nursing care may be necessary in some circumstances.

COMMENTS: Parents/guardians are responsible for supplying the required equipment. The facility should offer staff training and allow sufficient staff time to carry out the necessary procedures. Caring for children who require intermittent catheterization or maintaining supplemental oxygen is not as demanding as it first sounds, but the implication of this standard is that facilities serving children who have complex medical problems need special training, consultation, and monitoring.

Before enrolling a child who will need this type of care, caregivers/teachers can request and review fact sheets, instructions, and training by an appropriate health care professional that includes a return demonstration of competence of the caregivers/teachers for handling specific procedures. Often, the child's parents/guardians or clinicians have these materials and know where training is available. If possible, parents/guardians should be present and take part in the training. The primary care provider is responsible for providing the health care plan for the child; the plan can be communicated to the caregiver/teacher by the parent/guardian with the help of the child care health consultant who can then assist in training the staff. When the specifics are known, caregivers/teachers can make a more responsible decision about what would be required to serve the child. A caregiver/teacher should not assume care for a child with special medical needs unless comfortable with training received and approved for that role by the child care health consultant or consulting primary care provider.

Communication between parents/guardians, the child care program and the primary care provider (medical home) requires the free exchange of protected medical information (1). Confidentiality should be maintained at each step in compliance with any laws or regulations that are pertinent to all parties such as the Family Educational Rights and Privacy Act (commonly known as FERPA) and/or the Health Insurance Portability and Accountability Act (commonly known as HIPAA) (1).

TYPE OF FACILITY: Center; Large Family Child Care; Small Family Child Care Home

RELATED STANDARDS:
Standard 1.4.3.1: First Aid and CPR Training for Staff
Standard 1.6.0.1: Child Care Health Consultants
Standard 3.5.0.1: Care Plan for Children with Special Health Care Needs
Chapter 8: Children with Special Health Care Needs and Disabilities

REFERENCES:
1. Donoghue, E. A., C. A. Kraft, eds. 2010. *Managing chronic health needs in child care and schools: A quick reference guide.* Elk Grove Village, IL: American Academy of Pediatrics.

3.6 Management of Illness

3.6.1 Inclusion/Exclusion Due to Illness

STANDARD 3.6.1.1: Inclusion/Exclusion/Dismissal of Children

(Adapted from: Aronson, S. S., T. R. Shope, eds. 2009. *Managing infectious diseases in child care and schools: A quick reference guide,* 39-43. 2nd ed. Elk Grove Village, IL: American Academy of Pediatrics.)

Preparing for managing illness:

Caregivers/teachers should:

a) Encourage all families to have a backup plan for child care in the event of short or long term exclusion;
b) Review with families the inclusion/exclusion criteria and clarify that the program staff (not the families) will make the final decision about whether children who are ill may stay based on the program's inclusion/exclusion criteria and their ability to care for the child who is ill without compromising the care of other children in the program;
c) Develop, with a child care health consultant, protocols and procedures for handling children's illnesses, including care plans and an inclusion/exclusion policy;
d) Request the primary care provider's note to readmit a child if the primary care provider's advice is needed to determine whether the child is a health risk to others, or if the primary care provider's guidance is needed about any special care the child requires (1);
e) Rely on the family's description of the child's behavior to determine whether the child is well enough to return, unless the child's status is unclear from the family's report.

Daily health checks as described in Standard 3.1.1.1 should be performed upon arrival of each child each day. Staff should objectively determine if the child is ill or well. Staff should determine which children with mild illnesses can remain in care and which need to be excluded.

Staff should notify the parent/guardian when a child develops new signs or symptoms of illness. Parent/guardian notification should be immediate for emergency or urgent issues. Staff should notify parents/guardians of children who have symptoms that require exclusion and parents/guardians should remove the child from the child care setting as soon as possible. For children whose symptoms do not require exclusion, verbal or written notification of the parent/guardian at the end of the day is acceptable. Most conditions that require exclusion do not require a primary care provider visit before reentering care.

Conditions/symptoms that do not require exclusion:

a) Common colds, runny noses (regardless of color or consistency of nasal discharge);
b) A cough not associated with a infectious disease (such as pertussis) or a fever;

c) Watery, yellow or white discharge or crusting eye discharge without fever, eye pain, or eyelid redness;
d) Yellow or white eye drainage that is not associated with pink or red conjunctiva (i.e., the whites of the eyes);
e) Pink eye (bacterial conjunctivitis) indicated by pink or red conjunctiva with white or yellow eye mucous drainage and matted eyelids after sleep. Parents/guardians should discuss care of this condition with their child's primary care provider, and follow the primary care provider's advice. Some primary care providers do not think it is necessary to examine the child if the discussion with the parents/guardians suggests that the condition is likely to be self-limited. If two unrelated children in the same program have conjunctivitis, the organism causing the conjunctivitis may have a higher risk for transmission and a child health care professional should be consulted;
f) Fever without any signs or symptoms of illness in children who are older than six months regardless of whether acetaminophen or ibuprofen was given. Fever (temperature above 101°F [38.3°C] orally, above 102°F [38.9°C] rectally, or 100°F [37.8°C] or higher taken axillary [armpit] or measured by an equivalent method) is an indication of the body's response to something, but is neither a disease nor a serious problem by itself. Body temperature can be elevated by overheating caused by overdressing or a hot environment, reactions to medications, and response to infection. If the child is behaving normally but has a fever of below 102°F per rectum or the equivalent, the child should be monitored, but does not need to be excluded for fever alone;
g) Rash without fever and behavioral changes;
h) Lice or nits (exclusion for treatment of an active lice infestation may be delayed until the end of the day);
i) Ringworm (exclusion for treatment may be delayed until the end of the day);
j) Molluscum contagiosum (do not require exclusion or covering of lesions);
k) Thrush (i.e., white spots or patches in the mouth or on the cheeks or gums);
l) Fifth disease (slapped cheek disease, parvovirus B19) once the rash has appeared;
m) Methicillin-resistant Staphylococcus aureus, or MRSA, without an infection or illness that would otherwise require exclusion. Known MRSA carriers or colonized individuals should not be excluded;
n) Cytomegalovirus infection;
o) Chronic hepatitis B infection;
p) Human immunodeficiency virus (HIV) infection;
q) Asymptomatic children who have been previously evaluated and found to be shedding potentially infectious organisms in the stool. Children who are continent of stool or who are diapered with formed stools that can be contained in the diaper may return to care. For some infectious organisms, exclusion is required until certain guidelines have been met. Note: These agents are not common and caregivers/teachers will usually not know the cause of most cases of diarrhea;
r) Children with chronic infectious conditions that can be accommodated in the program according to the legal requirement of federal law in the Americans with Disabilities Act. The act requires that child care programs make reasonable accommodations for children with disabilities and/or chronic illnesses, considering each child individually.

Key criteria for exclusion of children who are ill:

When a child becomes ill but does not require immediate medical help, a determination must be made regarding whether the child should be sent home (i.e., should be temporarily "excluded" from child care). Most illnesses do not require exclusion. The caregiver/teacher should determine if the illness:

a) Prevents the child from participating comfortably in activities;
b) Results in a need for care that is greater than the staff can provide without compromising the health and safety of other children;
c) Poses a risk of spread of harmful diseases to others.

If any of the above criteria are met, the child should be excluded, regardless of the type of illness. The child should be removed from direct contact with other children and should be monitored and supervised by a single staff member known to the child until dismissed from care to the care of a parent/guardian or a primary care provider. The area should be where the toys, equipment, and surfaces will not be used by other children or adults until after the ill child leaves and after the surfaces and toys have been cleaned and disinfected.

Temporary exclusion is recommended when the child has any of the following conditions:

a) The illness prevents the child from participating comfortably in activities;
b) The illness results in a need for care that is greater than the staff can provide without compromising the health and safety of other children;
c) An acute change in behavior - this could include lethargy/lack of responsiveness, irritability, persistent crying, difficult breathing, or having a quickly spreading rash;
d) Fever (temperature above 101°F [38.3°C] orally, above 102°F [38.9°C] rectally, or 100°F [37.8°C] or higher taken axillary [armpit] or measured by an equivalent method) and behavior change or other signs and symptoms (e.g., sore throat, rash, vomiting, diarrhea). An unexplained temperature above 100°F (37.8°C) axillary (armpit) or 101°F (38.3°C) rectally in a child younger than six months should be medically evaluated. Any infant younger than two months of age with any fever should get urgent medical attention. See COMMENTS Below for important information about taking temperatures;
e) Diarrhea is defined by watery stools or decreased form of stool that is not associated with changes of

diet. Exclusion is required for all diapered children whose stool is not contained in the diaper and toilet-trained children if the diarrhea is causing soiled pants or clothing. In addition, diapered children with diarrhea should be excluded if the stool frequency exceeds two or more stools above normal for that child, because this may cause too much work for the caregivers/teachers. Readmission after diarrhea can occur when diapered children have their stool contained by the diaper (even if the stools remain loose) and when toilet-trained children are continent. Special circumstances that require specific exclusion criteria include the following (2):

1) Toxin-producing *E. coli* or *Shigella* infection, until stools are formed and the test results of two stool cultures obtained from stools produced twenty-four hours apart do not detect these organisms;
2) *Salmonella* serotype Typhi infection, until diarrhea resolves. In children younger than five years with *Salmonella* serotype Typhi, three negative stool cultures obtained with twenty-four-hour intervals are required; people five years of age or older may return after a twenty-four-hour period without a diarrheal stool. Stool cultures should be collected from other attendees and staff members, and all infected people should be excluded;

f) Blood or mucus in the stools not explained by dietary change, medication, or hard stools;
g) Vomiting more than two times in the previous twenty-four hours, unless the vomiting is determined to be caused by a non-infectious condition and the child remains adequately hydrated;
h) Abdominal pain that continues for more than two hours or intermittent pain associated with fever or other signs or symptoms of illness;
i) Mouth sores with drooling unless the child's primary care provider or local health department authority states that the child is noninfectious;
j) Rash with fever or behavioral changes, until the primary care provider has determined that the illness is not a infectious disease;
k) Active tuberculosis, until the child's primary care provider or local health department states child is on appropriate treatment and can return;
l) Impetigo, until treatment has been started;
m) Streptococcal pharyngitis (i.e., strep throat or other streptococcal infection), until twenty-four hours after treatment has been started;
n) Head lice until after the first treatment (note: exclusion is not necessary before the end of the program day);
o) Scabies, until after treatment has been given;
p) Chickenpox (varicella), until all lesions have dried or crusted (usually six days after onset of rash);
q) Rubella, until six days after the rash appears;
r) Pertussis, until five days of appropriate antibiotic treatment;
s) Mumps, until five days after onset of parotid gland swelling;
t) Measles, until four days after onset of rash;
u) Hepatitis A virus infection, until one week after onset of illness or jaundice if the child's symptoms are mild or as directed by the health department. (Note: immunization status of child care contacts should be confirmed; within a fourteen-day period of exposure, incompletely immunized or unimmunized contacts from one through forty years of age should receive the hepatitis A vaccine as post exposure prophylaxis, unless contraindicated.) Other individuals may receive immune globulin. Consult with a primary care provider for dosage and recommendations;
v) Any child determined by the local health department to be contributing to the transmission of illness during an outbreak.

Procedures for a child who requires exclusion:

The caregiver/teacher will:

a) Provide care for the child in a place where the child will be comfortable and supervised by someone who knows the child well and who will continue to observe the child for new or worsening symptoms. A potentially contagious child should be separated from other children by at least three feet. Each facility should have a predetermined physical location(s) where an ill child(ren) could be placed until care can be transferred to a parent/guardian or primary care provider;
b) Ask the family to pick up the child as soon as possible;
c) Discuss the signs and symptoms of illness with the parent/guardian who is assuming care. Review guidelines for return to child care. If necessary, provide the family with a written communication that may be given to the primary care provider. The communication should include onset time of symptoms, observations about the child, vital signs and times (e.g., temperature 101.5°F at 10:30 AM) and any actions taken and the time actions were taken (e.g., one children's acetaminophen given at 11:00 AM). The nature and severity of symptoms and or requirements of the local or state health department will determine the necessity of medical consultation. Telephone advice, electronic transmissions of instructions are acceptable without an office visit;
d) Follow the advice of the child's primary care provider;
e) Contact the local health department if there is a question of a reportable (harmful) infectious disease in a child or staff member in the facility. If there are conflicting opinions from different primary care providers about the management of a child with a reportable infectious disease, the health department has the legal authority to make a final determination;
f) Document actions in the child's file with date, time, symptoms, and actions taken (and by whom); sign and date the document;
g) In collaboration with the local health department, notify the parents of contacts to the child or staff

member with presumed or confirmed reportable infectious infection.

The caregiver/teacher should make the decision about whether a child meets or does not meet the exclusion criteria for participation and the child's need for care relative to the staff's ability to provide care. If parents/guardians and the child care staff disagree, and the reason for exclusion relates to the child's ability to participate or the caregiver's/teacher's ability to provide care for the other children, the caregiver/teacher should not be required to accept responsibility for the care of the child.

Reportable conditions:

The current list of infectious diseases designated as notifiable in the United States at the national level by the Centers for Disease Control and Prevention (CDC) are listed at http://www.cdc.gov/osels/ph_surveillance/.

The caregiver/teacher should contact the local health department:

a) When a child or staff member who is in contact with others has a reportable disease;
b) If a reportable illness occurs among the staff, children, or families involved with the program;
c) For assistance in managing a suspected outbreak. Generally, an outbreak can be considered to be two or more unrelated (e.g., not siblings) children with the same diagnosis or symptoms in the same group within one week. Clusters of mild respiratory illness, ear infections, and certain dermatological conditions are common and generally do not need to be reported.

Caregivers/teachers should work with their child care health consultants to develop policies and procedures for alerting staff and families about their responsibility to report illnesses to the program and for the program to report diseases to the local health authorities.

RATIONALE: Excluding children with mild illnesses is unlikely to reduce the spread of most infectious agents (germs) caused by bacteria, viruses, parasites and fungi. Most infections are spread by children who do not have symptoms. They spread the infectious agent (germs) before or after their illnesses and without evidence of symptoms. Exposure to frequent mild infections helps the child's immune system develop in a healthy way. As a child gets older s/he develops immunity to common infectious agents and will become ill less often. Since exclusion is unlikely to reduce the spread of disease, the most important reason for exclusion is the ability of the child to participate in activities and the staff to care for the child.

The terms contagious, infectious and communicable have similar meanings. A fully immunized child with a contagious, infectious or communicable condition will likely not have an illness that is harmful to the child or others. Children attending child care frequently carry contagious organisms that do not limit their activity nor pose a threat to their contacts. Hand and personal hygiene is paramount in preventing transmission of these organisms. Written notes should not be required for return to child care for common respiratory illnesses that are not specifically listed in the excludable condition list above.

For specific conditions, *Managing Infectious Diseases in Child Care and Schools: A Quick Reference Guide, 2nd Edition* has educational handouts that can be copied and distributed to parents/guardians, health professionals, and caregivers/teachers. This publication is available from the American Academy of Pediatrics (AAP) at http://www.aap.org.

For more detailed rationale regarding inclusion/exclusion, return to care, when a health visit is necessary, and health department reporting for children with specific symptoms, please see Appendix A, Signs and Symptoms Chart.

State licensing law or code defines the conditions or symptoms for which exclusion is necessary. States are increasingly using the criteria defined in *Caring for Our Children* and the *Managing Infectious Diseases in Child Care and Schools* publications. Usually, the criteria in these two sources are more detailed than the state regulations so can be incorporated into the local written policies without conflicting with state law.

In this edition of *Caring for Our Children*, the exclusion criteria for bacterial conjunctivitis (pink eye) and diarrhea have changed. Exclusion is no longer required for pink eye and treatment is not required. This change reflects the recognition that conjunctivitis is a self-limiting infection and there is not any evidence that treatment or exclusion reduces its spread. Children with diarrhea may remain in care as long as the stool is contained in the diaper or the child can maintain continence. If additional criteria are met, such as an inability to participate in activities or requiring more care than staff can provide, then a child should be excluded until the criteria for return of care are met. A provision was included that if the stool frequency is two or more stools per day above the normal then exclusion could be indicated. This accounts for the increased staff time involved in diaper changing. Infants should routinely receive rotavirus vaccine, which has been the most common cause of viral diarrhea in this age group.

COMMENTS: When taking a child's temperature, remember that:

a) The amount of temperature elevation varies at different body sites;
b) The height of fever does not indicate a more or less severe illness;
c) The method chosen to take a child's temperature depends on the need for accuracy, available equipment, the skill of the person taking the temperature, and the ability of the child to assist in the procedure;
d) Oral temperatures are difficult to take for children younger than four years of age;
e) Rectal temperatures should be taken only by persons with specific health training in performing this procedure and permission given by parents/guardians;
f) Axillary (armpit) temperatures are accurate only when the thermometer remains within the closed armpit for the time period recommended by the device;

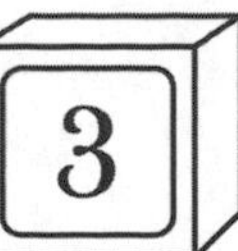

g) Electronic devices for measuring temperature require periodic calibration and specific training in proper technique;
h) Any device used improperly may give inaccurate results;
i) Mercury thermometers should not be used;
j) Aural (ear) devices may underestimate fever and should not be used in children less than four months.

TYPE OF FACILITY: Center; Large Family Child Care Home; Small Family Child Care Home

RELATED STANDARDS:
Standard 3.1.1.1: Conduct of Daily Health Check
Standard 3.6.1.2: Staff Exclusion for Illness
Standard 3.6.1.3: Thermometers for Taking Human Temperatures
Standard 3.6.1.4: Infectious Disease Outbreak Control
Chapter 7: Infectious Diseases
Appendix A: Signs and Symptoms Chart

REFERENCES:
1. Aronson, S. S., T. R. Shope, eds. 2009. *Managing infectious diseases in child care and schools: A quick reference guide.* 2nd ed. Elk Grove Village, IL: American Academy of Pediatrics.
2. Pickering, L. K., C. J. Baker, D. W. Kimberlin, S. S. Long, eds. 2009. *Red book: 2009 report of the Committee on Infectious Diseases.* 28th ed. Elk Grove Village, IL: American Academy of Pediatrics.

STANDARD 3.6.1.2: Staff Exclusion for Illness

Please note that if a staff member has no contact with the children, or with anything with which the children come into contact, this standard may not apply to that staff member.

A facility should not deny admission to or send home a staff member or substitute with illness unless one or more of the following conditions exists. The staff member should be excluded as follows:

a) Chickenpox, until all lesions have dried and crusted, which usually occurs by six days;
b) Shingles, only if the lesions cannot be covered by clothing or a dressing until the lesions have crusted;
c) Rash with fever or joint pain, until diagnosed not to be measles or rubella;
d) Measles, until four days after onset of the rash (if the staff member or substitute is immunocompetent);
e) Rubella, until six days after onset of rash;
f) Diarrheal illness, stool frequency exceeds two or more stools above normal for that individual or blood in stools, until diarrhea resolves; if *E. coli* 0157:H7 or *Shigella* is isolated, until diarrhea resolves and two stool cultures are negative, for *Salmonella* serotype Typhi, three stool cultures collected at twenty-four hour intervals and resolution of diarrhea is required;
g) Vomiting illness, two or more episodes of vomiting during the previous twenty-four hours, until vomiting resolves or is determined to result from non-infectious conditions;
h) Hepatitis A virus, until one week after symptom onset or as directed by the health department;
i) Pertussis, until after five days of appropriate antibiotic therapy;
j) Skin infection (such as impetigo), until treatment has been initiated; exclusion should continue if lesion is draining AND cannot be covered;
k) Tuberculosis, until noninfectious and cleared by a health department official or a primary care provider;
l) Strep throat or other streptococcal infection, until twenty-four hours after initial antibiotic treatment and end of fever;
m) Head lice, from the end of the day of discovery until after the first treatment;
n) Scabies, until after treatment has been completed;
o) Haemophilus influenzae type b (Hib), prophylaxis, until antibiotic treatment has been initiated;
p) Meningococcal infection, until appropriate therapy has been administered for twenty-four hours;
q) Respiratory illness, if the illness limits the staff member's ability to provide an acceptable level of child care and compromises the health and safety of the children.

Caregivers/teachers who have herpes cold sores should not be excluded from the child care facility, but should:

a) Cover and not touch their lesions;
b) Carefully observe hand hygiene policies.

RATIONALE: Adults are as capable of spreading infectious disease as children (1-3). See also the rationale for Standard 3.6.1.1 Inclusion/Exclusion/Dismissal of Children.

TYPE OF FACILITY: Center; Large Family Child Care Home; Small Family Child Care Home

RELATED STANDARDS:
Standard 3.6.1.1: Inclusion/Exclusion/Dismissal of Children
Standard 3.6.1.4: Infectious Disease Outbreak Control
Chapter 7: Infectious Diseases

REFERENCES:
1. Reves, R. R., L. K. Pickering. 1992. Impact of child day care on infectious diseases in adults. *Infect Dis Clin North Amer* 6:239-50.
2. Pickering, L. K., C. J. Baker, D. W. Kimberlin, S. S. Long, eds. 2009. *Red book: 2009 report of the Committee on Infectious Diseases.* 28th ed. Elk Grove Village, IL: American Academy of Pediatrics.
3. Murph, J. R., S. D. Palmer, D. Glassy, eds. 2005. *Health in child care: A manual for health professionals.* Elk Grove Village, IL: American Academy of Pediatrics.

STANDARD 3.6.1.3: Thermometers for Taking Human Temperatures

Digital thermometers should be used with infants and young children when there is a concern for fever. Tympanic (ear) thermometers may be used with children four months and older. However, while a tympanic thermometer gives quick results, it needs to be placed correctly in the child's ear to be accurate.

Glass or mercury thermometers should not be used. Mercury containing thermometers and any waste created from the cleanup of a broken thermometer should be disposed of at a household hazardous waste collection facility.

Rectal temperatures should be taken only by persons with specific health training in performing this procedure. Oral

(under the tongue) temperatures can be used for children over age four. Individual plastic covers should be used on oral or rectal thermometers with each use or thermometers should be cleaned and sanitized after each use according to the manufacturer's instructions. Axillary (under the arm) temperatures are less accurate, but are a good option for infants and young children when the caregiver/teacher has not been trained to take a rectal temperature.

RATIONALE: When using tympanic thermometers, too much earwax can cause the reading to be incorrect. Tympanic thermometers may fail to detect a fever that is actually present (1). Therefore, tympanic thermometers should not be used in children under four months of age, where fever detection is most important.

Mercury thermometers can break and result in mercury toxicity that can lead to neurologic injury. To prevent mercury toxicity, the American Academy of Pediatrics (AAP) encourages the removal of mercury thermometers from homes. This includes all child care settings as well (1).

Although not a hazard, temporal thermometers are not as accurate as digital thermometers (2).

COMMENTS: The site where a child's temperature is taken (rectal, oral, axillary, or tympanic) should be documented along with the temperature reading and the time the temperature was taken, because different sites give different results and affect interpretation of temperature.

More information about taking temperatures can be found on the AAP Website http://www.healthychildren.org/English/health-issues/conditions/fever/pages/How-to-Take-a-Childs-Temperature.aspx.

Safety and child abuse concerns may arise when using rectal thermometers. Caregivers/teachers should be aware of these concerns. If rectal temperatures are taken, steps must be taken to ensure that all caregivers/teachers are trained properly in this procedure and the opportunity for abuse is negligible (for example, ensure that more than one adult present during procedure). **Rectal temperatures should be taken only by persons with specific health training in performing this procedure and permission given by parents/guardians.**

Many state or local agencies operate facilities that collect used mercury thermometers. Typically, the service is free. For more information on household hazardous waste collections in your area, call your State environmental protection agency or your local health department.

TYPE OF FACILITY: Center; Large Family Child Care Home; Small Family Child Care Home

REFERENCES:

1. Healthy Children. 2010. Health issues: How to take a child's temperature. American Academy of Pediatrics. http://www.healthychildren.org/English/health-issues/conditions/fever/pages/How-to-Take-a-Childs-Temperature.aspx.

2. Dodd, S. R., G. A. Lancaster, J. V. Craig, R. L. Smyth, P. R. Williamson. 2006. In a systematic review, infrared ear thermometry for fever diagnosis in children finds poor sensitivity. *J Clin Epidemiol* 59:354-57.

STANDARD 3.6.1.4: Infectious Disease Outbreak Control

During the course of an identified outbreak of any reportable illness at the facility, a child or staff member should be excluded if the health department official or primary care provider suspects that the child or staff member is contributing to transmission of the illness at the facility, is not adequately immunized when there is an outbreak of a vaccine preventable disease, or the circulating pathogen poses an increased risk to the individual. The child or staff member should be readmitted when the health department official or primary care provider who made the initial determination decides that the risk of transmission is no longer present.

RATIONALE: Secondary spread of infectious disease has been proven to occur in child care. Control of outbreaks of infectious diseases in child care may include age-appropriate immunization, antibiotic prophylaxis, observing well children for signs and symptoms of disease and for decreasing opportunities for transmission of that may sustain an outbreak. Removal of children known or suspected of contributing to an outbreak may help to limit transmission of the disease by preventing the development of new cases of the disease (1).

TYPE OF FACILITY: Center; Large Family Child Care Home; Small Family Child Care Home

RELATED STANDARDS:

Standard 3.6.1.1: Inclusion/Exclusion/Dismissal of Children
Standard 3.6.1.2: Staff Exclusion for Illness
Standard 3.6.4.1: Procedure for Parent/Guardian Notification About Exposure of Children to Infectious Disease
Chapter 7: Infectious Diseases
Standard 9.2.4.4: Written Plan for Seasonal and Pandemic Influenza

REFERENCES:

1. Siegel, J. D., E. Rhinehart, M. Jackson, L. Chiarello, Healthcare Infection Control Practices Advisory Committee. 2007. 2007 guideline for isolation precautions: Preventing transmission of infectious agents in healthcare settings. http://www.cdc.gov/hicpac/pdf/isolation/Isolation2007.pdf.

STANDARD 3.6.1.5: Sharing of Personal Articles Prohibited

Combs, hairbrushes, toothbrushes, personal clothing, bedding, and towels should not be shared and should be labeled with the name of the child who uses these objects.

RATIONALE: Respiratory and gastrointestinal infections are common infectious diseases in child care. These diseases are transmitted by direct person-to-person contact or by sharing personal articles such as combs, brushes, towels, clothing, and bedding. Prohibiting the sharing of personal articles and providing space so that personal items may be stored separately helps prevent these diseases from spreading.

TYPE OF FACILITY: Center; Large Family Child Care Home; Small Family Child Care Home

RELATED STANDARDS:

Standard 5.5.0.1: Storage and Labeling of Personal Articles

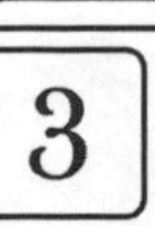

3.6.2 Caring for Children Who Are Ill

STANDARD 3.6.2.1: Exclusion and Alternative Care for Children Who Are Ill

At the discretion of the person authorized by the child care provider to make such decisions, children who are ill should be excluded from the child care facility for the conditions defined in Standard 3.6.1.1. When children are not permitted to receive care in their usual child care setting and cannot receive care from a parent/guardian or relative, they should be permitted to receive care in one of the following arrangements, if the arrangement meets the applicable standards:

a) Care in the child's usual facility in a special area for care of children who are ill;
b) Care in a separate small family child care home or center that serves only children with illness or temporary disabilities;
c) Care by a child care provider in the child's own home.

RATIONALE: Young children who are developing trust, autonomy, and initiative require the support of familiar caregivers and environments during times of illness to recover physically and avoid emotional distress (1). Young children enrolled in group care experience a higher incidence of mild illness (such as upper respiratory infections or otitis media) and other temporary disabilities (such as exacerbation of asthma) than those who have less interaction with other children. Sometimes, these illnesses preclude their participation in the usual child care activities. Most state regulations require that children with certain conditions be excluded from their usual care arrangement (2). To accommodate situations where parents/guardians cannot provide care for their own children who are ill, several types of alternative care arrangements have been established. The majority of viruses are spread by children who are asymptomatic, therefore, exposure of children to others with active symptoms or who have recently recovered, does not significantly raise the risk of transmission over the baseline (3).

TYPE OF FACILITY: Center; Large Family Child Care Home; Small Family Child Care Home

RELATED STANDARDS:
Standard 3.6.1.1: Inclusion/Exclusion/Dismissal of Children
Standards 3.6.2.2-3.6.2.10: Caring for Children Who are Ill

REFERENCES:
1. Crowley, A. 1994. Sick child care: A developmental perspective. *J Pediatric Health Care*. 8:261-67.
2. National Resource Center for Health and Safety in Child Care and Early Education. 2010. Individual states child care licensure regulations. http://nrckids.org/STATES/states.htm.
3. Aronson, S. S., T. R. Shope, eds. 2009. *Managing infectious diseases in child care and schools: A quick reference guide.* 2nd ed. Elk Grove Village, IL: American Academy of Pediatrics.

STANDARD 3.6.2.2: Space Requirements for Care of Children Who Are Ill

Environmental space utilized for the care of children who are ill with infectious diseases and cannot receive care in their usual child care group should meet all requirements for well children and include the following additional requirements:

a) If the program for children who are ill is in the same facility as the well-child program, well children should not use or share furniture, fixtures, equipment, or supplies designated for use with children who are ill unless it has been cleaned and sanitized before use by well children;
b) Indoor space that the facility uses for children who are ill, including hallways, bathrooms, and kitchens, should be separate from indoor space used with well children; this reduces the likelihood of mixing supplies, toys, and equipment. The facility may use a single kitchen for ill and well children if the kitchen is staffed by a cook who has no child care responsibilities other than food preparation and who does not handle soiled dishes and utensils until after food preparation and food service are completed for any meal;
c) Children whose symptoms indicate infections of the gastrointestinal tract (often with diarrhea) who receive care in special facilities for children who are ill should receive this care in a space separate from other children with other illnesses to reduce the likelihood of disease being transmitted between children by limiting child-to-child interaction, separating staff responsibilities, and not mixing supplies, toys, and equipment;
d) If the facility cares for children with chickenpox, these children require a room with separate ventilation with exhaust to, and air exchange with, the outside (3);
e) Each child care room should have a handwashing sink that can provide a steady stream of water, between 60°F and 120°F, at least for ten seconds. Soap and disposable paper towels should be available at the handwashing sink at all times. A hand sanitizing dispenser is an alternative to traditional handwashing;
f) Each room where children who wear diapers receive care should have its own diaper changing area adjacent to a handwashing sink and/or hand sanitizer dispenser.

RATIONALE: Transmission of infectious diseases in child care settings may be influenced by the design, construction, and maintenance of the physical environment (2). The population that uses centers should in time become less susceptible to chickenpox through immunization. Some children, however, are too young to be routinely immunized and may be susceptible; and, although universal immunization with varicella vaccine is recommended, full compliance with the recommendation has not been achieved.

Chickenpox is readily spread by airborne droplets (1) or direct contact.

Handwashing sinks should be stationed in each room, to promote hand hygiene and also to give the caregivers/teachers an opportunity for continuous supervision of the other children in care when washing their hands. The sink must deliver a consistent flow of water for ten seconds so that the user does not need to touch the faucet handles. Diaper changing areas should be adjacent to sinks to foster cleanliness and also to enable caregivers/teachers to provide continuous supervision of other children in care. The provision of alcohol-based hand sanitizing dispensers may be an alternative to traditional handwashing with soap and water.

COMMENTS: Some facilities have staffed "get well" rooms typically caring for fewer than six children who are ill.

TYPE OF FACILITY: Center; Large Family Child Care Home; Small Family Child Care Home

RELATED STANDARDS:
Chapter 7: Infectious Diseases

REFERENCES:

1. Pickering, L. K., C. J. Baker, D. W. Kimberlin, S. S. Long, eds. 2009. *Red book: 2009 report of the Committee on Infectious Diseases.* 28th ed. Elk Grove Village, IL: American Academy of Pediatrics.
2. Staes, C., S. Balk, K. Ford, R. J. Passantino, A. Torrice. 1994. Environmental factors to consider when designing and maintaining a child's day-care environment. *Pediatrics* 94:1048-50.
3. Aronson, S. S., T. R. Shope, eds. 2009. *Managing infectious diseases in child care and schools: A quick reference guide.* 2nd ed. Elk Grove Village, IL: American Academy of Pediatrics.

STANDARD 3.6.2.3: Qualifications of Directors of Facilities That Care for Children Who Are Ill

The director of a facility that cares for children who are ill should have the following minimum qualifications, in addition to the general qualifications described in Director's Qualifications, Standards 1.3.1.1 and 1.3.1.2:

a) At least forty hours of training in prevention and control of infectious diseases and care of children who are ill, including subjects listed in Standard 3.6.2.5;
b) At least two prior years of satisfactory performance as a director of a regular facility;
c) At least twelve credit hours of college-level training in child development or early childhood education.

RATIONALE: The director should be college-prepared in early childhood education and have taken college-level courses in illness prevention and control, since the director is the person responsible for establishing the facility's policies and procedures and for meeting the training needs of new staff members (1).

TYPE OF FACILITY: Center

RELATED STANDARDS:
Standards 1.3.1.1-1.3.1.2: Director's Qualifications
Standard 3.6.2.5: Caregiver/Teacher Qualifications for Facilities that Care for Children Who are Ill

REFERENCES:

1. Fiene, R. 2002. *13 indicators of quality child care: Research update.* Washington, DC: U.S. Department of Health and Human Services, Office of the Assistant Secretary for Planning and Evaluation. http://aspe.hhs.gov/hsp/ccquality-ind02/.

STANDARD 3.6.2.4: Program Requirements for Facilities That Care for Children Who Are Ill

Any facility that offers care for the child who is ill of any age should:

a) Provide a caregiver/teacher who is familiar to the child;
b) Provide care in a place with which the child is familiar and comfortable away from other children in care;
c) Involve a caregiver/teacher who has time to give individual care and emotional support, who knows of the child's interests, and who knows of activities that appeal to the level of child development age group and to a sick child;
d) Offer a program with trained personnel planned in consultation with qualified health care personnel and with ongoing medical direction.

RATIONALE: When children are ill, they are stressed by the illness itself. Unfamiliar places and caregivers/teachers add to the stress of illness when a child is sick. Since illness tends to promote regression and dependency, children who are ill need a person who knows and can respond to the child's cues appropriately.

COMMENTS: Because children are most comfortable in a familiar place with familiar people, the preferred arrangement for children who are ill will be the child's home or the child's regular child care arrangement, when the child care facility has the resources to adapt to the needs of such children.

TYPE OF FACILITY: Center; Large Family Child Care Home; Small Family Child Care Home

RELATED STANDARDS:
Standard 3.6.2.2: Space Requirements for Care of Children Who Are Ill
Standards 3.6.4.1-3.6.4.5: Reporting Illness and Death
Standard 10.5.0.1: State and Local Health Department Role

STANDARD 3.6.2.5: Caregiver/Teacher Qualifications for Facilities That Care for Children Who Are Ill

Each caregiver/teacher in a facility that cares for children who are ill should have at least two years of successful work experience as a caregiver/teacher in a regular well-child facility prior to employment in the special facility. In addition, facilities should document, for each caregiver/teacher, twenty hours of pre-service orientation training on care of children who are ill beyond the orientation training specified in Standards 1.4.2.1 through Standard 1.4.2.3. This training should include the following subjects:

a) Pediatric first aid and CPR, and first aid for choking;
b) General infection-control procedures, including:
    1) Hand hygiene;
    2) Handling of contaminated items;
    3) Use of sanitizing chemicals;
    4) Food handling;
    5) Washing and sanitizing of toys;
    6) Education about methods of disease transmission.

c) Care of children with common mild childhood illnesses, including:
   1) Recognition and documentation of signs and symptoms of illness including body temperature;
   2) Administration and recording of medications;
   3) Nutrition of children who are ill;
   4) Communication with parents/guardians of children who are ill;
   5) Knowledge of immunization requirements;
   6) Recognition of need for medical assistance and how to access;
   7) Knowledge of reporting requirements for infectious diseases;
   8) Emergency procedures.
d) Child development activities for children who are ill;
e) Orientation to the facility and its policies.

This training should be documented in the staff personnel files, and compliance with the content of training routinely evaluated. Based on these evaluations, the training on care of children who are ill should be updated with a minimum of six hours of annual training for individuals who continue to provide care to children who are ill.

RATIONALE: Because meeting the physical and psychological needs of children who are ill requires a higher level of skill and understanding than caring for well children, a commitment to children and an understanding of their general needs is essential (1). Work experience in child care facilities will help the caregiver/teacher develop these skills. States that have developed rules regulating facilities have recognized the need for training in illness prevention and control and management of medical emergencies. Staff members caring for children who are ill in special facilities or in a get well room in a regular center should meet the staff qualifications that are applied to child care facilities generally.

Caregivers/teachers have to be prepared for handling illness and must understand their scope of work. Special training is required of caregivers/teachers who work in special facilities for children who are ill because the director and the caregivers/teachers are dealing with infectious diseases and need to know how to prevent the spread of infection. Each caregiver/teacher should have training to decrease the risk of transmitting disease (1).

TYPE OF FACILITY: Center; Large Family Child Care Home; Small Family Child Care Home

RELATED STANDARDS:
Standards 1.4.2.1-1.4.2.3: Orientation Training
Standard 10.5.0.1: State and Local Health Department Role

REFERENCES:
1. Heymann, S. J., P. Hong Vo, C. A. Bergstrom. 2002. Child care providers' experiences caring for sick children: Implications for public policy. *Early Child Devel Care* 172:1-8.

STANDARD 3.6.2.6: Child-Staff Ratios for Facilities That Care for Children Who Are Ill

Each facility for children who are ill should maintain a child-to-staff ratio no greater than the following:

Age of Children	Child to Staff Ratio
3-35 months	3 children to 1 staff member
36-71 months	4 children to 1 staff member
72 months and older	6 children to 1 staff member

RATIONALE: Some states stipulate the ratios for caring for children who are ill in their regulations. The expert consensus is based on theories of child development including attachment theory and recognition of children's temporary emotional regression during times of illness (1-3); the lowest ratios used per age group seem appropriate.

COMMENTS: These ratios do not include other personnel, such as bus drivers, necessary for specialized functions such as transportation.

TYPE OF FACILITY: Center; Large Family Child Care Home; Small Family Child Care Home

REFERENCES:
1. Davies, D. 1999. *Child development: A practitioner's guide*. New York: The Guilford Press.
2. Schumacher, R. 2008. *Charting progress for babies in child care: CLASP center ratios and group sizes – Research based rationale.* http://www.clasp.org/admin/site/babies/make_the_case/files/cp_rationale6.pdf.
3. Crowley, A. A. 1994. Sick child care: A developmental perspective. *J Pediatric Health Care* 8:261-67.

STANDARD 3.6.2.7: Child Care Health Consultants for Facilities That Care for Children Who Are Ill

Each special facility that provides care for children who are ill should use the services of a child care health consultant for ongoing consultation on overall operation and development of written policies relating to health care. The child care health consultant should have the knowledge, skills and preparation as stated in Standard 1.6.0.1.

The facility should involve the child care health consultant in development and/or implementation, review, and sign-off of the written policies and procedures for managing specific illnesses. The facility staff and the child care health consultant should review and update the written policies annually.

The facility should assign the child care health consultant the responsibility for reviewing written policies and procedures for the following:

a) Admission and readmission after illness, including inclusion/exclusion criteria;
b) Health evaluation procedures on intake, including physical assessment of the child and other criteria used to determine the appropriateness of a child's attendance;
c) Plans for health care and for managing children with infectious diseases;

d) Plans for surveillance of illnesses that are admissible and problems that arise in the care of children with illness;
e) Plans for staff training and communication with parents/guardians and primary care providers;
f) Plans for injury prevention;
g) Situations that require medical care within an hour.

RATIONALE: Appropriate involvement of child care health consultants is especially important for facilities that care for children who are ill. Facilities should use the expertise of primary care providers to design and provide a child care environment with sufficient staff and facilities to meet the needs of children who are ill (2,3). The best interests of the child and family must be given primary consideration in the care of children who are ill. Consultation by primary care providers, especially those whose specialty is pediatrics, is critical in planning facilities for the care of children who are ill (1).

COMMENTS: Caregivers/teachers should seek the services of a child care health consultant through state and local professional organizations, such as:

a) Healthy Child Care Consultant Network Support Center (maintains a national registry of NTI-trained CCHCs);
b) Local chapters of the American Academy of Pediatrics (AAP);
c) Local Children's hospital;
d) American Nurses Association (ANA);
e) Visiting Nurse Association (VNA);
f) American Academy of Family Physicians (AAFP);
g) National Association of Pediatric Nurse Practitioners (NAPNAP);
h) National Association for the Education of Young Children (NAEYC);
i) National Association for Family Child Care (NAFCC);
j) National Association of School Nurses (NASN);
k) Emergency Medical Services for Children (EMSC) National Resource Center;
l) National Training Institute for Child Care Health Consultants (NTI);
m) State or local health department (especially public health nursing, infectious disease, and epidemiology departments).

TYPE OF FACILITY: Center; Large Family Child Care Home; Small Family Child Care Home

RELATED STANDARDS:

Standard 1.6.0.1: Child Care Health Consultants

REFERENCES:

1. Donowitz, L. G., ed. 1996. *Infection control in the child care center and preschool,* 18-19, 68. 2nd ed. Baltimore, MD: Williams and Wilkins.
2. Churchill, R. B., L. K. Pickering. 1997. Infection control challenges in child care centers. *Infect Dis Clin North Am* 11:347-65.
3. Crowley A. A. 2000. Child care health consultation: The Connecticut experience. *Matern Child Health J* 4:67-75.

STANDARD 3.6.2.8: Licensing of Facilities That Care for Children Who Are Ill

A facility may care for children with symptoms requiring exclusion provided that the licensing authority has given approval of the facility, written plans describing symptoms and conditions that are admissible, and procedures for daily care. In jurisdictions that lack regulations and licensing capacity for facilities that care for children who are ill, the child care health consultant with the local health authority should review these plans and procedures annually in an advisory capacity.

RATIONALE: Facilities for children who are ill generally are required to meet the licensing requirements that apply to all facilities of a specific type, for example, small or large family child care homes or centers. Additional requirements should apply when children who are ill will be in care.

This standard ensures that child care facilities are continually reviewed by an appropriate state authority and that facilities maintain appropriate standards in caring for children who are ill.

COMMENTS: If a child care health consultant is not available, than the local health authority should review plans and procedures annually.

TYPE OF FACILITY: Center; Large Family Child Care Home; Small Family Child Care Home

RELATED STANDARDS:

Standard 3.6.2.10: Inclusion and Exclusion of Children from Facilities that Serve Children Who Are Ill
Standard 10.2.0.1: Regulation of All Out-of-Home Child Care
Standard 10.3.1.1: Operation Permits

STANDARD 3.6.2.9: Information Required for Children Who Are Ill

For each day of care in a special facility that provides care for children who are ill, the caregiver/teacher should have the following information on each child:

a) The child's specific diagnosis and the individual providing the diagnosis (primary care provider, parent/guardian);
b) Current status of the illness, including potential for contagion, diet, activity level, and duration of illness;
c) Health care, diet, allergies (particularly to foods or medication), and medication and treatment plan, including appropriate release forms to obtain emergency health care and administer medication;
d) Communication with the parent/guardian on the child's progress;
e) Name, address, and telephone number of the child's source of primary health care;
f) Communication with the child's primary care provider.

Communication between parents/guardians, the child care program and the primary care provider (medical home) requires the free exchange of protected medical information (2). Confidentiality should be maintained at each step in compliance with any laws or regulations that are pertinent to all parties such as the Family Educational Rights and

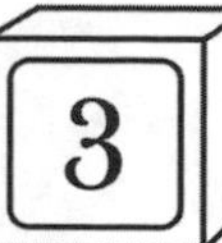

Privacy Act (commonly known as FERPA) and/or the Health Insurance Portability and Accountability Act (commonly known as HIPAA) (2).

RATIONALE: The caregiver/teacher must have child-specific information to provide optimum care for each child who is ill and to make appropriate decisions regarding whether to include or exclude a given child. The caregiver/teacher must have contact information for the child's source of primary health care or specialty health care (in the case of a child with asthma, diabetes, etc.) to assist with the management of any situation that arises.

COMMENTS: For school-age children, documentation of the care of the child during the illness should be provided to the parent to deliver to the school health program upon the child's return to school. Coordination with the child's source of health care and school health program facilitates the overall care of the child (1).

TYPE OF FACILITY: Center; Large Family Child Care Home; Small Family Child Care Home

REFERENCES:

1. Beierlein, J. G., J. E. Van Horn. 1995. Sick child care. National Network for Child Care. http://www.nncc.org/eo/emp.sick.child .care.html.

2. Donoghue, E. A., C. A. Kraft, eds. 2010. *Managing chronic health needs in child care and schools: A quick reference guide.* Elk Grove Village, IL: American Academy of Pediatrics.

STANDARD 3.6.2.10: Inclusion and Exclusion of Children from Facilities That Serve Children Who Are Ill

Facilities that care for children who are ill who have conditions that require additional attention from the caregiver/teacher, should arrange for or ask the child care health consultant to arrange for a clinical health evaluation, by a licensed primary care provider, for each child who is admitted to the facility. These facilities should include children with conditions listed in Standard 3.6.1.1 if their policies and plans address the management of these conditions, except for the following conditions which require exclusion from all types of child care facilities that are not medical care institutions (such as hospitals or skilled nursing facilities):

a) Fever (see COMMENTS section for definition of fever) and a stiff neck, lethargy, irritability, or persistent crying;
b) Diarrhea (loose stools, not contained in the diaper, that are two or more greater than normal frequency) and one or more of the following:
    1) Signs of dehydration, such as dry mouth, no tears, lethargy, sunken fontanelle (soft spot on the head);
    2) Blood or mucus in the stool until it is evaluated for organisms tha can cause dysentery;
    3) Diarrhea caused by *Salmonella*, *Campylobacter*, *Giardia*, *Shigella* or *E.coli* 0157:H7 until specific criteria for treatment and return to care are met.
c) Vomiting with signs of dehydration and inability to maintain hydration with oral intake;
d) Contagious stages of pertussis, measles, mumps, chickenpox, rubella, or diphtheria, unless the child is appropriately isolated from children with other illnesses and cared for only with children having the same illness;
e) Untreated infestation of scabies or head lice;
f) Untreated infectious tuberculosis;
g) Undiagnosed rash WITH fever or behavior change;
h) Abdominal pain that is intermittent or persistent and is accompanied by fever, diarrhea, or vomiting;
i) Difficulty in breathing;
j) An acute change in behavior;
k) Undiagnosed jaundice (yellow skin and whites of eyes);
l) Other conditions as may be determined by the director or child care health consultant;
m) Upper or lower respiratory infection in which signs or symptoms require a higher level of care than can be appropriately provided.

RATIONALE: These signs and symptoms may indicate a significant systemic infection that requires professional medical management and parental care (1). Diarrheal illnesses that require an intensity of care that cannot be provided appropriately by a caregiver/teacher could result in temporary exclusion.

COMMENTS: Fever is defined as a temperature above 101°F (38.3°C) orally, above 102°F (38.9°C) rectally, or 100°F (37.8°C) or higher taken axillary (armpit) or measured by an equivalent method.

TYPE OF FACILITY: Center; Large Family Child Care Home; Small Family Child Care Home

RELATED STANDARDS:

Standard 1.6.0.1: Child Care Health Consultants
Standard 3.6.1.1: Inclusion/Exclusion/Dismissal of Children
Standard 3.6.1.4: Infectious Disease Outbreak Control
Chapter 7: Infectious Diseases

REFERENCES:

1. Pickering, L. K., C. J. Baker, D. W. Kimberlin, S. S. Long, eds. 2009. *Red book: 2009 report of the Committee on Infectious Diseases.* 28th ed. Elk Grove Village, IL: American Academy of Pediatrics.

3.6.3 Medications

STANDARD 3.6.3.1: Medication Administration

The administration of medicines at the facility should be limited to:

a) Prescription or non-prescription medication (over-the-counter [OTC]) ordered by the prescribing health professional for a specific child with written permission of the parent/guardian. Written orders from the prescribing health professional should specify medical need, medication, dosage, and length of time to give medication;
b) Labeled medications brought to the child care facility by the parent/guardian in the original container (with a label that includes the child's name, date filled,

prescribing clinician's name, pharmacy name and phone number, dosage/instructions, and relevant warnings).

Facilities should not administer folk or homemade remedy medications or treatment. Facilities should not administer a medication that is prescribed for one child in the family to another child in the family.

No prescription or non-prescription medication (OTC) should be given to any child without written orders from a prescribing health professional and written permission from a parent/guardian. Exception: Non-prescription sunscreen and insect repellent always require parental consent but do not require instructions from each child's prescribing health professional.

Documentation that the medicine/agent is administered to the child as prescribed is required.

"Standing orders" guidance should include directions for facilities to be equipped, staffed, and monitored by the primary care provider capable of having the special health care plan modified as needed. Standing orders for medication should only be allowed for individual children with a documented medical need if a special care plan is provided by the child's primary care provider in conjunction with the standing order or for OTC medications for which a primary care provider has provided specific instructions that define the children, conditions and methods for administration of the medication. Signatures from the primary care provider and one of the child's parents/guardians must be obtained on the special care plan. Care plans should be updated as needed, but at least yearly.

RATIONALE: Medicines can be crucial to the health and wellness of children. They can also be very dangerous if the wrong type or wrong amount is given to the wrong person or at the wrong time. Prevention is the key to prevent poisonings by making sure medications are inaccessible to children.

All medicines require clear, accurate instruction and medical confirmation of the need for the medication to be given while the child is in the facility. Prescription medications can often be timed to be given at home and this should be encouraged. Because of the potential for errors in medication administration in child care facilities, it may be safer for a parent/guardian to administer their child's medicine at home.

Over the counter medications, such as acetaminophen and ibuprofen, can be just as dangerous as prescription medications and can result in illness or even death when these products are misused or unintentional poisoning occurs. Many children's over the counter medications contain a combination of ingredients. It is important to make sure the child isn't receiving the same medications in two different products which may result in an overdose. Facilities should not stock OTC medications (1).

Cough and cold medications are widely used for children to treat upper respiratory infections and allergy symptoms. Recently, concern has been raised that there is no proven benefit and some of these products may be dangerous (2,3,5). Leading organizations such as the Consumer Healthcare Products Association (CHPA) and the American Academy of Pediatrics (AAP) have recommended restrictions on these products for children under age six (4-7).

If a medication mistake or unintentional poisoning does occur, call your local poison center immediately at 1-800-222-1222.

Parents/guardians should always be notified in every instance when medication is used. Telephone instructions from a primary care provider are acceptable if the caregiver/teacher fully documents them and if the parent/guardian initiates the request for primary care provider or child care health consultant instruction. In the event medication for a child becomes necessary during the day or in the event of an emergency, administration instructions from a parent/guardian and the child's prescribing health professional are required before a caregiver/teacher may administer medication.

TYPE OF FACILITY: Center; Large Family Child Care Home; Small Family Child Care Home

RELATED STANDARDS:

Standard 3.4.5.1: Sun Safety Including Sunscreen
Standard 3.4.5.2: Insect Repellent and Protection from Vector-Borne Diseases
Standard 3.6.2.9: Information Required For Children Who Are Ill
Standard 3.6.3.1: Medication Administration
Standard 3.6.3.2: Labeling, Storage, and Disposal of Medication

REFERENCES:

1. American Academy of Pediatrics, Committee on Drugs. 2009. Policy statement: Acetaminophen toxicity in children. *Pediatrics* 123:1421-22.
2. Schaefer, M. K., N. Shehab, A. Cohen, D. S. Budnitz. 2008. Adverse events from cough and cold medications in children. *Pediatrics* 121:783-87.
3. Centers for Disease Control and Prevention. 2007. Infant deaths associated with cough and cold medications: Two states. *MMWR* 56:1-4.
4. Consumer Healthcare Products Association. Makers of OTC cough and cold medicines announce voluntary withdrawal of oral infant medicines. http://www.chpa-info.org/10_11_07_OralInfantMedicines.aspx.
5. U.S. Department of Health and Human Services, Food and Drug Administration. 2008. *Public Health advisory: FDA recommends that over-the-counter (OTC) cough and cold products not be used for infants and children under 2 years of age.* http://www.fda.gov/Drugs/DrugSafety/PostmarketDrugSafetyInformationforPatientsandProviders/DrugSafetyInformationforHeathcareProfessionals/PublicHealthAdvisories/ucm051137.htm.
6. Vernacchio, L., J. Kelly, D. Kaufman, A. Mitchell. 2008. Cough and cold medication use by U.S. children, 1999-2006: Results from the Slone Survey. *Pediatrics* 122: e323-29.
7. American Academy of Pediatrics. 2008. *AAP Urges caution in use of over-the-counter cough and cold medicines.* http://www.aap.org/advocacy/releases/jan08coughandcold.htm.

STANDARD 3.6.3.2: Labeling, Storage, and Disposal of Medications

Any prescription medication should be dated and kept in the original container. The container should be labeled by a pharmacist with:

- The child's first and last names;
- The date the prescription was filled;
- The name of the prescribing health professional who wrote the prescription, the medication's expiration date;
- The manufacturer's instructions or prescription label with specific, legible instructions for administration, storage, and disposal;
- The name and strength of the medication.

Over-the-counter medications should be kept in the original container as sold by the manufacturer, labeled by the parent/guardian, with the child's name and specific instructions given by the child's prescribing health professional for administration.

All medications, refrigerated or unrefrigerated, should:

- Have child-resistant caps;
- Be kept in an organized fashion;
- Be stored away from food;
- Be stored at the proper temperature;
- Be completely inaccessible to children.

Medication should not be used beyond the date of expiration. Unused medications should be returned to the parent/guardian for disposal. In the event medication cannot be returned to the parent or guardian, it should be disposed of according to the recommendations of the US Food and Drug Administration (FDA) (1). Documentation should be kept with the child care facility of all disposed medications. The current guidelines are as follows:

a) If a medication lists any specific instructions on how to dispose of it, follow those directions.
b) If there are community drug take back programs, participate in those.
c) Remove medications from their original containers and put them in a sealable bag. Mix medications with an undesirable substance such as used coffee grounds or kitty litter. Throw the mixture into the regular trash. Make sure children do not have access to the trash (1).

RATIONALE: Child-resistant safety packaging has been shown to significantly decrease poison exposure incidents in young children (1).

Proper disposal of medications is important to help ensure a healthy environment for children in our communities. There is growing evidence that throwing out or flushing medications into our sewer systems may have harmful effects on the environment (1-3).

COMMENTS: A small lock box can be kept in the refrigerator to hold medications. Programs may also consult with their local pharmacy regarding disposal. For more information on medication take back programs see Teleosis Institute at http://www.teleosis.org/gpp-national.php.

TYPE OF FACILITY: Center; Large Family Child Care Home; Small Family Child Care Home

REFERENCES:

1. U.S. Food and Drug Administration. 2010. Disposal by flushing of certain unused medicines: What you should know. http://www.fda.gov/Drugs/ResourcesForYou/Consumers/BuyingUsingMedicineSafely/EnsuringSafeUseofMedicine/SafeDisposalofMedicines/ucm186187.htm.
2. U.S. Environmental Protection Agency. 2009. Pharmaceuticals and personal care products as pollutants (PPCPs). http://www.epa.gov/ppcp/.
3. Fiene, R. 2002. *13 indicators of quality child care: Research update.* Washington, DC: U.S. Department of Health and Human Services, Office of the Assistant Secretary for Planning and Evaluation. http://aspe.hhs.gov/hsp/ccquality-ind02/.

STANDARD 3.6.3.3: Training of Caregivers/Teachers to Administer Medication

Any caregiver/teacher who administers medication should complete a standardized training course that includes skill and competency assessment in medication administration. The trainer in medication administration should be a licensed health professional. The course should be repeated according to state and/or local regulation. At a minimum, skill and competency should be monitored annually or whenever medication administration error occurs. In facilities with large numbers of children with special health care needs involving daily medication, best practice would indicate strong consideration to the hiring of a licensed health care professional. Lacking that, caregivers/teachers should be trained to:

a) Check that the name of the child on the medication and the child receiving the medication are the same;
b) Check that the name of the medication is the same as the name of the medication on the instructions to give the medication if the instructions are not on the medication container that is labeled with the child's name;
c) Read and understand the label/prescription directions or the separate written instructions in relation to the measured dose, frequency, route of administration (ex. by mouth, ear canal, eye, etc.) and other special instructions relative to the medication;
d) Observe and report any side effects from medications;
e) Document the administration of each dose by the time and the amount given;
f) Document the person giving the administration and any side effects noted;
g) Handle and store all medications according to label instructions and regulations.

The trainer in medication administration should be a licensed health professional: Registered Nurse, Advanced Practice Registered Nurse (APRN), MD, Physician's Assistant, or Pharmacist.

RATIONALE: Administration of medicines is unavoidable as increasing numbers of children entering child care take medications. National data indicate that at any one time, a significant portion of the pediatric population is taking medication, mostly vitamins, but between 16% and 40% are taking antipyretics/analgesics (5). Safe medication administration in child care is extremely important and training of caregivers/teachers is essential (1).

Caregivers/teachers need to know what medication the child is receiving, who prescribed the medicine and when, for what purpose the medicine has been prescribed and what the known reactions or side effects may be if a child has a negative reaction to the medicine (2,3). A child's reaction to medication can be occasionally extreme enough to initiate the protocol developed for emergencies. The medication record is especially important if medications are frequently prescribed or if long-term medications are being used (4).

COMMENTS: Caregivers/teachers need to know the state laws and regulations on training requirements for the administration of medications in out-of-home child care settings. These laws may include requirements for delegation of medication administration from a primary care provider. Training on medication administration for caregivers/teachers is available in several states. *Model Child Care Health Policies, 2nd Ed.* from Healthy Child Care Pennsylvania is available at http://www.ecels-healthychildcarepa.org/content/MHP4thEd Total.pdf, and contains sample polices and forms related to medication administration.

TYPE OF FACILITY: Center; Large Family Child Care Home; Small Family Child Care Home

RELATED STANDARDS:
Standard 3.6.3.1: Medication Administration
Standard 3.6.3.2: Labeling, Storage, and Disposal of Medications
Standard 9.2.3.9: Written Policy on Use of Medications
Appendix O: Care Plan for Children with Special Health Care Needs
Appendix AA: Medication Administration Packet

REFERENCES:
1. Heschel, R. T., A. A. Crowley, S. S. Cohen. 2005. State policies regarding nursing delegation and administration in child care settings: A case study. *Policy, Politics, and Nursing Practice* 6:86-98.
2. Qualistar Early Learning. 2008. Colorado Medication Administration Curriculum. 5th ed. http://www.qualistar.org/medication-administration.html.
3. Fiene, R. 2002. *13 indicators of quality child care: Research update*. Washington, DC: US Department of Health and Human Services, Office of the Assistant Secretary for Planning and Evaluation. http://aspe.hhs.gov/hsp/ccquality-ind02/.
4. Calder, J. 2004. Medication administration in child care programs. *Health and Safety Notes.* Berkeley, CA: California Childcare Health Program. http://www.ucsfchildcarehealth.org/pdfs/healthandsafety/medadminEN102004_adr.pdf.
5. Vernacchio, L., J. P. Kelly, D. W. Kaufman, A. A. Mitchell. 2009. Medication use among children <12 years of age in the United States: Results from the Slone Survey. *Pediatrics* 124:446-54.

3.6.4 Reporting Illness and Death

STANDARD 3.6.4.1: Procedure for Parent/Guardian Notification About Exposure of Children to Infectious Disease

Caregivers/teachers should work collaboratively with local and state health authorities to notify parents/guardians about potential or confirmed exposures of their child to a infectious disease. Notification should include the following information:

a) The names, both the common and the medical name, of the diagnosed disease to which the child was exposed, whether there is one case or an outbreak, and the nature of the exposure (such as a child or staff member in a shared room or facility);
b) Signs and symptoms of the disease for which the parent/guardian should observe;
c) Mode of transmission of the disease;
d) Period of communicability and how long to watch for signs and symptoms of the disease;
e) Disease-prevention measures recommended by the health department (if appropriate);
f) Control measures implemented at the facility;
g) Pictures of skin lesions or skin condition may be helpful to parents/guardians (i.e., chicken pox, spots on tonsils, etc.)

The notice should not identify the child who has the infectious disease.

RATIONALE: Effective control and prevention of infectious diseases in child care depends on affirmative relationships between parents/guardians, caregivers/teachers, public health authorities, and primary care providers.

COMMENTS: The child care health consultant can locate appropriate photographs of conditions for parent/guardian information use. Resources for fact sheets and photographs include: *Managing Infectious Diseases in Child Care and Schools, 2nd Edition* (1) and the Centers for Disease Control and Prevention Website on conditions and diseases at http://www.cdc.gov/DiseasesConditions/. For a sample letter to parents notifying them of illness of their child or other enrolled children, see Healthy Young Children, available from the National Association for the Education of Young Children (NAEYC) at http://www.naeyc.org.

TYPE OF FACILITY: Center; Large Family Child Care Home; Small Family Child Care Home

RELATED STANDARDS:
Standard 3.6.1.4: Infectious Disease Outbreak Control
Chapter 7: Infectious Diseases
Appendix A: Signs and Symptoms Chart

REFERENCES:
1. Aronson, S. S., T. R. Shope, eds. 2009. *Managing infectious diseases in child care and schools: A quick reference guide.* 2nd ed. Elk Grove Village, IL: American Academy of Pediatrics.

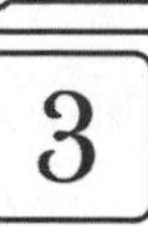

STANDARD 3.6.4.2: Infectious Diseases That Require Parent/Guardian Notification

In cooperation with the child care regulatory authority and health department, the facility or the health department should inform parents/guardians if their child may have been exposed to the following diseases or conditions while attending the child care program, while retaining the confidentiality of the child who has the infectious disease:

a) *Neisseria meningitidis* (meningitis);
b) Pertussis;
c) Invasive infections;
d) Varicella-zoster (Chickenpox) virus;
e) Skin infections or infestations (head lice, scabies, and ringworm);
f) Infections of the gastrointestinal tract (often with diarrhea) and hepatitis A virus (HAV);
g) *Haemophilus influenzae* type B (Hib);
h) Parvovirus B19 (fifth disease);
i) Measles;
j) Tuberculosis;
k) Two or more affected unrelated persons affiliated with the facility with a vaccine-preventable or infectious disease.

RATIONALE: Early identification and treatment of infectious diseases are important in minimizing associated morbidity and mortality as well as further reducing transmission (1). Notification of parents/guardians will permit them to discuss with their child's primary care provider the implications of the exposure and to closely observe their child for early signs and symptoms of illness.

TYPE OF FACILITY: Center; Large Family Child Care Home; Small Family Child Care Home

RELATED STANDARDS:
Standard 3.6.1.4: Infectious Disease Outbreak Control
Chapter 7: Infectious Diseases

REFERENCES:
1. Aronson, S. S., T. R. Shope, eds. 2009. *Managing infectious diseases in child care and schools: A quick reference guide.* 2nd ed. Elk Grove Village, IL: American Academy of Pediatrics.

STANDARD 3.6.4.3: Notification of the Facility About Infectious Disease or Other Problems by Parents

Upon registration of each child, the facility should inform parents/guardians that they must notify the facility within twenty-four hours after their child or any member of the immediate household has developed a known or suspected infectious or vaccine-preventable disease (1). When a child has a disease that may require exclusion, the parents/guardians should inform the facility of the diagnosis.

The facility should encourage parents/guardians to inform the caregivers/teachers of any other problems which may affect the child's behavior.

RATIONALE: This requirement will facilitate prompt reporting of disease and enable the caregiver/teacher to provide better care. Disease surveillance and reporting to local health authorities is crucial to preventing and controlling diseases in the child care setting. The major purpose of surveillance is to allow early detection of disease and prompt implementation of control measures. If it is known that the child attends another center or facility, all facilities should be informed (for example, if the child attends a Head Start program and a child care program that are separate–then both need to be notified and the notification of local health authority should name both facilities).

Ascertaining whether a child who is ill is attending a facility is important when evaluating childhood illnesses. Ascertaining whether an adult with illness is working in a facility or is a parent/guardian of a child attending a facility is important when considering infectious diseases that are more commonly manifest in adults. Cases of illness in family member such as infections of the gastrointestinal tract (with diarrhea), or infections of the liver may necessitate questioning about possible illness in the child attending child care. Information concerning infectious disease in a child care attendee, staff member, or household contact should be communicated to public health authorities, to the child care director, and to the child's parents/guardians.

TYPE OF FACILITY: Center; Large Family Child Care Home; Small Family Child Care Home

RELATED STANDARDS:
Standard 3.6.1.1: Inclusion/Exclusion/Dismissal of Children

REFERENCES:
1. Aronson, S. S., T. R. Shope, eds. 2009. *Managing infectious diseases in child care and schools: A quick reference guide.* 2nd ed. Elk Grove Village, IL: American Academy of Pediatrics.

STANDARD 3.6.4.4: List of Excludable and Reportable Conditions for Parents

The facility should give to each parent/guardian a written list of conditions for which exclusion and dismissal may be indicated (2).

For the following symptoms, the caregiver/teacher should ask parents to have the child evaluated by a primary care provider. The advice of the primary care provider should be documented for the caregiver/teacher in the following situations:

a) The child has any of the following conditions: fever, lethargy, irritability, persistent crying, difficult breathing, or other manifestations of possible severe illness;
b) The child has a rash with fever and behavioral change;
c) The child has tuberculosis that has not been evaluated;
d) The child has scabies;
e) The child has a persistent cough with inability to practice respiratory etiquette.

The facility should have a list of reportable diseases provided by the health department and should provide a copy to each parent/guardian.

RATIONALE: Vomiting with symptoms such as lethargy and/or dry skin or mucous membranes or reduced urine output may indicate dehydration, and the child should be medically evaluated. Diarrhea with fever or other symptoms usually indicates infection. Blood and/or mucus may indicate shigellosis or infection with *E. coli* 0157:H7, which should be evaluated. Effective control and prevention of infectious diseases in child care depend on affirmative relationships between parents, caregivers, health departments, and primary care providers (1).

COMMENTS: If there is more than one case of vomiting in the facility, it may indicate either contagious illness or food poisoning.

If a child with abdominal pain is drowsy, irritable, and unhappy, has no appetite, and is unwilling to participate in usual activities, the child should be seen by that child's primary care provider. Abdominal pain may be associated with viral, bacterial, or parasitic gastrointestinal tract illness, which is contagious, or with food poisoning. It also may be a manifestation of another disease or illness such as kidney disease. If the pain is severe or persistent, the child should be referred for medical consultation (by telephone, if necessary).

If the caregiver/teacher is unable to contact the parent/guardian, medical advice should be sought until the parents can be located.

The facility should post the health department's list of infectious diseases as a reference. The facility should inform parents/guardians that the program is required to report infectious diseases to the health department.

For information on assisting families in finding a medical home or primary care provider, consult the local chapter of the American Academy of Pediatrics (AAP), the facility's child care health consultant, Nurse Practitioner Central (3), the local public health department, or the American Academy of Family Physicians (AAFP). For more information, see also the AAP *Managing Infectious Diseases in Child Care and Schools, 2nd ed.*, available at http://www.aap.org.

TYPE OF FACILITY: Center; Large Family Child Care Home; Small Family Child Care Home

RELATED STANDARDS:

Standard 3.6.1.1: Inclusion/Exclusion/Dismissal of Children
Chapter 7: Infectious Diseases
Appendix P: Situations that Require Medical Attention Right Away

REFERENCES:

1. Pickering, L. K., C. J. Baker, D. W. Kimberlin, S. S. Long. 2009. *Red book: 2009 report of the Committee on Infectious Diseases.* 28th ed. Elk Grove Village, IL: American Academy of Pediatrics.
2. Donowitz, L. G., ed. 1996. *Infection control in the child care center and preschool,* 18-19, 68. 2nd ed. Baltimore, MD: Williams and Wilkins.
3. Nurse Practitioner Central. 2003. National nurse practitioner directory. http://www.npclinics.com.

STANDARD 3.6.4.5: Death

Each facility should have a plan in place for responding to any death relevant to children enrolled in the facility and their families. The plan should describe protocols the program will follow and resources available for children, families, and staff.

If a facility experiences the death of a child or adult, the following should be done:

a) If a child or adult dies while at the facility:
   1) The caregiver/teacher(s) responsible for any children who observed or were in the same room where the death occurred, should take the children to a different room, while other staff tend to appropriate response/follow-up. Minimal explanations should be provided until direction is received from the proper authorities. Supportive and reassuring comments should be provided to children directly affected;
   2) Designated staff should:
      i) Immediately notify emergency medical personnel;
      ii) Immediately notify the child's parents/guardians or adult's emergency contact;
      iii) Notify the Licensing agency and law enforcement the same day the death occurs;
      iv) Follow all law enforcement protocols regarding the scene of the death:
         a. Do not disturb the scene;
         b. Do not show the scene to others;
         c. Reserve conversation about the event until having completed all interviews with law enforcement.
      v) Provide age-appropriate information for children, parents/guardians and staff;
      vi) Make resources for support available to staff, parents and children;

b) For a suspected Sudden Infant Death Syndrome (SIDS) death or other unexplained deaths:
   1) Seek support and information from local, state, or national SIDS resources;
   2) Provide SIDS information to the parents/guardians of the other children in the facility;
   3) Provide age-appropriate information to the other children in the facility;
   4) Provide appropriate information for staff at the facility;

c) If a child or adult known to the children enrolled in the facility dies while not at the facility:
   1) Provide age-appropriate information for children, parents/guardians and staff;
   2) Make resources for support available to staff, parents and children.

Facilities may release specific information about the circumstances of the child or adult's death that the authorities and the deceased member's family agrees the facility may share.

If the death is due to suspected child maltreatment, the caregiver/teacher is mandated to report this to child protective services.

Depending on the cause of death (SIDS, suffocation or other infant death, injury, maltreatment etc.), there may be a need for updated education on the subject for caregivers/teachers and/or children as well as implementation of improved health and safety practices.

RATIONALE: Following the steps described in this standard would constitute prudent action (1-3). Accurate information given to parents/guardians and children will help them understand the event and facilitate their support of the caregiver/teacher (4-7).

COMMENTS: It is important that caregivers/teachers are knowledgeable about SIDS and that they take proper steps so that they are not falsely accused of child abuse and neglect. The licensing agency and/or a SIDS agency support group (e.g., CJ Foundation for SIDS at http://www.cjsids.org, the National Sudden and Unexpected Infant/Child Death and Pregnancy Loss Resource Center at http://www.sidscenter.org, and First Candle at http://www.firstcandle.org) can offer support and counseling to caregivers/teachers.

TYPE OF FACILITY: Center; Large Family Child Care Home; Small Family Child Care Home

RELATED STANDARDS:
Standard 3.1.4.1: Safe Sleep Practices and SIDS/Suffocation Risk Reduction
Standards 3.4.4.1-3.4.4.5: Child Abuse and Neglect

REFERENCES:
1. Moon, R. Y., K. M. Patel, S. J. M. Shaefer. 2000. Sudden infant death syndrome in child care settings. *Pediatrics* 106:295-300.
2. Moon, R. Y., T. Calabrese, L. Aird. 2008. Reducing the risk of sudden infant death syndrome in child care and changing provider practices: Lessons learned from a demonstration project. *Pediatrics* 122:788-98.
3. Moon, R. Y., L. Kotch, L. Aird. 2006. State child care regulations regarding infant sleep environment since the Healthy Child Care America – Back to Sleep Campaign. *Pediatrics* 118:73-83.
4. Boston Medical Center. Good grief program. http://www.bmc.org/pediatrics-goodgrief.htm.
5. Rivlin, D. The good grief program of Boston Medical Center: What do children need? Boston Medical Center. http://www.wayland.k12.ma.us/claypit_hill/GoodGriefHandout.pdf.
6. Trozzi, M. 1999. Talking with children about Loss: Words, strategies, and wisdom to help children cope with death, divorce, and other difficult times. New York: Berkley Publishing Group.
7. Knapp, J., D. Mulligan-Smith, Committee on Pediatric Emergency Medicine. 2005. Death of a child in the emergency department. *Pediatrics* 115:1432-37.

Chapter 4

4

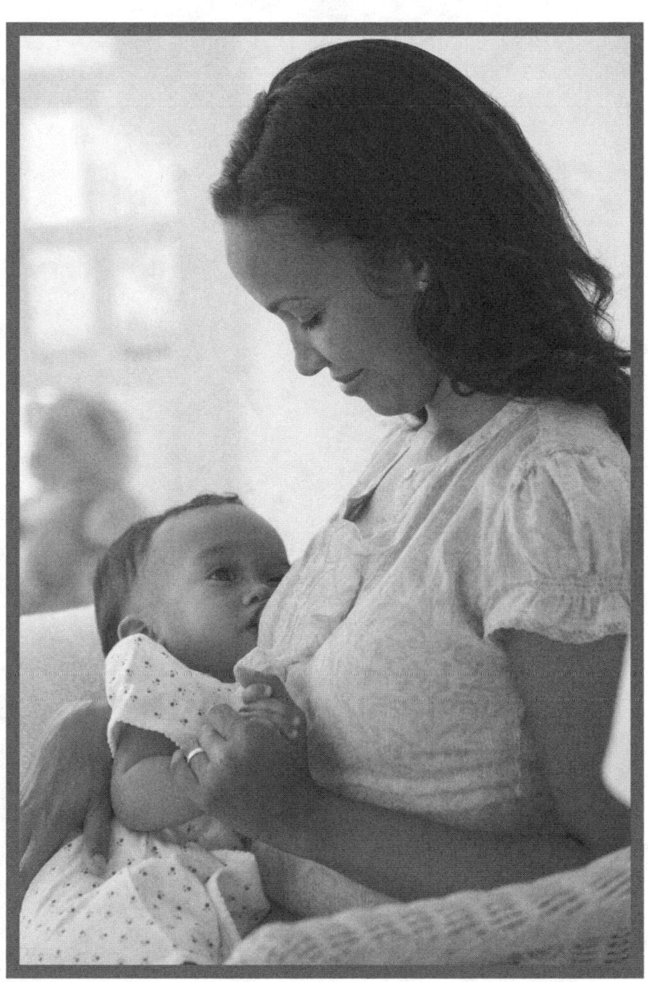

Nutrition and Food Service

4.1 Introduction

One of the basic responsibilities of every parent/guardian and caregiver/teacher is to provide nourishing food daily that is clean, safe, and developmentally appropriate for children. Food is essential in any early care and education setting to keep infants and children free from hunger. Children also need freely available, clean drinking water. Feeding should occur in a relaxed and pleasant environment that fosters healthy digestion and positive social behavior. Food provides energy and nutrients needed by infants and children during the critical period of their growth and development.

Feeding nutritious food everyday must be accompanied by offering appropriate daily physical activity and play time for the healthy physical, social, and emotional development of infants and young children. There is solid evidence that physical activity can prevent a rapid gain in weight which leads to childhood obesity early in life. The early care and education setting is an ideal environment to foster the goal of providing supervised, age-appropriate physical activity during the critical years of growth when health habits and patterns are being developed for life. The overall benefits of practicing healthy eating patterns, while being physically active daily are significant. Physical, social, and emotional habits are developed during the early years and continue into adulthood; thus these habits can be improved in early childhood to prevent and reduce obesity and a range of chronic diseases. Active play and supervised structured physical activities promote healthy weight, improved overall fitness, including mental health, improved bone development, cardiovascular health, and development of social skills. The physical activity standards outline the blueprint for practical methods of achieving the goal of promoting healthy bodies and minds of young children.

Breastfeeding sets the stage for an infant to establish healthy attachment. The American Academy of Pediatrics, the United States Breastfeeding Committee, the Academy of Breastfeeding Medicine, the American Academy of Family Physicians, the World Health Organization, and the United Nations Children's Fund (UNICEF) all recommend that women should breastfeed exclusively for about the first six months of the infant's life, adding age-appropriate solid foods (complementary foods) and continuing breastfeeding for at least the first year if not longer.

Human milk, containing all the nutrients to promote optimal growth, is the most developmentally appropriate food for infants. It changes during the course of each feeding and over time to meet the growing child's changing nutritional needs. All caregivers/teachers should be trained to encourage, support, and advocate for breastfeeding. Caregivers/teachers have a unique opportunity to support breastfeeding mothers, who are often daunted by the prospect of continuing to breastfeed as they return to work. Early care and education programs can reduce a breastfeeding mother's anxiety by welcoming breastfeeding families and providing a staff that is well-trained in the proper handling of human milk and feeding of breastfed infants.

Mothers who formula feed can also establish healthy attachment. A mother may choose not to breastfeed her infant for reasons that may include: human milk is not available, there is a real or perceived inadequate supply of human milk, her infant fails to gain weight, there is an existing medical condition for which human milk is contraindicated, or a mother desires not to breastfeed. Today there is a range of infant formulas on the market that vary in nutrient content and address specific needs of individual infants. A primary care provider should prescribe the specific infant formula to be used to meet the nutritional requirements of an individual infant. When infant formula is used to supplement an infant being breastfed, the mother should be encouraged to continue to breastfeed or to pump human milk since her milk supply will decrease if her milk production isn't stimulated by breastfeeding or pumping.

Given adequate opportunity, assistance, and age-appropriate equipment, children learn to self-feed as age-appropriate solid foods are introduced. Equally important to self-feeding is children's attainment of normal physical growth, motor coordination, and cognitive and social skills. Modeling of healthy eating behavior by early care and education staff helps a child to develop lifelong healthy eating habits. This period, beginning at six months of age, is an opportune time for children to learn more about the world around them by expressing their independence. Children pick and choose from different kinds and combinations of foods offered. To ensure programs are offering a variety of foods, selections should be made from these groups of food:

a) Grains – especially whole grains;

b) Vegetables – dark, green leafy and deep yellow;

c) Fruits – deep orange, yellow, and red whole fruits, 100% fruit juices limited to no more than four to six ounces per day for children one year of age and over;

d) Milk – whole milk, or reduced fat (2%) milk for children at risk for obesity or hypercholesterolemia, for children from one year of age up to two years of age; skim or 1% for children two years or older, unsweetened low-fat yogurt or low-fat cheese (e.g. cottage, farmer's);

e) Meats and Beans – baked or broiled chicken, fish, lean meats, dried peas and beans; and

f) Oils – vegetable.

Current research supports a diet based on a variety of nutrient dense foods which provide substantial amounts of essential nutrients – protein, carbohydrates, oils, and vitamins and minerals – with appropriate calories to meet the child's needs. For children, the availability of a variety of clean, safe, nourishing foods is essential during a period of rapid growth and development. The nutrition and food service standards, along with related appendices, address age-appropriate foods and feeding techniques beginning

with the very first food, preferably human milk and when not possible, infant formula based on the recommendation of the infant's primary care provider and family. As part of their developing growth and maturity, toddlers often exhibit changed eating habits compared to when they were infants. One may indulge in eating sprees, wanting to eat the same food for several days. Another may become a picky eater, picking or dawdling over food, or refusing to eat a certain food because it is new and unfamiliar with a new taste, color, odor, or texture. If these or other food behaviors persist, parents/guardians, caregivers/teachers, and the primary care provider together should determine the reason(s) and come up with a plan to address the issue. The consistency of the plan is important in helping a child to build sound eating habits during a time when they are focused on developing as an individual and often have erratic, unpredictable appetites. Family homes and center-based out-of-home early care and education settings have the opportunity to guide and support children's sound eating habits and food learning experiences (1-3).

Early food and eating experiences form the foundation of attitudes about food, eating behavior, and consequently, food habits. Responsive feeding, where the parents/guardians or caregivers/teachers recognize and respond to infant and child cues, helps foster trust and reduces overfeeding. Sound food habits are built on eating and enjoying a variety of healthful foods. Including culturally specific family foods is a dietary goal for feeding infants and young children. Current research documents that a balanced diet, combined with daily and routine age-appropriate physical activity, can reduce diet-related risks of overweight, obesity, and chronic disease later in life (1). Two essentials – eating healthy foods and engaging in physical activity on a daily basis – promote a healthy beginning during the early years and throughout the life span. *2010 Dietary Guidelines for Americans* and the U.S. Department of Agriculture's ChooseMyPlate.gov are designed to support lifestyle behaviors that promote health, including a diet composed of a variety of healthy foods and physical activity at two years of age and older (1-2,4-7).

TYPE OF FACILITY: Center; Large Family Child Care Home; Small Family Child Care Home

REFERENCES:

1. U.S. Department of Health and Human Services, U.S. Department of Agriculture. 2010. *Dietary guidelines for Americans, 2010*. 7th ed. Washington, DC: U.S. Government Printing Office. http://www.health.gov/dietaryguidelines/dga2010/DietaryGuidelines2010.pdf
2. U.S. Department of Agriculture. 2011. *MyPlate*. http://www.choosemyplate.gov.
3. Zero to Three. 2007. *Healthy from the start—How feeding nurtures your young child's body, heart, and mind*. Washington, DC: Zero to Three.
4. Pipes, P. L., C. M. Trahms, eds. 1997. *Nutrition in infancy and childhood*. 6th ed. New York: McGraw-Hill.
5. Marotz, L. R. 2008. *Health, safety, and nutrition for the young child*. 7th ed. Clifton Park, NY: Delmar Learning.
6. Herr, J. 2008. *Working with young children*. 4th ed. Tinley Park, IL: Goodheart-Willcox Company.
7. Dalton, S. 2004. *Our overweight children: What parents, schools, and communities can do to control the fatness epidemic*. Berkeley, CA: University of California Press.

4.2 General Requirements

STANDARD 4.2.0.1: Written Nutrition Plan

The facility should provide nourishing and attractive food for children according to a written plan developed by a qualified nutritionist/registered dietitian. Caregivers/teachers, directors, and food service personnel should share the responsibility for carrying out the plan. The administrator is responsible for implementing the plan but may delegate tasks to caregivers/teachers and food service personnel. Where infants and young children are involved, special attention to the feeding plan may include attention to supporting mothers in maintaining their human milk supply. The nutrition plan should include steps to take when problems require rapid response by the staff, such as when a child chokes during mealtime or has an allergic reaction to a food. The completed plan should be on file, easily accessible to staff, and available to parents/guardians upon request.

If the facility is large enough to justify employment of a full-time nutritionist/registered dietitian or child care food service manager, the facility should delegate to this person the responsibility for implementing the written plan.

Some children may have medical conditions that require special dietary modifications. A written care plan from the primary care provider, clearly stating the food(s) to be avoided and food(s) to be substituted should be on file. This information should be updated periodically if the modification is not a lifetime special dietary need. Staff should be trained about a child's dietary modification to ensure that no child in care ingests inappropriate foods while at the facility. The proper modifications should be implemented whether the child brings their own food or whether it is prepared on site. The facility needs to inform all families and staff if certain foods, such as nut products (example: peanut butter), should not be brought from home because of a child's life-threatening allergy. Staff should also know what procedure to follow if ingestion occurs. In addition to knowing ahead of time what procedures to follow, staff must know their designated roles during an emergency. The emergency plan should be dated and updated.

RATIONALE: Nourishing and attractive food is the cornerstone for children's health, growth, and development as well as developmentally appropriate learning experiences (1-9). Nutrition and feeding are fundamental and required in every facility. Because children grow and develop more rapidly during the first few years of life than at any other time, the child's home and the facility together must provide food that is adequate in amount and type to meet each child's growth and nutritional needs. Children can learn healthy eating habits and be better equipped to maintain a healthy weight if they eat nourishing food while attending early care and education settings and if they are allowed to feed themselves and determine the amount of food they will ingest at any

one sitting. The obesity epidemic makes this an important lesson today.

Meals and snacks provide the caregiver/teacher an opportunity to model appropriate mealtime behavior and guide the conversation, which aids in children's conceptual, sensory language development, and eye/hand coordination. In larger facilities, professional nutrition staff must be involved to assure compliance with nutrition and food service guidelines, including accommodation of children with special health care needs.

COMMENTS: *Making Food Healthy and Safe for Children, 2nd Ed.* (http://nti.unc.edu/course_files/curriculum/nutrition/making_food_healthy_and_safe.pdf) contains practical tips for implementing the standards for culturally diverse groups of infants and children.

TYPE OF FACILITY: Center; Large Family Child Care Home; Small Family Child Care Home

RELATED STANDARDS:

Standard 4.2.0.2: Assessment and Planning of Nutrition for Individual Children
Standard 4.2.0.8: Feeding Plans and Dietary Modifications
Standard 4.4.0.2: Use of Nutritionist/Registered Dietitian
Standard 4.7.0.1: Nutrition Learning Experiences for Children
Standard 9.2.3.11: Food and Nutrition Service Policies and Plans
Appendix C: Nutrition Specialist, Registered Dietitian, Licensed Nutritionist, Consultant, and Food Service Staff Qualifications

REFERENCES:

1. U.S. Department of Health and Human Services, Administration for Children and Families, Office of Head Start. 2009. *Head Start program performance standards*. Rev. ed. Washington, DC: U.S. Government Printing Office. http://eclkc.ohs.acf.hhs.gov/hslc/Head Start Program/Program Design and Management/Head Start Requirements/Head Start Requirements/45 CFR Chapter XIII/45 CFR Chap XIII_ENG.pdf.
2. Hagan, Jr., J. F., J. S. Shaw, P. M. Duncan, eds. 2008. *Bright futures: Guidelines for health supervision of infants, children, and adolescents*. 3rd ed. Elk Grove Village, IL: American Academy of Pediatrics.
3. Story, M., K. Holt, D. Sofka, eds. 2002. *Bright futures in practice: Nutrition*. 2nd ed. Arlington, VA: National Center for Education in Maternal and Child Health. http://www.brightfutures.org/nutrition/pdf/frnt_mttr.pdf.
4. Wardle, F., N. Winegarner. 1992. Nutrition and Head Start. *Child Today* 21:57.
5. Benjamin, S. E., ed. 2007. *Making food healthy and safe for children: How to meet the national health and safety performance standards – Guidelines for out of home child care programs*. 2nd ed. Chapel Hill, NC: National Training Institute for Child Care Health Consultants. http://nti.unc.edu/course_files/curriculum/nutrition/making_food_healthy_and_safe.pdf.
6. Dietz, W. H., L. Stern, eds. 1998. *American Academy of Pediatrics guide to your child's nutrition*. New York: Villard.
7. Kleinman, R. E., ed. 2009. *Pediatric nutrition handbook*. 6th ed. Elk Grove Village, IL: American Academy of Pediatrics.
8. Lally, J. R., A. Griffin, E. Fenichel, M. Segal, E. Szanton, B. Weissbourd. 2003. *Caring for infants and toddlers in groups: Developmentally appropriate practice*. Arlington, VA: Zero to Three.
9. Enders, J. B., R. E. Rockwell. 2003. *Food, nutrition, and the young child*. 4th ed. New York: Macmillan.

STANDARD 4.2.0.2: Assessment and Planning of Nutrition for Individual Children

As a part of routine health supervision by the child's primary care provider, children should be evaluated for nutrition-related medical problems such as failure to thrive, overweight, obesity, food allergy, reflux disease, and iron-deficiency anemia. The nutritional standards throughout this document are general recommendations that may not always be appropriate for some children with medically-identified special nutrition needs. Caregivers/teachers should communicate with the child's parent/guardian and primary care provider to adapt nutritional offerings to individual children as indicated and medically-appropriate. Caregivers/teachers should work with the parent/guardian to implement individualized feeding plans developed by the child's primary care provider to meet a child's unique nutritional needs. These plans could include, for instance, additional iron-rich foods to a child who has been diagnosed as having iron-deficiency anemia. For a child diagnosed as overweight, the plan would focus on controlling portion sizes. Also, calorie dense foods like sugar sweetened juices, nectars, and beverages should not be served. Denying a child food that others are eating is difficult to explain and difficult for some children to understand and accept. Attention should be paid to teaching about proper portion sizes and the average daily caloric intake of the child.

Some children require special feeding techniques such as thickened foods or special positioning during meals. Other children will require dietary modifications based on food intolerances such as lactose or wheat (gluten) intolerance. Some children will need dietary modifications based on cultural or religious preferences such as vegetarian or kosher diets.

RATIONALE: The early years are a critical time for children's growth and development. Nutritional problems must be identified and treated during this period in order to prevent serious or long-term medical problems. The early care and education setting may be offering a majority of a child's daily nutritional intake especially for children in full-time care. It is important that the facility ensures that food offerings are congruent with nutritional interventions or dietary modifications recommended by the child's primary care provider in consultation with the nutritionist/registered dietitian to make certain that intervention is child specific.

TYPE OF FACILITY: Center; Large Family Child Care Home; Small Family Child Care Home

RELATED STANDARDS:

Standard 3.1.2.1: Routine Health Supervision and Growth Monitoring
Standard 4.2.0.8: Feeding Plans and Dietary Modifications

STANDARD 4.2.0.3: Use of USDA - CACFP Guidelines

All meals and snacks and their preparation, service, and storage should meet the requirements for meals of the child care component of the U.S. Department of Agriculture

(USDA), Child and Adult Care Food Program (CACFP), and the 7 Code of Federal Regulations (CFR) Part 226.20 (1,5).

RATIONALE: The CACFP regulations, policies, and guidance materials on meal requirements provide the basic guidelines for sound nutrition and sanitation practices. Meals and snacks offered to young children should provide a variety of nourishing foods on a frequent basis to meet the nutritional needs of infants from birth to children age twelve (2-4). The CACFP guidance for meals and snack patterns ensures that the nutritional needs of infants and children, including school-age children up through age twelve, are met based on current scientific knowledge (5). Programs not eligible for reimbursement under the regulations of CACFP should use the CACFP food guidance.

COMMENTS: The staff should use information on the child's growth in developing individual feeding plans. For the current CACFP meal patterns, go to http://www.fns.usda.gov/cnd/care/ProgramBasics/Meals/Meal_Patterns.htm.

TYPE OF FACILITY: Center; Large Family Child Care Home; Small Family Child Care Home

RELATED STANDARDS:
Standard 3.1.2.1: Routine Health Supervision and Growth Monitoring
Standard 4.2.0.4: Categories of Foods
Standard 4.2.0.5: Meal and Snack Patterns
Standard 4.3.2.1: Meal and Snack Patterns for Toddlers and Preschoolers
Standard 4.3.3.1: Meal and Snack Patterns for School-Age Children

REFERENCES:

1. Lally, J. R., A. Griffin, E. Fenichel, M. Segal, E. Szanton, B. Weissbourd. 2003. *Caring for infants and toddlers in groups: Developmentally appropriate practice*. Arlington, VA: Zero to Three.
2. U.S. Department of Agriculture (USDA), Child and Adult Care Food Program (CACFP). 2002. *Menu magic for children: A menu planning guide for child care*. Washington, DC: USDA. http://www.fns.usda.gov/tn/resources/menu_magic.pdf.
3. U.S. Department of Agriculture (USDA), Team Nutrition. 2000. *Building blocks for fun and healthy meals: A menu planner for the child and adult care food program*. Washington, DC: USDA. http://teamnutrition.usda.gov/Resources/buildingblocks.html.
4. U.S. Department of Agriculture, Team Nutrition. 2010. Child care providers: Healthy meals resource system. http://healthymeals.nal.usda.gov/nal_display/index.php?tax_level=1&info_center=14&tax_subject=264/.
5. U.S. Department of Agriculture, Food and Nutrition Service. 2011. Child and Adult Care Food Program (CACFP). http://www.fns.usda.gov/cnd/care/.

STANDARD 4.2.0.4: Categories of Foods

Children in care should be offered items of food from the following categories:

Making Healthy Food Choices*		
Food Groups	**USDA**†	**CFOC Guidelines for Young Children**
Fruits	All fresh, frozen, canned, dried fruits, and fruit juices	• Eat a variety, especially whole fruits • Whole fruit, mashed or pureed, for infants seven months up to one year of age • No juice before twelve months of age • 4 to 6 oz juice /day for one- to six-year-olds • 8 to 12 oz juice/day for seven- to twelve-year-olds
Vegetables	Dark green, red, and orange; beans and peas (legumes); starchy vegetables; other vegetables	• Dark green, red, orange, deep yellow vegetables • Other vegetables, including starchy ones like potatoes • Other root vegetables, such as viandas • Dried peas and beans (legumes)
Grains	Whole grains and enriched grains	• Whole and enriched grains, breads, cereals, crackers, pasta, and rice
Protein Foods	Seafood, meat, poultry, eggs, nuts, seeds, and soy products	• Fish, chicken, lean meat, eggs • Nuts and seeds (if appropriate) • Avoid fried fish, meat, and chicken
Dairy	Milk	• Human milk, infant formula for infants at least up to one year of age • Whole milk for children ages on up to two years of age or reduced fat (2%) milk for those at risk for obesity or hypercholesterolemia • 1% or skim milk for children two years of age and older • Other milks such as soy when recommended • Other milk equivalent products such as yogurt and cottage cheese (low-fat for children two years of age and older)
Oils	Oils, soft margarines, includes vegetable, nut, and fish oils and soft vegetable oil table spreads that have no trans fats	• Choose monounsaturated and polyunsaturated fats (olive oil, safflower oil) • Soft margarines
Solid Fats and Added Sugar	Limit calories (% of calories) of these food groups	• Avoid concentrated sweets such as candy, sodas, sweetened drinks, fruit nectars, and flavored milk • Limit salty foods such as chips and pretzels
*All foods are assumed to be in nutrient-dense forms, lean or low-fat and prepared without added fats, sugars, or salt. Solid fats and added sugars may be included up to the daily maximum limit identified in the *Dietary Guidelines for Americans, 2010*. †Recommends: Find your balance between food and physical activity.		

Additional Resources:

- U.S. Department of Health and Human Services (DHHS). 2010. *The Surgeon General's vision for a healthy and fit nation*. Washington, DC: DHHS, Office of the Surgeon General. http://www.surgeongeneral.gov/library/obesityvision/obesityvision2010.pdf.
- U.S. Department of Health and Human Services, U.S. Department of Agriculture. 2011. *Dietary guidelines for Americans, 2010*. 7th ed. Washington, DC: U.S. Government Printing Office. http://www.health.gov/dietaryguidelines/dga2010/DietaryGuidelines2010.pdf.
- U.S. Department of Health and Human Services, Office of Disease Prevention and Health Promotion (ODPHP). 2008. *2008 physical activity guidelines for Americans*. Rockville, MD: ODPHP. http://www.health.gov/paguidelines/guidelines/default.aspx.
- Story, M., K. Holt, D. Sofka, eds. 2002. *Bright futures in practice: Nutrition*. 2nd ed. Arlington, VA: National Center for Education in Maternal and Child Health. http://www.brightfutures.org/nutrition/pdf/frnt_mttr.pdf.
- U.S. Department of Agriculture. 2011. *MyPlate*. http://www.choosemyplate.gov.

RATIONALE: The *Dietary Guidelines for Americans, 2010* and "The Surgeon General's Call to Action to Support Breast Feeding" support feeding nutritious foods and healthy lifestyles to prevent the onset of overweight and obesity and chronic diseases (1,2). From the very first feeding of an infant begins setting the stage for lifetime eating behavior. Using the food groups as a tool is a practical approach to select foods high in essential nutrients and moderate in calories/energy. Meals and snacks planned based on the five food groups promote normal growth and development of children as well as reduce their risk of overweight, obesity and related chronic diseases later in life. Age-specific guidance for meals and snacks is outlined in CACFP guidelines and accessible at http://www.fns.usda.gov/cnd/care/ProgramBasics/Meals/Meal_Patterns.htm (3). Early care and education settings provide the opportunity

for children to learn about the food they eat, to develop and strengthen their fine and gross motor skills, and to engage in social interaction at mealtimes (4).

COMMENTS: Early Care and education settings should encourage mothers to breastfeed their infants. Scientific evidence documents and supports the nutritional and health contributions of human milk (2). For more information on portion sizes and types of food, see CACFP Guidelines at http://www.fns.usda.gov/cnd/care/ProgramBasics/Meals/Meal_Patterns.htm.

TYPE OF FACILITY: Center; Large Family Child Care Home; Small Family Child Care Home

RELATED STANDARDS:

Standard 4.2.0.5: Meal and Snack Patterns
Standard 4.2.0.7: 100% Fruit Juice
Standard 4.2.0.8: Feeding Plans and Dietary Modifications
Standard 4.3.1.3: Preparing, Feeding, and Storing Human Milk
Standard 4.3.1.5: Preparing, Feeding, and Storing Infant Formula
Standard 4.3.1.7: Feeding Cow's Milk
Standard 4.3.2.1: Meal and Snack Patterns for Toddlers and Preschoolers
Standard 4.3.3.1: Meal and Snack Patterns for School-Age Children
Standard 4.7.0.1: Nutritional Learning Experiences for Children
Standard 4.7.0.2: Nutrition Education for Parents/Guardians
Appendix Q: Getting Started with MyPlate
Appendix R: Choose MyPlate: 10 Tips to a Great Plate

REFERENCES:

1. U.S. Department of Health and Human Services, U.S. Department of Agriculture. 2011. *Dietary guidelines for Americans, 2010*. 7th ed. Washington, DC: U.S. Government Printing Office. http://www.health.gov/dietaryguidelines/dga2010/DietaryGuidelines2010.pdf.
2. U.S. Department of Health and Human Services (HHS). 2011. *The Surgeon General's call to action to support breastfeeding*. Washington, DC: HHS, Office of the Surgeon General. http://www.surgeongeneral.gov/topics/breastfeeding/calltoactiontosupportbreastfeeding.pdf.
3. U.S. Department of Agriculture, Food and Nutrition Service. 2011. Child and adult care food program (CACFP). http://www.fns.usda.gov/cnd/care/.
4. Nemours Health and Prevention Services. 2008. *Best practices for healthy eating: A guide to help children grow up healthy*. Version 2. Newark, DE: Nemours Foundation. http://www.nemours.org/content/dam/nemours/www/filebox/service/preventive/nhps/heguide.pdf.

STANDARD 4.2.0.5: Meal and Snack Patterns

The facility should ensure that the following meal and snack pattern occurs:

a) Children in care for eight and fewer hours in one day should be offered at least one meal and two snacks or two meals and one snack.
b) Children in care more than eight hours in one day should be offered at least two meals and two snacks or three snacks and one meal.
c) A nutritious snack should be offered to all children in midmorning (if they are not offered a breakfast on-site that is provided within three hours of lunch) and in the middle of the afternoon.
d) Children should be offered food at intervals at least two hours apart and not more than three hours apart unless the child is asleep. Some very young infants may need to be fed at shorter intervals than every two hours to meet their nutritional needs, especially breastfed infants being fed expressed human milk. Lunch service may need to be served to toddlers earlier than the preschool-aged children due to their need for an earlier nap schedule. Children must be awake prior to being offered a meal/snack.
e) Children should be allowed time to eat their food and not be rushed during the meal or snack service. They should not be allowed to play during these times.
f) Caregivers/teachers should discuss the breastfed infant's feeding patterns with the parents/guardians because the frequency of breastfeeding at home can vary. For example, some infants may still be feeding frequently at night, while others may do the bulk of their feeding during the day. Knowledge about the infant's feeding patterns over twenty-four hours will help caregivers/teachers assess the infant's feeding during his/her time with the caregiver/teacher.

RATIONALE: Young children, under the age of six, need to be offered food every two to three hours. Appetite and interest in food varies from one meal or snack to the next. To ensure that the child's daily nutritional needs are met, small feedings of nourishing food should be scheduled over the course of a day (1-6). Snacks should be nutritious, as they often are a significant part of a child's daily intake. Children in care for more than eight hours need additional food because this period represents a majority of a young child's waking hours.

COMMENTS: Caloric needs vary greatly from one child to another. A child may require more food during growth spurts. Some states have regulations indicating suggested times for meals and snacks. By regulation, in the Child and Adult Care Food Program (CACFP), centers and family child care homes may be approved to claim up to two reimbursable meals (breakfast, lunch or supper) and one snack, or two snacks and one meal, for each eligible participant, each day. Many after-school programs provide before school care or full day care when elementary school is out of session. Many of these programs offer either a breakfast and/or a morning snack. After-school care programs may claim reimbursement for serving each child one snack, each day. In some states after-school programs also have the option of providing a supper. These are reimbursed by CACFP if they meet certain guidelines and timeframes. For more information on CACFP meal reimbursement see the CACFP Website at http://www.fns.usda.gov/cnd/care/CACFP/aboutcacfp.htm.

TYPE OF FACILITY: Center; Large Family Child Care Home; Small Family Child Care Home

RELATED STANDARDS:

Standard 4.3.2.1: Meal and Snack Patterns for Toddlers and Preschoolers
Standard 4.3.3.1: Meal and Snack Patterns for School-Age Children

REFERENCES:
1. U.S. Department of Health and Human Services, Administration for Children and Families, Office of Head Start. 2009. *Head Start program performance standards*. Rev. ed. Washington, DC: U.S. Government Printing Office. http://eclkc.ohs.acf.hhs.gov/hslc/Head Start Program/Program Design and Management/Head Start Requirements/Head Start Requirements/45 CFR Chapter XIII/45 CFR Chap XIII_ENG.pdf.
2. Benjamin, S. E., ed. 2007. *Making food healthy and safe for children: How to meet the national health and safety performance standards – Guidelines for out of home child care programs*. 2nd ed. Chapel Hill, NC: National Training Institute for Child Care Health Consultants. http://nti.unc.edu/course_files/curriculum/nutrition/making_food_healthy_and_safe.pdf.
3. Pipes, P. L., C. M. Trahms, eds. 1997. *Nutrition in infancy and childhood*. 6th ed. New York: McGraw-Hill.
4. Butte, N., S. K. Cobb. 2004. The Start Healthy feeding guidelines for infants and children. *J Am Diet Assoc* 104:442-54.
5. Kleinman, R. E., ed. 2009. *Pediatric nutrition handbook*. 6th ed. Elk Grove Village, IL: American Academy of Pediatrics.
6. Plemas, C., B. M. Popkin. 2010. Trends in snacking among U.S. children. *Health Affairs* 29:399-404.

STANDARD 4.2.0.6: Availability of Drinking Water

Clean, sanitary drinking water should be readily available, in indoor and outdoor areas, throughout the day. Water should not be a substitute for milk at meals or snacks where milk is a required food component unless it is recommended by the child's primary care provider.

On hot days, infants receiving human milk in a bottle can be given additional human milk in a bottle but should not be given water, especially in the first six months of life. Infants receiving formula and water can be given additional formula in a bottle. Toddlers and older children will need additional water as physical activity and/or hot temperatures cause their needs to increase. Children should learn to drink water from a cup or drinking fountain without mouthing the fixture. They should not be allowed to have water continuously in hand in a "sippy cup" or bottle. Permitting toddlers to suck continuously on a bottle or sippy cup filled with water, in order to soothe themselves, may cause nutritional or in rare instances, electrolyte imbalances. When tooth brushing is not done after a feeding, children should be offered water to drink to rinse food from their teeth.

RATIONALE: When children are thirsty between meals and snacks, water is the best choice. Encouraging children to learn to drink water in place of fruit drinks, soda, fruit nectars, or other sweetened drinks builds a beneficial habit. Drinking water during the day can reduce the extra caloric intake which is associated with overweight and obesity (1). Drinking water is good for a child's hydration and reduces acid in the mouth that contributes to early childhood caries (1,3,4). Water needs vary among young children and increase during times in which dehydration is a risk (e.g., hot summer days, during exercise, and in dry days in winter) (2).

COMMENTS: Clean, small pitchers of water and single-use paper cups available in the classrooms and on the playgrounds allow children to serve themselves water when they are thirsty. Drinking fountains should be kept clean and sanitary and maintained to provide adequate drainage.

TYPE OF FACILITY: Center; Large Family Child Care Home; Small Family Child Care Home

RELATED STANDARDS:
Standard 3.1.3.2: Playing Outdoors
Standard 4.3.1.3: Preparing, Feeding, and Storing Human Milk
Standard 4.3.1.5: Preparing, Feeding, and Storing Infant Formula

REFERENCES:
1. Kleinman, R. E., ed. 2009. *Pediatric nutrition handbook*. 6th ed. Elk Grove Village, IL: American Academy of Pediatrics.
2. Manz, F. 2007. Hydration in children. *J Am Coll Nutr* 26:562S-569S.
3. Casamassimo, P., K. Holt, eds. 2004. *Bright futures in practice: Oral health–pocket guide*. Washington, DC: National Maternal and Child Oral Health Resource Center. http://www.mchoralhealth.org/PDFs/BFOHPocketGuide.pdf.
4. Centers for Disease Control and Prevention. 2011. Community water fluoridation. http://www.cdc.gov/fluoridation/.

STANDARD 4.2.0.7: 100% Fruit Juice

The facility should serve only full-strength (100%) pasteurized fruit juice or full-strength fruit juice diluted with water from a cup to children twelve months of age or older. Juice should have no added sweeteners. The facility should offer juice at specific meals and snacks instead of continuously throughout the day. Juice consumption should be no more than a total of four to six ounces a day for children aged one to six years. This amount includes juice served at home. Children ages seven through twelve years of age should consume no more than a total of eight to twelve ounces of fruit juice per day. Caregivers/teachers should ask parents/guardians if they provide juice at home and how much. This information is important to know if and when to serve juice. Infants should not be given any fruit juice before twelve months of age. Whole fruit, mashed or pureed, is recommended for infants seven months up to one year of age.

RATIONALE: Whole fruit is more nutritious than fruit juice and provides dietary fiber. Fruit juice which is 100% offers no nutritional advantage over whole fruits.

Limiting the feeding of juice to specific meals and snacks will reduce acids produced by bacteria in the mouth that cause tooth decay. The frequency of exposure, rather than the quantity of food, is important in determining whether foods cause tooth decay. Although sugar is not the only dietary factor likely to cause tooth decay, it is a major factor in the prevalence of tooth decay (1,2).

Drinks that are called fruit juice drinks, fruit punches, or fruit nectars contain less than 100% fruit juice and are of a lower nutritional value than 100% fruit juice. Liquids with high sugar content have no place in a healthy diet and should be avoided. Continuous consumption of juice during the day has been associated with a decrease in appetite for other nutritious foods which can result in feeding problems and overweight/obesity. Infants should not be given juice from bottles or easily transportable, covered cups (e.g., sippy cups) that allow them to consume juice throughout the day.

The American Academy of Pediatrics (AAP) recommends that children aged one to six years drink no more than four to six ounces of fruit juice a day (3). This amount is the total quantity for the whole day, including both time at early care and education and at home. Caregivers/teachers should not give the entire amount while a child is in their care. For breastfed infants, AAP recommends that gradual introduction of iron-fortified foods may occur no sooner than around four months, but preferably six months to complement the human milk. Infants should not be given juice before they reach twelve months of age.

Overconsumption of 100% fruit juice can contribute to overweight and obesity (3-6). One study found that two- to five-year-old children who drank twelve or more ounces of fruit juice a day were more likely to be obese than those who drank less juice (2). Excessive fruit juice consumption may be associated with malnutrition (over nutrition and under nutrition), diarrhea, flatulence, and abdominal distention (3). Unpasteurized fruit juice may contain pathogens that can cause serious illnesses (3). The U.S. Food and Drug Administration requires a warning on the dangers of harmful bacteria on all unpasteurized juice or products (7).

COMMENTS: Caregivers/teachers, as well as many parents/guardians, should strive to understand the relationship between the consumption of sweetened beverages and tooth decay. Drinks with high sugar content should be avoided because they can contribute to childhood obesity (2,5,6), tooth decay, and poor nutrition.

TYPE OF FACILITY: Center; Large Family Child Care Home; Small Family Child Care Home

RELATED STANDARDS:
Standard 4.2.0.4: Categories of Food

REFERENCES:

1. Casamassimo, P., K. Holt, eds. 2004. *Bright futures in practice: Oral health–pocket guide*. Washington, DC: National Maternal and Child Oral Health Resource Center. http://www.mchoralhealth.org/PDFs/BFOHPocketGuide.pdf.
2. Dennison, B. A., H. L. Rockwell, S. L. Baker. 1997. Excess fruit juice consumption by preschool-aged children is associated with short stature and obesity. *Pediatrics* 99:15-22.
3. American Academy of Pediatrics, Committee on Nutrition. 2007. Policy statement: The use and misuse of fruit juice in pediatrics. *Pediatrics* 119:405.
4. Faith, M. S., B. A. Dennison, L. S. Edmunds, H. H. Stratton. 2006. Fruit juice intake predicts increased adiposity gain in children from low-income families: Weight status-by-environment interaction. *Pediatrics* 118:2066-75.
5. Dubois, L., A. Farmer, M. Girard, K. Peterson. 2007. Regular sugar-sweetened beverage consumption between meals increases risk of overweight among preschool-aged children. *J Am Diet Assoc* 107:924-34.
6. Dennison, B. A., H. L. Rockwell, M. J. Nichols, P. Jenkins. 1999. Children's growth parameters vary by type of fruit juice consumed. *J Am Coll Nutr* 18:346-52.
7. U.S. Food and Drug Administration. *Safe handling of raw produce and fresh-squeezed fruit and vegetable juices*. New York: JMH Education. http://www.fda.gov/Food/ResourcesForYou/Consumers/ucm114299.htm.

STANDARD 4.2.0.8: Feeding Plans and Dietary Modifications

Before a child enters an early care and education facility, the facility should obtain a written history that contains any special nutrition or feeding needs for the child, including use of human milk or any special feeding utensils. The staff should review this history with the child's parents/guardians, clarifying and discussing how parental/guardian home feeding routines may differ from the facility's planned routine. The child's primary care provider should provide written information about any dietary modifications or special feeding techniques that are required at the early care and education program and these plans should be shared with the child's parents/guardians upon request.

If dietary modifications are indicated, based on a child's medical or special dietary needs, the caregiver/teacher should modify or supplement the child's diet to meet the individual child's specific needs. Dietary modifications should be made in consultation with the parents/guardians and the child's primary care provider. Caregivers/teachers can consult with a nutritionist/registered dietitian.

Reasons for modification of a child's diet may be related to food sensitivity. Food sensitivity includes a range of conditions in which a child exhibits an adverse reaction to a food that, in some instances, can be life threatening. Modification of a child's diet may be related to a food allergy, inability to digest or to tolerate certain foods, need for extra calories, need for special positioning while eating, diabetes and the need to match food with insulin, food idiosyncrasies, and other identified feeding issues. Examples include celiac disease, phenylketonuria, diabetes, severe food allergy (anaphylaxis), and others. In some cases, a child may become ill if the child is unable to eat, so missing a meal could have a negative consequence, especially for diabetics.

For a child identified with special health care needs for dietary modification or special feeding techniques, written instructions from the child's parent/guardian and the child's primary care provider should be provided in the child's record and carried out accordingly. Dietary modifications should be recorded. These written instructions must identify:

a) The child's full name and date of instructions;
b) The child's special needs;
c) Any dietary restrictions based on the special needs;
d) Any special feeding or eating utensils;
e) Any foods to be omitted from the diet and any foods to be substituted;
f) Limitations of life activities;
g) Any other pertinent special needs information;
h) What, if anything, needs to be done if the child is exposed to restricted foods.

The written history of special nutrition or feeding needs should be used to develop individual feeding plans and, collectively, to develop facility menus. Disciplines related to special nutrition needs, including nutrition, nursing, speech, occupational therapy, and physical therapy, should participate when needed and/or when they are available to the

facility. The nutritionist/registered dietitian should approve menus that accommodate needed dietary modifications.

The feeding plan should include steps to take when a situation arises that requires rapid response by the staff, such as a child's choking during mealtime or a child with a known history of food allergies demonstrating signs and symptoms of anaphylaxis (severe allergic reaction, e.g., difficulty breathing or severe redness and swelling of the face or mouth). The completed plan should be on file and accessible to the staff and available to parents/guardians upon request.

RATIONALE: Children with special health care needs may have individual requirements related to diet and swallowing, involving special feeding utensils and feeding needs that will necessitate the development of an individual plan prior to their entry into the facility (1-3). A number of children with special health care needs have difficulty with feeding, including delayed attainment of basic chewing, swallowing, and independent feeding skills. Food, eating style, food utensils, and equipment, including furniture, may have to be adapted to meet the developmental and physical needs of individual children (1-3).

Some children have difficulty with slow weight gain and need their caloric intake monitored and supplemented. Others with special needs, such as those with diabetes, may need to have their diet matched to their medication (insulin if they are on a fixed dose of insulin). Some children are unable to tolerate certain foods because of their allergy to the food or their inability to digest it. In children, foods are the most common cause of anaphylaxis. Nuts, seeds, eggs, soy, milk, and seafood are among the most common allergens for food-induced anaphylaxis in children (3). Staff members must know ahead of time what procedures to follow, as well as their designated roles during an emergency.

As a safety and health precaution, the staff should know in advance whether a child has food allergies, inborn errors of metabolism, diabetes, celiac disease, tongue thrust, or special health care needs related to feeding, such as requiring special feeding utensils or equipment, nasogastric or gastric tube feedings, or special positioning. These situations require individual planning prior to the child's entry into early care and education and on an ongoing basis (3,4).

In some cases, dietary modifications are based on religious or cultural beliefs. Detailed information on each child's special needs whether stemming from dietary, feeding equipment, or cultural needs, is invaluable to the facility staff in meeting the nutritional needs of that child.

COMMENTS: Close collaboration between the home and the facility is necessary for children on special diets. Parents/guardians may have to provide food on a temporary or, even, a permanent basis, if the facility, after exploring all community resources, is unable to provide the special diet.

TYPE OF FACILITY: Center; Large Family Child Care Home; Small Family Child Care Home

RELATED STANDARDS:

Standard 4.2.0.2: Assessment and Planning of Nutrition for Individual Children

REFERENCES:

1. Samour, P. Q., K. King. 2005. *Handbook of pediatric nutrition*. 3rd ed. Lake Dallas, TX: Helm.
2. Dietz, W. H., L. Stern, eds. 1998. *American Academy of Pediatrics guide to your child's nutrition*. New York: Villard.
3. Kleinman, R. E., ed. 2009. *Pediatric nutrition handbook*. 6th ed. Elk Grove Village, IL: American Academy of Pediatrics.
4. Lally, J. R., A. Griffin, E. Fenichel, M. Segal, E. Szanton, B. Weissbourd. 2003. *Caring for infants and toddlers in groups: Developmentally appropriate practice*. Arlington, VA: Zero to Three.

STANDARD 4.2.0.9: Written Menus and Introduction of New Foods

Facilities should develop, at least one month in advance, written menus showing all foods to be served during that month and should make the menus available to parents/guardians. The facility should date and retain these menus for six months, unless the state regulatory agency requires a longer retention time. The menus should be amended to reflect any and all changes in the food actually served. Any substitutions should be of equal nutrient value.

To avoid problems of food sensitivity in very young children under eighteen months of age, caregivers/teachers should obtain from the child's parents/guardians a list of foods that have already been introduced (without any reaction), and then serve some of these foods to the child. As new foods are considered for serving, caregivers/teachers should share and discuss these foods with the parents/guardians prior to their introduction.

RATIONALE: Planning menus in advance helps to ensure that food will be on hand. Parents/guardians need to be informed about food served in the facility to know how to complement it with the food they serve at home. If a child has difficulty with any food served at the facility, parents/guardians can address this issue with appropriate staff members. Some regulatory agencies require menus as a part of the licensing and auditing process (2).

COMMENTS: Caregivers/teachers should be aware that new foods may need to be offered between eight to fifteen times before a food may be accepted (3,5). Posting menus in a prominent area and distributing them to parents/guardians helps to inform them about proper nutrition. Sample menus and menu planning templates are available from most state health departments, the state extension service, and the Child and Adult Care Food Program (CACFP).

Good communication between the caregiver/teacher and the parents/guardians is essential for successful feeding, in general, including when introducing age-appropriate solid foods (complementary foods). The decision to feed specific foods should be made in consultation with the parents/guardians. It is recommended that the caregiver/teacher be given written instructions on the introduction and feeding of foods from the parents/guardians and the infant's primary care provider. Caregivers/teachers should use or develop a

take-home sheet for parents/guardians on which the caregiver/teacher records the food consumed each day or, for breastfed infants, the number of breastfeedings, and other important notes on the infant. Caregivers/teachers should continue to consult with each infant's parents/guardians concerning foods they have introduced and are feeding. In this way, the caregiver/teacher can follow a schedule of introducing new foods one at a time and more easily identify possible food allergies or intolerances. Caregivers/teachers should let parents/guardians know what and how much their infant eats each day. Consistency between home and the early care and education setting is essential during the period of rapid change when infants are learning to eat age-appropriate solid foods (1,4,6).

TYPE OF FACILITY: Center; Large Family Child Care Home; Small Family Child Care Home

RELATED STANDARDS:
Standard 4.3.1.1: General Plan for Feeding Infants
Standard 4.3.1.11: Introduction of Age-Appropriate Solid Foods to Infants
Standard 4.5.0.8: Experience with Familiar and New Foods

REFERENCES:

1. Benjamin, S. E., ed. 2007. *Making food healthy and safe for children: How to meet the national health and safety performance standards – Guidelines for out-of-home child care programs*. 2nd ed. Chapel Hill, NC: National Training Institute for Child Care Health Consultants. http://nti.unc.edu/course_files/curriculum/nutrition/making_food_healthy_and_safe.pdf.
2. Benjamin, S. E., K. A. Copeland, A. Cradock, E. Walker, M. M. Slining, B. Neelon, M. W. Gillman. 2009. Menus in child care: A comparison of state regulations to national standards. *J Am Diet Assoc* 109:109-15.
3. Sullivan, S. A., L. L. Birch. 1990. Pass the sugar, pass the salt: Experience dictates preference. *Devel Psych* 26:546-51.
4. U.S. Department of Agriculture, Food and Nutrition Service (FNS). 2001. *Feeding infants: A guide for use in the child nutrition programs*. Rev ed. Alexandria, VA: FNS. http://www.fns.usda.gov/tn/resources/feeding_infants.pdf.
5. Pipes, P. L., C. M. Trahms, eds. 1997. *Nutrition in infancy and childhood*. 6th ed. New York: McGraw-Hill.
6. Grummer-Strawn, L. M., K. S. Scanlon, S. B. Fein. 2008. Infant feeding and feeding transitions during the first year of life. *Pediatrics* 122: S36-S42.

STANDARD 4.2.0.10: Care for Children with Food Allergies

When children with food allergies attend the early care and education facility, the following should occur:

a) Each child with a food allergy should have a care plan prepared for the facility by the child's primary care provider, to include:
   1) Written instructions regarding the food(s) to which the child is allergic and steps that need to be taken to avoid that food;
   2) A detailed treatment plan to be implemented in the event of an allergic reaction, including the names, doses, and methods of administration of any medications that the child should receive in the event of a reaction. The plan should include specific symptoms that would indicate the need to administer one or more medications;

b) Based on the child's care plan, the child's caregivers/teachers should receive training, demonstrate competence in, and implement measures for:
   1) Preventing exposure to the specific food(s) to which the child is allergic;
   2) Recognizing the symptoms of an allergic reaction;
   3) Treating allergic reactions;

c) Parents/guardians and staff should arrange for the facility to have necessary medications, proper storage of such medications, and the equipment and training to manage the child's food allergy while the child is at the early care and education facility;

d) Caregivers/teachers should promptly and properly administer prescribed medications in the event of an allergic reaction according to the instructions in the care plan;

e) The facility should notify the parents/guardians immediately of any suspected allergic reactions, the ingestion of the problem food, or contact with the problem food, even if a reaction did not occur;

f) The facility should recommend to the family that the child's primary care provider be notified if the child has required treatment by the facility for a food allergic reaction;

g) The facility should contact the emergency medical services system immediately whenever epinephrine has been administered;

h) Parents/guardians of all children in the child's class should be advised to avoid any known allergens in class treats or special foods brought into the early care and education setting;

i) Individual child's food allergies should be posted prominently in the classroom where staff can view and/or wherever food is served;

j) The written child care plan, a mobile phone, and the proper medications for appropriate treatment if the child develops an acute allergic reaction should be routinely carried on field trips or transport out of the early care and education setting.

RATIONALE: Food allergy is common, occurring in between 2% and 8% of infants and children (1). Food allergic reactions can range from mild skin or gastrointestinal symptoms to severe, life-threatening reactions with respiratory and/or cardiovascular compromise. Hospitalizations from food allergy are being reported in increasing numbers (5). A major factor in death from anaphylaxis has been a delay in the administration of life-saving emergency medication, particularly epinephrine (6). Intensive efforts to avoid exposure to the offending food(s) are therefore warranted. The maintenance of detailed care plans and the ability to implement such plans for the treatment of reactions are essential for all food-allergic children (2-4).

COMMENTS: Successful food avoidance requires a cooperative effort that must include the parents/guardians, the child, the child's primary care provider, and the early care and education staff. The parents/guardians, with the help

of the child's primary care provider, must provide detailed information on the specific foods to be avoided. In some cases, especially for children with multiple food allergies, the parents/guardians may need to take responsibility for providing all of the child's food. In other cases, the early care and education staff may be able to provide safe foods as long as they have been fully educated about effective food avoidance.

Effective food avoidance has several facets. Foods can be listed on an ingredient list under a variety of names, such as milk being listed as casein, caseinate, whey, and/or lactoglobulin. Food sharing between children must be prevented by careful supervision and repeated instruction to the child about this issue. Exposure may also occur through contact between children or by contact with contaminated surfaces, such as a table on which the food allergen remains after eating. Some children may have an allergic reaction just from being in proximity to the offending food, without actually ingesting it. Such contact should be minimized by washing children's hands and faces and all surfaces that were in contact with food. In addition, reactions may occur when a food is used as part of an art or craft project, such as the use of peanut butter to make a bird feeder or wheat to make play dough.

Some children with a food allergy will have mild reactions and will only need to avoid the problem food(s). Others will need to have an antihistamine or epinephrine available to be used in the event of a reaction. For all children with a history of anaphylaxis (severe allergic reaction), or for those with peanut and/or tree nut allergy (whether or not they have had anaphylaxis), epinephrine should be readily available. This will usually be provided as a pre-measured dose in an auto-injector, such as the EpiPen or EpiPen Junior. Specific indications for administration of epinephrine should be provided in the detailed care plan. Within the context of state laws, appropriate personnel should be prepared to administer epinephrine when needed. In virtually all cases, Emergency Medical Services (EMS) should be called immediately and children should be transported to the emergency room by ambulance after the administration of epinephrine. A single dose of epinephrine wears off in fifteen to twenty minutes and many experts will recommend that a second dose be available for administration.

For more information on food allergies, contact the Food Allergy and Anaphylaxis Network or visit their Website at http://www.foodallergy.org.

Some early care and education/school settings require that all foods brought into the classroom are store-bought in their original packaging so that a list of ingredients is included, in order to prevent exposure to allergens.

TYPE OF FACILITY: Center; Large Family Child Care Home; Small Family Child Care Home

RELATED STANDARDS:
Standard 4.2.0.2: Assessment and Planning of Nutrition for Individual Children
Standard 4.2.0.8: Feeding Plans and Dietary Modifications

REFERENCES:
1. Burks, A. W., J. S. Stanley. 1998. Food allergy. *Curr Opin Pediatrics* 10:588-93.
2. U.S. Department of Health and Human Services, Administration for Children and Families, Office of Head Start. 2009. *Head Start program performance standards*. Rev. ed. Washington, DC: U.S. Government Printing Office. http://eclkc.ohs.acf.hhs.gov/hslc/Head Start Program/Program Design and Management/Head Start Requirements/Head Start Requirements/45 CFR Chapter XIII/45 CFR Chap XIII_ENG.pdf.
3. Kleinman, R. E., ed. 2009. *Pediatric nutrition handbook*. 6th ed. Elk Grove Village, IL: American Academy of Pediatrics.
4. Samour, P. Q., K. King. 2005. *Handbook of pediatric nutrition*. 3rd ed. Lake Dallas, TX: Helm.
5. Branum, A. M., S. L. Lukacs. 2008. *Food allergy among U.S. children: Trends in prevalence and hospitalizations*. NCHS data brief, no. 10. Hyattsville, MD: National Center for Health Statistics.
6. Muraro, A., et al. 2010. The management of the allergic child at school: EAACI/GA2LEN Task Force on the allergic child at school. *Allergy* 65:681-89.

STANDARD 4.2.0.11: Ingestion of Substances that Do Not Provide Nutrition

All children should be monitored to prevent them from eating substances that do not provide nutrition (often referred to as Pica). The parents/guardians of children who repeatedly place non-nutritive substances in their mouths should be notified and informed of the importance of their child visiting their primary care provider.

RATIONALE: Children who ingest paint chips or contaminated soil can develop lead toxicity which can lead to developmental delays and neurodevelopmental disability. Children who regularly ingest non-nutritive substances can develop iron deficiency anemia. Eating soil or drinking contaminated water could result in an infection with a parasite.

In collaboration with the child's parent/guardian, an assessment of the child's eating behavior and dietary intake should occur along with any other health issues to begin an intervention strategy. Dietary intake plays an important role because certain nutrients such as a diet high in fat or lecithin increase the absorption of lead which can result in toxicity (1).

Currently there is consensus that repeated ingestion of some non-food items results in an increased lead burden of the body (1,2). Early detection and intervention in non-food ingestion can prevent nutritional deficiencies and growth/developmental disabilities.

The occasional ingestion of non-nutritive substances can be a part of everyday living and is not necessarily a concern. For example, ingestion of non-nutritive substances can occur from mouthing, placing dirty hands in the mouth, or eating dropped food. Pica involves the recurrent ingestion of substances that do not provide nutrition. Pica is most prevalent among children between the ages of one and three years (1). Among children with intellectual developmental disability and concurrent mental illness, the incidence exceeds 50% (1).

COMMENTS: Lead-based paint (old housing as well as lead water pipes), neighborhoods with heavy traffic (leaded fuel), and the storage of acidic foods in open cans or ceramic containers with a lead glaze are sources of lead and should be addressed concurrently with a nutritionally adequate diet as prevention strategies. Community water supply may be a source of lead and should be analyzed for its lead content and other metals. Once a child is identified with lead toxicity, it is important to control the child's exposure to the source of lead and promote a healthy and balanced diet. This health problem can be addressed through collaboration among the child's parents/guardians, primary care provider, local childhood lead poisoning prevention program, and the comprehensive child care team of health, education, and nutrition staff.

TYPE OF FACILITY: Center; Large Family Child Care Home; Small Family Child Care Home

REFERENCES:

1. Ekvall, S. W., V. K. Ekvall, eds. 2005. *Pediatric nutrition in chronic disease and developmental disorders: Prevention, assessment, and treatment*. 2nd ed. New York: Oxford University Press.

2. Mitchell, M. K. 2002. *Nutrition across the life span*. 2nd ed. Philadelphia: W. R. Saunders Co.

STANDARD 4.2.0.12: Vegetarian/Vegan Diets

Infants and children, including school-age children from families practicing any level of vegetarian diet, can be accommodated in an early care and education environment when there is:

a) Written documentation from parents/guardians on the detailed and accurate dietary history about food choices - foods eaten, levels of limitations/restrictions to foods, and frequency of foods offered;

b) An up-to-date health record of the child available to the caregivers/teachers, including information about linear growth and rate of weight gain, or consistent poor appetite (these indicators can be warning signs of growth deficiencies);

c) Collaboration among early care and education staff, especially the sharing of updated information on the child's health with the parents/guardians by the child care health consultant and the nutritionist/registered dietitian;

d) Sound health and nutrition information that is culturally relevant to the family to ensure that the child receives adequate calories and essential nutrients which promote adequate growth and development of the child.

RATIONALE: Infants and young children are at highest risk for nutritional deficiencies for energy levels and essential nutrients including protein, calcium, iron, zinc, vitamins B6, B12, and vitamin D (1-3). The younger the child the more critical it is to know about family food choices, limitations and restrictions because the child is dependent on family food (2). Also due to the rapid growth in the early years, it is imperative that a child's diet should consist of a variety of nourishing food to support growth during this critical period. All vegetarian/vegan children should receive multivitamins, especially vitamin D (400 IU of vitamin D are recommended for infants six months to adulthood unless there is certainty of having the daily allowance met by foods); infants under six months who are exclusively or partially breastfed and who receive less than sixteen ounces of formula per day should receive 400 IU of vitamin D (4).

COMMENTS: For older children who have more choice about what they chose to eat and drink, effort should be made to provide accurate nutrition information so they make the wisest food choices for themselves. Both the early care and education program/school and the caregiver/teacher have an opportunity to inform, teach, and promote sound eating practices along with the consequences when poor food choices are made (1). Sensitivity to cultural factors including beliefs and practices of a child's family should be maintained.

Changing lifestyles, convictions and beliefs about food and religion, what is eaten and what foods are restricted or never consumed, have some families with infants and children practicing several levels of vegetarian diets. Some parents/guardians indicate they are vegetarians, semi-vegetarian, or strict vegetarians because they do not or seldom eat meat. Others label themselves lacto-ovo vegetarians, eating or drinking foods such as eggs and dairy products. Still others describe themselves as vegans who restrict themselves strictly to ingesting only plant-based foods, avoiding all and any animal products.

TYPE OF FACILITY: Center; Large Family Child Care Home; Small Family Child Care Home

RELATED STANDARDS:

Standard 3.1.2.1: Routine Health Supervision and Growth Monitoring
Standard 4.2.0.2: Assessment and Planning of Nutrition for Individual Children
Standard 4.3.1.6: Use of Soy-Based Formula and Soy Milk

REFERENCES:

1. Kleinman, R. E., ed. 2009. *Pediatric nutrition handbook*. 6th ed. Elk Grove Village, IL: American Academy of Pediatrics.

2. Pipes, P. L., C. M. Trahms, eds. 1997. *Nutrition in infancy and childhood*. 6th ed. New York: McGraw-Hill.

3. Mitchell, M. K. 2002. *Nutrition across the life span*. 2nd ed. Philadelphia: W. R. Saunders Co.

4. Wagner, C. L., F. R. Greer. 2008. Prevention of rickets and vitamin D deficiency in infants, children, and adolescents. *Pediatrics* 122:1142-52

4.3 Requirements for Special Groups or Ages of Children

4.3.1 Nutrition for Infants

STANDARD 4.3.1.1: General Plan for Feeding Infants

At a minimum, meals and snacks the facility provides for infants should contain the food in the meal and snack patterns of the Child and Adult Care Food Program (CACFP).

Food should be appropriate for the infant's individual nutrition requirements and developmental stages as determined by written instructions obtained from the child's parent/guardian or primary care provider.

The facility should encourage, provide arrangements for, and support breastfeeding. The facility staff, with appropriate training, should be the mother's cheerleader and enthusiastic supporter for the mother's plan to provide her milk. Facilities should have a designated place set aside for breastfeeding mothers who want to come during work to breastfeed, as well as a private area with an outlet (not a bathroom) for mothers to pump their breast milk (2-8). A place that mothers feel they are welcome to breastfeed, pump, or bottle feed can create a positive environment when offered in a supportive way.

Infants may need a variety of special formulas such as soy-based formula or elemental formulas which are easier to digest and less allergenic. Elemental or special non-allergic formulas should be specified in the infant's care plan.

Age-appropriate solid foods (complementary foods) may be introduced no sooner than when the child has reached the age of four months, but preferably six months and as indicated by the individual child's nutritional and developmental needs. For breastfed infants, gradual introduction of iron-fortified foods may occur no sooner than around four months, but preferably six months to complement the human milk.

RATIONALE: Human milk, as an exclusive food, is best suited to meet the entire nutritional needs of an infant from birth until six months of age, with the exception of recommended vitamin D supplementation. In addition to nutrition, breastfeeding supports optimal health and development. Human milk is also the best source of milk for infants for at least the first twelve months of age and, thereafter, for as long as mutually desired by mother and child. Breastfeeding protects infants from many acute and chronic diseases and has advantages for the mother, as well (4).

Research overwhelmingly shows that exclusive breastfeeding for six months, and continued breastfeeding for at least a year or longer, dramatically improves health outcomes for children and their mothers. *Healthy People 2010* Objective 16 includes increasing the proportion of mothers who breastfeed their infants, and increasing the duration of breastfeeding and of exclusively breastfeeding (1).

Importance of breastfeeding to the infant includes reduction of some of the risks that are greater for infants in group care. Many advantages of breastfeeding are documented by research, including reduction in the incidence of diarrhea, respiratory disease, otitis media, bacteremia, bacterial meningitis, botulism, urinary tract infections, necrotizing enterocolitis, SIDS, insulin-dependent diabetes, lymphoma, allergic disease, ulcerative colitis, ear infections, and other chronic digestive diseases (4,13,15).Evidence suggests that breastfeeding is associated with enhanced cognitive development (6,10). Additionally, some evidence suggests that breastfeeding reduces the risk of childhood obesity (9,11). Breastfeeding also lowers the mother's risk of diabetes, breast cancer, and heart disease (17).

Except in the presence of rare medical conditions, the clear advantage of human milk over any formula should lead to vigorous efforts by caregivers/teachers to promote and sustain breastfeeding for mothers who are willing to nurse their infants whenever they can, and to pump and supply their milk to the early care and education facility when direct feeding from the breast is not possible. Even if infants receive formula during the child care day, some breastfeeding or expressed human milk from their mothers is beneficial (8).

Iron-fortified infant formula is an acceptable alternative to human milk as a food for infant feeding even though it lacks any anti-infective or immunological components. An adequately nourished infant is more likely to achieve normal physical and mental development, which will have long-term positive consequences on health (12,13).

COMMENTS: Some ways to help a mother to breastfeed successfully in the early care and education facility (3):

a) If she wishes to breastfeed her infant or child when she comes to the facility, offer or provide her a:
   1) Quiet, comfortable, and private place to breastfeed (this helps her milk to letdown);
   2) Place to wash her hands;
   3) Pillow to support her infant on her lap while nursing if requested;
   4) Nursing stool or stepstool if requested for her feet so she doesn't have to strain her back while nursing; and
   5) Glass of water or other liquid to help her stay hydrated;
b) Encourage her to get the infant used to being fed her expressed human milk by another person before the infant starts in early care and education, while continuing to breastfeed directly herself;
c) Discuss with her the infant's usual feeding pattern and whether she wants the caregiver/teacher to feed the infant by cue or on a schedule, also ask her if she wishes to time the infant's last feeding so that the infant is hungry and ready to breastfeed when she arrives, also, ask her to leave her availability schedule with the early care and education program and ask her to call if she is planning to miss a feeding or is going to be late;
d) Encourage her to provide a back-up supply of frozen or refrigerated expressed human milk with the infant's full name on the bottle or other clean storage container in case the infant needs to eat more often than usual or the mother's visit is delayed;
e) Share with her information about other places in the community that can answer her questions and concerns about breastfeeding, for example, local lactation consultants (14,16);
f) Ensure that all staff receive training in breastfeeding support and promotion;
g) Ensure that all staff are trained in the proper handling and feeding of each milk product, including human milk or infant formula;

h) Provide culturally appropriate breastfeeding materials including community resources for parents/guardians that include appropriate language and pictures of multicultural families to assist families to identify with them.

TYPE OF FACILITY: Center; Large Family Child Care Home; Small Family Child Care Home

RELATED STANDARDS:

Standard 4.2.0.9: Written Menus and Introduction of New Foods
Standard 4.3.1.3: Preparing, Feeding, and Storing Human Milk
Standard 4.3.1.5: Preparing, Feeding, and Storing Infant Formula
Standard 4.3.1.11: Introduction of Age-Appropriate Solid Foods to Infants
Standard 4.3.1.12: Feeding Age-Appropriate Solid Foods to Infants
Appendix JJ: Our Child Care Center Supports Breastfeeding

REFERENCES:

1. U.S. Department of Health and Human Services. 2000. *Healthy people 2010: Understanding and improving health*. 2nd ed. Washington, DC: U.S. Government Printing Office.
2. Dietitians of Canada, American Dietetic Association. 2000. *Manual of clinical dietetics*. 6th ed. Chicago: ADA.
3. U.S. Department of Agriculture, Food and Nutrition Service (FNS). 1993. *Breastfed babies welcome here!* Alexandria, VA: FNS.
4. American Academy of Pediatrics, Section on Breastfeeding. 2005. Policy statement: Breastfeeding and the use of human milk. *Pediatrics* 115:496-506.
5. Uauy, R., I. DeAndroca. 1995. Human milk and breast feeding for optimal brain development. *J Nutr* 125:2278-80.
6. Wang, Y. S., S. Y. Wu. 1996. The effect of exclusive breast feeding on development and incidence of infection in infants. *J Hum Lactation* 12:27-30.
7. Quasdt, S. 1998. Ecology of breast feeding in the US: An applied perspective. *Am J Hum Biol* 10:221-28.
8. Hammosh, M. 1996. Breast feeding and the working mother. *Pediatrics* 97:492-98.
9. Kramer M. S., L. Matush, I. Vanilovich, et al. 2007. Effects of prolonged and exclusive breastfeeding on child height, weight, adiposity, and blood pressure at age 6.5 y: Evidence from a large randomized trial. *Am J Clin Nutr* 86:1717–21.
10. Lawrence, R. A., R. Lawrence. 2005. *Breast feeding: A guide for the medical profession*. 6th ed. St. Louis: Mosby.
11. Birch, L., W. Dietz, eds. 2008. *Eating behaviors of the young child: Prenatal and postnatal influences on healthy eating*. Elk Grove Village, IL: American Academy of Pediatrics.
12. Dietz, W. H., L. Stern, eds. 1998. *American Academy of Pediatrics guide to your child's nutrition*. New York: Villard.
13. Kleinman, R. E., ed. 2009. *Pediatric nutrition handbook*. 6th ed. Elk Grove Village, IL: American Academy of Pediatrics.
14. U.S. Department of Agriculture, Food and Nutrition Service (FNS). 2002. *Feeding infants: A guide for use in the child nutrition programs*. Rev ed. Alexandria, VA: FNS. http://www.fns.usda.gov/tn/resources/feeding_infants.pdf.
15. Ip, S., M. Chung, G. Raman, P. Chew, N. Magula, D. DeVine, T. Trikalinos, J. Lau. 2007. *Breastfeeding and maternal and infant health outcomes in developed countries*. Rockville, MD: Agency for Healthcare Research and Quality.
16. U.S. Department of Agriculture, Food and Nutrition Service. Benefits and services: Breastfeeding promotion and support in WIC. http://www.fns.usda.gov/wic/breastfeeding/mainpage.HTM.
17. Stuebe, A. M., E. B. Schwarz. 2009. The risks and benefits of infant feeding practices for women and their children. *J Perinatology* (July 16).

STANDARD 4.3.1.2: Feeding Infants on Cue by a Consistent Caregiver/Teacher

Caregivers/teachers should feed infants on the infant's cue unless the parent/guardian and the child's primary care provider give written instructions otherwise (6). Whenever possible, the same caregiver/teacher should feed a specific infant for most of that infant's feedings. Cues such as opening the mouth, making suckling sounds, and moving the hands at random all send information from an infant to a caregiver/teacher that the infant is ready to feed. Caregivers/teachers should not feed infants beyond satiety, just as hunger cues are important in initiating feedings, observing satiety cues can limit overfeeding.

RATIONALE: Cue feeding meets the infant's nutritional and emotional needs and provides an immediate response to the infant, which helps ensure trust and feelings of security. Cues such as turning away from the nipple, increased attention to surroundings, keeping mouth closed, and saying no are all indications of satiation (1,2,6).

When the same caregiver/teacher regularly works with a particular child, that caregiver/teacher is more likely to understand that child's cues and to respond appropriately. Feeding infants on cue rather than on a schedule may help prevent childhood obesity (3,6). Early relationships between an infant and caregivers/teachers involving feeding set the stage for an infant to develop eating patterns for life (1,4).

COMMENTS: Caregivers/teachers should be gentle, patient, sensitive, and reassuring by responding appropriately to the infant's feeding cues (1). Waiting for an infant to cry to indicate hunger is not necessary or desirable. Crying may indicate that feeding cues have been missed and adequate attention has not been paid to the infant (5). Nevertheless, feeding children who are alert and interested in interpersonal interaction, but who are not showing signs of hunger, is not appropriate. Cues for hunger or interaction-seeking may vary widely in different infants. A pacifier should not be offered to a hungry infant, they need food first.

A series of trainings on infant cues can be found at NCAST-AVENUW, University of Washington at http://www.ncast.org/index.cfm?category=16.

TYPE OF FACILITY: Center; Large Family Child Care Home; Small Family Child Care Home

RELATED STANDARDS:

Standard 4.3.1.1: General Plan for Feeding Infants
Standard 4.3.1.8: Techniques for Bottle Feeding

REFERENCES:

1. Branscomb, K. R., C. B. Goble. 2008. Infants and toddlers in group care: Feeding practices that foster emotional health. *Young Children* 63:28-33.
2. Trahms, C. M., P. L. Pipes, eds. 1997. *Nutrition and infancy in childhood*. 6th ed. New York: McGraw-Hill.
3. Taveras, E. M., S. L. Rifas-Shiman, K. S. Scanlon, L. M. Grummer-Strawn, B. Sherry, M. W. Gillman. 2006. To what extent is the protective effect of breastfeeding on future overweight explained by decreased maternal feeding restriction? *Pediatrics* 118:2341-48.

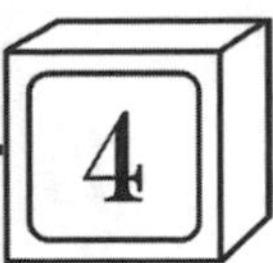

4. Hodges, E. A., S. O. Hughes, J. Hopkinson, J. O. Fisher. 2008. Maternal decisions about the initiation and termination of infant feeding. *Appetite* 50:333-39.
5. Hagan, Jr., J. F., J. S. Shaw, P. M. Duncan, eds. 2008. *Bright futures: Guidelines for health supervision of infants, children, and adolescents.* 3rd ed. Elk Grove Village, IL: American Academy of Pediatrics.
6. Satter, E. 2000. *Child of mine: Feeding with love and good sense*. 3rd ed. Boulder, CO: Bull Publishing.

STANDARD 4.3.1.3: Preparing, Feeding, and Storing Human Milk

Expressed human milk should be placed in a clean and sanitary bottle with a nipple that fits tightly or into an equivalent clean and sanitary sealed container to prevent spilling during transport to home or to the facility. Only cleaned and sanitized bottles, or their equivalent, and nipples should be used in feeding. The bottle or container should be properly labeled with the infant's full name and the date and time the milk was expressed. The bottle or container should immediately be stored in the refrigerator on arrival.

The mother's own expressed milk should only be used for her own infant. Likewise, infant formula should not be used for a breastfed infant without the mother's written permission.

Bottles made of plastics containing BPA or phthalates should be avoided (labeled with #3, #6, or #7). Glass bottles or plastic bottles labeled BPA-free or with #1, #2, #4, or #5 are acceptable.

Non-frozen human milk should be transported and stored in the containers to be used to feed the infant, identified with a label which will not come off in water or handling, bearing the date of collection and child's full name. The filled, labeled containers of human milk should be kept refrigerated. Human milk containers with significant amount of contents remaining (greater than one ounce) may be returned to the mother at the end of the day as long as the child has not fed directly from the bottle.

Frozen human milk may be transported and stored in single use plastic bags and placed in a freezer (not a compartment within a refrigerator but either a freezer with a separate door or a standalone freezer). Human milk should be defrosted in the refrigerator if frozen, and then heated briefly in bottle warmers or under warm running water so that the temperature does not exceed 98.6°F. If there is insufficient time to defrost the milk in the refrigerator before warming it, then it may be defrosted in a container of running cool tap water, very gently swirling the bottle periodically to evenly distribute the temperature in the milk. Some infants will not take their mother's milk unless it is warmed to body temperature, around 98.6°F. The caregiver/teacher should check for the infant's full name and the date on the bottle so that the oldest milk is used first. After warming, bottles should be mixed gently (not shaken) and the temperature of the milk tested before feeding.

Expressed human milk that presents a threat to an infant, such as human milk that is in an unsanitary bottle, is curdled, smells rotten, and/or has not been stored following the storage guidelines of the Academy of Breastfeeding Medicine as shown later in this standard, should be returned to the mother.

Some children around six months to a year of age may be developmentally ready to feed themselves and may want to drink from a cup. The transition from bottle to cup can come at a time when a child's fine motor skills allow use of a cup. The caregiver/teacher should use a clean small cup without cracks or chips and should help the child to lift and tilt the cup to avoid spillage and leftover fluid. The caregiver/teacher and mother should work together on cup feeding of human milk to ensure the child is receiving adequate nourishment and to avoid having a large amount of human milk remaining at the end of feeding. Two to three ounces of human milk can be placed in a clean cup and additional milk can be offered as needed. Small amounts of human milk (about an ounce) can be discarded.

Human milk can be stored using the following guidelines from the Academy of Breastfeeding Medicine:

Guidelines for Storage of Human Milk			
Location	**Temperature**	**Duration**	**Comments**
Countertop, table	Room temperature (up to 77°F or 25°C)	6-8 hours	Containers should be covered and kept as cool as possible; covering the container with a cool towel may keep milk cooler.
Insulated cooler bag	5°F – 39°F or -15°C – 4°C	24 hours	Keep ice packs in contact with milk containers at all times, limit opening cooler bag.
Refrigerator	39°F or 4°C	5 days	Store milk in the back of the main body of the refrigerator.
Freezer compartment of a refrigerator	5°F or -15°C	2 weeks	Store milk toward the back of the freezer, where temperature is most constant. Milk stored for longer durations in the ranges listed is safe, but some of the lipids in the milk undergo degradation resulting in lower quality.
Freezer compartment of refrigerator with separate doors	0°F or -18°C	3-6 months	
Chest or upright deep freezer	-4°F or -20°C	6-12 months	

Source: Academy of Breastfeeding Medicine Protocol Committee. 2010. Clinical protocol #8: Human milk storage information for home use for healthy full term infants, revised. *Breastfeeding Med* 5:127-30. http://www.bfmed.org/Resources/Download.aspx?filename=Protocol 8 - English.pdf.

From the Centers for Disease Control and Prevention Website: Proper handling and storage of human milk – Storage duration of fresh human milk for use with healthy full term infants. http://www.cdc.gov/breastfeeding/recommendations/handling_breastmilk.htm.

RATIONALE: Labels for containers of human milk should be resistant to loss of the name and date/time when washing and handling. This is especially important when the frozen bottle is thawed in running tap water. There may be several bottles from different mothers being thawed and warmed at the same time in the same place.

By following this standard, the staff is able, when necessary, to prepare human milk and feed an infant safely, thereby reducing the risk of inaccuracy or feeding the infant unsanitary or incorrect human milk (2,5). Written guidance for both staff and parents/guardians should be available to determine when milk provided by parents/guardians will not be served. Human milk cannot be served if it does not meet the requirements for sanitary and safe milk.

Excessive shaking of human milk may damage some of the cellular components that are valuable to the infant.

It is difficult to maintain 0°F consistently in a freezer compartment of a refrigerator or freezer, so caregivers/teachers should carefully monitor, with daily log sheets, temperature of freezers used to store human milk using an appropriate working thermometer. Human milk contains components that are damaged by excessive heating during or after thawing from the frozen state (1). Currently, there is nothing in the research literature that states that feedings must be warmed at all prior to feeding. Frozen milk should never be thawed in a microwave oven as 1) uneven hot spots in the milk may cause burns in the infant and 2) excessive heat may destroy beneficial components of the milk.

By following safe preparation and storage techniques, nursing mothers and caregivers/teachers of breastfed infants and children can maintain the high quality of expressed human milk and the health of the infant (3,4,6).

COMMENTS: Although human milk is a body fluid, it is not necessary to wear gloves when feeding or handling human milk. Unless there is visible blood in the milk, the risk of exposure to infectious organisms either during feeding or from milk that the infant regurgitates is not significant.

Returning unused human milk to the mother informs her of the quantity taken while in the early care and education program.

TYPE OF FACILITY: Center; Large Family Child Care Home; Small Family Child Care Home

RELATED STANDARDS:
Standard 4.3.1.1: General Plan for Feeding Infants
Standard 4.3.1.4: Feeding Human Milk to Another Mother's Child
Standard 4.3.1.7: Feeding Cow's Milk
Standard 4.3.1.8: Techniques for Bottle Feeding
Standard 4.3.1.9: Warming Bottles and Infant Foods

REFERENCES:
1. American Academy of Pediatrics, Section on Breastfeeding. 2005. Policy statement: Breastfeeding and the use of human milk. *Pediatrics* 115:496-506.
2. Clark, A., J. Anderson, E. Adams, S. Baker. 2008. Assessing the knowledge, attitudes, behaviors and training needs related to infant feeding, specifically breastfeeding, of child care providers. *Matern Child Health J* 12:128-35.
3. Kleinman, R. E., ed. 2009. *Pediatric nutrition handbook*. 6th ed. Elk Grove Village, IL: American Academy of Pediatrics.
4. Samour, P. Q., K. King. 2005. *Handbook of pediatric nutrition*. 3rd ed. Lake Dallas, TX: Helm.
5. Lawrence, R. A., R. Lawrence. 2005. *Breast feeding: A guide for the medical profession*. 6th ed. St. Louis: Mosby.
6. Endres, J. B., R. E. Rockwell. 2003. *Food, nutrition, and the young child*. 4th ed. New York: Macmillan.

STANDARD 4.3.1.4: Feeding Human Milk to Another Mother's Child

If a child has been mistakenly fed another child's bottle of expressed human milk, the possible exposure to hepatitis B, hepatitis C, or HIV should be treated as if an exposure to other body fluids had occurred. For possible exposure to hepatitis B, hepatitis C, or HIV, the caregiver/teacher should:

a) Inform the mother who expressed the human milk about the mistake and when the bottle switch occurred, and ask:
   1) When the human milk was expressed and how it was handled prior to being delivered to the caregiver/teacher or facility;
   2) Whether she has ever had a hepatitis B, hepatitis C, or HIV blood test and, if so, the date of the test and would she be willing to share the results with the parents/guardians of the child who was fed the incorrect milk;
   3) If she does not know whether she has ever been tested for hepatitis B, hepatitis C, or HIV, would she be willing to contact her primary care provider and find out if she has been tested;
   4) If she has never been tested for hepatitis B, hepatitis C, or HIV, would she be willing to be tested and share the results with the parents/guardians of the other child;
b) Discuss the mistake of giving the wrong milk with the parents/guardians of the child who was fed the wrong bottle:
   1) Inform them that their child was given another child's bottle of expressed human milk and the date it was given;
   2) Inform them that the risk of transmission of hepatitis B, hepatitis C, or HIV and other infectious diseases is low;
   3) Encourage the parents/guardians to notify the child's primary care provider of the exposure;
   4) Provide the family with information including the time at which the milk was expressed and how the milk was handled prior to its being delivered to the caregiver/teacher so that the parents/guardians may inform the child's primary care provider;
   5) Inform the parents/guardians that, depending upon the results from the mother whose milk was given mistakenly (1), their child may soon need to undergo a baseline blood test for hepatitis B (also see below), hepatitis C, or HIV;
c) Assess why the wrong milk was given and develop a prevention plan to be shared with the parents/guardians as well as the staff in the facility.

If the human milk given mistakenly to a child is from a woman who does not know her hepatitis B status, the caregiver/teacher should determine if the child has received the complete hepatitis B vaccine series. If the child has not been vaccinated or is incompletely vaccinated, then the parent/guardian of the child who received the milk should seek vaccination of the child. The child should complete the recommended childhood hepatitis B vaccine series as soon as possible. If human milk from a hepatitis B-positive woman is given mistakenly to a an unimmunized child, the child may receive HBIG (Hepatitis B Immune Globulin) as soon as possible within seven days, but it is not necessary because of the low risk of transmission (3). The hepatitis B vaccine series should be initiated and completed as soon as possible.

RATIONALE: The risk of hepatitis B, hepatitis C, or HIV transmission from expressed human milk consumed by another child is believed to be low because:

a) In the United States, women who are HIV-positive and aware of that fact are advised NOT to breastfeed their infants and therefore the potential for exposure to milk from an HIV-positive woman is low;
b) In the United States, women with high hepatitis C antiviral loads or who have cracked or bleeding nipples might transmit the infection through breastfeeding. Therefore, they are advised to refrain from breastfeeding (3,4);
c) Chemicals present in human milk act, together with time and cold temperatures, to destroy the HIV present in expressed human milk;
d) Transmission of HIV from a single human milk exposure has never been documented (1).

Because parents/guardians may express concern about the likelihood of transmitting these diseases through human milk, this issue is addressed in detail to assure there is a very small risk of such transmission occurring.

Among known HIV-positive women in Africa (where HIV-positive women are still advised to breastfeed only if they are located in areas where the water supply is unreliable), a study found that the transmission rate among infants who were fed infected human milk exclusively for several months was found to be 4%; thirteen infants out of 324 (2).

TYPE OF FACILITY: Center; Large Family Child Care Home; Small Family Child Care Home

RELATED STANDARDS:

Standard 4.3.1.3: Preparing, Feeding, and Storing Human Milk

REFERENCES:

1. Centers for Disease Control and Prevention. What to do if an infant or child is mistakenly fed another woman's expressed breast milk. http://www.cdc.gov/breastfeeding/recommendations/other_mothers_milk.htm.

2. Becquet, R., D. K. Ekouevi, H. Menan, C. Amani-Bosse, L. Bequet, I. Viho, F. Dabis, M. Timite-Konan, V. Leroy. 2008. Early mixed feeding and breastfeeding beyond 6 months increase the risk of postnatal HIV transmission. *Prev Med* 47:27-33.

3. Pickering, L. K., C. J. Baker, D. W. Kimberlin, S. J. Long, eds. 2009. *Red book: 2009 report of the Committee on Infectious Diseases*. Elk Grove Village, IL: American Academy of Pediatrics.

4. Philip Spradling, CDC, email message to the NRC, May 12, 2010.

STANDARD 4.3.1.5: Preparing, Feeding, and Storing Infant Formula

Formula provided by parents/guardians or by the facility should come in a factory-sealed container. The formula should be of the same brand that is served at home and should be of ready-to-feed strength or liquid concentrate to be diluted using water from a source approved by the health department. Powdered infant formula, though it is the least expensive formula, requires special handling in mixing because it cannot be sterilized. The primary source for proper and safe handling and mixing is the manufacturer's instructions that appear on the can of powdered formula. Before opening the can, hands should be washed. The can and plastic lid should be thoroughly rinsed and dried. Caregivers/teachers should read and follow the manufacturer's directions. If instructions are not readily available, caregivers/teachers should obtain information from the World Health Organization's *Safe Preparation, Storage and Handling of Powdered Infant Formula Guidelines* at http://www.who.int/foodsafety/publications/micro/pif2007/en/index.html (8). The local WIC program can also provide instructions.

Formula mixed with cereal, fruit juice, or any other foods should not be served unless the child's primary care provider provides written documentation that the child has a medical reason for this type of feeding.

Iron-fortified formula should be refrigerated until immediately before feeding. For bottles containing formula, any contents remaining after a feeding should be discarded.

Bottles of formula prepared from powder or concentrate or ready-to-feed formula should be labeled with the child's full name and time and date of preparation. Any prepared formula must be discarded within one hour after serving to an infant. Prepared powdered formula that has not been given to an infant should be covered, labeled with date and time of preparation and child's full name, and may be stored in the refrigerator for up to twenty-four hours. An open container of ready-to-feed, concentrated formula, or formula prepared from concentrated formula, should be covered, refrigerated, labeled with date of opening and child's full name, and discarded at forty-eight hours if not used (7,9). The caregiver/teacher should always follow manufacturer's instructions for mixing and storing of any formula preparation.

Some infants will require specialized formula because of allergy, inability to digest certain formulas, or need for extra calories. The appropriate formula should always be available and should be fed as directed. For those infants getting supplemental calories, the formula may be prepared in a different way from the directions on the container. In those circumstances, either the family should provide the prepared formula or the caregiver/teacher should receive special training, as noted in the infant's care plan, on how to prepare the formula.

RATIONALE: This standard promotes the feeding of infant formula that is familiar to the infant and supports family feeding practice. By following this standard, the staff is able, when necessary, to prepare formula and feed an infant safely, thereby reducing the risk of inaccuracy or feeding the infant unsanitary or incorrect formula. Written guidance for both staff and parents/guardians must be available to determine when formula provided by parents/guardians will not be served. Formula cannot be served if it does not meet the requirements for sanitary and safe formula.

If a child has a special health problem, such as reflux, or inability to take in nutrients because of delayed development of feeding skills, the child's primary care provider should provide a written plan for the staff to follow so that the child is fed appropriately. Some infants are allergic to milk and soy and need to be fed an elemental formula which does not contain allergens. Other infants need supplemental calories because of poor weight gain.

Infants should not be fed a formula different from the one the parents/guardians feed at home, as even minor differences in formula can cause gastrointestinal upsets and other problems (6).

Excessive shaking of formula may cause foaming that increases the likelihood of feeding air to the infant.

Formula should not be used beyond the stated shelf life period (1).

COMMENTS: The intent of this standard is to protect a child's health by ensuring safe and sanitary conditions for transporting and feeding infant formula prepared at home and brought to the facility, and by ensuring that all infants get the proper formula.

Parents/guardians should supply enough clean and sterilized bottles to be used throughout the day. The bottles must be sanitary, properly prepared and stored, and must be the same brand in the early care and education program and at home.

Staff preparing formula should thoroughly wash their hands prior to beginning preparation of infant feedings of any type. Water used for mixing infant formula must be from a safe water source as defined by the local or state health department. If the caregiver/teacher is concerned or uncertain about the safety of the tap water, s/he may use bottled water or bring cold tap water to a rolling boil for one minute (no longer), then cool the water to room temperature for no more than thirty minutes before it is used. Warmed water should be tested in advance to make sure it is not too hot for the infant. To test the temperature, the caregiver/teacher should shake a few drops on the inside of her/his wrist. A bottle can be prepared by adding powdered formula and room temperature water from the tap just before feeding. Bottles made in this way from powdered formula can be ready for feeding as no additional refrigeration or warming would be required.

Caregivers/teachers should only use the scoop that comes with the can and not interchange the scoop from one product to another, since the volume of the scoop may vary from manufacturer to manufacturer and product to product. Also, a scoop can be contaminated with a potential allergen from another type of formula. Although many infant formulas are made from powder, the liquid preparations are diluted with water at the factory. Concentrated infant formula, not ready-to feed, must be diluted with water. Sealed, ready-to-feed bottles are easy to use, however they are the most expensive approach to feeding formula.

If concentrated liquid or powdered infant formulas are used, it is very important to prepare them properly, with accurate dilution, according to the directions on the container. Adding too little water to formula puts a burden on an infant's kidneys and digestive system and may lead to dehydration (4). Adding too much water dilutes the formula. Diluted formula may interfere with an infant's growth and health because it provides inadequate calories and nutrients and can cause water intoxication. Water intoxication can occur in breastfed or formula-fed infants or children over one year of age who are fed an excessive amount of water. Water intoxication can be life-threatening to an infant or young child (5).

TYPE OF FACILITY: Center; Large Family Child Care Home; Small Family Child Care Home

RELATED STANDARDS:
Standard 4.3.1.1: General Plan for Feeding Infants
Standard 4.3.1.8: Techniques for Bottle Feeding
Standard 4.3.1.9: Warming Bottles and Infant Foods

REFERENCES:
1. Kleinman, R. E., ed. 2009. *Pediatric nutrition handbook*. 6th ed. Elk Grove Village, IL: American Academy of Pediatrics.
2. Dietitians of Canada, American Dietetic Association. 2000. *Manual of clinical dietetics*. 6th ed. Chicago: ADA.
3. Pipes, P. L., C. M. Trahms, eds. 1997. *Nutrition in infancy and childhood*. 6th ed. New York: McGraw-Hill.
4. Institute for Safe Medication Practices. Infant formula: Read and follow the label instructions! http://www.ismp.org/consumers/Formula.asp.
5. U.S. Department of Agriculture, Food and Nutrition Service (FNS). 2001. *Feeding infants: A guide for use in the child nutrition programs*. Rev ed. Alexandria, VA: FNS. http://www.fns.usda.gov/tn/resources/feeding_infants.pdf.
6. American Academy of Pediatrics, Section on Breastfeeding. 2005. Policy statement: Breastfeeding and the use of human milk. *Pediatrics* 115:496-506.
7. Fomon, S. J. 1993. *Nutrition of normal infants*. St. Louis: Mosby.
8. World Health Organization (WHO), Food and Agriculture Organization of the United Nations. 2007. *Safe preparation, storage and handling of powdered infant formula: Guidelines*. Geneva: WHO.
9. International Formula Council. Guidelines for traveling with infants: Keeping formula safe and sound. http://www.infantformula.org/for-parents/traveling-infants/.

STANDARD 4.3.1.6: Use of Soy-Based Formula and Soy Milk

Soy-based formula or soy milk should be provided to a child whose parents/guardians present a written request because of family dietary restrictions on foods produced from animals (i.e., cow's milk and other dairy products). Both soy-based formula and soy milk should be labeled with the infant's or child's full name and date and stored properly.

The caregiver/teacher should collaborate with parents/guardians in exploring community resources to secure soy-based formula. Soy milk should be available for the children of parents/guardians participating in the Women, Infants, and Children (WIC) Supplemental Food Program, Child and Adult Care Food Program (CACFP), or Food Stamp Program.

RATIONALE: The American Academy of Pediatrics (AAP) recommends use of hypoallergenic formula (not soy-based formula) for infants who are allergic to cow's milk proteins. Soy-based formulas are appropriate for children with galactosemia or congenital lactose intolerance (1). Because there is a lot of confusion in the public regarding cow's milk proteins and lactose intolerance, these indications should be documented by the child's primary care provider and not based on parental/guardian possible misinterpretation of symptoms. Soy-based formulas are made from soy meal (plant based) with added methionine, carbohydrates, and oils (soy or vegetable) and are fortified with vitamins and minerals (2). In the U.S., all soy-based formula is fortified with iron. Soy meal does not contain lactose, so it is used for feeding infants with primary care provider documented congenital lactose intolerance.

COMMENTS: The taste of soy milk is similar to cow's milk. Because soy formula and soy milk are derived from a plant source, parents/guardians may choose these products for dietary (e.g., vegan) or religious reasons. In such cases, soy-based formula is used for infant feeding and unflavored soy milk is the choice for young children.

Caregivers/teachers should encourage parents/guardians of children with primary care provider documented indications for soy formula, participating in WIC and/or Food Stamp Programs, to learn how they can obtain soy-based infant formula or soy milk/products.

Infants may need a variety of special or elemental formulas which are easier to digest and less allergenic. Elemental or special non-allergic formulas should be specified in the infant's care plan.

TYPE OF FACILITY: Center; Large Family Child Care Home; Small Family Child Care Home

RELATED STANDARDS:
Standard 4.2.0.12: Vegetarian/Vegan Diets
Standard 4.3.1.5: Preparing, Feeding, and Storing Infant Formula

REFERENCES:
1. Bhatia, J., F. Greer, Committee on Nutrition. 2008. Use of soy protein-based formulas for infant feeding. *Pediatrics* 121:1062-68.
2. Dietitians of Canada, American Dietetic Association (ADA). 2000. *Manual of clinical dietetics*. 6th ed. Chicago: ADA.

STANDARD 4.3.1.7: Feeding Cow's Milk

The facility should not serve cow's milk to infants from birth to twelve months of age, unless provided with a written exception and direction from the child's primary care provider and parents/guardians. Children between twelve and twenty-four months of age, who are not on human milk or prescribed formula, can be served whole pasteurized milk, or reduced fat (2%) pasteurized milk for those children who are at risk for hypercholesterolemia or obesity (1). Children two years of age and older should be served skim or 1% pasteurized milk.

RATIONALE: For children between twelve months and twenty-four months of age, for whom overweight or obesity is a concern or who have a family history of obesity, dyslipidemia, or early cardiovascular disease, the use of reduced fat (2%) milk is appropriate (1). The child's primary care provider may also recommend reduced fat (2%) milk for some children this age. Studies show no compromise in growth, and no difference in height, weight, or percentage of body fat and neurological development in toddlers fed reduced fat (2%) milk compared with those fed whole milk (2,8,9). The American Academy of Pediatrics recommends that cow's milk not be used during the first year of life (3-7).

COMMENTS: Sometimes early care and education programs have children ages eighteen months to three years of age in one classroom and staff report it is difficult to serve different types of milk (1% and 2%) to specific children. Programs can use a different color label for each type of milk on the container or pitcher. Caregivers/teachers can explain to the children the meaning of the color labels and identify which milk they are drinking.

TYPE OF FACILITY: Center; Large Family Child Care Home; Small Family Child Care Home

RELATED STANDARDS:
Standard 4.2.0.4: Categories of Foods
Standard 4.9.0.3: Precautions for a Safe Food Supply

REFERENCES:
1. Daniels, S. R., F. R. Greer, Committee on Nutrition. 2008. Lipid screening and cardiovascular health in childhood. *Pediatrics* 122:198-208.
2. Wosje, K. S., B. L. Specker, J. Giddens. 2001. No differences in growth or body composition from age 12 to 24 months between toddlers consuming 2% milk and toddlers consuming whole milk. *J Am Diet Assoc* 101:53-56.
3. Dietz, W. H., L. Stern, eds. 1998. *American Academy of Pediatrics guide to your child's nutrition*. New York: Villard.
4. Kleinman, R. E., ed. 2009. *Pediatric nutrition handbook*. 6th ed. Elk Grove Village, IL: American Academy of Pediatrics.
5. Dietitians of Canada, American Dietetic Association. 2000. *Manual of clinical dietetics*. 6th ed. Chicago: ADA.
6. Pipes, P. L., C. M. Trahms, eds. 1997. *Nutrition in infancy and childhood*. 6th ed. New York: McGraw-Hill.
7. American Academy of Pediatrics, Committee on Nutrition. 1992. The use of whole cow's milk in infancy. *Pediatrics* 89:1105-9.
8. Rask-Nissila, L., E. Jokinen, P. Terho, A. Tammi, H. Lapinleimu, T. Ronnemaa, J. Viikari, R. Seppanen, T. Korhonen, J. Tuominen, I. Valimaki, O. Simell. 2000. Neurological development of 5-year-old children receiving a low-saturated fat, low-cholesterol diet since infancy: A randomized controlled trial. *JAMA* 284:993-1000.
9. Niinikoski, H. Lapinleimu, , J. Viikari, H. Lapinleimu, T. Rönnemaa, E. Jokinen, R. Seppänen, P. Terho, J. Tuominen, I. Välimäki, O. Simell. 1997. Growth until 3 years of age in a prospective, randomized trial of a diet with reduced saturated fat and cholesterol. *Pediatrics* 99:687-94.

STANDARD 4.3.1.8: Techniques for Bottle Feeding

Infants should always be held for bottle feeding. Caregivers/teachers should hold infants in the caregiver's/teacher's arms or sitting up on the caregiver's/teacher's lap. Bottles should never be propped. The facility should not permit infants to have bottles in the crib. The facility should not permit an infant to carry a bottle while standing, walking, or running around.

Bottle feeding techniques should mimic approaches to breastfeeding:

a) Initiate feeding when infant provides cues (rooting, sucking, etc.);
b) Hold the infant during feedings and respond to vocalizations with eye contact and vocalizations;
c) Alternate sides of caregiver's/teacher's lap;
d) Allow breaks during the feeding for burping;
e) Allow infant to stop the feeding.

A caregiver/teacher should not bottle feed more than one infant at a time.

Bottles should be checked to ensure they are given to the appropriate child, have human milk, infant formula, or water in them.

When using a bottle for a breastfed infant, a nipple with a cylindrical teat and a wider base is usually preferable. A shorter or softer nipple may be helpful for infants with a hypersensitive gag reflex, or those who cannot get their lips well back on the wide base of the teat (22).

The use of a bottle or cup to modify or pacify a child's behavior should not be allowed (1,16).

RATIONALE: The manner in which food is given to infants is conducive to the development of sound eating habits for life. Caregivers/teachers should promote proper feeding practices and oral hygiene including proper use of the bottle for all infants and toddlers. Bottle propping can cause choking and aspiration and may contribute to long-term health issues, including ear infections (otitis media), orthodontic problems, speech disorders, and psychological problems (1-6). When infants and children are "cue fed", they are in control of frequency and amount of feedings. This has been found to reduce the risk of childhood obesity.

Any liquid except plain water can cause early childhood caries (7-18). Early childhood caries in primary teeth may hold significant short-term and long-term implications for the child's health (7-18). Frequently sipping any liquid besides plain water between feeds encourages tooth decay.

Children are at an increased risk for injury when they walk around with bottle nipples in their mouths. Bottles should not be allowed in the crib or bed for safety and sanitary reasons and for preventing dental caries. It is difficult for a caregiver/teacher to be aware of and respond to infant feeding cues when the child is in a crib or bed and when feeding more than one infant at a time.

COMMENTS: Caregivers/teachers and parents/guardians need to understand the relationship between bottle feeding and emotional security. Caregivers/teachers should hold infants who are bottle feeding whenever possible, even if the children are old enough to hold their own bottle.

Caregivers/teachers should offer children fluids from a cup as soon as they are developmentally ready. Some children may be able to drink from a cup around six months of age, while for others it is later (2). Weaning a child to drink from a cup is an individual process, which occurs over a wide range of time. The American Academy of Pediatric Dentistry

(AAPD) recommends weaning from a bottle by the child's first birthday (1-3,6-9). Instead of sippy cups, caregivers/teachers should use smaller cups and fill halfway or less to prevent spills as children learn to use a cup (19-21). If sippy cups are used, it should only be for a very short transition period.

Some children around six months to a year of age may be developmentally ready to feed themselves and may want to drink from a cup. The transition from bottle to cup can come at a time when a child's fine motor skills allow use of a cup. The caregiver/teacher should use a clean small cup without cracks or chips and should help the child to lift and tilt the cup to avoid spillage and leftover fluid. The caregiver/teacher and parent/guardian should work together on cup feeding of human milk to ensure the child's receiving adequate nourishment and to avoid having a large amount of human milk remaining at the end of feeding. Two to three ounces of human milk can be placed in a clean cup and additional milk can be offered as needed. Small amounts of human milk (about an ounce) can be discarded.

Infants should be burped after every feeding and preferably during the feeding as well.

TYPE OF FACILITY: Center; Large Family Child Care Home; Small Family Child Care Home

RELATED STANDARDS:
Standard 4.3.1.2: Feeding Infants on Cue by a Consistent Caregiver/Teacher
Standard 4.3.1.9: Warming Bottles and Infant Foods

REFERENCES:
1. Kleinman, R. E., ed. 2009. *Pediatric nutrition handbook*. 6th ed. Elk Grove Village, IL: American Academy of Pediatrics.
2. Casamassimo, P., K. Holt, eds. 2004. *Bright futures in practice: Oral health–pocket guide*. Washington, DC: National Maternal and Child Oral Health Resource Center. http://www.mchoralhealth.org/PDFs/BFOHPocketGuide.pdf.
3. Dietitians of Canada, American Dietetic Association. 2000. *Manual of clinical dietetics*. 6th ed. Chicago: ADA.
4. Wang, Y. S., S. Y. Wu. 1996. The effect of exclusive breast feeding on development and incidence of infection in infants. *J Hum Lactation* 12:27-30.
5. American Academy of Pediatric Dentistry. 1993. Recommendation for preventive pediatric dental care. *Pediatr Dent* 15:158-59.
6. American Academy of Pediatric Dentistry. 1994. Reference manual, 1994-1995. *Pediatr Dent* 16:196.
7. Schafer, T. E., S. M. Adair. 2000. Prevention of dental disease: The role of the pediatrician. *Pediatr Clin North Am* 47:1021-42.
8. Ramos-Gomez, F. J. 2005. Clinical considerations for an infant oral health care program. *Compend Contin Educ Dent* 26:17-23.
9. Ramos-Gomez, F. J., B. Jue, C. Y. Bonta. 2002. Implementing an infant oral care program. *J Calif Dent Assoc* 30:752-61.
10. U.S. Department of Health and Human Services (DHHS). 2000. *Oral health in America: A report of the surgeon general–Executive summary*. Rockville, MD: DHHS, National Institute of Dental and Craniofacial Research, National Institutes of Health.
11. Section on Pediatric Dentistry and Oral Health. 2008. Preventive oral health intervention for pediatricians. *Pediatrics* 122:1387-94.
12. New York State Department of Health. 2006. Oral health care during pregnancy and early childhood: Practice guidelines. Albany, NY: New York State Department of Health. http://www.health.state.ny.us/publications/0824.pdf.
13. American Dental Association. 2004. From baby bottle to cup: Choose training cups carefully, use them temporarily. *J Am Dent Assoc* 135:387.
14. American Dental Association. ADA statement on early childhood caries. http://www.ada.org/2057.aspx.
15. The American Academy of Pediatric Dentistry (AAPD). 2002. Policy on baby bottle tooth decay (BBTD)/early childhood caries (ECC). In *Reference manual 2002-2003,* 23. Chicago, IL: AAPD. http://www.aapd.org/members/referencemanual/pdfs/02-03/Baby Bottle Tooth Decay.pdf.
16. American Academy of Pediatrics. 2007. Brushing up on oral health: Never too early to start. *Healthy Children* (Winter): 14-15. http://www.healthychildren.org/english/healthy-living/oral-health/pages/Brushing-Up-on-Oral-Health-Never-Too-Early-to-Start.aspx.
17. Tinanoff, N., C. Palmer. 2000. Dietary determinants of dental caries and dietary recommendations for preschool children. *J Public Health Dent* 60:197-206.
18. Pipes, P. L., C. M. Trahms, eds. 1997. *Nutrition in infancy and childhood*. 6th ed. New York: McGraw-Hill.
19. Prolonged use of sippy cups under scrutiny. 2002. *Dentistry Today* 21:44.
20. Behrendt, A., F. Szlegoleit, V. Muler-Lessmann, G. Ipek-Ozdemir, W. F. Wetzel. 2001. Nursing-bottle syndrome caused by prolonged drinking from vessels with bill-shaped extensions. *ASDC J Dent Child* 68:47-54.
21. Satter, E. 2000. *Child of mine: Feeding with love and good sense*. 3rd ed. Boulder, CO: Bull Publishing.
22. Watson Genna, C. 2008. *Supporting sucking skills in breastfeeding infants*. Sudbury, MA: Jones and Bartlett.

STANDARD 4.3.1.9: Warming Bottles and Infant Foods

Bottles and infant foods can be served cold from the refrigerator and do not have to be warmed. If a caregiver/teacher chooses to warm them, bottles should be warmed under running, warm tap water or by placing them in a container of water that is no warmer than 120°F. Bottles should not be left in a pot of water to warm for more than five minutes. Bottles and infant foods should never be warmed in a microwave oven.

Infant foods should be stirred carefully to distribute the heat evenly. A caregiver/teacher should not hold an infant while removing a bottle or infant food from the container of warm water or while preparing a bottle or stirring infant food that has been warmed in some other way. Only BPA-free plastic, plastic labeled #1, #2, #4 or #5, or glass bottles should be used.

If a slow-cooking device, such as a crock pot, is used for warming infant formula, human milk, or infant food, this slow-cooking device should be out of children's reach, should contain water at a temperature that does not exceed 120°F, and should be emptied, cleaned, sanitized, and refilled with fresh water daily.

RATIONALE: Bottles of human milk or infant formula that are warmed at room temperature or in warm water for an extended time provide an ideal medium for bacteria to grow. Infants have received burns from hot water dripping from an infant bottle that was removed from a crock pot or by pulling the crock pot down on themselves by a dangling cord. Caution should be exercised to avoid raising the water temperature above a safe level for warming infant formula or infant food. Human milk, formula, or food fed to infants should never be heated in a microwave oven as uneven hot spots in milk and/or food may burn the infant (1,2).

TYPE OF FACILITY: Center; Large Family Child Care Home; Small Family Child Care Home

RELATED STANDARDS:

Standard 4.3.1.8: Techniques for Bottle Feeding
Standard 4.3.1.12: Feeding Age-Appropriate Solid Foods to Infants

REFERENCES:

1. Nemethy, M., E. R. Clore. 1990. Microwave heating of infant formula and breast milk. *J Pediatr Health Care* 4:131-35.
2. Dixon J. J., D. A. Burd, D. G. Roberts. 1997. Severe burns resulting from an exploding teat on a bottle of infant formula milk heated in a microwave oven. *Burns* 23:268-69.

STANDARD 4.3.1.10: Cleaning and Sanitizing Equipment Used for Bottle Feeding

Bottles, bottle caps, nipples and other equipment used for bottle feeding should not be reused without first being cleaned and sanitized by washing in a dishwasher or by washing, rinsing, and boiling them for one minute.

RATIONALE: Infant feeding bottles are contaminated by the child's saliva during feeding. Formula and milk promote growth of bacteria, yeast, and fungi. Bottles, bottle caps, and nipples that are reused should be washed and sanitized to avoid contamination from previous feedings.

COMMENTS: Excessive boiling of latex bottle nipples will damage them. Nipples that are discolored, thinning, tacky, or ripped should not be used.

TYPE OF FACILITY: Center; Large Family Child Care Home; Small Family Child Care Home

STANDARD 4.3.1.11: Introduction of Age-Appropriate Solid Foods to Infants

A plan to introduce age-appropriate solid foods (complementary foods) to infants should be made in consultation with the child's parent/guardian and primary care provider. Age-appropriate solid foods may be introduced no sooner than when the child has reached the age of four months, but preferably six months and as indicated by the individual child's nutritional and developmental needs.

For breastfed infants, gradual introduction of iron-fortified foods may occur no sooner than around four months, but preferably six months and to complement the human milk. Modification of basic food patterns should be provided in writing by the child's primary care provider.

Evidence for introducing complementary foods in a specific order or rate is not available. The current best practice is that the first solid foods should be single-ingredient foods and should be introduced one at a time at two- to seven-day intervals (1).

RATIONALE: Early introduction of age-appropriate solid food and fruit juice interferes with the intake of human milk or iron-fortified formula that the infant needs for growth. Age-appropriate solid food given before an infant is developmentally ready may be associated with allergies and digestive problems (2,8). Around about six months of age, breastfed infants may require an additional source of iron. Vitamin drops with iron may be needed. Infants who are not exclusively fed human milk should consume iron-fortified formula as the substitute for human milk (9). In the United States, major non-milk sources of iron in the infant diet are iron-fortified cereal and meats (2). Zinc is important for healthy growth and proper immune function. Infant stores of zinc may subsidize the intake from human milk for several months. Age-appropriate solid foods such as meat (a good source of zinc) are needed beginning at six months (2). A full daily allowance of vitamin C is found in human milk (3). The American Academy of Pediatrics (AAP) recommends that all breastfed or partially breastfed infants receive a minimum daily intake of 400 IU of vitamin D supplementation beginning soon after birth until they consume sufficient vitamin D fortified milk (about one quart per day) to meet the 400 IU daily requirements (4). These supplements should be given at home by the parents/guardians to take the burden off the caregiver/teacher.

The transitional phase of feeding age-appropriate solid foods which occurs no sooner than four months and preferably six months of age is a critical time for development of gross, fine, and oral motor skills. When an infant is able to hold his/her head steady, open her/his mouth, lean forward in anticipation of food offered, close the lips around a spoon, and transfer from front of the tongue to the back and swallow, s/he is ready to eat semi-solid foods. The process of learning a more mature style of eating begins because of physical growth occurring concurrently with social, cultural, sociological, and physiological development.

COMMENTS: Many infants find fruit juices appealing and may be satisfied by the calories in age-appropriate solid foods so that they subsequently drink less human milk or formula. When fruit juice is introduced at one year of age, it should be by cup rather than a bottle or other container (such as a box) to decrease the occurrence of dental caries. Infants, birth up to one year of age, should not be served juice. Whole fruit, mashed or pureed, is appropriate for infants seven months up to one year of age. Children one year of age through age six should be limited to a total of four to six ounces of juice per day.

Many people believe that infants sleep better when they start to eat age-appropriate solid foods, however research shows that longer sleeping periods are developmentally and not nutritionally determined in mid-infancy (2,5).

An important goal of early childhood nutrition is to ensure children's present and future health by fostering the development of healthy eating behaviors (2,9). Caregivers/teachers are responsible for providing a variety of nutritious foods, defining the structure and timing of meals and creating a mealtime environment that facilitates eating and social

exchange (7). Children are responsible for participating in choices about food selection and should be allowed to take responsibility for determining how much is consumed at each eating occasion (2).

Good communication between the caregiver/teacher and the parents/guardians cannot be over-emphasized and is essential for successful feeding in general, including when and how to introduce age-appropriate solid foods. The decision to feed specific foods should be made in consultation with the parent/guardian. Caregivers/teachers should be given written instructions on the introduction and feeding of foods from the infant's parent/guardian and primary care provider. Caregivers/teachers can use or develop a take-home sheet for parents/guardians in which the caregiver/teacher records the food consumed, how much, and other important notes on the infant, each day. Caregivers/teachers should continue to consult with each infant's parents/guardians concerning which foods they have introduced and are feeding. This schedule of introducing new foods one at a time, followed by waiting two to seven days before introducing another new food, enables parents and caregivers/teachers to pinpoint any problems a child might have with any specific food (10). Following this schedule for introducing new foods, the caregiver/teacher can more easily identify an infant's possible food allergy or intolerance. Consistency between home and the early care and education setting is essential during the period of rapid change when infants are learning to eat age-appropriate solid foods (6,8).

TYPE OF FACILITY: Center; Large Family Child Care Home; Small Family Child Care Home

RELATED STANDARDS:

Standard 4.2.0.7: 100% Fruit Juice
Standard 4.2.0.9: Written Menus and Introduction of New Foods
Standard 4.2.0.10: Care for Children with Food Allergies
Standard 4.3.1.12: Feeding Age-Appropriate Solid Foods to Infants
Standard 4.5.0.8: Experience with Familiar and New Foods

REFERENCES:

1. Hagan, Jr., J. F., J. S. Shaw, P. M. Duncan, eds. 2008. Promoting healthy nutrition. In *Bright futures: Guidelines for health supervision of infants, children, and adolescents.* 3rd ed. Elk Grove Village, IL: American Academy of Pediatrics. http://brightfutures.aap.org/pdfs/Guidelines_PDF/6-Promoting_Healthy_Nutrition.pdf.
2. Kleinman, R. E., ed. 2009. *Pediatric nutrition handbook*. 6th ed. Elk Grove Village, IL: American Academy of Pediatrics.
3. Lawrence, R. A., R. Lawrence. 2005. *Breast feeding: A guide for the medical profession*. 6th ed. St. Louis: Mosby.
4. Wagner, C. L., F. R. Greer, Section on Breastfeeding, Committee on Nutrition. 2008. Prevention of rickets and vitamin D deficiency in infants, children, and adolescents. *Pediatrics* 122:1142–52.
5. Lally, J. R., A. Griffin, E. Fenichel, M. Segal, E. Szanton, B. Weissbourd. 2003. *Caring for infants and toddlers in groups: Developmentally appropriate practice*. Arlington, VA: Zero to Three.
6. U.S. Department of Agriculture, Food and Nutrition Service (FNS). 2002. *Feeding infants: A guide for use in the child nutrition programs*. Rev ed. Alexandria, VA: FNS. http://www.fns.usda.gov/tn/resources/feeding_infants.pdf.
7. Branscomb, K. R., C. B. Goble. 2008. Infants and toddlers in group care: Feeding practices that foster emotional health. *Young Children* 63:28-33.
8. Grummer-Strawn, L. M., K. S. Scanlon, S. B. Fein. 2008. Infant feeding and feeding transitions during the first year of life. *Pediatrics* 122: S36-S42.
9. Griffiths, L. J., L. Smeeth, S. S. Hawkins, T. J. Cole, C. Dezateux. 2008. Effects of infant feeding practice on weight gain from birth to 3 years. *Arch Dis Child* (November): 1-17.
10. Pipes, P. L., C. M. Trahms, eds. 1997. *Nutrition in infancy and childhood*. 6th ed. New York: McGraw-Hill.

STANDARD 4.3.1.12: Feeding Age-Appropriate Solid Foods to Infants

Staff members should serve commercially packaged baby food from a dish, not directly from a factory-sealed container. They should serve age-appropriate solid food (complementary food) by spoon only. Age-appropriate solid food should not be fed in a bottle or an infant feeder unless written in the child's care plan by the child's primary care provider. Caregivers/teachers should discard uneaten food left in dishes from which they have fed a child. The facility should wash off all jars of baby food with soap and warm water before opening the jars, and examine the food carefully when removing it from the jar to make sure there are not glass pieces or foreign objects in the food.

Food should not be shared among children using the same dish or spoon. Unused portions in opened factory-sealed baby food containers or food brought in containers prepared at home should be stored in the refrigerator and discarded if not consumed after twenty-four hours of storage.

RATIONALE: Feeding of age-appropriate solid foods in a bottle to a child is often associated with premature feeding of age-appropriate solid foods (when the infant is not developmentally ready for them) (1-5).

The external surface of a commercial container may be contaminated with disease-causing microorganisms during shipment or storage and may contaminate the food product during feeding. The portion of the food that is touched by a utensil should be consumed or discarded. A dish should be cleaned and sanitized before use, thereby reducing the likelihood of surface contamination. Any food brought from home should not be served to other children. This will prevent cross-contamination and reinforce the policy that food sent to the facility is for the designated child only.

Uneaten food should not be put back into its original container for storage because it may contain potentially harmful bacteria from the infant's saliva. Age-appropriate solid food should not be fed in a bottle or an infant feeder apparatus because of the potential for choking. Additionally, this feeding method teaches the infant to eat age-appropriate solid foods incorrectly.

TYPE OF FACILITY: Center; Large Family Child Care Home; Small Family Child Care Home

RELATED STANDARDS:

Standard 4.3.1.11: Introduction of Age-Appropriate Solid Foods to Infants

REFERENCES:

1. Kleinman, R. E., ed. 2009. *Pediatric nutrition handbook*. 6th ed. Elk Grove Village, IL: American Academy of Pediatrics.

2. Dietitians of Canada, American Dietetic Association (ADA). 2000. *Manual of clinical dietetics*. 6th ed. Chicago: ADA.
3. Endres, J. B., R. E. Rockwell. 2003. *Food, nutrition, and the young child*. 4th ed. New York: Macmillan.
4. Samour, P. Q., K. King. 2005. *Handbook of pediatric nutrition*. 3rd ed. Lake Dallas, TX: Helm.
5. Lawrence, R. A., R. Lawrence. 2005. *Breast feeding: A guide for the medical profession*. 6th ed. St. Louis: Mosby.

4.3.2 Nutrition for Toddlers and Preschoolers

STANDARD 4.3.2.1: Meal and Snack Patterns for Toddlers and Preschoolers

Meals and snacks should contain at least the minimum amount of foods shown in the meal and snack patterns for toddlers and preschoolers described in the Child and Adult Care Food Program (CACFP) guidelines at http://www.fns.usda.gov/cnd/care/ProgramBasics/Meals/Meal_Patterns.htm.

RATIONALE: Even during periods of slower growth, children must continue to eat nutritious foods. With limited appetites and selective eating by toddlers and preschoolers, less nutritious foods should not be served as they can displace more nutritious foods from the child's diet.

COMMENTS: Children who are eating more than one snack and one meal may not want all the food offered at any one of these times. On the other hand, toddlers and preschoolers may eat only some meals or some snacks. The amount of food offered to them must be sufficient to meet their needs at that particular time but not too large to promote overeating.

TYPE OF FACILITY: Center; Large Family Child Care Home; Small Family Child Care Home

RELATED STANDARDS:
Standard 4.2.0.4: Categories of Food
Standard 4.2.0.5: Meal and Snack Patterns

STANDARD 4.3.2.2: Serving Size for Toddlers and Preschoolers

The facility should serve toddlers and preschoolers small-sized, age-appropriate portions and should permit children to have one or more additional servings of the nutritious foods that are low in fat, sugar, and sodium as needed to meet the caloric needs of the individual child. Serving dishes should contain the appropriate amount of food based on serving sizes or portions recommended for each child and adult as described in the Child and Adult Care Food Program (CACFP) guidelines at http://www.fns.usda.gov/cnd/care/ProgramBasics/Meals/Meal_Patterns.htm. Young children should learn what appropriate portion size is by being served in plates, bowls, and cups that are developmentally appropriate to their nutritional needs.

Food service staff and/or a caregiver/teacher is responsible for preparing the amount of food based on the recommended age-appropriate amount of food per serving for each child to be fed. Usually a reasonable amount of additional food is prepared to respond to a child or children requesting a second serving of the nutritious foods that are low in fat, sugar, and sodium.

RATIONALE: Gradual extension of the diet begun in infancy should continue throughout the preschool period. A child will not eat the same amount each day because appetites vary and food sprees are common (1-5). If normal variations in eating patterns are accepted without comment, feeding problems usually do not develop. Requiring that a child eat a specified food or amount of food may be counterproductive. Eating habits established in infancy and early childhood may contribute to suboptimal eating patterns later in life. Including nutritious snacks in the daily meal plan will help to ensure that the child's nutrient needs are met. The quality of snacks for young children and school-age children is especially important, and small, frequent feedings are recommended to achieve the total desired daily intake.

Strong evidence supports that larger plate, bowl, and cup sizes promote overeating in adults (6,7). It is likely that the same is true in children. Larger serving sizes and what is considered "normal" serving size (portion size distortion), at least in part is explained by increasing size of plates, bowls, and cups.

COMMENTS: Continuing to meet the child's needs for growth and activity is important. During the second and third years of life, the child grows much less rapidly than during the first year of life.

Standardized recipes for cooking for young children are available and are a valuable resource. Periodic training is also available from resources such as regional Head Start agencies, State Child Care agencies, resource and referral agencies, local health departments, local colleges, and universities.

Size appropriate plates, bowls, and cups in early care and education settings should help children and caregivers/teachers recognize and understand appropriate portion sizes. They may also help decrease the risk of overeating.

TYPE OF FACILITY: Center; Large Family Child Care Home; Small Family Child Care Home

RELATED STANDARDS:
Standard 4.3.2.1: Meal and Snack Patterns for Toddlers and Preschoolers
Standard 4.3.2.3: Encouraging Self-Feeding by Older Infants and Toddlers

REFERENCES:
1. Kleinman, R. E., ed. 2009. *Pediatric nutrition handbook*. 6th ed. Elk Grove Village, IL: American Academy of Pediatrics.
2. Endres, J. B., R. E. Rockwell. 2003. *Food, nutrition, and the young child*. 4th ed. New York: Macmillan.
3. U.S. Department of Agriculture, Food Service and Nutrition. 2010. Child and adult care food program. http://www.fns.usda.gov/CND/Care/CACFP/aboutcacfp.htm.
4. U.S. Department of Agriculture (USDA). 2002. *Making nutrition count for children – Nutrition guidance for child care homes*. Washington, DC: USDA. http://www.fns.usda.gov/tn/Resources/nutritioncount.html.

5. Pipes, P. L., C. M. Trahms, eds. 1997. *Nutrition in infancy and childhood*. 6th ed. New York: McGraw-Hill.
6. Wansink, B. 2004. Environmental factors that increase the food intake and consumption volume of unknowing consumers. *Annual Review of Nutrition* 24:455-79.
7. Wansink, B., J. E. Painter, J. North. 2005. Bottomless bowls: Why visual cues of portion size may influence intake. *Obesity Research* 13:93-100.

STANDARD 4.3.2.3: Encouraging Self-Feeding by Older Infants and Toddlers

Caregivers/teachers should encourage older infants and toddlers to hold and drink from an appropriate child-sized cup, to use a child-sized spoon (short handle with a shallow bowl like a soup spoon), a child-sized fork (short, blunt tines and broad handle similar to a salad fork), all of which are developmentally appropriate for young children to feed themselves, and to use their fingers for self-feeding.

RATIONALE: As children enter the second year of life, they are interested in doing things for themselves. Self-feeding appropriately separates the responsibilities of adults and children. The adult is responsible for providing nutritious food, and the child is responsible for deciding how much of it to eat (1-5). To allow for the proper development of motor skills and eating habits, children need to be allowed to practice learning to feed themselves (6-8). Children in group care should be provided with opportunities to serve and eat a variety of food for themselves. Children will continue to self-feed using their fingers even after mastering the use of a utensil.

COMMENTS: Foods served should be appropriate to the toddler's developmental ability and cut small enough to avoid choking hazards.

TYPE OF FACILITY: Center; Large Family Child Care Home; Small Family Child Care Home

RELATED STANDARDS:
Standard 4.3.2.2: Serving Size for Toddlers and Preschoolers
Standard 4.5.0.5: Numbers of Children Fed Simultaneously by One Adult
Standard 4.5.0.6: Adult Supervision of Children Who are Learning to Feed Themselves

REFERENCES:
1. Benjamin, S. E., ed. 2007. *Making food healthy and safe for children: How to meet the national health and safety performance standards – Guidelines for out of home child care programs*. 2nd ed. Chapel Hill, NC: National Training Institute for Child Care Health Consultants. http://nti.unc.edu/course_files/curriculum/nutrition/making_food_healthy_and_safe.pdf.
2. Kleinman, R. E., ed. 2009. *Pediatric nutrition handbook*. 6th ed. Elk Grove Village, IL: American Academy of Pediatrics.
3. Endres, J. B., R. E. Rockwell. 2003. *Food, nutrition, and the young child*. 4th ed. New York: Macmillan.
4. Pipes, P. L., C. M. Trahms, eds. 1997. *Nutrition in infancy and childhood*. 6th ed. New York: McGraw-Hill.
5. Briley, M. E., C. Roberts-Gray. 1999. Position of the American Dietetic Association: Nutrition standards for child-care programs. *J Am Diet Assoc* 99:981-88.
6. Branscomb, K. R., C. B. Goble. 2008. Infants and toddlers in group care: Feeding practices that foster emotional health. *Young Children* 63:28-33.
7. Hagan, Jr., J. F., J. S. Shaw, P. M. Duncan, eds. 2008. *Bright futures: Guidelines for health supervision of infants, children, and adolescents*. 3rd ed. Elk Grove Village, IL: American Academy of Pediatrics.
8. University of Idaho, College of Agricultural and Life Sciences. Feeding young children in group settings. http://www.cals.uidaho.edu/feeding/.

4.3.3 Nutrition for School-Age Children

STANDARD 4.3.3.1: Meal and Snack Patterns for School-Age Children

Meals and snacks should contain at a minimum the meal and snack patterns shown for school-age children in the Child and Adult Care Food Program (CACFP) guidelines found at http://www.fns.usda.gov/cnd/care/ProgramBasics/Meals/Meal_Patterns.htm.

Children attending facilities for two or more hours after school need at least one snack.

Breakfast is recommended for all children enrolled in an early care and education facility or in school. Depending on age, in-between eating such as a snack should occur about two hours after a meal based on the total length of time a child is in care. Child care facilities enrolled in the CACFP must allow at least one and a half hours between the end of a snack and the beginning of another meal and they must allow three hours between the end of one meal to the beginning of the next meal. CACFP requirements differ from state to state; see CACFP's Website for current recommendations.

RATIONALE: The principles of providing adequate, nourishing food for younger children apply to this group as well. This age is characterized by a rapid rate of growth that increases the need for energy and essential nutrients to support optimal growth. Food intake may vary considerably because this is a time when children express strong food likes and dislikes. The quantity and quality of food provided should contribute toward meeting nutritional needs for the day and should not dull the appetite (1-5).

COMMENTS: A nutrient analysis was conducted of the CACFP requirements, to ensure that a snack and lunch meet two-thirds of the Recommended Dietary Allowances (6).

TYPE OF FACILITY: Center; Large Family Child Care Home; Small Family Child Care Home

REFERENCES:
1. Hagan, Jr., J. F., J. S. Shaw, P. M. Duncan, eds. 2008. *Bright futures: Guidelines for health supervision of infants, children, and adolescents*. 3rd ed. Elk Grove Village, IL: American Academy of Pediatrics.
2. Story, M., K. Holt, D. Sofka, eds. 2002. *Bright futures in practice: Nutrition*. 2nd ed. Arlington, VA: National Center for Education in Maternal and Child Health. http://www.brightfutures.org/nutrition/pdf/frnt_mttr.pdf.

3. Benjamin, S. E., ed. 2007. *Making food healthy and safe for children: How to meet the national health and safety performance standards – Guidelines for out of home child care programs*. 2nd ed. Chapel Hill, NC: National Training Institute for Child Care Health Consultants. http://nti.unc.edu/course_files/curriculum/nutrition/making_food_healthy_and_safe.pdf.
4. Endres, J. B., R. E. Rockwell. 2003. *Food, nutrition, and the young child*. 4th ed. New York: Macmillan.
5. Pipes, P. L., C. M. Trahms, eds. 1997. *Nutrition in infancy and childhood*. 6th ed. New York: McGraw-Hill.
6. Briley, M. E., C. Roberts-Gray. 1999. Position of the American Dietetic Association: Nutrition standards for child-care programs. *J Am Diet Assoc* 99:981-88.

4.4 Staffing

STANDARD 4.4.0.1: Food Service Staff by Type of Facility and Food Service

Each center-based facility should employ trained staff and provide ongoing supervision and consultation in accordance with individual site needs as determined by the nutritionist/registered dietitian. In centers, prior work experience in food service should be required for the solitary worker responsible for food preparation without continuous on-site supervision of a food service manager. For facilities operating six or more hours a day or preparing and serving food on the premises, the following food service staff requirements should apply:

Setting	Food Service Staff
Small and large family child care homes	Caregiver/teacher and/or helper (note: some large homes must have a helper)
Centers serving up to 30 children	Full-time child care Food Service Worker (cook)
Centers serving up to 50 children	Full-time child care Food Service Worker (cook) and part-time child care Food Service Aide
Centers serving up to 125 children	Full-time child care Food Service Manager or full-time child care Food Service Worker (cook) and full-time child care Food Service Aide
Centers serving up to 200 children	Full-time child care Food Service Manager and full-time child care Food Service Worker (cook) and one full-time plus one part-time child care Food Service Aide
Vendor food service	One assigned staff member or one part-time staff member, depending on amount of food service preparation needed after delivery

RATIONALE: Trained personnel are essential workers in the food service of facilities to assure the maintenance of nutrition standards required in these facilities (1-6). Home cooking experience is not enough when large volumes of food must be served to children and adults. The type of food service, type of equipment, number of children to be fed, location of the facility, and food budget determine the staffing patterns. An adequate number of food service personnel is essential to ensure that children are fed according to the facility's daily schedule. If a facility that operates for six or more hours a day serves only food brought from home, food service staff is needed to oversee the appropriate use of such food.

COMMENTS: The food service staff may not necessarily consist of full-time or regular staff members but may include some workers hired on a consulting or contractual basis. Resources for food service staff include vocational high school food preparation programs, university and community college food preparation programs, and trade schools that train cooks and chefs.

TYPE OF FACILITY: Center, Large Family Child Care Home, Small Family Child Care Home

RELATED STANDARDS:
Appendix C: Nutrition Specialist, Registered Dietitian, Licensed Nutritionist, Consultant, and Food Service Staff Qualifications

REFERENCES:
1. Benjamin, S. E., ed. 2007. *Making food healthy and safe for children: How to meet the National health and safety performance standards – Guidelines for out of home child care programs*. 2nd ed. Chapel Hill, NC: National Training Institute for Child Care Health Consultants. http://nti.unc.edu/course_files/curriculum/nutrition/making_food_healthy_and_safe.pdf.
2. Enders, J. B. 1994. *Food, nutrition and the young child*. New York: Merrill.
3. Pipes, P. L., C. M. Trahms, eds. 1997. *Nutrition in infancy and childhood*. 6th ed. New York: McGraw-Hill.
4. Briley, M. E., C. Roberts-Gray. 1999. Position of the American Dietetic Association: Nutrition standards for child-care programs. *J Am Diet Assoc* 99:981-88.
5. U.S. Department of Agriculture (USDA), Food and Nutrition Service. 2009. *USDA recipes for child care*. http://teamnutrition.usda.gov/Resources/childcare_recipes.html.
6. U.S. Department of Agriculture, Food and Nutrition Service. 2008. *Food Buying Guide for Child Nutrition Programs*. Rev ed. http://www.fns.usda.gov/tn/Resources/foodbuyingguide.html.

STANDARD 4.4.0.2: Use of Nutritionist/ Registered Dietitian

A local nutritionist/registered dietitian, knowledgeable of the specific needs of infants and children, should work with the on-site food service expert and the architect or engineer on the design of the parts of the facility involved in food service. Additionally the nutritionist/registered dietitian should work with the food service expert and the early care and education staff to develop and to implement the facility's nutrition plan and to prepare the initial food service budget. The nutrition plan encompasses:

a) Kitchen layout;
b) Food budget and service;
c) Food procurement and food storage;
d) Menu and meal planning (including periodic review of menus);
e) Food preparation and service;
f) Child feeding practices and policies;
g) Kitchen and mealtime staffing;

h) Nutrition education for children, staff and parents/guardians (including the prevention of childhood obesity and other chronic diseases, food learning experiences, and knowledge of choking hazards);
i) Dietary modification plans.

RATIONALE: Efficient and cost-effective food service in a facility begins with a plan and evaluation of the physical components of the facility. Planning for the food service unit includes consideration of location and adequacy of space for receiving, storing, preparing, and serving areas; cleaning up; dish washing; dining areas, plus space for desk, telephone, records, and employee facilities (such as handwashing sinks, toilets, and lockers). All facets must be considered for new or existing sites, including remodeling or renovation of the unit (1-5).

COMMENTS: Nutritionists/registered dietitians assist food service staff/caregivers/teachers in planning menus for meals/snacks consisting of healthy foods which meet CACFP guidelines; ensuring use of age-appropriate eating utensils and suitable furniture (tables, chairs) for children to sit comfortably while eating; addressing any dietary modification needed; providing training for staff and nutrition education for children and their parents/guardians; consulting on meeting local health department regulations and meeting local regulations when using an off-site food vendor. This standard is primarily for Centers.

TYPE OF FACILITY: Center; Large Family Child Care Home; Small Family Child Care Home

RELATED STANDARDS:
Standard 3.1.2.1: Routine Health Supervision and Growth Monitoring
Standard 4.2.0.1: Written Nutrition Plan
Standard 4.2.0.2: Assessment and Planning of Nutrition for Individual Children
Standard 4.2.0.8: Feeding Plans and Dietary Modifications
Standard 9.2.3.11: Food and Nutrition Service Policies and Plans
Appendix C: Nutrition Specialist, Registered Dietitian, Licensed Nutritionist, Consultant, and Food Service Staff Qualifications

REFERENCES:

1. Endres, J. B., R. E. Rockwell. 2003. *Food, nutrition, and the young child*. 4th ed. New York: Macmillan.
2. U.S. Department of Agriculture (USDA). 2002. *Making nutrition count for children - Nutrition guidance for child care homes*. Washington, DC: USDA. http://www.fns.usda.gov/tn/Resources/nutritioncount.html.
3. Pipes, P. L., C. M. Trahms, eds. 1997. Nutrition in infancy and childhood. 6th ed. New York: McGraw-Hill.
4. Benjamin, S. E., K. A. Copeland, A. Cradock, E. Walker, M. M. Slining, B. Neelon, M. W. Gillman. 2009. Menus in child care: A comparison of state regulations to national standards. *J Am Diet Assoc* 109:109-15.
5. Kaphingst, K. M., M. Story. 2009. Child care as an untapped setting for obesity prevention: State child care licensing regulations related to nutrition, physical activity, and media use for preschool-aged children in the United States. *Prev Chronic Dis* 6(1).

4.5 Meal Service, Seating, and Supervision

STANDARD 4.5.0.1: Developmentally Appropriate Seating and Utensils for Meals

The child care staff should ensure that children who do not require highchairs are comfortably seated at tables that are between waist and mid-chest level and allow the seated child's feet to rest on a firm surface.

All furniture and eating utensils that a child care facility uses should make it possible for children to eat at their best skill level and to increase their eating skill.

RATIONALE: Proper seating while eating reduces the risk of food aspiration and improves comfort in eating (7,9).

Suitable furniture and utensils, in addition to providing comfort, enable the children to perform eating tasks they have already mastered and facilitate the development of skill and coordination in handling food and utensils (4-6,8,9).

COMMENTS: Eating utensils should be unbreakable, durable, attractive, and suitable in function, size, and shape for use by children. Dining areas, whether in a classroom or in a separate area, should be clean and cheerful (1-6).

Compliance can be measured by observing the fit of the furniture for children.

TYPE OF FACILITY: Center; Large Family Child Care Home; Small Family Child Care Home

RELATED STANDARDS:
Standard 4.5.0.2: Tableware and Feeding Utensils

REFERENCES:

1. U.S. Department of Health and Human Services, Administration for Children and Families (ACF). 2006. *Head Start Program Performance Standards and other Regulations*. Rev ed. Washington, DC: ACF, Head Start Bureau.
2. Story, M., K. Holt, D. Sofka, eds. 2002. *Bright futures in practice: Nutrition*. 2nd ed. Arlington, VA: National Center for Education in Maternal and Child Health. http://www.brightfutures.org/nutrition/pdf/frnt_mttr.pdf.
3. Benjamin, S. E., ed. 2007. *Making food healthy and safe for children: How to meet the National health and safety performance standards – Guidelines for out of home child care programs*. 2nd ed. Chapel Hill, NC: National Training Institute for Child Care Health Consultants. http://nti.unc.edu/course_files/curriculum/nutrition/making_food_healthy_and_safe.pdf.
4. Enders, J. B. 1994. *Food, nutrition and the young child*. New York: Merrill.
5. U.S. Department of Agriculture (USDA). 2002. *Making nutrition count for children - Nutrition guidance for child care homes*. Washington, DC: USDA. http://www.fns.usda.gov/tn/Resources/nutritioncount.html.
6. Pipes, P. L., C. M. Trahms, eds. 1997. *Nutrition in infancy and childhood*. 6th ed. New York: McGraw-Hill.
7. U.S. Department of Agriculture (USDA), Food and Nutrition Service. 2009. *USDA recipes for child care*. http://teamnutrition.usda.gov/Resources/childcare_recipes.html.
8. Hagan, Jr., J. F., J. S. Shaw, P. M. Duncan, eds. 2008. *Bright futures: Guidelines for health supervision of infants, children, and*

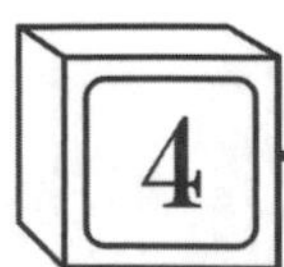

adolescents. 3rd ed. Elk Grove Village, IL: American Academy of Pediatrics.

9. Fletcher, J., L. Branen, E. Price. 2005. *Building mealtime environments and relationships: An inventory for feeding young children in group settings*. Moscow, ID: University of Idaho. http://www.cals.uidaho.edu/feeding/pdfs/BMER.pdf.

STANDARD 4.5.0.2: Tableware and Feeding Utensils

Tableware and feeding utensils should meet the following requirements:

a) Dishes should have smooth, hard, glazed surfaces and should be free from cracks or chips. Sharp-edged plastic utensils (intended for use in the mouth) or dishes that have sharp or jagged edges should not be used;

b) Imported dishes and imported ceramic dishware or pottery should be certified by the regulatory health authority to meet U.S. standards and to be safe from lead or other heavy metals before they can be used;

c) Disposable tableware (such as plates, cups, utensils made of heavy weight paper, food-grade medium-weight or BPA- or phthalates-free plastic) should be permitted for single service if they are discarded after use. The facility should not use foam tableware for children under four years of age;

d) Single-service articles (such as napkins, paper placemats, paper tablecloths, and paper towels) should be discarded after one use;

e) Washable bibs, placemats, napkins, and tablecloths, if used, should be laundered or washed, rinsed, and sanitized after each meal. Fabric articles should be sanitized by being machine-washed and dried after each use;

f) Highchair trays, plates, and all items used in food service that are not disposable should be washed, rinsed, and sanitized. Highchair trays that are used for eating should be washed, rinsed, and sanitized just before and immediately after they are used for eating. Children who eat at tables should have disposable or washed and sanitized plates for their food;

g) All surfaces in contact with food should be lead-free;

h) Tableware and feeding utensils should be child-sized and developmentally appropriate.

RATIONALE: Clean food service utensils, napkins, bibs, and tablecloths prevent the spread of microorganisms that can cause disease. The surfaces that are in contact with food must be sanitary.

Food should not be put directly on the table surface for two reasons. First, even washed and sanitized tables are more likely to be contaminated than disposable plates or washed and sanitized dishes. Second, eating from plates reduces contamination of the table surface when children put down their partially eaten food while they are eating.

Although highchair trays can be considered tables, they function as plates for seated children. The tray should be washed and sanitized before and after use (1-3). The use of disposable items eliminates the spread of contamination and disease and fosters safety and injury prevention. Single-service items are usually porous and should not be washed and reused. Items intended for reuse must be capable of being washed, rinsed, and sanitized.

Medium-weight plastic should be chosen because lighter-weight plastic utensils are more likely to have sharp edges and break off small pieces easily. Sharp-edged plastic spoons can cut soft oral tissues, especially when an adult is feeding a child and slides the spoon out of the child's closed mouth. Older children can cut their mouth tissues in the same way.

Foam can break into pieces that can become choking hazards for young children.

Imported dishware may be improperly fired and may release toxic levels of lead into food. U.S. government standards prevent the marketing of domestic dishes with lead in their glazes. There is no safe level of lead in dishware.

COMMENTS: Ideally, food should not be placed directly on highchair trays, as studies have shown that highchair trays can be loaded with infectious microorganisms. If the highchair tray is made of plastic, is in good repair, and is free from cracks and crevices, it can be made safe if it is washed and sanitized before placing a child in the chair for feeding and if the tray is washed and sanitized after each child has been fed. Food must not be placed directly on highchair trays made of wood or metal, other than stainless steel, to prevent contamination by infectious microorganisms or toxicity from metals.

If there is a question about whether tableware is safe and sanitary, consult the regulatory health authority or local health department.

TYPE OF FACILITY: Center; Large Family Child Care Home; Small Family Child Care Home

RELATED STANDARDS:
Standard 4.9.0.9: Cleaning of Food Areas and Equipment
Standard 5.2.9.9: Plastic Containers and Toys

REFERENCES:

1. U.S. Department of Health and Human Services, Administration for Children and Families (ACF). 2006. *Head Start Program Performance Standards and other Regulations*. Rev ed. Washington, DC: ACF, Head Start Bureau.

2. Benjamin, S. E., ed. 2007. *Making food healthy and safe for children: How to meet the National health and safety performance standards – Guidelines for out of home child care programs*. 2nd ed. Chapel Hill, NC: National Training Institute for Child Care Health Consultants. http://nti.unc.edu/course_files/curriculum/nutrition/making_food_healthy_and_safe.pdf.

3. Enders, J. B. 1994. *Food, nutrition and the young child*. New York: Merrill.

STANDARD 4.5.0.3: Activities that Are Incompatible with Eating

Children should be seated when eating. Caregivers/teachers should ensure that children do not eat when standing, walking, running, playing, lying down, watching TV, playing on the computer, or riding in vehicles.

Children should not be allowed to continue to feed themselves or continue to be assisted with feeding themselves if they begin to fall asleep while eating. Caregivers/teachers should check that no food is left in a child's mouth before laying a child down to sleep.

RATIONALE: Seating children, while they are eating, reduces the risk of aspiration (1-4). Eating while doing other activities (including playing, walking around, or sitting at a computer) limits opportunities for socialization during meals and snacks. Eating while watching television is associated with an increased risk of obesity (5-8). Continuing to eat while falling asleep puts the child at great risk for gagging or choking.

COMMENTS: Staff can role model appropriate eating behaviors by sitting down when they are eating and eating "family style" with the children when possible.

TYPE OF FACILITY: Center; Large Family Child Care Home; Small Family Child Care Home

RELATED STANDARDS:
Standard 4.5.0.4: Socialization During Meals

REFERENCES:
1. Benjamin, S. E., ed. 2007. *Making food healthy and safe for children: How to meet the national health and safety performance standards – Guidelines for out of home child care programs*. 2nd ed. Chapel Hill, NC: National Training Institute for Child Care Health Consultants. http://nti.unc.edu/course_files/curriculum/nutrition/making_food_healthy_and_safe.pdf.
2. Lally, J. R., A. Griffin, E. Fenichel, M. Segal, E. Szanton, B. Weissbourd. 2003. *Caring for infants and toddlers in groups: Developmentally appropriate practice*. Arlington, VA: Zero to Three.
3. Endres, J. B., R. E. Rockwell. 2003. *Food, nutrition, and the young child*. 4th ed. New York: Macmillan.
4. U.S. Department of Agriculture (USDA). 2002. *Making nutrition count for children - Nutrition guidance for child care homes*. Washington, DC: USDA. http://www.fns.usda.gov/tn/Resources/nutritioncount.html.
5. Briley, M., C. Roberts-Gray. 2005. Position of the American Dietetic Association: Benchmarks for nutrition programs in child care settings. *J Am Dietetic Association* 105:979–86.
6. Andersen, R. E., C. J. Crespo, S. J. Bartlett, L. J. Cheskin, M. Pratt. 1998. Relationship of physical activity and television watching with body weight and level of fatness among children. *J Am Med Assoc* 279:938-42.
7. Dennison, B. A., T. A. Erb, P. L. Jenkins. 2002. Television viewing and television in bedroom associated with overweight risk among low-income preschool children. *Pediatrics* 109:1028-35.
8. Mendoza, J. A., F. J. Zimmerman, D. A. Christakis. 2007. Television viewing, computer use, obesity, and adiposity in US preschool children. *Int J Behav Nutr Physical Activity* 4, no. 44 (September 25). http://ijbnpa.org/content/4/1/44/.

STANDARD 4.5.0.4: Socialization During Meals

Caregivers/teachers and children should sit at the table and eat the meal or snack together. Family style meal service, with the serving platters, bowls, and pitchers on the table so all present can serve themselves, should be encouraged, except for infants and very young children who require an adult to feed them. A separate utensil should be used for serving. Children should not handle foods that they will not be consuming. The adults should encourage, but not force, the children to help themselves to all food components offered at the meal. When eating meals with children, the adult(s) should eat items that meet nutrition standards. The adult(s) should encourage social interaction and conversation, using vocabulary related to the concepts of color, shape, size, quantity, number, temperature of food, and events of the day. Extra assistance and time should be provided for slow eaters. Eating should be an enjoyable experience at the facility and at home.

Special accommodations should be made for children who cannot have the food that is being served. Children who need limited portion sizes should be taught and monitored.

RATIONALE: "Family style" meal service promotes and supports social, emotional, and gross and fine motor skill development. Caregivers/teachers sitting and eating with children is an opportunity to engage children in social interactions with each other and for positive role-modeling by the adult caregiver/teacher. Conversation at the table adds to the pleasant mealtime environment and provides opportunities for informal modeling of appropriate eating behaviors, communication about eating, and imparting nutrition learning experiences (1-3,5-7). The presence of an adult or adults, who eat with the children, helps prevent behaviors that increase the possibility of fighting, feeding each other, stuffing food into the mouth and potential choking, and other negative behaviors. The future development of children depends, to no small extent, on their command of language. Richness of language increases as adults and peers nurture it (5). Family style meals encourage children to serve themselves which develops their eye-hand coordination (3-5). In addition to being nourished by food, infants and young children are encouraged to establish warm human relationships by their eating experiences. When children lack the developmental skills for self-feeding, they will be unable to serve food to themselves. An adult seated at the table can assist and be supportive with self-feeding so the child can eat an adequate amount of food to promote growth and prevent hunger.

COMMENTS: Compliance is measured by structured observation. Use of small pitchers, a limited number of portions on service plates, and adult assistance to enable children to successfully serve themselves helps to make family style service possible without contamination or waste of food.

TYPE OF FACILITY: Center; Large Family Child Care Home; Small Family Child Care Home

RELATED STANDARDS:
Standard 4.3.2.2: Serving Size for Toddlers and Preschoolers
Standard 4.3.2.3: Encouraging Self-Feeding by Older Infants and Toddlers
Standard 4.7.0.1: Nutrition Learning Experiences for Children

REFERENCES:
1. U.S. Department of Health and Human Services, Administration for Children and Families, Office of Head Start. 2009. *Head Start program performance standards*. Rev. ed. Washington, DC: U.S. Government Printing Office. http://eclkc.ohs.acf.hhs.gov/hslc/Head Start Program/Program Design and Management/Head Start

Requirements/Head Start Requirements/45 CFR Chapter XIII/45 CFR Chap XIII_ENG.pdf.
2. Benjamin, S. E., ed. 2007. *Making food healthy and safe for children: How to meet the national health and safety performance standards – Guidelines for out of home child care programs*. 2nd ed. Chapel Hill, NC: National Training Institute for Child Care Health Consultants. http://nti.unc.edu/course_files/curriculum/nutrition/making_food_healthy_and_safe.pdf.
3. Endres, J. B., R. E. Rockwell. 2003. *Food, nutrition, and the young child*. 4th ed. New York: Macmillan.
4. U.S. Department of Agriculture (USDA). 2002. *Making nutrition count for children - Nutrition guidance for child care homes*. Washington, DC: USDA. http://www.fns.usda.gov/tn/Resources/nutritioncount.html.
5. Pipes, P. L., C. M. Trahms, eds. 1997. *Nutrition in infancy and childhood*. 6th ed. New York: McGraw-Hill.
6. Branscomb, K. R., C. B. Goble 2008. Infants and toddlers in group care: Feeding practices that foster emotional health. *Young Children* 63:28-33.
7. Sigman-Grant, M., E. Christiansen, L. Branen, J. Fletcher, S. L. Johnson. 2008. About feeding children: Mealtimes in child-care centers in four western states. *J Am Diet Assoc* 108:340-46.

STANDARD 4.5.0.5: Numbers of Children Fed Simultaneously by One Adult

One adult should not feed more than one infant or three children who need adult assistance with feeding at the same time.

RATIONALE: Cross-contamination among children whom one adult is feeding simultaneously poses significant risk. In addition, mealtime should be a socializing occasion. Feeding more than three children at the same time necessarily resembles an impersonal production line. It is difficult for the caregiver/teacher to be aware of and respond to infant feeding cues when feeding more than one infant at a time. A child may need one-on-one feeding based on age or degree of ability. Feeding more than three children also presents a potential risk of injury and/or choking.

TYPE OF FACILITY: Center; Large Family Child Care Home; Small Family Child Care Home

RELATED STANDARDS:
Standard 4.3.1.2: Feeding Infants on Cue by a Consistent Caregiver/Teacher
Standard 4.3.2.2: Serving Size for Toddlers and Preschoolers
Standard 4.3.2.3: Encouraging Self-Feeding by Older Infants and Toddlers
Standard 4.5.0.4: Socialization During Meals
Standard 4.5.0.6: Adult Supervision of Children Who are Learning to Feed Themselves

STANDARD 4.5.0.6: Adult Supervision of Children Who Are Learning to Feed Themselves

Children in mid-infancy who are learning to feed themselves should be supervised by an adult seated within arm's reach of them at all times while they are being fed. Children over twelve months of age who can feed themselves should be supervised by an adult who is seated at the same table or within arm's reach of the child's highchair or feeding table. When eating, children should be within sight of an adult at all times.

RATIONALE: A supervising adult should watch for several common problems that typically occur when children in mid-infancy begin to feed themselves. "Squirreling" of several pieces of food in the mouth increases the likelihood of choking. A choking child may not make any noise, so adults must keep their eyes on children who are eating. Active supervision is imperative. Supervised eating also promotes the child's safety by discouraging activities that can lead to choking (1). For best practice, children of all ages should be supervised when eating. Adults can monitor age-appropriate portion size consumption.

COMMENTS: Adults can help children while they are learning, by modeling active chewing (i.e., eating a small piece of food, showing how to use their teeth to bite it) and making positive comments to encourage children while they are eating. Adults can demonstrate how to eat foods on the menu, how to serve food, and how to ask for more food as a way of helping children learn the names of foods (e.g., "please pass the bowl of noodles").

TYPE OF FACILITY: Center; Large Family Child Care Home; Small Family Child Care Home

RELATED STANDARDS:
Standard 4.3.2.3: Encouraging Self-Feeding by Older Infants and Toddlers
Standard 4.5.0.4: Socialization During Meals
Standard 4.5.0.5: Numbers of Children Fed Simultaneously by One Adult

REFERENCES:
1. American Academy of Pediatrics, Committee on Injury, Violence, and Poison Prevention. 2010. Policy statement: Prevention of choking among children. *Pediatrics* 125:601-7.

Standard 4.5.0.7: Participation of Older Children and Staff in Mealtime Activities

Both older children and staff should be actively involved in serving food and other mealtime activities, such as setting and cleaning the table. Staff should supervise and assist children with appropriate handwashing procedures before and after meals and sanitizing of eating surfaces and utensils to prevent cross contamination.

RATIONALE: Children develop social skills and new motor skills as well as increase their dexterity through this type of involvement. Children require close supervision by staff and other adults when they use knives and have contact with food surfaces and food that other children will use.

COMMENTS: Compliance is measured by structured observation.

TYPE OF FACILITY: Center; Large Family Child Care Home; Small Family Child Care Home

RELATED STANDARDS:
Standard 4.5.0.4: Socialization During Meals

STANDARD 4.5.0.8: Experience with Familiar and New Foods

In consultation with the family and the nutritionist/registered dietitian, caregivers/teachers should offer children familiar foods that are typical of the child's culture and religious preferences and should also introduce a variety of healthful foods that may not be familiar, but meet a child's nutritional needs. Experiences with new foods can include tasting and swallowing but also include engagement of all senses (seeing, smelling, speaking, etc.) to facilitate the introduction of these new foods.

RATIONALE: By learning about new food, children increase their knowledge of the world around them, and the likelihood that they will choose a more varied, better balanced diet in later life. Eating habits and attitudes about food formed in the early years often last a lifetime. New food acceptance may take eight to fifteen times of offering a food before it is eaten (1).

TYPE OF FACILITY: Center; Large Family Child Care Home; Small Family Child Care Home

RELATED STANDARDS:

Standard 4.2.0.9: Written Menus and Introduction of New Foods
Standard 4.3.1.11: Introduction of Age-Appropriate Solid Foods to Infants

REFERENCES:

1. Sullivan, S. A., L. L. Birch. 1990. Pass the sugar, pass the salt: Experience dictates preference. *Developmental Psychology* 26:546-51.

STANDARD 4.5.0.9: Hot Liquids and Foods

Adults should not consume hot liquids above 120°F in child care areas (3). Hot liquids and hot foods should be kept out of the reach of infants, toddlers, and preschoolers. Hot liquids and foods should not be placed on a surface at a child›s level, at the edge of a table or counter, or on a tablecloth that could be yanked down. Appliances containing hot liquids, such as coffee pots and crock pots, should be kept out of the reach of children. Electrical cords from any appliance, including coffee pots, should not be allowed to hang within the reach of children. Food preparers should position pot handles toward the back of the stove and use only back burners when possible.

RATIONALE: The most common burn suffered by young children is scalding from hot liquids tipped over in the kitchen (1). The skin of young children is much thinner than that of adults and can burn at temperatures that adults find comfortable (2). In a recent study, 90.4% of scald injuries to children under age five were related to hot cooking or drinking liquids (4).

COMMENTS: Hot liquids can cause burns to young children at the following rates of contact: one second at 156°F, two seconds at 149°F, five seconds at 140°F, fifteen seconds at 133°F, five minutes at 120°F (2).

TYPE OF FACILITY: Center; Large Family Child Care Home; Small Family Child Care Home

REFERENCES:

1. Ring, L. M. 2007. Kids and hot liquids-A burning reality. *J of Pediatric Health Care* 21:192-94.
2. Children's Safety Association of Canada. Safety fact sheet: Scald burns. http://www.safekid.org/scald.htm.
3. Turner, C., A. Spinks, R. J. McClure, J. Nixon. 2004. Community-based interventions for the prevention of burns and scalds in children. *Cochrane Database Systematic Rev* (2).
4. Lowell, G., K. Quinlan, L. J. Gottlieb. 2008. *Pediatrics* 122:799-804.

STANDARD 4.5.0.10: Foods that Are Choking Hazards

Caregivers/teachers should not offer to children under four years of age foods that are associated with young children's choking incidents (round, hard, small, thick and sticky, smooth, compressible or dense, or slippery). Examples of these foods are hot dogs and other meat sticks (whole or sliced into rounds), raw carrot rounds, whole grapes, hard candy, nuts, seeds, raw peas, hard pretzels, chips, peanuts, popcorn, rice cakes, marshmallows, spoonfuls of peanut butter, and chunks of meat larger than can be swallowed whole. Food for infants should be cut into pieces one-quarter inch or smaller, food for toddlers should be cut into pieces one-half inch or smaller to prevent choking. In addition to the food monitoring, children should always be seated when eating to reduce choking hazards. Children should be supervised while eating, to monitor the size of food and that they are eating appropriately (for example, not stuffing their mouths full).

RATIONALE: High-risk foods are those often implicated in choking incidents (1,9,10). Almost 90% of fatal choking occurs in children younger than four years of age (2-7). Peanuts may block the lower airway. A chunk of hot dog or a whole seedless grape may completely block the upper airway (2-8,10). The compressibility or density of a food item is what allows the food to conform to and completely block the airway. Hot dogs are the foods most commonly associated with fatal choking in children.

COMMENTS: To reduce the risk of choking, menus should reflect the developmental abilities of the age of children served. Because it is normal for children to get their first teeth at a widely variable age, menus must take into account not only the ages of children but also their teeth, or lack thereof. This becomes particularly important with those whose teeth come in late. Foods considered otherwise appropriate for one year-olds with a full complement of teeth may need to be reevaluated for the child whose first tooth has just emerged. Lists of high-risk foods should be made available. The presence of molars is a good indication of a healthy child's ability to chew hard foods that are likely to cause choking (such as raw carrot rounds). To date, raisins appear to be safe, but, as when eating all foods, children should be seated and supervised.

TYPE OF FACILITY: Center; Large Family Child Care Home; Small Family Child Care Home

REFERENCES:
1. Rimell, F. L., A. Thome Jr., S. Stool, et al. 1995. Characteristics of objects that cause choking in children. *JAMA* 274:1763-66.
2. Benjamin, S. E., ed. 2007. *Making food healthy and safe for children: How to meet the National health and safety performance standards – Guidelines for out of home child care programs*. 2nd ed. Chapel Hill, NC: National Training Institute for Child Care Health Consultants. http://nti.unc.edu/course_files/curriculum/nutrition/making_food_healthy_and_safe.pdf.
3. Dietz, W.H., L. Stern, eds. 1998. *Guide to your child's nutrition*. Elk Grove Village, IL: American Academy of Pediatrics.
4. Kleinman, R. E., ed. 2009. *Pediatric Nutrition Handbook*. 6th ed. Elk Grove Village, IL: American Academy of Pediatrics.
5. Enders, J. B. 1994. *Food, nutrition and the young child*. New York: Merrill.
6. U.S. Department of Agriculture (USDA). 2002. *Making nutrition count for children - Nutrition guidance for child care homes.* Washington, DC: USDA. http://www.fns.usda.gov/tn/Resources/nutritioncount.html.
7. U.S. Department of Agriculture (USDA), Child and Adult Care Food Program (CACFP). 2002. *Menu magic for children: A menu planning guide for child care*. Washington, DC: USDA. http://www.fns.usda.gov/tn/resources/menu_magic.pdf.
8. Baker, S. B., R. S. Fisher. 1980. Childhood asphyxiation by choking or suffocation. *JAMA* 244:1343-46.
9. Morley, R. E., J. P. Ludemann, J. P. Moxham, F. K. Kozak, K. H. Riding. 2004. Foreign body aspiration in infants and toddlers: Recent trends in British Columbia. *J Otolaryngology* 33:37-41.
10. American Academy of Pediatrics, Committee on Injury, Violence, and Poison Prevention. 2010. Policy statement: Prevention of choking among children. *Pediatrics* 125:601-7.

STANDARD 4.5.0.11: Prohibited Uses of Food

Caregivers/teachers should not force or bribe children to eat nor use food as a reward or punishment.

RATIONALE: Children who are forced to eat or, for whom adults use food to modify behavior, come to view eating as a tug-of-war and are more likely to develop lasting food dislikes and unhealthy eating behaviors. Offering food as a reward or punishment places undue importance on food and may have negative effects on the child by promoting "clean the plate" responses that may lead to obesity or poor eating behavior (1-5).

COMMENTS: All components of the meal should be offered at the same time, allowing children to select and enjoy all of the foods on the menu.

TYPE OF FACILITY: Center; Large Family Child Care Home; Small Family Child Care Home

REFERENCES:
1. U.S. Department of Health and Human Services, Administration for Children and Families, Office of Head Start. 2009. *Head Start program performance standards*. Rev. ed. Washington, DC: U.S. Government Printing Office. http://eclkc.ohs.acf.hhs.gov/hslc/Head Start Program/Program Design and Management/Head Start Requirements/Head Start Requirements/45 CFR Chapter XIII/45 CFR Chap XIII_ENG.pdf.
2. Kleinman, R. E., ed. 2009. *Pediatric nutrition handbook*. 6th ed. Elk Grove Village, IL: American Academy of Pediatrics.
3. Murph, J. R., S. D. Palmer, D. Glassy, eds. 2005. *Health in child care: A manual for health professionals*. Elk Grove Village, IL: American Academy of Pediatrics.
4. Benjamin, S. E., ed. 2007. *Making food healthy and safe for children: How to meet the national health and safety performance standards – Guidelines for out of home child care programs*. 2nd ed. Chapel Hill, NC: National Training Institute for Child Care Health Consultants. http://nti.unc.edu/course_files/curriculum/nutrition/making_food_healthy_and_safe.pdf.
5. Birch, L. L., J. O. Fisher, K. K. Davison. 2003. Learning to overeat: Maternal use of restrictive feeding practices promotes girls' eating in the absence of hunger. *Am J Clin Nutr* 78:215-20.

4.6 Food Brought From Home

STANDARD 4.6.0.1: Selection and Preparation of Food Brought From Home

The parent/guardian may provide meals for the child upon written agreement between the parent/guardian and the staff. Food brought into the facility should have a clear label showing the child's full name, the date, and the type of food. Lunches and snacks the parent/guardian provides for one individual child's meals should not be shared with other children. When foods are brought to the facility from home or elsewhere, these foods should be limited to those listed in the facility's written policy on nutritional quality of food brought from home. Potentially hazardous and perishable foods should be refrigerated and all foods should be protected against contamination.

RATIONALE: Food borne illness and poisoning from food is a common occurrence when food has not been properly refrigerated and covered. Although many such illnesses are limited to vomiting and diarrhea, sometimes they are life-threatening. Restricting food sent to the facility to be consumed by the individual child reduces the risk of food poisoning from unknown procedures used in home preparation, storage, and transport. Food brought from home should be nourishing, clean, and safe for an individual child. In this way, other children should not be exposed to unknown risk. Inadvertent sharing of food is a common occurrence in early care and education. The facility has an obligation to ensure that any food offered to children at the facility or shared with other children is wholesome and safe as well as complying with the food and nutrition guidelines for meals and snacks that the early care and education program should observe.

COMMENTS: The facility, in collaboration with parents/guardians and the food service staff/nutritionist/registered dietitian, should establish a policy on foods brought from home for celebrating a child's birthday or any similar festive occasion. Programs should inform parents/guardians about healthy food alternatives like fresh fruit cups or fruit salad for such celebrations. Sweetened treats are highly discouraged, but if provided by the parent/guardian, then the portion size of the treat served should be small.

TYPE OF FACILITY: Center; Large Family Child Care Home; Small Family Child Care Home

RELATED STANDARDS:
Standard 4.6.0.2: Nutritional Quality of Food Brought from Home
Standard 9.2.3.11: Food and Nutrition Service Policies and Plans

STANDARD 4.6.0.2: Nutritional Quality of Food Brought From Home

The facility should provide parents/guardians with written guidelines that the facility has established a comprehensive plan to meet the nutritional requirements of the children in the facility's care and suggested ways parents/guardians can assist the facility in meeting these guidelines. The facility should develop policies for foods brought from home, with parent/guardian consultation, so that expectations are the same for all families (1,2). The facility should have food available to supplement a child's food brought from home if the food brought from home is deficient in meeting the child's nutrient requirements. If the food the parent/guardian provides consistently does not meet the nutritional or food safety requirements, the facility should provide the food and refer the parent/guardian for consultation to a nutritionist/registered dietitian, to the child's primary care provider, or to community resources with trained nutritionists/registered dietitians (such as The Women, Infants and Children [WIC] Supplemental Food Program, extension services, and health departments).

RATIONALE: The caregiver/teacher/facility has a responsibility to follow feeding practices that promote optimum nutrition supporting growth and development in infants, toddlers, and children. Caregivers/teachers who fail to follow best feeding practices, even when parents/guardians wish such counter practices to be followed, negate their basic responsibility of protecting a child's health, social, and emotional well-being.

COMMENTS: Some local health and/or licensing jurisdictions prohibit any foods being brought from home.

TYPE OF FACILITY: Center; Large Family Child Care Home; Small Family Child Care Home

RELATED STANDARDS:
Standard 4.2.0.1: Written Nutrition Plan
Standard 4.6.0.1: Selection and Preparation of Food Brought from Home
Standard 9.2.3.11: Food and Nutrition Service Policies and Plans

REFERENCES:

1. Sweitzer, S., M. E. Briley, C. Robert-Gray. 2009. Do sack lunches provided by parents meet the nutritional needs of young children who attend child care? *J Am Diet Assn* 109:141-44.
2. Contra Costa Child Care Council, Child Health and Nutrition Program. 2006. *CHOICE: Creating healthy opportunities in child care environments*. Concord, CA: Contra Costa Child Care Council, Child Health and Nutrition Program. http://w2.cocokids.org/_cs/downloadables/cc-healthnutrition-choicetoolkit.pdf.

4.7 Nutrition Learning Experiences for Children and Nutrition Education for Parents/Guardians

STANDARD 4.7.0.1: Nutrition Learning Experiences for Children

The facility should have a nutrition plan that integrates the introduction of food and feeding experiences with facility activities and home feeding. The plan should include opportunities for children to develop the knowledge and skills necessary to make appropriate food choices.

For centers, this plan should be a written plan and should be the shared responsibility of the entire staff, including directors and food service personnel, together with parents/guardians. The nutrition plan should be developed with guidance from, and should be approved by, the nutritionist/registered dietitian or child care health consultant.

Caregivers/teachers should teach children about the taste, smell, texture of foods, and vocabulary and language skills related to food and eating. The children should have the opportunity to feel the textures and learn the different colors, sizes, and shapes of foods and the nutritional benefits of eating healthy foods. Children should also be taught about appropriate portion sizes. The teaching should be evident at mealtimes and during curricular activities, and emphasize the pleasure of eating. Caregivers/teachers need to be aware that children between the ages of two- and five-years-old are often resistant to trying new foods and that food acceptance may take eight to fifteen times of offering a food before it is eaten (14).

RATIONALE: Nourishing and attractive food is a foundation for developmentally appropriate learning experiences and contributes to health and well-being (1-13,15). Coordinating the learning experiences with the food service staff maximizes effectiveness of the education. In addition to the nutritive value of food, infants and young children are helped, through the act of feeding, to establish warm human relationships. Eating should be an enjoyable experience for children and staff in the facility and for children and parents/guardians at home. Enjoying and learning about food in childhood promotes good nutrition habits for a lifetime (17,18).

COMMENTS: Parents/guardians and caregivers/teachers should always be encouraged to sit at the table and eat the same food offered to young children as a way to strengthen family style eating which supports child's serving and feeding him or herself (19). Family style eating requires special training for the food service and early care and education staff since they need to monitor food served in a group setting. Portions should be age-appropriate as specified in Child and Adult Care Food Program (CACFP) guidelines. The use of serving utensils should be encouraged to minimize food handling by children. Children should not eat directly out of serving dishes or storage containers. The

presence of an adult at the table with children while they are eating is a way to encourage social interaction and conversation about the food such as its name, color, texture, taste, and concepts such as number, size, and shape; as well as sharing events of the day. These are some practical examples of age-appropriate information for young children to learn about the food they eat. The parent/guardian or adult can help the slow eater, prevent behaviors that might increase risk of fighting, of eating each others' food, and of stuffing food in the mouth in such a way that it might cause choking.

Several community-based nutrition resources can help caregivers/teachers with the nutrition and food service component of their programs (16-18). The key to identifying a qualified nutrition professional is seeking a record of training in pediatric nutrition (normal nutrition, nutrition for children with special health care needs, dietary modifications) and experience and competency in basic food service systems.

Local resources for nutrition education include:

a) Local and state nutritionists/RDs in health departments, in maternal and child health programs, and divisions of children with special health care needs;
b) Nutritionists/RDs at hospitals;
c) The Women, Infants, and Children (WIC) Supplemental Food Program and cooperative extension nutritionists/RDs;
d) School food service personnel;
e) State administrators of the Child and Adult Care Food Program;
f) National School Food Service Management Institute;
g) Healthy Meals Resource System of the Food and Nutrition Information System (National Agricultural Library, U.S. Department of Agriculture);
h) Nutrition consultants with local affiliates of the following organizations:
    1) American Dietetic Association;
    2) American Public Health Association;
    3) Society for Nutrition Education;
    4) American Association of Family and Consumer Sciences;
    5) Dairy Council;
    6) American Heart Association;
    7) American Cancer Society;
    8) American Diabetes Association;
    9) Professional home economists like teachers and those with consumer organizations;
    10) Nutrition departments of local colleges and universities.

Compliance is measured by structured observation.

Following are select resources for caregivers/teachers in providing ongoing opportunities for children and their families to learn about food and healthy eating:

a) Brieger, K. M. 1993. *Cooking up the Pyramid: An early childhood nutrition curriculum*. Pine Island, NY: Clinical Nutrition Services.
b) Cunningham, M. 1995. *Cooking with children: 15 lessons for children, age 7 and up, who really want to learn to cook*. New York: Alfred A. Knopf.
c) Goodwin, M. T., G. Pollen. 1980. *Creative food experiences for children*. Rev. ed. Washington, DC: Center for Science in the Public Interest.
d) King, M. 1993. *Healthy choices for kids: Nutrition and activity education program based on the US Dietary Guidelines*. Levels 1-3 and 4-5. Wenatchee, WA: The Growers of Washington State Apples.

TYPE OF FACILITY: Center; Large Family Child Care Home; Small Family Child Care Home

RELATED STANDARDS:

Standard 2.1.1.2: Health, Nutrition, Physical Activity, and Safety Awareness
Standard 4.2.0.1: Written Nutrition Plan
Standard 4.5.0.4: Socialization During Meals
Standard 4.5.0.7: Participation of Older Children and Staff in Mealtime Activities
Standard 4.5.0.8: Experience with Familiar and New Foods
Standard 4.7.0.2: Nutrition Education for Parents/Guardians
Standard 9.2.3.11: Food and Nutrition Service Policies and Plans
Appendix C: Nutrition Specialist, Registered Dietitian, Licensed Nutritionist, Consultant, and Food Service Staff Qualifications

REFERENCES:

1. U.S. Department of Health and Human Services, Administration for Children and Families, Office of Head Start. 2009. *Head Start program performance standards*. Rev. ed. Washington, DC: U.S. Government Printing Office. http://eclkc.ohs.acf.hhs.gov/hslc/Head Start Program/Program Design and Management/Head Start Requirements/Head Start Requirements/45 CFR Chapter XIII/45 CFR Chap XIII_ENG.pdf.
2. Hagan, Jr., J. F., J. S. Shaw, P. M. Duncan, eds. 2008. *Bright futures: Guidelines for health supervision of infants, children, and adolescents*. 3rd ed. Elk Grove Village, IL: American Academy of Pediatrics.
3. Story, M., K. Holt, D. Sofka, eds. 2002. *Bright futures in practice: Nutrition*. 2nd ed. Arlington, VA: National Center for Education in Maternal and Child Health. http://www.brightfutures.org/nutrition/pdf/frnt_mttr.pdf.
4. Wardle, F., N. Winegarner. 1992. Nutrition and Head Start. *Child Today* 21:57.
5. Benjamin, S. E., ed. 2007. *Making food healthy and safe for children: How to meet the national health and safety performance standards – Guidelines for out of home child care programs*. 2nd ed. Chapel Hill, NC: National Training Institute for Child Care Health Consultants. http://nti.unc.edu/course_files/curriculum/nutrition/making_food_healthy_and_safe.pdf.
6. Dietz, W. H., L. Stern, eds. 1998. *American Academy of Pediatrics guide to your child's nutrition*. New York: Villard.
7. Kleinman, R. E., ed. 2009. *Pediatric nutrition handbook*. 6th ed. Elk Grove Village, IL: American Academy of Pediatrics.
8. Lally, J. R., A. Griffin, E. Fenichel, M. Segal, E. Szanton, B. Weissbourd. 2003. *Caring for infants and toddlers in groups: Developmentally appropriate practice*. Arlington, VA: Zero to Three.
9. Endres, J. B., R. E. Rockwell. 2003. *Food, nutrition, and the young child*. 4th ed. New York: Macmillan.
10. Stang, J., C. T. Bayerl, M. M. Flatt. 2006. Position of the American Dietetic Association: Child and adolescent food and nutrition programs. *J American Dietetic Assoc* 106:1467-75.
11. Pipes, P. L., C. M. Trahms, eds. 1997. *Nutrition in infancy and childhood*. 6th ed. New York: McGraw-Hill.

12. William, C. O., ed. 1998. *Pediatric manual of clinical dietetics*. Chicago: American Dietetic Association.
13. Tamborlane, W. V., J. Warshaw, eds. 1997. *The Yale guide to children's nutrition*. New Haven, CT: Yale University Press.
14. Sullivan, S. A., L. L. Birch. 1990. Pass the sugar, pass the salt: Experience dictates preference. *Devel Psych* 26:546-51.
15. Murph, J. R., S. D. Palmer, D. Glassy, eds. 2005. *Health in child care: A manual for health professionals*. Elk Grove Village, IL: American Academy of Pediatrics.
16. Benjamin, S. E., D. F. Tate, S. I. Bangdiwala, B. H. Neelon, A. S. Ammerman, J. M. Dodds, D. S. Ward. 2008. Preparing child care health consultants to address childhood overweight: A randomized controlled trial comparing web to in-person training. *Maternal Child Health J* 12:662-69.
17. Ammerman, A. S., D. S. Ward, S. E. Benjamin, et al. 2007. An intervention to promote healthy weight: Nutrition and physical activity self-assessment for child care theory and design. *Public Health Research, Practice, Policy* 4:1-12.
18. Story, M., K. M. Kaphingst, S. French. 2006. The role of child care settings in the prevention of obesity. *The Future of Children* 16:143-68
19. Dietz, W., L. Birch. 2008. *Eating behaviors of young child: Prenatal and postnatal influences on healthy eating*. Elk Grove Village, IL: American Academy of Pediatrics.

STANDARD 4.7.0.2: Nutrition Education for Parents/Guardians

Parents/guardians should be informed of the range of nutrition learning activities provided in the facility. Formal nutrition information and education programs should be conducted at least twice a year under the guidance of the nutritionist/registered dietitian based on a needs assessment for nutrition information and education as perceived by families and staff. Informal programs should be implemented during the "teachable moments" throughout the year.

RATIONALE: One goal of a facility is to provide a positive environment for the entire family. Informing parents/guardians about nutrition, food, food preparation, and mealtime enhances nutrition and mealtime interactions in the home, which helps to mold a child's food habits and eating behavior (1-9). Because of the current epidemic of childhood obesity, prevention of childhood obesity through nutrition and physical activity is an appropriate topic for parents/guardians. Periodically providing families records of the food eaten and progress in physical activities by their children will help families coordinate home food preparation, nutrition, and physical activity with what is provided at the early care and education facility. Nutrition education directed at parents/guardians complements and enhances the nutrition learning experiences provided to their children.

COMMENTS: One method of nutrition education for parents/guardians is providing healthy recipes that are quick and inexpensive to prepare and sharing information regarding access to local sources of healthy foods (farmers' markets, grocery stores, healthier prepared foods and restaurant options). Also caregivers/teachers can provide parents/guardians ideas for healthy and inexpensive snacks including foods available and served at parents'/guardians' meetings. Education should be helpful, culturally relevant and incorporate the use of locally produced food. The educational programs may be supplemented by periodic distribution of newsletters and/or literature.

TYPE OF FACILITY: Center; Large Family Child Care Home; Small Family Child Care Home

RELATED STANDARDS:
Standard 4.7.0.1: Nutrition Learning Experiences for Children (contains resources for nutrition expertise)

REFERENCES:
1. U.S. Department of Health and Human Services, Administration for Children and Families, Office of Head Start. 2009. *Head Start program performance standards*. Rev. ed. Washington, DC: U.S. Government Printing Office. http://eclkc.ohs.acf.hhs.gov/hslc/ Head Start Program/Program Design and Management/Head Start Requirements/Head Start Requirements/45 CFR Chapter XIII/45 CFR Chap XIII_ENG.pdf.
2. Hagan, Jr., J. F., J. S. Shaw, P. M. Duncan, eds. 2008. *Bright futures: Guidelines for health supervision of infants, children, and adolescents*. 3rd ed. Elk Grove Village, IL: American Academy of Pediatrics.
3. Benjamin, S. E., ed. 2007. *Making food healthy and safe for children: How to meet the national health and safety performance standards – Guidelines for out of home child care programs*. 2nd ed. Chapel Hill, NC: National Training Institute for Child Care Health Consultants. http://nti.unc.edu/course_files/curriculum/nutrition/making_food_healthy_and_safe.pdf.
4. Dietz, W. H., L. Stern, eds. 1998. *American Academy of Pediatrics guide to your child's nutrition*. New York: Villard.
5. Endres, J. B., R. E. Rockwell. 2003. *Food, nutrition, and the young child*. 4th ed. New York: Macmillan.
6. U.S. Department of Agriculture. 2002. *Making nutrition count for children - Nutrition guidance for child care homes*. Washington, DC: USDA. http://www.fns.usda.gov/tn/Resources/nutritioncount.html.
7. Pipes, P. L., C. M. Trahms, eds. 1997. *Nutrition in infancy and childhood*. 6th ed. New York: McGraw-Hill.
8. Tamborlane, W. V., ed. 1997. *The Yale guide to children's nutrition*. New Haven, CT: Yale University Press.
9. Kleinman, R. E., ed. 2009. *Pediatric nutrition handbook*. 6th ed. Elk Grove Village, IL: American Academy of Pediatrics.

4.8 Kitchen and Equipment

STANDARD 4.8.0.1: Food Preparation Area

The food preparation area of the kitchen should be separate from eating, play, laundry, toilet, and bathroom areas and from areas where animals are permitted. The food preparation area should not be used as a passageway while food is being prepared. Food preparation areas should be separated by a door, gate, counter, or room divider from areas the children use for activities unrelated to food, except in small family child care homes when separation may limit supervision of children.

Infants and toddlers should not have access to the kitchen in child care centers. Access by older children to the kitchen of centers should be permitted only when supervised by staff members who have been certified by the nutritionist/registered dietitian or the center director as qualified to follow the facility's sanitation and safety procedures.

In all types of child care facilities, children should never be in the kitchen unless they are directly supervised by

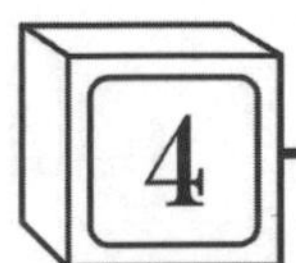

a caregiver/teacher. Children of preschool-age and older should be restricted from access to areas where hot food is being prepared. School-age children may engage in food preparation activities with adult supervision in the kitchen or the classroom. Parents/guardians and other adults should be permitted to use the kitchen only if they know and follow the food safety rules of the facility. The facility should check with local health authorities about any additional regulations that apply.

RATIONALE: The presence of children in the kitchen increases the risk of contamination of food and the risk of injury to children from burns. Use of kitchen appliances and cooking techniques may require more skill than can be expected for children's developmental level. The most common burn in young children is scalding from hot liquids tipped over in the kitchen (1).

The kitchen should be used only by authorized individuals who have met the requirements of the local health authority and who know and follow the food safety rules of the facility so they do not contaminate food and food surfaces for food-related activities. Under adult supervision, school-age children may be encouraged to help with developmentally appropriate food preparation, which increases the likelihood that they will eat new foods.

TYPE OF FACILITY: Center; Large Family Child Care Home; Small Family Child Care Home

RELATED STANDARDS:

Appendix C: Nutrition Specialist, Registered Dietitian, Licensed Nutritionist, Consultant, and Food Service Staff Qualifications

REFERENCES:

1. Ring, L. M. 2007. Kids and hot liquids–A burning reality. *J Pediatric Health Care* 21:192-94.

STANDARD 4.8.0.2: Design of Food Service Equipment

Food service equipment should be designed, installed, operated, and maintained according to the manufacturer's instructions and in a way that meets the performance, health, and safety standards of the National Sanitation Foundation (1) or applicable State or local public health authority, or the U.S. Department of Agriculture (USDA) food program and sanitation codes (3), as determined by the regulatory public health authority.

RATIONALE: The design, installation, operation, and maintenance of food service equipment must follow the manufacturer's instructions and meet the standards for such equipment to ensure that the equipment protects the users from injury and the consumers of foods prepared with this equipment from foodborne disease (1,2). The manufacturer's warranty that equipment will meet recognized standards is valid only if the equipment is properly maintained.

COMMENTS: Inspectors from state and local agencies with appropriate training should check food service equipment and provide technical assistance to facilities. The local public health department typically conducts such inspections. Manufacturers should attest to their compliance with equipment standards of the National Sanitation Foundation (NSF) and the Code of Federal Regulations, Part 200, Section 354.210 (revised January 1990). Testing labs such as Underwriters Laboratories (UL) also test food service equipment. Before making a purchase, child care facilities should check not only the warranty but also the maintenance instructions provided by the equipment manufacturer to be sure the required maintenance is feasible, given the facility's resources. If the facility receives inspections from the public health department, the facility may want to consult with them before making a purchase. The facility director or food service staff should retain maintenance instructions and check to be sure that all users of the equipment follow the instructions.

TYPE OF FACILITY: Center

REFERENCES:

1. National Sanitation Foundation. 2007. Commercial cooking, rethermalization and powered hot food holding, and transport equipment, ANSI/NSF 4. Ann Harbor, MI: National Sanitation Foundation.

2. National Restaurant Association. 2008. *ServSafe essentials*. 5th ed. Upper Saddle River, NJ: Prentice Hall.

3. U.S. Department of Health and Human Services, Public Health Service, Food and Drug Administration (FDA). 2009. *2009 Food code.* College Park, MD: FDA. http://www.fda.gov/downloads/Food/FoodSafety/RetailFoodProtection/FoodCode/FoodCode2009/UCM189448.pdf.

STANDARD 4.8.0.3: Maintenance of Food Service Surfaces and Equipment

All surfaces that come into contact with food, including tables and countertops, as well as floors and shelving in the food preparation area should be in good repair, free of cracks or crevices, and should be made of smooth, nonporous material that is kept clean and sanitized. All kitchen equipment should be clean and should be maintained in operable condition according to the manufacturer's guidelines for maintenance and operation. The facility should maintain an inventory of food service equipment that includes the date of purchase, the warranty date, and a history of repairs.

RATIONALE: Cracked or porous materials should be replaced because they trap food and other organic materials in which microorganisms can grow (1). Harsh scrubbing of these areas tends to create even more areas where organic material can lodge and increase the risk of contamination. Repairs with duct tape, package tapes, and other commonly used materials add surfaces that trap organic materials.

Food service equipment is designed by the manufacturer for specific types of use. The equipment must be maintained to meet those performance standards or food will become contaminated and spoil (1). An accurate and ongoing inventory of food service equipment tracks maintenance requirements and can provide important information when a breakdown occurs.

TYPE OF FACILITY: Center; Large Family Child Care Home; Small Family Child Care Home

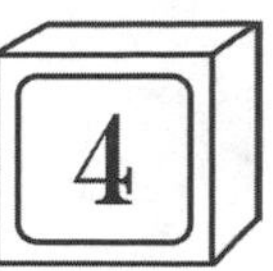

REFERENCES:
1. National Restaurant Association. 2008. *ServSafe essentials*. 5th ed. Upper Saddle River, NJ: Prentice Hall.

STANDARD 4.8.0.4: Food Preparation Sinks

The sink used for food preparation should not be used for handwashing or any other purpose. Handwashing sinks and sinks involved in diaper changing should not be used for food preparation. All food service sinks should be supplied with hot and cold running water under pressure.

RATIONALE: Separation of sinks used for handwashing or other potentially contaminating activities from those used for food preparation prevents contamination of food. Hot and cold running water are essential for thorough cleaning and sanitizing of equipment and utensils and cleaning of the facility.

TYPE OF FACILITY: Center; Large Family Child Care Home; Small Family Child Care Home

RELATED STANDARDS:
Standard 4.9.0.13: Method for Washing Dishes by Hand
Standard 5.2.1.14: Water Heating Devices and Temperatures Allowed

STANDARD 4.8.0.5: Handwashing Sink Separate from Food Zones

Centers should provide a separate handwashing sink in the food preparation area of the facility. It should have an eight-inch-high splash guard or have eighteen inches of space between the handwashing sink and any open food zones (such as preparation tables and food sink).

Where continuous warm water pressure is not available, handwashing sinks should have at least thirty seconds of continuous flow of warm water to initiate and complete handwashing.

RATIONALE: Separation of sinks used for handwashing or other potentially contaminating activities from those used for food preparation prevents contamination of food.

Proper handwashing requires a continuous flow of water, no less than 100°F and no more than 120°F, for at least thirty seconds to allow sufficient time for wetting and rinsing the hands (1).

TYPE OF FACILITY: Center

RELATED STANDARDS:
Standard 3.2.2.2: Handwashing Procedure

REFERENCES:
1. U.S. Department of Health and Human Services, Public Health Service, Food and Drug Administration (FDA). 2009. *2009 Food code.* College Park, MD: FDA. http://www.fda.gov/downloads/Food/FoodSafety/RetailFoodProtection/FoodCode/FoodCode2009/UCM189448.pdf.

STANDARD 4.8.0.6: Maintaining Safe Food Temperatures

The facility should use refrigerators that maintain food temperatures of 41°F or lower in all parts of the food storage areas, and freezers should maintain temperatures of 0°F or lower in food storage areas.

Thermometers with markings in no more than 2° increments should be provided in all refrigerators, freezers, ovens, and holding areas for hot and cold foods. Thermometers should be clearly visible, easy to read, and accurate, and should be kept in working condition and regularly checked. Thermometers should be mercury free.

RATIONALE: Storage of food at proper temperatures minimizes bacterial growth (1).

The use of accurate thermometers to monitor temperatures at which food is cooked and stored helps to ensure food safety. Hot foods must be checked to be sure they reach temperatures that kill microorganisms in that type of food. Cold foods must be checked to see that they are being maintained at temperatures that safely retard the growth of bacteria. Thermometers with larger than 2° increments, are hard to read accurately.

COMMENTS: Refrigerator and freezer thermometers are widely available in stores and over the Internet. They are available in both digital and analog forms. Providing thermometers with a dual scale in Fahrenheit and Celsius will avoid the necessity for a child care provider to convert temperature scales.

TYPE OF FACILITY: Center; Large Family Child Care Home; Small Family Child Care Home

RELATED STANDARDS:
Appendix U: Recommended Safe Minimum Internal Cooking Temperatures

REFERENCES:
1. Food Marketing Institute, U.S. Department of Agriculture, Food Safety and Inspection Service. 1996. *Facts about food and floods: A consumer guide to food quality and safe handling after a flood or power outage.* Washington, DC: Food Marketing Institute.

STANDARD 4.8.0.7: Ventilation Over Cooking Surfaces

In centers using commercial cooking equipment to prepare meals, ventilation should be equipped with an exhaust system in compliance with the applicable building, mechanical, and fire codes. These codes may vary slightly with each locale, and centers are responsible to ensure their facilities meet the requirements of these codes (1-2).

All gas ranges in centers should be mechanically vented and fumes filtered prior to discharge to the outside. All vents and filters should be maintained free of grease build-up and food spatters, and in good repair.

RATIONALE: Properly maintained vents and filters control odor, fire hazards, and fumes.

An exhaust system must collect fumes and grease-laden vapors properly at their source.

COMMENTS: The center should refer to the owner's manual of the exhaust system for a description of capture velocity. Commercial cooking equipment refers to the type of equip-

ment that is typically found in restaurants and other food service businesses.

Proper construction of the exhaust system duct-work assures that grease and other build-up can be easily accessed and cleaned.

If the odor of gas is present when the pilot lights are on, turn off gas and immediately call a qualified gas technician, commercial gas provider, or local gas, electric or utility provider. Never use an open flame to locate a gas leak.

TYPE OF FACILITY: Center

REFERENCES:

1. American Society of Heating, Refrigeration and Air Conditioning Engineers. 2007. *ASHRAE handbook: HVAC applications*. Atlanta, GA: ASHRAE.
2. Clark, J. 2003. Commercial kitchen ventilation design: What you need to know. http://www.esmagazine.com/Articles/Feature_Article/229549b01fca8010VgnVCM100000f932a8c0.

STANDARD 4.8.0.8: Microwave Ovens

Microwave ovens should be inaccessible to all children, with the exception of school-age children under close adult supervision. Any microwave oven in use in a child care facility should be manufactured after October 1971 and should be in good condition. While the microwave is being used, it should not be left unattended.

If foods need to be heated in a microwave:

a) Avoid heating foods in plastic containers;
b) Avoid transferring hot foods/drinks into plastic containers;
c) Do not use plastic wrap or aluminum foil in the microwave;
d) Avoid plastics for food and beverages labeled "3" (PVC), "6" (PS), and "7" (polycarbonate);
e) Stir food before serving to prevent burns from hot spots.

RATIONALE: Young children can be burned when their faces come near the heat vent. The issues involved with the safe use of microwave ovens (such as no metal and steam trapping) make use of this equipment by preschool-age children too risky. Older ovens made before the Federal standard went into effect in October 1971 can expose users or passers-by to microwave radiation. If adults or school-age children use a microwave, it is recommended that they do not heat food in plastic containers, plastic wrap or aluminum foil due to concerns of releasing toxic substances even if the container is specified for use in a microwave (1).

COMMENTS: If school-age children are allowed to use a microwave oven in the facility, this use should be closely supervised by an adult to avoid injury. See Standard 4.3.1.9 for prohibition of use of microwave ovens to warm infant feedings.

TYPE OF FACILITY: Center; Large Family Child Care Home; Small Family Child Care Home

RELATED STANDARDS:
Standard 4.3.1.9: Warming Bottles and Infant Foods
Standard 5.2.9.9: Plastic Containers and Toys

REFERENCES:

1. Institute for Agriculture and Trade Policy (IATP), Food and Health Program. 2005. *Smart plastics guide: Healthier food uses of plastics for parents and children*. Minneapolis, MN: IATP.

4.9 Food Safety

STANDARD 4.9.0.1: Compliance with U.S. Food and Drug Administration Food Sanitation Standards, State and Local Rules

The facility should conform to the applicable portions of the U.S. Food and Drug Administration model food sanitation standards (1) and all applicable state and local food service rules and regulations for centers and large and small family child care homes regarding safe food protection and sanitation practices. If federal model standards and local regulations are in conflict, the health authority with jurisdiction should determine which requirement the facility must meet.

RATIONALE: Minimum standards for food safety are based on current scientific data that demonstrate the conditions required to prevent contamination of food with infectious and toxic substances that cause foodborne illness. Many of these standards have been placed in statutes and must be complied with by law.

Federal, state, and local food safety codes, regulations, and standards may be in conflict. In these circumstances, the decision of the regulatory health authority should prevail.

COMMENTS: The U.S. Food and Drug Administration's (FDA) Model Food Code is a good resource to have on hand. The current Food Code is available at http://www.fda.gov/downloads/Food/FoodSafety/RetailFoodProtection/FoodCode/FoodCode2009/UCM189448.pdf.

TYPE OF FACILITY: Center; Large Family Child Care Home; Small Family Child Care Home

REFERENCES:

1. U.S. Department of Health and Human Services, Public Health Service, Food and Drug Administration (FDA). 2009. *2009 Food code*. College Park, MD: FDA. http://www.fda.gov/downloads/Food/FoodSafety/RetailFoodProtection/FoodCode/FoodCode2009/UCM189448.pdf.

STANDARD 4.9.0.2: Staff Restricted from Food Preparation and Handling

Anyone who has signs or symptoms of illness, including vomiting, diarrhea, and infectious skin sores that cannot be covered, or who potentially or actually is infected with bacteria, viruses or parasites that can be carried in food, should be excluded from food preparation and handling. Staff members may not contact exposed, ready-to-eat food with their bare hands and should use suitable utensils such as deli tissue, spatulas, tongs, single-use gloves, or dispensing equipment. No one with open or infected skin eruptions should work in the food preparation area unless the injuries are covered with nonporous (such as latex or vinyl), single use gloves.

In centers and large family child care homes, staff members who are involved in the process of preparing or handling food should not change diapers. Staff members who work with diapered children should not prepare or serve food for older groups of children. When staff members who are caring for infants and toddlers are responsible for changing diapers, they should handle food only for the infants and toddlers in their groups and only after thoroughly washing their hands. Caregivers/teachers who prepare food should wash their hands carefully before handling any food, regardless of whether they change diapers. When caregivers/teachers must handle food, staffing assignments should be made to foster completion of the food handling activities by caregivers/teachers of older children, or by caregivers/teachers of infants and toddlers before the caregiver/teacher assumes other caregiving duties for that day. Aprons worn in the food service area must be clean and should be removed when diaper changing or when using the toilet.

RATIONALE: Food handlers who are ill can easily transmit their illness to others by contaminating the food they prepare with the infectious agents they are carrying. Frequent and proper handwashing before and after using plastic gloves reduces food contamination (1,2,4).

Caregivers/teachers who work with infants and toddlers are frequently exposed to feces and to children with infections of the intestines (often with diarrhea) or of the liver. Education of child care staff regarding handwashing and other cleaning procedures can reduce the occurrence of illness in the group of children with whom they work (1,2,4).

The possibility of involving a larger number of people in a foodborne outbreak is greater in child care than in most households. Cooking larger volumes of food requires special caution to avoid contamination of the food with even small amounts of infectious materials. With larger volumes of food, staff must exercise greater diligence to avoid contamination because larger quantities of food take longer to heat or to cool to safe temperatures. Larger volumes of food spend more time in the danger zone of temperatures (between 41°F and 135°F) where more rapid multiplication of microorganisms occurs (3).

TYPE OF FACILITY: Center; Large Family Child Care Home; Small Family Child Care Home

RELATED STANDARDS:
Standards 3.2.2.1-3.2.2.5: Handwashing

REFERENCES:
1. Cowell, C., S. Schlosser. 1998. Food safety in infant and preschool day care. *Top Clin Nutr* 14:9-15.
2. U.S. Department of Agriculture (USDA), Food Safety and Inspection Service. 2000. *Keeping kids safe: A guide for safe handling and sanitation, for child care providers*. Rev ed. Washington, DC: USDA. http://teamnutrition.usda.gov/resources/appendj.pdf.
3. U.S. Department of Health and Human Services, Public Health Service, Food and Drug Administration (FDA). 2009. *2009 Food code.* College Park, MD: FDA. http://www.fda.gov/downloads/Food/FoodSafety/RetailFoodProtection/FoodCode/FoodCode2009/UCM189448.pdf.
4. U.S. Department of Health and Human Services, U.S. Department of Agriculture. 2010. *Dietary guidelines for Americans, 2010*. 7th ed. Washington, DC: U.S. Government Printing Office. http://www.health.gov/dietaryguidelines/dga2010/DietaryGuidelines2010.pdf.

STANDARD 4.9.0.3: Precautions for a Safe Food Supply

All foods stored, prepared, or served should be safe for human consumption by observation and smell (1-2). The following precautions should be observed for a safe food supply:

a) Home-canned food; food from dented, rusted, bulging, or leaking cans, and food from cans without labels should not be used;
b) Foods should be inspected daily for spoilage or signs of mold, and foods that are spoiled or moldy should be promptly and appropriately discarded;
c) Meat should be from government-inspected sources or otherwise approved by the governing health authority (3);
d) All dairy products should be pasteurized and Grade A where applicable;
e) Raw, unpasteurized milk, milk products; unpasteurized fruit juices; and raw or undercooked eggs should not be used. Freshly squeezed fruit or vegetable juice prepared just prior to serving in the child care facility is permissible;
f) Unless a child's health care professional documents a different milk product, children from twelve months to two years of age should be served only human milk, formula, whole milk or 2% milk (6). Note: For children between twelve months and two years of age for whom overweight or obesity is a concern or who have a family history of obesity, dyslipidemia, or CVD, the use of reduced-fat milk is appropriate only with written documentation from the child's primary health care professional (4). Children two years of age and older should be served skim or 1% milk. If cost-saving is required to accommodate a tight budget, dry milk and milk products may be reconstituted in the facility for cooking purposes only, provided that they are prepared, refrigerated, and stored in a sanitary manner, labeled with the date of preparation, and used or discarded within twenty-four hours of preparation;
g) Meat, fish, poultry, milk, and egg products should be refrigerated or frozen until immediately before use (5);
h) Frozen foods should be defrosted in one of four ways: In the refrigerator; under cold running water; as part of the cooking process, or by removing food from packaging and using the defrost setting of a microwave oven (5). Note: Frozen human milk should not be defrosted in the microwave;
i) Frozen foods should never be defrosted by leaving them at room temperature or standing in water that is not kept at refrigerator temperature (5);
j) All fruits and vegetables should be washed thoroughly with water prior to use (5);

k) Food should be served promptly after preparation or cooking or should be maintained at temperatures of not less than 135°F for hot foods and not more than 41°F for cold foods (12);

l) All opened moist foods that have not been served should be covered, dated, and maintained at a temperature of 41°F or lower in the refrigerator or frozen in the freezer, verified by a working thermometer kept in the refrigerator or freezer (12);

m) Fully cooked and ready-to-serve hot foods should be held for no longer than thirty minutes before being served, or promptly covered and refrigerated;

n) Pasteurized eggs or egg products should be substituted for raw eggs in the preparation of foods such as Caesar salad, mayonnaise, meringue, eggnog, and ice cream. Pasteurized eggs or egg products should be substituted for recipes in which more than one egg is broken and the eggs are combined, unless the eggs are cooked for an individual child at a single meal and served immediately, such as in omelets or scrambled eggs; or the raw eggs are combined as an ingredient immediately before baking and the eggs are fully cooked to a ready-to-eat form, such as a cake, muffin or bread;

o) Raw animal foods should be fully cooked to heat all parts of the food to a temperature and for a time of; 145°F or above for fifteen seconds for fish and meat; 160°F for fifteen seconds for chopped or ground fish, chopped or ground meat or raw eggs; or 165°F or above for fifteen seconds for poultry or stuffed fish, stuffed meat, stuffed pasta, stuffed poultry or stuffing containing fish, meat or poultry.

RATIONALE: Safe handling of all food is a basic principle to prevent and reduce foodborne illnesses (14). For children, a small dose of infectious or toxic material can lead to serious illness (13). Some molds produce toxins that may cause illness or even death (such as aflatoxin or ergot).

Keeping cold food below 41°F and hot food above 135°F prevents bacterial growth (1,6,12). Food intended for human consumption can become contaminated if left at room temperature.

Foodborne illnesses from *Salmonella* and *E. coli 0157:H7* have been associated with consumption of contaminated, raw, or undercooked egg products, meat, poultry, and seafood. Children tend to be more susceptible to *E. coli 0157:H7* infections from consumption of undercooked meats, and such infections can lead to kidney failure and death.

Home-canned food, food from dented, rusted, bulging or leaking cans, or leaking packages/bags of frozen foods, have an increased risk of containing microorganisms or toxins. Users of unlabeled food cans cannot be sure what is in the can and how long the can has been stored.

Excessive heating of foods results in loss of nutritional content and causes foods to lose appeal by altering color, consistency, texture, and taste. Positive learning activities for children, using their senses of seeing and smelling, help them to learn about the food they eat. These sensory experiences are counterproductive when food is overcooked. Children are not only shortchanged of nutrients, but are denied the chance to use their senses fully to learn about foods.

Caregivers/teachers should discourage parents/guardians from bringing home-baked items for the children to share as it is difficult to determine the quality of the ingredients used and the cleanliness of the environment in which the items are baked and transported. Parents/guardians should be informed why home baked items like birthday cake and cupcakes are not the healthiest choice and the facility should provide ideas for healthier alternatives such as fruit cups or fruit salad to celebrate birthdays and other festive events.

Several states allow the sale of raw milk or milk products. These products have been implicated in outbreaks of salmonellosis, listeriosis, toxoplasmosis, and campylobacteriosis and should never be served in child care facilities (7,8). Only pasteurized milk and fruit juices should be served. Foods made with uncooked eggs have been involved in a number of outbreaks of Salmonella infections. Eggs should be well-cooked before being eaten, and only pasteurized eggs or egg substitutes should be used in foods requiring raw eggs.

The American Academy of Pediatrics (AAP) recommends that children from twelve months to two years of age receive human milk, formula, whole milk, or 2% milk. For children between twelve months and two years of age for whom overweight or obesity is a concern or who have a family history of obesity, dyslipidemia, or CVD, the use of reduced-fat milk is appropriate only with written documentation from the child's primary health care professional (4). Children two years of age and older can drink skim, or 1%, milk (6,9-11).

Soil particles and contaminants that adhere to fruits and vegetables can cause illness. Therefore, all fruits or vegetables to be eaten and used to make fresh juice at the facility should be thoroughly washed first.

Thawing frozen foods under conditions that expose any of the food's surfaces to temperatures between 41°F and 135°F promotes the growth of bacteria that may cause illness if ingested. Storing perishable foods at safe temperatures in the refrigerator or freezer reduces the rate at which microorganisms in these foods multiply (12).

COMMENTS: The use of dairy products fortified with vitamins A and D is recommended (4).

The FDA provides the following Website for caregivers/teachers to check status of foods and food products that have been recalled, see http://www.fda.gov.

Temperatures come from the FDA *2009 Food Code* (12). Local or state regulations may differ. Caregivers/teachers should consult with the health department concerning questions on proper cooking temperatures for specific foods.

TYPE OF FACILITY: Center; Large Family Child Care Home; Small Family Child Care Home

RELATED STANDARDS:
Standard 4.3.1.7: Feeding Cow's Milk
Standard 4.8.0.6: Maintaining Safe Food Temperatures
Appendix U: Recommended Safe Minimum Internal Cooking Temperatures

REFERENCES:

1. Enders, J. B. 1994. *Food, nutrition and the young child*. New York: Merrill.
2. U.S. Department of Agriculture (USDA). 2002. *Making nutrition count for children - Nutrition guidance for child care homes.* Washington, DC: USDA. http://www.fns.usda.gov/tn/Resources/nutritioncount.html.
3. U.S. Department of Agriculture (USDA), Food Safety and Inspection Service. 2000. *Keeping kids safe: A guide for safe handling and sanitation, for child care providers*. Rev ed. Washington, DC: USDA. http://teamnutrition.usda.gov/Resources/appendj.pdf.
4. Daniels, S. R., F. R. Greer, Committee on Nutrition. 2008. Lipid screening and cardiovascular health in childhood. *Pediatrics* 122:198-208.
5. Food Marketing Institute (FMI), U.S. Department of Agriculture, Food Safety and Inspection Service. 1996. *Facts about food and floods: A consumer guide to food quality and safe handling after a flood or power outage*. Washington, DC: FMI.
6. Kleinman, R. E., ed. 2009. *Pediatric Nutrition Handbook*. 6th ed. Elk Grove Village, IL: American Academy of Pediatrics.
7. Potter, M. E. 1984. Unpasteurized milk: The hazards of a health fetish. *JAMA* 252:2048-52.
8. Sacks, J. J. 1982. Toxoplasmosis infection associated with raw goat's milk. *JAMA* 246:1728-32.
9. Dietz, W.H., L. Stern, eds. 1998. *Guide to your child's nutrition*. Elk Grove Village, IL: American Academy of Pediatrics.
10. Chicago Dietetic Association. 1996. *Manual of clinical dietetics*. 5th ed. Chicago, IL: American Dietetic Association.
11. Pipes, P. L., C. M. Trahms, eds. 1997. *Nutrition in infancy and childhood*. 6th ed. New York: McGraw-Hill.
12. U.S. Department of Health and Human Services, Public Health Service, Food and Drug Administration (FDA). 2009. *2009 Food code.* College Park, MD: FDA. http://www.fda.gov/downloads/Food/FoodSafety/RetailFoodProtection/FoodCode/FoodCode2009/UCM189448.pdf.
13. Cowell, C., S. Schlosser. 1998. Food safety in infant and preschool day care. *Top Clin Nutr* 14:9-15.
14. U.S. Department of Health and Human Services, U.S. Department of Agriculture. 2010. *Dietary guidelines for Americans, 2010*. 7th ed. Washington, DC: U.S. Government Printing Office. http://www.health.gov/dietaryguidelines/dga2010/DietaryGuidelines2010.pdf.

STANDARD 4.9.0.4: Leftovers

Food returned from individual plates and family style serving bowls, platters, pitchers, and unrefrigerated foods into which microorganisms are likely to have been introduced during food preparation or service, should be immediately discarded.

Unserved perishable food should be covered promptly for protection from contamination, should be refrigerated immediately, and should be used within twenty-four hours. "Perishable foods" include those foods that are subject to decay, spoilage or bacteria unless it is properly refrigerated or frozen (1).

Hot food can be placed directly in the refrigerator or it can be rapidly chilled in an ice or cold water bath before refrigerating. Hot foods should be promptly cooled first before they are fully covered in the refrigerator. Prepared perishable foods that have not been maintained at safe temperatures for two hours or more should be discarded immediately. If the air or room temperature is above 90°F, this time is reduced to one hour after which the food should be discarded (2). "Safe temperatures" mean keeping foods cold (below 41°F) or hot (above 135°F) (4).

RATIONALE: Served foods have a high probability of contamination during serving. Bacterial multiplication proceeds rapidly in perishable foods out of refrigeration, as much as doubling the numbers of bacteria every fifteen to twenty minutes.

The potential is high for perishable foods (food that is subject to decay, spoilage, or bacteria unless it is properly refrigerated or frozen) that have been out of the refrigerator for more than two hours to have substantial loads of bacteria. This time can be as short as one hour if the air temperature is above 90°F. When such food is stored and served again, it may cause foodborne illness.

COMMENTS: All food, once served or handled outside the food preparation area, should be discarded.

TYPE OF FACILITY: Center; Large Family Child Care Home; Small Family Child Care Home

RELATED STANDARDS:
Standard 4.8.0.6: Maintaining Safe Food Temperatures

REFERENCES:

1. U.S. Department of Agriculture, Food Safety and Inspection Service. Glossary: Perishable. http://www.fsis.usda.gov/Help/glossary-P/index.asp.
2. U.S. Department of Agriculture, Food Safety and Inspection Service. 2006. *Safe food handling, basics for handling food safely*. http://www.fsis.usda.gov/PDF/Basics_for_Safe_Food_Handling.pdf.
3. U.S. Department of Agriculture, Food Safety and Inspection Service. 2006. *Safe food handling, how temperatures affect food*. http://www.fsis.usda.gov/PDF/How_Temperatures_Affect_Food.pdf.
4. U.S. Department of Health and Human Services, Public Health Service, Food and Drug Administration (FDA). 2009. *2009 Food code.* College Park, MD: FDA. http://www.fda.gov/downloads/Food/FoodSafety/RetailFoodProtection/FoodCode/FoodCode2009/UCM189448.pdf.

STANDARD 4.9.0.5: Preparation for and Storage of Food in the Refrigerator

All food stored in the refrigerator should be tightly covered, wrapped, or otherwise protected from direct contact with other food. Hot foods to be refrigerated and stored should be transferred to shallow containers in food layers less than three inches deep and refrigerated immediately. These foods should be covered when cool. Any pre-prepared or leftover foods that are not likely to be served the following day should be labeled with the date of preparation before being placed in the refrigerator. The basic rule for serving food should be, "first food in, first food out" (1-3).

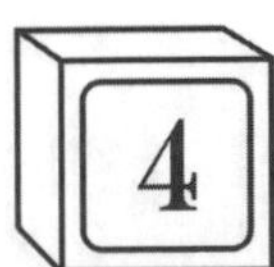

In the refrigerator, raw meat, poultry and fish should be stored below cooked or ready to eat foods.

RATIONALE: Covering food protects it from contamination and keeps other food particles from falling into it. Hot food cools more quickly in a shallow container, thereby decreasing the time when the food would be susceptible to contamination. Foods should be covered only after they have cooled. Leaving hot food uncovered allows it to cool more quickly, thereby decreasing the time when bacteria may be produced.

Labeling of foods will inform the staff about the duration of storage, which foods to use first, and which foods to discard because the period of safe storage has passed.

Storing raw meat, poultry and fish on a dish or in a pan below ready-to-eat foods reduces the possibility that spills or drips from raw animal foods might contaminate ready-to-eat food.

TYPE OF FACILITY: Center; Large Family Child Care Home; Small Family Child Care Home

RELATED STANDARDS:
Standard 4.8.0.6: Maintaining Safe Food Temperatures
Standard 4.9.0.3: Precautions for a Safe Food Supply
Appendix V: Food Storage Chart

REFERENCES:

1. Benjamin, S. E., ed. 2007. *Making food healthy and safe for children: How to meet the National health and safety performance standards – Guidelines for out of home child care programs*. 2nd ed. Chapel Hill, NC: National Training Institute for Child Care Health Consultants. http://nti.unc.edu/course_files/curriculum/nutrition/making_food_healthy_and_safe.pdf.
2. Enders, J. B. 1994. *Food, nutrition and the young child*. New York: Merrill.
3. U.S. Department of Agriculture (USDA). 2002. *Making nutrition count for children - Nutrition guidance for child care homes.* Washington, DC: USDA. http://www.fns.usda.gov/tn/Resources/nutritioncount.html.

STANDARD 4.9.0.6: Storage of Foods Not Requiring Refrigeration

Foods not requiring refrigeration should be stored at least six inches above the floor in clean, dry, well-ventilated storerooms or other approved areas (1,2). Food products should be stored in such a way (such as in nonporous containers off the floor) as to prevent insects and rodents from entering the products.

RATIONALE: Storage of food off the floor in a safe and sanitary manner helps prevent food contamination from cleaning chemicals or spills of other foods and keeps insects and rodents from entering the products.

COMMENTS: Storing food six inches or higher above the floor enables easier cleaning of the floor under the food.

TYPE OF FACILITY: Center; Large Family Child Care Home; Small Family Child Care Home

RELATED STANDARDS:
Standard 5.2.8.1: Integrated Pest Management

REFERENCES:

1. Food Marketing Institutes (FMI). 1996. Facts about food and floods: A consumer guide to food quality and safe handling after a flood or power outage. Washington, DC: FMI.
2 U.S. Department of Health and Human Services, Public Health Service, Food and Drug Administration (FDA). 2009. *2009 Food code.* College Park, MD: FDA. http://www.fda.gov/downloads/Food/FoodSafety/RetailFoodProtection/FoodCode/FoodCode2009/UCM189448.pdf.

STANDARD 4.9.0.7: Storage of Dry Bulk Foods

Dry, bulk foods that are not in their original, unopened containers should be stored off the floor in clean metal, glass, or food-grade plastic containers with tight-fitting covers. All bulk food containers should be labeled and dated, and placed out of children's reach. Children should be permitted to handle household-size food containers during adult-supervised food preparation and cooking activities and when the container holds a single serving of food intended for that child's consumption.

RATIONALE: Food-grade nonporous containers prevent insect infestations and contamination from other foods and cleaning chemicals. By labeling and dating food, the food service staff can rotate the oldest foods to be used next and discard foods that have gone beyond safe storage times. Keeping bulk food containers out of the children's reach prevents contamination and misuse. Young children cannot be expected to have learned safe food handling practices well enough to prevent contaminating the food supply of others.

TYPE OF FACILITY: Center

RELATED STANDARDS:
Standard 5.2.8.1: Integrated Pest Management

STANDARD 4.9.0.8: Supply of Food and Water for Disasters

In areas where natural disasters (such as earthquakes, blizzards, tornadoes, hurricanes, floods) occur, a seventy-two hour supply of food and water should be kept in stock for each child and staff member (1). For some areas, an additional thirty-six hour supply may be needed, for example those areas at risk during hurricane season. The supply of food and water should be dated to know by which time it should be used to avoid its expiration date.

RATIONALE: It may take seventy-two hours or longer for help to arrive in some areas after a natural disaster of great magnitude. The direct path of a hurricane or other natural disaster cannot always be anticipated and it is not possible for supplies to be brought into some disaster locations until: a) efforts to rescue/save lives are completed and b) needs of communities/populations are assessed.

COMMENTS: Child care providers should periodically use and replace the food and water supplies from the emergency supplies to ensure usage before expiration dates. A child care facility should consult with their local health authority or local emergency preparedness agency to integrate disaster planning within the community.

TYPE OF FACILITY: Center; Large Family Child Care Home; Small Family Child Care Home

RELATED STANDARDS:
Standard 9.2.4.3: Disaster Planning, Training, and Communication

REFERENCES:

1. American Public Health Association. Get ready. http://www.getreadyforflu.org/newsite.htm.

STANDARD 4.9.0.9: Cleaning Food Areas and Equipment

Areas and equipment used for storage, preparation, and service of food should be kept clean. All of the food preparation, food service, and dining areas should be cleaned and sanitized before and after use. Food preparation equipment should be cleaned and sanitized after each use and stored in a clean and sanitary manner, and protected from contamination.

Sponges should not be used for cleaning and sanitizing. Disposable paper towels should be used. If washable cloths are used, they should be used once, then stored in a covered container and thoroughly washed daily. Microfiber cloths are preferable to cotton or paper towels for cleaning tasks because of microfiber's numerous advantages, including its long-lasting durability, ability to remove microbes, ergonomic benefits, superior cleaning capability and reduction in the amount of chemical needed.

RATIONALE: Outbreaks of foodborne illness have occurred in child care settings. Many of these infectious diseases can be prevented through appropriate hygiene and sanitation methods. Keeping hands clean reduces soiling of kitchen equipment and supplies. Education of child care staff regarding routine cleaning procedures can reduce the occurrence of illness in the group of children with whom they work (1).

Sponges harbor bacteria and are difficult to clean and sanitize between cleaning surface areas.

COMMENTS: "Clean" means removing all visible soil. Routine cleaning of kitchen areas should comply with the cleaning schedule provided in Appendix K or local health authority regulations.

"Sanitize" means using a product to reduce germs on inanimate surfaces to levels considered safe by public health codes or regulations.

TYPE OF FACILITY: Center; Large Family Child Care Home; Small Family Child Care Home

RELATED STANDARDS:
Appendix J: Selecting an Appropriate Sanitizer or Disinfectant
Appendix K: Routine Schedule for Cleaning, Sanitizing, and Disinfecting

REFERENCES:

1. Cowell, C., S. Schlosser. 1998. Food safety in infant and preschool day care. *Top Clin Nutr* 14:9-15.

STANDARD 4.9.0.10: Cutting Boards

Cutting boards should be made of nonporous material and should be scrubbed with hot water and detergent and sanitized between uses for different foods or placed in a dishwasher for cleaning and sanitizing. The facility should not use porous wooden cutting boards, boards made with wood components, and boards with crevices and cuts. Only hard maple or an equivalently hard, close-grained wood (e.g. oak) may be used for cutting boards.

RATIONALE: Some wood boards and boards with cracks and crevices harbor food or organic material that can promote bacterial growth and contaminate the next food cut on the surface.

COMMENTS: Heavy duty plastic and Plexiglas cutting boards can be placed in dishwashers. Programs should check with their local health department with questions regarding the proper hard wood for an allowable wood cutting board in child care facilities.

TYPE OF FACILITY: Center; Large Family Child Care Home; Small Family Child Care Home

STANDARD 4.9.0.11: Dishwashing in Centers

Centers should provide a three-compartment dishwashing area with dual integral drain boards or an approved dishwasher capable of sanitizing multi-use utensils. If a dishwasher is installed, there should be at least a two-compartment sink with a spray unit. If a dishwasher or a combination of dish pans and sink compartments that yield the equivalent of a three-compartment sink is not used, paper cups, paper plates and plastic utensils should be used and should be disposed of after every use.

RATIONALE: These are minimum requirements for proper cleaning and sanitizing of dishes and utensils (1).

A three-compartment sink is ideal. If only a single- or double-compartment sink is available, three freestanding dish pans or two sinks and one dish pan may be used as the compartments needed to wash, rinse, and sanitize dishes.

An approved dishwasher is a dishwasher that meets the approval of the regulatory health authority. Dishwashers should be carefully chosen. Depending on the size of the child care center and the quantity of food prepared, a household dishwasher may be adequate. Because of the time required to complete a full wash, rinse, and dry cycle, household domestic dishwashers are recommended for centers that do only one load of dishes after a snack or meal. Commercial dishwashers are required for some sizes of centers in some locales. Centers are responsible to comply with the requirements of the local regulatory health agency.

The length of time to wash dishes in commercial dishwashers is three to four minutes. Commercial dishwashers that operate at low water temperatures (140°F to 150°F) are recommended because they are more energy-efficient. These would be equipped with automatic detergent and sanitizer injectors. When choosing a dishwasher, caregivers/teachers can consult with the local health authority or state/local

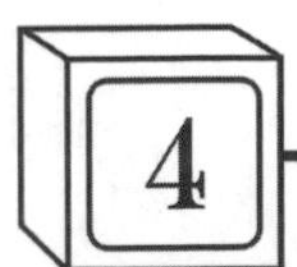

nutritionist/registered dietitian to ensure that they meet local health regulations.

COMMENTS: Household dishwashing machines can effectively wash and sanitize dishes and utensils provided that certain conditions are met. The three types of household dishwashers are:

a) Those that lack or operate without sanitizing wash or rinse cycles;
b) Those that have sanitizing wash or rinse cycles and a thermostat that senses a temperature of 150°F or higher before the machine advances to the next step in its cycle;
c) Those that have a sanitizing cycle and a thermostat as in (b) but advance to the next step in its cycle after fifteen minutes, if the temperature required to operate the thermostat is not reached.

All three types of household dishwashers are capable of producing the cumulative heat factor to meet the National Sanitation Foundation time-temperature standard for commercial, spray-type dishwashing machines. Dishwasher types (a) and (c) are capable of doing so only if the temperature of their inlet water is 155°F or higher.

The temperature of a hot water supply necessary for operating a dishwasher conflicts with what is considered a safe temperature to prevent scalding (no higher than 120°F). Installing a separate small hot water heater exclusively for dishwasher type (a) or (c) is a way to meet this requirement.

TYPE OF FACILITY: Center

RELATED STANDARDS:

Standard 5.2.1.14: Water Heating Devices and Temperatures Allowed

REFERENCES:

1. U.S. Department of Agriculture (USDA). 2002. *Making nutrition count for children - Nutrition guidance for child care homes.* Washington, DC: USDA. http://www.fns.usda.gov/tn/Resources/nutritioncount.html.

STANDARD 4.9.0.12: Dishwashing in Small and Large Family Child Care Homes

Small and large family child care homes should provide a three-compartment dishwashing arrangement or a dishwasher. At least a two-compartment sink or a combination of dish pans and sink compartments should be installed to be used in conjunction with a dishwasher to wash, rinse, and sanitize dishes. The dishwashing machine must incorporate a chemical or heat sanitizing process. If a dishwasher or a three-compartment dishwashing arrangement is not used, paper cups, paper plates and plastic utensils should be used and should be disposed of after every use.

RATIONALE: These are minimum requirements for proper cleaning and sanitizing of dishes and utensils (1). The purpose is to remove food particles and other soil, and to control bacteria.

TYPE OF FACILITY: Large Family Child Care Home; Small Family Child Care Home

RELATED STANDARDS:

Standard 4.9.0.11: Dishwashing in Centers
Appendix J: Selecting an Appropriate Sanitizer or Disinfectant
Appendix K: Routine Schedule for Cleaning, Sanitizing, and Disinfecting

REFERENCES:

1. U.S. Department of Agriculture (USDA). 2002. *Making nutrition count for children - Nutrition guidance for child care homes.* Washington, DC: USDA. http://www.fns.usda.gov/tn/Resources/nutritioncount.html.

STANDARD 4.9.0.13: Method for Washing Dishes by Hand

If the facility does not use a dishwasher, reusable food service equipment and eating utensils should be first scraped to remove any leftover food, washed thoroughly in hot water containing a detergent solution, rinsed, and then sanitized by one of the following methods:

a) Immersion for at least two minutes in a lukewarm (not less than 75°F) chemical sanitizing solution (bleach solution of a least 100 parts per million by mixing 1 1/2 teaspoons of domestic bleach per gallon of water). The sanitized items should be air-dried; or
b) Immersed in an EPA-registered sanitizer following the manufacturer's instructions for preparation and use; or
c) Complete immersion in hot water and maintenance at a temperature of 170 °F for not less than thirty seconds. The items should be air-dried (1);
d) Or, other methods if approved by the health department.

RATIONALE: These procedures provide for proper sanitizing and control of bacteria (2-4).

COMMENTS: To manually sanitize dishes and utensils in hot water at 170°F, a special hot water booster is usually required. To avoid burning the skin while immersing dishes and utensils in this hot water bath, special racks are required. Therefore, if dishes and utensils are being washed by hand, the chemical sanitizer method will be a safer choice.

Often, sponges are used in private homes when washing dishes. The structure of natural and artificial sponges provides an environment in which microorganisms thrive. This may contribute to the microbial load in the wash water. Nevertheless, the rinsing and sanitizing process should eliminate any pathogens contributed by a sponge. When possible, a cloth that can be laundered should be used instead of a sponge.

The concentration of bleach used for sanitizing dishes is much more diluted than the concentration recommended for disinfecting surfaces elsewhere in the facility. After washing and rinsing the dishes, the amount of infectious material on the dishes should be small enough so that the two minutes of immersion in the bleach solution (or treatment with an EPA-registered sanitizer) combined with air-drying will reduce the number of microorganisms to safe levels.

Air-drying of surfaces that have been sanitized using bleach leaves no residue, since chlorine evaporates when the solution dries. However, other sanitizers may need to be rinsed off to remove retained chemical from surfaces.

TYPE OF FACILITY: Center; Large Family Child Care Home; Small Family Child Care Home

RELATED STANDARDS:
Standard 4.9.0.12: Dishwashing in Small and Large Family Child Care Homes
Appendix J: Selecting an Appropriate Sanitizer or Disinfectant

REFERENCES:

1. Bryan, F. L., G. H. DeHart. 1975. Evaluation of household dishwashing machines, for use in small institutions. *J Milk Food Tech* 38:509-15.
2. Benjamin, S. E., ed. 2007. *Making food healthy and safe for children: How to meet the National health and safety performance standards – Guidelines for out of home child care programs*. 2nd ed. Chapel Hill, NC: National Training Institute for Child Care Health Consultants. http://nti.unc.edu/course_files/curriculum/nutrition/making_food_healthy_and_safe.pdf.
3. Enders, J. B. 1994. *Food, nutrition and the young child*. New York: Merrill.
4. U.S. Department of Agriculture (USDA). 2002. *Making nutrition count for children - Nutrition guidance for child care homes.* Washington, DC: USDA. http://www.fns.usda.gov/tn/Resources/nutritioncount.html.

4.10 Meals from Outside Vendors or Central Kitchens

STANDARD 4.10.0.1: Approved Off-Site Food Services

Food provided by a central kitchen or vendor to off-site locations should be obtained from sources approved and inspected by the local health authority.

RATIONALE: This standard ensures that the child care facility receives safe food.

TYPE OF FACILITY: Center; Large Family Child Care Home; Small Family Child Care Home

STANDARD 4.10.0.2: Food Safety During Transport

After preparation, food should be transported promptly in clean, covered, and temperature-controlled containers. Hot foods should be maintained at temperatures not lower than 135°F, and cold foods should be maintained at temperatures of 41°F or lower (1). Hot foods may be allowed to cool to 110°F or lower before serving to young children as long as the food is cooked to appropriate temperatures and the time at room temperature does not exceed two hours (or if room temperature is above 90°F then the time does not exceed one hour) (2). The temperature of foods should be checked with a working food-grade, metal probe thermometer.

RATIONALE: Served foods have a high probability of becoming contaminated during serving. Bacteria multiply rapidly in perishable foods out of refrigeration, as much as doubling every fifteen to twenty minutes (2).

Foods at more than 110°F are too hot for children's mouths.

A working food-grade, metal probe thermometer will determine accurately when foods are safe for consumption.

COMMENTS: If the temperature of hot foods is well below 135°F when it arrives, the caregiver/teacher should review delivery and storage practices and make any changes necessary to maintain proper food temperatures during storage and delivery.

The caregiver/teacher should record food temperatures in a log book to document the pattern of temperature control and spot shifts toward unsafe levels.

TYPE OF FACILITY: Center; Large Family Child Care Home; Small Family Child Care Home

RELATED STANDARDS:
Standard 4.8.0.6: Maintaining Safe Food Temperatures

REFERENCES:

1. U.S. Department of Health and Human Services, Public Health Service, Food and Drug Administration (FDA). 2009. *2009 Food code.* College Park, MD: FDA. http://www.fda.gov/downloads/Food/FoodSafety/RetailFoodProtection/FoodCode/FoodCode2009/UCM189448.pdf.
2. U.S. Department of Agriculture, Food Safety and Inspection Service. 2006. *Safe food handling, how temperatures affect food.* http://www.fsis.usda.gov/PDF/How_Temperatures_Affect_Food.pdf.

STANDARD 4.10.0.3: Holding of Food Prepared At Off-Site Food Service Facilities

Facilities receiving food from an off-site food service facility should have provisions for the proper holding and serving of food and washing of utensils to meet the requirements of the Food and Drug Administration's Model Food Code and the standards approved by the State or local health authority (1).

RATIONALE: Served foods have a high probability of becoming contaminated during serving. Bacteria multiply rapidly in perishable foods out of refrigeration, as much as doubling every fifteen to twenty minutes (2).

TYPE OF FACILITY: Center; Large Family Child Care Home; Small Family Child Care Home

REFERENCES:

1. U.S. Department of Health and Human Services, Public Health Service, Food and Drug Administration (FDA). 2009. *2009 Food code.* College Park, MD: FDA. http://www.fda.gov/downloads/Food/FoodSafety/RetailFoodProtection/FoodCode/FoodCode2009/UCM189448.pdf.
2. U.S. Department of Agriculture, Food Safety and Inspection Service. 2006. *Safe food handling, how temperatures affect food.* http://www.fsis.usda.gov/PDF/How_Temperatures_Affect_Food.pdf.

Chapter 5

5

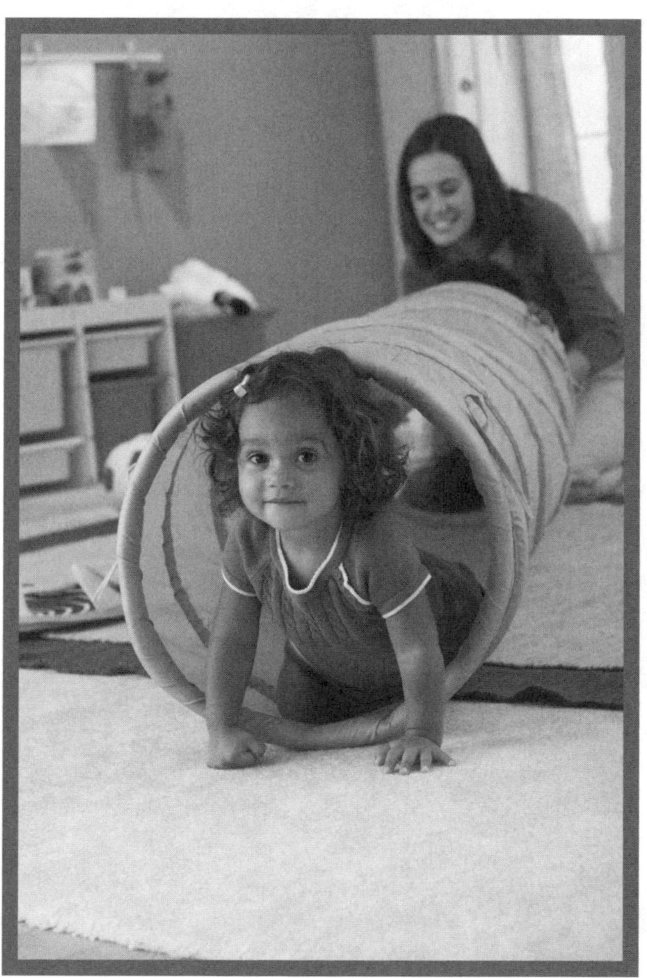

Facilities, Supplies, Equipment, and Environmental Health

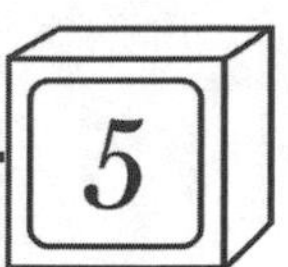

5.1 Overall Requirements

5.1.1 General Location, Layout, and Construction of the Facility

STANDARD 5.1.1.1: Location of Center

A center should not be located in a private residence unless that portion of the residence is used exclusively for the care of children during the hours of operation.

RATIONALE: Centers in these standards are generally defined as "providing care and education for any number of children in a non-residential setting or thirteen or more children in any setting." When there are a large number of children in care who may span the age groups of infants, toddlers, preschool, and school-age children, special sanitation and design are needed to protect children from injury and prevent transmission of disease. Undivided attention must be given to these purposes during child care operations.

COMMENTS: The portion of a private residence used as a child care facility is variable and unique to each specific situation. If other people will be using the private residence during the child care facility's hours of operation, then the caregiver/teacher must arrange the residence so that the activities of these people do not occur in the area designated for child care.

TYPE OF FACILITY: Center

RELATED STANDARDS:
Standard 5.1.1.9: Unrelated Business in a Child Care Area

STANDARD 5.1.1.2: Inspection of Buildings

Newly constructed, renovated, remodeled, or altered buildings should be inspected by a public inspector to assure compliance with applicable building and fire codes before the building can be made accessible to children.

RATIONALE: Building codes are designed to ensure that a building is safe for occupants. Environmental health recommendations are designed to ensure the building and property are free of health hazards for children and workers.

COMMENTS: Any building not used for child care for a period of time should be inspected for compliance with applicable building and fire codes. Review of environmental health hazards by county or city public health environmental offices can help to meet safety requirements.

TYPE OF FACILITY: Center

RELATED STANDARDS:
Standard 5.1.1.3: Compliance with Fire Prevention Code

STANDARD 5.1.1.3: Compliance with Fire Prevention Code

Every twelve months, the child care facility should obtain written documentation to submit to the regulatory licensing authority that the facility complies with a state-approved or nationally recognized Fire Prevention Code. If available, this documentation should be obtained from a fire prevention official with jurisdiction where the facility is located. Where fire safety inspections or a Fire Prevention Code applicable to child care centers is not available from local authorities, the facility should arrange for a fire safety inspection by an inspector who is qualified to conduct such inspections using the National Fire Protection Association's *NFPA 101: Life Safety Code*.

RATIONALE: Regular fire safety checks by trained officials will ensure that a child care facility continues to meet all applicable fire safety codes. *NFPA 101: Life Safety Code* addresses child care facilities in two chapters devoted exclusively to this occupancy – chapter 16, "New Day-Care Occupancies" and chapter 17, "Existing Day-Care Occupancies" (1).

TYPE OF FACILITY: Center

REFERENCES:
1. National Fire Protection Association (NFPA). 2009. *NFPA 101: Life Safety Code.* 2009 ed. Quincy, MA: NFPA.

STANDARD 5.1.1.4: Accessibility of Facility

The facility should be accessible for children and adults with disabilities, in accordance with Section 504 of the Rehabilitation Act of 1973 and the Americans with Disabilities Act (ADA). Accessibility includes access to buildings, toilets, sinks, drinking fountains, outdoor play areas, meal and snack areas, and all classroom and therapy areas.

RATIONALE: Accessibility has been detailed in full, in Section 504 of the Rehabilitation Act of 1973. It is also a key component of the ADA, barring discrimination against anyone with a disability.

COMMENTS: Any facility accepting children with motor disabilities must be accessible to all children served. Small family home caregivers/teachers may be limited in their ability to serve such children, but are not precluded from doing so if there is a reasonable degree of compliance with this standard. Accommodation of adaptive equipment for all children should be made to ensure access to all activities of the care setting. Access to public and most private facilities is a key to the implementation of the ADA. If toilet learning/training is a relevant activity, the facility may be required to provide adapted toilet equipment.

For more information on requirements regarding accessibility, consult the *Americans with Disabilities Act Accessibility Guidelines for Buildings and Facilities (ADAAG)*, available at http://www.access-board.gov/adaag/html/adaag.htm, and the U.S. Access Board's play area accessibility guidelines at http://www.access-board.gov/play/guide/intro.htm.

TYPE OF FACILITY: Center; Large Family Child Care Home; Small Family Child Care Home

RELATED STANDARDS:
Standard 5.4.1.7: Toilet Learning/Training Equipment
Standard 5.4.6.2: Space for Therapy Services
Standard 6.2.1.2: Play Equipment and Surfaces Meet ADA Requirements

STANDARD 5.1.1.5: Environmental Audit of Site Location

An environmental audit should be conducted before construction of a new building; renovation or occupation of an older building; or after a natural disaster, to properly evaluate and, where necessary, remediate or avoid sites where children's health could be compromised (1,3).

The environmental audit should include assessments of:

a) Potential air, soil, and water contamination on child care facility sites and outdoor play spaces;
b) Potential toxic or hazardous materials in building construction; and
c) Potential safety hazards in the community surrounding the site.

A written environmental audit report that includes any remedial action taken should be kept on file.

RATIONALE: Evaluation of potential health and safety risks associated with the physical site location of a child care facility will identify any remedial action required or whether the site should be avoided if children's health could be compromised.

Children are much more vulnerable to exposures of contaminated environmental media materials than adults because their bodies are developing; they eat more, drink more, and breathe more in proportion to their body size; and their behavior, such as crawling and hand-to-mouth activity, can expose them more to chemicals (4).

Awareness of remedial action required or sites to avoid will reduce exposure to conditions that cause injury or adversely affect health.

Epidemiological studies indicate a relationship between outdoor air pollution and adverse respiratory effects on children (2). Research suggests that exposure to air pollution is a function of proximity to roadways (5-7).

The soil in play areas should not contain hazardous levels of any toxic chemical or substance. Soil contaminated with toxic materials can poison children. For example, ensuring that soil in play areas is free of dangerous levels of lead helps prevent lead poisoning (8-10).

Existing buildings may contain potentially toxic or hazardous construction materials (e.g., lead paint, asbestos) that may be released during renovation work. Assessing the presence of such materials enables the management of potential exposures through removal, containment, or by other means (11).

COMMENTS: Potential safety hazards in the community surrounding the site location of a child care facility may include:

a) Proximity to hazardous industrial air emissions;
b) Proximity to toxic or hazardous substances in adjacent or nearby property;
c) Proximity to transportation hazards (e.g., local automobile traffic, major roadways, airports, railroads);
d) Proximity to utilities (e.g., drinking water reservoirs or storage tanks, electrical sub-stations, high-voltage power transmission lines, pressurized gas transmission lines);
e) Proximity to explosive or flammable products (e.g., propane tanks).

Possible options for reducing exposure to potential safety hazards in the community may include:

a) Locating the site of a child care facility at a safe distance from the hazard; and/or
b) Providing a physical barrier to prevent children from being exposed to the safety hazards (e.g., fencing).

TYPE OF FACILITY: Center; Large Family Child Care Home; Small Family Child Care Home

RELATED STANDARDS:
Standard 5.1.1.2: Inspection of Buildings
Standard 5.2.1.1: Fresh Air
Standard 5.2.3.1: Noise Levels
Standard 5.2.9.6: Preventing Exposure to Asbestos or Other Friable Materials
Standard 5.2.9.13: Testing for Lead

REFERENCES:
1. Etzel, R. A., S. J. Balk, eds. 2004. *Pediatric environmental health.* 2nd ed. Elk Grove Village, IL: American Academy of Pediatrics.
2. American Academy of Pediatrics, Committee on Environmental Health. 2004. Policy statement: Ambient air pollution: Health hazards to children. *Pediatrics* 114:1699-1707.
3. U.S. Environmental Protection Agency. 2010. Siting of school facilities. http://cfpub.epa.gov/schools/top_sub.cfm?t_id=45&s_id=64/.
4. U.S. Environmental Protection Agency. Human health risk assessment. http://www.epa.gov/risk/health-risk.htm.
5. Boothe V. L., D. G. Shendell. 2008. Potential health effects associated with residential proximity to freeways and primary roads: Review of scientific literature, 1999-2006. *J Environmental Health* 70:33-41, 55-56.
6. Zhou Y., J. I. Levy. 2007. Factors influencing the spatial extent of mobile source air pollution impacts: A meta-analysis. *BMC Public Health* 7:89. http://www.biomedcentral.com/content/pdf/1471-2458-7-89.pdf.
7. Zhua Y., W. C. Hinds, S. Kim, S. Shen, C. Sioutas. 2002. Study of ultrafine particles near a major highway with heavy-duty diesel traffic. *Atmospheric Environment* 36:4323–35.
8. U.S. Environmental Protection Agency. 2010. *The lead-safe certified guide to renovate right.* http://www.epa.gov/lead/pubs/renovaterightbrochure.pdf.
9. Burke, P., J. Ryan. 2001. *Providing solutions for a better tomorrow: Reducing the risks associated with lead in soil.* Washington, DC: U.S. Environmental Protection Agency. http://www.epa.gov/nrmrl/pubs/600f01014/600f01014.pdf.
10. Centers for Disease Control and Prevention (CDC). 2005. *Preventing lead poisoning in young children*. Atlanta, GA: CDC. http://www.cdc.gov/nceh/lead/publications/prevleadpoisoning.pdf.
11. Fiene, R. 2002. *13 indicators of quality child care: Research update.* Washington, DC: U.S. Department of Health and Human Services, Office of the Assistant Secretary for Planning and Evaluation. http://aspe.hhs.gov/hsp/ccquality-ind02/.

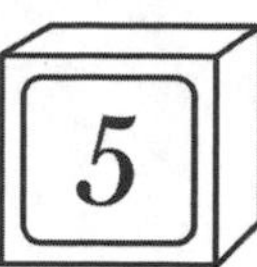

STANDARD 5.1.1.6: Structurally Sound Facility

Every exterior wall, roof, and foundation should be structurally sound, weather-tight, and water-tight to ensure protection from weather and natural disasters.

Every interior floor, wall, and ceiling should be structurally sound and should be finished in accordance with local building codes to control exposure of the occupants to levels of toxic fumes, dust, and mold.

RATIONALE: Both the design of structures and the lack of maintenance can lead to exposure of children to physical injury, mold, dust, pests, and toxic materials (1).

COMMENTS: Child care operations sometimes use older buildings or buildings designed for purposes other than child care.

TYPE OF FACILITY: Center; Large Family Child Care Home; Small Family Child Care Home

RELATED STANDARDS:
Standard 5.1.1.2: Inspection of Buildings
Standard 5.1.1.5: Environmental Audit of Site Location
Standard 5.7.0.7: Structure Maintenance

REFERENCES:
1. Whole Building Design Guide Secure/Safe Committee. 2010. Ensure occupant safety and health. National Institute of Building Sciences. http://www.wbdg.org/design/ensure_health.php.

STANDARD 5.1.1.7: Use of Basements and Below Grade Areas

Finished basements or areas that are partially below grade may be used for children who independently ambulate and who are two years of age or older, if the space is in compliance with applicable building and fire codes. Environmental health factors may be reviewed with county or city public health departments.

RATIONALE: Basement and partially below grade areas can be quite habitable and should be usable as long as building, fire safety (1), and environmental quality is satisfactory.

COMMENTS: To "independently ambulate" means that children are able to walk from place to place with or without the use of assistive devices.

TYPE OF FACILITY: Center; Large Family Child Care Home; Small Family Child Care Home

RELATED STANDARDS:
Standard 5.1.1.8: Buildings of Wood Frame Construction
Standard 5.1.2.1: Space Required Per Child
Standard 5.1.2.2: Floor Space Beneath Low Ceiling Heights
Standard 5.1.4.1: Alternate Exits and Emergency Shelter
Standard 5.1.4.2: Evacuation of Children with Special Health Care Needs and Children with Disabilities
Standard 5.2.1.1: Fresh Air
Standard 5.2.2.1: Levels of Illumination
Standard 5.2.9.4: Radon Concentrations
Standard 5.2.9.5: Carbon Monoxide Detectors
Standard 5.2.9.6: Preventing Exposure to Asbestos or Other Friable Materials

REFERENCES:
1. National Fire Protection Association (NFPA). 2009. *NFPA 101: Life Safety Code.* 2009 ed. Quincy, MA: NFPA.

STANDARD 5.1.1.8: Buildings of Wood Frame Construction

Infants and toddlers should be housed and cared for only on the ground floor in buildings of wood frame construction. Preschool-age and school-age children should be able to use floors other than the ground floor in a building of wood construction if the building has required exits and care is provided in:

a) A daylight-lit basement with exits that are no more than a half flight high;
b) A tri-level facility with half flights of stairs;
c) A facility that is protected throughout by an automatic sprinkler system, which has its exit stairs enclosed by minimum one-hour fire barriers with openings in those barriers protected by minimum one-hour fire doors;
d) Any door encountered along the egress route should be easy for caregivers/teachers and older preschool-age children to open.

RATIONALE: Fire and building safety experts recommend that children be permitted above ground level only in buildings of wood construction with certain exceptions (1).

COMMENTS: Infants and toddlers should always be on the main floor with access directly to the outdoors. Doors along the egress route need to be easy to open. Consult local or state fire safety codes and child care licensing laws for restrictions on floor occupancy by age groups.

TYPE OF FACILITY: Center; Large Family Child Care Home; Small Family Child Care Home

RELATED STANDARDS:
Standard 5.1.1.7: Use of Basements and Below Grade Areas

REFERENCES:
1. National Fire Protection Association (NFPA). 2009. *NFPA 101: Life Safety Code.* 2009 ed. Quincy, MA: NFPA.

STANDARD 5.1.1.9: Unrelated Business in a Child Care Area

Child care areas should not be used for any business or purpose unrelated to providing child care when children are present in these areas.

If unrelated business is conducted in child care areas when the child care facility is not in operation, activities associated with such business should not leave any residue in the air or on the surfaces, or leave behind materials or equipment, that could be harmful to children.

RATIONALE: Some activities that leave a harmful residue are smoking, ammunition reloading, soldering, woodworking, and welding (1). Examples of materials or equipment that could be harmful are small screws, nails, and electric tools with sharp blades. Child care requires child-oriented, child-safe areas where the child's needs are primary.

COMMENTS: Employers should inform caregivers/teachers about harmful residues or equipment that may potentially remain from unrelated business activity so that such residues or equipment can be removed.

TYPE OF FACILITY: Center; Large Family Child Care Home; Small Family Child Care Home

RELATED STANDARDS:
Standard 5.1.1.11: Separation of Operations from Child Care Areas
Standard 5.2.1.5: Ventilation of Recently Carpeted or Paneled Areas
Standard 5.2.9.1: Use and Storage of Toxic Substances
Standard 5.2.9.3: Informing Staff Regarding Presence of Toxic Substances
Standard 5.2.9.10: Prohibition of Poisonous Plants
Standard 5.2.9.15: Construction and Remodeling During Hours of Operation
Standard 5.7.0.2: Removal of Hazards from Outdoor Areas
Standard 5.7.0.4: Inaccessibility of Hazardous Equipment

REFERENCES:
1. U.S. Environmental Protection Agency, U.S. Consumer Product Safety Commission. 2010. The inside story: A guide to indoor air quality. http://www.epa.gov/iaq/pubs/insidest.html.

STANDARD 5.1.1.10: Office Space

Office space separate from child care areas should be provided for administration and staff in centers. Children should not have access to this area unless they are supervised by staff.

RATIONALE: For the efficient and effective operation of a center, office areas where activities incompatible with the care of young children are conducted should be separate from child care areas. These office areas can be expected to contain supplies, equipment and records/documents that should not be accessible to children. Office staff should be free from the distractions of child care (1,2).

COMMENTS: Child care staff should have access to an area that is separate from the child care areas where they can meet personal needs such as a break room, adult bathroom, resource library, etc.

TYPE OF FACILITY: Center

REFERENCES:
1. National Association for the Education of Young Children (NAEYC). 1977. *Planning environments for young children*. Washington, DC: NAEYC.
2. Murph, J. R., S. D. Palmer, D. Glassy, eds. 2005. *Health in child care: A manual for health professionals*. 4th ed. Elk Grove Village, IL: American Academy of Pediatrics.

STANDARD 5.1.1.11: Separation of Operations from Child Care Areas

Rooms or spaces that are used for the following activities or operations should be separated from the child care areas and the egress route should not pass through such spaces:

a) Commercial-type kitchen;
b) Boiler, maintenance shop;
c) Janitor closet and storage areas for cleaning products, pesticides, and other chemicals;
d) Laundry and laundering supplies;
e) Woodworking shop;
f) Flammable or combustible storage;
g) Painting operation;
h) Rooms that are used for any purpose involving the presence of toxic substances;
i) Area for medication storage.

Areas that have combustibles should be protected by fire-resistant barriers. The egress route and the fire-resistant separation should be approved by the appropriate regulatory agencies responsible for building and fire inspections. In small and large family child care homes, a fire-resistant separation should not be required where the food preparation kitchen contains only a domestic cooking range and the preparation of food does not result in smoke or grease-laden vapors escaping into indoor areas. Where separation is provided between the egress route and the hazardous area, it should be safe to use such route, but egress should not require passage through the hazardous area.

RATIONALE: Hazards and toxic substances must be kept separate in a locked closet or room from space used for child care to prevent children's and staff members' exposure to injury (1).

Cleaning agents must be inaccessible to children (out of reach and behind locked doors). Food preparation surfaces must be separate from diaper changing areas including sinks for handwashing. Children must be restricted from access to the stove when cooking surfaces are hot.

COMMENTS: In small family child care homes, mixed use of rooms is common (2). Some combined use of space for food preparation, storage of cleaning equipment and household tools, laundry, and diaper changing requires that each space within a room be defined according to its purpose and that exposure of children to hazards be controlled. Food preparation should be separate from all exposure to possible cross-contamination.

TYPE OF FACILITY: Center; Large Family Child Care Home; Small Family Child Care Home

REFERENCES:
1. National Fire Protection Association (NFPA). 2009. *NFPA 101: Life Safety Code.* 2009 ed. Quincy, MA: NFPA.
2. Olds, A. R. 2001. *Child care design guide*. New York: McGraw-Hill.

STANDARD 5.1.1.12: Multiple Use of Rooms

Playing, eating, and napping may occur in the same area (exclusive of diaper changing areas, toilet rooms, kitchens, hallways, and closets), provided that:

a) The room is of sufficient size to have a defined area for each of the activities allowed there at the time the activity is under way;
b) The room meets other building requirements;
c) Programming is such that use of the room for one purpose does not interfere with use of the room for other purposes.

RATIONALE: Except for toilet and diaper changing areas, which must have no other use, the use of common space

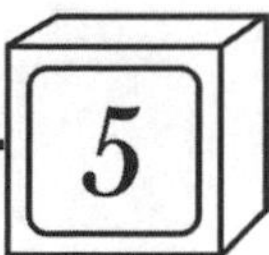

for different activities for children facilitates close supervision of a group of children, some of whom may be involved simultaneously in more than one of the activities listed in the standard (1).

COMMENTS: Compliance is measured by direct observation.

TYPE OF FACILITY: Center; Large Family Child Care Home; Small Family Child Care Home

REFERENCES:

1. Olds, A. 2001. Zoning a group room. In *Child care design guide,* 137-65. New York: McGraw-Hill.

5.1.2 Space per Child

STANDARD 5.1.2.1: Space Required per Child

In general, the designated area for children's activities should contain a minimum of forty-two square feet of usable floor space per child. A usable floor space of fifty square feet per child is preferred.

This excludes floor area that is used for:

a) Circulation (e.g., walkways around the activity area);
b) Classroom support (e.g., staff work areas and activity equipment storage that may be adjacent to the activity area);
c) Furniture (e.g., bookcases, sofas, lofts, block corners, tables and chairs);
d) Center support (e.g., administrative office, washrooms, etc.)

Usable, indoor floor space for the children's activity area depends on the design and layout of the child care facility, and whether there is an opportunity and space for outdoor activities.

RATIONALE: Numerous studies have explored child care space requirements that are necessary to:

a) Provide an environment that is highly functional for program delivery and to encourage strong, positive staff-to-child relationships;
b) Accommodate the recommended group size and staff-to-child ratio; and
c) Efficiently use space and incorporates ease of supervision.
d) Recommendations from research studies range between forty-two to fifty-four square feet per child (1).

Studies have shown that the quality of the physical designed environment of early child care centers is related to children's cognitive, social, and emotional development (e.g., size, density, privacy, well-defined activity settings, modified open-plan space, a variety of technical design features and the quality of outdoor play spaces). In addition to meeting the needs of children, caregivers/teachers require space to implement programs and facilitate interactions with children.

A review of the literature indicates that in the past ten years, there has been growing research and study into how the physical design of child care settings affects child development. Historically, a standard of thirty-five square feet was used. Recommendations from research studies range between forty-two to fifty-four square feet per child. Comments from researchers indicate that other factors must also be considered when assessing the context of usable floor space for child care activities (1,5-8).

Although each child's development is unique to that child, age groups are often used to categorize developmental needs. To meet these needs, the use of activity space for each age group will be inherently different.

Child behavior tends to be more constructive when sufficient space is organized to promote developmentally appropriate skills. Crowding has been shown to be associated with increased risk of developing upper respiratory infections (2). Also, having sufficient space will reduce the risk of injury from simultaneous activities.

Children with special health care needs may require more space than typically developing children (1).

COMMENTS: The usable floor space for children's activities in this standard refers to indoor space that is used as the primary play space. Consideration should also be given to the presence or absence of secondary indoor play space that might be shared between programs as well as to outdoor play space.

Staff-child ratios (i.e., the number of staff required per number of children) should also be taken into account since staff consumes floor area space as well as children. Group size for various age groups should also be considered. Since groups of infants are smaller than groups of preschoolers, "infant and toddler rooms tend to be small, while preschool and school-age rooms are a bit generous at full capacity" (1). Infant and toddler rooms often dedicate a considerable amount of inflexible space to cribs and diaper changing areas. Sufficient space to accommodate these activities, space for adult seating to care for infants, and space for safe mobility of infants and toddlers requires that the per child square foot requirements are applied for their areas also.

Square footage estimates should only be intended as guidelines. Especially in child care facilities with fewer than fifty children, "plugging in" the square footage into a formula to calculate space required usually does not work (1).

It is important to keep in mind that state licensing regulations specify minimum space requirements and that they must be legally adhered to. Such requirements vary from state to state (3). For Federal child care centers, the U.S. General Services Administration's (GSA) child care design standards require a minimum of forty-eight and one-half square feet per child in the classroom (4).

Although providing adequate space for implementing a program of activities that meets the developmental needs of children is important in providing quality child care, how that space is actually used is likely more critical (8). It has been observed that child care facilities operating in older buildings with less than ideal space can still deliver quality child care programs to meet the needs of children. Nevertheless, the amount of activity space required per child should take the known research into consideration.

TYPE OF FACILITY: Center; Large Family Child Care Home; Small Family Child Care Home

RELATED STANDARDS:
Standards 1.1.1.1-1.1.1.3: Ratios and Supervision
Standard 2.1.2.3: Space and Activity to Support Learning of Infants and Toddlers
Standard 2.1.4.2: Space for School-Age Activity

REFERENCES:

1. Olds, A. R. 2001. *Child care design guide*. New York: McGraw-Hill.
2. Fleming, D. W., S. L. Cochi, A. W. Hightower, et al. 1987. Childhood upper respiratory tract infections: To what degree is incidence affected by daycare attendance? *Pediatrics* 79:55-60.
3. National Child Care Information and Technical Assistance Center and the National Association for Regulatory Administration. 2009. *The 2007 licensing child care study*. http://www.naralicensing.org/associations/4734/files/2007 Licensing Study_full_report.pdf.
4. U.S. General Services Administration (GSA). 2003. *Child care center design guide*. New York: GSA Public Buildings Service, Office of Child Care. http://www.gsa.gov/graphics/pbs/designguidesmall.pdf.
5. Beach J., M. Friendly. 2005. Child care centre physical environments. Working Documents, Child Care Resource and Research Unit. http://www.childcarequality.ca/wdocs/QbD_PhysicalEnvironments.pdf.
6. Moore, G. T., T. Sugiyama, L. O'Donnell. 2003. Children's physical environments rating scale. Paper presented at the Australian Early Childhood Education 2003 Conference, Hobart, Australia. http://sydney.edu.au/architecture/documents/ebs/AECA_2003_paper.pdf.
7. White, R., V. Stoecklin. 2003. The great 35 square foot myth. http://www.whitehutchinson.com/children/articles/35footmyth.shtml.
8. The Family Child Care Accreditation Project, Wheelock College. 2005. *Quality standards for NAFCC accreditation.* 4th ed. Salt Lake City, UT: National Association for Family Child Care. http://www.nafcc.org/documents/QualStd.pdf.

STANDARD 5.1.2.2: Floor Space Beneath Low Ceiling Heights

In a room where the entire ceiling height is less than seven and a half feet above the floor, the floor area should not be counted in determining compliance with the space requirements specified in Standard 5.1.2.1.

In a room where the ceiling is at different levels at least two-thirds of the usable floor area should have a ceiling height of at least seven and one-half feet and one-third of the usable floor area should have a ceiling height of greater than six feet eight inches. Floor areas beneath ceiling heights less than six-feet eight-inches tall should not be considered (1).

RATIONALE: Ceiling height must be adequate for caregivers/teachers to supervise and reach children who require assistance.

TYPE OF FACILITY: Center; Large Family Child Care Home; Small Family Child Care Home

RELATED STANDARDS:
Standard 5.1.2.1: Space Required Per Child

REFERENCES:

1. National Fire Protection Association (NFPA). 2009. *NFPA 101: Life Safety Code.* 2009 ed. Quincy, MA: NFPA.

STANDARD 5.1.2.3: Areas for School-Age Children

When school-age children are in care for periods that exceed two hours before or after school, a separate area away from areas for younger children should be available for school-age children to do homework. Areas used for this purpose should, in addition to meeting the other facility standards have:

a) Table space;
b) Chairs;
c) Adequate ventilation;
d) Lighting of 40 to 50 foot-candles in the room;
e) Lighting of 50 to 100 foot-candles on the surface used as a desk (1).

RATIONALE: School-age children need a quiet space for reading and to do homework so they are not forced to work against the demands for attention that younger children pose. In family child care homes such an area might be within the same room and separated by a room dividing arrangement of furniture.

TYPE OF FACILITY: Center; Large Family Child Care Home; Small Family Child Care Home

RELATED STANDARDS:
Standard 5.1.2.1: Space Required Per Child
Standard 5.2.1.1: Fresh Air
Standard 5.2.1.2: Indoor Temperatures
Standard 5.2.2.1: Levels of Illumination

REFERENCES:

1. American Society of Heating, Refrigeration and Air-conditioning Engineers (ASHRAE), American Institute of Architects, Illuminating Engineering Society of North America, U.S. Green Building Council, U.S. Department of Energy. 2008. *Advanced energy design guide for K-12 school buildings*, 148. Atlanta, GA: ASHRAE.

5.1.3 Openings

STANDARD 5.1.3.1: Weather-Tightness and Water-Tightness of Openings

Each window, exterior door, and basement or cellar hatchway should be weather-tight and water-tight when closed.

RATIONALE: Children's environments must be protected from exposure to moisture, dust, and temperature extremes.

TYPE OF FACILITY: Center; Large Family Child Care Home; Small Family Child Care Home

STANDARD 5.1.3.2: Possibility of Exit from Windows

All windows in areas used by children under five years of age should be constructed, adapted, or adjusted to limit the exit opening accessible to children to less than four inches, or be otherwise protected with guards that prevent exit by a child, but that do not block outdoor light. Where such

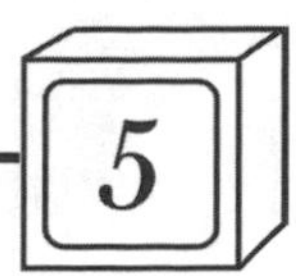

windows are required by building or fire codes to provide for emergency rescue and evacuation, the windows and guards, if provided, should be equipped to enable staff to release the guard and open the window fully when evacuation or rescue is required. Opportunities should be provided for staff to practice opening these windows, and such release should not require the use of tools or keys. Children should be given information about these windows, relevant safety rules, as well as what will happen if the windows need to be opened for an evacuation.

RATIONALE: To prevent children from falling out of windows, standards from the U.S. Consumer Product Safety Commission (CPSC) and the ASTM International (ASTM) require the opening size to be four inches to prevent the child from getting through or the head from being entrapped (1,2). Some children may be able to pass their body through a slightly larger opening but then get stuck and hang from the window opening with their head trapped inside. Caregivers/teachers must not depend on screens to keep children from falling out of windows. Windows to be used as fire exits must be immediately accessible. Staff should supervise children when they are near these windows, and incorporate safety information and relevant emergency procedures and drills into their day-to-day curriculum so that children will better understand the safety issues and what will happen if they need to leave the building through the windows.

COMMENT: "Screens" are intended to prevent flying insects from coming into the facility whereas window "guards" are the type of devices commonly used to provide building security and prevent intruders.

TYPE OF FACILITY: Center; Large Family Child Care Home; Small Family Child Care Home

REFERENCES:

1. U.S. Consumer Product Safety Commission (CPSC). 2000. New standards for window guards to help protect children from falls. Release #00-126. Washington, DC: CPSC. http://www.cpsc.gov/CPSCPUB/PREREL/prhtml00/00126.html.

2. ASTM International. ASTM F2090-08 *Standard specification for window fall prevention devices with emergency escape (egress) release mechanisms*. West Conshohocken, PA: ASTM.

STANDARD 5.1.3.3: Screens for Ventilation Openings

All openings used for ventilation should be screened against insect entry.

RATIONALE: Screens prevent the entry of insects, which may bite, sting, or carry disease.

TYPE OF FACILITY: Center; Large Family Child Care Home; Small Family Child Care Home

RELATED STANDARDS:

Standard 5.1.3.2: Possibility of Exit from Windows

STANDARD 5.1.3.4: Safety Guards for Glass Windows/Doors

Glass windows and glass door panels within thirty-six inches of the floor should have safety guards (such as rails or mesh) or be of safety-grade glass or polymer and equipped with a vision strip.

RATIONALE: Glass panels can be invisible to an active child or adult (1). When a child collides with a glass panel, serious injury can result from the collision impact or the broken glass.

COMMENTS: In areas where glass windows are repeatedly broken, installation of polymer material should be considered.

TYPE OF FACILITY: Center; Large Family Child Care Home; Small Family Child Care Home

RELATED STANDARDS:

Standard 5.1.3.2: Possibility of Exit from Windows

REFERENCES:

1. International Code Council (ICC). 2009. *2009 international building code*. Washington, DC: ICC.

STANDARD 5.1.3.5: Finger-Pinch Protection Devices

Finger-pinch protection devices should be installed wherever doors, cupboards/cabinets, and gates are accessible to children. These devices include:

a) Flexible plastic and rubber devices that cover the gap created at the front and rear hinge-sides of a door or gate when it is opened;
b) Other types of flexible coverings for these gaps;
c) Adjustable door closing devices that slow the rate of door closing. Slowing the door closing rate helps prevent finger pinching in the latch area of the door or abrupt closing of the door against a small child.

RATIONALE: Finger-pinch injuries in doors are a significant cause of injury among claims against liability insurance in child care. Closing doors and gates create significant exposure to children for bruised, cut, or smashed fingers, torn or cracked fingernails, broken bones, and even amputations. Finger-pinch injuries happen very quickly, often before staff can react. Finger-pinch protection devices ensure that this type of injury does not occur.

COMMENTS: A child doesn't have to pass through a door or gate to acquire a finger-trapping injury. A child can be on the outside of one of these doors and still get their fingers trapped while it is being closed. Young children are vulnerable to injury when they fall against the rear hinge-side of doors and gates, striking the projecting hinges. The installation of rear finger-pinch protection devices will eliminate this problem, too (1). Piano hinges are not recommended to alleviate this problem as they tend to sag over time with heavy use.

Costs of these devices vary significantly, as do method and extent of protection, product durability and warranty; the different products may not provide equally suitable protection. Whatever hardware is selected should prevent (not just discourage) the entry of a finger into the danger zone from both sides of the door or gate and should protect the door or gate through the full extent of its swing (i.e., it should be capable of protecting doors and gates that open 180 degrees). Attachment should use screws rather than glue for a stronger, more durable connection.

TYPE OF FACILITY: Center; Large Family Child Care Home; Small Family Child Care Home

REFERENCES:

1. Moseley, G. 2008. Closing the door on finger injuries. *Doors and Hardware* 72:38-41.

STANDARD 5.1.3.6: Directional Swing of Indoor Doors

Doors, other than exit stair enclosure doors, from a building area with fewer than fifty persons should swing in the direction of most frequent travel. Doors from a building area with more than fifty persons and exit stair enclosure doors should swing in the direction of egress travel (the path for going out). An exception is that boiler room doors should swing into the room.

RATIONALE: Proper door swings provide easy, quick passage and prevent injuries. Boiler room doors should swing inward to help contain explosions.

The *NFPA 101: Life Safety Code* from the National Fire Protection Association (NFPA), and the model building codes in wide use throughout the United States, require that doors serving an area with fifty or more persons swing in the direction of egress travel (1). This is important because large numbers of persons might push against each other leaving those up against a door without the ability to step back and allow the door to swing back into the room.

COMMENTS: Doors in homes usually open inward. The requirement for door swing may be addressed in local building codes.

TYPE OF FACILITY: Center

REFERENCES:

1. National Fire Protection Association (NFPA). 2009. *NFPA 101: Life Safety Code.* 2009 ed. Quincy, MA: NFPA.

5.1.4 Exits

STANDARD 5.1.4.1: Alternate Exits and Emergency Shelter

Each building or structure, new or old, should be provided with a minimum of two exits, at different sides of the building or home, leading to an open space at ground level. If the basement in a small family child care home is being used, one exit must lead directly to the outside. Exits should be unobstructed, allowing occupants to escape to an outside door or exit stair enclosure in case of fire or other emergency. Each floor above or below ground level used for child care should have at least two unobstructed exits that lead to an open area at ground level and thereafter to an area that meets safety requirements for a child care indoor or outdoor area. Children should remain there until their parents/guardians can pick them up, if reentry into the facility is not possible.

Entrance and exit routes should be reviewed and approved by the applicable fire inspector. Exiting should meet all the requirements of the current edition of the *NFPA 101: Life Safety Code* from the National Fire Protection Association (NFPA).

RATIONALE: Unobstructed exit routes are essential for prompt evacuation. The purpose of having two ways to exit when child care is provided on a floor above or below ground level is to ensure an alternative exit if fire blocks one exit (1).

COMMENTS: Using an outdoor playground as a safe place to exit to may not always be possible. Where the playground is fully surrounded by fencing, it is important that a gate that staff is trained, authorized, and equipped to open, be provided to permit travel away from the building should fire expose children and staff to radiant heat and smoke. Some authorities will permit a fenced area with sufficient accumulation space at least fifty feet from the building to serve in lieu of a gated opening. Some child care facilities do not have a playground located adjacent to the child care building and use local parks as the playground site. Access to these parks may require crossing a street at an intersection with a crosswalk. This would normally be considered safe, especially in areas of low traffic; however, when sirens go off, a route that otherwise may be considered safe becomes chaotic and dangerous. During evacuation or an emergency, children, as well as staff, become excited and may run into the street when the playground is not fenced or immediately adjacent to the center (1).

In the event of a fire, staff members and children should be able to get at least fifty feet away from the building or structure. If the children cannot return to their usual building, a suitable shelter containing all items necessary for child care must be available where the children can safely remain until their parents/guardians come for them. An evacuation plan should take into consideration all available open areas to which staff and children can safely retreat in an emergency (1).

For information about the *NFPA 101: Life Safety Code*, contact the NFPA.

TYPE OF FACILITY: Center; Large Family Child Care Home; Small Family Child Care Home

RELATED STANDARDS:

Standard 5.1.4.6: Labeled Emergency Exits
Standard 5.1.4.7: Access to Exits

REFERENCES:

1. National Fire Protection Association (NFPA). 2009. *NFPA 101: Life Safety Code.* 2009 ed. Quincy, MA: NFPA.

STANDARD 5.1.4.2: Evacuation of Children with Special Health Care Needs and Children with Disabilities

In facilities that include children who have physical disabilities or other developmental disabilities, all exits and steps necessary for evacuation should have ramps approved by the local building inspector and be clearly marked or identi-

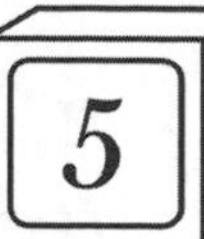

fied. Children who have ambulatory difficulty, mobility limitations or impairments, use wheelchairs or other equipment that must be transported with the child (such as an oxygen ventilator) should be located on the ground floor of the facility or provisions should be made for efficient emergency evacuation to a safe sheltered area. Children who have special medical or dietary needs should have their medical equipment brought along during an evacuation.

RATIONALE: The facility must meet building code standards for the community and also the requirements under the Americans with Disabilities Act (ADA) and their access guidelines (1). All children must be able to exit the building quickly in case of emergency. Locating children in wheelchairs or those with special equipment on the ground floor may eliminate the need for transporting these children down the stairs during an emergency evacuation. In buildings where the ground floor cannot be used for such children, arrangements must be made to move children to a safe location, such as a fire tower stairwell, during an emergency exit. Children with diabetes, asthma, or special medical diets may need medication or special foods brought along during an evacuation.

COMMENTS: Assuring physical access to a facility also requires that a means of evacuation meeting safety standards for exit accommodates any children with special health care needs in care.

TYPE OF FACILITY: Center; Large Family Child Care Home; Small Family Child Care Home

RELATED STANDARDS:
Standard 1.1.1.3: Ratios for Facilities Serving Children with Special Health Care Needs and Disabilities
Standard 5.1.1.4 Accessibility of Facility
Standard 5.1.1.8 Buildings of Wood Frame Construction

REFERENCES:
1. U.S. Architectural and Transportation Barriers Compliance Board (Access Board). 2002. *Americans with disabilities act accessibility guidelines for buildings and facilities (ADAAG)*. http://www.access-board.gov/adaag/ADAAG.pdf.

STANDARD 5.1.4.3: Path of Egress

The minimum width of any path of egress should be thirty-six inches. An exception is that doors should provide a minimum clear width of thirty-two inches. The width of doors should accommodate wheelchairs and the needs of individuals with physical disabilities.

Where exits are not immediately accessible from an open floor area, safe and continuous passageways, aisles, or corridors leading to every exit should be maintained and should be arranged to provide access for each occupant to at least two exits by separate ways of travel. Doorways, exit access paths, passageways, corridors and exits should be kept free of materials, furniture, equipment and debris to allow unobstructed egress travel from inside the child care facility to the outside.

RATIONALE: Unobstructed access to exits is essential to prompt evacuation (1). The hallways and door openings must be wide enough to permit easy exit in an emergency. The actual exit is the enclosed stair or the actual door to the outside; doors from most rooms and the travel along a corridor are considered exit access or the path of egress. The *NFPA 101: Life Safety Code* from the National Fire Protection Association (NFPA) permits the usual thirty-six inches minimum to be reduced to a clear opening of thirty-two inches for doors (1). This is consistent with *Americans with Disabilities Act Accessibility Guidelines for Buildings and Facilities (ADAAG)* as it affords enough width for a person in a wheelchair to maneuver through the door opening (2).

TYPE OF FACILITY: Center; Large Family Child Care Home; Small Family Child Care Home

REFERENCES:
1. National Fire Protection Association (NFPA). 2009. *NFPA 101: Life Safety Code*. 2009 ed. Quincy, MA: NFPA.
2. U.S. Architectural and Transportation Barriers Compliance Board (Access Board). 2002. *Americans with disabilities act accessibility guidelines for buildings and facilities (ADAAG)*. http://www.access-board.gov/adaag/ADAAG.pdf.

STANDARD 5.1.4.4: Locks

In centers, no door should have a lock or fastening device that prevents free egress from the interior. Free egress means that building occupants, without the use of a tool, key or special knowledge are able to operate the door, under all lighting conditions, using not more than one releasing operation. In all child care facilities, all door hardware in areas that school-age children use should be within the reach of the children. In centers, doors serving areas with more than 100 occupants should be permitted to be latched only if provided with panic hardware (latch release hardware that can be opened by pressure in the direction of travel).

In large or small family child day care homes, a double-cylinder deadbolt lock which requires a key to unlock the door from the inside should not be permitted on any door along the escape path from any child care except the exterior door, and then only if the key required to unlock the door is kept hanging at the door.

If emergency exits lead to potentially unsafe areas for children (such as a busy street), alarms or other signaling devices should be installed on these exit doors to alert the staff in case a child attempts to leave. An alarm or signaling system should also be in place in the case of a child with special behavior support needs who poses a risk for running out of a room or building.

RATIONALE: Children, as well as staff members, must be able to evacuate a building in the event of a fire or other emergency. Nevertheless, the caregiver/teacher must assure security from intruders and from unsupervised use of the exit by children.

COMMENTS: Double-cylinder deadbolt locks that require a key to unlock the door from the inside are often installed in private homes for added security. In such situations, these dead bolt locks should be present only on exterior doors and should be left in the unlocked position during the hours of child care operation. Locks that prevent opening from the outside, but can be opened without a key from the inside should be used for security during hours of child care operation. Double cylinder deadbolt locks should not be used on interior doors, such as closets, bathrooms, storage rooms, and bedrooms (1).

TYPE OF FACILITY: Center; Large Family Child Care Home; Small Family Child Care Home

REFERENCES:

1. National Fire Protection Association (NFPA). 2009. *NFPA 101: Life Safety Code*. 2009 ed. Quincy, MA: NFPA.

STANDARD 5.1.4.5: Closet Door Latches

Closet doors accessible to children should have an internal release for any latch so a child inside the closet can open the door.

RATIONALE: Closet doors that can be opened from the inside prevent entrapment (1).

TYPE OF FACILITY: Center; Large Family Child Care Home; Small Family Child Care Home

REFERENCES:

1. National Fire Protection Association (NFPA). 2009. *NFPA 101: Life Safety Code*. 2009 ed. Quincy, MA: NFPA.

STANDARD 5.1.4.6: Labeled Emergency Exits

In centers, required exits should be clearly identified and visible at all times during operation of the child care facility. The exits for egress should be arranged or marked so the path to safety outside is unmistakable.

RATIONALE: As soon as children can learn to recognize exit signs and pathway markings, they will benefit from having these paths of egress clearly marked. Adults who come into the building as visitors need these markings to direct them as well (1).

TYPE OF FACILITY: Center

REFERENCES:

1. National Fire Protection Association (NFPA). 2009. *NFPA 101: Life Safety Code*. 2009 ed. Quincy, MA: NFPA.

STANDARD 5.1.4.7: Access to Exits

Each room of a child care facility should be provided with direct access to:

a) An exit to the outside; or
b) A corridor or hallway providing direct access to an exit to the outside.

Where it is necessary to pass through an adjacent room for access to a corridor or exit, any doors providing passage to and through such room should not be latched or locked, or otherwise barricaded, to prevent access.

No obstructions should be placed in the corridors or passageways leading to the exits.

RATIONALE: A room that requires exit through another room to get to an exit path can entrap its occupants when there is a fire or emergency condition if passage can be impeded by a barrier or door that is latched (1).

An obstruction in the path of exit can lead to entrapment, especially in an emergency situation where groups of people may be exiting together.

TYPE OF FACILITY: Center; Large Family Child Care Home; Small Family Child Care Home

REFERENCES:

1. National Fire Protection Association (NFPA). 2009. *NFPA 101: Life Safety Code*. 2009 ed. Quincy, MA: NFPA.

5.1.5 Steps and Stairs

STANDARD 5.1.5.1: Balusters

Protective handrails and guardrails should have balusters/spindles at intervals of less than three and a half inches or have sufficient protective material to prevent a three and a half inch sphere from passing through if caring for children two years and over. If caring for children under the age of two years, balusters/spindles should be spaced at intervals less than two and three-eighths inches or have sufficient protective material to prevent a sphere with a diameter of two and three-eighths inches from passing through.

RATIONALE: A child's head may be small enough to be entrapped in a space more than three and a half inches wide (1). Infants and young toddlers may crawl or play close to railings around stairs. Because they may have access to railings, it is recommended to follow the same recommendation for the spacing of balusters/spindles for stair railings as the slats on a crib.

COMMENTS: Building codes vary from state to state and many regulations for balusters/spindles do not meet the recommendations for intervals less than three and a half inches. Some building codes are for intervals of four inches or greater. Because of this discrepancy and the expense of adding balusters/spindles, using a protective material may be the only option. Recommendations as stated above should be considered for remodeling or new construction.

TYPE OF FACILITY: Center; Large Family Child Care Home; Small Family Child Care Home

REFERENCES:

1. U.S. Consumer Product Safety Commission (CPSC). 2008. *Public playground safety handbook*. Bethesda, MD: CPSC. http://www.cpsc.gov/cpscpub/pubs/325.pdf.

STANDARD 5.1.5.2: Handrails

Handrails should be provided on both sides of stairways, be securely attached to the walls or stairs, and at a maximum height of thirty-eight inches.

The outside diameter of handrails should be between one and one-quarter inches and two inches.

When railings are installed on the side of stairs open to a stairwell, access to the stairwell should be prevented by a barrier so a child cannot use the railings as a ladder to jump or fall into the stairwell.

RATIONALE: Model codes, including the National Fire Protection Association's *NFPA 101: Life Safety Code,* require

handrails to be mounted in the height range of thirty-four to thirty-eight inches (1). Such handrails are equally usable by children. The stair researcher, Jake Pauls, has filmed small children effectively using handrails mounted as high as thirty-eight inches. This comes naturally to the children because they are used to reaching up to take an adult's hand while walking. There is no justification for forcing the center or home to incur the added expense of installing a second set of handrails closer to the floor.

Railings on both sides ensure a readily available handhold (whether right handed or left handed) in the event of a fall down the stairs. When handrails are installed to allow children a handhold, the stairwell should be designed so the railing does not provide the child with a ladder to climb.

COMMENTS: Open stairwells can be enclosed with rigid vertical materials to prevent children from climbing and falling over the rail. Handrails are for purposes of providing a graspable rail for help in arresting falls on stairs. Guards are for purposes of preventing falls over an open side where there is more than thirty inches vertical distance to fall.

TYPE OF FACILITY: Center; Large Family Child Care Home; Small Family Child Care Home

RELATED STANDARDS:
Standard 5.1.6.6: Guardrails and Protective Barriers

REFERENCES:
1. National Fire Protection Association (NFPA). 2009. *NFPA 101: Life safety code*. 2009 ed. Quincy, MA: NFPA.

STANDARD 5.1.5.3: Landings

Landings should be provided beyond each interior and exterior door that opens onto a stairway. Landing width should not be less than the width of stairway it serves and must be at least the width of stairway in direction of travel, but need not be more than forty-eight inches. When fully open, the door should not project more than seven inches into the landing. Dimensions (length and width) of the landing are equal to or greater than the width of the door.

RATIONALE: Landings are necessary to accommodate the swing of the door without pushing the person on the stairway into a precarious position while trying to leave the stairway (1).

TYPE OF FACILITY: Center; Large Family Child Care Home; Small Family Child Care Home

REFERENCES:
1. International Code Council (ICC). 2009. *2009 international building code*. Washington, DC: ICC.

STANDARD 5.1.5.4: Guards at Stairway Access Openings

Securely installed, effective guards (such as gates) should be provided at the top and bottom of each open stairway in facilities where infants and toddlers are in care. Gates should have latching devices that adults (but not children) can open easily in an emergency. "Pressure gates" or accordion gates should not be used. Gate design should not aid in climbing. Gates at the top of stairways should be hardware mounted (e.g., to the wall) for stability. Basement stairways should be shut off from the main floor level by a full door. This door should be self-closing and should be kept locked to entry when the basement is not in use. No door should be locked to prohibit exit at any time.

RATIONALE: Falls down stairs and escape upstairs can injure infants and toddlers. A gate with a difficult opening device can cause entrapment in an emergency (1).

TYPE OF FACILITY: Center; Large Family Child Care Home; Small Family Child Care Home

RELATED STANDARDS:
Standard 5.1.6.6: Guardrails and Protective Barriers

REFERENCES:
1. U.S. Consumer Product Safety Commission (CPSC). Old accordion style baby gates are dangerous. http://www.cpsc.gov/CPSCPUB/PUBS/5085.pdf.

5.1.6 Exterior Areas

Note to Reader: *See Chapter 6 for Outdoor Play Area Requirements*

STANDARD 5.1.6.1: Designated Walkways, Bike Routes, and Drop-Off and Pick-Up Points

Safe pedestrian crosswalks, drop-off and pick-up points, and bike routes in the vicinity of the facility should be identified, written in the facility's procedures, and communicated to all children, parents/guardians, and staff. Parking for drop-off and pick-up should not require street-side removal of children from a vehicle.

RATIONALE: In 2008, one-fifth (20%) of all children between the ages of five and nine who were killed in traffic crashes were pedestrians (1). Identification and communication of safe routes practices may reduce the potential of injuries resulting from children darting into traffic (2). Providing bike route information may encourage the use of this health-promoting, economical, and environmentally friendly mode of transportation.

TYPE OF FACILITY: Center; Large Family Child Care Home; Small Family Child Care Home

RELATED STANDARDS:
Standard 6.5.2.1: Drop-Off and Pick-Up

REFERENCES:
1. U.S. Department of Transportation, National Highway Traffic Safety Administration (NHTSA). 2008. *Traffic Safety Facts 2008: Pedestrians.* Washington, DC: NHTSA. http://www-nrd.nhtsa.dot.gov/Pubs/811163.PDF.
2. U.S. General Services Administration (GSA). 2003. *Child care center design guide*. New York: GSA Public Buildings Service, Office of Child Care. http://www.gsa.gov/graphics/pbs/designguidesmall.pdf.

STANDARD 5.1.6.2: Construction and Maintenance of Walkways

Inside and outside stairs, ramps, porches, and other walkways to the structure should be constructed for safe use as required by the local building code and should be

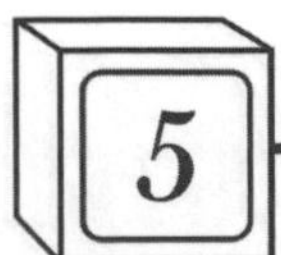

kept in sound condition, well-lighted, and in good repair (1). Walkways must be cleared and maintained during inclement weather to prevent falls.

RATIONALE: Prevention of slipping and tripping hazards is key to preventing injuries from falls.

TYPE OF FACILITY: Center; Large Family Child Care Home; Small Family Child Care Home

RELATED STANDARDS:
Standards 5.1.6.3-5.1.6.4: Surfaces

REFERENCES:
1. Whole Building Design Guide Secure/Safe Committee. 2010. Ensure occupant safety and health. National Institute of Building Sciences. http://www.wbdg.org/design/ensure_health.php.

STANDARD 5.1.6.3: Drainage of Paved Surfaces

All paved surfaces should be well-drained to avoid accumulation of water and ice.

RATIONALE: Well-drained paved surfaces help prevent injury and deterioration of the surface by discouraging the accumulation of water and ice (1).

TYPE OF FACILITY: Center; Large Family Child Care Home; Small Family Child Care Home

REFERENCES:
1. Whole Building Design Guide Secure/Safe Committee. 2010. Ensure occupant safety and health. National Institute of Building Sciences. http://www.wbdg.org/design/ensure_health.php.

STANDARD 5.1.6.4: Walking Surfaces

All walking surfaces, such as walkways, ramps, and decks, should have a non-slip finish and be free of loose material (e.g., gravel, sand), water, and ice. Sand may be used on walkways during ice and snow conditions.

All walking surfaces and other play surfaces should be free of holes and abrupt irregularities in the surface.

RATIONALE: Slippery and uneven walking surfaces can lead to injury even during activities of children and adults that do not involve play (1).

COMMENTS: An example of a non-slip finish is asphalt or asphalt with a covering of sand for icy walkways.

TYPE OF FACILITY: Center; Large Family Child Care Home; Small Family Child Care Home

REFERENCES:
1. Whole Building Design Guide Secure/Safe Committee. 2010. Ensure occupant safety and health. National Institute of Building Sciences. http://www.wbdg.org/design/ensure_health.php.

STANDARD 5.1.6.5: Areas Used by Children for Wheeled Vehicles

The area used by children for wheeled vehicles should have a flat, smooth, non-slippery surface. A physical barrier should separate this area from the following:

a) Traffic;
b) Streets;
c) Parking;
d) Delivery areas;
e) Driveways;
f) Stairs;
g) Hallways used as fire exits;
h) Balconies;
i) Pools and other areas containing water.

RATIONALE: Uneven or slippery riding surfaces can lead to injury (1). Physical separation from environmental obstacles is necessary to prevent potential collision, injuries, falls, and drowning.

TYPE OF FACILITY: Center

RELATED STANDARDS:
Standards 5.1.6.2-5.1.6.4: Surfaces

REFERENCES:
1. U.S. General Services Administration (GSA). 2003. *Child care center design guide*. New York: GSA Public Buildings Service, Office of Child Care. http://www.gsa.gov/graphics/pbs/designguidesmall.pdf.

STANDARD 5.1.6.6: Guardrails and Protective Barriers

Guardrails, a minimum of thirty-six inches in height, should be provided at open sides of stairs, ramps, and other walking surfaces (e.g., landings, balconies, porches) from which there is more than a thirty-inch vertical distance to fall. Spaces below the thirty-six inches height guardrail should be further divided with intermediate rails or balusters as detailed in the next paragraph.

For preschoolers, bottom guardrails greater than nine inches but less or equal to twenty-three inches above the floor should be provided for all porches, landings, balconies, and similar structures. For school age children, bottom guardrails should be greater than nine inches but less or equal to twenty inches above the floor, as specified above.

For infants and toddlers, protective barriers should be less than three and one-half inches above the floor, as specified above. All spaces in guardrails should be less than three and a half inches. All spaces in protective barriers should be less than three and one-half inches. If spaces do not meet the specifications as listed above, a protective material sufficient to prevent the passing of a three and one-half inch diameter sphere should be provided.

Where practical or otherwise required by applicable codes, guardrails should be a minimum of forty-two inches in height to help prevent falls over the open side by staff and other adults in the child care facility.

RATIONALE: Structures such as porches, landings, balconies, and other similar structures that are raised more than thirty inches above an adjacent ground or floor, pose increased risk for fall injuries. Spaces between three and one-half inches and nine inches are a head entrapment hazard (1).

Guardrails are designed to protect against falls from elevated surfaces, but do not discourage climbing or pro-

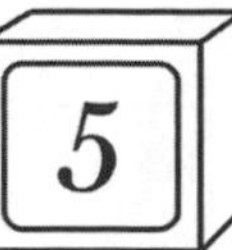

tect against climbing through or under. Protective barriers protect against all three and provide greater protection. Guardrails are not recommended to use for infants and toddlers; protective barriers should be used instead.

A top guardrail with a minimum height of forty-two inches serves the needs of all occupants – children as well as adults (2). The minimum thirty-six-inch guardrail height detailed in this standard is based solely on the needs of children.

TYPE OF FACILITY: Center; Large Family Child Care Home; Small Family Child Care Home

REFERENCES:

1. U.S. Consumer Product Safety Commission (CPSC). 2008. *Public playground safety handbook*. Bethesda, MD: CPSC. http://www.cpsc.gov/cpscpub/pubs/325.pdf.
2. National Fire Protection Association (NFPA). 2009. *NFPA 101: Life safety code*. 2009 ed. Quincy, MA: NFPA.

STANDARD 5.1.6.7: Location of Satellite Dishes

A satellite dish should not be located within playgrounds or other areas accessible to children. If a satellite dish is on the premises, it should be surrounded by a fence (at least four feet high) that prevents children from climbing and gaining access to the satellite dish.

RATIONALE: Children are at risk for injury if they are allowed to climb on or play near satellite dishes. Natural barriers are not recommended due to the fact that they can change with seasons and weather, affecting the effectiveness of the barrier.

COMMENTS: Satellite dishes come in many sizes. Smaller diameter satellite dishes between eighteen to thirty inches are often mounted on a rooftop or the side of a building. Older, large six-foot diameter satellite dishes may be mounted on the ground.

TYPE OF FACILITY: Center; Large Family Child Care Home; Small Family Child Care Home

REFERENCES:

1. Olds, A. R. 2001. *Child care design guide*. New York: McGraw-Hill.

5.2 Quality of the Outdoor and Indoor Environment

5.2.1 Ventilation, Heating, Cooling, and Hot Water

STANDARD 5.2.1.1: Fresh Air

As much fresh outdoor air as possible should be provided in rooms occupied by children. Windows should be opened whenever weather and the outdoor air quality permits or when children are out of the room (1). When windows are not kept open, rooms should be ventilated, as specified in Standards 5.2.1.1-5.2.1.6. The specified rates at which outdoor air must be supplied to each room within the facility range from fifteen to sixty cubic feet per minute per person (cfm/p). The rate depends on the activities that normally occur in that room.

RATIONALE: The health and well-being of both the staff and the children can be greatly affected by indoor air quality. The air people breathe inside a building is contaminated with organisms shared among occupants and sometimes the indoor air is more polluted than the outdoor air. Young children may be affected more than adults by air pollution. Air quality significantly impacts people's health. The health impacts from exposure to air pollution (indoor and outdoor) can include: decreased lung function, asthma, bronchitis, emphysema, and even some types of cancer. Children are particularly vulnerable to air pollution because their lungs are still developing and they breathe more air per pound of body weight than adults do. Indoor air pollution is often greater than outdoor levels of air pollution due to a general lack of adequate air filtration and ventilation (4). The presence of dirt, moisture, and warmth encourages the growth of mold and other contaminants, which can trigger allergic reactions and asthma (2). Children who spend long hours breathing contaminated or polluted indoor air are more likely to develop respiratory problems, allergies, and asthma (3-5).

Although insulation of a building is important in reducing heating or cooling costs, it is unwise to try to seal the building completely. Air circulation is essential to clear infectious disease agents, odors, and toxic substances in the air. Levels of carbon dioxide are an indicator of the quality of ventilation (6). Air circulation can be adjusted by a properly installed and adjusted heating, ventilation, air conditioning, and cooling (HVAC) system as well as by using fans and open windows.

COMMENTS: For further information on air quality and on ventilation standards related to type of room use, contact the American Society of Heating, Refrigerating, and Air-Conditioning Engineers (ASHRAE), the U.S. Environmental Protection Agency (EPA) Public Information Center, the American Gas Association (AGA), the Edison Electric Institute (EEI), the American Lung Association (ALA), the U.S. Consumer Product Safety Commission (CPSC), and the Safe Building Alliance (SBA).

For child care, ANSI/ASHRAE 62.1-2007 calls for 10 cfm/person plus 0.18 cfm/sq.ft. of space. ANSI/ASHRAE 62-1989 or ASHRAE Standard 55-2007 is information on Thermal Environmental Conditions for Human Occupancy.

Qualified engineers can ensure heating, ventilation, air conditioning (HVAC) systems are functioning properly and that applicable standards are being met. The American Society of Heating, Refrigerating, and Air-Conditioning Engineers (ASHRAE) Website (http://www.ashrae.org) includes the qualifications required of its members and the location of the local ASHRAE chapter. The contractor who services the child care HVAC system should provide evidence of successful completion of ASHRAE or comparable courses. Caregivers/teachers should understand enough about codes and standards to be sure the facility's building is a healthful place to be.

Indoor air quality is important to children who have asthma. A checklist from the National Heart, Lung and Blood Institute, *How Asthma Friendly is your Child Care Setting*? (available at http://www.nhlbi.nih.gov/health/public/lung/asthma/chc_chk.pdf), can help caregivers/teachers create a more asthma-friendly environment.

TYPE OF FACILITY: Center; Large Family Child Care Home; Small Family Child Care Home

RELATED STANDARDS:
Standard 3.1.3.2: Playing Outdoors
Standard 3.1.3.3: Protection from Air Pollution while Children are Outside
Standard 5.2.1.3: Heating and Ventilation Equipment Inspection and Maintenance
Standard 5.2.9.5: Carbon Monoxide Detectors

REFERENCES:
1. American Society of Heating, Refrigeration and Air-conditioning Engineers (ASHRAE), American Institute of Architects, Illuminating Engineering Society of North America, U.S. Green Building Council, U.S. Department of Energy. 2008. *Advanced energy design guide for K-12 school buildings*, 148. Atlanta, GA: ASHRAE.
2. U.S. Environmental Protection Agency. IAQ tools for schools program. http://www.epa.gov/iaq/schools/.
3. U.S. Environmental Protection Agency (EPA). 2008. *Care for your air: A guide to indoor air quality*. Washington, DC: EPA. http://www.epa.gov/iaq/pdfs/careforyourair.pdf.
4. U.S. Environmental Protection Agency, Consumer Product Safety Commission. 2010. The inside story: A guide to indoor air quality. http://www.epa.gov/iaq/pubs/insidest.html.
5. American Lung Association, American Lung Association, U.S. Consumer Product Safety Commission, U.S. Environmental Protection Agency (EPA). 1994. *Indoor air pollution: An introduction for health professionals*. Cincinnati: EPA National Service Center for Environmental Publications. http://www.epa.gov/iaq/pdfs/indoor_air_pollution.pdf.
6. Daneault, S., M. Beusoleil, K. Messing. 1992. Air quality during the winter in Quebec day-care centers. *Am J Public Health* 82:432-34.

STANDARD 5.2.1.2: Indoor Temperature

A draft-free temperature of 68°F to 75°F should be maintained at thirty to fifty percent relative humidity during the winter months. A draft-free temperature of 74°F to 82°F should be maintained at thirty to fifty percent relative humidity during the summer months (1,3). All rooms that children use should be heated and cooled to maintain the required temperatures and humidity.

RATIONALE: These requirements are based on the standards of the American Society of Heating, Refrigerating, and Air-Conditioning Engineers (ASHRAE), which take both comfort and health into consideration (1,3). High humidity can promote growth of mold, mildew, and other biological agents that can cause eye, nose, and throat irritation and may trigger asthma episodes in people with asthma (2). These precautions are essential to the health and well-being of both the staff and the children. When planning construction of a facility, it is healthier to build windows that open. Some people need filtered air that helps control pollen and other airborne pollutants found in raw outdoor air.

COMMENTS: Simple and inexpensive devices that measure the ambient relative humidity indoors may be purchased in hardware stores or toy stores that specialize in science products. The ASHRAE Website (http://www.ashrae.org) has a list of membership chapters, and membership criteria that help to establish expertise on which caregivers/teachers could rely in selecting a contractor.

TYPE OF FACILITY: Center; Large Family Child Care Home; Small Family Child Care Home

RELATED STANDARDS:
Standard 5.2.1.3: Heating and Ventilation Equipment Inspection and Maintenance

REFERENCES:
1. American Society of Heating, Refrigeration and Air-conditioning Engineers, American Institute of Architects, Illuminating Engineering Society of North America, U.S. Green Building Council, U.S. Department of Energy. 2008. *Advanced energy design guide for K-12 school buildings*, 148. Atlanta, GA: ASHRAE.
2. U.S. Environmental Protection Agency (EPA). 2008. *Care for your air: A guide to indoor air quality*. Washington, DC: EPA. http://www.epa.gov/iaq/pdfs/careforyourair.pdf.
3. American Society of Heating, Refrigerating and Air-conditioning Engineers (ASHRAE). 2007. Standard 55-2007: Thermal conditions for human occupancy. Atlanta: ASHRAE.

STANDARD 5.2.1.3: Heating and Ventilation Equipment Inspection and Maintenance

All heating and ventilating equipment, including heaters, stoves used for heating (or furnaces), stovepipes, boilers, and chimneys, should be inspected and cleaned before each cooling and heating season by a qualified heating/air conditioning contractor, who should verify in writing that the equipment is properly installed, cleaned, and maintained to operate efficiently and effectively. The system should be operated in accordance with operating instructions and be certified that it meets the local building code by a representative of the agency that administers the building code. Documentation of these inspections and certification of safety should be kept on file in the facility.

RATIONALE: Routinely scheduled inspections and proper operation ensure that equipment is working properly. Heating equipment is the second leading cause of ignition in fatal house fires (1). Heating equipment that is kept in good repair is less likely to cause fires.

COMMENTS: Qualified engineers can ensure heating, ventilation, air conditioning (HVAC) systems are functioning properly and that applicable standards are being met. The American Society of Heating, Refrigerating, and Air-Conditioning Engineers (ASHRAE) Website (http://www.ashrae.org) includes the qualifications required of its members and the location of the local ASHRAE chapter. The contractor who services the child care HVAC system should provide evidence of successful completion of ASHRAE or comparable courses. Caregivers/teachers should understand enough

about codes and standards to be sure the facility's building is a healthful place to be.

TYPE OF FACILITY: Center; Large Family Child Care Home; Small Family Child Care Home

RELATED STANDARDS:
Standard 5.2.1.1: Fresh Air
Standard 5.2.1.8: Maintenance of Air Filters
Standard 5.2.9.5: Carbon Monoxide Detectors

REFERENCES:
1. Chowdhury, R., M. Greene, D. Miller. 2008. *2003-2005 residential fire loss estimates*. Washington, DC: U.S. Consumer Product Safety Commission. http://www.cpsc.gov/library/fire05.pdf.

STANDARD 5.2.1.4: Ventilation When Using Art Materials

Areas where arts and crafts activities are conducted should be well-ventilated. Materials that create toxic fumes or gases such as spray adhesives and paints should not be used when children are present. Material Safety Data Sheets (MSDS) should be obtained and kept for all chemicals used.

RATIONALE: Some art and craft supplies contain toxic ingredients, including possible human carcinogens, creating a significant risk to the health and well-being of children. Art supplies containing toxic chemicals can also produce fumes that trigger asthma, allergies, headaches, and nausea (1). Art and craft materials should conform to all applicable ACMI safety standards. Materials should be labeled in accordance with the chronic hazard labeling standard, ASTM D4236-94(2005) (1). Children in grade six and lower should only use non-toxic art and craft materials (1,2). Labels are required on art supplies to identify any hazardous ingredients, risks associated with their use, precautions, first aid, and sources of further information.

COMMENTS: Staff should be educated to the possibility that some children may have special vulnerabilities to certain art materials (such as children with asthma or allergies). Not allowing food and drink near supplies prevents the possible cross contamination of materials and reduces potential injuries from poisoning. For more information on poisoning, contact the poison center at 1-800-222-1222.

See the *How Asthma Friendly is Your Child Care Setting?* checklist at http://www.nhlbi.nih.gov/health/public/lung/asthma/chc_chk.pdf to learn more about creating an asthma-friendly indoor environment.

TYPE OF FACILITY: Center; Large Family Child Care Home; Small Family Child Care Home

RELATED STANDARDS:
Standard 5.2.9.7: Proper Use of Art and Craft Materials

REFERENCES:
1. Art and Creative Materials Institute. 2010. Safety - what you need to know. http://www.acminet.org/Safety.htm.
2. Art and Creative Materials Institute, Arts, Crafts, and Theater Safety, Inc., National Art Education Association, U.S. Consumer Product Safety Commission (CPSC). *Art and craft safety guide*. Bethesda, MD: CPSC. http://www.cpsc.gov/cpscpub/pubs/5015.pdf.

STANDARD 5.2.1.5: Ventilation of Recently Carpeted or Paneled Areas

Doors and windows should be opened in areas that have been recently carpeted or paneled using adhesives until the odors are no longer present. Window fans, room air conditioners, or other means to exhaust emission to the outdoors should be used.

RATIONALE: Adhesives that contain toxic materials can cause significant symptoms in occupants of buildings where these materials are used. Many carpets contain polybrominated diphenyl ethers (PBDEs) to retard flames. PBDEs are associated with several adverse health effects in animal studies including changes in memory and learning, interference with thyroid function, endocrine disruption, and cancer (2). One study found that toddlers and preschoolers typically had three times more of these compounds in their blood as their mothers (1).

COMMENTS: Facilities should choose carpeting or other flooring options that are PBDE-free. Low-odor, water-based, non-toxic products should be encouraged.

For more information on "safe" levels of home indoor air pollutants, contact the U.S. Environmental Protection Agency (EPA) or the U.S. Consumer Product Safety Commission (CPSC).

TYPE OF FACILITY: Center; Large Family Child Care Home; Small Family Child Care Home

REFERENCES:
1. Lunder, S., A. Jacob. 2008. Fire retardants in toddlers and their mothers: Levels three times higher in toddlers than moms. Environmental Working Group. http://www.ewg.org/reports/pbdesintoddlers/.
2. U.S. Environmental Protection Agency. Pollution prevention and toxics: Polybrominated diphenylethers (PBDEs). http://www.epa.gov/oppt/pbde/.

STANDARD 5.2.1.6: Ventilation to Control Odors

Odors in toilets, bathrooms, diaper changing, and other inhabited areas of the facility should be controlled by ventilation and appropriate cleaning and disinfecting. Toilets and bathrooms, janitorial closets, and rooms with utility sinks or where wet mops and chemicals are stored should be mechanically ventilated to the outdoors with local exhaust mechanical ventilation to control and remove odors in accordance with local building codes. Chemical air fresheners or air sanitizers should not be used. Adequate ventilation should be maintained during any cleaning, sanitizing or disinfecting procedure to prevent children and caregivers/teachers from inhaling potentially toxic fumes.

RATIONALE: Chemical air fresheners and chemical air sanitizers may cause nausea or an allergic response in some children (2). Ventilation and sanitation help control and prevent the spread of disease and contamination. The Material Safety Data Sheet (MSDS) for every chemical product that the facility uses should be checked and available to anyone who uses or who might be exposed to the chemical in the

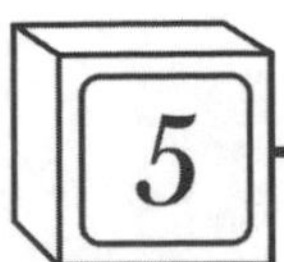

child care facility to be sure that the chemical does not pose a risk to children and adults.

COMMENTS: The MSDS gives legally required information about the presence of Volatile Organic Compounds (VOCs) and the risk of exposure from all the chemicals in the product. The Occupational Safety and Health Administration (OSHA) requires the availability of the MSDS to the workers who use chemicals (1). In addition these sheets should be available to anyone who might be exposed to the chemical in the child care facility.

TYPE OF FACILITY: Center; Large Family Child Care Home; Small Family Child Care Home

RELATED STANDARDS:
Standard 3.3.0.1: Routine Cleaning, Sanitizing, and Disinfecting

REFERENCES:
1. U.S. Occupational Safety and Health Administration. 2009. Hazard communication: Foundation of workplace chemical safety programs. http://www.osha.gov/dsg/hazcom/index.html.
2. Elliott, L., M. P. Longnecker, G. E. Kissling, S. J. London. 2006. Volatile organic compounds and pulmonary function in the Third National Health and Nutrition Examination Survey, 1988-1994. *Environmental Health Perspective* 114:1210-14.

STANDARD 5.2.1.7: Electric Fans

Electric fans, if used, should bear the safety certification mark of a nationally recognized testing laboratory and be inaccessible to children (1). The cords to fans should also be inaccessible to children.

RATIONALE: Children having access to electric fans might insert their fingers or objects and otherwise interfere with the safe operation of the fan. Access to the cords of electric fans could result in a child pulling the fan onto him/herself.

COMMENTS: The Occupational Safety and Health Administration (OSHA) has a program that recognizes Nationally Recognized Testing Laboratories. Private sector organizations are listed at http://www.osha.gov/dts/otpca/nrtl/index.html#nrtls.

TYPE OF FACILITY: Center; Large Family Child Care Home; Small Family Child Care Home

REFERENCES:
1. U.S. Occupational Safety and Health Administration. 2010. Certification of workplace products by nationally recognized testing laboratories. http://www.osha.gov/dts/shib/shib021610.html.

STANDARD 5.2.1.8: Maintenance of Air Filters

Filters in forced-air heating and cooling system equipment should be checked and cleaned or replaced according to the manufacturer's instructions on a regular basis, at least every three months (and more often if necessary) (1).

RATIONALE: Clogged filters will impede proper air circulation required for heating and ventilation. Poor air flow causes pressure imbalances in the system and can result in the premature failure of equipment. Low air flow can reduce heating and cooling performance of the system and cause cooling coils to freeze up.

TYPE OF FACILITY: Center; Large Family Child Care Home; Small Family Child Care Home

REFERENCES:
1. U.S. Environmental Protection Agency. 2009. *Indoor air quality for schools program: Update*. http://www.epa.gov/iaq/schools/pdfs/publications/iaqtfs_update17.pdf.

STANDARD 5.2.1.9: Type and Placement of Room Thermometers

Thermometers that will not easily break and that do not contain mercury should be placed on interior walls in every indoor activity area at children's height.

RATIONALE: The temperature of the room can vary between the floor and the ceiling. Because heat rises, the temperature at the level where children are playing can be much cooler than at the usual level of placement of interior thermometers (the standing, eye level of adults). Mercury, glass, or similar materials in thermometers can cause injury and poisoning of children and adults. Mercury is a potent neurotoxin that can damage the brain and nervous system (1). Placing a safe digital thermometer at the children's height allows proper monitoring of temperature where the children are in the room. A thermometer should not break easily if a child or adult bumps into it.

TYPE OF FACILITY: Center; Large Family Child Care Home; Small Family Child Care Home

RELATED STANDARDS:
Standard 5.2.1.2: Indoor Temperature

REFERENCES:
1. U.S. Environmental Protection Agency. 2010. Mercury: Health effects. http://www.epa.gov/mercury/effects.htm.

STANDARD 5.2.1.10: Gas, Oil, or Kerosene Heaters, Generators, Portable Gas Stoves, and Charcoal and Gas Grills

Unvented gas or oil heaters and portable open-flame kerosene space heaters should be prohibited. Gas cooking appliances, including portable gas stoves, should not be used for heating purposes. Charcoal grills should not be used for space heating or any other indoor purposes.

Heat in units that involve flame should be vented properly to the outside and should be supplied with a source of combustion air that meets the manufacturer's installation requirements.

RATIONALE: Due to improper ventilation, worn or faulty parts, or malfunctioning equipment, dangerous gases can accumulate and cause a fire or carbon monoxide poisoning. Carbon monoxide is a colorless, odorless, gas that is formed when carbon-containing fuel is not burned completely and can cause illness or death. See Standard 5.2.9.5 on installation of carbon monoxide detectors.

Many burns have been caused by contact with space heaters and other hot surfaces such as charcoal and gas grills (1). If charcoal grills are used outside, adequate staff

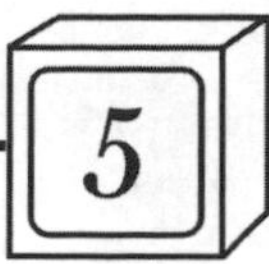

ratios must be maintained and the person operating the grill should not be counted in the ratio.

COMMENTS: For more information on carbon monoxide poisoning and poison prevention, contact your local poison center by calling 1-800-222-1222.

TYPE OF FACILITY: Center; Large Family Child Care Home; Small Family Child Care Home

RELATED STANDARDS:
Standard 5.2.1.13: Barriers/Guards for Heating Equipment and Units
Standard 5.2.9.5: Carbon Monoxide Detectors

REFERENCES:
1. Palmieri, T. L., D. G. Greenhalgh. 2002. Increased incidence of heater-related burn injury during a power crisis. *Arch Surg* 137:1106-8.

STANDARD 5.2.1.11: Portable Electric Space Heaters

Portable electric space heaters should:

a) Be attended while in use and be off when unattended;
b) Be inaccessible to children;
c) Have protective covering to keep hands and objects away from the electric heating element;
d) Bear the safety certification mark of a nationally recognized testing laboratory;
e) Be placed on the floor only and at least three feet from curtains, papers, furniture, and any flammable object;
f) Be properly vented, as required for proper functioning;
g) Be used in accordance with the manufacturer's instructions;
h) Not be used with an extension cord.

The heater cord should be inaccessible to children as well.

RATIONALE: Portable electric space heaters are a common cause of fires and burns resulting from very hot heating elements being too close to flammable objects and people (1).

COMMENTS: To prevent burns and potential fires, space heaters must not be accessible to children. Children can start fires by inserting flammable material near electric heating elements. Curtains, papers, and furniture must be kept away from electric space heaters to avoid potential fires. Some electric space heaters function by heating oil contained in a heat-radiating portion of the appliance. Even though the electrical heating element is inaccessible in this type of heater, the hot surfaces of the appliance can cause burns. Cords to electric space heaters should be inaccessible to the children. Heaters should not be placed on a table or desk. Children and adults can pull an active unit off or trip on the cord.

To prevent burns or potential fires, consideration must be given to the ages and activity levels of children in care and the amount of space in a room. Alternative methods of heating may be safer for children. Baseboard electric heaters are cooler than radiant portable heaters, but still hot enough to burn a child if touched.

If portable electric space heaters are used, electrical circuits must not be overloaded. Portable electric space heaters are usually plugged into a regular 120-volt electric outlet connected to a fifteen-ampere circuit breaker. A circuit breaker is an overload switch that prevents the current in a given electric circuit from exceeding the capacity of a line. Fuses perform the same function in older systems. If too many appliances are plugged into a circuit, calling for more power than the capacity of the circuit, the breaker reacts by switching off the circuit. Constantly overloaded electrical circuits can cause electrical fires. If a circuit breaker is continuously switching the electric power off, reduce the load to the circuit before manually resetting the circuit breaker (more than one outlet may be connected to a single circuit breaker). If the problem persists, stop using the circuit and consult an electrical inspector or electrical contractor.

The Occupational Safety and Health Administration (OSHA) has a program that recognizes Nationally Recognized Testing Laboratories. Private sector organizations are listed on their Website at http://www.osha.gov/dts/otpca/nrtl/index.html#nrtls.

Manufacturer's instructions should be kept on file.

TYPE OF FACILITY: Center; Large Family Child Care Home; Small Family Child Care Home

RELATED STANDARDS:
Standard 5.2.1.13: Barriers/Guards for Heating Equipment and Units

REFERENCES:
1. U.S. Consumer Product Safety Commission (CPSC). 2001. *What you should know about space heaters*. Washington, DC: CPSC. http://www.nnins.com/documents/WHATYOUSHOULDKNOWABOUTSPACEHEATERS.pdf.

STANDARD 5.2.1.12: Fireplaces, Fireplace Inserts, and Wood/Corn Pellet Stoves

Fireplaces, fireplace inserts, and wood/corn pellet stoves should be inaccessible to children. Fireplaces, fireplace inserts, and wood/corn pellet stoves should be certified to recognized national performance standards such as Underwriters Laboratories (UL) or the American National Standards Institute (ANSI) and Environmental Protection Agency (EPA) standards for air emissions. The front opening should be equipped with a secure and stable protective safety screen. Fireplaces, fireplace inserts, and wood/corn pellet stoves should be installed in accordance with the local or regional building code and the manufacturer's installation instructions. The facility should clean the chimney as necessary to prevent excessive build-up of burn residues or smoke products in the chimney.

RATIONALE: Fireplaces provide access to surfaces hot enough to cause burns. Children should be kept away from fire because their clothing can easily ignite. Children should be kept away from a hot surface because they can be burned simply by touching it. Improperly maintained

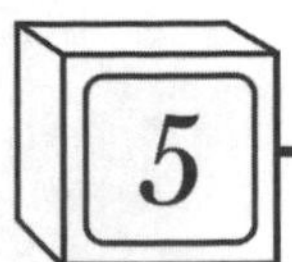

fireplaces, fireplace inserts, wood/corn pellet stoves, and chimneys can lead to fire and accumulation of toxic fumes.

A protective safety screen over the front opening of a fireplace will contain sparks and reduce a child's accessibility to an open flame.

Heating equipment is the second leading cause of ignition of fatal house fires (1). This equipment can become very hot when in use, potentially causing significant burns.

TYPE OF FACILITY: Center; Large Family Child Care Home; Small Family Child Care Home

RELATED STANDARDS:
Standard 5.2.1.10: Gas, Oil, or Kerosene Heaters, Generators, Portable Gas Stoves, and Charcoal and Gas Grills
Standard 5.2.1.13: Barriers/Guards for Heating Equipment and Units
Standard 5.2.9.5: Carbon Monoxide Detectors

REFERENCES:
1. Chowdhury, R., M. Greene, D. Miller. 2008. *2003-2005 residential fire loss estimates*. Washington, DC: U.S. Consumer Product Safety Commission. http://www.cpsc.gov/library/fire05.pdf.

STANDARD 5.2.1.13: Barriers/Guards for Heating Equipment and Units

Heating equipment and units, including hot water heating pipes and baseboard heaters with a surface temperature hotter than 120°F, should be made inaccessible to children by barriers such as guards, protective screens, or other devices.

RATIONALE: A mechanical barrier separating the child from the source of heat can reduce the likelihood of burns (1,2).

TYPE OF FACILITY: Center; Large Family Child Care Home; Small Family Child Care Home

RELATED STANDARDS:
Standard 5.2.1.3: Heating and Ventilation Equipment Inspection and Maintenance
Standard 5.2.1.11: Portable Electric Space Heaters
Standard 5.2.1.12: Fireplaces, Fireplace Inserts, and Wood/Corn Pellet Stoves

REFERENCES:
1. Ytterstad, B., G. S. Smith, C. A. Coggan. 1998. Harstad injury prevention study: Prevention of burns in young children by community based interventions. *Inj Prev* 4:176-80.
2. McLoughlin, E., C. J. Vince, A. M. Lee, et al. 1982. Project burn prevention: Outcomes and implications. *Am J Public Health* 72: 241-47.

STANDARD 5.2.1.14: Water Heating Devices and Temperatures Allowed

Facilities should have water heating devices connected to the water supply system as required by the regulatory authority. These facilities should be capable of heating water to at least 120°F. Hot water temperature at sinks used for handwashing, or where the hot water will be in direct contact with children, should be at a temperature of at least 60°F and not exceeding 120°F. Scald-prevention devices, such as special faucets or thermostatically controlled valves, should be permanently installed, if necessary, to provide this temperature of water at the faucet. Where a dishwasher is used, it should have the capacity to heat water to at least 140°F for the dishwasher (with scald preventing devices that prohibit the opening of the dishwasher during operation cycle).

RATIONALE: Hot water is needed to clean and sanitize dishes and food utensils adequately and sanitize laundry. Tap water burns are a common source of scald injuries in young children (1). Children under six years of age are the most frequent victims of non-fatal burns (1). Water heated to temperatures greater than 120°F takes less than thirty seconds to burn the skin (1). If the water is heated to 120°F it takes two minutes to burn the skin (2). That extra two minutes could provide enough time to remove the child from the hot water source and avoid a burn.

COMMENTS: Anti-scald aerators designed to fit on the end of a modern bathroom and kitchen faucets, and anti-scald bathtub spouts, are also available. Only devices approved by the American National Standards Institute (ANSI) or the Canadian Standards Association (CSA) should be considered. A number of other scald-prevention devices are available on the market. Consult a plumbing contractor for details.

TYPE OF FACILITY: Center; Large Family Child Care Home; Small Family Child Care Home

REFERENCES:
1. D'Souza, A. L., N. G. Nelson, L. B. McKenzie. 2009. Pediatric burn injuries treated in US emergency departments between 1990 and 2006. *Pediatrics* 124:1424-30.
2. Erdmann, T. C., K. W. Feldman, F. P. Rivara, D. M. Heimbach, H. A. Wall. 1991. Tap water burn prevention: The effect of legislation. *Pediatrics* 88:572-77.

STANDARD 5.2.1.15: Maintenance of Humidifiers and Dehumidifiers

If humidifiers or dehumidifiers are used to maintain humidity, as specified in Standard 5.2.1.2, the facility should follow the manufacturer's cleaning, drainage, and maintenance instructions to avoid growth of bacteria and mold and subsequent discharge into the air.

RATIONALE: Bacteria and mold often grow in the tanks and drainage hoses of portable and console room humidifiers and can be released in the mist. Breathing dirty mist may cause lung problems ranging from flu-like symptoms to serious infection, and is of special concern to children and staff with allergy or asthma (1). Humidifiers or dehumidifiers may be required to meet American National Standards Institute (ANSI) and Association of Home Appliance Manufacturers (AHAM) humidifier standards and must not introduce additional hazards.

COMMENTS: Improperly maintained humidifiers may become incubators of biological organisms and increase the risk of disease. Film or scum appearing on the water surface, on the sides or bottom of the tank, or on exposed motor parts may indicate that the humidifier tank contains bacteria or mold. Also, increased humidity enhances the

survival of dust mites, and many children are allergic to dust mites.

TYPE OF FACILITY: Center; Large Family Child Care Home; Small Family Child Care Home

RELATED STANDARDS:
Standard 5.2.1.2: Indoor Temperature

REFERENCES:
1. U.S. Consumer Product Safety Commission (CPSC). CPSC issues alert about care of room humidifiers: Safety alert–dirty humidifiers may cause health problems. Document #5046. Washington, DC: CPSC. http://www.cpsc.gov/cpscpub/pubs/5046.html.

5.2.2 Lighting

STANDARD 5.2.2.1: Levels of Illumination

Natural lighting should be provided in rooms where children work and play for more than two hours at a time. Wherever possible, windows installed at child's eye level should be provided to introduce natural lighting. All areas of the facility should have glare-free natural and/or artificial lighting that provides adequate illumination and comfort for facility activities. The following guidelines should be used for levels of illumination:

a) Reading, painting, and other close work areas: fifty to 100 foot-candles on the work surface;
b) Work and play areas: thirty to fifty foot-candles on the surface;
c) Stairs, walkways, landings, driveways, entrances: at least twenty foot-candles on the surface;
d) Sleeping and napping areas: no more than five foot-candles during sleeping or napping except for infants and children who are resting in the same room that other children are involved with activities.

RATIONALE: These levels of illumination facilitate cleaning, reading, comfort, completion of projects, and safety (3). Too little light, too much glare and confusing shadows are commonly experienced lighting problems. Inadequate artificial lighting has been linked to eyestrain, headache, and non-specific symptoms of illness (1).

Natural lighting is the most desirable lighting of all. Windows installed at children's eye level not only provide a source of natural light, they also provide a variety of perceptual experiences of sight, sound, and smell, which may serve as learning activities for children and a focus for conversation. The visual stimulation provided by a window is important to a young child's development (1,2). Natural lighting provided by sky lights exposes children to variations in light during the day that is less perceptually stimulating than eye-level windows, but is still preferable to artificial lighting.

A study on school performance shows that elementary school children seem to learn better in classrooms with substantial daylight and the opportunity for natural ventilation (4).

Lighting levels should be reduced during nap times to promote resting or napping behavior in children. During napping and rest periods, some degree of illumination must be allowed to ensure that staff can continue to observe children. While decreased illumination for sleeping and napping areas is a reasonable standard when all the children are resting, this standard must not prevent support of individualized sleep schedules that are essential for infants and may be required by other children from time to time.

COMMENTS: When providing artificial lighting, consider purchasing energy-efficient bulbs or lamps (e.g., compact fluorescent lights [CFL] or light emitting diode [LED] bulbs) to help benefit our children's environment (5-7). Saving electricity reduces carbon monoxide emissions, sulfur oxide, and high-level nuclear waste (8). CFLs contain very small amounts of mercury and care should be taken to ensure the lights are not at risk for breaking and are disposed of properly. In rooms that are used for many purposes, providing the ability to turn on and off different banks of lights in a room, or installation of light dimmers, will allow caregivers/teachers to adjust lighting levels that are appropriate to the activities that are occurring in the room.

Contact the lighting or home service department of the local electric utility company to have foot-candles measured.

TYPE OF FACILITY: Center; Large Family Child Care Home; Small Family Child Care Home

RELATED STANDARDS:
Standard 5.1.2.3: Areas for School-Age Children

REFERENCES:
1. Greiner, D., D. Leduc, eds. 2008. *Well beings: A guide to health in child care*. 3rd ed. Ottawa, ON: Canadian Paediatric Society.
2. Greenman, J. 1998. *Caring spaces, learning places: Children's environments that work*. Redmond, WA: Exchange Press.
3. IESNA School and College Lighting Committee. 2000. Recommended practice on lighting for educational facilities. ANSI/IESNA RP-3-00. New York: Illuminating Engineering Society of North America.
4. Heschong, L. 2002. Daylighting and human performance. *ASHRAE J* (June): 65-67.
5. American Society of Heating, Refrigeration and Air-conditioning Engineers, American Institute of Architects, Illuminating Engineering Society of North America, U.S. Green Building Council, U.S. Department of Energy. 2008. *Advanced energy design guide for K-12 school buildings*, 148. Atlanta, GA: ASHRAE.
6. Kats, G. 2006. *Greening America's schools: costs and benefits.* http://www.usgbc.org/ShowFile.aspx?DocumentID=2908.
7. Tanner, C. 2008. Explaining relationships among student outcomes and the school's physical environment. *J Advanced Academics* 19:444-71.
8. Maine Senate Democrats. 2007. Legislative leaders change to high-efficiency light bulbs. http://www.maine.gov/tools/whatsnew/index.php?topic=Senatedemsall&id=43036&v=Article.

STANDARD 5.2.2.2: Light Fixtures Including Halogen Lamps

Light fixtures containing shielded or shatterproof bulbs should be used throughout the child care facility. When portable halogen lamps are provided, they should be installed securely to prevent them from tipping over, and a safety screen must be installed over the bulb.

RATIONALE: Use of shielded or shatterproof bulbs prevents injury to people and contamination of food. Halogen lamps burn at a temperature of approximately 1200°F and are a potential burn or fire hazard (1). Halogen lighting provides a more energy-efficient alternative to illuminate a room. Halogen bulbs are incorporated into freestanding lamps. Many of the older-style lamps do not have a protective screen to prevent children from touching the hot bulb or placing flammable materials on the bulb. Some portable lamps have a design that places the halogen bulb on the top of a tall pole. Although the base of these lamps is relatively heavy in weight, children can easily tip the lamps on their side and cause a potential fire hazard.

COMMENTS: Halogen lamps are also incorporated into light fixtures that are mounted permanently on the ceiling or walls. The fixtures are usually placed out of the reach of children and, if properly installed, should not pose a safety hazard.

TYPE OF FACILITY: Center; Large Family Child Care Home; Small Family Child Care Home

RELATED STANDARDS:
Standard 5.2.2.1: Levels of Illumination

REFERENCES:
1. Lamp Section, National Electrical Manufacturers Association (NEMA). 2003. Tungsten-halogen lamps (bulbs): Ultraviolet, rupture, and high temperature risks. Rosslyn, VA: NEMA. http://www.nema.org/gov/env_conscious_design/lamps/upload/LSD 1 T-H Lamps v2_4 2003 C6.pdf.

STANDARD 5.2.2.3: High Intensity Discharge Lamps, Multi-Vapor, and Mercury Lamps

High intensity discharge lamps, multi-vapor, and mercury lamps should not be used for lighting the interior of buildings unless provided with special bulbs that self-extinguish if the outer glass envelope is broken.

RATIONALE: Multi-vapor and mercury lamps can be harmful when the outer bulb envelope is broken, causing serious skin burns and eye inflammation (1).

COMMENTS: High intensity lamps are not appropriate for internal illumination of child care facilities since the level of lighting generated is generally too strong for the size of a typical room and/or generates too much glare.

TYPE OF FACILITY: Center; Large Family Child Care Home; Small Family Child Care Home

RELATED STANDARDS:
Standard 5.2.2.1: Levels of Illumination

REFERENCES:
1. Balk, S. J., S. S. Aronson. 2003. Mercury in the environment: A danger to children. *Child Care Info Exch* (July/Aug): 58-60.

STANDARD 5.2.2.4: Emergency Lighting

Emergency lighting approved by the local authority should be provided in corridors, stairwells, and at building exits. Open flames should not be used as emergency lighting in child care facilities.

RATIONALE: Provision of emergency lighting in corridors and stairwells enables safe passage to emergency exits or shelter-in-place locations in the event of an electrical power outage (1). Open flames such as candles, flares, and lanterns are not safe.

COMMENTS: In many places, daylight hours end while child care is still in session, especially in the fall and winter seasons. If electric power outages are frequent, consideration should be given to providing emergency lighting in each room that is accessible to children. In child care homes, battery-powered household emergency lights that insert into electrical wall outlets (to remain charged) may be sufficient, depending on the location of the electrical outlets in corridors, stairwells, and near building exits.

A battery-operated flashlight is the preferred type of portable emergency lighting in child care facilities. In some jurisdictions, fixed mounted emergency lighting may be required. Ask the local fire marshal for fire safety code requirements. Although candles are sometimes recommended in emergency situations for portable lighting, they pose a significant fire hazard and should not be used.

TYPE OF FACILITY: Center; Large Family Child Care Home; Small Family Child Care Home

REFERENCES:
1. National Fire Protection Association (NFPA). 2009. *NFPA 101: Life Safety Code.* 2009 ed. Quincy, MA: NFPA.

5.2.3 Noise

STANDARD 5.2.3.1: Noise Levels

Measures should be taken in all rooms or areas accommodating children to maintain the decibel (db) level at or below thirty-five decibels for at least 80% of the time as measured by an acoustical engineer or, more practically, by the ability to be clearly heard and understood in a normal conversation without raising one's voice. These measures include noncombustible acoustical ceiling, rugs, wall covering, partitions, or draperies, or a combination thereof.

RATIONALE: Excessive sound levels can be damaging to hearing, reduce effective communication, and reduce psychosocial well-being. The level of noise that causes hearing loss commonly experienced by children with fluid in their middle ear space is thirty-five decibels (1). This level of hearing loss correlates with decreased understanding of language. By inference, this level of ambient noise may interfere with the ability of children to hear well enough to develop language normally (2,3).

Research on the effects of ambient noise levels in child care settings has focused on a) concern with damage to the child's auditory system and b) non-auditory effects such as physiological effects (e.g., elevated blood pressure levels), motivational effects, and cognitive effects (3). Although noise sources may be located outside the child care facility, sometimes the noise source is related to the design of the child care spaces within the facility. In the article "Design of Child Care Centers and Effects of Noise on Young Children,"

Maxwell states "spaces must allow for the fact that children need to make noise but the subsequent noise levels should not be harmful to them or others in the center" (3).

COMMENTS: When there is new construction or renovation of a facility, consideration should be given to a design that will reduce noise from outside. High ceiling heights may contribute to noise levels. Installing acoustical tile ceilings reduce noise levels as well as curtains or other soft window treatments over windows and wall-mounted cork boards (4).

While carpets can help reduce the level of noise, they can absorb moisture and serve as a place for microorganisms to grow. Area rugs should be considered instead of carpet because they can be taken up and washed often. Area rugs should be secured with a non-slip mat or other method to prevent tripping hazards.

Caregivers/teachers who need extensive help with sound abatement should consult a child care health consultant for additional ideas or with an acoustical engineer to measure noise levels within the facility. For further assistance on finding an acoustical engineer, contact the Acoustical Society of America.

TYPE OF FACILITY: Center; Large Family Child Care Home; Small Family Child Care Home

REFERENCES:

1. Lazaridis, E., J. C. Saunders. 2008. Can you hear me now? A genetic model of otitis media with effusion. *J Clin Invest* 118:471-74.
2. Newman, R. 2005. The cocktail party effect in infants revisited: Listening to one's name in noise. *Devel Psych* 41:352-62.
3. Maxwell, L. E., G. W. Evans. Design of child care centers and effects of noise on young children. Design Share. http://www.designshare.com/research/lmaxwell/noisechildren.htm.
4. Manlove, E. E., T. Frank. 2001. Why should we care about noise in classrooms and child care settings? *Child Youth Care Forum* 30:55-64.

5.2.4 Electrical Fixtures and Outlets

STANDARD 5.2.4.1: Electrical Service

Facilities should be supplied with electric service. Outlets and fixtures should be installed and connected to the source of electric energy in a manner that meets the National Electrical Code, as amended by local electrical codes (if any), and as certified by an electrical code inspector.

RATIONALE: Proper installation of outlets and fixtures helps to prevent injury.

COMMENTS: State or local electrical codes may apply. For further information, see the National Fire Protection Association's (NFPA) National Electrical Code and the *NFPA 101: Life Safety Code* from the NFPA (1).

TYPE OF FACILITY: Center; Large Family Child Care Home; Small Family Child Care Home

REFERENCES:

1. National Fire Protection Association (NFPA). 2009. *NFPA 101: Life Safety Code.* 2009 ed. Quincy, MA: NFPA.

STANDARD 5.2.4.2: Safety Covers and Shock Protection Devices for Electrical Outlets

All electrical outlets accessible to children who are not yet developmentally at a kindergarten grade level of learning should be a type called "tamper-resistant electrical outlets." These types of outlets look like standard wall outlets but contain an internal shutter mechanism that prevents children from sticking objects like hairpins, keys, and paperclips into the receptacle (2). This spring-loaded shutter mechanism only opens when equal pressure is applied to both shutters such as when an electrical plug is inserted (2,3).

In existing child care facilities that do not have "tamper-resistant electrical outlets," outlets should have "safety covers" that are attached to the electrical outlet by a screw or other means to prevent easy removal by a child. "Safety plugs" should not be used since they can be removed from an electrical outlet by children (2,3).

All newly installed or replaced electrical outlets that are accessible to children should use "tamper-resistant electrical outlets."

In areas where electrical products might come into contact with water, a special type of outlet called Ground Fault Circuit Interrupters (GFCIs) should be installed (2). A GFCI is designed to trip before a deadly electrical shock can occur (1). To ensure that GFCIs are functioning correctly, they should be tested at least monthly (2). GFCIs are also available in a tamper-resistant design.

RATIONALE: Tamper-resistant electrical outlets or securely attached safety covers prevent children from placing fingers or sticking objects into exposed electrical outlets and reduce the risk of electrical shock, electrical burns, and potential fires (2). GFCIs provide protection from electrocution when an electric outlet or electric product may come into contact with water (1).

Approximately 2,400 children are injured annually by inserting objects into the slots of electrical outlets (2,3). The majority of these injuries involve children under the age of six (2,3).

Plastic safety plugs inserted into electric outlets are not the safest option since they can easily be removed by children and, depending on their size, present a potential choking hazard if placed in a child's mouth (3).

COMMENTS: One type of outlet cover replaces the outlet face plate with a plate that has a spring-loaded outlet cover, which will stay in place when the receptacle is not in use. For receptacles where the facility does not intend to unplug the appliance, a more permanent cap-type cover that screws into the outlet receptacle is available. Several effective outlet safety devices are available in home hardware and infant/children stores (4).

TYPE OF FACILITY: Center; Large Family Child Care Home; Small Family Child Care Home

RELATED STANDARDS:

Standard 5.2.4.3: Ground-Fault Circuit-Interrupter for Outlets Near Water

REFERENCES:
1. National Fire Protection Association (NFPA). 2010. *NFPA 70: National electrical code.* 2011 ed. Quincy, MA: NFPA.
2. Electrical Safety Foundation International (ESFI). 2008. *Know the dangers in your older home*. Rosslyn, VA: ESFI. http://esfi.org/index.cfm/pk/download/id/10802/pid/3003/.
3. National Fire Protection Association. National electrical code fact sheet: Tamper-resistant electrical receptacles. http://www.nfpa.org/itemDetail.asp?categoryID=1508&itemID=36117&URL=Safety Information/For consumers/Causes/Electrical/Tamper-resistant electrical receptacles&cookie_test=1/.
4. National Electrical Manufacturers Association. Real safety with tamper-resistant receptacles. http://www.childoutletsafety.org.

STANDARD 5.2.4.3: Ground-Fault Circuit-Interrupter for Outlets Near Water

All electrical outlets located within six feet of a sink or other water source must have a ground-fault circuit-interrupter (GFCI), which should be tested at least once every three months using the test button located on the device.

RATIONALE: This provision eliminates shock hazards. GFCIs provide protection from electrocution when an electric outlet or electric product may come into contact with water (1).

COMMENTS: Electrical receptacles of the type often found in bathrooms of new homes have a GFCI built into the receptacle. The GFCI does not necessarily have to be near the sink. An electrical receptacle can be protected by a special type of circuit breaker (which has a built-in GFCI) in the electrical panel (1).

TYPE OF FACILITY: Center; Large Family Child Care Home; Small Family Child Care Home

RELATED STANDARDS:
Standard 5.2.4.2: Safety Covers and Shock Protection Devices for Electrical Outlets

REFERENCES:
1. National Fire Protection Association (NFPA). 2011. *NFPA 70: National electrical code.* 2011 ed. Quincy, MA: NFPA.

STANDARD 5.2.4.4: Location of Electrical Devices Near Water

No electrical device or apparatus accessible to children should be located so it could be plugged into an electrical outlet while a person is in contact with a water source, such as a sink, tub, shower area, water table, or swimming pool.

RATIONALE: Contact with a water source while using an electrical device provides a path for electricity through the person who is using the device (1,2). This can lead to electrical injury.

TYPE OF FACILITY: Center; Large Family Child Care Home; Small Family Child Care Home

REFERENCES:
1. National Fire Protection Association (NFPA). 2011. *NFPA 70: National electrical code.* 2011 ed. Quincy, MA: NFPA.
2. U.S. Consumer Product Safety Commission (CPSC). CPSC safety alert: Install Ground-Fault Circuit-Interrupter Protection for Pools, Spas and Hot Tubs. http://www.cpsc.gov/cpscpub/pubs/5039.html.

STANDARD 5.2.4.5: Extension Cords

The use of extension cords should be discouraged; however, when used, they should bear the listing mark of a nationally recognized testing laboratory, and should not be placed through doorways, under rugs or carpeting, behind wall-hangings, or across water-source areas. Electrical cords (extension and appliance) should not be frayed or overloaded.

RATIONALE: Electrical malfunction is a major cause of ignition of fatal house fires. The U.S. Consumer Product Safety Commission (CPSC) reports that from 2002-2004 extension cords and other electric cords were the ignition sources of fires that caused an average of sixty deaths and 150 burn injuries each year (1). Extension cords should not be accessible to children, whether in use or when temporarily not in use but plugged in. There is risk of electric shock to a child who may poke a metal object into the extension cord socket (2).

COMMENTS: The Occupational Safety and Health Administration (OSHA) has a Link to a list of Nationally Recognized Testing Laboratories at http://www.osha.gov/dts/otpca/nrtl/index.html#nrtls.

TYPE OF FACILITY: Center; Large Family Child Care Home; Small Family Child Care Home

REFERENCES:
1. Chowdhury, R., M. Greene, D. Miller. 2008. *2003-2005 residential fire loss estimates*. Washington, DC: U.S. Consumer Product Safety Commission. http://www.cpsc.gov/library/fire05.pdf.
2. U.S. Consumer Product Safety Commission. Extension cords fact sheet. http://www.cpsc.gov/cpscpub/pubs/16.html.

STANDARD 5.2.4.6: Electrical Cords

Electrical cords should be placed beyond children's reach.

RATIONALE: Severe injuries have occurred in child care when children have pulled appliances like crock-pots down onto themselves by pulling on the cord (1). Injuries have occurred in child care when children pulled appliances such as tape players down on themselves by pulling on the cord (2). When children chew on an appliance cord, they can reach the wires and suffer severe disfiguring mouth injuries (3).

TYPE OF FACILITY: Center; Large Family Child Care Home; Small Family Child Care Home

REFERENCES:
1. Lowell, G., K. Quinlan, L. J. Gottlieb. 2008. Preventing unintentional scald burns: Moving beyond tap water. *Pediatrics* 122:799-804.
2. U.S. Consumer Product Safety Commission. CPSC safety alert. *The tipping point: Preventing TV, furniture, and appliance tip-over deaths and injuries*. http://www.cpsc.gov/cpscpub/pubs/5004.pdf.
3. Healthy Children. 2010. Health issues: Electric shock. http://www.healthychildren.org/English/health-issues/injuries-emergencies/pages/Electric-Shock.aspx.

5.2.5 Fire Warning Systems

STANDARD 5.2.5.1: Smoke Detection Systems and Smoke Alarms

In centers with new installations, a smoke detection system (such as hard-wired system detectors with battery back-up system and control panel) or monitored wireless battery operated detectors that automatically signal an alarm through a central control panel when the battery is low or when the detector is triggered by a hazardous condition should be installed with placement of the smoke detectors in the following areas:

a) Each story in front of doors to the stairway;
b) Corridors of all floors;
c) Lounges and recreation areas;
d) Sleeping rooms.

In large and small family child care homes, smoke alarms that receive their operating power from the building electrical system or are of the wireless signal-monitored-alarm system type should be installed. Battery-operated smoke alarms should be permitted provided that the facility demonstrates to the fire inspector that testing, maintenance, and battery replacement programs ensure reliability of power to the smoke alarms and signaling of a monitored alarm when the battery is low and that retrofitting the facility to connect the smoke alarms to the electrical system would be costly and difficult to achieve.

Facilities with smoke alarms that operate using power from the building electrical system should keep a supply of batteries and battery-operated detectors for use during power outages.

RATIONALE: Because of the large number of children at risk in a center, up-to-date smoke detection system technology is needed. Wireless smoke alarm systems that signal and set off a monitored alarm are acceptable. In large and small family child care homes, single-station smoke alarms are acceptable. However, for all new building installations where access to enable necessary wiring is available, smoke alarms should be used that receive their power from the building's electrical system. These hard-wired detecting systems typically have a battery operated back-up system for times of power outage. The hard-wired and wireless smoke detectors should be interconnected so that occupants receive instantaneous alarms throughout the facility, not just in the room of origin. Single-station batteries are not reliable enough; single-station battery-operated smoke alarms should be accepted only where connecting smoke detectors to existing wiring would be too difficult and expensive as a retrofitted arrangement.

COMMENTS: Some state and local building codes specify the installation and maintenance of smoke detectors and fire alarm systems. For specific information, see the *NFPA 101: Life Safety Code* (1) and the *NFPA 72: National Fire Alarm and Signaling Code* from the National Fire Protection Association.

The Federal Emergency Management Agency (FEMA) has an online coloring book that can be printed and used to teach children about fire safety at https://www.usfa.dhs.gov/applications/publications/display.cfm?id=208/.

TYPE OF FACILITY: Center; Large Family Child Care Home; Small Family Child Care Home

RELATED STANDARDS:
Standard 5.1.1.3: Compliance with Fire Prevention Code

REFERENCES:
1. National Fire Protection Association (NFPA). 2009. *NFPA 101: Life Safety Code.* 2009 ed. Quincy, MA: NFPA.

STANDARD 5.2.5.2: Portable Fire Extinguishers

Portable fire extinguisher(s) should be installed and maintained and staff should be trained on their proper use as stated in Standard 3.4.3.2. The fire extinguisher should be of the A-B-C type. Size/number of fire extinguishers should be determined after a survey by the fire marshal or by an insurance company fire loss prevention representative. Instructions for the use of the fire extinguisher should be posted on or near the fire extinguisher. Fire extinguishers should not be accessible to children. Fire extinguishers should be inspected and maintained annually or more frequently as recommended by the manufacturer's instructions.

RATIONALE: All fire extinguishers are labeled, using standard symbols, for the classes of fires on which they can be used. A red slash through any of the symbols tells you the extinguisher cannot be used on that class of fire. Class A designates ordinary combustibles such as wood, cloth, and paper. Class B designates flammable liquids such as gasoline, oil, and oil-based paint. Class C designates energized electrical equipment, including wiring, fuse boxes, circuit breakers, machinery, and appliances.

COMMENTS: Staff should be trained that the first priority is to remove the children from the facility safely and quickly. Fighting a fire is secondary to the safe exit of the children and staff.

For information on automatic fire extinguishers, see the National Fire Protection Association's *NFPA 101: Life Safety Code* (1).

TYPE OF FACILITY: Center; Large Family Child Care Home; Small Family Child Care Home

RELATED STANDARDS:
Standard 3.4.3.2: Use of Fire Extinguishers
Standard 5.1.1.3: Compliance with Fire Prevention Code

REFERENCES:
1. National Fire Protection Association (NFPA). 2009. *NFPA 101: Life Safety Code.* 2009 ed. Quincy, MA: NFPA.

5.2.6 Water Supply and Plumbing

STANDARD 5.2.6.1: Water Supply

Every facility should be supplied with piped running water under pressure, from a source approved by the Environmental Protection Agency (EPA) and/or the regulatory health authority, to provide an adequate water supply to every fixture connected to the water supply and drainage system. The water should be sufficient in quantity and pressure to supply water for cooking, cleaning, drinking, toilets, and outside uses.

Water supplied by a well or other private source should meet all applicable health and safety federal, state, and local public health standards and should be approved by the local regulatory health authority. Well water should be tested annually for bacterial and chemical content (nitrates or other run-off chemicals) or according to local regulatory health authority (2). Any facility not served by a public water supply should keep on file documentation of approval, from the local regulatory health authority, of the water supply.

RATIONALE: A water supply that is safe and does not spread disease or filth or contain dangerous substances is essential to life and health (1).

COMMENTS: For more information on water supply standards, contact the local health authority or the EPA.

TYPE OF FACILITY: Center; Large Family Child Care Home; Small Family Child Care Home

RELATED STANDARDS:
Standards 5.2.6.2-5.2.6.4: Testing of Drinking Water

STANDARD 5.2.6.2: Testing of Drinking Water Not From Public System

If the facility's drinking water does not come from a public water system, or the facility gets the drinking water from a household well, programs should test the water every year or as required by the local health department, for bacteriological quality, nitrates, total dissolved solids, pH levels, and other water quality indicators as required by the local health department. Testing for nitrate is especially important if there are infants under six months of age in care.

RATIONALE: Drinking water sources should be approved by the local health department. If a child care facility does not receive drinking water from a public water system, the child care operator should ensure that the drinking water is safe. Unsafe water supplies may cause illness or other problems (1) and contain bacteria and parasites. Infants below the age of six months who drink water containing nitrate in excess of the maximum concentration limit of ten milligrams per liter could become seriously ill and, if untreated, may die. Symptoms include shortness of breath and blue-baby syndrome (methemoglobinia) (2). Even if a private water supply is safe, regular testing is valuable because it establishes a record of water quality.

COMMENTS: Public water systems are responsible for complying with all regulations, including monitoring, reporting, and performing treatment techniques. Testing of private water supplies should be completed by a state certified laboratory (1). Most testing laboratories or services supply their own sample containers. Samples for bacteriological testing must be collected in sterile containers and under sterile conditions. Laboratories may sometimes send a trained technician to collect the sample. For further information, contact the local health authority or the U.S. Environmental Protection Agency (EPA).

TYPE OF FACILITY: Center; Large Family Child Care Home; Small Family Child Care Home

RELATED STANDARDS:
Standard 5.2.6.1: Water Supply
Standard 5.2.6.3: Testing for Lead and Copper Levels in Drinking Water
Standard 5.2.6.4: Water Test Results

REFERENCES:
1. U.S. Environmental Protection Agency (EPA). 2005. Home water testing. Washington, DC: EPA, Office of Water. http://www.epa.gov/ogwdw000/faq/pdfs/fs_homewatertesting.pdf.
2. American Academy of Pediatrics. Policy statement: Drinking water from private wells and risks to children. *Pediatrics* 123:1599-1605.

STANDARD 5.2.6.3: Testing for Lead and Copper Levels in Drinking Water

Drinking water, including water in drinking fountains, should be tested and evaluated in accordance with the assistance of the local health authority or state drinking water program to determine whether lead and copper levels are safe.

RATIONALE: Lead and copper in pipes can leach into water in harmful amounts and present a potential serious exposure. Lead exposure can cause: lower IQ levels, hearing loss, reduced attention span, learning disabilities, hyperactivity, aggressive behavior, coma, convulsion, and even death (2,3). Copper exposure can cause stomach and intestinal distress, liver or kidney damage, and complications of Wilson's disease. Children's bodies absorb more lead and copper than the average adult because of their rapid development (2,3).

It is especially important to test and have safe water at child care facilities because of the amount of time children spend in these facilities.

Caregivers/teachers should always run cold water for fifteen to thirty seconds before using for drinking, cooking, and making infant formula (3). Cold water is less likely to leach lead from the plumbing.

COMMENTS: Lead is not usually found in water that comes from wells or public drinking water supply systems. More commonly, lead can enter the drinking water when the water comes into contact with plumbing materials that contain lead (2,4).

Child care facilities that have their own water supply and are considered non-transient, non-community water systems (NTNCWS) are subject to the Environmental Protection Agency's (EPA) Lead and Copper Rule (LCR) requirements, which include taking water samples for testing (1,2).

Contact your local health department or state drinking water program for information on how to collect samples and for advice on frequency of testing. See also the EPA references below.

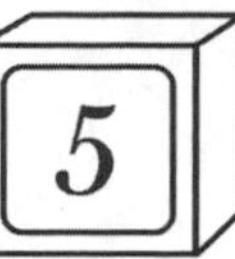

TYPE OF FACILITY: Center; Large Family Child Care Home; Small Family Child Care Home

RELATED STANDARDS:
Standard 5.2.6.1: Water Supply
Standard 5.2.6.2: Testing of Drinking Water Not From Public System
Standard 5.2.6.4: Water Test Results
Standard 5.2.9.13: Testing for Lead

REFERENCES:
1. U.S. Environmental Protection Agency (EPA). 2009. Drinking water in schools and child care facilities. http://water.epa.gov/infrastructure/drinkingwater/schools/index.cfm.
2. U.S. Environmental Protection Agency (EPA). 2005. *Lead and copper rule: A quick reference guide for schools and child care facilities that are regulated under the safe Drinking Water Act*. Washington, DC: EPA, Office of Water. http://www.epa.gov/safewater/schools/pdfs/lead/qrg_lcr_schools.pdf.
3. U.S. Environmental Protection Agency (EPA). 2005. *3Ts for reducing lead in drinking water in child care facilities: Revised guidance*. Washington, DC: EPA, Office of Water. http://www.epa.gov/safewater/schools/pdfs/lead/toolkit_leadschools_guide_3ts_childcare.pdf.
4. Zhang, Y., A. Griffin, M. Edwards. 2008. Nitrification in premise plumbing: Role of phosphate, pH and pipe corrosion. *Environ Sci Tech* 42:4280-84.

STANDARD 5.2.6.4: Water Test Results

All water test results should be in written form and kept with other required reports and documents in one central location in the facility, ready for immediate viewing by consumers and regulatory personnel. Early care and education programs should maintain photocopies of all water-testing results if the business is required to submit reports to the regulatory authority.

RATIONALE: Consumers and regulatory personnel can determine that testing has been done through written documentation (1).

COMMENTS: Some regulatory authorities prefer to review copies of water test results available for inspection on site; others that do not provide on-site inspections may prefer to have the reports submitted to them.

TYPE OF FACILITY: Center; Large Family Child Care Home; Small Family Child Care Home

RELATED STANDARDS:
Standard 5.2.6.2: Testing of Drinking Water Not From Public System
Standard 5.2.6.3: Testing for Lead and Copper Levels in Drinking Water
Standard 9.4.1.6: Availability of Documents to Parents/Guardians

REFERENCES:
1. U.S. Environmental Protection Agency (EPA). 2005. *3Ts for reducing lead in drinking water in child care facilities: Revised guidance*. Washington, DC: EPA, Office of Water. http://www.epa.gov/safewater/schools/pdfs/lead/toolkit_leadschools_guide_3ts_childcare.pdf.

STANDARD 5.2.6.5: Emergency Safe Drinking Water and Bottled Water

Emergency safe drinking water should be supplied during interruption of the regular approved water supply. Bottled water should be certified as chemically and bacteriologically potable by the Food and Drug Administration (FDA), local health department or its designee.

RATIONALE: Children must have constant access to fresh, potable water if the regular approved supply of drinking water is temporarily interrupted.

COMMENTS: The FDA regulates commercially bottled water and has established specific regulations for bottled water in Title 21 of the Code of Federal Regulations (21 CFR) (1). In addition to the FDA, state and local governments also regulate bottled water. Commercially-bottled water is considered to have an indefinite safety shelf life if it is produced in accordance with current good manufacturing practices (CGMP) and quality standard regulations and is stored in an unopened, properly sealed container. Therefore, FDA does not require an expiration date for bottled water. However, long-term storage of bottled water may result in aesthetic defects, such as off-odor and taste. Bottlers may voluntarily put expiration dates on their labels. The materials used to produce plastic containers for bottled water are regulated by the FDA as food contact substances. Food contact substances must be approved under FDA's food additive regulations. Commercial bottled water containers should not be used for any purpose other than to hold drinking water. Other liquids should not be stored in bottled-water containers. All drinking water containers must be thoroughly washed and sanitized prior to being refilled with drinking water. For information on safe plastics, see Standard 5.2.9.9.

Under FDA labeling rules, bottled water includes products labeled: bottled water, drinking water, artesian water, mineral water, sparkling bottled water, spring water, purified water, distilled, de-mineralized, de-ionized, or reverse osmosis water. Waters with added carbonation, soda water (or club soda), tonic water, and seltzer historically are regulated by FDA as soft drinks (1).

TYPE OF FACILITY: Center; Large Family Child Care Home; Small Family Child Care Home

RELATED STANDARDS:
Standard 4.9.0.8: Supply of Food and Water for Disasters
Standard 5.2.9.9: Plastic Containers and Toys

REFERENCES:
1. Posnick, L. M., H. Kim. 2002. Bottled water regulation and the FDA. *Food Safety Mag* (Aug/Sept).

STANDARD 5.2.6.6: Water Handling and Treatment Equipment

Newly installed water handling, treatment, filtering, or softening equipment should meet applicable National Sanitation Foundation (NSF) standards and should be approved by the local regulatory health authority.

RATIONALE: Adherence to NSF standards will help ensure a safe water supply. State and local codes vary, but they generally protect against toxins or sewage entering the water supply.

COMMENTS: Model codes are available from the NSF.

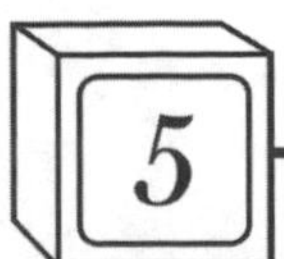

TYPE OF FACILITY: Center; Large Family Child Care Home; Small Family Child Care Home

REFERENCES:
1. NSF International. 2004. Home water treatment devices. http://www.nsf.org/consumer/drinking_water/dw_treatment.asp.

STANDARD 5.2.6.7: Cross-Connections

The facility should have no cross-connections that could permit contamination of the potable water supply:

a) Backflow preventers, vacuum breakers, or strategic air gaps should be provided for all boiler units in which chemicals are used. Backflow preventers should be tested annually;
b) Vacuum breakers should be installed on all threaded janitorial sink faucets and outdoor/indoor hose bibs;
c) Non-submersible, antisiphon ballcocks should be provided on all flush tank-type toilets.

RATIONALE: Pressure differentials may allow contamination of drinking water if cross-connections or submerged inlets exist. Water must be protected from cross-connections with possible sources of contamination (1).

COMMENTS: Short hoses are often attached to the faucets of janitorial sinks (and laundry sinks) and often extend below the top edge of the basin. The ends of a hose in a janitorial sink and a garden hose attached to an outside hose bibs are often found in a pool of potentially contaminated water. If the water faucet is not completely closed, a loss of pressure in the water system could result in the contaminated water being drawn up the hose like dirt is drawn into a vacuum cleaner, thus contaminating the drinking water supply.

Vacuum breakers may be installed as part of the plumbing fixture or are available to attach to the end of a faucet of hose bib.

TYPE OF FACILITY: Center; Large Family Child Care Home; Small Family Child Care Home

REFERENCES:
1. International Code Council (ICC). 2009. *2009 international plumbing code.* Washington, DC: ICC.

STANDARD 5.2.6.8: Installation of Pipes and Plumbing Fixtures

Each gas pipe, water pipe, gas-burning fixture, plumbing fixture and apparatus, or any other similar fixture and all connections to water, sewer, or gas lines should be installed and free from defects, leaks, and obstructions in accordance with the requirements of the state and/or local regulatory agency for buildings.

RATIONALE: This standard prevents injuries and hazardous and unsanitary conditions.

TYPE OF FACILITY: Center; Large Family Child Care Home; Small Family Child Care Home

STANDARD 5.2.6.9: Handwashing Sink Using Portable Water Supply

When plumbing is unavailable to provide a handwashing sink, the facility should provide a handwashing sink using a portable water supply and a sanitary catch system approved by a local public health department. A mechanism should be in place to prevent children from gaining access to soiled water or more than one child from washing in the same water.

RATIONALE: The best way to clean hands is to wash with soap and running water or use a hand sanitizer, with supervision. Ideally, properly equipped handwashing sinks should be provided (see Standard 5.4.1.10). However, in emergency situations when a supply of running water or hand sanitizer may not be realistically available, sinks with a portable water supply can be used.

COMMENTS: A variety of portable hand sinks are available for purchase. Before purchasing, facilities should consult with their local health department on what types of portable sinks are allowed or approved for use.

The handling of waste water poses sanitation hazards for children and staff. Portable systems often require staff to lift the water containers. Such lifting may pose an occupational health risk.

TYPE OF FACILITY: Center; Large Family Child Care Home; Small Family Child Care Home

RELATED STANDARDS:
Standard 3.2.2.2: Handwashing Procedure
Standard 3.2.2.5: Hand Sanitizers
Standard 5.2.1.14: Water Heating Devices and Temperatures Allowed
Standards 5.4.1.10-5.4.1.12: Sinks

STANDARD 5.2.6.10: Drinking Fountains

Drinking fountains should have an angled jet and orifice guard above the rim of the fountain. The pressure should be regulated so the water stream does not contact the orifice guard or splash on the floor, but should rise at least two inches above the orifice guard.

Drinking fountains should be cleaned and disinfected at least daily and whenever visibly dirty.

At least eighteen inches of space should be provided between a drinking fountain and any kind of towel dispenser.

RATIONALE: Access to water provides for fluid maintenance essential to body health. The water must be protected from contamination to avoid the spread of disease. Space between a drinking fountain and sink or towel dispenser helps prevent contamination of the drinking fountain by organisms being splashed or deposited during use.

Moist surfaces such as drinking fountains in child care centers can be sources of rotavirus contamination during an outbreak (1).

TYPE OF FACILITY: Center

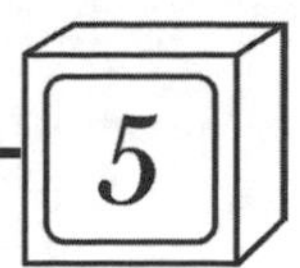

REFERENCES:
1. Butz, A. M., P. Fosarelli, J. Dick, T. Cusack, R. Yolken. 1993. Prevalence of rotavirus on high risk fomites in day-care facilities. *Pediatrics* 92:202-5.

5.2.7 Sewage and Garbage

STANDARD 5.2.7.1: On-Site Sewage Systems

A sewage system should be provided and inspected in accordance with state and local regulations. Whenever a public sewer is available, the facility should be connected to it. Where public sewers are not available, an on-site sewage system or other method approved by the local public health department should be installed. Raw or treated wastes should not be discharged on the surface of the ground.

The wastewater or septic system drainage field should not be located within the outdoor play area of a child care program, unless the drainage field has been designed by a sanitation engineer with the presence of an outdoor play area in mind and meets the approval of the local health authority.

The exhaust vent from a wastewater or septic system and drainage field should not be located within the children's outdoor play area.

RATIONALE: Sewage must not be allowed to contaminate drinking water or ground water. It must be carried from the facility to a place where sanitary treatment equipment is available. Raw sewage is a health hazard and usually has an offensive odor.

The weight of children or the combined weight of children and playground equipment may cause the drainage field to become compacted, resulting in failure of the system. Some structures are anchored in concrete, which adds weight. The legs of some equipment, such as swing sets, can puncture the surface of drainage fields. In areas where frequent rains are coupled with high water tables, poor drainage, and flooding, the surface of drainage fields often becomes contaminated with untreated sewage.

COMMENTS: Whether the presence of an outdoor play area would adversely affect the operation of an on-site sewage system will depend on the type of playground equipment and method of anchoring, the type of resilient surface placed beneath playground equipment to reduce injury from falls, the soil type where the field would be placed (some soils are more compactable than others), the type of ground cover present (a cover of good grass underlain by a good sandy layer is much better than packed clay or some impermeable or slowly impermeable surface layer), and the design of the drainage field itself. Septic systems are now most commonly called "on-site sewage systems" or "on-site systems" because they treat and dispose of household wastewater on the household's own property (1).

Staff should consult with the local public health department regarding sewage storage and disposal. The national/international organization representing on-site wastewater/sewage interests is the National On-Site Wastewater Recycling Association, Inc. (NOWRA).

TYPE OF FACILITY: Center; Large Family Child Care Home; Small Family Child Care Home

REFERENCES:
1. National Onsite Wastewater Recycling Association (NOWRA). *Homeowner's onsite system guide and record keeping folder*. http://www.nowra.org/documents/HomeownerOnsiteSystemGuide.pdf.

STANDARD 5.2.7.2: Removal of Garbage

Garbage and rubbish should be removed from rooms occupied by children, staff, parents/guardians, or volunteers on a daily basis and removed from the premises at least twice weekly or at other frequencies required by the regulatory health authority.

RATIONALE: This practice provides proper sanitation and protection of health, prevents infestations by rodents, insects, and other pests, and prevents odors and injuries.

COMMENTS: Compliance can be tested by checking for evidence of infestation and odors.

TYPE OF FACILITY: Center; Large Family Child Care Home; Small Family Child Care Home

STANDARD 5.2.7.3: Containment of Garbage

Garbage should be kept in containers approved by the regulatory health authority. Such containers should be constructed of durable metal or other types of material, designed and used so wild and domesticated animals and pests do not have access to the contents, and so they do not leak or absorb liquids. Waste containers should be kept covered with tight-fitting lids or covers when stored.

The facility should have a sufficient number of waste and diaper containers to hold all of the garbage and diapers that accumulate between periods of removal from the premises. Plastic garbage bag liners should be used in such containers. Exterior garbage containers should be stored on an easily cleanable surface. Garbage areas should be free of litter and waste that is not contained. Children should not be allowed access to garbage, waste, and refuse storage areas.

If a compactor is used, the surface should be graded to a suitable drain, as approved by the regulatory health authority.

RATIONALE: Containers for garbage attract animals and insects. When trash contains organic material, decomposition creates unpleasant odors. Therefore, child care facilities must choose and use garbage containers that control sanitation risks, pests, and offensive odors. Lining the containers with plastic bags reduces the contamination of the container itself and the need to wash the containers, which hold a concomitant risk of spreading the contamination into the environment.

TYPE OF FACILITY: Center; Large Family Child Care Home; Small Family Child Care Home

RELATED STANDARDS:
Standard 5.2.8.1: Integrated Pest Management

STANDARD 5.2.7.4: Containment of Soiled Diapers

Soiled diapers should be stored inside the facility in containers separate from other waste. Washable, plastic-lined, tightly covered receptacles, with a firmly fitting cover that does not require touching with contaminated hands or objects, should be provided, within arm's reach of diaper changing tables, to store soiled diapers. The container for soiled diapers should be designed to prevent the user from contaminating any exterior surfaces of the container or the user when inserting the soiled diaper. Soiled diapers do not have to be individually bagged before placing them in the container for soiled diapers. Soiled cloth diapers and soiled clothing that are to be sent home with a parent/guardian, however, should be individually bagged.

The following types of diaper containers should not be used;

a) Those that require the user's hand to push the diaper through a narrow opening;
b) Those with exterior surfaces that must be touched with the hand;
c) Those with exterior surfaces that are likely to be touched with the soiled diaper while the user is discarding the soiled diaper;
d) Those that have lids with handles.

Separate containers should be used for disposable diapers, cloth diapers (if used), and soiled clothes and linens. All containers should be inaccessible to children and should be tall enough to prevent children reaching into the receptacle or from falling headfirst into containers. The containers should be placed in an area that children cannot enter without close adult supervision.

RATIONALE: Separate, plastic-lined waste receptacles that do not require touching with contaminated hands or objects and that children cannot access enclose odors within, and prevent children from coming into contact with body fluids. Anything that increases handling increases potential for contamination (1). Step cans or other hands-free cans with tightly fitted lids provide protection against odor and hand contamination.

COMMENTS: Fecal material and urine should not be mixed with regular trash and garbage. Where possible, soiled disposable diapers should be disposed of as biological waste rather than in the local landfill. In some areas, recycling depots for disposable diapers may be available. The facility should not use the short, poorly made domestic step cans that require caregivers/teachers to use their hands to open the lids because the foot pedals don't work. Caregivers/teachers will find it worthwhile to invest in commercial-grade step cans of sufficient size to hold the number of soiled diapers the facility collects before someone can remove the contents to an outside trash receptacle. These are the types used by doctor's offices, hospitals, and restaurants. A variety of sizes and types are available from restaurant and medical wholesale suppliers. Other types of hands-free containers can be used as long as the user can place the soiled diaper into the receptacle without increasing contact of the user's hands and the exterior of the container with the soiled diaper.

TYPE OF FACILITY: Center; Large Family Child Care Home; Small Family Child Care Home

RELATED STANDARDS:
Standard 3.2.3.4: Prevention of Exposure to Blood and Bodily Fluids

REFERENCES:
1. Pickering, L. K., C. J. Baker, D. W. Kimberlin, S. S. Long, eds. 2009. *Red book: 2009 report of the Committee on Infectious Diseases.* Elk Grove Village, IL: American Academy of Pediatrics.

STANDARD 5.2.7.5: Labeling, Cleaning, and Disposal of Waste and Diaper Containers

Each waste and diaper container should be labeled to show its intended contents. These containers should be cleaned daily to keep them free from build-up of soil and odor. Wastewater from these cleaning operations should be disposed of by pouring it down a toilet or floor drain. Wastewater should not be poured onto the ground, into handwashing sinks, laundry sinks, kitchen sinks, or bathtubs.

RATIONALE: This standard prevents noxious odors and spread of disease.

TYPE OF FACILITY: Center; Large Family Child Care Home; Small Family Child Care Home

STANDARD 5.2.7.6: Storage and Disposal of Infectious and Toxic Wastes

Infectious and toxic wastes should be stored separately from other wastes, and should be disposed of in a manner approved by the regulatory health authority.

RATIONALE: This practice provides for safe storage and disposal of infectious and toxic wastes.

TYPE OF FACILITY: Center; Large Family Child Care Home; Small Family Child Care Home

RELATED STANDARDS:
Standards 5.2.9.1-5.2.9.15: Prevention and Management of Toxic Substances

5.2.8 Integrated Pest Management

STANDARD 5.2.8.1: Integrated Pest Management

Facilities should adopt an integrated pest management program (IPM) to ensure long-term, environmentally sound pest suppression through a range of practices including pest exclusion, sanitation and clutter control, and elimination of conditions that are conducive to pest infestations. IPM is a simple, common-sense approach to pest management that eliminates the root causes of pest problems, providing safe and effective control of insects, weeds, rodents, and other pests while minimizing risks to human health and the environment (2,4).

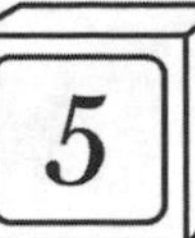

Pest Prevention: Facilities should prevent pest infestations by ensuring sanitary conditions. This can be done by eliminating pest breeding areas, filling in cracks and crevices; holes in walls, floors, ceilings and water leads; repairing water damage; and removing clutter and rubbish on the premises (5).

Pest Monitoring: Facilities should establish a program for regular pest population monitoring and should keep records of pest sightings and sightings of indicators of the presence of pests (e.g., gnaw marks, frass, rub marks).

Pesticide Use: If physical intervention fails to prevent pest infestations, facility managers should ensure that targeted, rather than broadcast applications of pesticides are made, beginning with the products that pose least exposure hazard first, and always using a pesticide applicator who has the licenses or certifications required by state and local laws.

Facility managers should follow all instructions on pesticide product labels and should not apply any pesticide in a manner inconsistent with label instructions. Material Safety Data Sheets (MSDS) are available from the product manufacturer or a licensed exterminator and should be on file at the facility Facilities should ensure that pesticides are never applied when children are present and that re-entry periods are adhered to.

Records of all pesticides applications (including type and amount of pesticide used), timing and location of treatment, and results should be maintained either on-line or in a manner that permits access by facility managers and staff, state inspectors and regulatory personnel, parents/guardians, and others who may inquire about pesticide usage at the facility.

Facilities should avoid the use of sprays and other volatilizing pesticide formulations. Pesticides should be applied in a manner that prevents skin contact and any other exposure to children or staff members and minimizes odors in occupied areas. Care should be taken to ensure that pesticide applications do not result in pesticide residues accumulating on tables, toys, and items mouthed or handled by children, or on soft surfaces such as carpets, upholstered furniture, or stuffed animals with which children may come in direct contact (3).

Following the use of pesticides, herbicides, fungicides, or other potentially toxic chemicals, the treated area should be ventilated for the period recommended on the product label.

Notification: Notification should be given to parents/guardians and staff before using pesticides, to determine if any child or staff member is sensitive to the product. A member of the child care staff should directly observe the application to be sure that toxic chemicals are not applied on surfaces with which children or staff may come in contact.

Registry: Child care facilities should provide the opportunity for interested staff and parents/guardians to register with the facility if they want to be notified about individual pesticide applications before they occur.

Warning Signs: Child care facilities must post warning signs at each area where pesticides will be applied. These signs must be posted forty-eight hours before and seventy-two hours after applications and should be sufficient to restrict uninformed access to treated areas.

Record Keeping: Child care facilities should keep records of pesticide use at the facility and make the records available to anyone who asks. Record retention requirements vary by state, but federal law requires records to be kept for two years (7). It is a good idea to retain records for a minimum of three years.

Pesticide Storage: Pesticides should be stored in their original containers and in a locked room or cabinet accessible only to authorized staff. No restricted-use pesticides should be stored or used on the premises except by properly licensed persons. Banned, illegal, and unregistered pesticides should not be used.

RATIONALE: Children must be protected from exposure to pesticides (1). To prevent contamination and poisoning, child care staff must be sure that these chemicals are applied by individuals who are licensed and certified to do so. Direct observation of pesticide application by child care staff is essential to guide the pest management professional away from surfaces that children can touch or mouth and to monitor for drifting of pesticides into these areas. The time of toxic risk exposure is a function of skin contact, the efficiency of the ventilating system, and the volatility of the toxic substance. Spraying the grounds of a child care facility exposes children to toxic chemicals. Studies and a recent consensus statement address the risk of neurodevelopmental effects from exposure to pesticides (6). Exposure to pesticides has been linked to learning and developmental disorders. Children are more vulnerable as their metabolic, enzymatic, and immunological systems are immature. Pesticides should only be used as an emergency application to eliminate threats to human health (6).

COMMENTS: Manufacturers of pesticides usually provide product warnings that exposure to these chemicals can be poisonous.

Child care staff should ask to see the license of the pest management professional and should be certain that the individual who applies the toxic chemicals has personally been trained and preferably, individually licensed, i.e., not working in the capacity of a technician being supervised by a licensed pest management professional. In some states only the owner of a pest management company is required to have this training, and s/he may then employ unskilled workers. Child care staff should ensure that the pest management professional is familiar with the pesticide s/he is applying.

Child care staff should contact their state pesticide office and request that their child care facility be added to the state pesticide sensitivity list, in states where such a list exists. When a child care facility is placed on the state pesticide sensitivity list, the child care staff will be notified if there are plans for general pesticide application occurring near the child care facility.

For further information about pest control, contact the state pesticide regulatory agency, the Environmental Protection Agency (EPA), or the National Pesticide Information Center. For possible poison exposure, contact the local poison center at 1-800-222-1222.

TYPE OF FACILITY: Center; Large Family Child Care Home; Small Family Child Care Home

REFERENCES:

1. Tulve, N. S., P. A. Jones, M. G. Nishioka, R. C. Fortmann, C. W. Croghan, J. Y. Zhou, A. Fraser, C. Cave, W. Friedman. 2006. Pesticide measurements from the First National Environmental Health Survey of Child Care Centers using a multi-residue GC/MS analysis method. *Environ Sci Tech* 40:6269-74.
2. U.S. Environmental Protection Agency. Integrated pest management (IPM) in schools. http://www.epa.gov/pesticides/ipm/index.htm.
3. U.S. Environmental Protection Agency. Integrated pest management (IPM) in child care. http://www.epa.gov/pesticides/controlling/childcare-ipm.htm.
4. The IPM Institute of North America. IPM standards for schools. http://ipminstitute.org/school.htm.
5. University of California, Agriculture and Natural Resources. UC IPM online: Statewide integrated pest management program. How to manage pests. http://www.ipm.ucdavis.edu.
6. Gilbert, S. G. 2007. *Scientific consensus statement on environmental agents associated with neurodevelopmental disorders*. Bolinas, CA: Collaborative on Health and the Environment (CHE). http://www.neep.org/uploads/NEEPResources/id27/lddistatement.pdf.
7. South Dakota State University, Department of Plant Science. Restricted use pesticide record keeping: Pesticide recordkeeping is more than just a good idea -- it's the law! http://www.sdstate.edu/ps/extension/pat/pesticide-record.cfm.

STANDARD 5.2.8.2: Insect Breeding Hazard

No facility should maintain or permit to be maintained any receptacle or pool, whether natural or artificial, containing water in such condition that insects breeding therein may become a public health issue.

RATIONALE: Collection of water in tin cans, children's toys, flower pots, rain gutters, discarded tires and other refuse, and natural pools of water can provide breeding sites for mosquitoes. Elimination of mosquito breeding sites is one of the basic environmental control methods.

Mosquitoes are responsible for transmitting a variety of diseases. Mosquito-borne viruses such as West Nile virus, eastern equine encephalitis, western equine encephalitis, and St. Louis encephalitis have occurred in the United States and Canada (1). Children can develop allergic reactions to mosquito and fire ant bites and bee and wasp stings.

COMMENTS: Regular surveillance for stinging insect nests is important.

TYPE OF FACILITY: Center; Large Family Child Care Home; Small Family Child Care Home

RELATED STANDARDS:
Standard 3.4.5.2: Insect Repellent and Protection from Vector-Borne Diseases
Standard 5.2.8.1: Integrated Pest Management

REFERENCES:

1. Heymann, D. L. 2008. *Control of communicable diseases manual*. 19th ed. Washington, DC: American Public Health Association.

5.2.9 Prevention and Management of Toxic Substances

STANDARD 5.2.9.1: Use and Storage of Toxic Substances

The following items should be used as recommended by the manufacturer and should be stored in the original labeled containers:

a) Cleaning materials;
b) Detergents;
c) Automatic dishwasher detergents;
d) Aerosol cans;
e) Pesticides;
f) Health and beauty aids;
g) Medications;
h) Lawn care chemicals;
i) Other toxic materials.

Material Safety Data Sheets (MSDS) must be available on-site for each hazardous chemical that is on the premises.

These substances should be used only in a manner that will not contaminate play surfaces, food, or food preparation areas, and that will not constitute a hazard to the children or staff. When not in active use, all chemicals used inside or outside should be stored in a safe and secure manner in a locked room or cabinet, fitted with a child-resistive opening device, inaccessible to children, and separate from stored medications and food.

Chemicals used in lawn care treatments should be limited to those listed for use in areas that can be occupied by children.

Medications can be toxic if taken by the wrong person or in the wrong dose. Medications should be stored safely (see Standard 3.6.3.1) and disposed of properly (see Standard 3.6.3.2).

The telephone number for the poison center should be posted in a location where it is readily available in emergency situations (e.g., next to the telephone). Poison centers are open twenty-four hours a day, seven days a week, and can be reached at 1-800-222-1222.

RATIONALE: There are over two million human poison exposures reported to poison centers every year. Children under six years of age account for over half of those potential poisonings. The substances most commonly involved in poison exposures of children are cosmetics and personal care products, cleaning substances, and medications (1).

The MSDS explains the risk of exposure to products so that appropriate precautions may be taken.

COMMENTS: Many child-resistant types of closing devices can be installed on doors to prevent young children from accessing poisonous substances. Many of these devices are self-engaging when the door is closed and require an adult hand size or skill to open the door. A locked cabinet or room where children cannot gain access is best but must be used consistently. Child-resistant containers provide another level of protection.

TYPE OF FACILITY: Center; Large Family Child Care Home; Small Family Child Care Home

RELATED STANDARDS:

Standard 3.6.3.1: Medication Administration
Standard 3.6.3.2: Labeling, Storage, and Disposal of Medications
Standard 5.2.8.1: Integrated Pest Management
Standard 5.2.9.3: Informing Staff Regarding Presence of Toxic Substances
Standard 6.3.2.3: Pool Equipment and Chemical Storage Rooms
Standard 6.3.4.2: Chlorine Pucks

REFERENCES:

1. Bronstein, A. C., D. A. Spyker, L. R. Cantilena, Jr., J. L. Green, B. H. Rumack, S. E. Heard. 2008. 2007 annual report of the American Association of Poison Control Centers' National Poison Data System (NPDS): 25th annual report. *Clin Toxicol* 46:927-1057.

STANDARD 5.2.9.2: Use of a Poison Center

The poison center should be called for advice about any exposure to toxic substances, or any potential poisoning emergency. The national help line for the poison center is 1-800-222-1222, and specialists will link the caregiver/teacher with their local poison center. The advice should be followed and documented in the facility's files. The caregiver/teacher should be prepared for the call by having the following information for the poison center specialist:

a) The child's age and sex;
b) The substance involved;
c) The estimated amount;
d) The child's condition;
e) The time elapsed since ingestion or exposure.

The caregiver/teacher should not induce vomiting unless instructed by the poison center.

RATIONALE: Toxic substances, when ingested, inhaled, or in contact with skin, may react immediately or slowly, with serious symptoms occurring much later (1). It is important for the caregiver/teacher to call the poison center after the exposure and not "wait and see." Symptoms vary with the type of substance involved. Some common poisoning symptoms include dermatitis, nausea, vomiting, diarrhea, and congestion.

COMMENTS: Any question on possible risks for exposure should be referred to poison center professionals for proper first aid and treatment. Regional poison centers have access to the latest information on emergency care of the poisoning victim.

Caregivers/teachers can go to http://www.aapcc.org to find their local poison center or for additional information on poisoning and poison safety. They can also access a variety of services that poison centers have: poison prevention, poison control, information about toxic substances including lead and chemicals that may be found in consumer products, and even assistance with disaster planning. Caregivers/teachers should feel comfortable calling the poison center about medication dosing errors. Poison centers provide free, confidential advice on how to handle the situation.

TYPE OF FACILITY: Center; Large Family Child Care Home; Small Family Child Care Home

REFERENCES:

1. American Academy of Pediatrics, Committee on Injury, Violence, and Poison Prevention. 2007. Policy statement: Poison treatment in the home. *Pediatrics* 119:1031.

STANDARD 5.2.9.3: Informing Staff Regarding Presence of Toxic Substances

Employers should provide staff with hazard information, including access to and review of the Material Safety Data Sheets (MSDS) as required by the Occupational Safety and Health Administration (OSHA), about the presence of toxic substances such as formaldehyde, cleaning and sanitizing supplies, insecticides, herbicides, and other hazardous chemicals in use in the facility. Staff should always read the label prior to use to determine safety in use. For example, toxic products regulated by the Environmental Protection Agency (EPA) will have an EPA signal word of CAUTION, WARNING, or DANGER. Where nontoxic substitutes are available, these nontoxic substitutes should be used instead of toxic chemicals. If a nontoxic product is not available, caregivers/teachers should use the least toxic product for the job. A CAUTION label is safer than a WARNING label, which is safer than a DANGER label.

RATIONALE: These precautions are essential to the health and well-being of the staff and the children alike. Many cleaning products and art materials contain ingredients that may be toxic. Regulations require employers to make the complete identity of these materials known to users. Because nontoxic substitutes are available for virtually all necessary products, exchanging them for toxic products is required.

COMMENTS: The U.S. Department of Labor, which oversees OSHA, is responsible for protection of workers and is listed in the phone books of all large cities. Because standards change frequently, the facility should seek the latest standards from the EPA. Information on toxic substances in the environment is available from the EPA. For information on consumer products contact the U.S. Consumer Product Safety Commission (CPSC). For information on art and craft materials, contact the Art and Creative Materials Institute (ACMI). The local health jurisdiction can also be a resource for information on hazardous chemicals in child care.

The MSDS explains the risk of exposure to products so that appropriate precautions may be taken.

TYPE OF FACILITY: Center; Large Family Child Care Home

RELATED STANDARDS:

Standard 5.2.8.1: Integrated Pest Management
Standard 5.2.9.1: Use and Storage of Toxic Substances

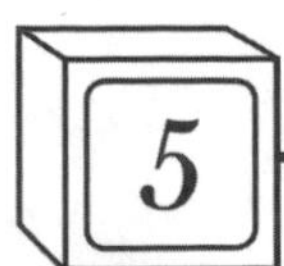

Standard 5.2.9.7: Proper Use of Art and Craft Materials
Standard 6.3.2.3: Pool Equipment and Chemical Storage Rooms
Standard 6.3.4.2: Chlorine Pucks

REFERENCES:

1. Wargo, J. 2004. *The physical school environment: An essential component of a health-promoting school*. WHO Information series on School Health, document 2. Geneva: WHO. http://www.who.int/school_youth_health/media/en/physical_sch_environment.pdf.
2. Fiene, R. 2002. *13 indicators of quality child care: Research update*. Washington, DC: U.S. Department of Health and Human Services, Office of the Assistant Secretary for Planning and Evaluation. http://aspe.hhs.gov/hsp/ccquality-ind02/.

STANDARD 5.2.9.4: Radon Concentrations

Radon concentrations inside a home or building used for child care must be less than four picocuries per liter of air. All facilities must be tested for the presence of radon, according to U.S. Environmental Protection Agency (EPA) testing protocols for long-term testing (i.e., greater than ninety days in duration using alpha-track or electret test devices).

RATIONALE: Radon is a colorless, odorless, radioactive gas that occurs naturally. It can be found in soil, water, building materials, and natural gas. Radon from the soil is the main cause of radon problems. Radon typically moves up through the ground to the air above and into a home or building through cracks and other holes in the foundation. Radon can get trapped inside the home or building where it can build up. In a small number of homes, the building materials can give off radon but the materials themselves rarely cause problems by themselves. If radon is present in the water supply, most of the risk is related to radon released into the air when water is used for showering or other household purposes (1). When radon gas is inhaled, it can damage lung tissue and lead to lung cancer. Radon levels can be easily measured to determine if acceptable levels have been exceeded. There is no known safe level of radon so there can always be some risk. The risk can be reduced by lowering the levels of radon in the home or building. Fixing buildings to reduce radon exposure may entail sealing cracks in the foundation or ventilating the area under the foundation.

COMMENTS: The average indoor radon level is estimated to be about 1.3 picocuries per liter of air, and about 0.4 picocuries per liter is normally found in the outside air. Most homes today can be reduced to two picocuries per liter or below (1).

Common test kits include: charcoal canisters, e-perm, alpha track detectors, and charcoal liquid scintillation devices. For more information on EPA and American Association of Radon Scientists and Technologists' (AARST) testing protocols, see http://www.aarst.org. For material and information on radon, contact the EPA.

TYPE OF FACILITY: Center; Large Family Child Care Home; Small Family Child Care Home

RELATED STANDARDS:
Standard 5.1.1.7: Use of Basements and Below Grade Areas

REFERENCES:

1. U.S. Environmental Protection Agency (EPA). 2009. *A citizen's guide to radon: The guide to protecting yourself and your family from radon*. http://www.epa.gov/radon/pdfs/citizensguide.pdf.
2. Fiene, R. 2002. *13 indicators of quality child care: Research update*. Washington, DC: U.S. Department of Health and Human Services, Office of the Assistant Secretary for Planning and Evaluation. http://aspe.hhs.gov/hsp/ccquality-ind02/.

STANDARD 5.2.9.5: Carbon Monoxide Detectors

Carbon monoxide detector(s) should be installed in child care settings if one of the following guidelines is met:

a) The child care program uses any sources of coal, wood, charcoal, oil, kerosene, propane, natural gas, or any other product that can produce carbon monoxide indoors or in an attached garage;
b) If detectors are required by state/local law or state licensing agency.

Facilities must meet state or local laws regarding carbon monoxide detectors. Detectors should be tested monthly. Batteries should be changed at least yearly. Detectors should be replaced at least every five years.

RATIONALE: Carbon monoxide (CO) is a deadly, colorless, odorless, poisonous gas. It is produced by the incomplete burning of various fuels, including coal, wood, charcoal, oil, kerosene, propane, and natural gas. Products and equipment powered by internal combustion engine-powered equipment such as portable generators, cars, lawn mowers, and power washers also produce carbon monoxide. Carbon monoxide detectors are the only way to detect this substance.

Carbon monoxide poisoning causes symptoms that mimic the flu; mild symptoms are typically headache, dizziness, fatigue, nausea, and diarrhea. Prolonged exposure can cause confusion, shortness of breath, unconsciousness, and even death.

On average, about 170 people in the United States die every year from carbon monoxide produced by non-automotive consumer products (1). These products include malfunctioning fuel-burning appliances such as furnaces, ranges, water heaters, and room heaters; engine-powered equipment such as portable generators; fireplaces; and charcoal that is burned in homes and other enclosed areas. In 2005 alone, the U.S. Consumer Product Safety Commission (CPSC) staff was aware of at least ninety-four generator-related carbon monoxide poisoning deaths (1). Still others die from carbon monoxide produced by non-consumer products, such as cars left running in attached garages. The Centers for Disease Control and Prevention (CDC) estimate that several thousand people go to hospital emergency rooms every year to be treated for carbon monoxide poisoning (1).

COMMENTS: Carbon monoxide detectors should be installed according to the manufacturer's instructions. One carbon monoxide detector should be installed in the hallway outside the bedrooms in each separate sleeping area. Carbon monoxide detectors may be installed into a plug-in

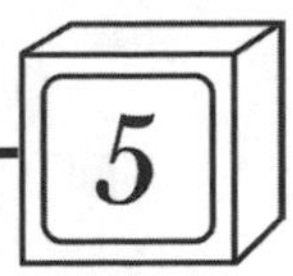

receptacle or high on the wall. Hard-wired or plug-in carbon monoxide detectors should have battery backup. Installing carbon monoxide detectors near heating vents, locations that can be covered by furniture or draperies, above fuel-burning appliances or in kitchens should be avoided (1).

There are a number of safety steps that child care programs can do to help prevent carbon monoxide exposure (1-3):

a) Make sure major appliances are professionally installed and inspected according to local building codes and have older appliances checked for malfunctions and leaks;
b) Choose vented appliances when possible;
c) Have heating systems inspected and cleaned by a qualified technician annually and make sure the chimney is clean and with a proper draft control to ensure a proper vent for flue gases;
d) Check the color of the flame in the burner and pilot light (a yellow-colored flame indicates the fuel is not burning efficiently and could be releasing more carbon monoxide) (4);
e) Never use a gas oven to heat your facility;
f) Do not burn charcoal indoors;
g) Never operate gasoline-powered engines or generators in confined areas in or near the building;
h) Never leave a vehicle running in a garage or closed area. Even if the garage door is open, normal circulation will not supply enough fresh air to prevent a buildup of CO gas;
i) If the CO alarm goes off or if you have symptoms of CO poisoning, exit the building and call 9-1-1.

For other questions on CO poisoning call the poison center.

TYPE OF FACILITY: Center; Large Family Child Care Home; Small Family Child Care Home

REFERENCES:

1. U.S. Consumer Product Safety Commission (CPSC). 2008. *Carbon monoxide questions and answers*. Document #466. Bethesda, MD: CPSC. http://www.cpsc.gov/CPSCPUB/PUBS/466.html.
2. Cowling, T. 2007. Safety first: Carbon monoxide poisoning. *Healthy Child Care* 10(5): 6-7. http://www.healthychild.net/SafetyFirst.php?article_id=402/.
3. Safe Kids USA. *Carbon monoxide fact sheet*. http://www.safekids.org/our-work/research/fact-sheets/carbon-monoxide-fact-sheet.html.
4. Tremblay, K. R., Jr. 2006. *Preventing carbon monoxide problems*. Colorado State University Extension. http://www.ext.colostate.edu/pubs/consumer/09939.html.

STANDARD 5.2.9.6: Preventing Exposure to Asbestos or Other Friable Materials

Any asbestos, fiberglass, or other friable material or any material that is in a dangerous condition found within a facility or on the grounds of the facility should be repaired or removed. Repair usually involves either sealing (encapsulating) or covering asbestos material. Any repair or removal of asbestos should be done by a contractor certified to do in accordance with existing regulations of the U.S. Environmental Protection Agency (EPA). No children or staff should be present until the removal and cleanup of the hazardous condition have been completed.

Pipe and boiler insulation should be sampled and examined in an accredited laboratory for the presence of asbestos in a friable or potentially dangerous condition.

Non-friable asbestos should be identified to prevent disturbance and/or exposure during remodeling or future activities.

RATIONALE: Removal of significant hazards will protect the staff, children, and families who use the facility. Asbestos dust and fibers that are inhaled and reach the lungs can cause lung disease (1,2).

COMMENTS: The mere presence of asbestos in a child care facility, home, or a building is not hazardous. The danger is that asbestos materials may become damaged over time. Damaged asbestos may release asbestos fibers and become a health hazard (2,3). The best thing to do with asbestos material that is in good condition is to leave it alone. Disturbing it may create a health hazard where none existed before (1).

Asbestos that is in a friable condition means that it is easily crumbled (2).

The National Asbestos School Hazard Abatement Act of 1984 specifies requirements for removal of asbestos. Contact your local health department for additional information on asbestos regulations in your area. For more information regarding asbestos and applicable EPA regulations, contact regional offices of the EPA.

TYPE OF FACILITY: Center; Large Family Child Care Home; Small Family Child Care Home

REFERENCES:

1. U.S. Consumer Product Safety Commission (CPSC). *Asbestos in the home*. http://www.cpsc.gov/cpscpub/pubs/453.html.
2. U.S. Department of Health and Human Services, Agency for Toxic Substances and Disease Registry. 2001. Toxicological profile for asbestos.
http://www.atsdr.cdc.gov/ToxProfiles/tp61-p.pdf.
3. Fiene, R. 2002. *13 indicators of quality child care: Research update*. Washington, DC: U.S. Department of Health and Human Services, Office of the Assistant Secretary for Planning and Evaluation. http://aspe.hhs.gov/hsp/ccquality-ind02/.

STANDARD 5.2.9.7: Proper Use of Art and Craft Materials

Only art and craft materials that are approved by the Art and Creative Materials Institute (ACMI) should be used in the child care facility. Art and craft materials should conform to all applicable ACMI safety standards. Materials should be labeled in accordance with the chronic hazard labeling standard, ASTM D4236.

The facility should prohibit use of unlabeled, improperly labeled old, or donated materials with potentially harmful ingredients.

Caregivers/teachers should closely supervise all children using art and craft materials and should make sure art and

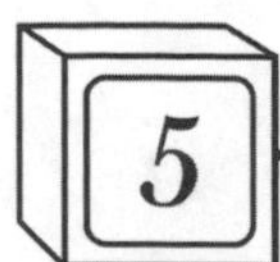

craft materials are properly used, cleaned up, and stored in original containers that are fully labeled. Materials should be age-appropriate. Children should not eat or drink while using art and craft materials.

Caregivers/teachers should have emergency protocols in place in the event of an injury, poisoning, or allergic reaction. If caregivers/teachers suspect a poisoning may have occurred they should call their poison center at 1-800-222-1222. Rooms should be well ventilated while using art and craft materials.

Only ACMI-approved unscented water-based markers should be used for children's art projects and work.

RATIONALE: Contamination and injury may occur if art and craft materials are improperly used or labeled. Labels are required on art supplies to identify any hazardous ingredients, risks associated with their use, precautions, first aid, and sources of further information (1).

Art material, approved by the ACMI, has been tested for both chronic and acute health hazards. The ACMI AP (Approved Product) Seal, with or without Performance Certification, identifies art materials that are safe and that are certified in a toxicological evaluation by a medical expert to contain no materials in sufficient quantities to be toxic or injurious to humans, including children, or to cause acute or chronic health problems. This seal is currently replacing the previous non-toxic seals: CP (Certified Product), AP (Approved Product), and HL Health Label (Non-Toxic) over a ten-year phase-in period. Such products are certified by ACMI to be labeled in accordance with the chronic hazard labeling standard, ASTM D4236, and the U.S. Labeling of Hazardous Art Materials Act (LHAMA). Additionally, products bearing the AP Seal with Performance Certification or the CP Seal are certified to meet specific requirements of material, workmanship, working qualities, and color developed by ACMI and others through recognized standards organizations, such as the American National Standards Institute (ANSI) and ASTM International. Some products cannot attain this performance certification because no quality standard currently exists for certain types of products (1).

Children have been known to try and eat fruit-scented markers. Solvent-based/permanent markers can trigger headaches and/or asthma (3).

COMMENTS: Non-toxic art and craft supplies intended for children are readily available.

Some products labeled "non-toxic" are not necessarily a safer alternative; thus the need to check for the proper labeling.

TYPE OF FACILITY: Center; Large Family Child Care Home; Small Family Child Care Home

RELATED STANDARDS:
Standard 5.2.1.4: Ventilation When Using Art Materials

REFERENCES:

1. Art and Creative Materials Institute. 2010. Safety - what you need to know. http://www.acminet.org/Safety.htm.
2. Fiene, R. 2002. 13 *indicators of quality child care: Research update.* Washington, DC: U.S. Department of Health and Human Services, Office of the Assistant Secretary for Planning and Evaluation. http://aspe.hhs.gov/hsp/ccquality-ind02/.
3. U.S. Consumer Product Safety Commission (CPSC). *Art and craft safety guide.* Bethesda, MD: CPSC. http://www.cpsc.gov/cpscpub/pubs/5015.pdf.

STANDARD 5.2.9.8: Use of Play Dough and Other Manipulative Art or Sensory Materials

The child care program should have the following procedures on the use and life span of manipulative art or sensory materials such as clay, play dough, etc:

a) If handmade, these materials should be made fresh each week, labeled, dated and stored in airtight containers;
b) If purchased, these products should be stored in their original packaging;
c) Products that are labeled as toxic are prohibited;
d) The surface upon which they are used and the tools used with these materials should be cleaned and sanitized before and after use;
e) Children should practice hand hygiene before and after each use;
f) Material should be discarded if it is sneezed upon, put into a child's mouth, or in any other way possibly contaminated;
g) Children with latex or gluten allergies should be given their own portion of the material and that individual portion should be stored separately if for repeat use.
h) Children with cuts, sores, scratches and colds with sneezing and runny noses should be given their own portion of the material and that individual portion should be stored separately if for repeat use.

RATIONALE: Hand hygiene, supervision of children, and discarding material that is contaminated are appropriate hygienic practices when using these materials. Providing children with their own portion of modeling material helps prevent cross-contamination (1).

TYPE OF FACILITY: Center; Large Family Child Care Home; Small Family Child Care Home

RELATED STANDARDS:
Standard 3.2.2.1: Situations that Require Hand Hygiene

REFERENCES:

1. Life Tips. Cutting down on playdough germs. http://parent.lifetips.com/tip/43479/day-care-and-babysitters/concerns-and-coping/cutting-down-on-playdough-germs.html.

STANDARD 5.2.9.9: Plastic Containers and Toys

The facility should use infant bottles, plastic containers, and toys that do not contain Polyvinyl chloride (PVC), Bisphenol A (BPA), or phthalates. When possible, caregivers/teachers should substitute materials such as paper, ceramic, glass, and stainless steel for plastics.

RATIONALE: Plastics can contain chemicals and metals, which are used as additives and stabilizers. Some of these additives and stabilizers can be toxic, such as lead (e.g., toys, vinyl lunchboxes). Plastics can release chemicals into

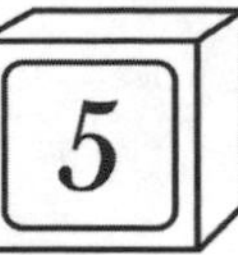

food and drink; some types of plastics are more likely to do so than others (polycarbonate, PVC, polystyrene). Effects are not fully studied or understood, but in animal studies, some plastics have been tied to a wide range of negative health effects including endocrine (hormone) disruption and cancer (1,11).

PVC, also known as vinyl, is one of the most commonly used types of plastics today. PVC is present in many things used daily, from water bottles and containers, to wallpaper, wall paneling, credit cards, and children's toys. Some of the substances added to PVC are among the hormone-disrupting chemicals that may pose hazards to human health and child development. PVC products, including certain toys, may have chemicals such as lead, cadmium, and phthalates, which can flake, leach, or off-gas, causing the release of these chemicals into the surroundings (2).

Phthalates is a class of chemicals used to make plastics flexible (3,4,11). Phthalates are used in many products: vinyl flooring, plastic clothing (e.g., raincoats), detergents, adhesives, personal-care products (fragrances, nail polish, soap), and is commonly found in vinyl (PVC) plastic products (toys, plastic bags) (13). In a national study, some phthalates have been found in 97% (5) of the people tested with generally higher concentrations found in children (6). In animal studies, health effects range from developmental and reproductive toxicity to damage to the liver (7,8).

Bisphenol A (BPA) is used when making polycarbonate and other plastic products. BPA is widely used in consumer products (infant bottles, protective coating in food cans, toys, containers, and personal care products) (13). It can leach from these products and potentially cause harm to those in contact with them. It can also have estrogen (female hormone)-like effects, which may impact biological systems at very low doses. Children may be exposed via: ingestion (diet and sucking/mouthing plastics), inhalation (of dust), and dermal contact. A national study found BPA in the urine of over 90% of people tested; children were found to have higher levels than adults (9). BPA has been found in pregnant women, umbilical cord blood, and placentas at levels demonstrated in animals to alter development (10).

COMMENTS: The Consumer Product Safety Improvement Act (CPSIA) empowers the U.S. Consumer Product Safety Commission (CPSC) to set regulations protecting consumers of these products with testing and labeling. As of this writing new CPSC requirements are under development. Consumers of products for children should look for products that state "phthalate-free" or "BPA-free" or certification by Toy Safety Certification Program (TSCP) or American National Standards Institute (ANSI).

Following are guidelines by which caregivers/teachers may reduce exposure to phthalates and BPA:

a) When possible, opt for glass, porcelain or stainless steel containers, particularly for hot food or liquids (12);
b) If using plastic, do not use plastic or plastic wrap for heating in microwave (try substituting a paper towel or waxpaper for covering foods) (12);
c) Check the symbol on the bottom of the plastic items including toys before buying. The plastics industry has developed identification codes to label different types of plastic. The identification system divides plastic into seven distinct types and uses a number code generally found on the bottom of containers. For a table that explains the seven code system, go to http://www.natureworksllc.com/the-ingeo-journey/end-of-life-options/recycling/plastic-codes.aspx. Contact the manufacturer if there is a question about the chemical content of a plastic item;
d) Best plastic choices are 1 (PETE), 2 (HDPE), 4 (LDPE), 5 (PP) and plastics labeled "phthalate-free" or "BPA-free";
e) Avoid plastics labeled 3 (V), 6 (PS), and 7 (PC). Polycarbonate containers that contain BPA usually have a number 7 on the bottom;
f) Use alternatives to polycarbonate "7" infant bottles. Alternatives include glass infant bottles, BPA free, and products made of safer plastics such as polyethylene and polypropylene that are less likely to release harmful plasticizers (12) (safer non-polycarbonate bottles are usually cloudy and squeezable);
g) Do not use latex rubber nipples or plastic bottle liners;
h) Avoid canned foods when possible;
i) If infant formula is used, it is best to use powdered formula in a can;
j) Do not place plastics in the dishwasher;
k) If using hard polycarbonate plastics (PC) such as water bottles/infant bottles, do not use for warm/hot liquids;
l) Dispose of plastic bottles when they are old and scratched;
m) Toys should be certified by the Toy Safety Certification Program (TSCP) or American National Standards Institute (ANSI).

For more tips on safer food use of plastics, see the Institute for Agriculture and Trade Policy (IATP) Website: Smart Plastics Guide: Healthier Food Uses of Plastics, available at http://www.iatp.org/foodandhealth/.

For more tips on safer alternatives to PVC plastics, see the Center for Health, Environment, and Justice (CHEJ) Website: The Campaign for Safe Healthy Consumer Products, available at http://www.besafenet.com/pvc/.

For general information on plastics and on how to recycle them, see the U.S. Environmental Protection Agency (EPA) Website: Common Wastes and Materials: Plastics, at http://www.epa.gov/osw/conserve/materials/plastics.htm.

TYPE OF FACILITY: Center; Large Family Child Care Home; Small Family Child Care Home

RELATED STANDARDS:

Standard 5.3.1.2: Product Recall Monitoring

REFERENCES:

1. Eco-Healthy Child Care. 2010. Plastics and plastic toys. Children's Environmental Health Network. http://www.cehn.org/files/Plastics_Plastic_Toys_Dec2010.pdf.

2. Healthy Building Network. PVC plastic: PVC facts. http://www.healthybuilding.net/pvc/facts.html.
3. Huff, J. 1982. Di(2-ethylhexyl) adipate: Condensation of the carcinogenesis bioassay, technical report. *Environ Health Perspectives* 45:205-7.
4. Kluwe, W. M. 1986. Carcinogenic potential of phthalic acid esters and related compounds: Structure-activity relationships. *Environ Health Perspectives* 65:271-78.
5. Silva, M. J., D. B. Barr, J. A. Reidy, et al. 2004. Urinary levels of seven phthalate metabolites in the U.S. population from the National Health and Nutrition Examination Survey (NHANES), 1999-2000. *Environ Health Perspectives* 112:331-38.
6. Kolarik, B., K. Naydenov, M. Larsson, et al. 2008. The association between phthalates in dust and allergic diseases among Bulgarian children. *Environ Health Perspectives* 116:98-103.
7. Centers for Disease Control and Prevention (CDC). 2009. *Fourth national report on human exposure to environmental chemicals.* Atlanta, GA: CDC. http://www.cdc.gov/exposurereport/pdf/FourthReport.pdf.
8. Blount, B. C., M. Silva, S. Caudill, et al. 2000. Levels of seven urinary phthalate metabolites in a human reference population. *Environ Health Perspectives* 108:979-82.
9. Calafat, A. M., X. Ye, L. Wong, et al. 2008. Exposure of the U.S. population to bisphenol A and 4-tertiary-octylphenol: 2003-2004. *Environ Health Perspectives* 116:39-44.
10. Ikezuki, Y., O. Tsutsumi, Y. Takai, Y. Kamei, Y. Taketani. 2002. Determination of bisphenol A concentrations in human biological fluids reveals significant early prenatal exposure. *Human Reproduction* 17:2839-41.
11. American Academy of Pediatrics. 2007. Technical report: Pediatric exposure and potential toxicity of phthalate plasticizers. *Pediatrics* 119:1031.
12. California Childcare Health Program (CCHP). 2008. *Banning chemicals called phthalates in childhood products*. Berkeley, CA: CCHP. http://www.ucsfchildcarehealth.org/pdfs/factsheets/BannedChem_0308.pdf.
13. U.S. Consumer Product Safety Commission. 2009. Prohibition on the sale of certain products containing specified phthalates. http://www.cpsc.gov/about/cpsia/108rfc.pdf.

STANDARD 5.2.9.10: Prohibition of Poisonous Plants

Poisonous or potentially harmful plants are prohibited in any part of a child care facility that is accessible to children. All plants not known to be nontoxic should be identified and checked by name with the local poison center (1-800-222-1222) to determine safe use.

RATIONALE: Plants are important to our health and well-being and are a great lesson in learning to understand and respect our environment. However, some plants can be harmful when eaten or touched (1,2). Plants are among the most common household substances that children ingest. Determining the toxicity of every commercially available household plant is difficult. A more reasonable approach is to keep any unknown plant out of the environment that children use. All outdoor plants and their leaves, fruit, and stems should be considered potentially toxic (1).

COMMENTS: Cuttings, trimmings, and leaves from potentially harmful plants must be disposed of safely so children do not have access to them.

For toxic, frequently ingested products and plants, see the American Academy of Pediatrics' (AAP) *Handbook of Common Poisonings in Children,* available at http://www.aap.org.

TYPE OF FACILITY: Center; Large Family Child Care Home; Small Family Child Care Home

RELATED STANDARDS:
Appendix Y: Non-Poisonous and Poisonous Plants

REFERENCES:
1. American Academy of Pediatrics. 2011. *Handbook of common poisonings in children*. 4th ed. Elk Grove Village, IL: AAP.
2. Fiene, R. 2002. *13 indicators of quality child care: Research update*. Washington, DC: U.S. Department of Health and Human Services, Office of the Assistant Secretary for Planning and Evaluation. http://aspe.hhs.gov/hsp/ccquality-ind02/.

STANDARD 5.2.9.11: Chemicals Used to Control Odors

The use of the following should be prohibited:
a) Incense;
b) Moth crystals or moth balls;
c) Chemical air fresheners; and
d) Toilet/urinal deodorizer blocks.

RATIONALE: Many chemicals are sold to cover up noxious odors or ward off pests. Many of these chemicals are hazardous (1). As an alternative, caregivers/teachers should remove the source of noxious odors to the extent possible by dissipating noxious odors through cleaning and ventilation (e.g., opening windows) and controlling pests using nontoxic methods.

Toilet/urinal deodorizer blocks commonly contain paradichlorobenzene (PDCB), a toxic chemical, designated as a possible human carcinogen (2), that has no cleaning function. These deodorizers only serves to mask odors that should be eliminated by proper cleaning.

COMMENTS: Contact the poison center at 1-800-222-1222 or the U.S. Environmental Protection Agency (EPA) Regional offices listed in the federal agency section of the telephone directory for assistance in identifying hazardous products.

TYPE OF FACILITY: Center; Large Family Child Care Home; Small Family Child Care Home

RELATED STANDARDS:
Standard 5.2.8.1: Integrated Pest Management

REFERENCES:
1. Fiene, R. 2002. *13 indicators of quality child care: Research update*. Washington, DC: U.S. Department of Health and Human Services, Office of the Assistant Secretary for Planning and Evaluation. http://aspe.hhs.gov/hsp/ccquality-ind02/.
2. Suhua, W., L. Rongzhu, Y. Changqing, X. Guangwei, H. Fangan, J. Junjie, X. Wenrong, M. Aschner. 2010. Lipid peroxidation and changes of trace elements in mice treated with paradichlorobenzene. *Biol Trace Elem Res* 136:320-36.

STANDARD 5.2.9.12: Treatment of CCA Pressure-Treated Wood

A penetrating coating (e.g., oil-based, semi-transparent stain) should be applied every six months to all chromated

copper arsenate (CCA)-treated surfaces to which a child may have access.

RATIONALE: The Consumer Product Safety Commission advises that arsenic exposure in children from contact with CCA-treated wood playground structures is estimated to be about 3.5 micrograms each day that includes a playground visit (1).The health effects related to arsenic include irritation of the stomach and intestines, birth or developmental effects, cancer, and infertility and miscarriages in women (1,2,3). Children can be exposed to the arsenic in CCA-treated wood by touching surfaces made from this material (1). Based on limited data, applying certain penetrating coatings may reduce the amount of arsenic that comes out of the wood (1).

COMMENTS: CCA-treated wood is found extensively in outdoor structures, furniture, and play equipment built prior to December 31, 2003 when manufacturers of CCA reached a voluntary agreement with the Environmental Protection Agency (EPA) to end the manufacture of CCA-treated wood for most consumer applications. EPA has indicated that some stocks of wood treated with CCA before this date might have been found on shelves until mid-2004. If a wooden structure was built prior to December 31, 2003 and is not of a rot-resistant type of wood (e.g., redwood, cedar) it is safe to assume it does contain arsenic. If the date the equipment was built is unknown or was built shortly after December 31, 2003, test kits are available from many common retailers.

Caregivers/teachers should be aware that children are exposed to arsenic through their hand-to-mouth activity while and after playing on CCA-treated wood playsets. To minimize the risk of exposure to arsenic from CCA-treated playsets, caregivers/teachers and children should thoroughly wash their hands with soap and water immediately after outdoor play, especially before eating (4). Children should also be discouraged from eating while on CCA-treated playsets. These precautions should be followed even if a protective coating has been applied to CCA-treated wood.

While available data are very limited, some studies suggest that applying certain penetrating coatings (e.g., oil-based, semi-transparent stains) on a regular basis may reduce the migration of wood preservative chemicals from CCA-treated wood (2). In selecting a finish, caregivers/teachers should be aware that, in some cases, "film-forming" or non-penetrating stains on outdoor surfaces such as decks and fences are not recommended, as subsequent peeling and flaking may ultimately have an impact on durability as well as exposure to the preservatives in the wood.

To eliminate the risk of children's exposure to arsenic from CCA-treated wood it is recommended it be replaced. If this is not feasible, replacing the components children come in contact with the most (e.g., handrails, retaining walls) will limit their exposure.

TYPE OF FACILITY: Center; Large Family Child Care Home; Small Family Child Care Home

RELATED STANDARDS:
Standard 6.1.0.8: Enclosures for Outdoor Play Areas
Standard 6.2.1.1: Play Equipment Requirements
Standard 6.2.5.1: Inspection of Indoor and Outdoor Play Areas and Equipment

REFERENCES:
1. U.S. Consumer Product Safety Commission (CPSC). Fact sheet: Chromated copper arsenate (CCA)-treated wood used in playground equipment. http://www.cpsc.gov/phth/ccafact.html.
2. U.S. Environmental Protection Agency. 2008. Chromated copper arsenate (CCA): Consumer advice related to CCA-treated wood. http://www.epa.gov/oppad001/reregistration/cca/cca_consumer_doc.htm.
3. U.S. Environmental Protection Agency. 2008. Chromated Copper Arsenate (CCA): Final probabilistic risk assessment for children who contact CCA-treated playsets and decks. http://www.epa.gov/oppad001/reregistration/cca/final_cca_factsheet.htm.
4. Gray, S., J. Houlihan. 2002. *All hands on deck: Nationwide consumer testing of backyard decks and playsets shows high levels of arsenic on old wood*. Washington, DC: Environmental Working Group. http://www.ewg.org/files/allhandsondeck.pdf.

STANDARD 5.2.9.13: Testing for Lead

In all centers, both exterior and interior surfaces covered by paint with lead levels of 0.06% and above, or equal to or greater than 1.0 milligram per square centimeter and accessible to children, should be removed by a safe chemical or physical means or made inaccessible to children, regardless of the condition of the surface.

In large and small family child care homes, flaking or deteriorating lead-based paint on any surface accessible to children should be removed or abated according to health department regulations. Where lead paint is removed, the surface should be refinished with lead-free paint or nontoxic material. Sanding, scraping, or burning of lead-based paint surfaces should be prohibited. Children and pregnant women should not be present during lead renovation or lead abatement activities.

Any surface and the grounds around and under surfaces that children use at a child care facility, including dirt and grassy areas should be tested for excessive lead in a location designated by the health department. Caregivers/teachers should check the U.S. Consumer Product Safety Commission's Website, http://www.cpsc.gov, for warnings of potential lead exposure to children and recalls of play equipment, toys, jewelry used for play, imported vinyl mini-blinds and food contact products. If they are found to have toxic levels, corrective action should be taken to prevent exposure to lead at the facility. Only nontoxic paints should be used.

RATIONALE: Ingestion of lead paint can result in high levels of lead in the blood, which affects the central nervous system and can cause mental retardation (2,3). Paint and other surface coating materials should comply with lead content provisions of the Code of Federal Regulations, Title 16, Part 1303.

Some imported vinyl mini-blinds contain lead and can deteriorate from exposure to sunlight and heat and form lead dust on the surface of the blinds (1). The U.S. Consumer Product Safety Commission (CPSC) recommends that consumers with children six years of age and younger remove old vinyl mini-blinds and replace them with new mini-blinds made without added lead or with alternative window coverings. See Comments for resources.

Lead is a neurotoxin. Even at low levels of exposure, lead can cause reduction in a child's IQ and attention span, and result in reading and learning disabilities, hyperactivity, and behavioral difficulties. Lead poisoning has no "cure." These effects cannot be reversed once the damage is done, affecting a child's ability to learn, succeed in school, and function later in life. Other symptoms of low levels of lead in a child's body are subtle behavioral changes, irritability, low appetite, weight loss, sleep disturbances, and shortened attention span (2,3).

COMMENTS: House paints made before 1978 may contain lead. If there is any doubt about the presence of lead in existing paint, contact the health department for information regarding testing. Lead is used to make paint last longer. The amount of lead in paint was reduced in 1950 and further reduced again in 1978. Houses built before 1950 likely contain lead paint, and houses built after 1950 have less lead in the paint. House paint sold today has little or no lead. Lead is prohibited in contemporary paints. Lead-based paint is the most common source of lead poisoning in children (3).

In buildings where lead has been removed from the surfaces, lead paint may have contaminated surrounding soil. Therefore, the soil in play areas around these buildings should be tested. Outdoor play equipment was commonly painted with lead-based paints, too. These structures and the soil around them should be checked if they are not known to be lead-free.

The danger from lead paint depends on:

a) Amount of lead in the painted surface;
b) Condition of the paint;
c) Amount of lead (from paint, chips, soil, or dust) that gets into the child.

Children nine months through five years of age are at the greatest risk for lead poisoning. Most children with lead poisoning do not look or act sick. A blood lead test is the only way to know if children are being lead poisoned. Children should have a test result below 10 ug/dL (2,4).

A booklet called *Protect Your Family from Lead in Your Home* is available from the U.S. Environmental Protection Agency (EPA), the CPSC, and U.S. Department of Housing and Urban Development (HUD). The EPA also has a pamphlet called *Finding a Qualified Lead Professional for Your Home*, which provides information on how to identify qualified lead inspectors and risk assessors. Before starting a renovation project on a facility built before 1978, the contractor or property owner is required to have parents/guardians sign a pre-renovation disclosure form, which indicates that the parents/guardians received *Renovate Right: Important Lead Hazard Information for Families, Child Care Providers, and Schools*, available at http://www.epa.gov/lead/pubs/renovaterightbrochure.pdf. The contractor must also make renovation information available to the parents/guardians of children under age six that attend child care centers or homes, and provide to owners and administrators of pre-1978 child care facilities to be renovated a copy of *Renovate Right: Important Lead Hazard Information for Families, Child Care Providers, and Schools* (5).

TYPE OF FACILITY: Center; Large Family Child Care Home; Small Family Child Care Home

RELATED STANDARDS:

Standard 5.2.6.3: Testing for Lead and Copper Levels in Drinking Water
Standard 5.2.9.15: Construction and Remodeling During Hours of Operation
Standard 5.3.1.2: Product Recall Monitoring

REFERENCES:

1. U.S. Consumer Product Safety Commission (CPSC). 1996. CPSC finds lead poisoning hazard for young children in imported vinyl miniblinds. http://www.cpsc.gov/CPSCPUB/PREREL/PRHTML96/96150.html.
2. Centers for Disease Control and Prevention (CDC). 2005. *Preventing lead poisoning in young children*. Atlanta, GA: CDC. http://www.cdc.gov/nceh/lead/publications/PrevLeadPoisoning.pdf.
3. U.S. Environmental Protection Agency (EPA). 2010. *The lead-safe certified guide to renovate right*. Washington, DC: EPA. http://www.epa.gov/lead/pubs/renovaterightbrochure.pdf.
4. Binns, H. J., C. Campbell, M. J. Brown. 2007. Interpreting and managing blood lead levels of less than 10 mg/dL in children and reducing childhood exposure to lead: Recommendations of the Centers for Disease Control and Prevention Advisory Committee on Childhood Lead Poisoning Prevention. *Pediatrics* 120: e1285-98.
5. U.S. Environmental Protection Agency. 2010. Lead in paint, dust, and soil: Renovation, repair and painting (RRP). http://www.epa.gov/lead/pubs/renovation.htm.

STANDARD 5.2.9.14: Shoes in Infant Play Areas

Adults and children should remove or cover shoes before entering a play area used by a specific group of infants. These individuals, as well as the infants playing in that area, may wear shoes, shoe covers, or socks that are used only in the play area for that group of infants.

RATIONALE: When infants play, they touch the surfaces on which they play with their hands, and then put their hands in their mouths. Lead and other toxins in soil around a facility can be a hazard when tracked into a facility on shoes (1).

COMMENTS: Facilities can meet this standard in several ways. The facility can designate contained play surfaces for infant play on which no one walks with shoes. Individuals can wear shoes or slippers that are worn only to walk in the infant play area or they can wear clean cloth or disposable shoe covers over shoes that have been used to walk outside the infant play area.

This standard applies to shoes that have been worn outdoors, in the play areas of other groups of children, and in toilet and diaper changing areas. All of these locations are potential sources of contamination.

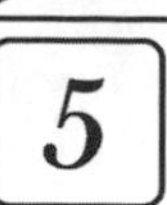

TYPE OF FACILITY: Center; Large Family Child Care Home; Small Family Child Care Home

REFERENCES:

1. U.S. Environmental Protection Agency. 2009. Lead in paint, dust and soil: Basic information. http://www.epa.gov/lead/pubs/leadinfo.htm.

STANDARD 5.2.9.15: Construction and Remodeling During Hours of Operation

Construction, remodeling, painting, or alterations of structures during child care operations should be isolated from areas where children are present and done in a manner that will prevent hazards or unsafe conditions (such as fumes, dust, safety, and fire hazards).

Low volatile organic compounds (VOC) paints should be used in child care areas. Painted areas should be ventilated until they are fully dry and odor-free before children are permitted to occupy them.

RATIONALE: Children should be protected from activities and equipment associated with construction and renovation of the facility that may cause injury or illness.

Volatile organic compounds (VOCs) are emitted as gases from certain solids or liquids. VOCs include a variety of chemicals, some of which may have short- and long-term adverse health effects. Some organic compounds can cause cancer in animals; some are suspected or known to cause cancer in humans. Key signs or symptoms associated with exposure to VOCs include conjunctival irritation, nose and throat discomfort, headache, allergic skin reaction, dyspnea, declines in serum cholinesterase levels, nausea, emesis, epistaxis, fatigue, and dizziness (2).

COMMENTS: Ideally, construction and renovation work should be done when the facility is not in operation and when there are no children present. Many facilities arrange to schedule such work on weekends. If this is not possible, temporary barriers can be constructed to restrict access of children to those areas under construction. A plastic vapor barrier sheet could be temporarily hung to prevent dust and fumes from drifting into those areas where children are present. However, the minimum number of egress/escape paths should be maintained without compromise during the rehabilitation work.

Common renovation activities like sanding, cutting, and demolition can create hazardous lead dust and chips by disturbing lead-based paint, which can be harmful to adults and children. U.S. Environmental Protection Agency (EPA) regulations require persons performing renovation, repair, and painting activities in homes, child care facilities, and schools built before 1978 to give a renovation-specific lead hazard information pamphlet to the owners and occupants of the building. Persons performing these activities in child care facilities and schools must also provide general information about the renovation to the parents/guardians of children using the facility. The renovation-specific pamphlet, called *Renovate Right: Important Lead Hazard Information for Families, Child Care Providers, and Schools,* is available at http://www.epa.gov/lead/pubs/renovaterightbrochure.pdf (1).

EPA regulations require training and certification of renovation contractors and building maintenance personnel performing renovation, repair and painting projects that disturb lead-based paint in homes, child care facilities, and schools built before 1978. They are required to follow specific work practices to prevent lead contamination. The EPA recommends that anyone performing renovation, repair, and painting projects in pre-1978 homes, child care facilities and schools follow lead-safe work practices, which include containing the work area to keep dust and debris inside the area, minimizing the creation of dust, and cleaning the work area thoroughly after the project has been completed.

The two most effective counter-measures against VOCs are to avoid VOC-emitting products and to ventilate areas when using VOC-emitting products. Caregivers/teachers can choose from many high quality latex-based paints that emit low levels of VOCs. Some major paint manufacturers offer special odorless VOC-free products (3).

When planning or beginning new construction, consideration should be given to using the least toxic or non-toxic materials.

TYPE OF FACILITY: Center; Large Family Child Care Home; Small Family Child Care Home

RELATED STANDARDS:

Standard 5.2.9.13: Testing for Lead
Standard 5.3.1.4: Surfaces of Equipment, Furniture, Toys, and Play Materials

REFERENCES:

1. U.S. Environmental Protection Agency (EPA). 2010. *The lead-safe certified guide to renovate right*. Washington, DC: EPA. http://www.epa.gov/lead/pubs/renovaterightbrochure.pdf.
2. U.S. Environmental Protection Agency. 2010. An introduction to indoor air quality: Volatile organic compounds (VOCs). http://www.epa.gov/iaq/voc.html.
3. American Academy of Pediatrics Pennsylvania Chapter, Health Child Care Pennsylvania. Indoor air pollution. *Health Link Online* 21:3. http://www.ecels-healthychildcarepa.org/content/9-4-09%20v8vol%2021%20fall%20%202009%20HL%20ONLINE.pdf.

5.3 General Furnishings and Equipment

Note to Reader: See Chapter 6 for Play Area/Playground Equipment Requirements

5.3.1 General Furnishings and Equipment Requirements

STANDARD 5.3.1.1: Safety of Equipment, Materials, and Furnishings

Equipment, materials, furnishings, and play areas should be sturdy, safe, and in good repair and should meet the recommendations of the U.S. Consumer Product Safety Commission (CPSC) for control of the following safety hazards:

a) Openings that could entrap a child's head or limbs;
b) Elevated surfaces that are inadequately guarded;
c) Lack of specified surfacing and fall zones under and around climbable equipment;
d) Mismatched size and design of equipment for the intended users;
e) Insufficient spacing between equipment;
f) Tripping hazards;
g) Components that can pinch, sheer, or crush body tissues;
h) Equipment that is known to be of a hazardous type;
i) Sharp points or corners;
j) Splinters;
k) Protruding nails, bolts, or other components that could entangle clothing or snag skin;
l) Loose, rusty parts;
m) Hazardous small parts that may become detached during normal use or reasonably foreseeable abuse of the equipment and that present a choking, aspiration, or ingestion hazard to a child;
n) Strangulation hazards (e.g., straps, strings, etc.);
o) Flaking paint;
p) Paint that contains lead or other hazardous materials;
q) Tip-over hazards, such as chests, bookshelves, and televisions.

RATIONALE: The hazards listed in this standard are those found by CPSC to be most commonly associated with injury (1).

A study conducted by the Center for Injury Research and Policy of The Research Institute at Nationwide Children's Hospital found that from 1990-2007 an average of nearly 15,000 children younger than eighteen years of age visited emergency departments annually for injuries received from furniture tip-overs (2).

COMMENTS: Equipment and furnishings that are not sturdy, safe, or in good repair, may cause falls, entrap a child's head or limbs, or contribute to other injuries. Disrepair may expose objects that are hazardous to children. Freedom from sharp points, corners, or edges should be judged according to the Code of Federal Regulations, Title 16, Section 1500.48, and Section 1500.49. Freedom from small parts should be judged according to the Code of Federal Regulations, Title 16, Part 1501. To obtain these publications, contact the Superintendent of Documents of the U.S. Government Printing Office. For assistance in interpreting the federal regulations, contact the CPSC; the CPSC also has regional offices.

Used equipment and furnishings should be closely inspected to determine whether they meet this standard before allowing them to be placed in a child care facility. If equipment and furnishings have deteriorated to a state of disrepair, where they are no longer sturdy or safe, they should be removed from all areas of a child care facility to which children have access. Staff should check on a regular basis to ensure that toys and equipment used by children have not been recalled. A list of recalls can be accessed at http://www.cpsc.gov, or facilities can subscribe to an email notification list from the CPSC (see also, RELATED STANDARDS).

TYPE OF FACILITY: Center; Large Family Child Care Home; Small Family Child Care Home

RELATED STANDARDS:
Standard 3.4.6.1: Strangulation Hazards
Standard 5.1.3.5: Finger-Pinch Protection Devices
Standard 5.1.6.6: Guardrails and Protective Barriers
Standard 5.4.5.2: Cribs
Standard 5.3.1.2: Product Recall Monitoring
Chapter 6: Play Areas/Playgrounds and Transportation

REFERENCES:
1. U.S. Consumer Product Safety Commission (CPSC). 2008. *Public playground safety handbook*. Bethesda, MD: CPSC. http://www.cpsc.gov/cpscpub/pubs/325.pdf.
2. Gottesman, B. L., L. B. McKenzie, K. A. Conner, G. A. Smith. 2009. Injuries from furniture tip-overs among children and adolescents in the United States, 1990-2007. *Clin Pediatrics* 48:851.

STANDARD 5.3.1.2: Product Recall Monitoring

Staff should, on a monthly basis, seek information on recalls of juvenile products that may be in use at the facility. Of particular importance are recalls related to cribs, bassinets, and portable play yards that may be used for infant sleep. Additionally, caregivers/teachers should be aware of recalls of toys, playground equipment, strollers, and any other product routinely used by children in the child care facility.

RATIONALE: Product recalls are often ineffective at removing hazardous products from use because the owners/users are not aware of the recall. Children have died in child care settings from injury related to sleep equipment that had been recalled.

COMMENTS: The U.S. Consumer Product Safety Commission (CPSC) offers a free subscription email service for product recall notices at http://www.cpsc.gov/cpsclist.aspx. Subscribers can note that they only want to receive recalls related to juvenile products.

TYPE OF FACILITY: Center; Large Family Child Care Home; Small Family Child Care Home

RELATED STANDARDS:
Standard 5.3.1.1: Safety of Equipment, Materials, and Furnishings
Standard 5.4.5.2: Cribs
Standard 6.4.1.2: Inaccessibility of Toys or Objects to Children Under Three Years of Age

STANDARD 5.3.1.3: Size of Furniture

Furniture should be durable and child-sized or adapted for children's use. Tables should be between waist and mid-chest level of the intended child-user and allow the child's feet to rest on a firm surface while seated for eating.

RATIONALE: Children cannot safely or comfortably use furnishings that are not sized for their use. When children eat or work at tables that are above mid-chest level, they must reach up to get their food or do their work instead of bringing the food from a lower level to their mouth and having

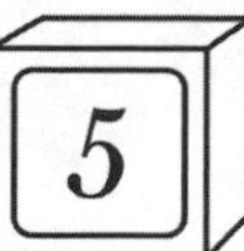

a comfortable arrangement when working to develop their fine-motor skills. When eating, this leads to scooping food into the mouth instead of eating more appropriately. When working, this leads to difficulty succeeding with hand-eye coordination. When children do not have a firm surface on which to rest their feet, they cannot reposition themselves easily if they slip down. This can lead to poor posture and increased risk of choking. When children use chairs that are too high for them, they are at risk for falling.

TYPE OF FACILITY: Center; Large Family Child Care Home; Small Family Child Care Home

STANDARD 5.3.1.4: Surfaces of Equipment, Furniture, Toys, and Play Materials

Equipment, furnishings, toys, and play materials should have smooth, nonporous surfaces or washable fabric surfaces that are easy to clean and sanitize, or be disposable.

Walls, ceilings, floors, furnishings, equipment, and other surfaces should be suitable to the location and the users. They should be maintained in good repair, free from visible soil and in a clean condition. Programs should choose materials with the least probability of containing materials that off-gas toxic elements such as volatile organic compounds (VOCs), formaldehyde, or toxic flame retardants (polybrominated diphenylethers [PBDE]). Carpets, porous fabrics, and other surfaces that trap soil and potentially contaminated materials should not be used in toilet rooms, diaper change areas, and areas where food handling occurs (1).

Areas used by staff or children who have allergies to dust mites or components of furnishings or supplies should be maintained according to the recommendations of primary care providers.

RATIONALE: Few young children practice good hygiene. Messy play is developmentally appropriate in all age groups, and especially among very young children, the same group that is most susceptible to infectious disease. These factors lead to soiling and contamination of equipment, furnishings, toys, and play materials. To avoid transmission of disease within the group, these materials must be easy to clean and sanitize.

Formaldehyde and toxic flame retardants are the toxins of most concern in household furnishings, as they are both commonly found in furniture and carpets. Formaldehyde is a flammable, colorless gas that has a pungent odor. It is a human carcinogen, an asthma trigger, and a suspected neurological, reproductive, and liver toxin. People are exposed by breathing contaminated air from pressed wood furniture, flooring, and after application of certain paints, fabrics, and household cleaners. Toxic Flame Retardants (PBDEs) are widely used in furniture foam, carpet padding, back coatings for draperies and upholstery, plastics, building materials, and electrical appliances. It is believed that more than 80% of PBDE exposure is from house dust. PBDEs persist in the environment and accumulate in living things. Health concerns associated with PBDE exposure include liver, thyroid, and neurodevelopmental toxicity.

Carpets and porous fabrics are not appropriate for some areas because they are difficult to clean and sanitize. Disease-causing microorganisms have been isolated from carpets. Caregivers/teachers must remove illness-causing materials. Many allergic children have allergies to dust mites, which are microscopic insects that ingest the tiny particles of skin that people shed normally every day. Dust mites live in carpeting and fabric but can be killed by frequent washing and use of a clothes dryer or mechanical, heated dryer. Restricting the use of carpeting and furnishings to types that can be laundered regularly helps. Other children may have allergies to animal products such as those with feathers, fur, or wool, while some may be allergic to latex.

COMMENTS: Toys that can be washed in a mechanical dishwasher that meets the standard for cleaning and sanitizing dishes can save labor, if the facility has a dishwasher. Otherwise, after the children have used them, these toys can be placed in a tub of detergent water to soak until the staff has time to scrub, rinse, and sanitize the surfaces of these items. Except for fabric surfaces, nonporous surfaces are best because porous surfaces can trap organic material and soil. Fabric surfaces that can be laundered provide the softness required in a developmentally appropriate environment for young children. If these fabrics are laundered when soiled, the facility can achieve cleanliness and sanitation. When a material cannot be cleaned and sanitized it should be discarded.

One way to measure compliance with the standard for cleanliness is to wipe the surface with a clean mop or clean rag, and then insert the mop or rag in cold rinse water. If the surface is clean, no residue will appear in the rinse water.

Disposable gloves are commonly made of latex or vinyl. If latex-sensitive individuals are present in the facility, only vinyl or nitrile disposable gloves should be used.

Tips for Reducing Exposure to Formaldehyde and PBDEs:

a) Avoid wall-to-wall carpets;
b) Limit use of pressed wood products that are made with adhesives that contain urea-formaldehyde (UF) resins; choose solid-wood furniture;
c) Do not leave foam exposed (this includes furniture and toys, such as stuffed animals);
d) Keep dust levels down;
e) Vacuum often – use a high efficiency particulate air (HEPA) filter vacuum cleaner;
f) Ventilate while cleaning;
g) Except in emergency situations, remove shoes prior to going indoors;
h) Clean area rugs with biodegradable cleaners;
i) Choose floor coverings that are made with natural fibers (cotton, hemp, and wool) that are naturally fire-resistant and contain fewer chemicals (2).

TYPE OF FACILITY: Center; Large Family Child Care Home; Small Family Child Care Home

RELATED STANDARDS:

Standard 5.2.9.15: Construction and Remodeling During Hours of Operation

REFERENCES:

1. U.S. Environmental Protection Agency. Polybrominated diphenylethers (PBDEs). http://www.epa.gov/oppt/pbde/.
2. Eco-Healthy Child Care (EHCC). *Furniture and carpets*. Washington, DC: EHCC. http://www.oeconline.org/resources/publications/factsheetarchive/Furniture and carpets.pdf.

STANDARD 5.3.1.5: Placement of Equipment and Furnishings

Equipment and furnishings should be placed to help prevent collisions and injuries, ensure proper supervision while meeting the objectives of the curriculum, and permit freedom of movement by the children. Televisions should be anchored or mounted to prevent tipping over.

RATIONALE: The placement of furnishings plays a significant role in the way space is used. If the staff places furnishings in such a way that they create large runways, children will run in this area. If the staff places furnishings that children can climb in locations where climbing is unsafe, this adds risk to the environment. Placement of furnishings should address the needs of the children for stimulation and development and at the same time help to prevent collisions and injury. Equipment and furnishings should be arranged so that a caregiver/teacher can easily view the children from different positions in the room.

From 2000 through 2006, the U.S. Consumer Product Safety Commission (CPSC) reported 134 tip-over related deaths involving children five years old or younger (1). Additionally, CPSC estimates that in 2006 at least 16,300 children five years old and younger were treated in U.S. hospital emergency rooms because of injuries associated with TV, furniture, and appliance tip-overs (1).

Industry standards require that TV stands, chests, bureaus, and dressers pass a stability test. If a piece of furniture violates these standards, the product can be subject to a safety recall.

COMMENTS: To prevent children from falling out of windows, the safest place for chairs and other furniture is away from windows. Chairs and other furnishings that children can easily climb should be kept away from cabinets and shelves to discourage children from climbing to a dangerous height or reaching for something hazardous.

To help prevent tip-over hazards, CPSC offers the following safety tips:

a) Verify that furniture is stable on its own (for added security, anchor to the floor or attach to the wall all entertainment units, TV stands, bookcases, shelving, and bureaus using appropriate hardware, such as brackets, screws, or toggle bolts);
b) Place televisions on sturdy furniture appropriate for the size of the TV or on a low-rise base;
c) Push the TV as far back as possible from the front of its stand;
d) Place electrical cords out of a child's reach, and teach children not to play with the cords;
e) Remove items that might tempt kids to climb, such as toys and remote controls, from the top of the TV and furniture (1).

TYPE OF FACILITY: Center; Large Family Child Care Home; Small Family Child Care Home

RELATED STANDARDS:
Standard 5.1.3.2: Possibility of Exit from Windows

REFERENCES:

1. U.S. Consumer Product Safety Commission (CPSC). *The tipping point: Preventing TV, furniture, and appliance tip-over deaths and injuries*. http://www.cpsc.gov/cpscpub/pubs/5004.pdf.

STANDARD 5.3.1.6: Floors, Walls, and Ceilings

Floors, walls, and ceilings should be in good repair, and easy to clean when soiled. Only smooth, nonporous surfaces should be permitted in areas that are likely to be contaminated by body fluids or in areas used for activities involving food. The hand contact and splash areas of doors and walls should be covered with a finish that is at least as cleanable as an epoxy finish or enamel paint.

Floors should be free from cracks, bare concrete, dampness, splinters, sliding rugs, and uncovered telephone jacks or electrical outlets.

Carpeting should be clean, in good repair, nonflammable, and nontoxic.

Each bathroom, toilet room, and shower room floor and wall should be impervious to water up to a height of five feet and capable of being kept in a clean and sanitary condition.

All public bathrooms should be constructed of materials that are impervious to moisture, bacteria, mold, or fungus growth. The floor-to-wall joints should be constructed to provide a sanitary cove with a minimum radius of three-eighths inch. Flooring material should be appropriate for bathroom use (e.g., vinyl sheet, ceramic tile, fiber-reinforced plastic, epoxy products). All wall surfaces within twenty-four inches of a water closet or urinal should be ceramic tile to a height of forty-eight inches (1).

RATIONALE: Messy play and activities that lead to soiling of floors and walls is developmentally appropriate in all age groups, but especially among very young children, the same group that is most susceptible to infectious disease. These factors lead to soiling and contamination of floors and walls. A smooth, nonporous surface prevents deterioration and mold and is easier to clean and sanitize; therefore, helps prevent the spread of infectious diseases. To avoid transmission of disease within the group, and to maintain an environment that supports learning cleanliness as a value, all surfaces should be kept clean.

Cracked or porous floors cannot be kept clean and sanitary. Dampness promotes the growth of mold. Rugs without friction backing or underlayment and uncovered telephone jacks or electrical outlets in floors are tripping hazards. Damaged floors, walls or ceilings can expose underlying hazardous structural elements and materials. Surface materials must not pose health, safety, or fire hazards.

COMMENTS: Carpeted floors are not smooth, and therefore, carpeting is not consistent with this standard, except for area carpets for activities that do not involve food or contact with body fluids. Many family child care homes and indoor playrooms of centers use wall-to-wall carpeting on the floor. Although carpeted floors may be more comfortable to walk and play on, smooth floor surfaces provide a better environment for children with allergies (2).

Washable rugs can be placed on smooth floor surfaces. By using friction backings or underlayment, removable and washable carpeting can be used on smooth floor surfaces safely.

When facilities use carpeting or sound-absorbing materials on walls and ceilings, these materials must not be used in areas where contamination with body fluids or food is likely because they are difficult to clean. Thus, carpeted walls should not be present around the diaper change areas, in toilet rooms, in food preparation areas, or where food is served.

Obtain ASTM D2859-06 Standard Test Method for Flammability of Finished Textile Floor Covering Materials, for flammability of finished materials from ASTM International. Ask the local fire marshal for fire safety code requirements.

TYPE OF FACILITY: Center; Large Family Child Care Home; Small Family Child Care Home

REFERENCES:

1. City of Edina, MN. 2000. City Code § 455. http://www.ci.edina.mn.us/CityCode/L5-01_CityCodeSect0455.htm.
2. Davis, J. L. Breathe easy: 5 ways to improve indoor air quality. http://www.webmd.com/health-ehome-9/indoor-air-quality.

STANDARD 5.3.1.7: Facility Arrangements to Minimize Back Injuries

The child care setting should be organized to reduce the risk of back injuries for adults provided that such measures do not pose hazards for children or affect the implementation of developmentally appropriate practice. Furnishings and equipment should enable caregivers/teachers to hold and comfort children and enable their activities while minimizing the need for bending and for lifting and carrying heavy children and objects. Caregivers/teachers should not routinely be required to use child-sized chairs, tables, or desks.

RATIONALE: Back strain can arise from adult use of child-sized furniture. Analysis of worker compensation claims shows that employees in the service industries, including child care, have an injury rate as great as or greater than that of workers employed in factories. Back injuries are the leading type of injury (1). Appropriate design of work activities and training of workers can prevent most back injuries. The principles to support these recommendations (see Comments) are standard principles of ergonomics, in which jobs and workplaces are designed to eliminate biomechanical hazards.

In a statewide (Wisconsin) survey of health status, behaviors, and concerns, 446 randomly selected early childhood professionals, directors, center teachers, and family providers, reported dramatic changes in frequency of backache and fatigue symptoms since working in child care (2).

COMMENTS: Some approaches to reduce risk are:

a) Adult-height changing tables;
b) Small, stable stepladders, stairs, and similar equipment to enable children to climb to the changing table or other places to which they would otherwise be lifted, without creating a fall hazard;
c) Convenient equipment for moving children, reducing the necessity of carrying them;
d) Adult furniture that eliminates awkward sitting or working positions in all areas where adults work.

This standard is not intended to interfere with child-adult interactions or to create hazards for children. Modifications can be made in the environment to minimize hazards and injuries for both children and adults. Adult furniture has to be available at least for break times, staff meetings, etc.

TYPE OF FACILITY: Center; Large Family Child Care Home; Small Family Child Care Home

RELATED STANDARDS:

Standards 1.7.0.1-1.7.0.5: Staff Health

REFERENCES:

1. Brown, M. Z., S. G. Gerberich. 1993. Disabling injuries to childcare workers in Minnesota, 1985 to 1990: An analysis of potential risk factors. *J Occup Med* 1993 35:1236-43.
2. Grantz, R. R., A. Claffey. 1996. Adult health in child care: Health status, behaviors, and concerns of teachers, directors, and family child care providers. *Early Child Res Q*. 11:243-67.

STANDARD 5.3.1.8: High Chair Requirements

High chairs, if used, should have a wide base and a securely locking tray, along with a crotch bar/guard to prevent a child from slipping down and becoming entrapped between the tray and the seat. High chairs should also be equipped with a safety strap to prevent a child from climbing out of the chair. The safety strap should be fastened with every use. Caps or plugs on tubing should be firmly attached. Folding high chairs should have a locking device that prevents the high chair from collapsing. High chairs should be labeled or warranted by the manufacturer in documents provided at the time of purchase or verified thereafter by the manufacturer as meeting the ASTM International current Standard F404-08 Consumer Safety Specification for High Chairs. High chairs should be used in accordance with manufacturer's instructions including following restrictions based on age and minimum/maximum weight of children.

Highchairs should be kept far enough away from a table, counter, wall or other surface so that the child can't use them to push off or to grab potentially dangerous cords or objects.

RATIONALE: High chairs offer potential for entrapment, falls and other injuries. Current ASTM Standard F404-08 Consumer Safety Specifications for High Chairs covers:

a) Sharp edges;
b) Locking devices;
c) Drop tests of the tray;
d) Disengagement of the tray;

e) Load and stability of the chair;
f) Protection from coil springs and scissoring;
g) Maximum size of holes;
h) Restraining system tests;
i) Labeling;
j) Instructional literature.

COMMENTS: The general age of high chair users is about six-months- to three-years-old (1). Caregivers/teachers should transition children from high chairs to small tables and chairs as soon as they are capable of using them.

Manufacturers and vendors also may indicate a weight restriction for use by children who do not exceed thirty-seven pounds (2). The Juvenile Products Manufacturers Association (JPMA) has a testing and certification program for highchairs, play yards, carriages, strollers, walkers, gates, and expandable enclosures. When purchasing such equipment, consumers can look for labeling that certifies that these products meet the standards. ASTM also maintains a Website at http://www.astm.org with the latest standards on high chair specifications.

TYPE OF FACILITY: Center; Large Family Child Care Home; Small Family Child Care Home

REFERENCES:

1. U.S. Consumer Product Safety Commission (CPSC). Tips for your baby's safety. http://www.cpsc.gov/cpscpub/pubs/200.html.
2. Lerner, N. D., R. W. Huey, B. M. Kotwal. 2001. *Product profile report*, 19. Rockville, MD: Westat.

STANDARD 5.3.1.9: Carriage, Stroller, Gate, Enclosure, and Play Yard Requirements

Each carriage, stroller, gate, enclosure, and play yard used should meet the corresponding ASTM International standard and should be so labeled on the equipment.

a) Carriages/strollers: ASTM F833-10 Standard Consumer Safety Performance Specification for Carriages and Strollers;
b) Gates/enclosures: ASTM F1004-10 Consumer Safety Specification for Expansion Gates and Expandable Enclosures;
c) Play yards: ASTM F406-10 Consumer Safety Specification for Non-Full-Size Baby Cribs/Play Yards.

RATIONALE: The presence of a Juvenile Products Manufacturers Association (JPMA) certification seal on products that are made for children ensures that the product is in compliance with the requirements of the current safety standard for that product at the time of manufacture.

COMMENTS: ASTM also maintains a website at http://www.astm.org with the latest standards on high chair specifications. For more information, contact the JPMA or the ASTM.

TYPE OF FACILITY: Center; Large Family Child Care Home; Small Family Child Care Home

STANDARD 5.3.1.10: Restrictive Infant Equipment Requirements

Restrictive infant equipment such as swings, stationary activity centers (e.g., exersaucers), infant seats (e.g., bouncers), molded seats, etc., if used, should only be used for short periods of time (a maximum of fifteen minutes twice a day) (1). Infants should not be placed in equipment until they are developmentally ready. Infants should be supervised when using equipment. Safety straps should be used if provided by the manufacturer of the equipment. Equipment should not be placed on elevated surfaces, uneven surfaces, near the top of stairs, or within reach of safety hazards. Stationary activity centers should be used with the stabilizing legs down in a locked position. Infants should not be allowed to sleep in equipment that was not manufactured as infant rest/sleep equipment. The use of jumpers (attached to a door frame or ceiling) and infant walkers is prohibited.

RATIONALE: Keeping an infant confined in a piece of infant equipment prevents an infant from active movement. Infants need the opportunity to play on the floor in a safe open area to develop their gross motor skills. If infants are not given the opportunity for floor time, their development can be hindered or delayed (2). The shape of an infant's head can be affected if pressure is applied often and for long periods of time. This molding of the skull is called plagiocephaly. Due to the recommendation for back sleeping, an infant's skull already experiences a great amount of time with pressure on the back of the head. When an infant is kept in a piece of infant equipment such as an infant seat or a swing, the pressure again is applied to the back of an infant's head; thus, increasing the likelihood of plagiocephaly. To prevent plagiocephaly and to promote normal development, infants should spend time on their tummies when awake and supervised (3).

Infants are not well-protected in restrictive infant equipment and can be injured by animals or other children. Other children or animals can hang, climb, or jump on or into the equipment; therefore, supervision is required during use. Safety straps must be used to prevent injuries and deaths of infants; infants have fallen out of equipment or have been strangled when safety straps have not been used (10).

Equipment must always be placed on the floor and away from the top of stairs to prevent falls; infants have been injured when equipment has been pushed or pulled off an elevated surface or the top of stairs. The surface or floor under the equipment needs to be level to prevent the risk of the equipment tipping over. It is imperative for equipment to be placed out of the reach of potential safety hazards such as furniture, dangling appliance cords, curtain pulls, blind cords, hot surfaces, etc., so infants cannot reach them. The guideline of twenty minutes twice a day was designated so that use could be clearly measured and monitored (1).

Infants should not be placed in equipment, such as stationary activity centers, that require them to support their heads on their own unless they have mastered this skill. Allowing infants to sleep in infant equipment is not recommended

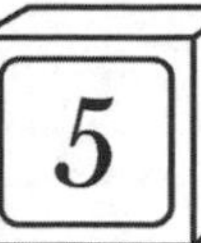

due to the documented decrease in an infant's oxygen saturation caused by the downward flexion of an infant's head and neck due to an infant's underdeveloped head and neck muscles (8,9). If an infant falls asleep in a piece of equipment, the infant should be promptly removed and placed flat on the infant's back in a safety approved crib.

If the stabilizing legs on stationary activity centers are not down and locked in place, this puts an infant at risk of tipping over in the equipment as well as creates an unstable piece of equipment for a mobile infant to use to pull himself up.

Infant walkers are dangerous because they move children around too fast and to hazardous areas, such as stairs. The upright position also can cause children in walkers to "tip over" or can bring children close to objects that they can pull down onto themselves. In addition, walkers can run over or run into others, causing pain or injury. Many injuries, some fatal, have been associated with infant walkers (4-7). There have been several reports of spring/clamp breaking on various models of jumpers (jump-up seats) according to the CPSC (7).

TYPE OF FACILITY: Center; Large Family Child Care Home; Small Family Child Care Home

RELATED STANDARDS:

Standard 3.1.3.4: Caregivers'/Teachers' Encouragement of Physical Activity

REFERENCES:

1. National Association for Family Child Care, The Family Child Care Accreditation Project, Wheelock College. 2005. *Quality standards for NAFCC accreditation,* standard 4.5. 4th ed. Salt Lake City, UT: NAFCC. http://www.nafcc.org/documents/QualStd.pdf.
2. American Physical Therapy Association (APTA). 2008. Lack of time on tummy shown to hinder achievement of developmental milestones, say physical therapists. Press release.
3. American Academy of Pediatrics (AAP), Healthy Child Care America. 2008. *Back to sleep, tummy to play*. Elk Grove Village, IL: AAP. http://www.healthychildcare.org/pdf/SIDStummytime.pdf.
4. American Academy of Pediatrics, Committee on Injury and Poison Prevention. 2008. Policy statement: Injuries associated with infant walkers. *Pediatrics* 122:450.
5. DiLillo, D., A. Damashek, L. Peterson. 2001. Maternal use of baby walkers with young children: Recent trends and possible alternatives. *Injury Prevention* 7:223-27.
6. Shields, B. J., G. A. Smith. 2006. Success in the prevention of infant walker-related injuries: An analysis of national data, 1990-2001. *Pediatrics* 117: e452-59.
7. Chowdhury, R. T. 2009. *Nursery product-related injuries and deaths among children under age five*. Washington, DC: U.S. Consumer Product Safety Commission. http://www.cpsc.gov/library/nursery07.pdf.
8. Kinane, T. B., J. Murphy, J. L. Bass, M. J. Corwin. 2006. Comparison of respiratory physiologic features when infants are placed in car safety seats or car beds. *Pediatrics* 118:522-27.
9. Kornhauser, C. L., C. V. Scirica, I. S. Gantar, D. Osredkar, D. Neubauer, T. B. Kinane. 2009. A comparison of respiratory patterns in healthy term infants placed in car safety seats and beds. *Pediatrics* 124: e396-e402.
10. Warda, L., G. Griggs. 2006. *Childhood Falls in Manitoba: CHIRPP Report: An assessment of injury severity and fall events by age group*. Winnipeg: The Injury Prevention Centre of Children's Hospital. http://www.mpeta.ca/documents/IOI/Falls.pdf.

STANDARD 5.3.1.11: Exercise Equipment

Children should not be permitted to have access to equipment intended for adult exercise.

RATIONALE: Exercise equipment can be potentially hazardous to young children especially if unsupervised. The U.S. Consumer Product Safety Commission (CPSC) estimates that each year about 8,700 children under five years of age are injured with exercise equipment. There are an additional 16,500 injuries per year to children ages five to fourteen. Types of equipment identified in these cases include stationary bicycles, treadmills, and stair climbers. Fractures and even amputations were reported in about 20% of exercise equipment-related injuries (1,2). These types of equipment may be attractive to young children because of their size and the inability to store after use (3). Equipment should be placed or stored in rooms that can be secured from children's access.

TYPE OF FACILITY: Center; Large Family Child Care Home; Small Family Child Care Home

REFERENCES:

1. U.S. Consumer Product Safety Commission (CPSC). Prevent injuries to children from exercise equipment. Document #5028. Washington, DC: CPSC. http://www.cpsc.gov/CPSCPUB/PUBS/5028.html.
2. U.S. Consumer Product Safety Commission (CPSC). 2000. *National electronic injury surveillance system: Exercise equipment estimate report, 1999*. Washington, DC: CPSC.
3. Jones, C. S., J. Freeman, T. M. Penhollow. 2006. Epidemiology of exercise equipment-related injuries to young children. *Pediatr Emergency Care* 22:160-63.

STANDARD 5.3.1.12: Availability and Use of a Telephone or Wireless Communication Device

The facility should provide at all times at least one working non-pay telephone or wireless communication device for general and emergency use:

a) On the premises of the child care facility;
b) In each vehicle used when transporting children;
c) On field trips.

Drivers, while transporting children should not operate a motor vehicle while using a mobile telephone or wireless communications device when the vehicle is in motion or a part of traffic, with the exception of use of a navigational system or global positioning system device.

RATIONALE: A telephone must be available to all caregivers/teachers in an emergency (1).

TYPE OF FACILITY: Center; Large Family Child Care Home; Small Family Child Care Home

RELATED STANDARDS:

Standard 6.5.1.1: Competence and Training of Transportation Staff
Standard 6.5.2.5: Distractions While Driving

REFERENCES:

1. Walsh, E. 2004. *Health and safety notes: Field trip safety tips*. Berkeley, CA: California Childcare Health Program. http://www

.ucsfchildcarehealth.org/pdfs/healthandsafety/fieldtripsen070604_adr.pdf.

5.3.2 Additional Equipment Requirements for Facilities Serving Children with Special Health Care Needs

Note to Reader: See Standard 3.6.3.2 for medication storage.

STANDARD 5.3.2.1: Therapeutic and Recreational Equipment

The facility should have therapeutic and recreational equipment to enhance the educational and developmental progress of children with special health care needs, to the extent that they can be safely and reasonably furnished. Some therapeutic equipment such as trampolines will need to have proper supervision for safety. Such equipment must be securely stored and inaccessible to children when not being used.

RATIONALE: Children with special health care needs may require special equipment of various types. For the individual child, the equipment should be available to meet the goals and methods outlined in the service plan. This equipment, if accessible, may pose a hazard to children in the facility.

COMMENTS: Devices and assisted technology that individual children require is unique to them, based on their own specific needs.

The Americans with Disabilities Act (ADA) does not require personal equipment (e.g., eyeglasses, wheelchairs, etc.) to be furnished by the child care program.

TYPE OF FACILITY: Center; Large Family Child Care Home; Small Family Child Care Home

STANDARD 5.3.2.2: Special Adaptive Equipment

Special adaptive equipment (such as toys, augmentative communication devices, and wheelchairs) for children with special health care needs should be available in and correctly utilized by the facility as part of their reasonable accommodations for the child.

Staff should be instructed and trained in use of communication devices and other adaptive equipment.

RATIONALE: If a facility serves one or more children with special health care needs, adaptive equipment necessary for the child's participation in all activities is needed.

COMMENTS: Most adaptive equipment can be created by making simple adaptation of typically used items such as eating utensils, cups, plates, etc.

Caregivers/teachers are not responsible for providing personal equipment (such as hearing aids, eyeglasses, braces, and wheelchairs), but should be aware of how they should be used and if repairs are necessary.

TYPE OF FACILITY: Center; Large Family Child Care Home; Small Family Child Care Home

RELATED STANDARDS:
Appendix X: Adaptive Equipment for Children with Special Health Care Needs

STANDARD 5.3.2.3: Storage for Adaptive Equipment

The facility should provide storage space for all adaptive equipment (such as equipment for physical therapy, occupational therapy, or adaptive physical education) separate and apart from classroom floor space. The storage space should be easily accessible to the staff. Equipment should be stored safely and in an organized way.

RATIONALE: Frequently, storing adaptive equipment is a problem in centers. This equipment should be stored outside of classroom space to maximize floor space and minimize distracting clutter.

TYPE OF FACILITY: Center

STANDARD 5.3.2.4: Orthotic and Prosthetic Devices

A trained, designated staff member should check prosthetic devices (upper and lower extremity), including hearing aids, processors for cochlear implants, eyeglasses, braces, and wheelchairs, daily to ensure that these appliances are in good working order, cleaned correctly, and have been applied properly.

RATIONALE: Battery-driven devices such as hearing aids require close monitoring because the batteries have a short life and young children require adult assistance to replace them. Eyeglasses scratch and break, as do other assistive appliances. Staff members should be adequately trained to perform orthotic and prosthetic device monitoring.

COMMENTS: The facility should have parents/guardians supply extra batteries for hearing aids. Facilities should store and discard the batteries in such a manner that children cannot ingest them. With the parents'/guardians' permission, the staff may perform minor repairs on equipment if they are trained but should not attempt major repairs.

Upper extremity and lower extremity orthotics and/or eyeglasses are not effective if they are not applied correctly to the child. Instruction from parents/guardians or professionals may be necessary to ensure proper application of devices.

TYPE OF FACILITY: Center; Large Family Child Care Home; Small Family Child Care Home

5.4 Space and Equipment in Designated Areas

5.4.1 Toilet and Handwashing Areas

STANDARD 5.4.1.1: General Requirements for Toilet and Handwashing Areas

Clean toilet and handwashing facilities should be located in the best place to meet the developmental needs of children.

For infant areas, toilets and handwashing facilities are for adult rather than child use. They should be located within the infant area to reduce staff absence.

For toddler areas, toilet and handwashing facilities should be located in or adjacent to the toddler rooms.

For preschool and school-age children, toilet and handwashing facilities should be located near the entrance to the group room and near the entrance to the playground. If both entrances are close to each other, then only one set of toilet and handwashing facilities is needed.

RATIONALE: Young children have poor bowel and bladder control and cannot wait long when they have to use the toilet (1). Young children must be able to get to toilet facilities quickly. Staff must have easy access to hand washing facilities to wash their hands at the times when it is appropriate and still maintain supervision of the children.

TYPE OF FACILITY: Center; Large Family Child Care Home; Small Family Child Care Home

RELATED STANDARDS:
Standard 3.2.2.3: Assisting Children with Hand Hygiene

REFERENCES:
1. Olds, A. R. 2001. *Child care design guide*. New York: McGraw-Hill.

STANDARD 5.4.1.2: Location of Toilets and Privacy Issues

Toilets should be located in rooms separate from those used for cooking or eating. If toilets are not on the same floor as the child care area and not within sight or hearing of a caregiver/teacher, an adult should accompany children younger than five years of age to and from the toilet area. In centers, males and females who are six years of age and older should have separate and private toilet facilities. Younger children who request privacy and have shown capability to use toilet facilities properly should be given permission to use separate and private toilet facilities.

RATIONALE: It is important to prevent contamination of food and to eliminate unpleasant odors from the food areas.

Supervision and assistance are necessary for young children. Although cultures differ in privacy needs, sex-separated toileting among people who are not relatives is the norm for adults. Children should be allowed the opportunity to practice modesty when independent toileting behavior is well-established in the majority of the group. By six years of age, most children can use the toilet by themselves (1).

COMMENTS: Compliance is monitored by observation.

TYPE OF FACILITY: Center; Large Family Child Care Home; Small Family Child Care Home

RELATED STANDARDS:
Standard 2.4.1.3: Gender and Body Awareness

REFERENCES:
1. Shelov, S. P., R. E. Hannemann, eds. 1998. *Caring for your baby and young child: Birth to age 5*. 2nd ed. Elk Grove Village, IL: American Academy of Pediatrics.

STANDARD 5.4.1.3: Ability to Open Toilet Room Doors

Children should be able to easily open every toilet room door from the inside, and caregivers/teachers should be able to easily open toilet room doors from the outside if adult assistance is required.

RATIONALE: Doors that can be opened easily will prevent entrapment.

COMMENTS: Inside latches that children can easily manage will allow the child to ensure privacy when using the toilet. The latch or lock available for use, must be of a type that the staff can easily open from the outside in case a child requires adult assistance.

TYPE OF FACILITY: Center; Large Family Child Care Home; Small Family Child Care Home

STANDARD 5.4.1.4: Preventing Entry to Toilet Rooms by Infants and Toddlers

Toilet rooms should have barriers that prevent entry by infants and toddlers who are unattended. Infants and toddlers should be supervised by sight and sound at all times.

RATIONALE: Infants and toddlers can drown in toilet bowls, play in the toilet, have contact with contaminated items or surfaces, or otherwise engage in potentially injurious behavior if they are not supervised in toilet rooms.

TYPE OF FACILITY: Center; Large Family Child Care Home; Small Family Child Care Home

STANDARD 5.4.1.5: Chemical Toilets

Chemical toilets should not be used in child care facilities unless they are provided as a temporary measure in the event that the facility's normal plumbed toilets are not functioning. Constant supervision should be required for young children using a chemical toilet. In the event that chemical toilets may be required on a temporary basis, the caregiver/teacher should seek approval for use from the regulatory health agency.

RATIONALE: Chemical toilets can pose a safety hazard to young children. Young children climbing on the toilet seat could fall through the opening and into the chemical that is contained in the waste receptacle.

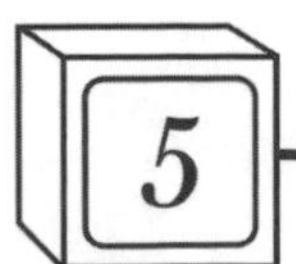

COMMENTS: A chemical toilet is a toilet consisting of a seat or bowl attached to a container holding a chemical solution that changes waste into sludge (1).

TYPE OF FACILITY: Center; Large Family Child Care Home; Small Family Child Care Home

REFERENCES:

1. Dictionary.com. 2000. Chemical toilets. *The American heritage dictionary of the English language*. 4th ed. http://dictionary.reference.com/browse/chemical toilets.

STANDARD 5.4.1.6: Ratios of Toilets, Urinals, and Hand Sinks to Children

Toilets and hand sinks should be easily accessible to children and facilitate adult supervision. The number of toilets and hand sinks should be subject to the following minimums:

a) Toddlers:
   1) If each group size is less than ten children, provide one sink and one toilet per group.
b) Preschool-age children:
   1) If each group size is less than ten children, provide one sink and one toilet per group;
   2) If each group size is between ten to sixteen children, provide two sinks and two flush toilets for each group.
c) School-age children:
   1) If each group size is less than ten children, provide one sink and one toilet per group;
   2) If each group size is between ten to twenty children, provide two sinks and two toilets per group. Provide separation of male and female toilets.

For toddlers and preschoolers, the maximum toilet height should be eleven inches, and maximum height for hand sinks should be twenty-two inches. Urinals should not exceed 30% of the total required toilet fixtures and should be used by one child at a time. For school-age children, standard height toilet, urinal, and hand sink fixtures are appropriate.

Non-flushing equipment in toilet learning/training should not be counted as toilets in the toilet:child ratio.

RATIONALE: The environment can become contaminated more easily with multiple simultaneous users of urinals, because at least one of the children must assume an off-center position in relationship to the fixture during voiding.

Young children use the toilet frequently and cannot wait long when they have to use the toilet. The ratio of 1:10 is based on best professional experience of early childhood educators who are facility operators (1). This ratio also limits the group that will be sharing facilities (and infections).

COMMENTS: The ratios of toilets and hand sinks to children provided above takes into consideration the maximum group size specified under Standard 1.1.1.2. Local building codes also dictate toilet and sink requirements based on number of children utilizing them.

State licensing regulations have often applied a ratio of 1:10 for toddlers and preschool children, and 1:15 for school-age children. The ratios used in this standard correspond to the maximum group sizes for each age group specified in Standard 1.1.1.2.

A ratio of one toilet to every ten children may not be sufficient if only one toilet is accessible to each group of ten, so a minimum of two toilets per group is preferable when the group size approaches ten. However, a large toilet room with many toilets used by several groups is less desirable than several small toilet rooms assigned to specific groups, because of the opportunities such a large room offers for transmitting infectious disease agents.

When providing bathroom fixtures for a mixed group of preschool and school-age children, requiring a school-age child to use bathroom fixtures designed for preschoolers may negatively impact the self-esteem of the school-age child.

TYPE OF FACILITY: Center; Large Family Child Care Home

RELATED STANDARDS:

Standard 1.1.1.2: Ratios for Large Family Child Care Homes and Centers

REFERENCES:

1. Olds, A. R. 2001. *Child care design guide*. New York: McGraw-Hill.

STANDARD 5.4.1.7: Toilet Learning/Training Equipment

Equipment used for toilet learning/training should be provided for children who are learning to use the toilet. Child-sized toilets or safe and cleanable step aids and modified toilet seats (where adult-sized toilets are present) should be used in facilities. Non-flushing toilets (i.e., potty chairs) should be strongly discouraged.

If child-sized toilets, step aids, or modified toilet seats cannot be used, non-flushing toilets (potty chairs) meeting the following criteria should be provided for toddlers, preschoolers, and children with disabilities who require them. Potty chairs should be:

a) Easily cleaned and disinfected;
b) Used only in a bathroom area;
c) Used over a surface that is impervious to moisture;
d) Out of reach of toilets or other potty chairs;
e) Cleaned and disinfected after each use in a sink used only for cleaning and disinfecting potty chairs.

Equipment used for toilet learning/training should be accessible to children only under direct supervision.

The sink used to clean and disinfect the potty chair should also be cleaned and disinfected after each use.

RATIONALE: Child-sized toilets that are flushable, steps, and modified toilet seats provide for easier use and maintenance. Sanitary handling of potty chairs is difficult. Flushable toilets are superior to any type of device that exposes the staff to contact with feces or urine. Many infectious diseases can be prevented through appropriate hygiene and disinfection methods. Surveys of environmental surfaces

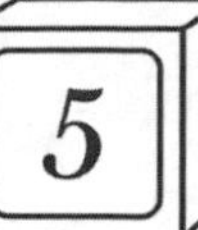

in child care settings have demonstrated evidence of fecal contamination (1). Fecal contamination has been used to gauge the adequacy of disinfection and hygiene.

COMMENTS: If potty chairs are used, they should be constructed of plastic or similar nonporous synthetic products. Wooden potty chairs should not be used, even if the surface is coated with a finish. The finished surface of wooden potty chairs is not durable and, therefore, may become difficult to wash and disinfect effectively.

TYPE OF FACILITY: Center; Large Family Child Care Home; Small Family Child Care Home

REFERENCES:

1. Gorski, P. A. 1999. Toilet training guidelines: Day care providers-the role of the day care provider in toilet training. *Pediatrics* 103:1367-68.

STANDARD 5.4.1.8: Cleaning and Disinfecting Toileting Equipment

Utility gloves and equipment designated for cleaning and disinfecting toilet learning/training equipment and flush toilets should be used for each cleaning and should not be used for other cleaning purposes. Utility gloves should be washed with soapy water and dried after each use.

RATIONALE: Contamination of hands and equipment in a child care room has played a role in the transmission of disease (1,2).

TYPE OF FACILITY: Center; Large Family Child Care Home; Small Family Child Care Home

RELATED STANDARDS:

Appendix D: Gloving
Appendix J: Selecting an Appropriate Sanitizer or Disinfectant
Appendix K: Routine Schedule for Cleaning, Sanitizing, and Disinfecting

REFERENCES:

1. Churchill, R. B., L. K. Pickering. 1997. Infection control challenges in child-care centers. *Infect Dis Clin North Am* 11:347-65.
2. Van, R., A. L. Morrow, R. R. Reves, L. K. Pickering. 1991. Environmental contamination in child day-care centers. *Am J Epidemiol* 133:460-70.

STANDARD 5.4.1.9: Waste Receptacles in the Child Care Facility and in Child Care Facility Toilet Room(s)

Waste receptacles in the facility should be kept clean, in good repair, and emptied daily. Toilet rooms should have at least one plastic-lined waste receptacle with a foot-pedal operated lid.

RATIONALE: This practice prevents the spread of disease and filth. In toilet rooms, users may need to dispose of waste that is contaminated with body fluids. Sanitary disposal of this material requires a lidded container that does not have to be handled to be opened.

TYPE OF FACILITY: Center; Large Family Child Care Home; Small Family Child Care Home

RELATED STANDARDS:

Standard 5.2.8.1: Integrated Pest Management
Standards 5.4.1.1-5.4.1.9: Toilets and Toilet Learning/Training Equipment
Standard 5.4.2.4: Use, Location, and Setup of Diaper Changing Areas

STANDARD 5.4.1.10: Handwashing Sinks

A handwashing sink should be accessible without barriers (such as doors) to each child care area. In areas for infants, toddlers, and preschoolers, the sink should be located so the caregiver/teacher may visually supervise the group of children while carrying out routine handwashing or having children wash their hands. Sinks should be placed at the child's height or be equipped with a stable step platform to make the sink available to children. If a platform is used, it should have slip-proof steps and platform surface. Also, each sink should be equipped so that the user has access to:

a) Water, at a temperature at least 60°F and no hotter than 120°F;
b) A foot-pedal operated, electric-eye operated, open, self-closing, slow-closing, or metering faucet that provides a flow of water for at least thirty seconds without the need to reactivate the faucet;
c) A supply of hand-cleansing non-antibacterial, unscented liquid soap;
d) Disposable single-use cloth or paper towels or a heated-air hand-drying device with heat guards to prevent contact with surfaces that get hotter than 120°F.

A steam tap or a water tap that provides hot water that is hotter than 120°F may not be used at a handwashing sink.

RATIONALE: Transmission of many infectious diseases can be prevented through handwashing (1). To facilitate routine handwashing at the many appropriate times, sinks must be close at hand and permit caregivers/teachers to provide continuous supervision while they wash their hands. The location, access, and supporting supplies to enable adequate handwashing are important to the successful integration of this key routine. Foot-pedaled operated or electric-eye operated handwashing sinks and liquid soap dispensers are preferable because they minimize hand contamination during and after handwashing. The flow of water must continue long enough for the user to wet the skin surface, get soap, lather for at least twenty seconds, and rinse completely.

Comfortably warm water helps to release soil from hand surfaces and provides comfort for the person who is washing the hands. When the water is too cold or too hot for comfort, the person is less likely to wet and rinse long enough to lather and wash off soil. Having a steam tap or a super-heated hot water tap available at a handwashing sink poses a significant risk of scald burns.

COMMENTS: Shared access to soap and disposable towels at more than one sink is acceptable if the location of these is fully accessible to each person. There is no

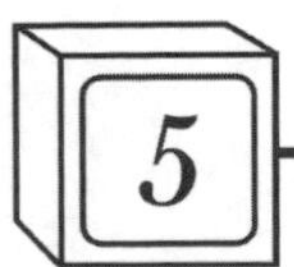

evidence that antibacterial soap reduces the incidence of illness among children in child care.

TYPE OF FACILITY: Center

RELATED STANDARDS:
Standard 4.8.0.4: Food Preparation Sinks
Standard 4.8.0.5: Handwashing Sink Separate from Food Zones
Standard 5.2.1.14: Water Heating Devices and Temperatures Allowed

REFERENCES:
1. Centers for Disease Control and Prevention (CDC). Wash your hands. http://www.cdc.gov/features/handwashing/.

STANDARD 5.4.1.11: Prohibited Uses of Handwashing Sinks

Handwashing sinks should not be used for rinsing soiled clothing, for cleaning equipment that is used for toileting, or for the disposal of any waste water used in cleaning the facility.

RATIONALE: The sink used to wash/rinse soiled clothing or equipment used for toileting becomes contaminated during this process and can be a source of transmission of disease to those who wash their hands in that sink (1).

TYPE OF FACILITY: Center; Large Family Child Care Home

REFERENCES:
1. Laborde, D. J., K. A. Weigle, D. J. Weber, J. B. Kotch. 1993. Effect of fecal contamination on the diarrheal illness rates in day-care centers. *Am J Epidemiol* 138:243-55.

STANDARD 5.4.1.12: Mop Sinks

Centers with more than thirty children should have a mop sink. Large and small family child care homes should have a means of obtaining clean water for mopping and disposing of it in a toilet or in a sink used only for such purposes.

RATIONALE: Handwashing and food preparation sinks must not be contaminated by wastewater. Contamination of hands, toys, and equipment in the room plays a role in the transmission of diseases in child care settings (1,2).

COMMENTS: Mop sinks are installed on the floor, similar to a shower pan, and are usually located in janitor's closets or laundry facilities.

TYPE OF FACILITY: Center; Large Family Child Care Home; Small Family Child Care Home

RELATED STANDARDS:
Standard 4.8.0.4: Food Preparation Sinks
Standard 4.8.0.5: Handwashing Sink Separate from Food Zones
Standard 5.2.6.9: Handwashing Sink Using Portable Water Supply

REFERENCES:
1. Churchill, R. B., L. K. Pickering. 1997. Infection control challenges in child-care centers. *Infect Dis Clin North Am* 11:347-65.
2. Van, R., A. L. Morrow, R. R. Reves, L. K. Pickering. 1991. Environmental contamination in child day-care centers. *Am J Epidemiol* 133:460-70.

5.4.2 Diaper Changing Areas

STANDARD 5.4.2.1: Diaper Changing Tables

The facility should have at least one diaper changing table per infant group or toddler group to allow sufficient time for changing diapers and for cleaning and sanitizing between children. Diaper changing tables and sinks should be used only by the children in the group whose routine care is provided together throughout their time in child care. The facility should not permit shared use of diaper changing tables and sinks by more than one group.

RATIONALE: Diaper changing requires time, as does cleaning the changing surfaces. When caregivers/teachers from different groups use the same diaper changing surface, disease spreads more easily from group to group. Child care facilities should not put the diaper changing tables and sinks in a buffer zone between two classrooms, because doing so effectively joins the groups from the perspective of cross-contamination.

TYPE OF FACILITY: Center; Large Family Child Care Home

RELATED STANDARDS:
Standards 1.1.1.1-1.1.1.2: Supervision According to Group Size
Standard 5.4.2.4: Use, Location, and Setup of Diaper Changing Areas

STANDARD 5.4.2.2: Handwashing Sinks for Diaper Changing Areas in Centers

Handwashing sinks in centers should be provided within arm's reach of the caregiver/teacher to diaper changing tables and toilets. A minimum of one handwashing sink should be available for every two changing tables. Where infants and toddlers are in care, sinks and diaper changing tables should be assigned for use to a specific group of children and used only by children and adults who are in the assigned group as defined by Standard 5.4.2.1. Handwashing sinks should not be used for bathing or removing smeared fecal material.

RATIONALE: Sinks must be close to where the diapering takes place to avoid transfer of contaminants to other surfaces en route to washing the hands of staff and children. Having sinks close by will help prevent the spread of contaminants and disease.

When sinks are shared by multiple groups, cross-contamination occurs. Many child care centers put the diaper changing tables and sinks in a buffer zone between two classrooms, effectively joining the groups through cross-contamination.

COMMENTS: Shared access to soap and disposable towels at more than one sink is acceptable if the location of these is fully accessible to each person.

TYPE OF FACILITY: Center

RELATED STANDARDS:
Standard 5.4.2.1: Diaper Changing Tables
Standard 5.4.2.4: Use, Location, and Setup of Diaper Changing Areas

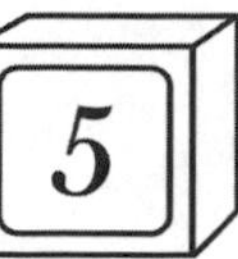

REFERENCES:

1. Fiene, R. 2002. *13 indicators of quality child care: Research update.* Washington, DC: U.S. Department of Health and Human Services, Office of the Assistant Secretary for Planning and Evaluation. http://aspe.hhs.gov/hsp/ccquality-ind02/.

STANDARD 5.4.2.3: Handwashing Sinks for Diaper Changing Areas in Homes

Handwashing sinks in large and small family child care homes should be supplied for diaper changing, as specified in Standard 5.4.2.2, except that they should be within ten feet of the changing table if the diapering area cannot be set up so the sink is adjacent to the changing table. If diapered toddlers and preschool-age children are in care, a stepstool should be available at the handwashing sink, as specified in Standard 5.4.1.10, so smaller children can stand at the sink to wash their hands. Handwashing sinks should not be used for bathing or removing smeared fecal material.

RATIONALE: When children from more than one family are in care, the diaper changing area should be arranged to be as close as possible to a non-food sink to avoid fecal-oral transmission of infection.

Sinks must be close to where the diapering takes place to avoid transfer of contaminants to other surfaces en route to washing the hands of staff and children. Having sinks close by will help prevent the spread of contaminants and disease.

TYPE OF FACILITY: Large Family Child Care Home; Small Family Child Care Home

RELATED STANDARDS:

Standard 5.4.1.10: Handwashing Sinks
Standard 5.4.2.2: Handwashing Sinks For Diaper Changing Areas in Centers
Standard 5.4.2.4: Use, Location, and Setup of Diaper Changing Areas

STANDARD 5.4.2.4: Use, Location, and Setup of Diaper Changing Areas

Infants and toddlers should be diapered only in the diaper changing area. Children should be discouraged from remaining in or entering the diaper changing area. The contaminated surfaces of waste containers should not be accessible to children.

Diaper changing areas and food preparation areas should be physically separated. Diaper changing should not be conducted in food preparation areas or on surfaces used for other purposes. Food and drinking utensils should not be washed in sinks located in diaper changing areas.

The diaper changing area should be set up so that no other surface or supply container is contaminated during diaper changing. Bulk supplies should not be stored on or brought to the diaper changing surface. Instead, the diapers, wipes, gloves, a thick layer of diaper cream on a piece of disposable paper, a plastic bag for soiled clothes, and disposable paper to cover the table in the amount needed for a specific diaper change will be removed from the bulk container or storage location and placed on or near the diaper changing surface before bringing the child to the diaper changing area.

Conveniently located, washable, plastic-lined, tightly covered, hands-free receptacles, should be provided for soiled cloths and linen containing body fluids.

Where only one staff member is available to supervise a group of children, the diaper changing table should be positioned to allow the staff member to maintain constant sight and sound supervision of children.

RATIONALE: The use of a separate area for diaper changing or changing of soiled underwear reduces contamination of other parts of the child care environment (1-2). Children cannot be expected to avoid contact with contaminated surfaces in the diaper changing area. They should be in this area only for diaper changing and be protected as much as possible from contact with contaminated surfaces. The separation of diaper changing areas and food preparation areas prevents transmission of disease. Using diaper changing surfaces for any other purpose increases the likelihood of contamination and spreading of infectious disease agents.

Bringing storage containers for bulk supplies to the diaper changing table is likely to result in their contamination during the diaper changing process. When these containers stay on the table or are replaced in a storage location, they become conduits for transmitting disease agents. Bringing to the table only the amount of each supply that will be consumed in that specific diaper changing will prevent contamination of diapering supplies and the environment.

Hands-free receptacles prevent environmental contamination so the children do not come into contact with disease-bearing body fluids.

Often, only one staff person is supervising children when a child has to be changed. Orienting the diaper changing table so the staff member can maintain direct observation of all children in the room allows adequate supervision.

TYPE OF FACILITY: Center; Large Family Child Care Home; Small Family Child Care Home

RELATED STANDARDS:

Standard 3.2.1.4: Diaper Changing Procedure
Standard 5.4.2.5: Changing Table Requirements
Standard 5.2.7.4: Containment of Soiled Diapers

REFERENCES:

1. Aronson, S. S. 1999. The ideal diaper changing station. *Child Care Information Exchange* 130:92.
2. Fiene, R. 2002. *13 indicators of quality child care: Research update*. Washington, DC: U.S. Department of Health and Human Services, Office of the Assistant Secretary for Planning and Evaluation. http://aspe.hhs.gov/hsp/ccquality-ind02/.

STANDARD 5.4.2.5: Changing Table Requirements

Changing tables should meet the following requirements:

a) Have impervious, nonabsorbent, smooth surfaces that do not trap soil and are easily disinfected;
b) Be sturdy and stable to prevent tipping over;

c) Be at a convenient height for use by caregivers/teachers (between twenty-eight and thirty-two inches high);
d) Be equipped with railings or barriers that extend at least six inches above the change surface.

RATIONALE: This standard is designed to prevent disease transmission and falls and to provide safety measures during diapering. Commercial diaper change tables vary as much as ten inches in height. Many standard-height thirty-six inch counters are used as the diaper change area. When a railing or barrier is attached, shorter staff members cannot change diapers without standing on a step.

Back injury is a common occupational injury for caregivers/teachers (3,5). Using changing tables that are sized for caregiver/teacher comfort and convenience can help prevent back injury (1,3-4). Railings of two inches or less in height have been observed in some diaper change areas and when combined with a moisture-impervious diaper changing pad approximately one inch thick, render the railing ineffective. A change table height of twenty-eight inches to thirty-two inches (standard table height) plus a six-inch barrier will reduce back strain on staff members and provide a safe barrier to prevent children from falling off the changing table.

Data from the U.S. Consumer Product Safety Commission (CPSC) show that falls are a serious hazard associated with infant changing tables (2). Safety straps on changing tables are provided to prevent falls but they trap soil and they are not easily disinfected. Therefore, diaper changing tables should not have safety straps.

COMMENTS: An impervious surface is defined as a smooth surface that does not absorb liquid or retain soil. While changing a child, the adult must hold onto the child at all times.

The activity of diaper changing presents an opportunity for adult interaction with the child whose diaper is being changed.

TYPE OF FACILITY: Center; Large Family Child Care Home; Small Family Child Care Home

REFERENCES:

1. Aronson, S. S. 1999. The ideal diaper changing station. *Child Care Info Exch* 130:92.
2. U.S. Consumer Product Safety Commission (CPSC). 1997. *The safe nursery*. Washington, DC: CPSC. http://www.cpsc.gov/cpscpub/pubs/202.pdf.
3. ASTM International. 2008. ASTM F2388-08. *Baby changing tables for domestic use*. West Conshohocken, PA: ASTM.
4. Gratz, R., A. Claffey, P. King, G. Scheuer. 2002. The physical demands and ergonomics of working with young children. *Early Child Devel Care* 172:531-37.
5. Fiene, R. 2002. *13 indicators of quality child care: Research update*. Washington, DC: U.S. Department of Health and Human Services, Office of the Assistant Secretary for Planning and Evaluation. http://aspe.hhs.gov/hsp/ccquality-ind02/.

STANDARD 5.4.2.6: Maintenance of Changing Tables

Changing tables should be nonporous, kept in good repair, and cleaned and disinfected after each use to remove visible soil and germs.

RATIONALE: Many infectious diseases can be prevented through appropriate cleaning and disinfection procedures. It is difficult, if not impossible, to disinfect porous surfaces, broken edges, and surfaces that cannot be completely cleaned. Bacterial cultures of environmental surfaces in child care facilities have shown fecal contamination, which has been used to gauge the adequacy of sanitation and hygiene measures practiced at the facility (1).

One study has demonstrated that "diapering, handwashing, and food preparation equipment that is specifically designed to reduce the spread of infectious agents significantly reduced diarrheal illness among the children and absence as a result of illness among staff in out-of-home child care centers" (2).

COMMENTS: Caregivers/teachers should be reminded that many disinfectants leave residues that can cause skin irritation or other symptoms. Caregivers/teachers should always follow the manufacturer's instructions for preparation and use.

A U.S. Environmental Protection Agency (EPA)-registered product labeled for use as a disinfectant suitable for the surface material should be used to disinfect the changing table after use. Some bleach products are EPA-registered disinfectants.

TYPE OF FACILITY: Center; Large Family Child Care Home; Small Family Child Care Home

RELATED STANDARDS:

Appendix J: Selecting an Appropriate Sanitizer or Disinfectant
Appendix K: Routine Schedule for Cleaning, Sanitizing, and Disinfecting

REFERENCES:

1. Pickering, L. K., C. J. Baker, D. W. Kimberlin, S. S. Long, eds. 2009. *Red Book: 2009 report of the Committee on Infectious Diseases*. Elk Grove Village, IL: American Academy of Pediatrics.
2. Kotch, J. B., P. Isbell, D. J. Weber, V. Nguyen, E. Gunn, S. Fowlkes, J. Virk, J. Allen. 2007. Hand-washing and diapering equipment reduces disease among children in out-of-home child care centers. *Pediatrics* 120: e29-e36.

5.4.3 Bathtubs and Showers

STANDARD 5.4.3.1: Ratio and Location of Bathtubs and Showers

The facility should have one bathtub or shower for every six children receiving overnight care. If the facility is caring for infants, it should have age-appropriate bathing facilities for them. Bathtubs and showers, when required or used as part of the daily program, should be located within the facility or in an approved building immediately adjacent to it.

RATIONALE: A sufficient number of age-appropriate bathing tubs and showers must be available to permit separate bathing for every child.

COMMENTS: Assuming that each bath takes ten to fifteen minutes, a ratio of one tub to six children with time to wash the tub between children means that bathing would require about one and one-half hours.

TYPE OF FACILITY: Center; Large Family Child Care Home; Small Family Child Care Home

STANDARD 5.4.3.2: Safety of Bathtubs and Showers

All bathing facilities should have a conveniently located grab bar that is mounted at a height appropriate for a child to use. Nonskid surfaces should be provided in all tubs and showers. Bathtubs should be equipped with a mechanism to guarantee that drains are kept open at all times, except during supervised use. Water temperature should not exceed 120°F and anti-scald devices should be permanently installed in the faucet and shower head.

RATIONALE: Falls in tubs are a well-documented source of injury according to the National Electronic Injury Surveillance System (NEISS) data collected by the U.S. Consumer Product Safety Commission (CPSC) (2). Grab bars and nonslip surfaces reduce this risk (2). Drowning and falls in bathtubs are also a significant cause of injury for young children and children with disabilities (1,2). An open drain will prevent a pool of water from forming if a child turns on a water faucet and, therefore, will prevent a potential drowning situation. Bathtub water comprises the leading cause of scalds for young children (2). Water heated to temperatures greater than 120°F takes less than thirty seconds to burn the skin (2).

COMMENTS: Various inexpensive devices to check water temperature are available at stores and on the Internet.

TYPE OF FACILITY: Center

REFERENCES:

1. Gipson, K. 2009. *Submersions related to non-pool and non-spa products, 2008 report.* Washington, DC: CPSC. http://www.cpsc.gov/library/FOIA/FOIA09/OS/nonpoolsub2008.pdf.
2. D'Souza, A. L., N. G. Nelson, L. B. McKenzie. 2009. Pediatric burn injuries treated in US emergency departments between 1990 and 2006. *Pediatrics* 124:1424-30.

5.4.4 Laundry Area

STANDARD 5.4.4.1: Laundry Service and Equipment

Centers should have a mechanical washing machine and dryer on site or should contract with a laundry service. Where laundry equipment is used in a large or small family child care home (or the large or small family home caregiver/teacher uses an off-site laundry facility), the equipment should comply with Standard 5.4.4.2.

RATIONALE: Bedding and towels that are not thoroughly cleaned pose a health threat to users of these items.

TYPE OF FACILITY: Center; Large Family Child Care Home; Small Family Child Care Home

RELATED STANDARDS:
Standard 5.4.4.2: Location of Laundry Equipment and Water Temperature for Laundering

STANDARD 5.4.4.2: Location of Laundry Equipment and Water Temperature for Laundering

Laundry equipment should be located in an area separate from the kitchen and child care areas and inaccessible to children. The water temperature for the laundry should be maintained above 140°F unless one of the following conditions exists:

a) The product labeled by the manufacturer as a sanitizer is applied according to the manufacturer's instructions, in which case the temperature should be as specified by the manufacturer of the product;
b) A dryer is used that the manufacturer attests heats the clothes above 140°F;
c) The clothes are completely ironed (1).

Dryers should be vented to the outside. Dryer hoses and vent connections should be checked periodically for proper alignment and connection. Lint must be removed with each use and periodically cleaned from the hose to avoid fires. If a commercial laundry service is used, its performance should meet or exceed the requirements listed above.

RATIONALE: Chemical sanitizers are temperature-dependent. Ironing or heating the clothing above 140°F will sanitize. Bent dryer hoses can cause lint to catch in dryers, which is a potential fire hazard. Disconnected dryer hoses will vent lint, dust, and particles indoors, which may cause respiratory problems.

TYPE OF FACILITY: Center; Large Family Child Care Home; Small Family Child Care Home

RELATED STANDARDS:
Standard 5.4.4.1: Laundry Service and Equipment

REFERENCES:

1. Witt, C. S., J. Warden. 1971. Can home laundries stop the spread of bacteria in clothing? *Textile Chemist Colorist* 3:55-57.

5.4.5 Sleep and Rest Areas

STANDARD 5.4.5.1: Sleeping Equipment and Supplies

Facilities should have an individual crib, cot, sleeping bag, bed, mat, or pad that has not been recalled for each child who spends more than four hours a day at the facility. No child should simultaneously share a crib, bed, or bedding with another child. Facilities should ensure that toddler beds are in compliance with the current U.S. Consumer Product Safety Commission (CPSC) and ASTM safety standards (1). Clean linens should be provided for each child. Beds and bedding should be washed between uses if used by different children. Regardless of age group, bed linens should not be used as rest equipment in place of cots, beds, pads, or similar approved equipment. Bed linens used under children on cots, cribs, futons, and playpens should be tight-fitting. Sheets for an adult bed should not be used on a crib mattress. See Standard 5.4.5.2 for crib specifications.

When pads are used, they should be enclosed in washable covers and should be long enough so the child's head or feet do not rest off the pad. Mats and cots should be made with a waterproof material that can be easily washed and sanitized. Plastic bags or loose plastic material should never be used as a covering.

No child should sleep on a bare, uncovered surface. Seasonally appropriate covering, such as sheets, sleep garments, or blankets that are sufficient to maintain adequate warmth, should be available and should be used by each child below school-age. Pillows, blankets, and sleep positioners should not be used with infants. If pillows are used by toddlers and older children, pillows should have removable cases that can be laundered, be assigned to a child, and used by that child only while s/he is enrolled in the facility. Each child's pillow, blanket, sheet, and any special sleep item should be stored separately from those of other children.

Pads and sleeping bags should not be placed directly on any floor that is cooler than 65°F when children are resting. Cribs, cots, sleeping bags, beds, mats, or pads in/on which children are sleeping should be placed at least three feet apart. If the room used for sleeping cannot accommodate three feet of spacing between children, it is recommended for caregivers/teachers to space children as far as possible from one another and/or alternate children head to feet. Screens used to separate sleeping children are not recommended because screens can affect supervision, interfere with immediate access to a child, and could potentially injure a child if pushed over on a child. If unoccupied sleep equipment is used to separate sleeping children, the arrangement of such equipment should permit the staff to observe and have immediate access to each child. The ends of cribs do not suffice as screens to separate sleeping children.

The sleeping surfaces of one child's rest equipment should not come in contact with the sleeping surfaces of another child's rest equipment during storage.

Caregivers/teachers should never use strings to hang any object, such as a mobile, or a toy or a diaper bag, on or near the crib where a child could become caught in it and strangle.

Infant monitors and their cords and other electrical cords should never be placed in the crib or sleeping equipment.

Crib mattresses should fit snugly and be made specifically for the size crib in which they are placed. Infants should not be placed on an inflatable mattress due to potential of entrapment or suffocation.

RATIONALE: Separate sleeping and resting, even for siblings, reduces the spread of disease from one child to another.

Droplet transmission occurs when droplets containing microorganisms generated from an infected person, primarily during coughing, sneezing, or talking are propelled a short distance (three feet) and deposited on the conjunctivae, nasal mucosa, or mouth (2).

Because respiratory infections are transmitted by large droplets of respiratory secretions, a minimum distance of three feet should be maintained between cots, cribs, sleeping bags, beds, mats, or pads used for resting or sleeping (2). A space of three feet between cribs, cots, sleeping bags, beds, mats, or pads will also provide access by the staff to a child in case of emergency. If the facility uses screens to separate the children, their use must not hinder observation of children by staff or access to children in an emergency.

Lice infestation, scabies, and ringworm are among the most common infectious diseases in child care. These diseases are transmitted by direct person-to-person contact. Ringworm is transmitted by the sharing of personal articles such as combs, brushes, towels, clothing, and bedding. Prohibiting the sharing of personal articles helps prevent the spread of these diseases.

The use of tight-fitting bed linens prevents suffocation and strangling. Adult bed sheets can become loose and entangle an infant (3).

From time to time, children drool, spit up, or spread other body fluids on their sleeping surfaces. Using cleanable, waterproof, nonabsorbent rest equipment enables the staff to wash and sanitize the sleeping surfaces. Plastic bags may not be used to cover rest and sleep surfaces/equipment because they contribute to suffocation if the material clings to the child's face.

Canvas cots are not recommended for infants and toddlers. The end caps require constant replacement and the cots are a cutting/pinching hazard when end caps are not in place. A variety of cots are made with washable sleeping surfaces that are designed to be safe for children.

COMMENTS: Although children freely interact and can contaminate each other while awake, reducing the transmission of infectious disease agents on large airborne droplets during sleep periods will reduce the dose of such agents to which the child is exposed overall. In small family child care homes, the caregiver/teacher should consider the home to be a business during child care hours and is expected to abide by regulatory expectations that may not apply outside of child care hours. Therefore, child siblings related to the caregiver/teacher may not sleep in the same bed during the hours of operation.

Caregivers/teachers may ask parents/guardians to provide bedding that will be sent home for washing at least weekly or sooner if soiled.

Pillows are not required for older children.

Many caregivers/teachers find that placing children in alternate positions so that one child's head is across from the other's feet reduces interaction and promotes settling during

rest periods. This positioning may be beneficial in reducing transmission of infectious agents as well.

The use of solid crib ends as barriers between sleeping children can serve as a barrier if they are three feet away from each other (2).

TYPE OF FACILITY: Center; Large Family Child Care Home; Small Family Child Care Home

RELATED STANDARDS:

Standard 3.1.4.1: Safe Sleep Practices and SIDS/Suffocation Risk Reduction
Standard 3.4.6.1: Strangulation Hazards
Standard 5.4.5.2: Cribs
Standard 9.2.4.5: Emergency and Evacuation Drills/Exercises Policy

REFERENCES:

1. U.S. Consumer Product Safety Commission (CPSC). 2011. CPSC approves new mandatory standard for toddler beds. http://www.cpsc.gov/cpscpub/prerel/prhtml11/11199.html.
2. Pickering, L. K., C. J. Baker, D. W. Kimberlin, S. S. Long, eds. 2009. *Red book: 2009 report of the Committee on Infectious Diseases*, **153**. Elk Grove Village, IL: American Academy of Pediatrics.
3. American Academy of Pediatrics. 2010. Ages and stages: A parent's guide to safe sleep. Healthy Children. http://www.healthychildren.org/English/ages-stages/baby/sleep/Pages/A-Parents-Guide-to-Safe-Sleep.aspx.

STANDARD 5.4.5.2: Cribs

Facilities should check each crib before its purchase and use to ensure that it is in compliance with the current U.S. Consumer Product Safety Commission (CPSC) and ASTM safety standards.

Recalled or "second-hand" cribs should not be used or stored in the facility. When it is determined that a crib is no longer safe for use in the facility, it should be dismantled and disposed of appropriately.

Staff should only use cribs for sleep purposes and should ensure that each crib is a safe sleep environment. No child of any age should be placed in a crib for a time-out or for disciplinary reasons. When an infant becomes large enough or mobile enough to reach crib latches or potentially climb out of a crib, they should be transitioned to a different sleeping environment (such as a cot or sleeping mat).

Each crib should be identified by brand, type, and/or product number and relevant product information should be kept on file (with the same identification information) as long as the crib is used or stored in the facility.

Staff should inspect each crib before each use to ensure that hardware is tightened and that there are not any safety hazards. If a screw or bolt cannot be tightened securely, or there are missing or broken screws, bolts, or mattress support hangers, the crib should not be used.

Safety standards document that cribs used in facilities should be made of wood, metal, or plastic. Crib slats should be spaced no more than two and three-eighths inches apart, with a firm mattress that is fitted so that no more than two fingers can fit between the mattress and the crib side in the lowest position. The minimum height from the top of the mattress to the top of the crib rail should be twenty inches in the highest position. Cribs with drop sides should not be used. The crib should not have corner post extensions (over one-sixteenth inch). The crib should have no cutout openings in the head board or footboard structure in which a child's head could become entrapped. The mattress support system should not be easily dislodged from any point of the crib by an upward force from underneath the crib. All cribs should meet the ASTM F1169-10a Standard Consumer Safety Specification for Full-Size Baby Cribs, F406-10b Standard Consumer Safety Specification for Non-Full-Size Baby Cribs/Play Yards, or the CPSC 16 CFR 1219, 1220, and 1500 – Safety Standards for Full-Size Baby Cribs and Non-Full-Size Baby Cribs; Final Rule.

Cribs should be placed away from window blinds or draperies.

As soon as a child can stand up, the mattress should be adjusted to its lowest position. Once a child can climb out of his/her crib, the child should be moved to a bed. Children should never be kept in their crib by placing, tying, or wedging various fabric, mesh, or other strong coverings over the top of the crib.

Cribs intended for evacuation purpose should be of a design and have wheels that are suitable for carrying up to five non-ambulatory children less than two years of age to a designated evacuation area. This crib should be used for evacuation in the event of fire or other emergency. The crib should be easily moveable and should be able to fit through the designated fire exit.

RATIONALE: Standards have been developed to define crib safety, and staff should make sure that cribs used in the facility meet these standards to protect children and prevent injuries or death (1-3). Significant changes to the ATSM and CPSC standards for cribs were published in December 2010. As of June 28, 2011 all cribs being manufactured, sold or leased must meet the new stringent requirements. Effective December 28, 2012 all cribs being used in early care and education facilities including family child care homes must also meet these standards. For the most current information about these new standards please go to http://www.cpsc.gov/info/cribs/index.html.

More infants die every year in incidents involving cribs than with any other nursery product (4). Children have become trapped or have strangled because their head or neck became caught in a gap between slats that was too wide or between the mattress and crib side.

An infant can suffocate if its head or body becomes wedged between the mattress and the crib sides (6).

Corner posts present a potential for clothing entanglement and strangulation (5). Asphyxial crib deaths from wedging the head or neck in parts of the crib and hanging by a necklace or clothing over a corner post have been well-documented (6).

Children who are thirty-five inches or taller in height have outgrown a crib and should not use a crib for sleeping (4). Turning a crib into a cage (covering over the crib) is not a

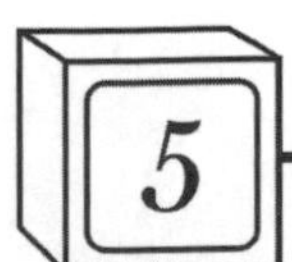

safe solution for the problems caused by children climbing out. Children have died trying to escape their modified cribs by getting caught in the covering in various ways and firefighters trying to rescue children from burning homes have been slowed down by the crib covering (6).

CPSC has received numerous reports of strangulation deaths on window blind cords over the years (7).

COMMENTS: For more information on articles in cribs, see Standard 5.4.5.1: Sleeping Equipment and Supplies and Standard 6.4.1.3: Crib Toys.

A "safety-approved crib" is one that has been certified by the Juvenile Product Manufacturers Association (JPMA).

If portable cribs and those that are not full-size are substituted for regular full-sized cribs, they must be maintained in the condition that meets the ASTM F406-10b Standard Consumer Safety Specification for Non-Full-Size Baby Cribs/Play Yards. Portable cribs are designed so they may be folded or collapsed, with or without disassembly. Although portable cribs are not designed to withstand the wear and tear of normal full-sized cribs, they may provide more flexibility for programs that vary the number of infants in care from time to time.

Cribs designed to be used as evacuation cribs, can be used to evacuate infants, if rolling is possible on the evacuation route(s).

To keep window blind cords out of the reach of children, staff can use tie-down devices or take the cord loop and cut it in half to make two separate cords. Consumers can call 1-800-506-4636 or visit the Window Covering Safety Council Website at http://windowcoverings.org to receive a free repair kit for each set of blinds.

TYPE OF FACILITY: Center; Large Family Child Care Home; Small Family Child Care Home

RELATED STANDARDS:
Standard 3.1.4.1: Safe Sleep Practices and SIDS/Suffocation Risk Reduction
Standard 5.4.5.1: Sleeping Equipment and Supplies
Standard 5.4.5.3: Stackable Cribs
Standard 6.4.1.3: Crib Toys

REFERENCES:

1. ASTM International. 2010. ASTM F1169-10a: *Standard consumer safety specification for full-size baby cribs*. West Conshohocken, PA: ASTM.
2. ASTM International. 2010. ASTM F406-10b*: Standard consumer safety specification for non-full-size baby cribs/play yards*. West Conshohocken, PA: ASTM.
3. U.S. Consumer Product Safety Commission (CPSC). 2010. Safety standards for full-size baby cribs and non-full-size baby cribs; final rule. 16 CFR 1219, 1220, and 1500. http://www.cpsc.gov/businfo/frnotices/fr11/cribfinal.pdf.
4. U.S. Consumer Product Safety Commission (CPSC). 1997. *The safe nursery*. Washington, DC: CPSC. http://www.cpsc.gov/cpscpub/pubs/202.pdf.
5. Juvenile Products Manufacturers Association. 2007. *Safe and sound for baby: A guide to juvenile product safety, use, and selection*. 9th ed. Moorestown, NJ: JPMA. http://www.jpma.org/content/retailers/safe-and-sound/.
6. U.S. Consumer Product Safety Commission (CPSC). 1996. CPSC warns parents about infant strangulations caused by failure of crib hardware. Document #5025. http://www.cpsc.gov/cpscpub/pubs/5025.html.
7. U.S. Consumer Product Safety Commission (CPSC). *Are your window coverings safe?* http://www.cpsc.gov/cpscpub/pubs/5009a.pdf.

STANDARD 5.4.5.3: Stackable Cribs

Use of stackable cribs (i.e., cribs that are built in a manner that there are two or three cribs above each other that do not touch the ground floor) in facilities is not advised. In older facilities, where these cribs are already built into the structure of the facility, staff should develop a plan for phasing out the use of these cribs.

If stackable cribs are used, they must meet the current Consumer Product Safety Commission's (CPSC) federal standard for non-full-size cribs, 16 CFR 1220. In addition they should be three feet apart and staff placing or removing a child from a crib that cannot reach from standing on the floor, should use a stable climbing device such as a permanent ladder rather than climbing on a stool or chair. Infants who are able to sit, pull themselves up, etc. should not be placed in stackable cribs.

RATIONALE: Stackable cribs are designed to save space by having one crib built on top of another. Although they may be practical from the standpoint of saving space, infants on the top level of stackable cribs will be positioned at a height that will be several feet from the floor. Infants who fall from several feet or more can have an intracranial hemorrhage (i.e., serious bleed inside of the skull). While no injury reports have been filed, there is a potential for injury as a result of either latch malfunction or a caregiver/teacher who slips or falls while placing or removing a child from a crib. It is best practice to place an infant to sleep in a safe sleep environment (safety-approved crib with a firm mattress and a tight-fitting sheet) at a level that is close to the floor.

A minimum distance of three feet between cribs is required because respiratory infections are transmitted by large droplets of respiratory secretions, which usually are limited to a range of less than three feet from the infected person. (1).

Young children placed to sleep in stackable cribs may have difficulties falling asleep because they may not be used to sleeping in this type of equipment. In addition, requiring staff to use stackable cribs may cause them concern and fear regarding their liability if an injury occurs.

COMMENTS: Many state child care licensing regulations prohibit the use of stackable cribs (2). If stackable cribs are not prohibited in the caregiver's/teacher's state and they are used, parents/guardians should be informed and extreme care should be taken to ensure that no infant falls from the higher level cribs due to the potential for injury. Any injury that is suspected to be related to the use of stackable cribs should be reported to the U.S. Consumer Product Safety Commission (CPSC) at 1-800-638-2772 or http://www.cpsc.gov.

TYPE OF FACILITY: Center; Large Family Child Care Home; Small Family Child Care Home

RELATED STANDARDS:
Standard 5.4.5.1: Sleeping Equipment and Supplies
Standard 5.4.5.2: Cribs

REFERENCES:
1. Pickering, L. K., C. J. Baker, D. W. Kimberlin, S. S. Long, eds. 2009. *Red book: 2009 report of the Committee on Infectious Diseases, 153*. Elk Grove Village, IL: American Academy of Pediatrics.
2. National Resource Center for Health and Safety in Child Care and Early Education (NRC). 2010. NRC Website. Individual states' child care licensure regulations. http://nrckids.org/STATES/states.htm.

STANDARD 5.4.5.4: Futons

Child-sized futons should be used only if they meet the following requirements:

a) Not on a frame;
b) Easily cleanable;
c) Encased in a tight-fitting waterproof cover;
d) Meet all other standards on sleep and rest areas (Section 5.4.5).

RATIONALE: Frames pose an entrapment hazard. Futons that are easy to clean can be kept sanitary. Supervision is necessary to maintain adequate spacing of futons and ensure that bedding is not shared, thereby reducing transmission of infectious diseases and keeping children out of traffic areas.

TYPE OF FACILITY: Center; Large Family Child Care Home; Small Family Child Care Home

STANDARD 5.4.5.5: Bunk Beds

Children younger than six years of age should not use the upper levels of double-deck beds (or "bunk beds"). Bunk beds must conform to the U.S. Consumer Product Safety Commission (CPSC) Facts Document #071, Bunk Beds and the ASTM F1427-07 Standard Consumer Safety Specification for Bunk Beds (1).

RATIONALE: Falls and entrapment between mattress and guardrails, bed structure and wall, or between slats from bunk beds are a well-documented cause of injury in young children (1).

COMMENTS: Consult the CPSC, the manufacturer's label, or the consumer safety information provided by the American Furniture Manufacturer's Association (AFMA) for advice. Check the ASTM Website, http://www.astm.org, for up to date Standards.

TYPE OF FACILITY: Center; Large Family Child Care Home; Small Family Child Care Home

REFERENCES:
1. ASTM International. ASTM F1427-07: *Standard consumer safety specification for bunk beds*. West Conshohocken, PA: ASTM International.

5.4.6 Space for Children Who Are Ill, Injured, or Need Special Therapies

STANDARD 5.4.6.1: Space for Children Who Are Ill

Each facility should have a separate room or designated area within a room for the temporary or ongoing care of a child who needs to be separated from the group because of injury or illness. This room or area should be located so the child may be supervised and may be within the child's usual child care room. Toilet and lavatory facilities should be readily accessible. If the child under care is suspected of having an infectious disease, all equipment the child uses should be cleaned and sanitized after use. This room or area may be used for other purposes when it is not needed for the separation and care of a child or if the uses do not conflict.

RATIONALE: Children who are injured or ill may need to be separated from other children to provide for rest and to minimize the spread of potential infectious disease (1). It is best practice for toilet and lavatory facilities to be readily available to permit frequent handwashing when children are well and even more so when they are ill. Proximity should provide rapid access in the event of vomiting or diarrhea to avoid contaminating the environment. Handwashing sinks should be stationed in each room not only to provide the opportunity to maintain cleanliness but also to permit the caregiver/teacher to maintain continuous supervision of the other children in care.

TYPE OF FACILITY: Center; Large Family Child Care Home; Small Family Child Care Home

RELATED STANDARDS:
Standard 3.6.1.1: Inclusion/Exclusion/Dismissal of Children
Standards 3.6.2.2-3.6.2.10: Care of Children Who are Ill
Standard 9.2.3.2: Content and Development of the Plan for Care of Children and Staff Who Are Ill

REFERENCES:
1. Pickering, L. K., C. J. Baker, D. W. Kimberlin, S. S. Long, eds. 2009. *Red book: 2009 report of the Committee on Infectious Diseases, 153*. Elk Grove Village, IL: American Academy of Pediatrics.

STANDARD 5.4.6.2: Space for Therapy Services

In addition to accessible classrooms, in facilities where some but fewer than fifteen children need occupational or physical therapy and some but fewer than twenty children need individual speech therapy, centers should provide a quiet, private, accessible area within the child care facility for therapy. No other activities should take place in this area at the time therapy is being provided.

Family child care homes and facilities integrating children who need therapy services should receive these services in a space that is separate and private during the time the child is receiving therapy.

Additional space may be needed for equipment according to a child's needs.

RATIONALE: Quiet, private space is necessary for physical, occupational, and speech therapies (1). Most caregivers/teachers also indicate that the other children in the facility are disrupted less if the therapies are provided in a separate area. For speech therapy, working with the child in a quiet location is especially important. Caregivers/teachers should attempt to incorporate therapeutic principles into the child's general child care activities. Doing so will achieve maximum benefit for the child receiving therapy and promote understanding on the part of the child's peers and caregivers/teachers about how to address the child's disability when the therapist is not present.

TYPE OF FACILITY: Center; Large Family Child Care Home; Small Family Child Care Home

REFERENCES:

1. Olds, A. R. 2001. Zoning a group room. In *Child care design guide*, 137-165. New York: McGraw-Hill.

5.5 Storage Areas

Note to Reader: *See Standard 3.6.3.2 for medication storage.*

STANDARD 5.5.0.1: Storage and Labeling of Personal Articles

The facility should provide separate storage areas for each child's and staff member's personal articles and clothing. Personal effects and clothing should be labeled with the child's name. Bedding should be labeled with the child's full name, stored separately for each child, and not touching other children's personal items.

If children use the following items at the child care facility, those items should be stored in separate, clean containers and should be labeled with the child's full name:

a) Individual cloth towels for bathing purposes;
b) Toothbrushes;
c) Washcloths;
d) Combs and brushes.

Toothbrushes, towels, and washcloths should be allowed to dry when they are stored and not touching.

RATIONALE: This standard prevents the spread of organisms that cause disease and promotes organization of a child's personal possessions. Lice infestation, scabies, and ringworm are common infectious diseases in child care. Providing space so personal items may be stored separately helps to prevent the spread of these diseases.

TYPE OF FACILITY: Center; Large Family Child Care Home; Small Family Child Care Home

RELATED STANDARDS:

Standard 3.6.1.5: Sharing of Personal Articles Prohibited
Standard 3.6.3.2: Labeling, Storage, and Disposal of Medications
Standard 5.4.5.1: Sleeping Equipment and Supplies

STANDARD 5.5.0.2: Coat Hooks/Cubicles

Coat hooks should be spaced so coats will not touch each other, or individual cubicles or lockers of the child's height should be provided for storing children's clothing and personal possessions.

RATIONALE: Ringworm is a common infectious disease in child care and can be transmitted by sharing personal articles such as combs, towels, clothing, and bedding (1). Providing space so personal items may be stored separately helps prevent the spread of disease.

COMMENTS: Whenever possible, coat hooks should not be placed at children's eye level because of potential risk of injury to eyes. Safety hooks should be used instead.

TYPE OF FACILITY: Center; Large Family Child Care Home; Small Family Child Care Home

REFERENCES:

1. Pickering, L. K., C. J. Baker, D. W. Kimberlin, S. S. Long, eds. 2009. *Red book: 2009 report of the Committee on Infectious Diseases, 661-662*. Elk Grove Village, IL: American Academy of Pediatrics.

STANDARD 5.5.0.3: Storage of Play and Teaching Equipment and Supplies

The facility should provide and use space to store play and teaching equipment, supplies, records and files, cots, mats, and bedding. Children should not have unsupervised access to storage areas.

RATIONALE: This practice enhances safety and provides a good example of an orderly environment.

TYPE OF FACILITY: Center; Large Family Child Care Home; Small Family Child Care Home

STANDARD 5.5.0.4: Storage for Soiled and Clean Linens

Child care facilities should provide separate storage areas for soiled linen and clean linen. Children should not have unsupervised access to storage areas.

RATIONALE: This practice discourages contamination of clean areas and children from soiled and contaminated linen. Providing separate storage areas reduces fire load and helps contain fire, if spontaneous combustion occurs in soiled linens.

TYPE OF FACILITY: Center; Large Family Child Care Home; Small Family Child Care Home

STANDARD 5.5.0.5: Storage of Flammable Materials

Gasoline, hand sanitizers*** in volume, and other flammable materials should be stored in a separate building, in a locked area, away from high temperatures and ignition sources***, and inaccessible to children.

RATIONALE: Flammable materials such as chemicals and cleaners account for the majority of burns to the head and face of children (1). These materials are also involved in unintentional ingestion by children.

TYPE OF FACILITY: Center; Large Family Child Care Home; Small Family Child Care Home

***Addition to Standard in second printing, August 2011

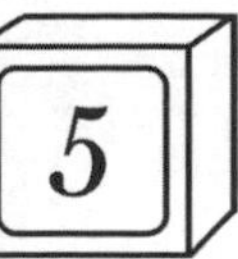

REFERENCES:
1. D'Souza, A. L., N. G. Nelson, L. B. McKenzie. 2009. Pediatric burn injuries treated in US emergency departments between 1990 and 2006. *Pediatrics* 124:1424-30.

STANDARD 5.5.0.6: Inaccessibility to Matches, Candles, and Lighters

Matches, candles, and lighters should not be accessible to children.

RATIONALE: The U.S. Consumer Product Safety Commission (CPSC) estimates that 150 deaths occur each year from fires started by children playing with lighters. Children under five-years-old account for most of these fatalities (1). A child playing with candles or near candles is one of the biggest contributors to candle fires (2). Matches have also been the source of some fire-related deaths. Children may hide in a closet or under a bed when faced with fire, leading to fatalities (2).

TYPE OF FACILITY: Center; Large Family Child Care Home; Small Family Child Care Home

REFERENCES:
1. U.S. Consumer Product Safety Commission (CPSC). *Child-resistant lighters protect young children*. Document #5021. Bethesda, MD: CPSC. http://www.cpsc.gov/cpscpub/pubs/5021.html.
2. Miller, D., R. Chowdhury, M. Greene. 2009. *2004-2006 residential fire loss estimates*. Washington, DC: U.S. Consumer Product Safety Commission (CPSC). http://www.cpsc.gov/LIBRARY/fire06.pdf.

STANDARD 5.5.0.7: Storage of Plastic Bags

Plastic bags, whether intended for storage, trash, diaper disposal, or any other purpose, should be stored out of reach of children.

RATIONALE: Plastic bags have been recognized for many years as a cause of suffocation. Warnings regarding this risk are printed on diaper-pail bags, dry-cleaning bags, and so forth. The U.S. Consumer Product Safety Commission (CPSC) has received average annual reports of twenty-five deaths per year to children due to suffocation from plastic bags. Nearly 90% of the reported deaths were to children under the age of one (1).

TYPE OF FACILITY: Center; Large Family Child Care Home; Small Family Child Care Home

REFERENCES:
1. U.S. Consumer Product Safety Commission (CPSC). *Children still suffocating with plastic bags*. Document #5064. Bethesda, MD: CPSC. http://www.cpsc.gov/CPSCPUB/PUBS/5064.html.

STANDARD 5.5.0.8: Firearms

Centers should not have any firearms, pellet or BB guns (loaded or unloaded), darts, bows and arrows, cap pistols, stun guns, paint ball guns, or objects manufactured for play as toy guns within the premises at any time. If present in a small or large family child care home, these items must be unloaded, equipped with child protective devices, and kept under lock and key with the ammunition locked separately in areas inaccessible to the children. Parents/guardians should be informed about this policy.

RATIONALE: The potential for injury to and death of young children due to firearms is apparent (1-5). These items should not be accessible to children in a facility (2,3).

COMMENTS: Compliance is monitored via inspection.

TYPE OF FACILITY: Center; Large Family Child Care Home; Small Family Child Care Home

REFERENCES:
1. American Academy of Pediatrics, Committee on Injury and Poison Prevention. 2004. Policy statement: Firearm-related injuries affecting the pediatric population. *Pediatrics* 114:1126.
2. DiScala, C., R. Sege. 2004. Outcomes in children and young adults who are hospitalized for firearms-related injuries. *Pediatrics* 113:1306-12.
3. Grossman, D. C., B. A. Mueller, C. Riedy, et al. 2005. Gun storage practices and risk of youth suicide and unintentional firearm injuries. *JAMA* 296:707-14.
4. Katcher, M. L., A. N. Meister., C. A. Sorkness, A. G. Staresinic, S. E. Pierce, B. M. Goodman, N. M. Peterson, P. M. Hatfield, J. A. Schirmer. 2006. Use of the modified Delphi technique to identify and rate home injury hazard risks and prevention methods for young children. *Injury Prev* 12:189-94.
5. Hemenway, D., D. Weil. 1990. Phasers on stun: The case for less lethal weapons. *J Policy Analysis Management* 9:94-98.

5.6 Supplies

STANDARD 5.6.0.1: First Aid and Emergency Supplies

The facility should maintain first aid and emergency supplies in each location where children are cared for. The first aid kit or supplies should be kept in a closed container, cabinet, or drawer that is labeled and stored in a location known to all staff, accessible to staff at all times, but locked or otherwise inaccessible to children. When children leave the facility for a walk or to be transported, a designated staff member should bring a transportable first aid kit. In addition, a transportable first aid kit should be in each vehicle that is used to transport children to and from a child care facility.

First aid kits or supplies should be restocked after use. An inventory of first aid supplies should be conducted at least monthly. A log should be kept that lists the date that each inventory was conducted, verification that expiration dates of supplies were checked, location of supplies (i.e., in the facility supply, transportable first aid kit(s), etc.), and the legal name/signature of the staff member who completed the inventory.

The first aid kit should contain at least the following items:

a) Disposable nonporous, latex-free or non-powdered latex gloves (latex-free recommended);
b) Scissors;
c) Tweezers;
d) Non-glass, non-mercury thermometer to measure a child's temperature;
e) Bandage tape;
f) Sterile gauze pads;

g) Flexible roller gauze;
h) Triangular bandages;
i) Safety pins;
j) Eye patch or dressing;
k) Pen/pencil and note pad;
l) Cold pack;
m) Current American Academy of Pediatrics (AAP) standard first aid chart or equivalent first aid guide such as the AAP *Pediatric First Aid For Caregivers and Teachers (PedFACTS) Manual*;
n) Coins for use in a pay phone and cell phone;
o) Water (two liters of sterile water for cleaning wounds or eyes);
p) Liquid soap to wash injury and hand sanitizer, used with supervision, if hands are not visibly soiled or if no water is present;
q) Tissues;
r) Wipes;
s) Individually wrapped sanitary pads to contain bleeding of injuries;
t) Adhesive strip bandages, plastic bags for cloths, gauze, and other materials used in handling blood;
u) Flashlight;
v) Whistle;
w) Battery-powered radio (1).

When children walk or are transported to another location, the transportable first aid kit should include ALL items listed above AND the following emergency information/items:

a) List of children in attendance (organized by caregiver/teacher they are assigned to) and their emergency contact information (i.e., parents/guardian/emergency contact home, work, and cell phone numbers);
b) Special care plans for children who have them;
c) Emergency medications or supplies as specified in the special care plans;
d) List of emergency contacts (i.e., location information and phone numbers for the Poison Center, nearby hospitals or other emergency care clinics, and other community resource agencies);
e) Maps;
f) Written transportation policy and contingency plans.

RATIONALE: Facilities must place emphasis on safeguarding each child and ensuring that the staff members are able to handle emergencies (2).

COMMENTS: Many centers simply leave a first aid kit in all vehicles used to transport children, regardless of whether the vehicle is used to take a child to or from a center, or for outings. Maps are required in case transporting staff need to find an alternate way back to the facility or another route to emergency services when roads are closed and/or communication and power systems are inaccessible. Programs may want to have access to hand-held or stationary electronic/cellular, or satellite devices (e.g., GIS systems or phones that include relevant features) when transporting to help locate alternative routes during an emergency.

Syrup of Ipecac should not be used to induce vomiting and should not be included in first aid kits or available at a child care program (1). Contact the local poison center at 1-800-222-1222 for instructions if needed.

Hand sanitizers may be used under supervision as an alternative to washing hands with soap and water if wipes are used to remove visible soil before the hand sanitizer is applied.

TYPE OF FACILITY: Center; Large Family Child Care Home; Small Family Child Care Home

RELATED STANDARDS:

Standard 3.2.2.5: Hand Sanitizers
Standard 3.6.1.3: Thermometers for Taking Human Temperatures

REFERENCES:

1. American Academy of Pediatrics. 2007. *Pediatric first aid for caregivers and teachers*. Rev ed. Elk Grove Village, IL: AAP. http://www.pedfactsonline.com/.
2. Fiene, R. 2002. *13 indicators of quality child care: Research update*. Washington, DC: U.S. Department of Health and Human Services, Office of the Assistant Secretary for Planning and Evaluation. http://aspe.hhs.gov/hsp/ccquality-ind02/.

STANDARD 5.6.0.2: Single Service Cups

Single service cups should be dispensed by staff or in a cup dispenser approved by the regulatory health authority. Single service cups should not be reused.

RATIONALE: Reusing cups, even by the same person, allows growth of organisms in the cup between uses.

TYPE OF FACILITY: Center; Large Family Child Care Home; Small Family Child Care Home

STANDARD 5.6.0.3: Supplies for Bathrooms and Handwashing Sinks

Bathrooms and handwashing sinks should be supplied with:

a) Liquid soap, hand sanitizer, hand lotion, and paper towels or other hand-drying devices approved by the regulatory health authority, within arm's reach of the user of each sink;
b) Toilet paper, within arm's reach of the user of each toilet.

The facility should permit the use of only single-use cloth or disposable paper towels. The shared use of a towel should be prohibited. All tissues and disposable towels should be discarded into an appropriate waste container after use.

RATIONALE: Lack of supplies discourages necessary handwashing. Cracks in the skin and excessive dryness from frequent handwashing discourage the staff from complying with necessary hygiene and may lead to increased bacterial accumulation on hands. The availability of hand lotion to prevent dryness encourages staff members to wash their hands more often. Supplies must be within arm's reach of the user to prevent contamination of the environment with waste, water, or excretion.

Shared cloth towels can transmit infectious disease. Even though a child may use a cloth towel that is solely for that child's use, preventing shared use of towels is difficult. Disposable towels prevent this problem, but once used, must

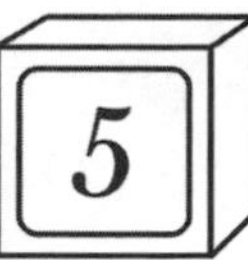

be discarded. Many infectious diseases can be prevented through appropriate hygiene and sanitation.

COMMENTS: Bar soap should not be used by children or staff. Liquid soap is widely available, economical, and easily used by staff and children. If anyone is sensitive to the type of product used, a substitute product that accommodates this special need should be used.

A disposable towel dispenser that dispenses the towel without having to touch the container or the fresh towel supply is better than towel dispensers in which the person must use a lever to get a towel, or handle the towel supply to remove one towel. Some roller devices dispense one towel at a time from a paper towel roll; some commercial dispensers hold either a large roll or a pile of folded towels inside the dispenser, with the towel intended for next use sticking out of the opening of the dispenser.

TYPE OF FACILITY: Center; Large Family Child Care Home; Small Family Child Care Home

RELATED STANDARDS:
Standard 3.2.2.5: Hand Sanitizers

STANDARD 5.6.0.4: Microfiber Cloths, Rags, and Disposable Towels and Mops Used for Cleaning

Microfiber cloths should be preferred for cleaning. They should be laundered between each use. If microfiber cloths are not appropriate for use, disposable towels should be preferred for cleaning. If clean reusable rags are used, they should be laundered separately between each one-time use for cleaning. Disposable towels should be sealed in a plastic bag and removed to outside garbage. Cloth rags should be placed in a closed, foot-operated, plastic-lined receptacle until laundering. When a mop is needed, microfiber mops should be considered as a preferred cleaning method over conventional loop mops. Use of sponges in child care facilities for cleaning purposes is not recommended.

RATIONALE: Microfiber cloths are superior at picking up bacteria and holding it in the fibers. The microfiber mopping system offers many health and safety benefits. The microfiber mopping system is as effective as using the traditional loop mop method, yet there is a reduction in the use of and exposure to harsh disinfectant chemicals (2). Additionally, the microfiber mops are lighter and easier to use than conventional mops thus lessening the potential for worker muscle sprains (1). The system leaves only a light film of water on the floor that dries quickly, thus lessening the potential for worker injury for slips and falls on a wet floor. Materials used for cleaning become contaminated in the process and must be handled so they do not spread potentially infectious material (3).

COMMENTS: Sponges generally are contaminated with bacteria and are difficult to clean.

For more detailed information on microfiber cloths and mopping, see Sustainable Hospitals Project EPA Best Practices Publication *Using Microfiber Mops in Hospitals,* available at http://www.epa.gov/region9/waste/p2/projects/hospital/mops.pdf.

TYPE OF FACILITY: Center; Large Family Child Care Home; Small Family Child Care Home

REFERENCES:
1. Sustainable Hospitals Project, University of Massachusetts–Lowell. 2003. *10 reasons to use microfiber mopping*. http://www.sustainablehospitals.org/PDF/tenreasonsmop.pdf.
2. Sustainable Hospitals Project, University of Massachusetts–Lowell. 2003. *Are microfiber mops beneficial for hospitals?* http://www.sustainablehospitals.org/PDF/MicrofiberMopCS.pdf.
3. Hoyle, M., B. Slezak. 2008. Understanding microfiber's role in infection. *Infection Control Today* (May). http://www.infectioncontroltoday.com/articles/2008/11/understanding-microfiber-s-role-in-infection-prev.aspx.

5.7 Maintenance

STANDARD 5.7.0.1: Maintenance of Exterior Surfaces

Porches, steps, stairs, and walkways should:

a) Be maintained free from accumulations of water, ice, or snow;
b) Have a non-slip surface;
c) Be kept free of loose objects;
d) Be in good repair;
e) Be free of flaking paint.

RATIONALE: Trip surfaces lead to injury. Flaking lead-based paint can be ingested in sufficient quantities to cause lead poisoning (1,2,3).

TYPE OF FACILITY: Center; Large Family Child Care Home; Small Family Child Care Home

RELATED STANDARDS:
Standard 5.2.9.13: Testing for Lead

REFERENCES:
1. U.S. Consumer Product Safety Commission (CPSC). What you should know about lead based paint in your home: Safety alert. http://www.cpsc.gov/cpscpub/pubs/5054.html.
2. Centers for Disease Control and Prevention (CDC). 2005. *Preventing lead poisoning in young children*. Atlanta, GA: CDC. http://www.cdc.gov/nceh/lead/publications/PrevLeadPoisoning.pdf.
3. U.S. Environmental Protection Agency (EPA). 2010. *The lead-safe certified guide to renovate right*. Washington, DC: EPA. http://www.epa.gov/lead/pubs/renovaterightbrochure.pdf.

STANDARD 5.7.0.2: Removal of Hazards From Outdoor Areas

All outdoor activity areas should be maintained in a clean and safe condition by removing:

a) Debris;
b) Dilapidated structures;
c) Broken or worn play equipment;
d) Building supplies and equipment;
e) Glass;
f) Sharp rocks;
g) Stumps and roots;
h) Branches;

i) Animal excrement;
j) Tobacco waste (cigarette butts);
k) Garbage;
l) Toxic plants;
m) Anthills;
n) Beehives and wasp nests;
o) Unprotected ditches;
p) Wells;
q) Holes;
r) Grease traps;
s) Cisterns;
t) Cesspools;
u) Unprotected utility equipment;
v) Other injurious material.

Holes or abandoned wells within the site should be properly filled or sealed. The area should be well-drained, with no standing water.

A maintenance policy for playgrounds and outdoor areas should be established and followed.

RATIONALE: Proper maintenance is a key factor when trying to ensure a safe play environment for children. Each playground is unique and requires a routine maintenance check program developed specifically for that setting.

TYPE OF FACILITY: Center; Large Family Child Care; Small Family Child Care Home

RELATED STANDARDS:
Standard 6.2.5.1: Inspection of Indoor and Outdoor Play Areas and Equipment
Standard 6.2.5.2: Inspection of Play Area Surfacing
Standard 9.2.6.1: Policy on Use and Maintenance of Play Areas

STANDARD 5.7.0.3: Removal of Allergen Triggering Materials From Outdoor Areas

Outdoor areas should be kept free of excessive dust, weeds, brush, high grass, and standing water.

RATIONALE: Dust, weeds, brush, and high grass are potential allergens (1). Standing water breeds insects.

TYPE OF FACILITY: Center; Large Family Child Care Home; Small Family Child Care Home

REFERENCES:
1. Asthma and Allergy Foundation of America. 2005. Allergy overview. http://www.aafa.org/display.cfm?id=9&cont=82/.

STANDARD 5.7.0.4: Inaccessibility of Hazardous Equipment

Any hazardous equipment should be made inaccessible to children by barriers, or removed until rendered safe or replaced. The barriers should not pose any hazard.

RATIONALE: Limiting access to hazardous equipment can prevent injuries to children and staff in child care.

COMMENTS: Examples of barriers to equipment that pose a safety hazard are structures (including fences) that children can climb, prickly bushes, and standing bodies of water. Barriers such as plastic orange construction site fencing could be used to block access. While not child proof, it is conspicuous and sends a message that it is there to prevent access to the equipment it surrounds.

TYPE OF FACILITY: Center; Large Family Child Care Home; Small Family Child Care Home

STANDARD 5.7.0.5: Cleaning Schedule for Exterior Areas

A cleaning schedule for exterior areas should be developed and assigned to appropriate staff members. Delegated staff members should actively look for flaking or peeling paint while cleaning the exterior areas. If flaking/peeling paint is found, it should be tested for lead. If the paint is found to contain lead, the area should be covered by latex-based paint to create a barrier between the lead-based paint and the children in care.

RATIONALE: Developing a cleaning schedule that delegates responsibility to specific staff members helps ensure that the child care facility is appropriately cleaned. Proper cleaning reduces the risk of injury and the transmission of disease.

Lead paint chips may be ingested by young children and lead to neurological and behavioral problems. Covering the lead paint with latex paint reduces toxic exposure (1-3).

TYPE OF FACILITY: Center; Large Family Child Care Home; Small Family Child Care Home

RELATED STANDARDS:
Standard 5.2.9.13: Testing for Lead

REFERENCES:
1. U.S. Consumer Product Safety Commission (CPSC). What you should know about lead based paint in your home: Safety alert. http://www.cpsc.gov/cpscpub/pubs/5054.html.
2. Centers for Disease Control and Prevention (CDC). 2005. *Preventing lead poisoning in young children*. Atlanta, GA: CDC. http://www.cdc.gov/nceh/lead/publications/PrevLeadPoisoning.pdf.
3. U.S. Environmental Protection Agency (EPA). 2010. *The lead-safe certified guide to renovate right*. Washington, DC: EPA. http://www.epa.gov/lead/pubs/renovaterightbrochure.pdf.

STANDARD 5.7.0.6: Storage Area Maintenance and Ventilation

Storage areas should have appropriate lighting and be kept clean. If the area is a storage room, the area should be mechanically ventilated to the outdoors when chemicals or a janitorial sink are present.

RATIONALE: Spilled items must be removed to promote health and safety. Spilled dry foods could attract rodent and insects. Chemicals and janitorial supplies can build up toxic fumes that can leak into occupied areas if they are not ventilated to the outdoors (1).

TYPE OF FACILITY: Center; Large Family Child Care Home; Small Family Child Care Home

REFERENCES:
1. U.S. Environmental Protection Agency. An introduction to indoor air quality. http://www.epa.gov/iaq/voc.html.

STANDARD 5.7.0.7: Structure Maintenance

The structure should be kept in good repair and safe condition.

Each window, exterior door, and basement or cellar hatchway should be kept in sound condition and in good repair.

RATIONALE: Older preschool-age and younger school-age children readily engage in play and explore their environments. The physical structure where children spend each day can present caregivers/teachers with special safety concerns if the structure is not kept in good repair and maintained in a safe condition. For example, peeling paint in an older building may be ingested, floor surfaces in disrepair could cause falls and other injury, and broken glass windows could cause severe cuts or other glass injury (1).

Children's environments must be protected from exposure to moisture, dust, and excessive temperatures.

TYPE OF FACILITY: Center; Large Family Child Care Home; Small Family Child Care Home

RELATED STANDARDS:
Standard 5.1.1.6: Structurally Sound Facility

REFERENCES:
1. Whole Building Design Guide Secure/Safe Committee. 2010. Ensure occupant safety and health. National Institute of Building Sciences. http://www.wbdg.org/design/ensure_health.php.

STANDARD 5.7.0.8: Electrical Fixtures and Outlets Maintenance

Electrical fixtures and outlets should be maintained in safe condition and good repair.

RATIONALE: Unsafe or broken electrical fixtures and outlets could expose children to serious electrical shock or electrocution. Loose or frayed wires are also unsafe.

COMMENTS: Running an appliance or extension cord underneath a carpet or rug is not recommended because the cord could fray or become worn and cause a fire (1).

TYPE OF FACILITY: Center; Large Family Child Care Home; Small Family Child Care Home

RELATED STANDARDS:
Standard 5.2.4.2: Safety Covers and Shock Protection Devices for Electrical Outlets
Standard 5.2.4.5: Extension Cords
Standard 5.2.4.6: Electrical Cords

REFERENCES:
1. Greiner, D., D. Leduc, eds. 2008. *Well beings: A guide to health in child care*. 3rd ed. Ottawa, ON: Canadian Paediatric Society.

STANDARD 5.7.0.9: Plumbing and Gas Maintenance

Each gas pipe, water pipe, gas-burning fixture, plumbing fixture and apparatus, or any other similar fixture, and all connections to water, sewer, or gas lines should be maintained in good, sanitary working condition.

RATIONALE: Pipe maintenance prevents injuries from hazardous and unsanitary conditions.

TYPE OF FACILITY: Center; Large Family Child Care Home; Small Family Child Care Home

RELATED STANDARDS:
Standard 5.2.6.8: Installation of Pipes and Plumbing Fixtures

STANDARD 5.7.0.10: Cleaning of Humidifiers and Related Equipment

Humidifiers, dehumidifiers, and air-handling equipment that involve water should be cleaned and disinfected according to manufacturers' instructions.

RATIONALE: These appliances provide comfort by controlling the amount of moisture in the indoor air. To get the most benefit, the facility should follow all instructions. If the facility does not follow recommended care and maintenance guidelines, microorganisms may be able to grow in the water and become airborne, which may lead to respiratory problems (1).

COMMENTS: For additional information, contact the U.S. Consumer Product Safety Commission (CPSC) and the Association of Home Appliance Manufacturers (AHAM).

TYPE OF FACILITY: Center; Large Family Child Care Home; Small Family Child Care Home

REFERENCES:
1. U.S. Consumer Product Safety Commission (CPSC). CPSC issues alert about care of room humidifiers: Safety alert. Dirty humidifiers may cause health problems. http://www.cpsc.gov/cpscpub/pubs/5046.html.

Chapter 6

6

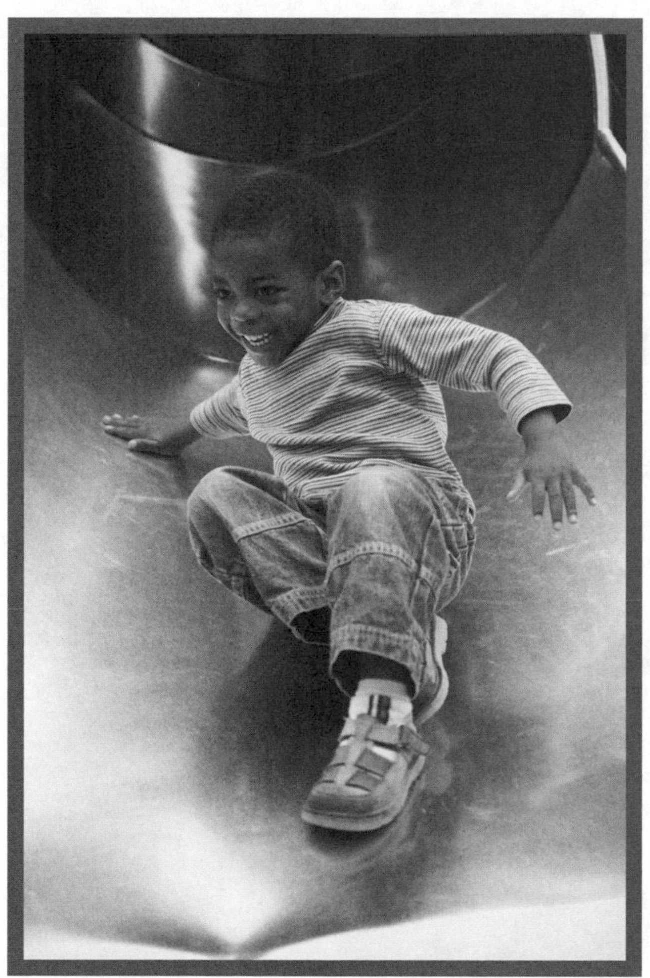

Play Areas/Playgrounds and Transportation

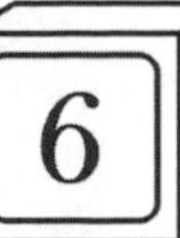

6.1 Play Area/Playground Size and Location

NOTE: The play spaces discussed in the following standards are assumed to be those at the site and thus are the facility's responsibility. Facilities that do not have on-site play areas but that use playgrounds and equipment in adjacent parks and/or schools may not be able to ensure that children in their facility are playing on equipment or in play space in absolute conformance with the standards presented here.

STANDARD 6.1.0.1: Size and Location of Outdoor Play Area

The facility or home should be equipped with an outdoor play area that directly adjoins the indoor facilities or that can be reached by a route that is free of hazards and is no farther than one-eighth mile from the facility. The playground should comprise a minimum of seventy-five square feet for each child using the playground at any one time.

The following exceptions to the space requirements should apply:

a) A minimum of thirty-three square feet of accessible outdoor play space is required for each infant;
b) A minimum of fifty square feet of accessible outdoor play space is required for each child from eighteen to twenty-four months of age.

There should be separated areas for play for the following ages of children:

a) Ages six through twenty-three months
b) Ages two to five years*
c) Ages five to twelve years**

*These areas may be further sub-divided into ages two to three years and four to five years.

** These areas may be further sub-divided into grades K-1, 2-3, and 4-6.

The outdoor playground should include an open space for running that is free of other equipment (4).

RATIONALE: Play areas must be sufficient to allow freedom of movement without collisions among active children.

Providing more square feet per child may correspond to a decrease in the number of injuries associated with gross motor play equipment (1). An aggregate size of greater than 4,200 square feet that includes all of a facility's playgrounds has been associated with significantly greater levels of children's physical activity (5).

In addition, meeting proposed Americans with Disabilities Act (ADA) outdoor play area requirements for accessible routes, and developing natural, outdoor play yards with variety and shade can only be achieved if sufficient outdoor play space is provided.

The space **exceptions** are based on early childhood and playground professionals' experience (2). This follows the developmental ages used for the development of the Standards for play equipment for children.

COMMENTS: Children benefit from being outside as much as possible and it is important to provide sufficient outdoor space to accommodate the full enrollment of children (2). If a facility has less than seventy-five square feet of outdoor space per child, then the facility should augment the outdoor space by providing a large indoor play area (see Standard 6.1.0.2).

Additional space beyond the standard of seventy-five square feet per child may be required to meet ADA outdoor play area requirements, depending on the layout and terrain (3). A Certified Playground Safety Inspector (CPSI) can be utilized for guidance in assisting with outdoor play areas. To locate a CPSI, check the National Park and Recreation Association (NPRA) registry at https://ipv.nrpa.org/CPSI_registry/.

Children may play in older children's areas if the equipment is appropriate for the youngest child present.

TYPE OF FACILITY: Center; Large Family Child Care Home; Small Family Child Care Home

RELATED STANDARDS:
Standard 3.1.3.1: Active Opportunities for Physical Activity
Standard 3.1.3.2: Playing Outdoors
Standard 3.1.3.4: Caregivers'/teachers' Encouragement of Physical Activity
Standard 5.1.1.5: Environmental Audit of Site Location
Standard 6.1.0.2: Size and Requirements of Indoor Play Area

REFERENCES:

1. Ruth, L. C. 2008. Playground design and equipment. Whole Building Design Guide. http://www.wbdg.org/resources/playground.php.
2. Olds, A. R. 2001. *Child care design guide*. New York: McGraw-Hill.
3. Architectural and Transportation Barriers Compliance Board (U.S. Access Board). 2005. *Accessible play areas: A summary of accessibility guidelines for play areas*. http://www.access-board.gov/play/guide/guide.pdf.
4. Brown, W. H., K. A. Pfeiffer, K. L. McIver, M. Dowda, C. L. Addy, R. R. Pate. 2009. Social and environmental factors associated with preschoolers' nonsedentary physical activity. *Child Devel* 80:45-58.
5. Dowda, M., W. H. Brown, C. Addy, K. A. Pfeiffer, K. L. McIver, R. R. Pate. 2009. Policies and characteristics of the preschool environment and physical activity of young children. *Pediatrics* 123: e261-66.

STANDARD 6.1.0.2: Size and Requirements of Indoor Play Area

If a facility has less than seventy-five square feet of accessible outdoor space per child or provides active play space indoors for other reasons, a large indoor activity room that meets the requirement for seventy-five square feet per child may be used if it meets the following requirements:

a) It provides for types of activities equivalent to those performed in an outdoor play space;
b) The area is ventilated with fresh, temperate air at a minimum of five cubic feet per minute per occupant when open windows are not possible;
c) The surfaces and finishes are shock-absorbing, as required for outdoor installations in Standard 6.2.3.1;

d) The play equipment meets the requirements for outdoor installation as stated in Standards 6.2.1.3-6.2.1.6 and Standards 6.2.2.3-6.2.2.4.

There should be separated areas for play for the following ages of children:

a) Ages six through twenty-three months
b) Ages two to five years*
c) Ages five to twelve years**

*These areas may be further sub-divided into ages two to three years and four to five years.

** These areas may be further sub-divided into grades K-1, 2-3, and 4-6.

RATIONALE: This standard provides facilities located in inner-city areas or areas with extreme weather with an alternative that allows gross motor play when outdoor spaces are unavailable or unusable. Indoor gross motor play must provide an experience like outdoor play, with safe and healthful environmental conditions that match the benefits of outdoor play as closely as possible. These spaces may be interior if ventilation is adequate to prevent undue concentration of organisms, odors, carbon dioxide, humidity and other substances consistent with ASHRAE's "Standard 62: Ventilation for Acceptable Indoor Air Quality." This follows the developmental ages used for the development of the Standards for play equipment for children (1,2).

COMMENTS: For days in which weather does not permit outdoor play, the facility is encouraged to provide an alternate place for gross motor activities indoors for children of all ages. This space could be a dedicated gross motor room or a gym, a large hallway, or even a classroom in which furniture has been pushed aside. The room should provide adequate space for children to do vigorous activities including running.

Qualified heating and air conditioning contractors should have a meter to measure the rate of airflow. Before indoor areas are used for gross motor activity, a heating and air conditioning contractor should be called in to make airflow measurements.

TYPE OF FACILITY: Center

RELATED STANDARDS:
Standard 3.1.3.1: Active Opportunities for Physical Activity
Standard 3.1.3.2: Playing Outdoors
Standard 3.1.3.4: Caregivers'/teachers' Encouragement of Physical Activity
Standards 6.2.1.3-6.2.2.2: Play Equipment
Standards 6.2.2.3-6.2.2.5: Location and Clearance for Outdoor Play Equipment
Standard 6.2.3.1: Surfaces for Placing Climbing Equipment

REFERENCES:
1. Olds, A. R. 2001. *Child care design guide*. New York: McGraw-Hill.
2. U.S. Consumer Product Safety Commission (CPSC). 2008. *Public playground safety handbook*. Bethesda, MD: CPSC. http://www.cpsc.gov/cpscpub/pubs/325.pdf.

STANDARD 6.1.0.3: Rooftops as Play Areas

A rooftop used as a play area should be enclosed with a fence from four to six feet high, in accordance with local ordinance, and the bottom edge should be less than three and one-half inches from the base (1). The fence should be designed to prevent children from climbing it. An approved fire escape should lead from the roof to an open space at the ground level that meets the safety standards for outdoor play areas.

RATIONALE: Rooftop spaces used for play must have safeguards to prevent children from falling off (1).

COMMENTS: Caregivers/teachers should check with local jurisdictions on required fence heights. Jurisdictions vary between four- and six-foot fence heights.

TYPE OF FACILITY: Center; Large Family Child Care Home; Small Family Child Care Home

RELATED STANDARDS:
Standards 5.1.4.1-5.1.4.7: Exits
Standard 6.1.0.8: Enclosures for Outdoor Play Areas

REFERENCES:
1. ASTM International (ASTM). 2009. *Standard guide for fences/barriers for public, commercial, and multi-family residential use outdoor play areas*. ASTM F2049-09b. West Conshohocken, PA: ASTM.

STANDARD 6.1.0.4: Elevated Play Areas

Elevated play areas that have been created using a retaining wall should have a guardrail, protective barrier, or fence running along the top of the retaining wall.

If the exposed side of the retaining wall is higher than two feet, a fence not less than six feet high should be installed. The bottom edge of the fence should be less than three and one-half inches from the base and should be designed to prevent children from climbing it. Fences should be designed so all spaces are less than three and one-half inches (1). If the height of the exposed side of the retaining wall is two feet or lower, a guardrail should be installed if caring for preschool and school-age children. The space between the bottom of the guardrail and the ground should be more than nine inches but less than or equal to twenty-three inches. For school-age children, the space between the bottom of the guardrail and the ground should be more than nine inches but less than or equal to twenty-eight inches. If caring for infants or toddlers, a protective barrier should be installed. The space between the barrier and the ground should be less than three and one-half inches and should be from four to six feet in height.

RATIONALE: Children falling from elevated play areas may suffer fatal head injuries. All spaces in fences or barriers are recommended to be less than three and one-half inches to prevent head entrapment (1,4) and climbing.

Guardrails are designed to protect against falls from elevated surfaces, but do not discourage climbing or protect against climbing through or under. Protective barriers protect against all three and provide greater protection.

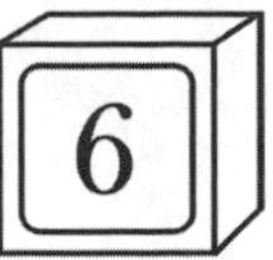

Guardrails are not recommended to use for infant and toddlers; protective barriers should be used instead.

COMMENTS: If the exposed side of the retaining wall is less than two feet high, additional safety can be provided by placing shock-absorbing material at the base of the exposed side of the retaining wall. A Certified Playground Safety Inspector (CPSI) can be utilized for guidance in assisting with elevated play areas.

According to the U.S. Consumer Product Safety Commission (CPSC), guardrails are not recommended for use with infants and toddlers because they do not discourage climbing or protect against climbing under or through (1). Protective barriers are recommended for infants and toddlers because they provide better protection and protect against all three risks (1).

For a list of shock-absorbing materials, see Appendix Z, the CPSC *Public Playground Safety Handbook*, and the ASTM International (ASTM) standards "F2223-09: Standard Guide for ASTM Standards on Playground Surfacing" and "F1292-09: Standard Specification for Impact Attenuation of Surfacing Materials within the Use Zone of Playground Equipment" (2,3). To locate a CPSI, check the National Park and Recreation Association (NPRA) registry at https://ipv.nrpa.org/CPSI_registry/.

TYPE OF FACILITY: Center; Large Family Child Care Home; Small Family Child Care Home

RELATED STANDARDS:
Standard 6.1.0.8: Enclosures for Outdoor Play Areas
Standard 6.2.3.1: Prohibited Surfaces for Placing Climbing Equipment
Appendix Z: Depth of Surface Materials

REFERENCES:
1. U.S. Consumer Product Safety Commission (CPSC). 2008. *Public playground safety handbook*. Bethesda, MD: CPSC. http://www.cpsc.gov/cpscpub/pubs/325.pdf.
2. ASTM International (ASTM). 2009. *Standard guide for ASTM standards on playground surfacing.* ASTM F2223-09. West Conshohocken, PA: ASTM.
3. ASTM International (ASTM). 2009. *Standard specification for impact attenuation of surfacing materials within the use zone of playground equipment.* ASTM F1292-09. West Conshohocken, PA: ASTM.
4. ASTM International (ASTM). 2009. *Standard safety performance specification for fences/barriers for public, commercial, and multi-family residential use outdoor play areas*. ASTM F2049-09b. West Conshohocken, PA: ASTM.

STANDARD 6.1.0.5: Visibility of Outdoor Play Area

The outdoor play area should be arranged so all areas are visible to the staff and easily supervised at all times (1). When a group of children are outdoors, the child care staff member responsible for the group should be able to summon another adult without leaving the group alone or unsupervised.

RATIONALE: This arrangement promotes the prevention of injury and abuse.

COMMENTS: Compliance can be ascertained by inspection. One tool to facilitate communication among caregivers/teachers is a walkie-talkie or cell phone.

TYPE OF FACILITY: Center; Large Family Child Care Home; Small Family Child Care Home

REFERENCES:
1. U.S. Consumer Product Safety Commission (CPSC). 2008. *Public playground safety handbook*. Bethesda, MD: CPSC. http://www.cpsc.gov/cpscpub/pubs/325.pdf.

STANDARD 6.1.0.6: Location of Play Areas Near Bodies of Water

Outside play areas should be free from the following bodies of water:

a) Unfenced swimming and wading pools;
b) Ditches;
c) Quarries;
d) Canals;
e) Excavations;
f) Fish ponds;
g) Water retention or detention basins;
h) Other bodies of water.

RATIONALE: Drowning is one of the leading causes of unintentional death in children one to fourteen years of age (1).

TYPE OF FACILITY: Center; Large Family Child Care Home; Small Family Child Care Home

REFERENCES:
1. Centers for Disease Control and Prevention. 2008. Water-related injuries. http://www.cdc.gov/HomeandRecreationalSafety/Water-Safety/.

STANDARD 6.1.0.7: Shading of Play Area

Children should be provided shade in play areas (not just playgrounds). Shading may be provided by trees, buildings, or shade structures. Metal equipment (especially slides) should be placed in the shade (1,2). Sun exposure should be reduced by timing children's outdoor play to take place before ten o'clock in the morning or after four o'clock in the afternoon standard time (3).

RATIONALE: The shade will provide comfort and prevent sunburn or burning because the structures or surfacing are hot. Access to sun and shade is beneficial to children while they play outdoors. Light exposure of the skin to sunlight promotes the production of vitamin D that growing children require for bone development and immune system health (8). Additionally, research shows sun may play an important role in alleviating depression. Exposure to sun is needed, but children must be protected from excessive exposure. Individuals who suffer severe childhood sunburns are at increased risk for skin cancer. Practicing sun-safe behavior during childhood is the first step in reducing the chances of getting skin cancer later in life (4). Placing metal equipment (such as slides) in the shade prevents the buildup of heat on play surfaces. Hot play surfaces can cause burns on children (5,7).

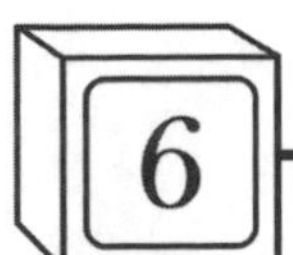

COMMENTS: A tent with sides up, awning, or other simple shelter from the sun can be available. Parents/guardians can be encouraged to supply protective clothing and age-appropriate sunscreen with written permission to apply to specified children, as necessary (6).

For more information on appropriate clothing and footwear when playing outdoors, see Standard 9.2.3.1.

TYPE OF FACILITY: Center; Large Family Child Care Home; Small Family Child Care Home

RELATED STANDARDS:
Standard 3.1.3.2: Playing Outdoors
Standard 3.4.5.1: Sun Safety Including Sunscreen
Standard 5.1.3.2: Appropriate Temperatures for Outdoor Play
Standard 9.2.3.1: Policies and Practices that Promote Physical Activity

REFERENCES:
1. U.S. Consumer Product Safety Commission (CPSC). 2008. *Public playground safety handbook*. Bethesda, MD: CPSC. http://www.cpsc.gov/cpscpub/pubs/325.pdf.
2. National Program for Playground Safety. Tips for limiting sun exposure. http://www.playgroundsafety.org/safety/sunexposure.htm.
3. Healthy Children. 2010. Safety and prevention: Sun safety. American Academy of Pediatrics. http://www.healthychildren.org/english/safety-prevention/at-play/pages/Sun-Safety.aspx.
4. U.S. Environmental Protection Agency. 2009. Sunwise kids. http://www.epa.gov/sunwise/kids/index.html.
5. Healthy Childcare Consultants. 2005. Safe fun in the sun. http://www.childhealthonline.org/Safe Fun in the Sun Booklet color.pdf.
6. California Department of Public Health. Skin cancer prevention program. http://www.cdph.ca.gov/programs/SkinCancer/Documents/Skin-Cancer-Mission.pdf.
7. Fiene, R. 2002. *13 indicators of quality child care: Research update*. Washington, DC: U.S. Department of Health and Human Services, Office of the Assistant Secretary for Planning and Evaluation. http://aspe.hhs.gov/hsp/ccquality-ind02/.

STANDARD 6.1.0.8: Enclosures for Outdoor Play Areas

The outdoor play area should be enclosed with a fence or natural barriers. Fences and barriers should not prevent the observation of children by caregivers/teachers. If a fence is used, it should conform to applicable local building codes in height and construction. Fence posts should be outside the fence where allowed by local building codes. These areas should have at least two exits, with at least one being remote from the buildings.

Gates should be equipped with self-closing and positive self-latching closure mechanisms. The latch or securing device should be high enough or of a type such that children cannot open it. The openings in the fence and gates should be no larger than three and one-half inches. The fence and gates should be constructed to discourage climbing. Play areas should be secured against inappropriate use when the facility is closed.

Wooden fences and playground structures created out of wood should be tested for chromated copper arsenate (CCA). Wooden fences and playground structures created out of wood that is found to contain CCA should be sealed with an oil-based outdoor sealant annually.

RATIONALE: This standard helps to ensure proper supervision and protection, prevention of injuries, and control of the area (3). An effective fence is one that prevents a child from getting over, under, or through it and keeps children from leaving the fenced outdoor play area, except when supervising adults are present. Although fences are not childproof, they provide a layer of protection for children who stray from supervision. Small openings in the fence (no larger than three and one-half inches) prevent entrapment and discourage climbing (1,2). Fence posts should be on the outside of the fence to prevent injuries from children running into the posts or climbing on horizontal supports (2).

Fences that prevent the child from obtaining a proper toe hold will discourage climbing. Chain link fences allow for climbing when the links are large enough for a foothold. Children are known to scale fences with diamonds or links that are two inches wide. One-inch diamonds are less of a problem.

CCA is a wood preservative and insecticide that is made up of 22% arsenic, a known carcinogen. In 2004, CCA was phased-out for residential uses; however, older, treated wood is a still a health concern, particularly for children. For more information on CCA-treated wood products, see Standard 5.2.9.12.

COMMENTS: Picket fences with V spaces at the top of the fencing are a potential entrapment hazard.

Some fence designs have horizontal supports on the side of the fence that is outside the play area which may allow intruders to climb over the fence. Facilities should consider selecting a fence design that prevents the ability to climb on either side of the fence.

For additional information on fencing, consult the ASTM International “Standard F2049-09b: Standard Guide for Fences/Barriers for Public, Commercial, and Multi-family Residential use Outdoor Play Areas” (2).

TYPE OF FACILITY: Center; Large Family Child Care Home; Small Family Child Care Home

RELATED STANDARDS:
Standard 5.2.9.12: Treatment of CCA Pressure-Treated Wood

REFERENCES:
1. U.S. Consumer Product Safety Commission (CPSC). 2008. *Public playground safety handbook*. Bethesda, MD: CPSC. http://www.cpsc.gov/cpscpub/pubs/325.pdf.
2. ASTM International (ASTM). 2009. *Standard guide for fences/barriers for public, commercial, and multi-family residential use outdoor play areas*. ASTM F2049-09b. West Conshohocken, PA: ASTM.
3. Fiene, R. 2002. *13 indicators of quality child care: Research update*. Washington, DC: U.S. Department of Health and Human Services, Office of the Assistant Secretary for Planning and Evaluation. http://aspe.hhs.gov/hsp/ccquality-ind02/.

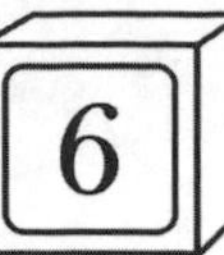

6.2 Play Area/Playground Equipment

6.2.1 General Requirements

STANDARD 6.2.1.1: Play Equipment Requirements

Play equipment and materials in the facility should meet the recommendations of the U.S. Consumer Product Safety Commission (CPSC) and the ASTM International (ASTM) for public playground equipment. Equipment and materials intended for gross-motor (active) play should conform to the recommendations in the CPSC Public Playground Safety Handbook and the provisions in the ASTM "Standard F1487-07ae1: Consumer Safety Performance Specifications for Playground Equipment for Public Use."

All play equipment should be constructed, installed, and made available to the intended users in such a manner that meets CPSC guidelines and ASTM standards, as warranted by the manufacturers' recommendations. A Certified Playground Safety Inspector (CPSI) who has been certified by the National Recreation and Park Association (NRPA) should conduct an inspection of playground plans for new installations. Previously installed playgrounds should be inspected at least once each year, by a CPSI or local regulatory agency, and whenever changes are made to the equipment or intended users.

Inspectors should specifically test wooden play equipment structures for chromated copper arsenate (CCA). The wood in many playground sets can contain potentially hazardous levels of arsenic due to the use of CCA as a wood preservative.

Play equipment and materials should be deemed appropriate to the developmental needs, individual interests, abilities, and ages of the children, by a person with at least a master's degree in early childhood education or psychology, or identified as age-appropriate by a manufacturer's label on the product package. Enough play equipment and materials should be available to avoid excessive competition and long waits.

The facility should offer a wide variety of age-appropriate portable play equipment (e.g., balls, jump ropes, hoops, ribbons, scarves, push/pull toys, riding toys, rocking and twisting toys, sand and water play toys) in sufficient quantities that multiple children can play at the same time (1-5).

Children should always be supervised when playing on playground equipment.

RATIONALE: The active play areas of a child care facility are associated with frequent and severe injuries (8). Many technical design and installation safeguards are addressed in the ASTM and CPSC standards. Manufacturers who guarantee that their equipment meets these standards and provide instructions for use to the purchaser ensure that these technical requirements will be met under threat of product liability. Certified Playground Safety Inspectors (CPSI) receive training from the NPRA in association with the National Playground Safety Institute (NPSI). Since the training received by CPSIs exceeds that of most child care personnel, obtaining a professional inspection to detect playground hazards before they cause injury is highly worthwhile.

Playgrounds designed for older children might present intrinsic hazards to preschool-age children. Equipment that is sized for larger and more mature children poses challenges that younger, smaller, and less mature children may not be able to meet.

The health effects related to arsenic include: irritation of the stomach and intestines, birth or developmental effects, cancer, infertility, and miscarriages in women. CCA is a wood preservative and insecticide that is made up of 22% arsenic, a known carcinogen. Much of the wood in playground equipment contains high levels of this toxic substance. In 2004, CCA was phased-out for residential uses; however, older, treated wood is a still a health concern, particularly for children (6).

COMMENTS: Compliance should be measured by structured observation.

A general guideline for establishing play equipment heights is one foot per year of age of the intended users. In some states, height limitations for playground equipment are:

a) Thirty-two inches for infants and toddlers (six months to twenty-three months) (7);
b) Forty-eight inches for preschoolers (thirty months to five years of age);
c) Six and one-half feet for school-age children (six through twelve years of age).

Consult with your regulatory health authority for any local or state requirements.

Check the ASTM Website – http://www.astm.org – for up-to-date standards. To obtain the publications listed above, contact the ASTM or the CPSC.

To locate a CPSI, check the NPRA registry at https://ipv.nrpa.org/CPSI_registry/.

TYPE OF FACILITY: Center; Large Family Child Care Home; Small Family Child Care Home

RELATED STANDARDS:
Standard 2.2.0.1: Methods of Supervision of Children
Standard 3.3.0.2: Cleaning and Sanitizing Toys
Standard 6.2.3.1: Prohibited Surfaces for Placing Climbing Equipment
Standard 6.2.5.1: Inspection of Indoor and Outdoor Play Areas and Equipment

REFERENCES:

1. Ammerman, A., S. E. Benjamin, et al. 2004. The nutrition and physical activity self assessment for child care (NAP SACC). Raleigh and Chapel Hill, NC: Division of Public Health, Center for Health Promotion and Disease Prevention.
2. Ammerman, A. S., D. S. Ward, et al. 2007. An intervention to promote healthy weight: Nutrition and physical activity self-assessment for child care (NAP SACC) theory and design. *Prev Chronic Dis* 4 (July).
3. Bower, J. K., D. P. Hales, et al. 2008. The childcare environment and children's physical activity. *Am J Prev Med* 34:23-29.

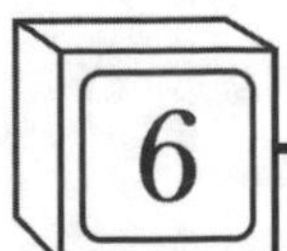

4. Brown, W. H., K. A. Pfeiffer, et al. 2009. Social and environmental factors associated with preschoolers' nonsedentary physical activity. *Child Development* 80:45-58.
5. Dowda, M., W. H. Brown, et al. 2009. Policies and characteristics of the preschool environment and physical activity of young children. *Pediatrics* 123: e261-66.
6. American Academy of Pediatrics (AAP), Committee on Environmental Health. 2003. Arsenic. In *Pediatric environmental health*, ed. R. A. Etzel. Elk Grove Village, IL: AAP.
7. ASTM International (ASTM). 2007. Standard consumer safety performance specification for playground equipment for public use. ASTM F1487-07ae1. West Conshohocken, PA: ASTM.
8. Fiene, R. 2002. 13 indicators of quality child care: Research update. Washington, DC: U.S. Department of Health and Human Services, Office of the Assistant Secretary for Planning and Evaluation. http://aspe.hhs.gov/hsp/ccquality-ind02/.

STANDARD 6.2.1.2: Play Equipment and Surfaces Meet ADA Requirements

Play equipment and play surfaces should conform to recommendations from the Americans with Disabilities Act (ADA) (1).

RATIONALE: Play equipment and play surfaces that are safe and accessible to children with disabilities will encourage all children to play together (2).

COMMENTS: For additional information regarding playground equipment and play surfaces accessible to children with disabilities, review the *Americans with Disabilities Act Accessibility Guidelines* (*ADAAG*) and the U.S. Access Board's *Summary of Accessibility Guidelines for Play Areas* at http://www.access-board.gov/play/guide/guide.pdf.

TYPE OF FACILITY: Center; Large Family Child Care Home; Small Family Child Care Home

REFERENCES:

1. Architectural and Transportation Barriers Compliance Board (U.S. Access Board). 2005. *Accessible play areas: A summary of accessibility guidelines for play areas*. http://www.access-board.gov/play/guide/guide.pdf.
2. Fiene, R. 2002. *13 indicators of quality child care: Research update*. Washington, DC: U.S. Department of Health and Human Services, Office of the Assistant Secretary for Planning and Evaluation. http://aspe.hhs.gov/hsp/ccquality-ind02/.

STANDARD 6.2.1.3: Design of Play Equipment

Play equipment should be of safe design and in good repair. Outdoor climbing equipment and swings should be assembled, anchored and maintained in accordance with the manufacturer's instructions. Swings should have soft and flexible seats. Access to play equipment should be limited to age groups for which the equipment is developmentally appropriate.

RATIONALE: Having well-designed, age-appropriate play equipment lessens injuries (1-3). Equipment that is sized for larger and more mature children poses challenges that younger, smaller, and less mature children may not be able to meet.

COMMENTS: The method of anchoring play equipment should take into consideration ground conditions and seasonal changes in ground condition.

TYPE OF FACILITY: Center; Large Family Child Care Home; Small Family Child Care Home

RELATED STANDARDS:
Standard 5.2.9.12: Treatment of CCA Pressure-Treated Wood
Standard 6.2.1.1: Play Equipment Requirements

REFERENCES:

1. U.S. Consumer Product Safety Commission (CPSC). 2008. *Public playground safety handbook*. Bethesda, MD: CPSC. http://www.cpsc.gov/cpscpub/pubs/325.pdf.
2. U.S. Consumer Product Safety Commission (CPSC). 2005. *Outdoor home playground safety handbook*. Bethesda, MD: CPSC. http://www.cpsc.gov/CPSCPUB/PUBS/324.pdf.
3. Fiene, R. 2002. *13 indicators of quality child care: Research update*. Washington, DC: U.S. Department of Health and Human Services, Office of the Assistant Secretary for Planning and Evaluation. http://aspe.hhs.gov/hsp/ccquality-ind02/.

STANDARD 6.2.1.4: Installation of Play Equipment

All pieces of play equipment should be installed as directed by the manufacturer's instructions and specifications of ASTM International/U.S. Consumer Product Safety Commission (ASTM/CPSC) standards. The equipment should be able to withstand the maximum anticipated forces generated by active use that might cause it to overturn, tip, slide, or move in any way.

RATIONALE: Secure anchoring is a key factor in stable installation, and because the required footing sizes and depths may vary according to type of equipment, the anchoring process should be completed in strict accordance with the manufacturer's specifications (1,2).

COMMENTS: If active play equipment is installed indoors, the same requirements for installation and use apply as in the outdoor setting, including surfacing, spacing, and arrangement. CPSC recommends anchoring for both public and residential playground equipment (1).

TYPE OF FACILITY: Center; Large Family Child Care Home; Small Family Child Care Home

RELATED STANDARDS:
Standard 6.2.1.5: Play Equipment Connecting and Linking Devices

REFERENCES:

1. U.S. Consumer Product Safety Commission (CPSC). 2008. *Public playground safety handbook*. Bethesda, MD: CPSC. http://www.cpsc.gov/cpscpub/pubs/325.pdf.
2. Fiene, R. 2002. *13 indicators of quality child care: Research update*. Washington, DC: U.S. Department of Health and Human Services, Office of the Assistant Secretary for Planning and Evaluation. http://aspe.hhs.gov/hsp/ccquality-ind02/.

STANDARD 6.2.1.5: Play Equipment Connecting and Linking Devices

All bolts, hooks, eyes, shackles, rungs, and other connecting and linking devices of all pieces of playground equipment should be designed and secured to prevent loosening or unfastening, except by authorized individuals with special tools. All connecting and linking devices should be maintained according to the manufacturer's instructions so not to cause sharp edges, entanglement, or impalement hazards.

RATIONALE: Children may be injured by protruding, incorrectly installed, or malfunctioning devices on play equipment (1).

TYPE OF FACILITY: Center; Large Family Child Care Home; Small Family Child Care Home

RELATED STANDARDS:
Standard 6.2.1.4: Installation of Play Equipment

REFERENCES:

1. Fiene, R. 2002. *13 indicators of quality child care: Research update*. Washington, DC: U.S. Department of Health and Human Services, Office of the Assistant Secretary for Planning and Evaluation. http://aspe.hhs.gov/hsp/ccquality-ind02/.

STANDARD 6.2.1.6: Size and Anchoring of Crawl Spaces

Crawl spaces in all pieces of playground equipment, such as pipes or tunnels, should be securely anchored to the ground to prevent movement and should have a diameter of twenty-three inches or greater to permit easy access to the space by adults in an emergency or for maintenance. Crawl tubes should have holes with less than three and one-half inches diameter in them so that adults can supervise the children and see them in the spaces (1).

RATIONALE: Playground equipment components must be secure to prevent sudden falls or collisions by children (1,2). Adequate access space permits adult assistance and first aid measures.

TYPE OF FACILITY: Center; Large Family Child Care Home; Small Family Child Care Home

REFERENCES:

1. U.S. Consumer Product Safety Commission (CPSC). 2008. *Public playground safety handbook*. Bethesda, MD: CPSC. http://www.cpsc.gov/cpscpub/pubs/325.pdf.
2. Fiene, R. 2002. *13 indicators of quality child care: Research update*. Washington, DC: U.S. Department of Health and Human Services, Office of the Assistant Secretary for Planning and Evaluation. http://aspe.hhs.gov/hsp/ccquality-ind02/.

STANDARD 6.2.1.7: Enclosure of Moving Parts on Play Equipment

All pieces of play equipment should be designed so moving parts (swing components, teeter-totter mechanism, spring-ride springs, and so forth) will be shielded or enclosed. Teeter-totters should not be used by preschool-age children unless they are equipped with a spring centering device and have an appropriate shock-absorbing material underneath the seats. Use of teeter totters is prohibited for infants and toddlers (1-3).

RATIONALE: Playground injuries often involve pinching, catching, or crushing of body parts or clothing by equipment mechanisms (4).

COMMENTS: For more information on play equipment with moving parts, see the U.S. Consumer Product Safety Commission (CPSC) *Public Playground Safety Handbook* and ASTM International (ASTM) standards "F1487-07ae1: Standard Consumer Safety Performance Specification for Playground Equipment for Public Use" and "F2373-08: Standard Consumer Safety Performance Specification for Public Use Play Equipment for Children 6 Months through 23 Months."

TYPE OF FACILITY: Center; Large Family Child Care Home; Small Family Child Care Home

REFERENCES:

1. ASTM International (ASTM). 2008. *Standard consumer safety performance specification for public use play equipment for children 6 months through 23 months*. ASTM F2373-08. West Conshohocken, PA: ASTM.
2. ASTM International (ASTM). 2007. *Standard consumer safety performance specification for playground equipment for public use*. ASTM F1487-07ae1. West Conshohocken, PA: ASTM.
3. U.S. Consumer Product Safety Commission (CPSC). 2008. *Public playground safety handbook*. Bethesda, MD: CPSC. http://www.cpsc.gov/cpscpub/pubs/325.pdf.
4. Fiene, R. 2002. *13 indicators of quality child care: Research update*. Washington, DC: U.S. Department of Health and Human Services, Office of the Assistant Secretary for Planning and Evaluation. http://aspe.hhs.gov/hsp/ccquality-ind02/.

STANDARD 6.2.1.8: Material Defects and Edges on Play Equipment

All pieces of play equipment should be free of sharp edges, protruding parts, weaknesses, and flaws in material construction. Sharp edges in wood, metal, or concrete should be rounded on all edges. All corners and edges on rigid materials should have a minimum radius of one-quarter inch unless the material thickness is less than one-half inch, in which case the radius should be half the thickness of the material. This requirement does not apply to swing seats, straps, ropes, chains, connectors, and other flexible components. Wood materials should be free of chromated copper arsenate (CCA), sanded smooth, and should be inspected regularly for splintering.

RATIONALE: Any sharp or protruding surface presents a potential for lacerations and contusions to the child's body (1-4).

TYPE OF FACILITY: Center; Large Family Child Care Home; Small Family Child Care Home

RELATED STANDARDS:
Standard 5.2.9.12: Treatment of CCA Pressure-Treated Wood

REFERENCES:

1. U.S. Consumer Product Safety Commission (CPSC). 2008. *Public playground safety handbook*. Bethesda, MD: CPSC. http://www.cpsc.gov/cpscpub/pubs/325.pdf.
2. ASTM International (ASTM). 2008. *Standard consumer safety performance specification for public use play equipment for children 6 months through 23 months*. ASTM F2373-08. West Conshohocken, PA: ASTM.
3. ASTM International (ASTM). 2007. *Standard consumer safety performance specification for playground equipment for public use*. ASTM F1487-07ae1. West Conshohocken, PA: ASTM.

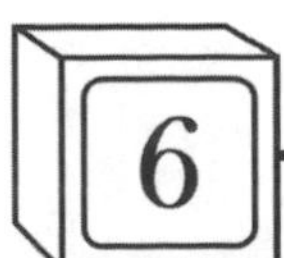

4. Fiene, R. 2002. *13 indicators of quality child care: Research update*. Washington, DC: U.S. Department of Health and Human Services, Office of the Assistant Secretary for Planning and Evaluation. http://aspe.hhs.gov/hsp/ccquality-ind02/.

STANDARD 6.2.1.9: Entrapment Hazards of Play Equipment

All openings in pieces of play equipment should be designed too large for a child's head to get stuck in or too small for a child's body to fit into, in order to prevent entrapment and strangulation. Openings in exercise rings (overhead hanging rings such as those used in a ring trek or ring ladder) should be smaller than three and one-half inches or larger than nine inches in diameter. Rings on long chains are prohibited. A play structure should have no openings with a dimension between three and one-half inches and nine inches. In particular, side railings, stairs, and other locations where a child might slip or try to climb through should be checked for appropriate dimensions.

Protrusions such as pipes, wood ends, or long bolts that may catch a child's clothing are prohibited. Distances between two vertical objects that are positioned near each other should be less than three and one-half inches to prevent entrapment of a child's head. No opening should have a vertical angle of less than fifty-five degrees. To prevent entrapment of fingers, openings should not be larger than three-eighths inch or smaller than one inch. A Certified Playground Safety Inspector (CPSI) is specially trained to find and measure various play equipment hazards.

RATIONALE: Any equipment opening between three and one-half inches and nine inches in diameter presents the potential for head entrapment. Similarly, openings between three-eighths inch and one inch can cause entrapment of the child's fingers (1-2).

COMMENTS: To locate a CPSI, check the National Park and Recreation Association (NPRA) registry at https://ipv.nrpa.org/CPSI_registry/.

TYPE OF FACILITY: Center; Large Family Child Care Home; Small Family Child Care Home

REFERENCES:

1. U.S. Consumer Product Safety Commission (CPSC). 2008. *Public playground safety handbook*. Bethesda, MD: CPSC. http://www.cpsc.gov/cpscpub/pubs/325.pdf.
2. Fiene, R. 2002. *13 indicators of quality child care: Research update*. Washington, DC: U.S. Department of Health and Human Services, Office of the Assistant Secretary for Planning and Evaluation. http://aspe.hhs.gov/hsp/ccquality-ind02/.

6.2.2 Use Zones and Clearance Requirements

STANDARD 6.2.2.1: Use Zone for Fixed Play Equipment

All fixed play equipment should have a minimum of six feet use zone (clearance space) from walkways, buildings, and other structures that are not used as part of play activities (1,3). For fixed play equipment only used by children six months to twenty-three months, a minimum three-foot use zone is required (2).

RATIONALE: Injuries from falls are more likely to occur when equipment spacing is inadequate (1).

TYPE OF FACILITY: Center; Large Family Child Care Home; Small Family Child Care Home

RELATED STANDARDS:

Standard 6.2.2.2: Arrangement of Play Equipment
Standard 6.2.2.4: Clearance Requirements of Playground Areas
Appendix HH: Use Zones and Clearance Dimensions for Single- and Multi-Axis

REFERENCES:

1. U.S. Consumer Product Safety Commission (CPSC). 2008. *Public playground safety handbook*. Bethesda, MD: CPSC. http://www.cpsc.gov/cpscpub/pubs/325.pdf.
2. ASTM International (ASTM). 2008. *Standard consumer safety performance specification for public use play equipment for children 6 months through 23 months*. ASTM F2373-08. West Conshohocken, PA: ASTM.
3. ASTM International (ASTM). 2007. *Standard consumer safety performance specification for playground equipment for public use*. ASTM F1487-07ae1. West Conshohocken, PA: ASTM.

STANDARD 6.2.2.2: Arrangement of Play Equipment

All equipment should be arranged so that children playing on one piece of equipment will not interfere with children playing on or running to another piece of equipment. All equipment should be arranged to facilitate proper supervision by sight and sound.

RATIONALE: Collisions between children utilizing different pieces of equipment more often occur when equipment is inappropriately placed (1).

TYPE OF FACILITY: Center; Large Family Child Care Home; Small Family Child Care Home

RELATED STANDARDS:

Standard 6.1.0.1: Size and Location of Outdoor Play Area
Standard 6.2.2.1: Use Zone for Fixed Play Equipment
Standard 6.2.2.3: Location of Moving Play Equipment
Standard 6.2.2.4: Clearance Requirements of Playground Areas
Appendix HH: Use Zones and Clearance Dimensions for Single- and Multi-Axis

REFERENCES:

1. U.S. Consumer Product Safety Commission (CPSC). 2008. *Public playground safety handbook*. Bethesda, MD: CPSC. http://www.cpsc.gov/cpscpub/pubs/325.pdf.

STANDARD 6.2.2.3: Location of Moving Play Equipment

Moving play equipment, such as swings and merry-go-rounds, should be located toward the edge or corner of a play area, or should be placed in such a way as to discourage children from running into the path of the moving equipment (see Appendix HH, Use Zones and Clearance Dimensions for Single- and Multi-Axis Swings).

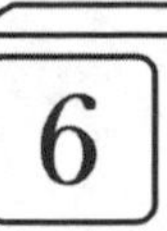

RATIONALE: Placing moving equipment around the perimeter of the play area will reduce the number of traffic paths around this equipment (1).

TYPE OF FACILITY: Center; Large Family Child Care Home; Small Family Child Care Home

RELATED STANDARDS:
Standard 6.2.2.1: Use Zone for Fixed Play Equipment
Standard 6.2.2.2: Arrangement of Play Equipment
Standard 6.2.2.4: Clearance Requirements of Playground Areas
Appendix HH: Use Zones and Clearance Dimensions for Single- and Multi-Axis Swings

REFERENCES:
1. U.S. Consumer Product Safety Commission (CPSC). 2008. *Public playground safety handbook*. Bethesda, MD: CPSC. http://www.cpsc.gov/cpscpub/pubs/325.pdf.

STANDARD 6.2.2.4: Clearance Requirements of Playground Areas

Playgrounds should be laid out to ensure clearance in accordance with the ASTM standards "F2373-08: Standard Consumer Safety Performance Specification for Public Use Play Equipment for Children 6 Months through 23 Months" and "F1487-07ae1: Standard Consumer Safety Performance Specification for Playground Equipment for Public Use" and the U.S. Consumer Product Safety Commission (CPSC) *Public Playground Safety Handbook*.

Equipment should be situated so that clearance space, called use zones, allocated to one piece of equipment does not encroach on that of another piece of equipment.

RATIONALE: Ample space to enable movement around and use of equipment also helps to restrict the number of pieces of equipment within the play area, thus preventing overcrowding and reducing the potential for injury (1-3).

TYPE OF FACILITY: Center; Large Family Child Care Home; Small Family Child Care Home

RELATED STANDARDS:
Standard 6.2.2.1: Use Zone for Fixed Play Equipment
Standard 6.2.2.3: Location of Moving Play Equipment
Appendix HH: Use Zones and Clearance Dimensions for Single- and Multi-Axis Swings

REFERENCES:
1. U.S. Consumer Product Safety Commission (CPSC). 2008. *Public playground safety handbook*. Bethesda, MD: CPSC. http://www.cpsc.gov/cpscpub/pubs/325.pdf.
2. ASTM International (ASTM). 2008. *Standard consumer safety performance specification for public use play equipment for children 6 months through 23 months*. ASTM F2373-08. West Conshohocken, PA: ASTM.
3. ASTM International (ASTM). 2007. *Standard consumer safety performance specification for playground equipment for public use*. ASTM F1487-07ae1. West Conshohocken, PA: ASTM.

STANDARD 6.2.2.5: Clearance Space for Swings

Swings should have a use zone (clearance space) on the sides of the swing of six feet. The use zone to the front and rear of the swings should extend a minimum distance of twice the height of the pivot point measured from a point directly beneath the pivot to the protective surface. Swings should be arranged in accordance with the ASTM International (ASTM) standards "F1487-07ae1: Consumer Safety Performance Specifications for Playground Equipment for Public Use" and "F2373-08: Consumer Safety Performance Specification for Public Use Play Equipment for Children 6 Months through 23 Months," and the U.S. Consumer Product Safety Commission (CPSC) *Public Playground Safety Handbook*.

RATIONALE: A use zone area is necessary to avoid body contact with children in swings (1-3).

COMMENTS: To calculate use zone: [height of the top pivot point of the swing from the ground] x 2 = "use zone" in front of the swing and [height of the top pivot point of the swing from the ground] x 2 = "use zone" behind the swing. There should be no objects or persons within the "use zone," other than the child on the swing.

TYPE OF FACILITY: Center; Large Family Child Care Home; Small Family Child Care Home

RELATED STANDARDS:
Standard 6.2.2.3: Location of Moving Play Equipment
Appendix HH: Use Zones and Clearance Dimensions for Single- and Multi-Axis Swings

REFERENCES:
1. U.S. Consumer Product Safety Commission (CPSC). 2008. *Public playground safety handbook*. Bethesda, MD: CPSC. http://www.cpsc.gov/cpscpub/pubs/325.pdf.
2. ASTM International (ASTM). 2008. *Standard consumer safety performance specification for public use play equipment for children 6 months through 23 months*. ASTM F2373-08. West Conshohocken, PA: ASTM.
3. ASTM International (ASTM). 2007. *Standard consumer safety performance specification for playground equipment for public use*. ASTM F1487-07ae1. West Conshohocken, PA: ASTM.

6.2.3 Play Area and Playground Surfacing

STANDARD 6.2.3.1: Prohibited Surfaces for Placing Climbing Equipment

Equipment used for climbing should not be placed over, or immediately next to, hard surfaces such as asphalt, concrete, dirt, grass, or flooring covered by carpet or gym mats not intended for use as surfacing for climbing equipment.

All pieces of playground equipment should be placed over and surrounded by a shock-absorbing surface. This material may be either the unitary or the loose-fill type, as defined by the U.S. Consumer Product Safety Commission (CPSC) guidelines and ASTM International (ASTM) standards, extending at least six feet beyond the perimeter of the stationary equipment (1,2). These shock-absorbing surfaces must conform to the standard stating that the impact of falling from the height of the structure will be less than or equal to peak deceleration of 200G and a Head Injury Criterion (HIC) of 1000 and should be maintained at all times (3). Organic materials that support colonization of molds and bacteria should not be used. All loose fill materials must be raked to retain their proper distribution, shock-absorbing properties and to remove foreign material. This standard applies whether the equipment is installed outdoors or indoors.

RATIONALE: Head-impact injuries present a significant danger to children. Falls into a shock-absorbing surface are less likely to cause serious injury because the surface is yielding, so peak deceleration and force are reduced (1). The critical issue of surfaces, both under equipment and in general, should receive the most careful attention (1).

COMMENTS: Children should not dig in sand used under swings. It is not safe and the sand could be contaminated. If sand is provided in a play area for the purpose of digging, it should be in a covered box. Sand used as surfacing does not need to be covered. Staff should realize that sand used as surfacing may be used as a litter box for animals. Also, sand compacts and becomes less shock-absorbing when wet and it can become very hard when temperatures drop below freezing. Two scales are used for measuring the potential severity of falls. One is known as the G-max, and the other is known as the HIC. G-max measures the peak force at the time of impact; HIC measures total force during impact. Levels of 200 G-max or 1000 HIC have been accepted as thresholds for risk of life-threatening injuries. G-max and HIC levels of playground surfaces can be tested in various ways. The easiest one to use is the instrumented hemispherical triaxial headform. The individual conducting the test should use a process that conforms to the ASTM standard "F1292-09: Standard Specification for Impact Attenuation of Surfacing Materials within the Use Zone of Playground Equipment" (2).

For guidelines on play equipment and surfacing, contact the CPSC or a Certified Playground Safety Inspector (CPSI).

TYPE OF FACILITY: Center; Large Family Child Care Home; Small Family Child Care Home

RELATED STANDARDS:
Standard 6.2.4.1: Sandboxes
Appendix Z: Depth of Surface Materials

REFERENCES:
1. U.S. Consumer Product Safety Commission (CPSC). 2008. *Public playground safety handbook*. Bethesda, MD: CPSC. http://www.cpsc.gov/cpscpub/pubs/325.pdf.
2. ASTM International (ASTM). 2009. *Standard specification for impact attenuation of surfacing materials within the use zone of playground equipment.* ASTM F1292-09. West Conshohocken, PA: ASTM.
3. Sushinsky, G. F. 2005. *Surfacing materials for indoor play areas: Impact attenuation test report.* Bethesda, MD: U.S. Consumer Product Safety Commission. http://www.cpsc.gov/LIBRARY/FOIA/foia06/os/surfacing.pdf.

6.2.4 Specific Play Equipment

STANDARD 6.2.4.1: Sandboxes

The facility should adhere to the following requirements for sand play areas:

a) Sandboxes should be constructed to permit drainage;
b) Sandboxes should be covered with a lid or other covering when they are not in use;
c) Sandboxes should be kept free from cat and other animal excrement;
d) Sandboxes should be regularly cleaned of foreign matter;
e) Sandboxes should be located away from prevailing winds, if this is not possible, windbreaks using bushes, trees, or fences should be provided;
f) Sand used in the box should be washed, free of organic, toxic, or harmful materials, and fine enough to be shaped easily;
g) Sand should be replaced as often as necessary to keep the sand visibly clean and free of extraneous materials;
h) Sand play areas should be distinct from landing areas for slides or other equipment;
i) Sand play area covers should be adequately secured when they are lifted or moved to allow children to play in the sandbox.

RATIONALE: Wet sand can be a breeding ground for insects and can promote mold and bacterial growth (2).

Uncovered sand is subject to contamination and transmission of disease from animal feces (such as toxoplasmosis from cat feces) and insects breeding in sandboxes (1). Replacement of sand may is required to keep it free of foreign material that could cause injury.

There is potential for used sand to contain toxic or harmful ingredients such as tremolite, an asbestos-like substance. Sand that is used as a building material or is harvested from a site containing toxic substances may contain potentially harmful substances. Sand can come from many sources. Caregivers/teachers should be sure they are using sand labeled as a safe play material or sand that is specifically prepared for sandbox use.

COMMENTS: Sand already installed in play areas cannot be safely cleaned without leaving residues that could harm children.

TYPE OF FACILITY: Center; Large Family Child Care Home; Small Family Child Care Home

RELATED STANDARDS:
Standard 3.3.0.2: Cleaning and Sanitizing Toys
Standard 5.2.8.1: Integrated Pest Management
Standard 5.2.8.2: Insect Breeding Hazard

REFERENCES:
1. Villar, R. G., M. Connick, L. L. Barton, F. J. Meaney, M. F. Davis. 1998. Parent and pediatrician knowledge, attitudes, and practices regarding pet-associated hazards. *Arch Pediatr Adolesc Med* 152:1035-37.
2. Warren, N. 2007. How to build a sandbox. Articles Base. http://www.articlesbase.com/home-improvement-articles/how-to-build-a-sandbox-115888.html.

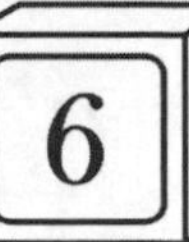

STANDARD 6.2.4.2: Water Play Tables

Communal, unsupervised water play tables should be prohibited. Communal water tables should be permitted if children are supervised and the following conditions apply:

a) The water tables should be filled with fresh potable water immediately before designated children begin a water play activity at the table, and changed when a new group begins a water play activity at the table even if all the child-users are from a single group in the space where the water table is located; or, the table should be supplied with freely flowing fresh potable water during the play activity;
b) The basin and toys should be washed and sanitized at the end of the day;
c) If the basin and toys are used by another classroom, the basin and toys should be washed and sanitized prior to use;
d) Only children without cuts, scratches, and sores on their hands should be permitted to use a communal water play table;
e) Children should wash their hands before and after they use a communal water play table;
f) Caregivers/teachers should ensure that no child drinks water from the water table;
g) Floor/surface under and around the water table should be dried during and after play;
h) Avoid use of bottles, cups, and glasses in water play, as these items encourage children to drink from them.

As an alternative to a communal water table, separate basins with fresh potable water for each child to engage in water play should be permitted. If separate basins of water are used and placed on the floor, close supervision is crucial to prevent drowning.

RATIONALE: Contamination of hands, toys, and equipment in the room in which play tables are located seems to play a role in the transmission of diseases in child care settings (1,2). Proper handwashing, supervision of children, and cleaning and sanitizing of the water table will help prevent the transmission of disease (3).

Children have drowned in very shallow water (4).

COMMENTS: A designated group of children is defined as the children in a classroom in a center or the children in a family child care setting.

To avoid splashing chemical solutions around the child care environment, the addition of bleach to the water is not recommended.

Keeping the floor/surface dry with towels and/or wiping up water on the floor during and after play is recommended to reduce the potential for children and staff slipping/falling.

Another way to use water play tables is to use the table to hold a personal basin of potable water for each child who is engaged in water play. With this approach, supervision must be provided to be sure children confine their play to their own basin. Wherever a suitable inlet and outlet of water can be arranged, safe communal water play can involve free-flowing potable water by attaching a hose to the table that connects to the water source and attaching a hose to the table's drain that connects to a water drain or suitable run-off area.

TYPE OF FACILITY: Center; Large Family Child Care Home; Small Family Child Care Home

RELATED STANDARDS:
Standard 3.2.2.1: Situations that Require Hand Hygiene
Standard 3.3.0.2: Cleaning and Sanitizing Toys
Standard 6.3.5.2: Water in Containers

REFERENCES:
1. Churchill, R. B., L. K. Pickering. 1997. Infection control challenges in child-care centers. *Infect Dis Clin North Am* 11:347-65.
2. Van, R., A. L. Morrow, R. R. Reves, L. K. Pickering. 1991. Environmental contamination in child day-care centers. *Am J Epidemiol* 133:460-70.
3. American Academy of Pediatrics (AAP), Committee on Environmental Health. 2003. Child care centers. In *Pediatric environmental health*, ed. R. A. Etzel. Elk Grove Village, IL: AAP.
4. U.S. Consumer Product Safety Commission (CPSC). 2009. CPSC warns of in-home drowning dangers with bathtubs, bath seats, buckets. Release #10-008. http://www.cpsc.gov/cpscpub/prerel/prhtml10/10008.html.

STANDARD 6.2.4.3: Sensory Table Materials

All materials used in a sensory table should be nontoxic and should not be of a size or material that could cause choking. Sensory table activities should not be used with children under eighteen months of age. For toddlers, materials should be limited to water, sand and fixed plastic objects. All sensory table activities should be supervised for toddlers and preschool children. When water is used in a sensory table, the requirements of Standard 6.2.4.2, Water Play Tables should be met.

RATIONALE: According to the federal government's small parts standard on safe-size toys for children under three years of age, a prohibited small part is any object that fits completely into a specially designed test cylinder two and one-quarter inches long by one and one-quarter inches wide, which approximates the size of the fully expanded throat of a child under three-years-old. Since round objects are more likely to choke children because they can completely block a child's airway, balls and toys with parts that are spheroid, ovoid, or elliptical with a diameter smaller than one and three-quarter inches should be banned for children under three years old (4,5); any part smaller than this is a potential choking hazard (5). Injury and fatality from aspiration of small parts is well-documented (4). Eliminating small parts from children's environment will greatly reduce this risk.

According to the U.S. Food and Drug Administration (FDA), eating as few as four or five uncooked kidney beans can cause severe nausea, vomiting, and diarrhea. In addition to their toxicity, raw kidney beans are small objects that could be inserted by a child into his nose or ear; beans can potentially get stuck, swell, and be difficult to remove (1). Styrofoam peanuts could cause choking. Flour could be aspirated and affect breathing; if spilled on the floor, flour could cause slipping. If soil is used, it must be free from chemicals such as fertilizer or pesticides.

Sensory table activities/materials are not developmentally appropriate for children under the age of eighteen months; the potential health and safety hazards outweigh the benefits for use with this age group. Supervision is required for toddlers and preschool-age children to ensure that they are using materials appropriately (2,3).

Sand used in sensory tables should be new "sterilized" natural sand that is labeled for use in children's sandboxes or labeled as play sand. Water used in sensory tables must be potable and clean.

COMMENTS: Children's hands should be washed before and after using the sensory table. Children with open areas (cuts/sores) should not be allowed to use the sensory table.

TYPE OF FACILITY: Center; Large Family Child Care Home; Small Family Child Care Home

RELATED STANDARDS:
Standard 3.2.2.1: Situations that Require Hand Hygiene
Standard 3.3.0.2: Cleaning and Sanitizing Toys
Standard 6.2.4.1: Sandboxes
Standard 6.2.4.2: Water Play Tables
Standard 6.4.1.2: Inaccessibility of Toys or Objects to Children Under Three Years of Age

REFERENCES:

1. California Childcare Health Program, University of California San Francisco School of Nursing. Health and safety tip. *Child Care Health Connections* 16:1. http://www.ucsfchildcarehealth.org/pdfs/newsletters/2003/CCHPJul_Aug03.pdf.
2. Harms, T., D. Cryer, R. M. Clifford. 2006. *Infant/toddler environment rating scale.* Rev ed. New York: Teachers College Press. http://ers.fpg.unc.edu/infanttoddler-environment-rating-scales-iters-r/.
3. Cryer, D., T. Harms, C. Riley. 2004. *All about the ITERS-R.* Lewisville, NC: Kaplan Early Learning.
4. U.S. Consumer Product Safety Commission (CPSC). 2004. CPSC warns parents about choking hazards to young children, announces new recall of toys posing choking hazards. Release #04-216. http://www.cpsc.gov/cpscpub/prerel/prhtml04/04216.html.
5. American Academy of Pediatrics, Committee on Injury, Violence, and Poison Prevention. 2010. Policy statement: Prevention of choking among children. *Pediatrics* 125:601-7.

STANDARD 6.2.4.4: Trampolines

Trampolines, both full and mini-size, should be prohibited from being used as part of the child care program activities both on-site and during field trips.

RATIONALE: Both the American Academy of Pediatrics (AAP) and American Academy of Orthopedic Surgeons (AAOS) Policy Statements recommend the prohibition of trampolines for children younger than six years of age (1,2). The U.S. Consumer Product Safety Commission (CPSC) also supports this position (3). The numbers of injuries incurred on trampolines is large and growing (4-8). Even if one accepts that the rates of injury are uncertain due to increasing sales as well as injuries, the severity of injury incurred (number of injuries requiring admission for surgery, small but documented number of deaths) all have supported those recommendations. Given the risk reflected in the recommendations of national health and safety groups, there are documented cases where insurance companies have refused to issue or to continue insurance to the home or child care center in which a trampoline was found.

COMMENTS: The AAP recommends: "Despite all currently available measures to prevent injury, the potential for serious injury while using a trampoline remains. The need for supervision and trained personnel at all times makes home use extremely unwise" (1). The trampoline should not be used at home, inside or outside. During anticipatory guidance, health care professionals should advise parents/guardians never to purchase a home trampoline or allow children to use home trampolines (2). The trampoline should not be part of routine physical education classes in schools (3). The trampoline has no place in outdoor playgrounds and should never be regarded as play equipment (1).

TYPE OF FACILITY: Center; Large Family Child Care Home; Small Family Child Care Home

REFERENCES:

1. American Academy of Pediatrics, Committee on Injury and Poison Prevention, and Committee on Sports Medicine and Fitness. 2006. Policy statement: Trampolines at home, school, and recreational centers. *Pediatrics* 117:1846-47.
2. American Academy of Orthopedic Surgeons (AAOS). 2005. *Trampolines and trampoline safety*. Position Statement no. 1135. Rosemont, IL: AAOS.
3. U.S. Consumer Product Safety Commission (CPSC). *Consumer product safety alert: Trampoline safety alert*. Washington, DC: CPSC. http://www.cpsc.gov/cpscpub/pubs/085.pdf.
4. Shields, B. J., S. A. Fernandez, G. A. Smith. 2005. Comparison of mini-trampoline and full-sized trampoline injuries in the United States. *Pediatrics* 116:96-103.
5. Linakis, J. G., M. J. Mello, J. Machan, S. Amanullah, L. M. Palmisciano. 2007. Emergency department visits for pediatric trampoline-related injuries: An update. *Academic Emergency Med* 14:539-44.
6. Levine, D. 2006. All-terrain vehicle, trampoline, and scooter injuries and their prevention in children. *Current Ops Pediatrics* 18:260-65.
7. Smith, G. A. 1998. Injuries to children in the United States related to trampolines, 1990-1995: A national epidemic. *Pediatrics* 101:406-12.
8. Bond, A. 2008. Trampolines unsafe for children at any age. *AAP News* 29:29.

STANDARD 6.2.4.5: Ball Pits

Children should be prohibited from playing in ball pits.

RATIONALE: Ball pits are hard to sanitize and disinfect (1). Supervision is difficult to monitor. Children can bury themselves making it possible for others to jump on them and cause injury (2).

COMMENTS: Although not common in child care facilities, caregivers/teachers should take caution in not allowing play in ball pits when using public play areas.

TYPE OF FACILITY: Center; Large Family Child Care Home; Small Family Child Care Home

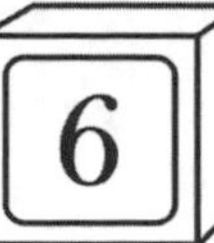

REFERENCES:

1. Davis, S. G., A. M. Corbitt, V. M. Everton, C. A. Grano, P. A. Kiefner, A. S. Wilson, M. Gray. 1999. Are ball pits the playground for potentially harmful bacteria? *Pediatric Nursing* 25:151-55.

2. Fiocchi, A., P. Restani, C. Ballabio, G. R. Bouygue, A. Serra, M. Travaini, L. Terracciano. 2001. Severe anaphylaxis induced by latex as a contaminant of plastic balls in play pits. *J Allergy Clin Immunol* 108:298-300.

6.2.5 Inspection of Play Areas/ Playgrounds and Equipment

STANDARD 6.2.5.1: Inspection of Indoor and Outdoor Play Areas and Equipment

The indoor and outdoor play areas and equipment should be inspected daily for the following:

a) Missing or broken parts;
b) Protrusion of nuts and bolts;
c) Rust and chipping or peeling paint;
d) Sharp edges, splinters, and rough surfaces;
e) Stability of handholds;
f) Visible cracks;
g) Stability of non-anchored large play equipment (e.g., playhouses);
h) Wear and deterioration.

Observations should be documented and filed, and the problems corrected.

Facilities should conduct a monthly inspection as outlined in Appendix EE, America's Playgrounds Safety Report Card.

RATIONALE: Regular outdoor inspections are critical to prevent deterioration of equipment and accumulation of hazardous materials within the play site, and to ensure that appropriate repairs are made as soon as possible (1,2). Pools of water may cause children to slip and fall.

A monthly safety check of all the equipment within the facility as a focused task provides an opportunity to notice wear and tear that requires maintenance.

COMMENTS: Regularity of inspections can be assured by assigning a staff member to check all play equipment to make certain that it is safe for children. Observations should be made while the children are playing, too, to spot any maintenance problems and correct them as soon as possible.

If an off-site play area is used, a safety check for hazardous materials within the play area should be done upon arrival to the off-site playground. Hazardous materials may have been left in the play area by other people before the arrival of children from the child care facility.

If the playground is not safe, then alternate gross motor activities should be offered rather than allowing children to use equipment that is not safe for them because of hazards.

TYPE OF FACILITY: Center; Large Family Child Care Home; Small Family Child Care Home

RELATED STANDARDS:

Standard 5.2.8.1: Integrated Pest Management
Standard 6.2.3.1: Prohibited Surfaces for Placing Climbing Equipment
Standard 9.2.6.1: Policy on Use and Maintenance of Play Areas
Standards 9.2.6.2-9.2.6.3: Reports/Records of Play Area and Equipment
Appendix EE: America's Playgrounds Safety Report Card

REFERENCES:

1. U.S. Consumer Product Safety Commission (CPSC). 2008. *Public playground safety handbook*. Bethesda, MD: CPSC. http://www.cpsc.gov/cpscpub/pubs/325.pdf.

2. U.S. Consumer Product Safety Commission (CPSC). *For kids' sake: Think toy safety*. Washington, DC: CPSC. http://www.cpsc.gov/cpscpub/pubs/281.pdf.

STANDARD 6.2.5.2: Inspection of Play Area Surfacing

Loose-fill surfacing materials used to provide impact absorption beneath play equipment should be checked frequently to ensure surfacing is of sufficient depth and has not shifted or displaced significantly, especially in areas under swings and slide exits. Missing or displaced loose-fill surfacing should be raked back into proper place or replaced so that a constant depth is maintained throughout the playground.

All loose-fill surfacing material, particularly sand, should be inspected daily for:

a) Debris (such as glass);
b) Animal excrement, and other foreign material;
c) Depth and compaction of surface;
d) Standing water, ice, or snow.

Loose fill surfaces should be hosed down for cleaning and raked or sifted to remove hazardous debris as often as needed to keep the surface free of dangerous, unsanitary materials. Surfacing should be raked to fill in areas of wear (e.g., under swings, bottom of slides, etc.) on a daily basis before use.

Check for packing as a result of rain or ice, and if found to be compressed, material should be turned over or raked up to increase resilience capacity. Play should not be permitted on structures in the area if a packed surface cannot be raked up or turned over.

RATIONALE: The number one cause of injury on playgrounds is falls to the surface. Maintaining the correct depth of loose-fill material is crucial for safety. Surfaces should be shock-absorbing (1-3). Cold temperatures may cause "packing," which causes the surface material to lose shock-absorbing capacity. Other materials, such as glass, debris, and animal excrement, present potential sources of injury or infection. Maintaining loose fill surfaces provides for proper sanitation

COMMENTS: Surfacing is not tested with ice or snow on it and thus its shock-absorbing and injury-preventing ability is unrated. Therefore, surfacing with ice or snow cannot be relied upon to absorb falls and prevent injuries. Sand is not an appropriate playground covering in areas where pets or animals are a problem. Contact a Certified Playground Safety Inspector (CPSI) for further guidance. To locate a

CPSI, check the National Park and Recreation Association (NPRA) registry at https://ipv.nrpa.org/CPSI_registry/.

TYPE OF FACILITY: Center; Large Family Child Care Home; Small Family Child Care Home

REFERENCES:

1. ASTM International (ASTM). 2009. *Standard guide for ASTM standards on playground surfacing.* ASTM F2223-09. West Conshohocken, PA: ASTM.

2. ASTM International (ASTM). 2009. *Standard specification for impact attenuation of surfacing materials within the use zone of playground equipment.* ASTM F1292-09. West Conshohocken, PA: ASTM.

3. U.S. Consumer Product Safety Commission (CPSC). 2008. *Public playground safety handbook*. Bethesda, MD: CPSC. http://www.cpsc.gov/cpscpub/pubs/325.pdf.

6.3 Water Play Areas (Pools, Etc.)

6.3.1 Access to and Safety Around Bodies of Water

STANDARD 6.3.1.1: Enclosure of Bodies of Water

All water hazards, such as pools, swimming pools, stationary wading pools, ditches, fish ponds, and water retention or detention basins should be enclosed with a fence that is four to six feet high or higher and comes within three and one-half inches of the ground. Openings in the fence should be no greater than three and one-half inches. The fence should be constructed to discourage climbing and kept in good repair.

If the fence is made of horizontal and vertical members (like a typical wooden fence) and the distance between the tops of the horizontal parts of the fence is less than forty-five inches, the horizontal parts should be on the swimming pool side of the fence. The spacing of the vertical members should not exceed one and three-quarters inches.

For a chain link fence, the mesh size should not exceed one and one-quarter square inches.

Exit and entrance points should have self-closing, positive latching gates with locking devices a minimum of fifty-five inches from the ground.

A wall of the child care facility should not constitute one side of the fence unless the wall has no openings capable of providing direct access to the pool (such as doors, windows, or other openings).

If the facility has a water play area, the following requirements should be met:

a) Water play areas should conform to all state and local health regulations;
b) Water play areas should not include hidden or enclosed spaces;
c) Spray areas and water-collecting areas should have a non-slip surface, such as asphalt;
d) Water play areas, particularly those that have standing water, should not have sudden changes in depth of water;
e) Drains, streams, water spouts, and hydrants should not create strong suction effects or water-jet forces;
f) All toys and other equipment used in and around the water play area should be made of sturdy plastic or metal (no glass should be permitted);
g) Water play areas in which standing water is maintained for more than twenty-four hours should be treated according to Standard 6.3.4.1, and inspected for glass, trash, animal excrement, and other foreign material.

RATIONALE: Most drownings happen in fresh water, often in home swimming pools (1). Most children drown within a few feet of safety and in the presence of a supervising adult (1). Small fence openings (three and one-half inches or smaller) prevent children from passing through the fence (4). All areas must be visible to allow adequate supervision.

An effective fence is one that prevents a child from getting over, under, or through it and keeps the child from gaining access to the pool or body of water except when supervising adults are present. Fences are not childproof, but they provide a layer of protection for a child who strays from supervision.

Fence heights are a matter of local ordinance but it is recommended that it should be at least five feet. A house exterior wall can constitute one side of a fence if the wall has no openings providing direct access to the pool.

With fences made up of horizontal and vertical members, children should not be allowed to use the horizontal members as a form of ladder to climb into a swimming pool area. If the distance between horizontal members is less than forty-five inches, placing the horizontal members on the pool side of the fence will prevent children using this to climb over and into the pool area. However, if the horizontal members are greater than forty-five inches apart, it is more difficult for a child to climb and therefore the horizontal members could be placed on the side of the fence facing away from the pool (2).

COMMENTS: See the American National Standards Institute (ANSI) and ASTM International standards for pool safety (2,3).

TYPE OF FACILITY: Center; Large Family Child Care Home; Small Family Child Care Home

RELATED STANDARDS:

Standard 6.2.5.1: Inspection of Indoor and Outdoor Play Areas and Equipment
Standard 6.2.5.2: Inspection of Play Area Surfacing

REFERENCES:

1. U.S. Consumer Product Safety Commission (CPSC). *How to plan for the unexpected: Preventing child drownings*. Washington, DC: CPSC. http://www.cpsc.gov/CPSCPUB/PUBS/359.pdf.

2. American National Standards Institute (ANSI). 2005. *Model barrier code for residential swimming pools, spas, and hot tubs*. ANSI/IAF-8. New York: ANSI.

3. ASTM International (ASTM). 2008. *Standard guide for fences*

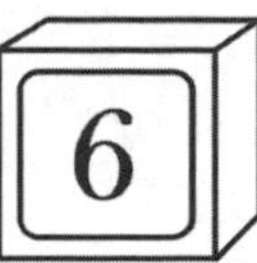

for residential outdoor swimming pools, hot tubs, and spas. ASTM F1908-08. West Conshohocken, PA: ASTM.
4. American Academy of Pediatrics, Committee on Injury, Violence, and Poison Prevention. 2010. Policy statement: Prevention of drowning. *Pediatrics* 126:178-85.

STANDARD 6.3.1.2: Accessibility to Above-Ground Pools

Above-ground pools should have non-climbable sidewalls that are at least four feet high or should be enclosed with an approved fence, as specified in Standard 6.3.1.1 (1,2). When the pool is not in use, steps should be removed from the pool or otherwise protected to ensure that they cannot be accessed.

RATIONALE: The U. S. Consumer Product Safety Commission (CPSC) has estimated that each year about 300 children under five-years-old drown in swimming pools (3).

COMMENTS: CPSC has published an illustrated guideline (*Safety barrier guidelines for home pools*) to explain barriers around and access to home swimming pools (3). The document is available online at http://www.cpsc.gov/cpscpub/pubs/pool.pdf.

TYPE OF FACILITY: Center; Large Family Child Care Home; Small Family Child Care Home

RELATED STANDARDS:
Standard 6.3.1.1: Enclosure of Bodies of Water

REFERENCES:
1. ASTM International (ASTM). 2008. *Standard guide for fences for residential outdoor swimming pools, hot tubs, and spas.* ASTM F1908-08. West Conshohocken, PA: ASTM.
2. ASTM International (ASTM). 2009. *Standard guide for fences/barriers for public, commercial, and multi-family residential use outdoor play areas.* ASTM F2049-09b. West Conshohocken, PA: ASTM.
3. U. S. Consumer Product Safety Commission (CPSC). *Safety barrier guidelines for home pools.* Pub. no. 362. Washington, DC: CPSC. http://www.cpsc.gov/cpscpub/pubs/pool.pdf.

STANDARD 6.3.1.3: Sensors or Remote Monitors

Sensors or remote monitors should not be used in lieu of a fence or proper supervision (1).

RATIONALE: A temporary power outage negates the protection of sensors. Response to an emergency is delayed if a remote monitor is used to replace direct supervision.

TYPE OF FACILITY: Center; Large Family Child Care Home; Small Family Child Care Home

RELATED STANDARDS:
Standard 1.1.1.5: Ratios and Supervision for Swimming, Wading, and Water Play

REFERENCES:
1. American Academy of Pediatrics, Committee on Injury, Violence, and Poison Prevention. 2010. Policy statement: Prevention of drowning. *Pediatrics* 126:178-85.

STANDARD 6.3.1.4: Safety Covers for Swimming Pools

When not in use, in-ground and above-ground swimming pools should be covered with a safety cover that meets or exceeds the ASTM International (ASTM) standard "F1346-03: Standard performance specification for safety covers and labeling requirements for all covers for swimming pools, spas, and hot tubs" (2).

RATIONALE: Fatal injuries have occurred when water has collected on top of a secured pool cover. The depression caused by the water, coupled with the smoothness of the cover material, has proved to be a deadly trap for some children (1). The ASTM standard now defines a safety cover "as a barrier (intended to be completely removed before water use) for swimming pools, spas, hot tubs, or wading pools, attendant appurtenances and/or anchoring mechanisms which reduces--when properly labeled, installed, used and maintained in accordance with the manufacturer's published instructions--the risk of drowning of children under five years of age, by inhibiting their access to the contained body of water, and by providing for the removal of any substantially hazardous level of collected surface water" (2).

Safety covers reduce the possibility of contamination by animals, birds, and insects.

COMMENTS: Facilities should check whether the manufacturers warrant their pool covers as meeting ASTM standards. See ASTM standard "F1346-03." Some jurisdictions require four-sided fencing around swimming pools; the facility should follow the requirements of their jurisdiction. Best practice is four-sided fencing.

TYPE OF FACILITY: Center; Large Family Child Care Home; Small Family Child Care Home

RELATED STANDARDS:
Standard 6.3.1.1: Enclosure of Bodies of Water

REFERENCES:
1. U.S. Consumer Product Safety Commission (CPSC). 2005. *Guidelines for entrapment hazards: Making pools and spas safer.* Washington, DC: CPSC. http://www.cdph.ca.gov/HealthInfo/injviosaf/Documents/DrowningEntrapmentHazards.pdf.
2. ASTM International (ASTM). 2003. *Standard performance specification for safety covers and labeling requirements for all covers for swimming pools, spas, and hot tubs.* ASTM F1346-03. West Conshohocken, PA: ASTM.

STANDARD 6.3.1.5: Deck Surface

A swimming pool should be surrounded by at least a four-foot wide, nonskid surface in good repair, free of tears or breaks (1).

RATIONALE: This standard is to prevent slipping and injury of children and adults and to allow supervising caregivers/teachers to walk around all sides of the pool.

TYPE OF FACILITY: Center; Large Family Child Care Home; Small Family Child Care Home

RELATED STANDARDS:
Standard 6.4.1.1: Pool Toys

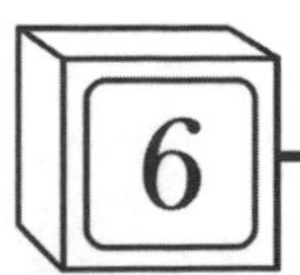

REFERENCES:

1. ASTM International (ASTM). 2009. *Standard practice for manufacture, construction, operation, and maintenance of aquatic play equipment*. ASTM F2461-09. West Conshohocken, PA: ASTM.

STANDARD 6.3.1.6: Pool Drain Covers

All covers for the main drain and other suction ports of swimming and wading pools should be listed by a nationally recognized testing laboratory in accordance with ASME/ANSI standard "A112.19.8: Standard for Suction Fittings for Use in Swimming Pools, Wading Pools, Spas and Hot Tubs," and should be used under conditions that do not exceed the approved maximum flow rate, be securely anchored using manufacturer-supplied parts installed per manufacturer's specifications, be in good repair, and be replaced at intervals specified by manufacturer. Facilities with one outlet per pump, or multiple outlets per pump with less than thirty-six inches center-to-center distance for two outlets, must be equipped with a Safety Vacuum Release System (SVRS) meeting the ASME/ANSI standard "A112.19.17: Manufactured Safety Vacuum Release Systems for Residential and Commercial Swimming Pool, Spas, Hot Tub and Wading Pool Suction Systems" or ASTM International (ASTM) standard "F2387-04: Standard Specification for Manufactured SVRS for Swimming Pools, Spas, and Hot Tubs" standards, as required by the *Virginia Graeme Baker Pool and Spa Safety Act*, Section 1404(c)(1)(A)(I) (1,2).

RATIONALE: In some instances, children have drowned as a result of their body or hair being entrapped or seriously injured by sitting on drain grates (3). Drain covers mitigate the five types of entrapment: hair, body, limb, evisceration, and mechanical (jewelry). Use of flat- or flush-mount covers/grates is prohibited. Use of drain covers under conditions that exceed the maximum flow rate can pose a hazard for entrapment. When drain covers are broken or missing, the body can be entrapped. When a child is playing with an open drain (one with the cover missing), a child can be entrapped by inserting a hand or foot into the pipe and being trapped by the resulting suction. Hair entrapment typically involves females with long, fine hair who are underwater with the head near the suction inlet; they become entrapped when their hair sweeps into and around the cover, and not because of the strong suction forces. Use of a SVRS will not mitigate hair, limb, and mechanical entrapment.

TYPE OF FACILITY: Center; Large Family Child Care Home; Small Family Child Care Home

REFERENCES:

1. American National Standards Institute (ANSI), American Society of Mechanical Engineers (ASME). 2007. *Standard for suction fittings for use in swimming pools, wading pools, spas and hot tubs.* ANSI/ASME A112.19.8. Washington, DC: ANSI.
2. U.S. Congress. 2007. *Virginia Graeme Baker Pool and Spa Safety Act.* 15 USC 8001. http://www.cpsc.gov/businfo/vgb/pssa.pdf.
3. U.S. Consumer Product Safety Commission (CPSC). 2005. *Guidelines for entrapment hazards: Making pools and spas safer.* Washington, DC: CPSC. http://www.cdph.ca.gov/HealthInfo/injviosaf/Documents/DrowningEntrapmentHazards.pdf.

STANDARD 6.3.1.7: Pool Safety Rules

Legible safety rules for the use of swimming and built-in wading pools should be posted in a conspicuous location, and each caregiver/teacher responsible for the supervision of children should read and review them often enough so s/he is able to cite the rules when asked. The facility should develop and review an emergency plan, as specified in Written Plan and Training for Handling Urgent Medical Care or Threatening Incidents, Standard 9.2.4.1.

RATIONALE: This standard is based on state and local regulations and ASTM International (ASTM) standard "F2518-06: Standard Guide for Use of a Residential Swimming Pool, Spa, and Hot Tub Safety" (1).

COMMENTS: Compliance can be assessed by interviewing caregivers/teachers to determine if they know the rules and by observing if the rules are followed.

TYPE OF FACILITY: Center; Large Family Child Care Home; Small Family Child Care Home

RELATED STANDARDS:

Standard 1.1.1.5: Ratios and Supervision for Swimming, Wading, and Water Play
Standards 2.2.0.4-2.2.0.5: Water Safety
Standard 9.2.4.1: Written Plan and Training for Handling Urgent Medical Care or Threatening Incidents

REFERENCES:

1. ASTM International (ASTM). 2006. *Standard guide for use of a residential swimming pool, spa, and hot tub safety: Audit to prevent unintentional drowning*. ASTM F2518-06. West Conshohocken, PA: ASTM.

STANDARD 6.3.1.8: Supervision of Pool Pump

The adult in the pool should be aware of the location of the pump shut-off switch and be able to turn it off in case a child is caught in the drain. Unobstructed access should be provided to an electrical switch that controls the pump. This adult should also have immediate access to a working telephone located at the pool.

RATIONALE: The power of suction of a pool drain often requires that the pump be turned off before a child can be removed. The adult supervisor needs immediate access to the pump shut-off switch (1,2).

TYPE OF FACILITY: Center; Large Family Child Care Home; Small Family Child Care Home

RELATED STANDARDS:

Standard 1.1.1.5: Ratios and Supervision for Swimming, Wading, and Water Play
Standard 6.3.1.6: Pool Drain Covers

REFERENCES:

1. National Fire Protection Association (NFPA). 2011. NFPA 70: *National Electrical Code*. 2011 ed. Quincy, MA: NFPA.
2. U.S. Consumer Product Safety Commission (CPSC). 2005. *Guidelines for entrapment hazards: Making pools and spas safer.* Washington, DC: CPSC. http://www.cdph.ca.gov/HealthInfo/injviosaf/Documents/DrowningEntrapmentHazards.pdf.

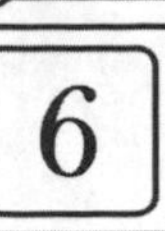

6.3.2 Pool Equipment

STANDARD 6.3.2.1: Lifesaving Equipment

Each swimming pool more than six feet in width, length, or diameter should be provided with a ring buoy and rope, a rescue tube, or a throwing line and a shepherd's hook that will not conduct electricity. This equipment should be long enough to reach the center of the pool from the edge of the pool, should be kept in good repair, and should be stored safely and conveniently for immediate access. Caregivers/teachers should be trained on the proper use of this equipment so that in emergencies, caregivers/teachers will use equipment appropriately. Children should be familiarized with the use of the equipment based on their developmental level.

RATIONALE: Drowning accounts for the highest rate of unintentional injury-related death in children one to four years of age; this lifesaving equipment is essential (1).

TYPE OF FACILITY: Center; Large Family Child Care Home; Small Family Child Care Home

RELATED STANDARDS:
Standard 1.4.3.3: CPR Training for Swimming and Water Play

REFERENCES:
1. National SAFE KIDS Campaign (NSKC). 2004. *Drowning fact sheet*. Washington, DC: NSKC. http://www.preventinjury.org/PDFs/DROWNING.pdf.

STANDARD 6.3.2.2: Lifeline in Pool

A lifeline (rope and float line) should be provided at the five-foot break in grade between the shallow and deep portions of the swimming pool.

RATIONALE: For children's safety, the five-foot depth boundary should be known to caregivers/teachers assisting children in the pool (1).

TYPE OF FACILITY: Center; Large Family Child Care Home; Small Family Child Care Home

RELATED STANDARDS:
Standard 6.3.2.1: Lifesaving Equipment

REFERENCES:
1. Association of Pool and Spa Professionals (APSA). *Layers of protection to help protect pool, spa, and hot tub users, especially children under five years of age*. Alexandria, VA: APSA. http://www.nespapool.org/pdf/consumer_pdf/LayersofProtectionAug05.pdf.

STANDARD 6.3.2.3: Pool Equipment and Chemical Storage Rooms

Pool equipment and chemical storage rooms should be locked, ventilated, and used only for pool equipment and pool chemicals.

RATIONALE: Pool chemicals are kept in concentrated forms that are hazardous to children. Access to these hazards must be carefully controlled (1).

TYPE OF FACILITY: Center; Large Family Child Care Home; Small Family Child Care Home

REFERENCES:
1. U.S. Environmental Protection Agency (EPA), Office of Solid Waste and Emergency Response. 2001. *Safe storage and handling of swimming pool chemicals*. Chemical Safety Alert. http://www.epa.gov/osweroe1/docs/chem/spalert.pdf.

6.3.3 Pool Maintenance

STANDARD 6.3.3.1: Pool Performance Requirements

Where applicable, swimming pools and built-in wading pool equipment and materials should meet the health effects and performance standards of the National Sanitation Foundation or equivalent standards as determined by the local regulatory health authority (1).

RATIONALE: Proper pool operation and maintenance minimizes injuries.

COMMENTS: The National Sanitation Foundation (NSF) standard "NSF/ANSI 50-2009: Equipment for Swimming Pools, Spas, Hot Tubs and other Recreational Water Facilities" provides evaluation criteria for materials, components, products, equipment, and systems for use at recreational water facilities.

TYPE OF FACILITY: Center; Large Family Child Care Home; Small Family Child Care Home

REFERENCES:
1. National Sanitation Foundation International (NSF). 2009. *Equipment for swimming pools, spas, hot tubs and other recreational water facilities*. NSF/ANSI 50-2009. Ann Arbor, MI: NSF.

STANDARD 6.3.3.2: Construction, Maintenance, and Inspection of Pools

If swimming pools or built-in wading pools are on the premises and children use them, the pools should be constructed, maintained, and used in accordance with applicable state or local regulations and should be inspected by the health department to ensure compliance as legally required

When indoor pools are used, they should have adequate ventilation to reduce indoor air pollution.

RATIONALE: Data indicate inadequate ventilation is a source of air pollution experienced by children because of the containment of fumes from chemicals used to treat the water (1).

This standard is based on state and local regulations.

COMMENTS: In the United States, all pool codes are created, reviewed, and approved by state and/or local public health officials. As a result, there are no uniform national standards governing design, construction, operation, and maintenance of swimming pools and other treated recreational water venues (2).

TYPE OF FACILITY: Center; Large Family Child Care Home; Small Family Child Care Home

REFERENCES:
1. Centers for Disease Control and Prevention. 2010. Irritants (chloramines) and indoor pool air quality. http://www.cdc.gov/

healthywater/swimming/pools/irritants-indoor-pool-air-quality.html.
2. Centers for Disease Control and Prevention. 2010. Model aquatic health code (MAHC). http://www.cdc.gov/healthywater/swimming/pools/mahc/.

STANDARD 6.3.3.3: Electrical Safety for Pool Areas

Electrical equipment should be installed and inspected at and around the pool at intervals as required by the regulatory electrical inspector.

No electrical wires or electrical equipment should be located over or within ten feet of the pool area, except as permitted by the National Electrical Code.

RATIONALE: Safety equipment and proper location of electrical equipment prevents electrical hazards that could be life-threatening (1,2). Electrical wires and equipment can produce electrical shock or electrocution.

COMMENTS: For electrical safety, a ground-fault circuit-interrupter is mandatory. The National Electrical Code (NEC) code prohibits electrical installations closer than five feet from water and requires GFCI protection for all electrical equipment, including 240-volt equipment located five to ten feet from the water and for receptacles within a twenty-foot perimeter (1,2).

The National Electrical Code is available from the Institute of Electrical and Electronics Engineers (IEEE).

TYPE OF FACILITY: Center; Large Family Child Care Home; Small Family Child Care Home

RELATED STANDARDS:
Standard 5.2.4.3: Ground-Fault Circuit-Interrupter for Outlets Near Water

REFERENCES:
1. National Fire Protection Association. 2011. *NFPA 70: National Electrical Code.* 2011 ed. Quincy, MA: NFPA.
2. U.S. Consumer Product Safety Commission (CPSC). 2003. CPSC safety alert: Install ground-fault circuit-interrupter protection for pools, spas and hot tubs. http://www.cpsc.gov/cpscpub/pubs/5039.html.

STANDARD 6.3.3.4: Pool Water Temperature

Water temperatures should be maintained at no less than 82°F and no more than 88°F while the pool is in use.

RATIONALE: Because of their relatively larger surface area to body mass, young children can lose or gain body heat more easily than adults. Water temperature for swimming and wading should be warm enough to prevent excess loss of body heat and cool enough to prevent overheating.

COMMENTS: Learner pools in public swimming centers are usually at least two degrees warmer than the main pool.

Caregivers/teachers should be advised about the length of time infants should usually spend in the water and how to recognize when an infant is cold so that temperature control should not be problem (1). Signs that an infant is cold are that the infant has cold skin, becomes unhappy, has low energy or becomes less responsive.

TYPE OF FACILITY: Center; Large Family Child Care Home; Small Family Child Care Home

REFERENCES:
1. Coleman, H., F. D. Finlay. 1995. When is it safe for babies to swim? *Profess Care Mother Child* 5:85-86.

6.3.4 Water Quality of Pools

STANDARD 6.3.4.1: Pool Water Quality

Water in swimming pools and built-in wading pools that children use should be maintained between pH 7.2 and pH 7.8. The water should be disinfected by available free chlorine between 1.0 ppm and 3.0 ppm, or bromine between 1.0 ppm and 6.0 ppm, or by an equivalent agent approved by the health department. The pool should be cleaned, and the chlorine or equivalent disinfectant level and pH level should be tested every two hours during periods of use.

Equipment should be available to test for and maintain a measurable residual disinfectant content in the water and to check the pH of the water. Water should be sampled and a bacteriological analysis conducted to determine absence of fecal coliforms (e.g., *Escherichia coli*, *Pseudomonas aeruginosa*, and *Giardia intestinalis*) at least monthly or at intervals required by the local health authority.

RATIONALE: This practice provides control of bacteria and algae and enhances the participants' comfort and safety. Maintaining pH and disinfectant levels within the prescribed range suppresses bacterial growth to tolerable levels.

Bacteriologic water safety must be ensured to prevent the spread of disease via ingestion of pool water. The chemicals a pool needs to maintain the required standards differ from pool to pool – and day to day. Keeping records of the pool chemistry over time can help interpret its characteristics and aid in performing the correct task (1,3).

COMMENTS: If a stabilized chlorine compound is used, the pH should be maintained between 7.2 and 7.7, and the free available chlorine residual should be at least 1.50 ppm.

For further information, see the Model Aquatic Health Code from the Centers for Disease Control and Prevention (2).

TYPE OF FACILITY: Center; Large Family Child Care Home; Small Family Child Care Home

REFERENCES:
1. Association of Pool and Spa Professionals (APSP), Recreational Water Quality Committee. 2009. *Standard for water quality in public pools and spas*. ANSI/APSP-11 2009. Alexandria, VA: APSP.
2. Centers for Disease Control and Prevention. 2010. Model aquatic health code. http://www.cdc.gov/healthywater/swimming/pools/mahc/.
3. American Chemistry Council, Chlorine Chemistry Division. Pool treatment 101: Introduction to chlorine sanitizing. http://www.americanchemistry.com/s_chlorine/sec_content.asp?CID=1167&DID=4529&CTYPEID=109/.

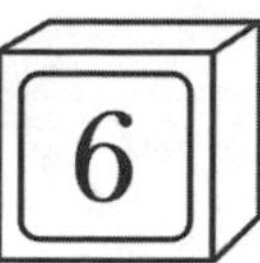

STANDARD 6.3.4.2: Chlorine Pucks

"Chlorine Pucks" must not be placed in skimmer baskets or placed anywhere in pools when children are present. If pucks are used, they must be dissolved before children enter the pool.

RATIONALE: Although this practice can keep chlorine disinfectant levels high, it can be dangerous because the "puck" is a concentrated form of chlorine and is very caustic. Curious children may take out a puck and handle it, causing serious skin irritations or burns (1). Contact with eyes can cause serious injury. Lung damage can occur if children inhale vapors, or children could ingest the poison.

TYPE OF FACILITY: Center; Large Family Child Care Home; Small Family Child Care Home

REFERENCES:

1. U.S. Environmental Protection Agency. 2010. Swimming pool chemicals, chlorine. http://www.epa.gov/kidshometour/products/cjug.htm.

6.3.5 Other Water Play Areas

STANDARD 6.3.5.1: Hot Tubs, Spas, and Saunas

Children should not be permitted in hot tubs, spas, or saunas in child care. Areas should be secured to prevent any access by children.

RATIONALE: Any body of water, including hot tubs, pails, and toilets, presents a drowning risk to young children (1-3). Toddlers and infants are particularly susceptible to overheating.

TYPE OF FACILITY: Center; Large Family Child Care Home; Small Family Child Care Home

RELATED STANDARDS:

Standard 6.3.1.1: Enclosure of Bodies of Water
Standard 6.3.1.4: Safety Covers For Swimming Pools
Standard 6.3.1.6: Pool Drain Covers

REFERENCES:

1. Gipson, K. 2008. *Pool and spa submersion: Estimated injuries and reported fatalities, 2008 report*. Atlanta: U.S. Consumer Product Safety Commission. http://www.cpsc.gov/LIBRARY/poolsub2008.pdf.
2. U.S. Consumer Product Safety Commission (CPSC). 2009. CPSC warns of in-home drowning dangers with bathtubs, bath seats, buckets. Release #10-008. http://www.cpsc.gov/cpscpub/prerel/prhtml10/10008.html.
3. American Academy of Pediatrics, Committee on Injury, Violence, and Poison Prevention. 2010. Policy statement: Prevention of drowning. *Pediatrics* 126:178-85.

STANDARD 6.3.5.2: Water in Containers

Bathtubs, buckets, diaper pails, and other open containers of water should be emptied immediately after use.

RATIONALE: In addition to home swimming and wading pools, young children drown in bathtubs and pails (4). Bathtub drownings are equally distributed in both sexes. Any body of water, including hot tubs, pails, and toilets, presents a drowning risk to young children (1,2,4,5).

From 2003-2005, eleven children under the age of five died from drowning in buckets or containers that were being used for cleaning (4). Of all buckets, the five-gallon size presents the greatest hazard to young children because of its tall straight sides and its weight with even just a small amount of liquid. It is nearly impossible for top-heavy infants and toddlers to free themselves when they fall into a five-gallon bucket head first (3).

TYPE OF FACILITY: Center; Large Family Child Care Home; Small Family Child Care Home

REFERENCES:

1. U.S. Consumer Product Safety Commission (CPSC). 1994. *How to plan for the unexpected: Preventing child drownings*. Document #359. Washington, DC: CPSC. http://www.cpsc.gov/CPSCPUB/PUBS/359.pdf.
2. Rivera, F. P. 1999. Pediatric injury control in 1999: Where do we go from here? *Pediatrics* 103:883-88.
3. U.S. Consumer Product Safety Commission (CPSC). Infants and toddlers can drown in 5-gallon buckets. Document #5006. http://www.cpsc.gov/cpscpub/pubs/5006.html.
4. Gipson, K. 2008. *Submersions related to non-pool and non-spa products, 2008 report.* Washington, DC: U.S. Consumer Product Safety Commission. http://www.cpsc.gov/library/FOIA/FOIA09/OS/nonpoolsub2008.pdf.
5. American Academy of Pediatrics, Committee on Injury, Violence, and Poison Prevention. 2010. Policy statement: Prevention of drowning. *Pediatrics* 126:178-85.

STANDARD 6.3.5.3: Portable Wading Pools

Portable wading pools should not be permitted.

RATIONALE: Small portable wading pools do not permit adequate control of sanitation and safety, and they promote transmission of infectious diseases (1,2).

COMMENTS: Sprinklers, hoses, or small individual water buckets are safe alternatives as a cooling or play activity, under close supervision.

TYPE OF FACILITY: Center; Large Family Child Care Home; Small Family Child Care Home

REFERENCES:

1. Murph, J. R., S. D. Palmer, D. Glassy, eds. 2005. *Health in child care: A manual for health professionals*. 4th ed. Elk Grove Village, IL: American Academy of Pediatrics.
2. American Academy of Pediatrics, Committee on Injury, Violence, and Poison Prevention. 2010. Policy statement: Prevention of drowning. *Pediatrics* 126:178-85.

6.4 Toys

6.4.1 Selected Toys

STANDARD 6.4.1.1: Pool Toys

Tricycles, wagons, and other non-water toys should not be permitted on the pool deck. Use of flotation devices such as inflatable items (e.g., water wings), kick boards, etc. should be prohibited. Use of properly fitted and age-appropriate life jackets according to the manufacturer's instructions should be permitted with close supervision. All toys appropriate for water play should be removed from the pool after use so children are not tempted to reach for them.

RATIONALE: Playing with non-water toys, such as tricycles or wagons, on the pool deck may result in unintentional injuries or falls into the water. Reliance on flotation devices may give children false confidence in their ability to protect themselves in deep water. Flotation devices also may promote complacency in caregivers/teachers who believe the child is safe (1). Toys left near the pool may be tempting for a child who could reach for it and fall into the water.

TYPE OF FACILITY: Center; Large Family Child Care Home; Small Family Child Care Home

RELATED STANDARDS:
Standard 6.3.1.5: Deck Surface

REFERENCES:
1. American Academy of Pediatrics, Committee on Injury, Violence, and Poison Prevention. 2010. Policy statement: Prevention of drowning. *Pediatrics* 126:178-85.

STANDARD 6.4.1.2: Inaccessibility of Toys or Objects to Children Under Three Years of Age

Small objects, toys, and toy parts available to children under the age of three years should meet the federal small parts standards for toys. The following toys or objects should not be accessible to children under three years of age:

a) Toys or objects with removable parts with a diameter less than one and one-quarter inches and a length between one inch and two and one-quarter inches;
b) Balls and toys with spherical, ovoid (egg shaped), or elliptical parts that are smaller than one and three-quarters inches in diameter;
c) Toys with sharp points and edges;
d) Plastic bags;
e) Styrofoam objects;
f) Coins;
g) Rubber or latex balloons;
h) Safety pins;
i) Marbles;
j) Magnets;
k) Foam blocks, books, or objects;
l) Other small objects;
m) Latex gloves;
n) Bulletin board tacks;
o) Glitter.

RATIONALE: Injury and fatality from aspiration of small parts is well-documented (1,2). Eliminating small parts from children's environment will greatly reduce the risk (2). Objects should not be small enough to fit entirely into a child's mouth.

According to the federal government's small parts standard on a safe-size toy for children under three years of age, a small part should be at least one and one-quarter inches in diameter and between one inch and two and one-quarter inches long; any part smaller than this has a potential choking hazard.

Magnets generally are small enough to pass through the digestive tract, however, they can attach to each other across intestinal walls, causing obstructions and perforations within the gastrointestinal tract (5).

Glitter, inadvertently rubbed in eyes, has been known to scratch the surface of the eye and is especially hazardous in children under three years of age (3).

Toys can also contain many chemicals of concern such as lead, phthalates found in many polyvinylchloride (PVC) plastics, cadmium, chlorine, arsenic, bromine, and mercury. When children put toys in their mouths, they may be exposed to these chemicals.

COMMENTS: Toys or games intended for use by children three to five years of age and that contain small parts should be labeled "CHOKING HAZARD--Small Parts. Not for children under three." Because choking on small parts occurs throughout the preschool years, small parts should be kept away from children at least up to three years of age. Also, children occasionally have choked on toys or toy parts that meet federal standards, so caregivers/teachers must constantly be vigilant (2).

The federal standard that applies is Code of Federal Regulations, Title 16, Part 1501 – "Method for Identifying Toys and Other Articles Intended for Use by Children Under 3 Years of Age Which Present Choking, Aspiration, or Ingestion Hazards Because of Small Parts" – which defines the method for identifying toys and other articles intended for use by children under three years of age that present choking, aspiration, or ingestion hazards because of small parts. To obtain this publication, contact the Superintendent of Documents of the U.S. Government Printing Office or access online at http://www.access.gpo.gov/nara/cfr/waisidx_04/16cfr1501_04.html. This information also is described in the U.S. Consumer Product Safety Commission (CPSC) document, "Small Parts Regulations: Toys and Products Intended for Use by Children Under 3 Years Old," available online at http://www.cpsc.gov/businfo/regsumsmallparts.pdf. Also note the ASTM International (ASTM) standard "F963-08: Standard Consumer Safety Specification on Toy Safety." To obtain this publication, contact the ASTM at http://www.astm.org.

CPSC has produced several useful resources regarding safety and toys based on age group, see: "Which Toy for Which Child Ages Birth to Five" at http://www.cpsc.gov/cpscpub/pubs/285.pdf and "Which Toy for Which Child Ages Six through Twelve" at http://www.cpsc.gov/cpscpub/pubs/286.pdf.

New technologies have become smaller and smaller. Caregivers/teachers should be aware of items such as small computer components, batteries in talking books, mobile phones, portable music players, etc. that fall under item a) in the list of prohibited items.

HealthyToys.org is a good resource for information on chemical contents in toys (4).

TYPE OF FACILITY: Center; Large Family Child Care Home; Small Family Child Care Home

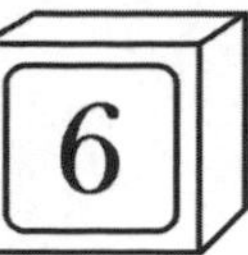

REFERENCES:

1. Chowdhury, R. T., U.S. Consumer Product Safety Commission. 2008. *Toy-related deaths and injuries, calendar year 2007*. Washington, DC: CPSC. http://www.cpsc.gov/LIBRARY/toymemo07.pdf.
2. American Academy of Pediatrics, Committee on Injury, Violence, and Poison Prevention. 2010. Policy statement: Prevention of choking among children. *Pediatrics* 125:601-7.
3. Southern Daily Echo. 2009. Dr. John Heyworth from Southampton General Hospital warns about festive injuries. http://www.dailyecho.co.uk/news/4814667.City_doctor_warns_about_bizarre_Christmas_injuries/.
4. HealthyStuff.org. Chemicals of concern: Introduction. http://www.healthystuff.org/departments/toys/chemicals.introduction.php.
5. Centers for Disease Control and Prevention. 2006. Gastrointestinal injuries from magnet ingestion in children — United States, 2003-2006. *MMWR* 55:1296-1300.

STANDARD 6.4.1.3: Crib Toys

Crib gyms, crib toys, mobiles, mirrors, and all objects/toys are prohibited in or attached to an infant's crib. Items or toys should not be hung from the ceiling over an infant's crib.

RATIONALE: Falling objects could cause injury to an infant lying in a crib.

The presence of crib gyms presents a potential strangulation hazard for infants who are able to lift their head above the crib surface. These children can fall across the crib gym and not be able to remove themselves from that position (1).

The presence of mobiles, crib toys, mirrors, etc. present a potential hazard if the objects can be reached and/or pulled down by an infant (1). Some stuffed animals and other objects that dangle from strings can wrap around a child's neck (2).

Soft objects/toys can cause suffocation.

COMMENTS: Ornamental or small toys are often hung over an infant to provide stimulation; however, the crib should be used for sleep only. The crib is not recommended as a place to entertain an infant or to "contain" an infant. If an infant is not content in a crib, the infant should be removed.

Even though this is best practice for infants in any environment, the recommendation for prohibiting all crib gyms, mobiles, and all toys/objects in or attached to cribs may differ from what is done at an infant's home. Caregivers/teachers have a professional responsibility to ensure a safe environment for children; therefore, child care settings are held at a higher standard, warranting the removal of these potential hazards.

TYPE OF FACILITY: Center; Large Family Child Care Home; Small Family Child Care Home

RELATED STANDARDS:
Standard 3.1.4.1: Safe Sleep Practices and SIDS/Suffocation Risk Reduction

REFERENCES:

1. U.S. Consumer Product Safety Commission (CPSC). CPSC warns of strangulation with crib toys. Consumer Product Safety Alert. http://www.cpsc.gov/cpscpub/pubs/5024.pdf.
2. American Academy of Pediatrics, Task Force on Sudden Infant Death Syndrome. 2005. Policy statement: The changing concept of sudden infant death syndrome: Diagnostic coding shifts, controversies regarding the sleeping environment, and new variables to consider in reducing risk. *Pediatrics* 116:1245-55.

STANDARD 6.4.1.4: Projectile Toys

Projectile toys should be prohibited.

RATIONALE: These types of toys present high risks for aspiration, eye injuries, and other types of injuries (1).

COMMENTS: Examples of projectile toys are: darts, arrows, air-pumped ball launchers, and sling shots.

TYPE OF FACILITY: Center; Large Family Child Care Home; Small Family Child Care Home

REFERENCES:

1. U.S. Consumer Product Safety Commission. 2007. CPSC delivers the ABC's of toy safety. Release no. 08-086. http://www.cpsc.gov/cpscpub/prerel/prhtml08/08086.html.

STANDARD 6.4.1.5: Balloons

Infants, toddlers, and preschool children should not be permitted to inflate balloons, suck on or put balloons in their mouths nor have access to uninflated or underinflated balloons. Children under eight should not have access to latex balloons or inflated latex objects that are treated as balloons and these objects should not be permitted in the child care facility.

RATIONALE: Balloons are an aspiration hazard (1). The U.S. Consumer Product Safety Commission (CPSC) reported eight deaths from balloon aspiration with choking between 2006 and 2008 (1). Aspiration injuries occur from latex balloons or other latex objects treated as balloons, such as inflated latex gloves. Latex gloves are commonly used in child care facilities for diaper changing, but they should not be inflated (2). When children bite inflated latex balloons or gloves, these objects may break suddenly and blow an obstructing piece of latex into the child's airway. Exposure to latex balloons could trigger an allergic reaction in children with latex allergies.

Underinflated or uninflated balloons of all types could be chewed or sucked and pieces potentially aspirated.

TYPE OF FACILITY: Center; Large Family Child Care Home; Small Family Child Care Home

RELATED STANDARDS:
Standard 6.4.1.2: Inaccessibility of Toys or Objects to Children Under Three Years of Age

REFERENCES:

1. Garland, S. 2009. *Toy-related deaths and injuries, calendar year 2008*. Bethesda, MD: U.S. Consumer Product Safety Commission. http://www.cpsc.gov/library/toymemo08.pdf.
2. American Academy of Pediatrics, Committee on Injury, Violence, and Poison Prevention. 2010. Policy statement: Prevention of choking among children. *Pediatrics* 125:601-7.

6.4.2 Riding Toys and Helmets

STANDARD 6.4.2.1: Riding Toys with Wheels and Wheeled Equipment

Riding toys (such as tricycles) and wheeled equipment (such as scooters) used in the child care setting should:

a) Be spokeless;
b) Be capable of being steered;
c) Be of a size appropriate for the child;
d) Have a low center of gravity;
e) Be in good condition, work properly, and free of sharp edges or protrusions that may injure the children;
f) Be non-motorized (excluding wheelchairs).

All riders should wear properly fitting helmets. See Standard 6.4.2.2 Helmets, regarding proper usage and type of helmet. Helmets should be removed once children are no longer using wheeled riding toys or wheeled equipment. Children should wear knee and elbow pads in addition to helmets when using wheeled equipment such as scooters, skateboards, rollerblades, etc.

Children should be closely supervised when using riding toys or wheeled equipment.

When not in use, riding toys with wheels and wheeled equipment should be stored in a location where they will not present a physical obstacle to the children and caregivers/teachers. The staff should inspect riding toys and wheeled equipment at least monthly for loose or missing hardware/parts, protrusions, cracks, or rough edges that can lead to injury.

RATIONALE: Riding toys can provide much enjoyment for children. However, because of their high center of gravity and speed, they often cause injuries in young children. Wheels with spokes can potentially cause entrapment injuries. Wearing helmets when children are learning to use riding toys or wheeled equipment teaches children the practice of wearing helmets while using any riding toy or wheeled equipment. Children should remove their helmets when they are no longer using a riding toy or wheeled equipment because helmets can be a potential strangulation hazard if they are worn for other activities (such as playing on playground equipment, climbing trees, etc.) and/or worn incorrectly.

Motorized wheeled equipment (excluding wheelchairs) used by children in a child care setting does not promote good physical activity (2). Vehicles used by children in child care need to be child propelled rather than battery propelled.

The U.S. Consumer Product Safety Commission (CPSC) and Centers for Disease Control and Prevention (CDC) reported in 2000 that 23% of children treated in emergency departments for scooter-related injuries were age eight or under (1).

Helmet use is associated with a reduction in the risk of any head injury by 69%, brain injury by 65%, and severe brain injuries by 74%, and recommended for all children one year of age and over (3).

COMMENTS: Concern regarding the spreading of head lice in sharing helmets should not override the practice of using helmets. The prevention of a potential brain injury heavily outweighs a possible case of head lice. While it is best practice for each child to have his/her own helmet, this may not be possible. If helmets need to be shared, it is recommended to clean the helmet between users. Wiping the lining with a damp cloth should remove any head lice, nits, or fungal spores. More vigorous washing of helmets, using detergents, cleaning chemicals, and sanitizers, is not recommended because these chemicals may cause the physical structure of the impact-absorbing material to deteriorate inside the helmet. The use of these chemicals can also deteriorate the straps used to hold the helmet on the head.

TYPE OF FACILITY: Center; Large Family Child Care Home; Small Family Child Care Home

RELATED STANDARDS:
Standards 3.3.0.2-3.3.0.3: Cleaning and Sanitizing Toys and Objects Intended for the Mouth
Standards 6.4.1.2-6.4.1.5: Special Play Equipment Requirements for Infants, Toddlers, and Preschoolers
Standard 6.4.2.2: Helmets
Appendix II: Bike Helmets: Quick-Fit Check

REFERENCES:
1. Kubiak, R., T. Slongo. 2003. Unpowered scooter injuries in children. *Acta Paediatrics* 92:50-54.
2. Griffin, R., C. T. Parks, L. W. Rue, III, G. McGwin, Jr. 2008. Comparison of severe injuries between powered and nonpowered scooters among children age 2 to 12 in the United States. *Academic Pediatrics* 8:379-82.
3. Thompson, D. C., F. P. Rivara, R. S. Thompson. 1996. Effectiveness of bicycle safety helmets in preventing head injuries: A case-control study. *JAMA* 276:1968-73.

STANDARD 6.4.2.2: Helmets

All children one year of age and over should wear properly fitted and approved helmets while riding toys with wheels (tricycles, bicycles, etc.) or using any wheeled equipment (rollerblades, skateboards, etc.). Helmets should be removed as soon as children stop riding the wheeled toys or using wheeled equipment. Approved helmets should meet the standards of the U.S. Consumer Product Safety Commission (CPSC) (5). The standards sticker should be located on the bike helmet. Bike helmets should be replaced if they have been involved in a crash, the helmet is cracked, when straps are broken, the helmet can no longer be worn properly, or according to recommendations by the manufacturer (usually after three years).

RATIONALE: Injuries occur when riding tricycles, bicycles, and other riding toys or wheeled equipment. Helmet use is associated with a reduction in the risk of any head injury by 69%, brain injury by 65%, and severe brain injuries by 74%, and recommended for all children one year of age and over (1-3).

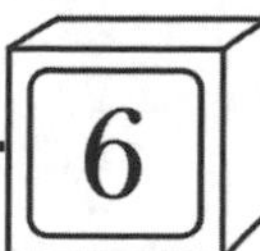

Helmets can be a potential strangulation hazard if they are worn for activities other than when using riding toys or wheeled equipment and/or when worn incorrectly.

It is not recommended that infants (children under the age of one year) wear helmets or ride as a passenger on wheeled equipment. Infants are just learning to sit unsupported at about nine months of age. Until this age, infants have not developed sufficient bone mass and muscle tone to enable them to sit unsupported with their backs straight. Pediatricians advise against having infants sitting in a slumped or curled position for prolonged periods due to the underdevelopment of their neck muscles (4). This situation may even be exacerbated by the added weight of a bicycle helmet on the infant's head. Because pediatricians recommend against having children under age one as passengers on bicycles, the CPSC does not want the certification label to imply that children under age one can ride safely.

COMMENTS: The CPSC helmet standard became effective in February 1999 (5). Bike helmets manufactured or imported for sale in the U.S. after January 1999 must meet the CPSC standard. Helmets made before this date will not have a CPSC approval label. However, helmets made before this date should have an ASTM International (ASTM) approval label. The American National Standard Institute (ANSI) standard for helmet approval has been withdrawn, and ANSI approval labels will no longer appear on helmets. The Snell Memorial Foundation also no longer certifies bike helmets.

Concern regarding the spreading of head lice when sharing helmets should not override the practice of using helmets. The prevention of a potential brain injury heavily outweighs a possible case of head lice. While it is best practice for each child to have his/her own helmet, this may not be possible. If helmets need to be shared, it is recommended to clean the helmet between users. Wiping the lining with a damp cloth should remove any head lice, nits, or fungal spores. More vigorous washing of helmets, using detergents, cleaning chemicals, and sanitizers, is not recommended because these chemicals may cause the physical structure of the impact-absorbing material to deteriorate inside the helmet as well as deteriorate the straps.

TYPE OF FACILITY: Center; Large Family Child Care Home; Small Family Child Care Home

RELATED STANDARDS:
Standard 6.4.2.1: Riding Toys with Wheels and Wheeled Equipment

REFERENCES:

1. Thompson, D. C., F. P. Rivara, R. S. Thompson. 1996. Effectiveness of bicycle safety helmets in preventing head injuries: A case-control study. *JAMA* 276:1968-73.
2. National Highway Traffic Safety Administration. Tip #7: Play it safe: Walking and biking safely. http://www.buckleupnc.org/pdf/NHTSA_ChildSafetyTip07.pdf.
3. U.S. Consumer Product Safety Commission. 2005. CPSC guidelines for age-related activities. Bicycle Helmet Safety Institute. http://www.helmets.org/ageguide.htm.
4. Bicycle Helmet Safety Institute. 2010. Should you take your baby along? http://www.helmets.org/little1s.htm.
5. U.S. Consumer Product Safety Commission (CPSC). 1999. CPSC issues new safety standard for bike helmets. http://www.cpsc.gov/cpscpub/prerel/prhtml98/98062.html.

STANDARD 6.4.2.3: Bike Routes

For facilities providing care for school-age children and permitting bicycling as an activity, the bike routes allowed should be reviewed and approved in writing by the local police and taught to the children in the facility. Children should wear safety helmets as described in Standard 6.4.2.2.

RATIONALE: School-age children who use bicycles for transportation should use bike routes that present the lowest potential for injury. Review and approval of bike routes by the local police minimizes the potential danger (1).

TYPE OF FACILITY: Center; Large Family Child Care Home; Small Family Child Care Home

RELATED STANDARDS:
Standard 6.4.2.2: Helmets

REFERENCES:

1. National Highway Traffic Safety Administration. Tip #7: Play it safe: Walking and biking safely. http://www.buckleupnc.org/pdf/NHTSA_ChildSafetyTip07.pdf.

6.5 Transportation

6.5.1 Transportation Staff

STANDARD 6.5.1.1: Competence and Training of Transportation Staff

At least one adult who accompanies or drives children for field trips and out-of-facility activities should receive training by a professional knowledgeable about child development and procedures, to ensure the safety of all children. The caregiver should hold a valid pediatric first aid certificate, including rescue breathing and management of blocked airways, as specified in First Aid and CPR Standards 1.4.3.1-1.4.3.3. Any emergency medications that a child might require, such as self-injecting epinephrine for life-threatening allergy, should also be available at all times as well as a mobile phone to call for medical assistance. Child:staff ratios should be maintained on field trips and during transport, as specified in Standards 1.1.1.1-1.1.1.5; the driver should not be included in these ratios. No child should ever be left alone in the vehicle.

All drivers, passenger monitors, chaperones, and assistants should receive instructions in safety precautions. Transportation procedures should include:

a) Use of developmentally appropriate safety restraints;
b) Proper placement of the child in the motor vehicle in accordance with state and federal child restraint laws and regulations and recognized best practice;
c) Training in handling of emergency medical situations. If a child has a chronic medical condition or special health care needs that could result in an emergency (such as asthma, diabetes, or seizures), the driver or chaperone should have written instructions including parent/guardian emergency contacts, child summary

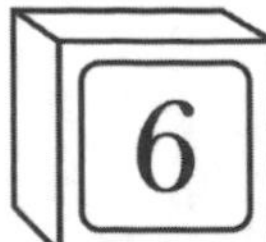

health information, special needs and treatment plans, and should:
1) Recognize the signs of a medical emergency;
2) Know emergency procedures to follow (3);
3) Have on hand any emergency supplies or medications necessary, properly stored out of reach of children;
4) Know specific medication administration (ex. a child who requires EpiPen or diazepam);
5) Know about water safety when field trip is to a location with a body of water.

d) Knowledge of appropriate routes to emergency facility;
e) Defensive driving;
f) Child supervision during transport, including never leaving a child unattended in or around a vehicle;
g) Issues that may arise in transporting children with behavioral issues (e.g., temper tantrums or oppositional behavior).

The receipt of such instructions should be documented in a personnel record for any paid staff or volunteer who participates in field trips or transportation activities.

Vehicles should be equipped with a first aid kit, fire extinguisher, seat belt cutter, and maps. At least one adult should have a functioning cell phone at hand. Information, names of the children and parent/guardian contact information should be carried in the vehicle along with identifying information (name, address, and telephone number) about the child care center.

RATIONALE: Injuries are more likely to occur when a child's surroundings or routine changes. Activities outside the facility may pose increased risk for injury. When children are excited or busy playing in unfamiliar areas, they are more likely to forget safety measures unless they are closely supervised at all times.

Children have died from heat stress from being left unattended in closed vehicles. Temperatures in hot motor vehicles can reach dangerous levels within fifteen minutes. Due to this danger, vehicles should be locked when not in use and checked after use to make sure no child is left unintentionally in a vehicle. Children left unattended also can be victims of backovers (when an unseen child is run over by being behind a vehicle that is backing up), power window strangulations, and other preventable injuries (1,2).

All adults cannot be assumed to be knowledgeable about the various developmental levels or special needs of children. Training by someone with appropriate knowledge and experience is needed to appropriately address these issues. This is particularly important with high incidence disabilities such as autistic spectrum disorders and ADHD.

COMMENTS: When field trips are planned, all field trip sites should be visited by a member of the child care staff and all potential hazards identified. The child care staff should be knowledgeable about location and any emergency plans of the location. For example, if the children are taken to the zoo, the zoo will have its own emergency procedures that the child care would be expected to follow. This standard also applies when caregivers/teachers are walking with children to and from a destination.

A designated staff person should check to ensure all children safely exit the vehicle when it arrives at the designated location. This may include use of an attendance list of all children being transported so it can be checked against those who get out of the vehicle. Also, have another staff member do a thorough and complete inspection of the vehicle to see that the vehicle is empty before locking.

The National Highway Traffic Safety Administration has materials on child passenger safety at: http://www.nhtsa.gov/Safety/CPS as well as materials from the American Academy of Pediatrics at http://www.aap.org/healthtopics/carseatsafety.cfm.

TYPE OF FACILITY: Center; Large Family Child Care Home; Small Family Child Care Home

RELATED STANDARDS:
Standards 1.1.1.1-1.1.1.5: Child:Staff Ratio and Group Size
Standards 1.4.3.1-1.4.3.3: First Aid and CPR
Standards 2.2.0.4-2.2.0.5: Water Safety
Standard 5.3.1.12: Availability and Use of a Telephone or Wireless Communication Device
Standard 6.5.2.1: Drop-Off and Pick-Up
Standard 6.5.2.4: Interior Temperature of Vehicles

REFERENCES:

1. Guard, A., S. S. Gallagher. 2005. Heat related deaths to young children in parked cars: An analysis of 171 fatalities in the United States, 1995-2002. *Injury Prevention* 11:33-37.
2. Babcock-Dunning, L., A. Guard, S. S. Gallagher, E. Streit-Kaplan. 2008. *Guidelines for developing educational materials to address children unattended in vehicles*. Newton, MA: Health and Human Development Programs, Education Development Center. http://www.hhd.org/sites/hhd.org/files/Children Unattended in Vehicles.pdf.
3. American Academy of Pediatrics, Committee on Injury, Violence, and Poison Prevention, and Council on School Health. 2007. Policy statement: School transportation safety. *Pediatrics* 120:213-20.

STANDARD 6.5.1.2: Qualifications for Drivers

Any driver who transports children for a child care program should be at least twenty-one years of age and should have:

a) A valid commercial driver's license that authorizes the driver to operate the vehicle being driven;
b) Evidence of a safe driving record for more than five years, with no crashes where a citation was issued;
c) No alcohol, prescription or over-the-counter medications, or other drugs associated with impaired ability to drive, within twelve hours prior to transporting children. Drivers should ensure that any prescription or over-the-counter drugs taken will not impair their ability to drive;
d) No tobacco, alcohol, or drug use while driving;
e) No criminal record of crimes against or involving children, child neglect or abuse, substance abuse, or any crime of violence;
f) No medical condition that would compromise driving, supervision, or evacuation capability including fatigue and sleep deprivation;

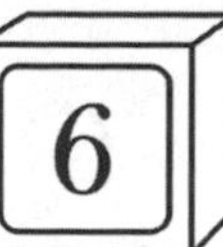

g) Valid pediatric CPR and first aid certificate if transporting children alone.

The driver's license number and date of expiration, vehicle insurance information, and verification of current state vehicle inspection should be on file in the facility.

The child care program should require drug testing when noncompliance with the restriction on the use of alcohol or other drugs is suspected.

RATIONALE: Driving children is a significant responsibility. Child care programs must assure that anyone who drives the children is competent to drive the vehicle being driven.

Patients treated with benzodiazepines, GABAergic compounds, or tricyclic antidepressants (TCAs) should be cautioned when driving a car. Studies have shown significant impairment after administration of these medications. Driving a car when treated with buspirone, venlafaxine, 5HT-antagonists, and SSRIs seems relatively safe (1).

COMMENTS: The driver should advise his/her primary care provider of his/her job and question whether it is safe to drive children while on medication(s) prescribed. Compliance can be measured by testing blood or urine levels for drugs. Refusal to permit such testing should preclude continued employment.

TYPE OF FACILITY: Center; Large Family Child Care Home; Small Family Child Care Home

RELATED STANDARDS:
Standard 6.5.2.5: Distractions While Driving
Standards 9.2.5.1-9.2.5.2: Transportation Policies

REFERENCES:
1. Verster, J. C., D. S. Veldhuijzen, E. R. Volkerts. 2005. Is it safe to drive a car when treated with anxiolytics? Evidence from on the road driving studies during normal traffic. *Current Psychiatry Reviews* 1:215-25.

6.5.2 Transportation Safety

STANDARD 6.5.2.1: Drop-Off and Pick-Up

The facility should have, and communicate to staff and parents/guardians, a plan for safe, supervised drop-off and pick-up points and pedestrian crosswalks in the vicinity of the facility. The plan should require drop off and pick up only at the curb or at an off-street location protected from traffic. The facility should assure that any adult who supervises drop-off and loading can see and assure that children are clear of the perimeter of all vehicles before any vehicle moves. The staff will keep an accurate attendance and time record of all children picked up and dropped off. The facility should assure that a staff member or adult parent/guardian is observing the process of dropping off and picking up children. The adult who is supervising the child should be required to stay with each child until the responsibility for that child has been accepted by the individual designated in advance to care for that child.

RATIONALE: Injuries and fatalities have occurred during the loading and unloading process, especially in situations where vans or school buses are used to transport children. Increased supervision and interactions between adults and children promotes safety and helps children learn to be aware of their surroundings.

COMMENTS: The staff should examine the parking area and determine the safest way to drop off and pick up children (1). Plans for loading and unloading should be discussed and demonstrated with the children, families, caregivers/teachers, and drivers.

TYPE OF FACILITY: Center; Large Family Child Care Home; Small Family Child Care Home

REFERENCES:
1. U.S. General Services Administration (GSA). 2003. *The child care center design guide*. New York: GSA. http://www.gsa.gov/graphics/pbs/designguidesmall.pdf.

STANDARD 6.5.2.2: Child Passenger Safety

When children are driven in a motor vehicle other than a bus, school bus, or a bus operated by a common carrier, the following should apply:

a) A child should be transported only if the child is restrained in developmentally appropriate car safety seat, booster seat, seat belt, or harness that is suited to the child's weight, age, and/or psychological development in accordance with state and federal laws and regulations and the child is securely fastened, according to the manufacturer's instructions, in a developmentally appropriate child restraint system.
b) Age and size-appropriate vehicle child restraint systems should be used for children under eighty pounds and under four-feet-nine-inches tall and for all children considered too small, in accordance with state and federal laws and regulations, to fit properly in a vehicle safety belt. The child passenger restraint system must meet the federal motor vehicle safety standards contained in the Code of Federal Regulations, Title 49, Section 571.213 (especially Federal Motor Vehicle Safety Standard 213), and carry notice of such compliance.
c) For children who are obese or overweight, it is important to find a car safety seat that fits the child properly. Caregivers/teachers should not use a car safety seat if the child weighs more than the seat's weight limit or is taller than the height limit. Caregivers/teachers should check the labels on the seat or manufacturer's instructions if they are unsure of the limits. Manufacturer's instructions that include these specifications can also be found on the manufacturer's Website.
d) Child passenger restraint systems should be installed and used in accordance with the manufacturer's instructions and should be secured in back seats only.
e) All children under the age of thirteen should be transported in the back seat of a car and each child not riding in an appropriate child restraint system (i.e.,

a child seat, vest, or booster seat), should have an individual lap-and-shoulder seat belt (2).

f) For maximum safety, infants and toddlers should ride in a rear-facing orientation (i.e., facing the back of the car) until they are two years of age or until they have reached the upper limits for weight or height for the rear-facing seat, according to the manufacturer's instructions (1). Once their seat is adjusted to face forward, the child passenger must ride in a forward-facing child safety seat (either a convertible seat or a combination seat) until reaching the upper height or weight limit of the seat, in accordance with the manufacturer's instructions (10). Plans should include limiting transportation times for young infants to minimize the time that infants are sedentary in one place.

g) A booster seat should be used when, according to the manufacturer's instructions, the child has outgrown a forward-facing child safety seat, but is still too small to safely use the vehicle seat belts (for most children this will be between four feet nine inches tall and between eight and twelve years of age) (1).

h) Car safety seats, whether provided by the child's parents/guardians or the child care program, should be labeled with the child passenger's name and emergency contact information.

i) Car safety seats should be replaced if they have been recalled, are past the manufacturer's "date of use" expiration date, or have been involved in a crash that meets the U.S. Department of Transportation crash severity criteria or the manufacturer's criteria for replacement of seats after a crash (3,11).

j) The temperature of all metal parts of vehicle child restraint systems should be checked before use to prevent burns to child passengers.

If the child care program uses a vehicle that meets the definition of a school bus and the school bus has safety restraints, the following should apply:

a) The school bus should accommodate the placement of wheelchairs with four tie-downs affixed according to the manufactures' instructions in a forward-facing direction;

b) The wheelchair occupant should be secured by a three-point tie restraint during transport;

c) At all times, school buses should be ready to transport children who must ride in wheelchairs;

d) Manufacturers' specifications should be followed to assure that safety requirements are met.

RATIONALE: According to the National Center for Health Statistics, motor vehicle crashes are the leading cause of death among children ages three to fourteen in the United States (4). Safety restraints are effective in reducing death and injury when they are used properly. The best car safety seat is one that fits in the vehicle being used, fits the child being transported, has never been in a crash, and is used correctly every time. The use of restraint devices while riding in a vehicle reduces the likelihood of any passenger suffering serious injury or death if the vehicle is involved in a crash. The use of child safety seats reduces risk of death by 71% for children less than one year of age and by 54% for children ages one to four (4). In addition, booster seats reduce the risk of injury in a crash by 45%, compared to the use of an adult seat belt alone (5).

The safest place for all infants and children under thirteen years of age is to ride in the back seat. Head-on crashes cause the greatest number of serious injuries. A child sitting in the back seat is farthest away from the impact and less likely to be injured or killed. Additionally, new cars, trucks and vans have had air bags in the front seats for many years. Air bags inflate at speeds up to 200 mph and can injure small children who may be sitting too close to the air bag or who are positioned incorrectly in the seat. If the infant is riding in the front seat, a rapidly inflating air bag can hit the back of a rear-facing infant seat behind a baby's head and cause severe injury or death. For this reason, a rear-facing infant must NEVER be placed in the front seat of a vehicle with active passenger air bags.

Infants under one year of age have less rigid bones in the neck. If an infant is placed in a child safety seat facing forward, a collision could snap the infant's head forward, causing neck and spinal cord injuries. If an infant is placed in a child safety seat facing the rear of the car, the force of a collision is absorbed by the child restraint and spread across the infant's entire body. The rigidity of the bones in the neck, in combination with the strength of connecting ligaments, determines whether the spinal cord will remain intact in the vertebral column. Based on physiologic measures, immature and incompletely ossified bones will separate more easily than more mature vertebrae, leaving the spinal cord as the last link between the head and the torso (6). After twelve months of age, more moderate consequences seem to occur than before twelve months of age (7). However, rear-facing positioning that spreads deceleration forces over the largest possible area is an advantage at any age. Newborns seated in seat restraints or in car beds have been observed to have lower oxygen levels than when placed in cribs, as observed over a period of 120 minutes in each position (8).

As of March 1, 2010, all but three states required booster seat use for children up to as high as nine years of age. Child passenger restraints are recommended increasingly for older children. State child restraint requirements are listed by state at: http://www.iihs.org/laws/ChildRestraint.aspx. Booster seats are recommended for use only with both lap and shoulder belts; NEVER install a booster seat with the lap belt only. When the vehicle safety belts fit properly, the lap belt lies low and tightly across the child's upper thighs (not the abdomen) and the shoulder belt lies flat across the chest and shoulder, away from the neck and face.

COMMENTS: A Child Passenger Safety Technician may be able to help find a car safety seat that fits a larger child. Car safety seat manufacturers increasingly are making car safety seats that fit larger children. To locate a Child Passenger Safety Technician see https://ssl13.cyzap.net/dzapps/dbzap.bin/apps/assess/webmembers/tool?pToolCode=TAB

9&pCategory1=TAB9_CERTSEARCH&Webid=SAFEKIDSCERTSQL. See http://www.healthychildren.org/English/safety-prevention/on-the-go/pages/Car-Safety-Seats-Product-Listing-2010.aspx for a list of available car safety seats. For toddlers or young children whose behavior will not yet allow safe use of a booster seat but who are too large for a forward-facing seat with a harness, caregivers/teachers can consider using a travel vest (9).

When school buses meet current standards for the transport of school-age children, containment design features help protect children from injury, although the use of seat belts would provide additional protection. The U.S. Department of Transportation and U.S. Federal Motor Vehicle Safety standards for school buses apply only to vehicles equipped with factory-installed seat belts after 1967. To obtain the Federal Regulations, contact the Superintendent of Documents at the Government Printing Office.

Written transportation policy that is communicated to parents/guardians, staff, and all who transport children can help assure understanding of requirements/recommendations for child passenger safety as well as decisions about the value/necessity of the trip.

Car seat manufacturer's the National Highway Traffic Safety Administration (NHTSA) guidance on car seat replacement after a crash is available at http://www.nhtsa.gov/people/injury/childps/ChildRestraints/ReUse/index.htm.

TYPE OF FACILITY: Center; Large Family Child Care Home; Small Family Child Care Home

RELATED STANDARDS:
Standard 2.2.0.2: Limiting Infant/Toddler Time in Crib, High Chair, Car Seat, Etc.
Standard 6.5.3.1: Passenger Vans
Standards 9.2.5.1-9.2.5.2: Transportation Policies

REFERENCES:
1. Durbin, D. R., American Academy of Pediatrics, Committee on Injury, Violence, and Poison Prevention. 2011. Policy statement: Child passenger safety. *Pediatrics* 127:788-93.
2. National Highway Traffic Safety Administration. Questions and answers about air bag safety. Safe and Sober Campaign. http://www.nhtsa.gov/people/outreach/safesobr/12qp/airbag.html.
3. National Highway Traffic Safety Administration. Child restraint re-use after minor crashes. http://www.nhtsa.dot.gov/people/injury/childps/ChildRestraints/ReUse/index.htm.
4. National Highway Traffic Safety Administration's National Center for Statistics and Analysis 2008. *Traffic safety facts, 2008, Children*. http://www-nrd.nhtsa.dot.gov/Pubs/811157.PDF.
5. Arbogast, K. B., J. S. Jermakian, M. J. Kallan, D. R. Durbin. 2009. Effectiveness of belt positioning booster seats: An updated assessment. *Pediatrics* 124:1281-86
6. Huelke, D. F., G. M. Mackay, A. Morris, M. Bradford. 1993. *Car crashes and non-head impact cervical spine injuries in infants and children*. Warrendale, PA: Society of Automotive Engineers.
7. Weber, K., D. Dalmotas, B. Hendrick. 1993. *Investigation of dummy response and restraint configuration factors associated with upper spinal cord injury in a forward-facing child restraint*. Warrendale, PA: Society of Automotive Engineers.
8. Cerar, L. K., C. V. Scirica, I. S. Gantar, D. Osredkar, D. Neubauer, T. B. Kinane. 2009. A comparison of respiratory patterns in healthy term infants placed in car safety seats and beds. *Pediatrics* 124: e396-e402.
9. American Academy of Pediatrics. Obese children and car safety seats: Suggestions for parents. http://www.aap.org/obesity/ObesityCarSeatSafety.html.
10. American Academy of Pediatrics. 2010. Car safety seats: Information for families for 2010. http://www.healthychildren.org/english/safety-prevention/on-the-go/pages/car-safety-seats-information-for-families-2010.aspx.
11. Child Restraint Safety. Manufacture and expiration. http://www.childrestraintsafety.com/manufacture-expiration.html.

STANDARD 6.5.2.3: Child Behavior During Transportation

Children, as both passengers and pedestrians, should be instructed in safe transportation behavior using terms and concepts appropriate for their age and stage of development.

RATIONALE: Teaching passenger safety to children reduces injury from motor vehicle crashes to young children (2). Young children need to develop skills that will aid them in assuming responsibility for their own health and safety, and these skills can be developed through health and safety education implemented during the early years (1,3). Supervision of children will help to reinforce appropriate behaviors.

COMMENTS: Examples of safe behavior training include wearing seat belts and staying in position. Curricula and materials can be obtained from state departments of transportation, the American Automobile Association (AAA), the American Academy of Pediatrics (AAP), the American Red Cross, and the National Association for the Education of Young Children (NAEYC).

TYPE OF FACILITY: Center; Large Family Child Care Home; Small Family Child Care Home

REFERENCES:
1. Lehman, G. R., E. S. Geller. 1990. Participative education for children: An effective approach to increase safety belt use. *J Appl Behav Anal* 23:219-25.
2. Windome, M. D., ed. 1997. *Injury prevention and control for children and youth*. 3rd ed. Elk Grove Village, IL: American Academy of Pediatrics.
3. Kane, W. M., K. E. Herrera. 1993. *Safety is no accident: Children's activities in injury prevention*. Santa Cruz, CA: ETR Associates.

STANDARD 6.5.2.4: Interior Temperature of Vehicles

The interior of vehicles used to transport children should be maintained at a temperature comfortable to children. When the vehicle's interior temperature exceeds 82°F and providing fresh air through open windows cannot reduce the temperature, the vehicle should be air-conditioned. When the interior temperature drops below 65°F and when children are feeling uncomfortably cold, the interior should be heated. To prevent hyperthermia, all vehicles should be locked when not in use, head counts of children should be taken after transporting to prevent a child from being left unintentionally in a vehicle, and children should never be intentionally left in a vehicle unattended.

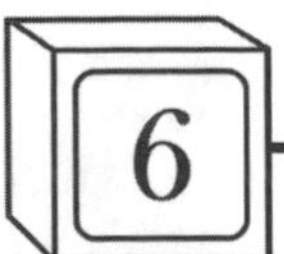

RATIONALE: Some children have problems with temperature variations. Whenever possible, opening windows to provide fresh air to cool a hot interior is preferable before using air conditioning. Over-use of air conditioning can increase problems with respiratory infections and allergies. Excessively high temperatures in vehicles can cause neurological damage in children (1).

Children's bodies overheat three to five times faster than adults because the hypothalamus regions of their brains, which control body temperature, are not as developed (1).

About thirty-seven children die every year from hyperthermia when they're left in cars and the cars quickly heat up. Even with comfortable temperatures outdoors, the temperature in an enclosed car climbs rapidly.

Temperature increase inside a car with an outside temperature of 80°F (elapsed time in minutes) (2):

a) After ten minutes: 99°F inside car;
b) After twenty minutes: 109°F;
c) After thirty minutes 114°F;
d) After forty minutes: 118°F;
e) After fifty minutes: 120°F;
f) After sixty minutes: 123°F.

COMMENTS: In geographical areas that are prone to very cold or very hot weather, a small thermometer should be kept inside the vehicle. In areas that are very cold, adults tend to wear very warm clothing and children tend to wear less clothing than might actually be required. Adults in a vehicle, then, may be comfortable while the children are not. When air conditioning is used, adults might find the cool air comfortable, but the children may find that the cool air is uncomfortably cold. To determine whether the interior of the vehicle is providing a comfortable temperature to children, a thermometer should be used and children in the vehicle should be asked if they are comfortable. Non-verbal children and infants should be assessed by an adult for signs of hypo- or hyperthermia. Signs of hypothermia include: cold skin, very low energy, and may be non-responsive. Young infants do not shiver when cold. Signs of hyperthermia include: dizziness, disorientation, agitation, confusion, sluggishness, seizure, hot dry skin that is flushed but not sweaty, loss of consciousness, rapid heartbeat, hallucinations (2).

TYPE OF FACILITY: Center; Large Family Child Care Home; Small Family Child Care Home

REFERENCES:

1. Guard, A., S. S. Gallagher. 2005. Heat related deaths to young children in parked cars: An analysis of 171 fatalities in the United States, 1995-2002. *Injury Prevention* 11:33-37.
2. McLaren, C., J. Null, J. Quinn. 2005. Heat stress from enclosed vehicles: Moderate ambient temperatures cause significant temperature rise in enclosed vehicles. *Pediatrics* 116: e109-12.

STANDARD 6.5.2.5: Distractions While Driving

The driver should not play the radio or CD player or use ear phones to listen to music or other distracting sounds while children are in the vehicles operated by the facility. The use of portable telephones or other devices to send or receive text messages, check email, etc. should be prohibited at all times while the vehicle is in motion or on an active road or highway (1,2,4). These devices should be used only when the vehicle is stopped and in emergency situations only.

In each vehicle from a center, a sign should be posted stating "NO RADIOS, TAPES, OR CDs."

RATIONALE: Loud noise interferes with normal conversation and may be especially disturbing to certain children. It is also distracting to the driver and the passenger monitor or assistant attending to the children in the vehicle (3).

COMMENTS: A driver's use of a portable radio, tape, mp3, or CD player with earphones is unacceptable.

TYPE OF FACILITY: Center; Large Family Child Care Home; Small Family Child Care Home

RELATED STANDARDS:

Standard 5.3.1.12: Availability and Use of a Telephone or Wireless Communication Device

REFERENCES:

1. Kalkhoff, W., G. W. Stanford, Jr., D. Melamed. 2009. Effects of dichotically enhanced electronic communication on crash risk and performance during simulated driving. *Perceptual Motor Skills* 108:449-64.
2. Al-Darrab, I. A., Z. A. Kahn, S. I. Ishrat. 2009. An experimental study on the effect of mobile phone conversation on drivers' reaction time in braking response. *J Safety Research* 40:185-89.
3. Chisholm, S. L., J. K. Caird, J. Lockhart. 2007. The effects of practice with mp3 players on driving performance. *Accident Analysis Prev* 40:704-13.
4. National Highway Traffic Safety Administration. Policy statement and compiled FAQs on distracted driving. http://www.nhtsa.gov/Driving+Safety/Distracted+Driving/Policy+Statement+and+Compiled+FAQs+on+Distracted+Driving.

STANDARD 6.5.2.6: Route to Emergency Medical Services

Any driver who transports children for a child care program should keep in the vehicle instructions for the quickest route to the nearest emergency medical facility from any point on the route.

RATIONALE: Driving children is a significant responsibility. Child care programs must assure that anyone who transports children can obtain emergency care promptly.

COMMENTS: Some hospitals in rural areas do not have emergency rooms. The driver must be knowledgeable of this fact and know where the nearest emergency facility is located. Maps are required in case transporting staff need to find an alternate way to emergency services when roads are closed and/or communication and power systems are inaccessible. Programs may want to have access to hand-held or stationary electronic/cellular, or satellite devices (e.g., GIS systems or devices that include relevant features) when transporting to help locate alternative routes during an emergency.

TYPE OF FACILITY: Center; Large Family Child Care Home; Small Family Child Care Home

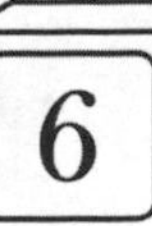

6.5.3 Vehicles

STANDARD 6.5.3.1: Passenger Vans

Child care facilities that provide transportation to children, parents/guardians, staff, and others should avoid the use of fifteen-passenger vans whenever possible. Other vehicles, such as vehicles meeting the definition of a "school bus," should be used to fulfill transportation of child passengers in particular. Conventional twelve- to fifteen-passenger vans cannot be certified as school buses by the National Highway Traffic Safety Administration (NHTSA) standards (2,4), and thus cannot be sold or leased, as new vehicles, to carry students on a regular basis. Caregivers/teachers should be knowledgeable about the laws of the state(s) in which their vehicles, including passenger vans, will be registered and used.

RATIONALE: Fifteen-passenger vans are more likely to be involved in a single-vehicle rollover crash than any other type of vehicle (1). Fifteen-passenger vans typically have seating positions for a driver and fourteen passengers. The risk of a rollover crash is greatly increased when ten or more people ride in a fifteen-passenger van (1). This increased risk occurs because the passenger weight raises the vehicle's center of gravity and causes it to shift rearward. As a result, the van has less resistance to rollover and handles differently from other commonly driven passenger vehicles, making it more difficult to control in an emergency situation (3). Occupant restraint use is especially critical because large numbers of people die in rollover crashes when they are partially or completely thrown from the vehicle. The National Highway Traffic Safety Administration (NHTSA) estimates that people who wear their seat belts are about 75% less likely to be killed in a rollover crash than people who do not.

The NHTSA has the authority to regulate the first sale or lease of a new vehicle by a dealer. The applicable statute requires any person selling or leasing a new vehicle to sell or lease a vehicle that meets all applicable standards (6). Under NHTSA's regulations, a "bus" is any vehicle, including a van, which has a seating capacity of eleven persons or more. The statute defines a "school bus" as any bus which is likely to be "used significantly" to transport "pre-primary, primary, and secondary" students to or from school or related events (5). A twelve- to fifteen-passenger van that is likely to be used significantly to transport students is a "school bus" by this definition, but cannot be certified as such.

COMMENTS: State law may require school bus equipment not specified in NHTSA regulations. Each state regulates how school buses are to be used and which agencies are responsible for developing and enforcing school bus regulations. In some states, requirements for transporting public school children differ from requirements for transporting children attending private schools and non-school organizations (e.g., Head Start programs, child care agencies, etc.)

For further information about state school bus regulations, contact the applicable State Director of Pupil Transportation. A list of State Directors can be obtained at http://www.nasdpts.org or by calling 1-800-585-0340.

Organizations that use fifteen-passenger vans to transport children, students, seniors, sports groups, or others, need to be informed about how to reduce rollover risks, avoid potential dangers, and better protect occupants in the event of a rollover crash. Drivers should be alert to these vehicles' high center of gravity – particularly when fully loaded – and their increased chance of rollover. The following are the NHTSA's official recommendations (1):

a) Caregivers/teachers should keep passenger load light. NHTSA research has shown that fifteen-passenger vans have a rollover risk that increases dramatically as the number of occupants increases from fewer than five to more than ten. In fact, fifteen-passenger vans (with ten or more occupants) had a rollover rate in single vehicle crashes that is nearly three times the rate of those that were lightly loaded.
b) The van's tire pressure should be checked frequently — at least once a week. A just-released NHTSA study found that 74% of all fifteen-passenger vans had improperly inflated tires. By contrast, 39% of passenger cars had improperly inflated tires. Improperly inflated tires can change handling characteristics, increasing the prospect of a rollover crash in fifteen-passenger vans.
c) Require all occupants to use their seat belts or the appropriate child restraint. Nearly 80% of those who have died nationwide in fifteen-passenger vans were not buckled up. Wearing seat belts dramatically increases the chances of survival during a rollover crash.
d) If at all possible, seat passengers and place cargo forward of the rear axle — and avoid placing any loads on the roof. By following these guidelines, you'll lower the vehicle's center of gravity and lower the chance of a rollover crash.
e) Be mindful of speed and road conditions. The analysis of fifteen-passenger van crashes also shows that the risk of rollover increases significantly at speeds over fifty miles per hour and on curved roads (1).
f) Only qualified drivers should be behind the wheel. Special training and experience are required to properly operate a fifteen-passenger van. Drivers should only operate these vehicles when well rested and fully alert.

For more information on fifteen-passenger vans, see http://www.nhtsa.gov/CA/10-14-2010/ and http://www.nhtsa.gov/people/injury/buses/choosing_schoolbus/pre-school-bus_01.html.

TYPE OF FACILITY: Center; Large Family Child Care Home; Small Family Child Care Home

RELATED STANDARDS:
Standards 9.2.5.1-9.2.5.2: Transportation Policies

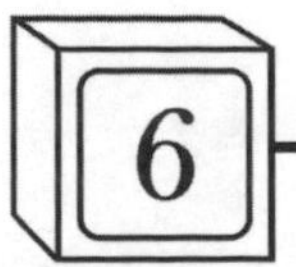

REFERENCES:

1. National Highway Traffic Safety Administration. *Reducing the risk of rollover crashes in 15-passenger vans*. http://www.safercar.gov/staticfiles/DOT/safercar/Equipment and Safety/Vans/documents/NHTSA_FLYER.pdf.
2. National Highway Traffic Safety Administration. School Buses. http://www.nhtsa.gov/School-Buses.
3. Aird, L. 2007. Moving kids safely in child care: A refresher course. *Exchange* (Jan/Feb): 25-28. http://www.childcareexchange.com/library/5017325.pdf.
4. American Academy of Pediatrics, Committee on Injury, Violence, and Poison Prevention, and Council on School Health. 2007. Policy statement: School transportation safety. *Pediatrics* 120:213-20.
5. Transportation. 1994. 49 U.S.C. §30125.
6. Transportation. 1994. 49 U.S.C. §30112.

Chapter 7

7

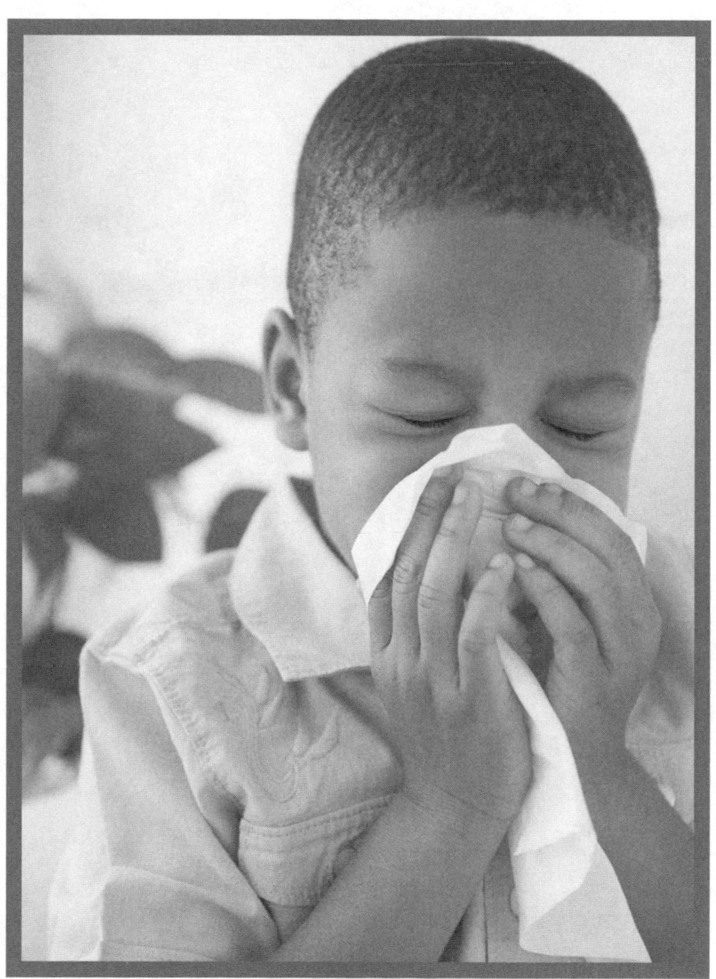

Infectious Diseases

7.1 How Infections Spread

Attendance at a child care facility may expose a child to the risk of acquiring infectious diseases for several reasons. Young children readily exchange secretions and frequently are not able to perform adequate hand hygiene or cough etiquette. In addition, children and adults with potentially infectious diseases are not always excluded from child care. Staff members face challenges in terms of enforcing recommended hygiene measures including hand hygiene and in maintaining environmental sanitation in child care settings.

There are three primary modes of transmission for spread of microorganisms in child care settings: contact, droplet, and airborne.

Many common infections encountered in the child care setting are transmitted by direct or indirect contact. Direct contact refers to person-to-person spread of an organism through direct physical contact. Indirect contact refers to spread that occurs by means of contact with a contaminated intermediate object (which could include objects such as shared toys), including hands. Contaminated hands are the most common means of transmission of infections in child care settings.

The majority of common viral respiratory and gastrointestinal tract infections and skin infections among young children, including those due to rhinoviruses, respiratory syncytial virus (RSV), rotavirus, noroviruses, hepatitis A virus, and scabies are transmitted by contact. Bacterial and parasitic intestinal tract infections (such as Shiga toxin-producing *E. coli* (STEC), Shigella, Clostridium difficile, Giardia, and Cryptosporidium) also are transmitted by contact. Cytomegalovirus (CMV) is transmitted by contact with urine and saliva containing CMV.

Transmission via the droplet route occurs when an infected person coughs, sneezes, or talks, generating large droplets. These droplets are propelled a short distance (generally less than three feet) and are deposited on the eyes, nasal mucosa, or mouth of a susceptible host (person). Infections and organisms transmitted by the droplet route include influenza, mumps, pertussis, RSV, and group A streptococcal (GAS) pharyngitis.

Airborne transmission occurs when small droplet nuclei, dust particles, or skin cells containing microorganisms are transmitted to a susceptible host (person) by air currents. Infections that are transmitted by the airborne route may be spread to others who are quite distant in space from the source infection. Varicella (chicken pox), tuberculosis, and measles are examples of infections transmitted by the airborne route.

Bloodborne transmission of infection through blood or blood containing material in child care is rare, but hepatitis B, C, and D, and HIV are viruses that may be transmitted via bloodborne exposures.

For a complete list of the routes of transmission for various infections, caregivers/teachers may refer to the published Healthcare Infection Control Practices Advisory Committee's 2007 Guideline for Isolation Precautions: Preventing Transmission of Infectious Agents in Healthcare Settings (also available at http://www.cdc.gov/hicpac/pdf/isolation/Isolation2007.pdf) or the current edition of the American Academy of Pediatrics' Red Book: Report of the Committee on Infectious Diseases (Red Book).

COMMENTS: As always, an experienced child care health consultant can be very helpful when dealing with issues around infectious diseases.

REFERENCES:

1. Siegel, J. D., E. Rhinehart, M. Jackson, L. Chiarello, Healthcare Infection Control Practices Advisory Committee. 2007 guideline for isolation precautions: Preventing transmission of infectious agents in health care settings. Am J Infect Control 35: S65-S164.

7.2 Immunizations

STANDARD 7.2.0.1: Immunization Documentation

Child care facilities should require that all parents/guardians of children enrolled in child care provide written documentation of receipt of immunizations appropriate for each child's age. Infants, children, and adolescents should be immunized as specified in the "Recommended Immunization Schedules for Persons Aged 0 Through 18 Years – United States, 2011" developed by the Advisory Committee on Immunization Practices (ACIP) of the Centers for Disease Control and Prevention (CDC), the American Academy of Pediatrics (AAP), and the American Academy of Family Physicians (AAFP). Children whose immunizations are not up-to-date or have not been administered according to the recommended schedule should receive the required immunizations, unless contraindicated or for legal exemptions (1,2).

An updated immunization schedule is published annually in the AAP's *Pediatrics* and in the CDC's *MMWR* and should be consulted for current information. In addition to print versions of the recommended immunization schedules, the current child, adolescent, and catch-up schedules are posted on the Websites of the CDC at http://www.cdc.gov/vaccines/ and the AAP at http://www.aap.org/immunization/.

RATIONALE: Routine immunizations at the appropriate age are the best means of protecting children against vaccine-preventable diseases. Legal requirements for age-appropriate immunizations of children attending licensed facilities exist in almost all states (see http://www.immunize.org/laws/). Parents/guardians of children who attend unregulated child care facilities should be encouraged to comply with the most recent "Recommended Immunization Schedules" (2).

Immunization is particularly important for children in child care because preschool-aged children have the highest age-specific incidence or are at high risk of complications from many vaccine-preventable diseases (specifically, measles, pertussis, rubella, influenza, varicella [chickenpox], rotavirus, and diseases due to *Haemophilus influenzae* type b (Hib) and pneumococcus) (3).

COMMENTS: Early education and child care settings present unique challenges for infection control due to the highly vulnerable population, close interpersonal contact, shared toys and other objects, and limited ability of young children to understand or practice good respiratory etiquette and hand hygiene. Parents/guardians, early childhood caregivers/teachers, and public health officials should be aware that, even under the best of circumstances, transmission of infectious diseases cannot be completely prevented in early childhood or other settings. No policy can keep everyone who is potentially infectious out of these settings (4).

TYPE OF FACILITY: Center; Large Family Child Care Home; Small Family Child Care Home

RELATED STANDARDS:
Standard 1.7.0.1: Pre-Employment and Ongoing Adult Health Appraisals, Including Immunization
Standard 9.2.3.5: Documentation of Exemptions and Exclusion of Children Who Lack Immunizations
Appendix G: Recommended Immunization Schedules for Persons Aged 0 Through 18 Years–United States, 2011

REFERENCES:
1. American Academy of Pediatrics, Committee on Infectious Diseases. 2011. Policy statement: Recommended childhood and adolescent immunization schedules – United States, 2011. *Pediatrics* 127:387-88.
2. Centers for Disease Control and Prevention. 2011. Recommended immunization schedules for persons aged 0-18 years – United States, 2011. *MMWR* 60 (5). http://www.cdc.gov/vaccines/recs/schedules/downloads/child/mmwr-child-schedule.pdf.
3. Fiene, R. 2002. *13 indicators of quality child care: Research update*. Washington, DC: U.S. Department of Health and Human Services, Office of the Assistant Secretary for Planning and Evaluation. http://aspe.hhs.gov/hsp/ccquality-ind02/.
4. Centers for Disease Control and Prevention (CDC). 2009. *CDC guidance on helping child care and early childhood programs respond to influenza during the 2009–2010 influenza season*. Atlanta: CDC. http://www.cdc.gov/h1n1flu/childcare/pdf/guidance.pdf.

STANDARD 7.2.0.2: Unimmunized Children

If immunizations have not been or are not to be administered because of a medical condition (contraindication), a statement from the child's primary care provider documenting the reason why the child is temporarily or permanently medically exempt from the immunization requirements should be on file. If immunizations are not to be administered because of the parents/guardians' religious or philosophical beliefs, a legal exemption with notarization, waiver or other state-specific required documentation signed by the parent/guardian should be on file (1,2).

The parent/guardian of a child who has not received the age-appropriate immunizations prior to enrollment and who does not have documented medical, religious, or philosophical exemptions from routine childhood immunizations should provide documentation of a scheduled appointment or arrangement to receive immunizations. This could be a scheduled appointment with the primary care provider or an upcoming immunization clinic sponsored by a local health department or health care organization. An immunization plan and catch-up immunizations should be initiated upon enrollment and completed as soon as possible according to the "Recommended Immunization Schedules for Persons Aged 0 Through 18 Years – United States, 2011" from the Advisory Committee on Immunization Practices (ACIP), the American Academy of Pediatrics (AAP), and the American Academy of Family Physicians (AAFP). Parents/guardians of children who attend an unlicensed child care facility should be encouraged to comply with the "Recommended Immunization Schedules" (6).

If a vaccine-preventable disease to which children are susceptible occurs in the facility and potentially exposes the unimmunized children who are susceptible to that disease, the health department should be consulted to determine whether these children should be excluded for the duration of possible exposure or until the appropriate immunizations have been completed. The local or state health department will be able to provide guidelines for exclusion requirements.

RATIONALE: Routine immunization at the appropriate age is the best means of protecting children against vaccine-preventable diseases. Mandates requiring age-appropriate immunization of children attending licensed facilities exist in all states (1).

Exclusion of an unimmunized (susceptible) or underimmunized child from the child care facility in the event of a risk of exposure to an outbreak of a vaccine-preventable disease protects the health of the unimmunized or underimmunized child and minimizes potential for further spread of that disease to other children, staff, family, and community members (2).

COMMENTS: A sample statement excluding a child from immunizations is: "This is to inform you that [NAME] should not be immunized with [VACCINE] because of [CONDITION, such as immunosuppression]. I expect this condition to persist for _______. [SIGNED], [PRIMARY CARE PROVIDER] [DATE]"

Vaccine Safety and Parental Choice – Some parents/guardians question the safety of routinely recommended vaccines. Sometimes they choose not to have their children fully vaccinated or to delay particular vaccinations. Unfortunately, this leaves the unimmunized child at risk for serious diseases and puts other children and caregivers/teachers who spend time with the unimmunized child at risk (2). Illness and death from vaccine-preventable diseases, including whooping cough and measles, have occurred in communities where there are unimmunized children who spread these diseases (3,4).

Vaccines are tested to establish safety and effectiveness before they are licensed by the U.S. Food and Drug Administration (FDA). The ACIP, a non-Federal advisory committee makes evidence-based recommendations to the Centers for Disease Control and Prevention (CDC) following review of all data before a new vaccine is recommended. ACIP is one of

many reputable sources of information. The Committee on Infectious Diseases makes evidence-based vaccine recommendations to the board of directors of the AAP. There are biased, inaccurate sources of vaccine information which are not based on evidence and often can confuse parents.

Autism allegedly has been associated with specific vaccines or ingredients in vaccines or combinations of vaccines. There is no evidence-based literature to support this association (5). Hesitant parents/guardians should be referred to reputable sources where evidence-based information is provided to assist them in making informed decisions about the benefits of immunization. Sites where reputable information can be found are shown below.

Since 1999, the mission of the AAP's Childhood Immunization Support Program (CISP) has been to improve the immunization delivery system for children across the nation by developing an infrastructure within the Academy to support its members and provide education and resources for parents and pediatricians on immunization and immunization-related issues (6).

Three sources of accurate information about immunizations are shown below. Each of the sites provides additional sources of information.

a) http://www.aap.org/immunization/about/programfacts.html -- CISP provides education and resources for parents/guardians and pediatricians on immunizations; CISP Goals are:
   1) Promote quality improvement and best immunization practices in community- and office-based primary care settings and other identified medical homes;
   2) Enable pediatricians and pediatric primary care providers to communicate effectively with parents/guardians;
   3) Promote system-wide improvements in the national immunization delivery system;
   4) Provide accurate and up-to-date resources to parents/guardians that address their most frequent immunization concerns (6).

b) http://www.cdc.gov/vaccines/ -- This CDC site provides information for health care professionals and parents/guardians about all aspects of immunization including vaccine recommendations, understanding vaccines and their purpose, vaccine misconceptions, and answers to commonly asked questions about vaccines (7).

c) http://www.immunizationinfo.org -- The mission of the National Network for Immunization Information (NNii) is to provide the public, health care professionals, policy makers, and the media with up-to-date, scientifically valid information related to immunization to assist with understanding the issues so that informed decisions can be made (8).

TYPE OF FACILITY: Center; Large Family Child Care Home; Small Family Child Care Home

RELATED STANDARDS:

Standard 9.2.3.5: Documentation of Exemptions and Exclusion of Children Who Lack Immunizations

Appendix G: Recommended Immunization Schedules for Persons Aged 0 Through 18 Years–United States, 2011

REFERENCES:

1. Immunization Action Commission. State mandates on immunization and vaccine-preventable diseases. http://www.immunize.org/laws/.
2. Omer, S. B., D. A. Salmon, W. A. Orenstein, M. P. deHart, N. Halsey. 2009. Vaccine refusal, mandatory immunization, and the risks of vaccine-preventable diseases. *New Eng J Med* 360:1981-88.
3. Centers for Disease Control and Prevention. 2009. Invasive *Haemophilus influenzae* type B disease in five young children – Minnesota, 2008. *MMWR* 58 (03): 58-60. http://www.cdc.gov/mmwr/preview/mmwrhtml/mm5803a4.htm.
4. Centers for Disease Control and Prevention. 2008. Update: Measles – United States, January-July 2008. *MMWR* 57 (33): 893-96. http://www.cdc.gov/mmwr/preview/mmwrhtml/mm5733a1.htm.
5. Institute of Medicine Immunization Safety Review Committee. Immunization safety review. http://iom.edu/Activities/PublicHealth/ImmunizationSafety.aspx.
6. American Academy of Pediatrics. Immunization. Childhood Immunization Support Program (CISP). http://www.aap.org/immunization/about/programfacts.html.
7. Centers for Disease Control and Prevention. Vaccines and immunizations. http://www.cdc.gov/vaccines/.
8. National Network for Immunization Information. NNii. http://www.immunizationinfo.org.

STANDARD 7.2.0.3: Immunization of Caregivers/Teachers

Caregivers/teachers should be current with all immunizations routinely recommended for adults by the Advisory Committee on Immunization Practices (ACIP) of the Centers for Disease Control and Prevention (CDC) as shown in the "Recommended Adult Immunization Schedule" at http://www.cdc.gov/vaccines/recs/schedules/default.htm#adult/. This schedule is updated annually at the beginning of the calendar year and can be found in Appendix H.

Caregivers/teachers should have received the recommended vaccines in the following categories: (1,2)

a) Vaccines recommended for all adults who meet the age requirements and who lack evidence of immunity (i.e., lack documentation of vaccination or have no evidence of prior infection):
   1) Tdap/Td;
   2) Varicella-zoster;
   3) MMR (measles, mumps, and rubella);
   4) Seasonal influenza;
   5) Human papillomaviruses (HPV) (eleven through twenty-six years of age);
   6) Others as determined by the ACIP and state and local public health authorities.

b) Recommended if a specific risk factor is present:
   1) Pneumococcal;
   2) Hepatitis A;
   3) Hepatitis B;
   4) Meningococcal;

5) Others as determined by the ACIP and state and local public health authorities.

c) If a staff member is not appropriately immunized for medical, religious or philosophical reasons, the child care facility should require written documentation of the reason.

d) If a vaccine-preventable disease to which adults are susceptible occurs in the facility and potentially exposes the unimmunized adults who are susceptible to that disease, the health department should be consulted to determine whether these adults should be excluded for the duration of possible exposure or until the appropriate immunizations have been completed. The local or state health department will be able to provide guidelines for exclusion requirements.

RATIONALE: Routine immunization of adults is the best means of preventing vaccine-preventable diseases. Vaccine-preventable diseases of adults represent a continuing cause of morbidity and mortality and a source of transmission of infectious organisms. Vaccines, which are safe and effective in preventing these diseases, need to be used in adults to minimize disease and to eliminate potential sources of transmission (1-3).

COMMENTS: Several of the vaccines recommended routinely for adults will prevent diseases that can be transmitted to children in the child care setting, including pertussis, varicella, measles, mumps, rubella and influenza. One dose of Tdap is a new recommendation for all adults and is especially important for those in close contact with infants. Adults often spread pertussis (whooping cough) to vulnerable infants and young children. Yearly influenza vaccination of adults in contact with children is also an especially important way to protect young infants. Hepatitis A vaccine is not recommended for routine administration to caregivers/teachers; however, hepatitis A vaccine can be administered to any person seeking protection from hepatitis A virus (HAV). Hepatitis A is an illness that often spreads to caregivers/teachers in early education and child care settings. Caregivers/teachers should be aware of the availability of hepatitis A vaccine. As of the printing of this edition, hepatitis A and B, pneumococcal and meningococcal vaccines are only recommended for adults with high risk conditions or in high risk settings unless requested.

Caregivers/teachers who do not complete the recommended immunization series put themselves, and children for whom they care, at risk. For additional information on adult immunization, visit the CDC Website on immunizations and vaccines at http://www.cdc.gov/vaccines/.

TYPE OF FACILITY: Center; Large Family Child Care Home; Small Family Child Care Home

RELATED STANDARDS:
Standard 1.7.0.1: Pre-Employment and Ongoing Adult Health Appraisals, Including Immunization
Appendix H: Recommended Adult Immunization Schedule–United States, 2011

REFERENCES:

1. Centers for Disease Control and Prevention. 2011. Recommended adult immunization schedule – United States, 2011. *MMWR* 60 (4). http://www.cdc.gov/vaccines/recs/schedules/downloads/adult/mmwr-adult-schedule.pdf.
2. Advisory Committee on Immunization Practices. 2011. Recommended adult immunization schedule – United States, 2011. *Ann Intern Med* 154:168-73.
3. Centers for Disease Control and Prevention. 2011. General recommendations on immunization: Recommendations of the Advisory Committee on Immunization Practices. *MMWR* 60 (RR02). http://www.cdc.gov/mmwr/pdf/rr/rr6002.pdf.

7.3 Respiratory Tract Infections

7.3.1 Group A Streptococcal (GAS) Infections

STANDARD 7.3.1.1: Exclusion for Group A Streptococcal (GAS) Infections

Children with symptomatic group A streptococcal (GAS) respiratory tract infections should be excluded from child care until twenty-four hours after antimicrobial therapy targeting GAS has been initiated, and until the child has no fever for twenty-four hours and is able to participate in activities. For skin infections, children do not need to be sent home early, but should not return until treatment is started and the child is able to participate in activities (3).

RATIONALE: Streptococcal respiratory tract infections and scarlet fever resulting from GAS have been reported in children in child care, but are not a major occurrence (1). GAS respiratory tract infections may resolve without treatment; however, symptomatic GAS respiratory tract infections can be complicated by pneumonia, arthritis, rheumatic fever, and glomerulonephritis (2). Invasive GAS disease and streptococcal toxic shock syndrome are designated as notifiable diseases at the national level (4). A notifiable disease is any disease that is required by law to be reported to state or local health departments.

Early identification ("strep" throat, fever, headache, rash) and treatment of GAS infection in children and adults are important in reducing the likelihood of complications of the infection and transmission of disease to others. Consultation with the local health department is advised when one case of invasive disease (e.g., toxic shock, necrotizing fasciitis) or two or more cases of localized streptococcal infection occurs in the same room in a child care facility. Parents/guardians of children exposed to a child with documented GAS infection should be notified of the exposure and observe their child for signs or symptoms of disease (4). Since the risk of secondary transmission is so low, chemoprophylaxis for contacts after a GAS infection in child care facilities generally is not recommended.

COMMENTS: For additional information regarding GAS respiratory tract infection, consult the current edition of the *Red Book* from the American Academy of Pediatrics (AAP).

TYPE OF FACILITY: Center; Large Family Child Care Home; Small Family Child Care Home

RELATED STANDARDS:
Standards 3.6.1.1-3.6.1.4: Child and Staff Inclusion/Exclusion/Dismissal
Standard 3.6.2.1: Exclusion and Alternative Care for Children Who are Ill

REFERENCES:

1. Agüero, J., M. Ortega-Mendi, M. Eliecer Cano, et al. 2008. Outbreak of invasive group A streptococcal disease among children attending a day-care center. *Pediatr Infect Dis J* 27:602-4.
2. Gerber, M., R. Baltimore, C. Eaton, et al. 2009. Prevention of rheumatic fever and diagnosis and treatment of acute streptococcal pharyngitis. *Circulation* 119:1541-51.
3. Aronson, S. S., T. R. Shope, eds. 2009. Strep throat and scarlet fever. In *Managing infectious diseases in child care and schools: A quick reference guide.* 2nd ed. Elk Grove Village, IL: American Academy of Pediatrics.
4. Pickering, L. K., C. J. Baker, D. W. Kimberlin, S. S. Long, eds. 2009. Group A streptococcal infections. In *Red book: 2009 report of the Committee on Infectious Diseases*. 28th ed. Elk Grove Village, IL: American Academy of Pediatrics.

STANDARD 7.3.1.2: Informing Caregivers/Teachers of Group A Streptococcal (GAS) Infection

Parents/guardians who become aware that their child is infected with group A streptococci (GAS), has strep throat, or has scarlet fever, should inform caregivers/teachers within twenty-four hours.

When exposure to GAS infection occurs and when appropriate, caregivers/teachers, in cooperation with health department officials, should inform parents/guardians of other children who attend the facility, that their children may have been exposed. GAS is a notifiable disease. A notifiable disease is any disease that is required by law to be reported to state or local health departments.

RATIONALE: Periodically, the incidence of rheumatic fever appears to increase. Identification and treatment of streptococcal infections of the respiratory tract are central to preventing rheumatic fever (1). Therefore, awareness of the occurrence of GAS infection in child care is important. Adult child care staff members are not immune to GAS infections and may be carriers of organisms that cause disease in children. When two or more cases of GAS disease occur, interventions are available to limit transmission of GAS infection. Consultation with health department authorities is advised when outbreaks of GAS infection occur in child care facilities. This information may be useful to the exposed child's primary care provider if the exposed child develops illness.

COMMENTS: Sample letters of notification to parents/guardians that their child may have been exposed to an infectious disease are contained in the publication of the American Academy of Pediatrics (AAP), *Managing Infectious Diseases in Child Care and Schools, 2nd Ed.* For additional information regarding GAS infections, consult the current edition of the *Red Book* from the American Academy of Pediatrics (AAP).

TYPE OF FACILITY: Center; Large Family Child Care Home; Small Family Child Care Home

RELATED STANDARDS:
Section 2.4: Health Education
Standard 3.6.4.3: Notification of the Facility About Infectious Disease or Other Problems by Parents

REFERENCES:

1. Gerber, M., R. Baltimore, C. Eaton, et al. 2009. Prevention of rheumatic fever and diagnosis and treatment of acute streptococcal pharyngitis. *Circulation* 119:1541-51.

7.3.2 *Haemophilus Influenzae* Type B (HIB)

STANDARD 7.3.2.1: Immunization for *Haemophilus Influenzae* Type B (HIB)

All children in a child care facility should have received age-appropriate immunizations with a *Haemophilus influenzae* type b (Hib) conjugate containing vaccine (1). Children in child care who are not immunized or not age-appropriately immunized against invasive Hib disease should be excluded from care immediately if the child care facility has been notified of a documented case of an invasive Hib infection. These children should be allowed to return when the risk of infection is no longer present, as determined by the health department.

RATIONALE: Appropriate immunization of children with a Hib conjugate-containing vaccine prevents the occurrence of disease and decreases the rate of carriage of this organism, thereby decreasing the risk of transmission to others (2). Since introduction of Hib conjugate-containing vaccines, the number of cases of invasive Hib disease has decreased from over 20,000 annually in the pre-vaccine era to less than 200 annually (3,4).

COMMENTS: Transmission of Hib may occur among unimmunized young children in group child care, especially children younger than twenty-four months of age. Hib causes pneumonia, meningitis, joint and bone infection, heart infection, and epiglottitis. In an outbreak of invasive Hib disease in child care, rifampin prophylaxis may be indicated for all non-pregnant contacts, especially when unimmunized or incompletely immunized children attend the child care facility (2).

TYPE OF FACILITY: Center; Large Family Child Care Home; Small Family Child Care Home

RELATED STANDARDS:
Appendix G: Recommended Immunization Schedules for Persons Aged 0 Through 18 Years–United States, 2011

REFERENCES:

1. American Academy of Pediatrics, Committee on Infectious Diseases. 2011. Policy statement: Recommended childhood and adolescent immunization schedules – United States, 2011. *Pediatrics* 127:387-88.
2. Pickering, L. K., C. J. Baker, D. W. Kimberlin, S. S. Long, eds.

2009. *Haemophilus influenzae* infections. In *Red book: 2009 report of the Committee on Infectious Diseases*. 28th ed. Elk Grove Village, IL: American Academy of Pediatrics.
3. Adams, W. G., K. A. Deaver, S. L. Cochi, et al. 1993. Decline of childhood *Haemophilus influenzae* type b (Hib) disease in the Hib vaccine era. *JAMA* 269:221-26.
4. Murphy, T. V., K. E. White, P. Pastor, et al. 1993. Declining incidence of *Haemophilus influenzae* type b disease since introduction of vaccination. *JAMA* 269:246-48.

STANDARD 7.3.2.2: Informing Parents/ Guardians of *Haemophilus Influenzae* Type B (HIB) Exposure

If a child with invasive *Haemophilus influenzae* type b (Hib) infection has been in care, the facility should inform parents/ guardians of other children who attend the facility, after consultation with health department authorities, that their children may have been exposed to the Hib bacteria and may have risk of developing serious Hib disease if their child is unimmunized or incompletely immunized. The facility should recommend that parents/guardians of unimmunized or under-immunized children contact their child's primary care provider.

Children in child care, who are not immunized or not age-appropriately immunized against invasive Hib disease, should be excluded from care immediately if the child care facility has been notified of a documented case of an invasive Hib infection. These children should be allowed to return when the risk of infection is no longer present, as determined by health department authorities.

RATIONALE: There is a risk of secondary cases of invasive Hib disease occurring among child care contacts of a child with invasive Hib disease. Risk of secondary cases of invasive Hib disease occurring among child care attendees is greatest among, and may be limited to, children younger than two years of age who are not immunized, not age-appropriately immunized, or have certain immune deficiencies. In settings with more than one classroom, increased risk has been shown only for children in the classroom of the infected child (1,2).

COMMENTS: Since introduction of the conjugated Hib-containing vaccines, invasive Hib disease has been remarkably reduced and is rare in child care facilities where all children should be appropriately immunized.

Sample letters of notification to parents/guardians that their child may have been exposed to an infectious disease are contained in the publication of the American Academy of Pediatrics (AAP), *Managing Infectious Diseases in Child Care and Schools, 2nd Ed.*

TYPE OF FACILITY: Center; Large Family Child Care Home; Small Family Child Care Home

RELATED STANDARDS:
Section 2.4: Health Education
Standard 7.3.2.1: Immunization for *Haemophilus Influenzae* Type B (HIB)

REFERENCES:

1. Murphy, T. V., J. F. Clements, J. A. Breedlove, et al. 1987. Risk of subsequent disease among daycare contacts of patients with systemic *Haemophilus influenzae* type b disease. *N Engl J Med* 316:5-10.
2. Fleming, D. W., M. H. Leibenhaut, D. Albanes, et al. 1985. Secondary *Haemophilus influenzae* type b in day care facilities: Risk factors and prevention. *JAMA* 254:509-14.

STANDARD 7.3.2.3: Informing Public Health Authorities of Invasive *Haemophilus Influenzae* Type B Cases

Invasive disease due to *Haemophilus influenza* type b (Hib) is designated as a notifiable disease at the national level and local and/or state public health department authorities should be notified immediately about cases of invasive Hib infections involving children or caregivers/teachers in the child care setting. Facilities should cooperate with health department officials in notifying parents/guardians of children who attend the facility about exposure to children with invasive Hib disease. This may include providing local health department officials with names and telephone numbers of parents/guardians of children in classrooms or facilities involved.

The health department may recommend rifampin, an antimicrobial agent taken to prevent infection, for children and staff members, to prevent secondary spread of invasive Hib disease in the facility (1). Antimicrobial prophylaxis is not recommended for pregnant women because the effect of rifampin on the fetus has not been established.

RATIONALE: There is a risk of secondary cases of invasive Hib disease among susceptible child care contacts of children with invasive Hib disease. Rifampin treatment of children exposed to a child with Hib disease can reduce the prevalence of Hib respiratory tract colonization in treated children and reduce the subsequent risk of invasive Hib infection, particularly in children under two years of age (1). Prophylaxis should be initiated as soon as possible, when two or more cases of invasive disease have occurred within sixty days in the same child care facility and when unimmunized or incompletely immunized children attend the child care facility.

In addition, children who are not immunized or are not age-appropriately immunized should receive a dose of Hib vaccine and should be scheduled for completion of the "Recommended Immunization Schedules for Persons Aged 0 Through 18 Years–United States, 2011" (2,3). (See Appendix G.)

COMMENTS: For additional information regarding Hib disease, consult the current edition of the *Red Book* from the American Academy of Pediatrics (AAP).

TYPE OF FACILITY: Center; Large Family Child Care Home; Small Family Child Care Home

RELATED STANDARDS:
Standards 3.6.4.3-3.6.4.4: Reporting Requirements for Infectious Diseases

Appendix G: Recommended Immunization Schedules for Persons Aged 0 Through 18 Years–United States, 2011

REFERENCES:

1. Shane, A. L., L. K. Pickering. 2008. Infections associated with group child care. In *Principles and practice of pediatric infectious diseases,* eds. S. S. Long, L. K. Pickering, C. G. Prober. 3rd ed. Philadelphia: Churchill Livingstone.
2. American Academy of Pediatrics, Committee on Infectious Diseases. 2011. Policy statement: Recommended childhood and adolescent immunization schedules – United States, 2011. *Pediatrics* 127:387-88.
3. Centers for Disease Control and Prevention. 2011. Recommended immunization schedules for persons aged 0-18 years – United States, 2011. *MMWR* 60 (5). http://www.cdc.gov/vaccines/recs/schedules/downloads/child/mmwr-child-schedule.pdf.

7.3.3 Influenza

STANDARD 7.3.3.1: Influenza Immunizations for Children and Caregivers/Teachers

The parent/guardian of each child six months of age and older should provide written documentation of current annual vaccination against influenza unless there is a medical contraindication or philosophical or religious objection. Children who are too young to receive influenza vaccine before the start of influenza season should be immunized annually beginning when they reach six months of age.

Staff caring for all children should receive annual vaccination against influenza. Ideally people should be vaccinated before the start of the influenza season (as early as August or September) and immunization should continue through March or April.

RATIONALE: The American Academy of Pediatrics (AAP) and the Advisory Committee on Immunization Practices (ACIP) recommend that influenza vaccination of all children, begins at six months of age, and adolescents and adults begin before or during the influenza season. Children who are at high risk of influenza complications and respiratory tract infections such as influenza commonly are scattered in out-of-home child care settings. The risk of complications from influenza is greater among children less than two years of age. Infants less than six months of age represent a particularly vulnerable group because they are too young to receive the vaccine. Therefore, people responsible for caring for these children should be immunized (1,2).

Seasonal influenza vaccine should be offered to all children as soon as the vaccine is available, even as early as August or September; a protective response to immunization remains throughout the influenza season. Immunization efforts should continue throughout the entire influenza season, even after influenza activity has been documented in a community. Each influenza season often extends well into March and beyond, and there may be more than one peak of activity in the same season. Thus, immunization through at least May 1st can still protect recipients during that particular season and also provide ample opportunity to administer a second dose of vaccine to children requiring two doses in that season (1).

Children who are too young to receive the influenza vaccine before the start of influenza season should be immunized when they reach six months of age, if influenza vaccination is still recommended at that time. Child contacts who are vaccine-eligible should be vaccinated.

TYPE OF FACILITY: Center; Large Family Child Care Home; Small Family Child Care Home

RELATED STANDARDS:
Standard 7.3.3.2: Influenza Control
Standard 7.3.3.3: Influenza Prevention Education

REFERENCES:

1. American Academy of Pediatrics, Committee on Infectious Disease. 2010. Recommendations for prevention and control of influenza in children, 2010-2011. *Pediatrics* 126:816-28.
2. Centers for Disease Control and Prevention. 2010. Update: Recommendations of the ACIP regarding use of CSL seasonal influenza vaccine (Afluria) in the United States during 2010-2011. *MMWR* 59 (31): 989-92. http://www.cdc.gov/mmwr/preview/mmwrhtml/mm5931a4.htm.

STANDARD 7.3.3.2: Influenza Control

When influenza is circulating in the community, facilities should encourage parents/guardians to keep children with symptoms of acute respiratory tract illness with fever at home until their fever has subsided for at least twenty-four hours without use of fever reducing medication.

Caregivers/teachers with symptoms of acute respiratory tract illness with fever also should remain at home until their fever subsides for at least twenty-four hours.

RATIONALE: The Centers for Disease Control and Prevention (CDC) recommends that caregivers/teachers encourage parents/guardians of sick children to keep the children home and away from their regular child care setting until the children have been without fever for twenty-four hours, to prevent spreading illness to others (1).

TYPE OF FACILITY: Center; Large Family Child Care Home; Small Family Child Care Home

RELATED STANDARDS:
Standard 7.3.3.1: Influenza Immunizations for Children and Caregivers/Teachers
Standard 7.3.3.3: Influenza Prevention Education
Standard 9.2.4.4: Written Plan for Seasonal and Pandemic Influenza

REFERENCES:

1. Centers for Disease Control and Prevention. 2010. Update: Recommendations of the ACIP regarding use of CSL seasonal influenza vaccine (Afluria) in the United States during 2010-2011. *MMWR* 59 (31): 989-92. http://www.cdc.gov/mmwr/preview/mmwrhtml/mm5931a4.htm.

STANDARD 7.3.3.3: Influenza Prevention Education

The child care facility should provide refresher training for all staff and children to include emphasis on the value of influenza vaccine, respiratory hygiene, cough etiquette, and hand hygiene at the beginning of each influenza season (usually considered to be September or October with a peak in February and March). Staff and children should be encouraged to practice these behaviors. Necessary equipment and supplies (e.g., disposable tissues and hand hygiene materials) should be made available.

RATIONALE: Although immunization is the single best way to prevent influenza, appropriate hygiene including respiratory hygiene, cough etiquette, and hand hygiene have been shown to reduce spread of respiratory tract infections.

In order to be effective, hygiene-based interventions need to be periodically reinforced. Influenza immunizations are recommended for healthy children and adolescents six months through eighteen years of age, for all adults including household contacts and caregivers/teachers of all children younger than five years and health care professionals (1).

COMMENTS: For more information, see the Centers for Disease Control and Prevention's (CDC) "Preventing the Spread of Influenza (the Flu) in Child Care Settings: Guidance for Administrators, Care Providers, and Other Staff" at http://www.cdc.gov/flu/professionals/infectioncontrol/childcaresettings.htm.

TYPE OF FACILITY: Center; Large Family Child Care Home; Small Family Child Care Home

RELATED STANDARDS:
Standard 7.3.3.2: Influenza Control

REFERENCES:

1. Centers for Disease Control and Prevention. 2010. Update: Recommendations of the ACIP regarding use of CSL seasonal influenza vaccine (Afluria) in the United States during 2010-2011. *MMWR* 59 (31): 989-92. http://www.cdc.gov/mmwr/preview/mmwrhtml/mm5931a4.htm.

7.3.4 Mumps

STANDARD 7.3.4.1: Mumps

Mumps is a contagious viral disease characterized by swelling of one or more salivary glands, usually the parotid glands. Any child or caregiver/teacher with suspected mumps should be excluded until the diagnosis of mumps or another infectious disease requiring exclusion is ruled out. Children or caregivers/teachers with proven mumps infection should be excluded for five days following the onset of parotid gland swelling (1).

Due to the risk of transmission and to control outbreaks of mumps, consider excluding children without documentation of vaccination with one or more doses of MMR vaccine or laboratory evidence of immunity including those children who have been exempted from this immunization. Excluded children can be readmitted immediately after immunization. Children who continue to be exempted from mumps immunization because of medical, religious, or other reasons should be excluded until at least twenty-six days after the onset of parotitis in the last person with mumps in the affected child care facility. Adults born during or after 1957 should have received one dose of MMR vaccine unless they have a medical contraindication or can provide laboratory evidence of immunity.

During an outbreak, a second dose of MMR (measles, mumps, and rubella) should be offered to the following groups:

a) Inadequately immunized people for whom two doses are recommended (preschool-aged children, school and college students, health care professionals, international travelers);
b) Adults born during or after 1957 without evidence of immunity who previously have received one dose of mumps vaccine. Adults born before 1957 generally are considered immune to mumps.

Mumps is designated as a notifiable disease at the national level, and local and/or state public health officials should be notified immediately about suspected cases of mumps involving children or caregivers/teachers in the child care setting. Facilities should cooperate with health department officials in notifying parents/guardians of children who attend the facility about exposures to children or staff with mumps.

RATIONALE: Mumps is a vaccine-preventable disease which is uncommon in children who receive at least two doses of live-attenuated MMR vaccine. The virus typically causes a systemic infection with swelling of the salivary glands, usually one or more of the parotid glands. In up to one-third of infections, the person is asymptomatic or has only a mild upper respiratory tract illness. Mumps can cause an infection of the central nervous system (e.g., encephalitis, meningitis), kidneys, and other organs. Involvement of the ovaries (in females) and testes (males) can occur, especially in those beyond puberty.

Mumps is spread typically by respiratory tract droplets or contact with respiratory tract secretions. The incubation period ranges from twelve to twenty-five days after exposure, typically sixteen to eighteen days. Infected people are contagious from one to two days before parotid swelling until five days after parotid swelling.

Mumps is an infectious disease and, therefore, routine exclusion of infected children is warranted. The American Academy of Pediatrics (AAP) and the Centers for Disease Control and Prevention (CDC) have revised the period of communicability to five days after the onset of parotid swelling (1).

Several mumps outbreaks have occurred since 2006 (2,3). Experience with outbreak control for other vaccine-preventable diseases indicates that the control strategy stated in the standard is effective.

COMMENTS: For more information on mumps, consult the current edition of the *Red Book* from the AAP.

TYPE OF FACILITY: Center; Large Family Child Care Home; Small Family Child Care Home.

REFERENCES:

1. Centers for Disease Control and Prevention. 2008. Updated recommendations for isolation of persons with mumps. *MMWR*

57:1103-5. http://www.cdc.gov/mmwr/preview/mmwrhtml/mm5740a3.htm.
2. Centers for Disease control and Prevention. 2010. Update: Mumps outbreak-New York and New Jersey, June 2009-January 2010. *MMWR* 59:125-29. http://www.cdc.gov/mmwr/preview/mmwrhtml/mm5905a1.htm.
3. Centers for Disease Control and Prevention. 2006. Updated recommendations of the ACIP for the control and elimination of mumps. *MMWR* 55:629-30. http://www.cdc.gov/mmwr/preview/mmwrhtml/mm5522a4.htm.

7.3.5 *Neisseria Meningitidis* (Meningococcus)

STANDARD 7.3.5.1: Recommended Control Measures for Invasive Meningococcal Infection in Child Care

Identification of an individual with invasive meningococcal infection in the child care setting should result in the following:

a) Immediate notification of the local or state health department;
b) Notification of parents/guardians about child care contacts to the person with invasive meningococcal infection;
c) Assistance with provision of antibiotic prophylaxis and vaccine receipt, as advised by the local or state health department, to child care contacts;
d) Frequent updates and communication with parents/guardians, health care professionals, and local health authorities.

RATIONALE: Due to the increased transmissibility of meningococcal infections following close personal contact with oral and respiratory tract secretions of a person with infection, institution of antibiotic prophylaxis within twenty-four hours of diagnosis of the index case is advised. Younger age and close contact with an infected person increases the attack rate of meningococcal disease among child care attendees to several hundred fold greater than the general population. As outbreaks may occur in child care settings, chemoprophylaxis with oral rifampin is the prophylaxis of choice for exposed child contacts. In some cases, intramuscular ceftriaxone may be used as an alternative if a contraindication to oral rifampin exists in the contact (1,3). In contacts over eighteen years of age, oral rifampin, ciprofloxacin, or intramuscular ceftriaxone, are effective (2,3). Rifampin is not recommended for pregnant women.

In addition to chemoprophylaxis with an oral antimicrobial agent, immunoprophylaxis with a meningococcal vaccination of age-eligible contacts in an outbreak setting, if the infection is due to a serogroup contained in the vaccine, may be recommended by the local or state health department (1,3).

COMMENTS: For facilities that care for older school-age children, meningococcal vaccine is recommended at eleven or twelve years of age with a second dose administered at sixteen years of age.

For additional information regarding meningococcal disease, consult the current edition of the *Red Book* from the American Academy of Pediatrics (AAP).

TYPE OF FACILITY: Center; Large Family Child Care Home; Small Family Child Care Home

REFERENCES:

1. Pickering, L. K., C. J. Baker, D. W. Kimberlin, S. S. Long, eds. 2009. Meningococcal infections. In *Red book: 2009 report of the Committee on Infectious Diseases*. 28th ed. Elk Grove Village, IL: American Academy of Pediatrics.
2. American Academy of Pediatrics, Committee on Infectious Diseases. 2009. Prevention and control of meningococcal disease: Recommendations for use of meningococcal vaccines in pediatric patients. *Pediatrics* 123:1421-22.
3. Centers for Disease Control and Prevention. 2007. Revised recommendations of the Advisory Committee on Immunization Practices to vaccinate all persons aged 11-18 years with meningococcal conjugate vaccine. *MMWR* 56:749-95. http://www.cdc.gov/mmwr/preview/mmwrhtml/mm5631a3.htm.

STANDARD 7.3.5.2: Informing Public Health Authorities of Meningococcal Infections

Meningococcal disease is designated as notifiable at the national level, and local and/or state public health department authorities should be notified immediately about the occurrence of invasive meningococcal disease in a child care facility. Timely reporting results in early recognition of outbreaks and prevention of additional infections. Facilities should cooperate with their local or state health department officials in notifying parents/guardians of children who attend the facility about exposures to children with invasive meningococcal infections. Early intervention minimizes anxiety and concern that may result from identification of an attendee with an invasive meningococcal infection. This may include providing local health officials with the names and telephone numbers of parents/guardians of children in involved classrooms or facilities.

RATIONALE: *Neisseria meningitidis* is a cause of serious infections, including meningitis, in young children and adolescents. Infection is spread from person to person by direct contact with respiratory tract droplets that contain *N. meningitidis* organisms (1,2).

COMMENTS: Sample letters of notification to parents/guardians that their child may have been exposed to an infectious disease are contained in the publication of the American Academy of Pediatrics (AAP), *Managing Infectious Diseases in Child Care and Schools, 2nd Ed*. For additional information regarding meningococcal disease, consult the current edition of the *Red Book* from the AAP.

TYPE OF FACILITY: Center; Large Family Child Care Home; Small Family Child Care Home

RELATED STANDARDS:

Section 2.4: Health Education
Standards 3.6.4.3-3.6.4.4: Reporting Requirements for Infectious Diseases

REFERENCES:

1. Centers for Disease Control and Prevention. 2007. Revised recommendations of the Advisory Committee on Immunization

Practices to vaccinate all persons aged 11-18 years with meningococcal conjugate vaccine. *MMWR* 56:749-95. http://www.cdc.gov/mmwr/preview/mmwrhtml/mm5631a3.htm.
2. American Academy of Pediatrics, Committee on Infectious Diseases. 2009. Prevention and control of meningococcal disease: Recommendations for use of meningococcal vaccines in pediatric patients. *Pediatrics* 123:1421-22.

7.3.6 Parvovirus B19

STANDARD 7.3.6.1: Attendance of Children with Erythema Infectiosum (EI) (Parvovirus B19)

Children who develop Erythema Infectiosum (EI), also known as fifth disease, following infection with parvovirus B19, should be allowed to attend child care because they are no longer contagious when signs and symptoms appear.

RATIONALE: EI is caused by parvovirus B19. EI begins with fever, headache, and muscle aches, followed by an intensely red rash on the cheeks with a "slapped cheek" appearance. A lace-like rash appears on the rest of the body. Isolation or exclusion of an immunocompetent person with parvovirus B19 infection in the child care setting is not necessary because little to no virus is present in respiratory tract secretions at the time of occurrence of the rash (1).

COMMENTS: Parvovirus B19 infections may be more serious in people with certain immune deficiencies and in people with hemolytic anemia such as sickle cell anemia. Parvovirus B19 infection in pregnancy may cause fetal loss or intrauterine growth retardation.

For additional information regarding parvovirus B19, consult the current edition of the *Red Book* from the American Academy of Pediatrics (AAP).

TYPE OF FACILITY: Center; Large Family Child Care Home; Small Family Child Care Home

REFERENCES:

1. Pickering, L. K., C. J. Baker, D. W. Kimberlin, S. S. Long, eds. 2009. Parvovirus B19. In *Red book: 2009 report of the Committee on Infectious Diseases*. 28th ed. Elk Grove Village, IL: American Academy of Pediatrics.

7.3.7 Pertussis

STANDARD 7.3.7.1: Informing Public Health Authorities of Pertussis Cases

Local and/or state public health authorities should be notified immediately about suspected or confirmed cases of pertussis (whooping cough) involving children or caregivers/teachers in the child care setting. Facilities should cooperate with their local or state health department officials in notifying parents/guardians of children who attend the facility about exposures to children or adults with pertussis. This may include providing health department officials with the names and telephone numbers of parents/guardians of children in the classrooms or facilities involved.

Guidelines for use of antibiotics and immunization for prevention of pertussis in people who have been in contact with children or adults who have pertussis should be implemented in cooperation with public health department officials. Children and staff who have been exposed to pertussis, especially those who are incompletely immunized, should be observed for respiratory tract symptoms for twenty-one days after the last contact with the infected person.

RATIONALE: Notification of health department officials when suspected or confirmed pertussis occurs in a child or staff member in a child care center will help ensure the following (1-3):

a) All children have received age-appropriate immunization;
b) Appropriate antibiotic prophylaxis is provided to children and adults exposed to the child first infected with pertussis;
c) Children and adults are observed for respiratory tract symptoms.

COMMENTS: Sample letters of notification to parents/guardians that their child may have been exposed to an infectious disease are contained in the publication of the American Academy of Pediatrics (AAP), *Managing Infectious Diseases in Child Care and Schools, 2nd Ed*. For additional information regarding pertussis, consult the current edition of the *Red Book,* also from the AAP.

TYPE OF FACILITY: Center; Large Family Child Care Home; Small Family Child Care Home

RELATED STANDARDS:
Section 2.4: Health Education
Standards 3.6.4.3-3.6.4.4: Reporting Requirements for Infectious Diseases

REFERENCES:

1. Pickering, L. K., C. J. Baker, D. W. Kimberlin, S. S. Long, eds. 2009. Pertussis (whooping cough). In *Red book: 2009 report of the Committee on Infectious Diseases*. 28th ed. Elk Grove Village, IL: American Academy of Pediatrics.
2. Centers for Disease Control and Prevention. 2006. Preventing tetanus, diphtheria, and pertussis among adolescents: Use of tetanus toxoid, reduced diphtheria toxoid and acellular pertussis vaccines. *MMWR* 55 (RR03). http://www.cdc.gov/mmwr/pdf/rr/rr5503.pdf.
3. Centers for Disease Control and Prevention. 2006. Preventing tetanus, diphtheria, and pertussis among adults: Use of tetanus toxoid, reduced diphtheria toxoid and acellular pertussis vaccine. *MMWR* 55 (RR17). http://www.cdc.gov/mmwr/preview/mmwrhtml/rr5517a1.htm.

STANDARD 7.3.7.2: Prophylactic Treatment for Pertussis

When there is a known or suspected occurrence of pertussis (whooping cough) in a child care facility, all exposed staff members and children in care regardless of prior immunization status should begin chemoprophylaxis (usually administration of azithromycin, erythromycin, or clarithromycin) and any additional treatment deemed medically necessary by a health care professional before they are allowed to return to the facility (1).

Adults and children who have been in contact with a person infected with pertussis should be monitored closely for respiratory tract symptoms for twenty-one days after the last contact with the infected person.

All adults who will be around children in out-of-home care, should have Tdap as their next tetanus booster. However, if the adults will be working with infants less than twelve months they should have the Tdap regardless of when they received their last tetanus booster (2).

RATIONALE: Even if outbreaks of pertussis in child care facilities have not been reported, children and staff who attend out-of-home child care occasionally contract pertussis. The spread of infection to contacts who are incompletely immunized can be reduced by treating the primary case and susceptible contacts with prophylactic antibiotics, usually azithromycin, erythromycin, or clarithromycin (1-4). Erythromycin is not recommended in children less than one month of age due to increased risk for hypertrophic pyloric stenosis (1-3).

COMMENTS: For additional information regarding pertussis, consult the current edition of the *Red Book* from the American Academy of Pediatrics (AAP).

TYPE OF FACILITY: Center; Large Family Child Care Home; Small Family Child Care Home

REFERENCES:

1. Centers for Disease Control and Prevention. 2006. Preventing tetanus, diphtheria, and pertussis among adolescents: Use of tetanus toxoid, reduced diphtheria toxoid and acellular pertussis vaccines. Recommendations of the Advisory Committee on Immunization Practices. *MMWR* 55 (RR03). http://www.cdc.gov/mmwr/pdf/rr/rr5503.pdf.
2. Centers for Disease Control and Prevention. 2006. Preventing tetanus, diphtheria, and pertussis among adults: Use of tetanus toxoid, reduced diphtheria toxoid and acellular pertussis vaccine. *MMWR* 55 (RR17). http://www.cdc.gov/mmwr/preview/mmwrhtml/rr5517a1.htm.
3. Centers for Disease Control and Prevention. 2005. Recommended antimicrobial agents for treatment and postexposure prophylaxis of pertussis: 2005 CDC Guidelines. *MMWR* 54 (RR14). http://www.cdc.gov/mmwr/preview/mmwrhtml/rr5414a1.htm.
4. Centers for Disease Control and Prevention. 2010. Vaccines and preventable diseases: Pretussis (whooping cough) vaccination. http://www.cdc.gov/vaccines/vpd-vac/pertussis/.

STANDARD 7.3.7.3: Exclusion for Pertussis

Children and staff members with characteristic symptoms of pertussis (whooping cough) should be excluded from child care pending evaluation by a primary care provider. A symptomatic child or staff member with pertussis or suspected pertussis may not return to the facility until:

a) Five days after initiation of a course of any of the following antibiotics: azithromycin (full course of treatment is five days), erythromycin (full course of treatment is fourteen days), or clarithromycin (full course of treatment is seven days) antimicrobial therapy;
b) The medical condition allows;
c) The child's need for care does not compromise the caregiver's/teacher's ability to provide for the health and safety of the other children in the group.

Untreated adults should be excluded until twenty-one days after onset of cough.

RATIONALE: Even if outbreaks of pertussis in child care facilities have not been reported, children and staff who attend out-of-home child care occasionally contract pertussis. The spread of infection to contacts who are incompletely immunized can be reduced by treating the primary case and susceptible contacts with prophylactic antibiotics (1-4).

COMMENTS: For additional information regarding pertussis, consult the current edition of the *Red Book* from the American Academy of Pediatrics (AAP).

TYPE OF FACILITY: Center; Large Family Child Care Home; Small Family Child Care Home

RELATED STANDARDS:

Standards 3.6.1.1-3.6.1.4: Child and Staff Inclusion/Exclusion/Dismissal
Standard 3.6.2.1: Exclusion and Alternative Care for Children Who are Ill

REFERENCES:

1. Centers for Disease Control and Prevention. 2006. Preventing tetanus, diphtheria, and pertussis among adolescents: Use of tetanus toxoid, reduced diphtheria toxoid and acellular pertussis vaccines. *MMWR* 55 (RR03). http://www.cdc.gov/mmwr/pdf/rr/rr5503.pdf.
2. Centers for Disease Control and Prevention. 2006. Preventing tetanus, diphtheria, and pertussis among adults: Use of tetanus toxoid, reduced diphtheria toxoid and acellular pertussis vaccine. *MMWR* 55 (RR17). http://www.cdc.gov/mmwr/preview/mmwrhtml/rr5517a1.htm.
3. Centers for Disease Control and Prevention. 2005. Recommended antimicrobial agents for treatment and postexposure prophylaxis of pertussis: 2005 CDC guidelines. *MMWR* 54 (RR14). http://www.cdc.gov/mmwr/preview/mmwrhtml/rr5414a1.htm.
4. Centers for Disease Control and Prevention. 2010. Vaccines and preventable diseases: Pretussis (whooping cough) vaccination. http://www.cdc.gov/vaccines/vpd-vac/pertussis/.

7.3.8 Respiratory Syncytial Virus (RSV)

STANDARD 7.3.8.1: Attendance of Children with Respiratory Syncytial Virus (RSV) Respiratory Tract Infection

Respiratory syncytial virus (RSV) is a common cause of respiratory tract infection in infants and young children, although infection in all ages may occur. Children with known RSV infection may return to child care once symptoms have resolved, temperature has returned to normal, the child can participate in child care activities and the child's care does not result in more care than the staff can provide without compromising the health and safety of other children.

Parents/guardians and staff need to be aware that the period of RSV shedding is usually three to eight days but shedding may last longer, especially in young infants from

whom virus can be shed in nasal secretions and saliva for three to four weeks following infection.

RATIONALE: RSV is a well-known cause of respiratory tract illness in children. Almost all children are infected at least once with RSV by two years of age and reinfection is common. In contrast to older children and adults who develop upper respiratory tract infections, RSV is one of the most frequent causes of lower respiratory tract infections including bronchiolitis (fever, cough, wheezing, and increased respiratory rate) or pneumonia in infants and young children less than two years of age.

RSV is responsible for greater than one hundred twenty-five thousand hospitalizations, mostly in infants and young children each year. Some 1% to 2% of previously healthy infants require hospitalization for bronchiolitis and up to 5% of these infants may require mechanical ventilation. Infants and children with weakened immune systems, specific types of heart problems, and those born prematurely have even greater difficulty with this infection (1,2).

Because RSV circulation is most common in the U.S. during a defined time period (generally November to March), and increased levels of RSV-specific antibody have been shown to decrease disease severity and/or prevent lower respiratory tract involvement, some infants and young children who meet specific criteria as outlined by the American Academy of Pediatrics (AAP) may benefit from receiving monthly injections (prophylaxis to prevent disease) of a monoclonal antibody (palivizumab) (2). Palivizumab does not treat someone already infected with RSV. For most patients infected with RSV, the disease is self-limited; no anti-viral therapy is available.

During an outbreak of RSV in a child care setting, most children and staff will be exposed before the occurrence of specific symptoms. Most viral respiratory tract illnesses, including RSV infections, are self-limited and go undiagnosed.

Transmission of virus occurs through close contact with respiratory tract secretions (2). Infants with chronic heart and lung problems and immunocompromised children may be at high risk for complications. Parents/guardians of such children should be alerted that a child with RSV has been diagnosed in their group.

Limiting the spread of RSV by using good hand hygiene practices, prohibiting sharing of food; bottles; toothbrushes; or toys, and disinfecting surfaces will be important to reducing the risk of RSV transmission in such situations.

COMMENTS: RSV is a major viral illness in children, especially children two years of age and younger. A critical aspect of RSV prevention among high risk infants is education of parents/guardians and other care providers about the importance of decreasing exposure to and transmission of RSV. Preventive measures may include limiting, where feasible, exposure to contagious settings, hand hygiene and avoidance of contact with people with respiratory tract infections.

For additional information regarding RSV, consult the current edition of the *Red Book* from the AAP.

TYPE OF FACILITY: Center; Large Family Child Care Home; Small Family Child Care Home.

RELATED STANDARDS:
Appendix A: Signs and Symptoms Chart

REFERENCES:

1. Peters, T. R., J. E. Crowe, Jr. 2008. Respiratory syncytial virus. In *Principles and practice of pediatric infectious diseases*, eds. S. S. Long, L. K. Pickering, C. G. Prober, 1112-16. 3rd ed. Philadelphia: Churchill Livingstone.
2. American Academy of Pediatrics, Committee on Infectious Diseases. 2009. Policy statement: Modified recommendations for use of palivizumab for prevention of respiratory syncytial virus infections. *Pediatrics* 124:1694-1701.

7.3.9 *Streptococcus Pneumoniae*

STANDARD 7.3.9.1: Immunization with *Streptococcus Pneumoniae* Conjugate Vaccine (PCV13)

Pneumococcal conjugate (PCV13) vaccine is recommended for all children from two through fifty-nine months of age, including children in child care facilities. The vaccine is recommended to be administered at two, four, six, and twelve through fifteen months of age (1-3,5). Healthy children between twenty-four and fifty-nine months of age who are not immunized completely for their age should be administered one dose of PCV13 (3,5).

Children two years of age or older at high risk of invasive disease caused by *Streptococcus pneumoniae* (including sickle cell disease, asplenia, HIV, chronic illness, cochlear implant or immunocompromised) who have received their recommended doses of PCV should receive *S. pneumoniae* polysaccharide vaccine two or more months after receipt of the last dose of PCV (1-3,5).

RATIONALE: Appropriate immunization of children with *S. pneumoniae* conjugate vaccine prevents the occurrence of invasive disease and decreases transmission to others.

Pneumococcal disease among children including children in out-of-home child care due to strains in the PCV7 vaccine has decreased since introduction of PCV7 vaccine that was used until the licensure of PCV13 by the U.S. Food and Drug Administration (FDA) and recommended for use by the Advisory Committee on Immunization Practices (ACIP) and the American Academy of Pediatrics (AAP) (3-5). PCV13 provides protection from invasive disease from six additional pneumococcal serotypes. The risk of contacting invasive pneumococcal disease is highest in children less than sixty months of age. The risk for invasive disease is greatest in infants, young children, elderly people and children of some American Indian populations (2,3).

COMMENTS: The pneumococcal conjugate vaccine containing thirteen pneumococcal serotypes (PCV13) will expand coverage against six additional serotypes of *S. pneumonia* not contained in PCV7 (5).

For additional information regarding *S. pneumoniae* disease, consult the current edition of the *Red Book* from the AAP.

TYPE OF FACILITY: Center; Large Family Child Care Home; Small Family Child Care Home

RELATED STANDARDS:
Appendix G: Recommended Immunization Schedules for Persons Aged 0 Through 18 Years–United States, 2011

REFERENCES:
1. American Academy of Pediatrics, Committee on Infectious Diseases. 2000. Technical report: Prevention of pneumococcal infections, including the use of pneumococcal conjugate and polysaccharide vaccines and antibiotic prophylaxis. *Pediatrics* 106:367-76.
2. Centers for Disease Control and Prevention. 2000. Preventing pneumococcal disease among infants and young children: Recommendations of the Advisory Committee on Immunization Practices. *MMWR* 49 (RR09). http://www.cdc.gov/mmwr/pdf/rr/rr4909.pdf.
3. Centers for Disease Control and Prevention. 2008. Updated recommendation from the Advisory Committee on Immunization Practices for use of 7-valent pneumococcal conjugate vaccine (PCV7) in children aged 24-59 months who are not completed vaccinated. *MMWR* 57:343-44. http://www.cdc.gov/mmwr/preview/mmwrhtml/mm5713a4.htm.
4. Centers for Disease Control and Prevention. 2010. Licensure of a 13-valent pneumococcal conjugate vaccine (PCV13) and recommendations for use among children – Advisory Committee on Immunization Practices, 2010. *MMWR* 59:258-61. http://www.cdc.gov/mmwr/preview/mmwrhtml/mm5909a2.htm.
5. American Academy of Pediatrics, Committee on Infectious Diseases. 2010. Policy statement: Recommendations for the prevention of *Streptococcus pneumoniae* infections in infants and children: Use of 13-valent pneumococcal conjugate vaccine (PCV13) and pneumococcal polysaccharide vaccine (PPSV23). *Pediatrics* 126:186-90.

STANDARD 7.3.9.2: Informing Public Health Authorities of Invasive *Streptococcus Pneumoniae*

Drug resistant invasive *Streptococcus pneumoniae* in all ages and all invasive (including non-drug resistant) *S. pneumoniae* in children younger than five years of age are designated as notifiable diseases at the national level. Local and/or state public health authorities should be notified about cases of invasive *S. pneumoniae* infections involving: children less than five years of age, caregivers/teachers in the child care setting, or drug resistant invasive *S. pneumoniae* disease in a person of any age.

Facilities should cooperate with their local or state health department officials in notifying parents/guardians of children who attend the facility about exposure to children with invasive *S. pneumoniae* disease. This may include providing local health officials with names and telephone numbers of parents/guardians of children in classrooms or facilities involved.

RATIONALE: Secondary spread of *S. pneumoniae* in child care has been reported, but the degree of risk of secondary spread in child care facilities is unknown (1). Prophylaxis of contacts after the occurrence of a single case of invasive *S. pneumoniae* disease is not recommended.

Infants and young children who are not immunized or who are not age-appropriately immunized should receive a dose of PCV13 and should be scheduled for completion of the "Recommended Childhood Immunization Schedules" from the American Academy of Pediatrics (AAP), Centers for Disease Control and Prevention (CDC), and American Academy of Family Physicians (AAFP) to provide protection from invasive pneumococcal disease (2-6). (See Appendix G.)

COMMENTS: For additional information regarding *S. pneumoniae* disease, consult the current edition of the *Red Book* from the AAP.

TYPE OF FACILITY: Center; Large Family Child Care Home; Small Family Child Care Home

RELATED STANDARDS:
Section 2.4: Health Education
Standards 3.6.4.3-3.6.4.4: Reporting Requirements for Infectious Diseases
Appendix G: Recommended Immunization Schedules for Persons Aged 0 Through 18 Years–United States, 2011

REFERENCES:
1. Rauch, A. M., M. O'Ryan, R. Van, et al. 1990. Invasive disease due to multiply resistant *Streptococcus pneumoniae* in Houston, Texas day-care centers. *Am J Dis Child* 144:933-27.
2. American Academy of Pediatrics, Committee on Infectious Diseases. 2000. Prevention of pneumococcal infections, including the use of pneumococcal conjugate and polysaccharide vaccines and antibiotic prophylaxis. *Pediatrics* 106:367-76.
3. Centers for Disease Control and Prevention. 2000. Preventing pneumococcal disease among infants and young children. *MMWR* 49 (RR09). http://www.cdc.gov/mmwr/pdf/rr/rr4909.pdf.
4. Centers for Disease Control and Prevention. 2008. Updated recommendation from the Advisory Committee on Immunization Practices for use of 7-valent pneumococcal conjugate vaccine (PCV7) in children aged 24-59 months who are not completed vaccinated. *MMWR* 57:343-44. http://www.cdc.gov/mmwr/preview/mmwrhtml/mm5713a4.htm.
5. Centers for Disease Control and Prevention. 2010. Licensure of a 13-valent pneumococcal conjugate vaccine (PCV13) and recommendations for use among children, 2010. *MMWR* 59:258-61. http://www.cdc.gov/mmwr/preview/mmwrhtml/mm5909a2.htm.
6. American Academy of Pediatrics, Committee on Infectious Diseases. 2010. Policy statement: Recommendations for the prevention of *Streptococcus pneumoniae* infections in infants and children: Use of 13-valent pneumococcal conjugate vaccine (PCV13) and pneumococcal polysaccharide vaccine (PPSV23). *Pediatrics* 126:186-90.

7.3.10 Tuberculosis

STANDARD 7.3.10.1: Measures for Detection, Control, and Reporting of Tuberculosis

Tuberculosis is designated as a notifiable disease at the national level and local and/or state public health authorities should be notified immediately about suspected or confirmed cases of tuberculosis infection or disease involving children or caregivers/teachers in the child care setting. Facilities should collaborate with local or state health department officials to notify parents/guardians about potential exposures to people with tuberculosis disease. This may include providing the health department officials with identifying information from children in the child care facilities as well as adolescents and adults who may have had contact with child care attendees.

Transmission of tuberculosis infection should be controlled by requiring all adolescents and adults who are present while children are in care to have their tuberculosis status assessed with a tuberculin skin test (TST) or interferon-gamma release assay (IGRA) blood test before caregiving activities are initiated. In people with a reactive TST or positive IGRA, chest radiography without evidence of active pulmonary disease and/or documentation of completion of therapy for latent tuberculosis infection (LTBI) or completion of therapy for active disease should be required. These people should be cleared for employment by their primary care provider or a health department official. Review of the health status of any adolescent or adult with a child care contact with a reactive TST, a positive IGRA or tuberculosis disease in the past should be part of routine annual health appraisal (1,2).

Tuberculosis screening by TST or IGRA of staff members with previously negative skin tests should not be repeated on a regular basis unless a caregiver/teacher is at risk of acquiring a new infection or required by the local or state health department recommendations. Anyone who develops an illness consistent with tuberculosis should be evaluated promptly by a primary care provider. The need for additional testing beyond placement of a TST or IGRA in immunosupressed people and adults over sixty years of age will be at the recommendation of an individual's primary care provider or the local or state health department. Staff members with previously reactive TSTs or positive IGRA should be under the care of a primary care provider who, annually, will document the risk of contagion related to the person's tuberculosis status by performing a symptom review including asking about chronic cough, unintentional weight loss, unexplained fever, and other potential risk factors.

RATIONALE: Young children acquire tuberculosis infection usually from adults and rarely from adolescents (1,2). Tuberculosis organisms are spread by inhalation of a small particle aerosol produced by coughing or sneezing by an adult or adolescent with contagious (active) pulmonary tuberculosis. Transmission usually occurs in an indoor environment. Infants and children under twelve months of age are more susceptible to invasive tuberculosis disease (3). Tuberculosis is not spread via contact with objects such as clothes, dishes, floors, and furniture.

COMMENTS: The two stages of tuberculosis are:

a) Latent tuberculosis infection (LTBI), reflected by a reactive TST or IGRA and the absence of symptoms;
b) Active tuberculosis (tuberculosis disease), reflected by a reactive TST or IGRA and the presence of symptoms, including but not limited to cough, fever, and weight loss.

Virtually all tuberculosis is transmitted from adults and adolescents with tuberculosis disease. Infants and young children with active tuberculosis are not likely to transmit the infection to other children or adults because they generally are unable to forcefully cough out organisms into the air.

A TST should be placed and interpreted by an experienced health care professional. IGRA is only recommended for immunocompetent children four years of age and older, adolescents, and adults.

For additional information regarding tuberculosis, consult the current edition of the *Red Book* from the American Academy of Pediatrics (AAP).

TYPE OF FACILITY: Center; Large Family Child Care Home; Small Family Child Care Home

REFERENCES:

1. Leggiadro, R. T., B. Callery, S. Dowdy, et al. 1989. An outbreak of tuberculosis in a family day care home. *Pediatr Infect Dis J* 8:52-54.
2. Dewan, P. K., H. Banouvong, N. Abernethy, T. Hoynes, L. Diaz, M. Woldemariam, T. Ampie, J. Grinsdale, L. M. Kawamura. 2006. A tuberculosis outbreak in a private-home family child care center in San Francisco, 2002 to 2004. *Pediatrics* 117:863-69.
3. Pickering, L. K., C. J. Baker, D. W. Kimberlin, S. S. Long, eds. 2009. Mycobacterium tuberculosis. In *Red book: 2009 report of the Committee on Infectious Diseases*. 28th ed. Elk Grove Village, IL: American Academy of Pediatrics.

STANDARD 7.3.10.2: Attendance of Children with Latent Tuberculosis Infection or Active Tuberculosis Disease

Children with active tuberculosis disease may attend group child care once effective therapy has been instituted, adherence to therapy has been documented, and clinical symptoms are absent. Local health officials or a primary care provider may recommend return to out-of-home child care once a child is considered non-infectious to others.

Children, adolescents, and adults with latent tuberculosis infection (LTBI) (reactive tuberculin skin test [TST] or a positive interferon-gamma release assay [IGRA] without evidence of active tuberculosis disease) may attend group child care. Appropriate therapy in consultation with a primary care provider is recommended to prevent progression to active tuberculosis disease (1).

RATIONALE: Efforts to prevent transmission of tuberculosis in child care should focus on permitting children with active tuberculosis disease to attend group child care only after the child is considered non-infectious to others. Children with latent tuberculosis are not infectious to others and may attend group child care but should receive appropriate therapy.

COMMENTS: For additional information regarding tuberculosis, consult the current edition of the *Red Book* from the American Academy of Pediatrics (AAP).

TYPE OF FACILITY: Center; Large Family Child Care Home; Small Family Child Care Home

REFERENCES:

1. Pickering, L. K., C. J. Baker, D. W. Kimberlin, S. S. Long, eds. 2009. Mycobacterium tuberculosis. In *Red book: 2009 report of the*

Committee on Infectious Diseases. 28th ed. Elk Grove Village, IL: American Academy of Pediatrics.

7.3.11 Unspecified Respiratory Tract Infection

STANDARD 7.3.11.1: Attendance of Children with Unspecified Respiratory Tract Infection

Children without fever who have mild symptoms associated with the common cold, sore throat, croup, bronchitis, rhinitis, rhinorrhea (runny nose), or otitis media (ear infection) should not be denied admission to child care, sent home from child care, or separated from other children in the facility unless their illness is characterized by one or more of the following conditions:

a) The illness has a specified cause that requires exclusion, as determined by other specific performance standards in Child and Staff Inclusion/Exclusion/Dismissal, Standards 3.6.1.1-3.6.1.4;
b) The illness limits the child's comfortable participation in child care activities;
c) The illness results in a need for more care than the staff can provide without compromising the health and safety of other children.

Treatment with antimicrobial agents should not be required or otherwise encouraged as a condition for attendance of children with mild respiratory tract infections unless directed by local health officials.

RATIONALE: The incidence of acute diseases of the respiratory tract, including the common cold, croup, bronchitis, pneumonia, and otitis media, is common in infants and young children, whether they are cared for at home or attend out-of-home facilities. Studies suggest that children who attend out-of-home child care facilities have more frequent episodes of upper and lower respiratory tract infections compared to children who are cared for at home. Infants and young children may have more upper respiratory infections when they first enter out-of-home group child care. In a national register-based study in Denmark, in children under one year of age, the first six months of enrollment in the first child care facility was associated with a 69% higher incidence of hospitalizations for acute respiratory tract infection compared with age-matched counterparts cared for at home. The incidence of hospitalizations for acute respiratory tract infections decreased after six months of enrollment in an out-of-home child care facility and by twelve months of out-of-home child care enrollment, the incidence of hospitalization for acute respiratory tract infection was comparable to age-matched children cared for at home (1).

Children under three years of age experience an average of five to ten respiratory tract infections each year, most of which are not severe and are caused by viruses that infect the respiratory tract (2). Routine hand hygiene and cough etiquette may reduce the incidence of most acute upper respiratory tract infections among children in child care. Frequently, infected children shed viruses before they are symptomatic, and some infected children never become overtly ill. Therefore, exclusion criteria based on symptomology will not reduce transmission of upper respiratory tract infections among child care attendees.

Inappropriate antibiotic use is common in child care enrollees with mild respiratory tract infections, the majority of which are caused by viruses. Parents/guardians may pressure their primary care provider to prescribe antibiotics because they believe that antibiotics will shorten the duration of exclusion from child care. Primary care providers and caregivers/teachers should reinforce an understanding of the ineffectiveness of antibiotics on duration of viral upper respiratory tract infection and should attempt to retain enrollees unless they meet exclusion criteria (3).

COMMENTS: Symptoms including uncontrolled coughing, difficult or rapid breathing, and wheezing (if associated with difficult breathing) may represent severe illness requiring medical evaluation before readmission to the facility.

For additional information regarding unspecified respiratory tract infections, consult the current edition of the *Red Book* from the American Academy of Pediatrics (AAP). For guidance and reproducible handouts about the management of infectious diseases, consult the most recent edition of *Managing Infectious Diseases in Child Care and Schools,* also from the AAP.

TYPE OF FACILITY: Center; Large Family Child Care Home; Small Family Child Care Home

RELATED STANDARDS:
Standards 3.6.1.1-3.6.1.4: Child and Staff Inclusion/Exclusion/Dismissal

REFERENCES:
1. Kamper-Jørgensen, M., J. Wohlfhart, J. Simonsen, M. Grønbaek, C. S. Benn. 2006. Population-based study of the impact of childcare attendance on hospitalizations for acute respiratory infections. *Pediatrics* 118:1439-46.
2. Fleming, D. W., S. L. Cochi, A. W. Hightower, C. V. Broome. 1987. Childhood upper respiratory tract infections: To what degree is incidence affected by daycare attendance? *Pediatrics* 79:55-60.
3. Dowell, S. F., B. Schwartz, W. R. Phillips, et al. 1998. Principles of judicious use of antimicrobial agents for pediatric upper respiratory tract infections. *Pediatrics* 101:163-65.

7.4 Enteric (Diarrheal) Infections and Hepatitis A Virus (HAV)

STANDARD 7.4.0.1: Control of Enteric (Diarrheal) and Hepatitis A Virus (HAV) Infections

Facilities should employ the following procedures, in addition to those stated in Child and Staff Inclusion/Exclusion/Dismissal, Standards 3.6.1.1-3.6.1.4, to prevent and control infections of the gastrointestinal tract (including diarrhea) or hepatitis A (1-3):

a) Toilet trained children who cannot use a toilet for all bowel movements while attending the facility and who develop diarrhea, as defined in Standard 3.6.1.1, should be removed from the facility by their parent/guardian. Exclude diapered children if stool is not contained in the diaper, stool frequency exceeds two or more stools above normal for that child, blood or mucus in the stool, abnormal color of stool, no urine output in eight hours, jaundice, fever with behavior change, or looks or acts ill. Pending arrival of the parent/guardian, the child should not be permitted to have contact with other children or be placed in areas used by adults who have contact with children in the facility. This should be accomplished by removing the child who is ill to a separate area of the child care program or, if not possible, to a separate area of the child's room. The area should be one where the child is supervised by an adult known to the child, and where the toys, equipment, and surfaces will not be used by other children or adults until after the child who is ill leaves and after the surfaces and toys have been disinfected. When moving a child to a separate area of the facility creates problems with supervision of the other children, as occurs in small family child care homes, the child who is ill should be kept as comfortable as possible, with minimal contact between children who are ill and well children, until the parent/guardian arrives. Caregivers/teachers with diarrhea as defined in Standard 3.6.1.2 should be excluded. Separation and exclusion of children or caregivers/teachers should not be deferred pending health assessment or laboratory testing to identify an enteric pathogen.

b) A child who develops jaundice (when skin and white parts of the eye are yellow) while attending child care should be separated from other children and the child's parent/guardian should be contacted to remove the child. The child should remain separated from other children as described above until the parent/guardian arrives and removes the child from the facility.
c) Exclusion for diarrhea should continue until either the diarrhea stops or the continued loose stools are deemed not to be infectious by a licensed health care professional. Exclusion for hepatitis A virus (HAV) should continue for one week after onset of jaundice.
d) Alternate care for children with diarrhea or hepatitis A in special facilities for children who are ill should be provided in facilities that can provide separate care for children with infections of the gastrointestinal tract (including diarrhea) or hepatitis A.
e) Children and caregivers/teachers who excrete intestinal pathogens but no longer have diarrhea generally may be allowed to return to child care once the diarrhea resolves, except for the case of infections with *Shigella*, Shiga toxin-producing *E. coli* (STEC),or Salmonella enterica serotype Typhi. For *Shigella* and STEC, resolution of symptoms and two negative stool cultures are required for readmission, unless state requirements differ. For *Salmonella* serotype Typhi, resolution of symptoms and three negative stool cultures are required for return to child care. For Salmonella species other than serotype Typhi, documentation of negative stool cultures are not required from asymptomatic people for readmission to child care.
f) The local health department should be informed immediately of the occurrence of HAV infection or an increased frequency of diarrheal illness in children or staff in a child care facility.
g) Recommended post-exposure prophylaxis for hepatitis A includes administration of hepatitis A vaccine or immune globulin to all previously unimmunized staff members and attendees of a child care facility in which a person with hepatitis A is identified.
h) If there has been an exposure to a person with hepatitis A or diarrhea in the child care facility, caregivers/teachers should inform parents/guardians, in cooperation with the health department, that their children may have been exposed to children with HAV infection or to another person with a diarrheal illness.

RATIONALE: Intestinal organisms, including HAV, cause disease in children, caregivers/teachers, and close family members (4-6). The primary age groups involved are children younger than three years of age who wear diapers. Disease has occurred in outbreaks within centers and as sporadic episodes. Although many intestinal agents can cause diarrhea in children in child care, rotavirus, other enteric viruses, *Giardia intestinalis*, *Shigella*, and *Cryptosporidium* have been the main organisms implicated in outbreaks. In addition, excretion of intestinal agents, particularly *Giardia intestinalis* and rotavirus, has been shown to occur in children who show no symptoms (3). The significance of this phenomenon in transmission is unknown. Caregivers/teachers should observe children for signs of disease to permit early detection and implementation of control measures. Facilities should consult the local health department to determine whether the increased frequency of diarrheal illness requires public health intervention.

The most important characteristic of child care facilities associated with increased frequencies of diarrhea or hepatitis A is the presence of young children who are not toilet trained. Contamination of hands, communal toys, and other classroom objects is common and plays a role in transmission of enteric pathogens in child care facilities.

Studies frequently find that fecal contamination of the environment is common in centers and is highest in infant and toddler areas, where diarrhea or hepatitis A are known to occur most often. Studies indicate that the risk of diarrhea is significantly higher for children in centers than for age-matched children cared for at home or in small family child care homes. The spread of infection from children who are not toilet trained to other children in child care facilities, or to their household contacts is common, particularly when *Shigella*, rotavirus, and other enteric viruses such as *Giardia intestinalis, Cryptosporidium*, or HAV are the causal agents (5).

With recommendations for administration of rotavirus vaccine between two and six months of age (7) and hepatitis A vaccine at twelve months of age (1,2) followed by a second dose six months later, rates of disease due to rotavirus and hepatitis A have decreased.

To decrease diarrheal disease in child care due to all pathogens, staff and parents/guardians must be educated about modes of transmission as well as practical methods of prevention and control. Staff training in hand hygiene, combined with close monitoring of compliance, is associated with a significant decrease in infant and toddler diarrhea (8). Staff training on a single occasion, without close monitoring, does not result in a decrease in diarrhea rates; this finding emphasizes the importance of monitoring as well as education. Therefore, appropriate hygienic practices, hygiene monitoring, and education are important in limiting diarrheal infections and hepatitis A in child care.

The Centers for Disease Control and Prevention (CDC) recommends excluding children with diarrhea (for any reason) from child care until diarrhea has resolved. The *Caring for Our Children* standard is more lenient than the CDC recommendation by allowing children who are continent to remain in care. Because outbreaks of diarrheal diseases are less common among continent children, a more lenient approach may be taken.

COMMENTS: Sample letters of notification to parents/guardians that their child may have been exposed to an infectious disease are contained in the publication of the American Academy of Pediatrics (AAP), *Managing Infectious Diseases in Child Care and Schools, 2nd Ed*. For additional information regarding enteric (diarrheal) and HAV infections, consult the current edition of the *Red Book,* also from the AAP.

TYPE OF FACILITY: Center; Large Family Child Care Home; Small Family Child Care Home

RELATED STANDARDS:
Section 2.4: Health Education
Standards 2.1.2.5: Toilet Learning/Training
Standards 3.2.1.1-3.2.1.5: Diapering
Standards 3.2.2.1-3.2.2.5: Hand Hygiene
Standards 3.3.0.1-3.3.0.5: Cleaning, Sanitizing, and Disinfecting
Standards 3.4.2.1-3.4.2.3: Animals
Standards 3.6.1.1-3.6.1.4: Child and Staff Inclusion/Exclusion/Dismissal
Standards 3.6.2.2-3.6.2.10: Caring for Children Who are Ill
Standards 4.9.0.1-4.9.0.9: Food Safety
Standards 9.2.3.11-9.2.3.12: Nutrition and Feeding Policies
Standards 9.4.2.1-9.4.2.8: Child Records

REFERENCES:
1. Centers for Disease Control and Prevention. 2006. Prevention of hepatitis A through active or passive immunization. *MMWR* 55 (RR07). http://www.cdc.gov/mmwr/preview/mmwrhtml/rr5507a1.htm.
2. American Academy of Pediatrics, Committee on Infectious Diseases. 2007. Policy statement: Hepatitis A vaccine recommendations. *Pediatrics* 120:189-99.
3. Shane, A. L., L. K. Pickering. 2008. Infections associated with group child care. In *Principles and practice of pediatric infectious diseases,* eds. S. S. Long, L. K. Pickering, C. G. Prober. 3rd ed. Philadelphia: Churchill Livingstone.
4. Centers for Disease Control and Prevention. 2007. Update: Prevention of hepatitis A after exposure to hepatitis A and in international travelers. *MMWR* 56:1080-84. http://www.cdc.gov/mmwr/preview/mmwrhtml/mm5641a3.htm.
5. Pickering, L. K., D. G. Evans, H. L. Dupont, et al. 1981. Diarrhea caused by *Shigella*, rotavirus and *Giardia* in day care centers; prospective study. *J Pediatr* 99:51-56.
6. Hadler, S. C., H. M. Webster, J. J. Erben, et al. 1980. Hepatitis A in day care centers: A community-wide assessment. *N Engl J Med* 302:1222-27.
7. Centers for Disease Control and Prevention. 2009. Prevention of rotavirus gastroenteritis among infants and children: Recommendations of the ACIP. *MMWR* 58 (RR02). http://www.cdc.gov/mmwr/preview/mmwrhtml/rr5802a1.htm.
8. Bartlett, A. V., B. A. Jarvis, V. Ross, et al. 1988. Diarrheal illness among infants and toddlers in day care centers: Effects of active surveillance and staff training without subsequent monitoring. *Am J Epidemiol* 127:808-17.

STANDARD 7.4.0.2: Staff Education and Policies on Enteric (Diarrheal) and Hepatitis A Virus (HAV) Infections

Facilities should adhere to the following staff educational policies to prevent and control infections of the gastrointestinal tract (mainly diarrhea) and hepatitis A:

a) The facility should conduct ongoing continuing education for staff members, to include the following:
   1) Methods of transmission of pathogens that cause diarrhea and hepatitis A;
   2) Recognition and prevention of diarrhea and disease associated with hepatitis A virus (HAV) infection.

b) All caregivers/teachers, food handlers, and maintenance staff should receive ongoing education and monitoring concerning hand hygiene and cleaning of environmental surfaces as specified in the facility's plan.

c) At least annually, the director should review all procedures related to preventing diarrhea and HAV infections. Each caregiver/teacher, food handler, and maintenance person should review a written copy of these procedures or view a video, which should include age-specific criteria for inclusion and exclusion of children who have a diarrheal illness or HAV infection and infection control procedures.

d) Guidelines for administration of immunization against HAV should be enforced to prevent infection in contacts of children and adults with hepatitis A disease (1).

RATIONALE: Routine immunization of infants with rotavirus vaccine (2) and of toddlers and older children with hepatitis A vaccine has decreased rates of these diseases in child care centers (3,4). In addition, staff training in hygiene and monitoring of staff compliance have been shown to reduce the spread of diarrhea (5). These studies suggest that training combined with outside monitoring of child care practices can modify staff behavior as well as the occurrence of disease.

Caregivers/teachers should observe children for signs of disease to permit early detection and implementation of control measures. Facilities should consult the local health department to determine whether the increased frequency of diarrheal illness requires public health intervention.

COMMENTS: Hepatitis A vaccine is not recommended for routine administration to caregivers/teachers; however, it can be administered to any person seeking protection from HAV. Hepatitis A vaccine is recommended for all children beginning at twelve months of age. However, children less than twelve months of age and children who are not immunized against hepatitis A can develop infection with HAV. Unimmunized infants and toddlers who develop infection with HAV are usually asymptomatic or mildly ill and can easily transmit infection to susceptible adults who often develop signs and symptoms of disease including jaundice and who may become seriously ill. Caregivers/teachers should be aware of the availability of hepatitis A vaccine.

For additional information regarding enteric (diarrheal) and HAV infections, consult the current edition of the *Red Book* from the American Academy of Pediatrics (AAP).

TYPE OF FACILITY: Center; Large Family Child Care Home; Small Family Child Care Home

RELATED STANDARDS:
Standards 3.2.2.1-3.2.2.5: Hand Hygiene
Standards 3.3.0.1-3.3.0.5: Cleaning, Sanitizing, and Disinfecting
Standards 3.6.1.1-3.6.1.4: Child and Staff Inclusion/Exclusion/Dismissal

REFERENCES:

1. Centers for Disease Control and Prevention. 2007. Update: Prevention of hepatitis A after exposure to hepatitis A and in international travelers. *MMWR* 56:1080-84. http://www.cdc.gov/mmwr/preview/mmwrhtml/mm5641a3.htm.
2. Centers for Disease Control and Prevention. 2009. Prevention of rotavirus gastroenteritis among infants and children. *MMWR* 58 (RR02). http://www.cdc.gov/mmwr/preview/mmwrhtml/rr5802a1.htm.
3. Centers for Disease Control and Prevention. 2006. Prevention of hepatitis A through active or passive immunization. *MMWR* 55 (RR07). http://www.cdc.gov/mmwr/preview/mmwrhtml/rr5507a1.htm.
4. American Academy of Pediatrics, Committee on Infectious Diseases. 2007. Policy statement: Hepatitis A vaccine recommendations. *Pediatrics* 120:189-99.
5. Bartlett, A. V., B. A. Jarvis, V. Ross, et al. 1988. Diarrheal illness among infants and toddlers in day care centers: Effects of active surveillance and staff training without subsequent monitoring. *Am J Epidemiol* 127:808-17.

STANDARD 7.4.0.3: Disease Surveillance of Enteric (Diarrheal) and Hepatitis A Virus (HAV) Infections

The child care facility should cooperate with local health authorities in notifying all staff and parents/guardians of other children who attend the facility of possible exposure to hepatitis A, and diarrheal agents including Shiga toxin-producing *E. coli* (STEC), *Shigella, Salmonella, Campylobacter, Giardia intestinalis*, and *Cryptosporidium*.

RATIONALE: Intestinal organisms, including hepatitis A virus (HAV), cause disease in children, caregivers/teachers, and others in the household including close family members (1-7). Disease has occurred in outbreaks within centers and as sporadic episodes. Although many intestinal agents can cause diarrhea in children in child care, rotavirus, other enteric viruses, *Giardia intestinalis*, *Shigella*, and *Cryptosporidium* have been the main organisms implicated in outbreaks.

Caregivers/teachers should observe children for signs of disease to permit early detection and implementation of control measures. Facilities should consult the local health department to determine whether the increased frequency of diarrheal illness requires public health intervention.

COMMENTS: Children who have completed the immunization series for rotavirus and HAV are likely to be protected against infections with these pathogens (1,2).

Sample letters of notification to parents/guardians that their child may have been exposed to an infectious disease in the publication of the American Academy of Pediatrics (AAP), *Managing Infectious Diseases in Child Care and Schools, 2nd Ed*. For more information, consult the current edition of the *Red Book* from the American Academy of Pediatrics (AAP).

TYPE OF FACILITY: Center; Large Family Child Care Home; Small Family Child Care Home

RELATED STANDARDS:
Section 2.4: Health Education

REFERENCES:

1. Centers for Disease Control and Prevention. 2006. Prevention of hepatitis A through active or passive immunization. *MMWR* 55 (RR07). http://www.cdc.gov/mmwr/preview/mmwrhtml/rr5507a1.htm.
2. American Academy of Pediatrics, Committee on Infectious Diseases. 2007. Policy statement: Hepatitis A vaccine recommendations. *Pediatrics* 120:189-99.
3. Shane, A. L., L. K. Pickering. 2008. Infections associated with group child care. In *Principles and practice of pediatric infectious diseases,* eds. S. S. Long, L. K. Pickering, C. G. Prober. 3rd ed. Philadelphia: Churchill Livingstone.
4. Pickering, L. K., D. G. Evans, H. L. Dupont, et al. 1981. Diarrhea caused by *Shigella*, rotavirus and *Giardia* in day care centers; prospective study. *J Pediatr* 99:51-56.
5. Hadler, S. C., H. M. Webster, J. J. Erben, et al. 1980. Hepatitis A in day care centers: A community-wide assessment. *N Engl J Med* 302:1222-27.
6. Centers for Disease Control and Prevention. 2009. Prevention of rotavirus gastroenteritis among infants and children. *MMWR* 58 (RR02). http://www.cdc.gov/mmwr/preview/mmwrhtml/rr5802a1.htm.
7. Bartlett, A. V., B. A. Jarvis, V. Ross, et al. 1988. Diarrheal illness among infants and toddlers in day care centers: Effects of active surveillance and staff training without subsequent monitoring. *Am J Epidemiol* 127:808-17.

STANDARD 7.4.0.4: Maintenance of Records on Incidents of Diarrhea

The facility should maintain a record of children and caregivers/teachers who have diarrhea while at home or at the facility. This record should include:

a) The child or caregiver's/teacher's name;
b) Dates the child or caregiver/teacher is ill;
c) Reason for diarrhea, if known;
d) Whether the child or caregiver/teacher was in attendance at the child care facility during the diarrhea episode;
e) Any leakage of feces from the diaper while the child was in attendance at the child care facility.

Infection with certain enteric diseases or pathogens (cryptosporidiosis, giardiasis, hepatitis A virus [HAV], salmonellosis, Shiga toxin-producing *E. coli* [STEC], shigellosis) is designated as notifiable at the national level. The facility should notify the local health department authorities whenever there have been two or more children with diarrhea in a given classroom or three or more unrelated children (not siblings) with diarrhea within the facility within a two-week period or occurrence of an enteric agent which is notifiable at the national level.

RATIONALE: Disease surveillance and reporting to the local health department authorities are critical in preventing and controlling diseases in the child care setting. A major purpose of surveillance is to allow early detection of disease and prompt implementation of control measures. Ascertaining whether a child who attends a facility is ill is important when evaluating childhood illnesses; ascertaining whether an adult who works in a facility or is a parent/guardian of a child attending a facility is ill is important when considering a diagnosis of hepatitis A and other diseases transmitted by the fecal-oral route. Cases of these infections in household contacts may require questioning about illness in the child attending child care, testing the child for infection, and possible use of hepatitis A vaccine or immune globulin in contacts. Information concerning infectious disease in a child care attendee, staff member, or household contact should be communicated to public health authorities, to the child care director, to all staff, and to all parents/guardians with children in the facility.

TYPE OF FACILITY: Center; Large Family Child Care Home; Small Family Child Care Home

RELATED STANDARDS:
Standards 3.6.4.3-3.6.4.4: Reporting Requirements for Infectious Diseases

7.5 Skin and Mucous Membrane Infections

7.5.1 Conjunctivitis

STANDARD 7.5.1.1: Conjunctivitis

Children and staff with conjunctivitis should not be excluded from child care unless:
a) They are unable to participate in activities;
b) Care for other children would be compromised because of the care that the child with conjunctivitis requires;
c) The person with conjunctivitis has fever or a change in behavior;
d) A health care professional or health department recommends exclusion of the person with conjunctivitis.

Note: Recommendations for the approach to children with conjunctivitis have changed since publication of the last edition of Caring for Our Children.

Children and staff in close contact with a person with conjunctivitis should be observed for symptoms and referred for evaluation, if indicated. If two or more children in a group care setting develop conjunctivitis in the same period, advice from the program's child care health consultant or public health authority should be obtained.

Conjunctivitis, defined as redness and swelling of the covering of the white part of the eye, may result from a number of causes. Bacteria, viruses, allergies, chemical reactions, and immunological conditions may manifest as redness and discharge from one or both eyes. Management of conjunctivitis should involve frequent hand hygiene to prevent spread and evaluation by the primary care provider of children who have severe or prolonged symptoms.

RATIONALE: Conjunctivitis may be caused by both infectious and non-infectious conditions. The length of time that a person is considered contagious due to a bacterial or viral conjunctivitis depends on the organism. Hand contact with eye, nose, and oral secretions is the most common way that organisms causing conjunctivitis are spread from person to person. Careful hand hygiene and sanitizing of surfaces and objects exposed to infectious secretions are the best ways to prevent spread. Antibiotic eye drops and oral medications may decrease the time that a person is considered to be contagious from a bacterial conjunctivitis. However, recovery time is not decreased with antibiotic treatment. The presence of people with conjunctivitis should be noted by caregivers/teachers, and parents/guardians of the child should be notified to seek care, if indicated (1).

COMMENTS: Occasionally, conjunctivitis might occur in several children at the same time or within a few days of each other. Some children with conjunctivitis may have other symptoms including fever, nasal congestion, respiratory, and gastrointestinal tract symptoms. Outbreaks of these symptoms may occur as a result of adenovirus infections. Consultation with a health care professional should be sought in this situation.

For more information on conjunctivitis, consult the current edition of the *Red Book* or *Managing Infectious Diseases in Child Care and Schools,* both from the American Academy of Pediatrics (AAP).

TYPE OF FACILITY: Center; Large Family Child Care Home; Small Family Child Care Home

REFERENCES:
1. Aronson, S. S., T. R. Shope, eds. 2009. Conjunctivitis. In *Managing infectious diseases in child care and schools: A quick reference guide*. 2nd ed. Elk Grove Village, IL: American Academy of Pediatrics.

7.5.2 Enteroviruses

STANDARD 7.5.2.1: Enterovirus Infections

Children and staff with enterovirus infections should not be excluded from child care unless:

a) They are unable to participate in activities;
b) Care for others would be compromised because of the care that the child with enterovirus requires;
c) The person infected with enterovirus has fever or a change in behavior;
d) A health care professional or health department recommends exclusion of the individual(s) with enterovirus infections.

Children and staff in close contact with an affected person should be observed for symptoms of enterovirus infections and referred for evaluation, if indicated.

Enteroviruses may cause one or more symptoms including cough, pharyngitis, mouth sores or ulcers, chest pain, rashes, headaches, diarrhea, muscle aches, and conjunctivitis. These symptoms usually are accompanied by fever. A common enterovirus infection in young children is "hand-foot-and-mouth disease" in which fever and blister-like eruptions in the mouth and/or a rash (usually on the palms and soles) may occur. Enterovirus infections occur commonly in children and may be spread by fecal-oral contact and contact with body fluids and secretions. Enteroviruses may survive for prolonged periods on environmental surfaces. There is no specific treatment for enterovirus infections. Supportive care and frequent hand hygiene to prevent spread are the mainstays of management. In people with severe or prolonged symptoms, evaluation by a primary care provider may be indicated.

RATIONALE: Enterovirus infections are common, especially among young children in whom hand hygiene may be poor. Infections are more common during the summer and early autumn months. Shedding of enteroviruses in respiratory and gastrointestinal tract secretions may occur after symptoms have resolved. Shedding from the gastrointestinal tract of previously infected individuals may be prolonged. Therefore meticulous hand hygiene following toilet use and diaper changing activities should be practiced. Careful hand hygiene and sanitization of surfaces and objects potentially exposed to infectious secretions are the best ways to prevent spread (1,2). The presence of individuals with symptoms suggestive of enterovirus infections should be noted by caregivers/teachers and parents/guardians of the child should be notified to seek the advice of a primary care provider if the child seems ill.

COMMENTS: Occasionally, enterovirus infections might occur in several children at the same time or within a few of days of each other. Consultation with a health care professional and the local health department may be sought when several children have signs and symptoms of an enterovirus infection.

For more information, consult the current edition of the *Red Book* from the American Academy of Pediatrics (AAP) and the Centers for Disease Control and Prevention (CDC) Web-page "Non-Polio Enterovirus Infections" at http://www.cdc.gov/ncidod/dvrd/revb/enterovirus/non-polio_entero.htm.

TYPE OF FACILITY: Center; Large Family Child Care Home; Small Family Child Care Home

REFERENCES:

1. Pickering, L. K., C. J. Baker, D. W. Kimberlin, S. S. Long, eds. Enterovirus (nonpoliovirus) infections. In *Red book: 2009 report of the Committee on Infectious Diseases*. 28th ed. Elk Grove Village, IL: American Academy of Pediatrics.
2. Aronson, S. S., T. R. Shope, eds. 2009. *Managing infectious diseases in child care and schools: A quick reference guide*. 2nd ed. Elk Grove Village, IL: American Academy of Pediatrics.

7.5.3 Human Papillomaviruses (Warts)

STANDARD 7.5.3.1: Human Papillomaviruses (HPV) (Warts)

Children and staff with warts should not be excluded from child care.

Human papillomaviruses (HPV) cause a number of skin and mucous membrane infections; the most common infection is the skin wart. These dome shaped, sometimes conical lesions generally appear on fingers, hands, feet, and face. HPV that causes these lesions are spread via person to person contact. However they are not very contagious. Warts do not require covering with an occlusive dressing. Hand hygiene should be regularly practiced to reduce opportunities for transmission of HPV (1).

RATIONALE: The length of time that an individual with a skin wart is considered contagious varies. However the presence of a wart likely represents an opportunity for transmission. The time from contact to the appearance of a wart may vary from months to years. In addition to hand hygiene after contact with warts, sharing of clothing and towels should be avoided. People with warts should be discouraged from touching and scratching warts.

COMMENTS: The HPV that causes skin warts differs from the HPV that causes genital warts and cervical cancer. Treatments of skin warts including liquid nitrogen and topical antiviral agents may result in earlier clearance of warts; however, warts may reappear, requiring additional treatments. Over time, most warts disappear without treatment. The appearance of skin warts is a common occurrence; immunocompromised people may have more lesions that may be present for an extended duration. The HPV vaccine does not prevent or treat skin warts.

For more information, consult the current edition of the *Red Book* from the American Academy of Pediatrics (AAP).

TYPE OF FACILITY: Center; Large Family Child Care Home; Small Family Child Care Home

REFERENCES:

1. Pickering, L. K., C. J. Baker, D. W. Kimberlin, S. S. Long, eds. 2009. Human papillomaviruses. In *Red book: 2009 report of the Committee on Infectious Diseases*. 28th ed. Elk Grove Village, IL: American Academy of Pediatrics.

7.5.4 Impetigo

STANDARD 7.5.4.1: Impetigo

The following should be instituted when children or staff with lesions suspicious for impetigo are identified:

a) Lesions should be covered with a dressing;
b) The individual should be excluded from child care at the end of the day until the child is treated. The child does not need to be sent home prior to the end of the day if the lesions can be covered and kept dry;
c) Consultation from a primary care provider should be sought to initiate antimicrobial therapy;
d) An individual may return to child care following receipt of antibiotic treatment for twenty-four hours if the sores can be covered and kept dry;
e) Hand hygiene should be emphasized after contact with lesions, administration of topical medication, or changing of dressings.

Exclusion should continue if:

a) Care for others would be compromised because of the care required by the child with impetigo;
b) The child with impetigo has fever or a change in behavior;
c) The sores cannot be kept covered and dry;
d) A health care professional or health department official recommends exclusion of the individual with impetigo.

Children and staff in close contact with an affected person should be observed for symptoms of impetigo and referred for evaluation, if indicated. The local health department should be notified if several children develop impetigo.

RATIONALE: Impetigo is a common skin infection, usually caused by either of two different types of bacteria – streptococci and staphylococci. Fluid filled blisters with "honey-colored" scabs often form. Some skin lesions also may appear as red-colored pimples. The lesions may be found on the face, extremities, or other areas of the body. The bacteria may be acquired from contact with another person with impetigo lesions, from sores on one's own skin at another location, or from contact with surfaces containing bacteria. The bacteria generally enter the skin at an opening or abrasion. Treatment of impetigo may consist of a topical, an oral, or an intravenous medication. Lesions are considered to be infectious until treatment has been administered for twenty-four hours. Lesions are less likely to be infectious once the crusting lesions have healed. Lesions should be kept covered and frequent hand hygiene should be practiced to prevent spread. Evaluation by a primary care provider for people with severe or prolonged symptoms may be indicated (1).

COMMENTS: Impetigo is common, especially among young children in whom hand hygiene may not be adequate. Infections may be more common during the warmer months when skin exposure to trauma may be increased. Impetigo also may occur in cooler months in chapped and wind-burned skin. Shedding of bacteria from wound secretions may occur until crusting of lesions has resolved. Meticulous hand hygiene following contact with lesions should be practiced. Careful hand hygiene and sanitizing of surfaces and objects potentially exposed to infectious material are the best methods to prevent spread. The presence of children with impetigo infections should be noted by caregivers/teachers and parents/guardians of the child should be notified to seek care, if indicated.

For more information, consult the current edition of the *Red Book* from the American Academy of Pediatrics (AAP).

TYPE OF FACILITY: Center; Large Family Child Care Home; Small Family Child Care Home

REFERENCES:

1. Aronson, S. S., T. R. Shope, eds. 2009. Impetigo. In *Managing infectious diseases in child care and schools: A quick reference guide*. 2nd ed. Elk Grove Village, IL: American Academy of Pediatrics.

7.5.5 Lymphadenitis

STANDARD 7.5.5.1: Lymphadenitis

When children or staff with lymphadenitis are identified:

a) They should undergo evaluation by a primary care provider to attempt to assess an infectious etiology, if one has not been defined previously;
b) The child should be excluded from child care, if care for others would be compromised by the care required by the child with lymphadenitis;
c) If the child with lymphadenitis has fever or a change in behavior, the child should be excluded until evaluated;
d) Exclusion should occur if a health care professional or health department official recommends this action.

Children and staff in close contact with an affected child should be observed for symptoms of infection and referred for evaluation, if indicated. The local health department should be notified if a caregiver/teacher has a concern that several children have symptoms of lymphadenitis.

Lymphadenitis, an inflammation and generally an enlargement of one or more lymph nodes (glands), may result from both non-infectious and infectious causes. Lymphadenopathy is an enlargement of a lymph node without inflammation. The most common infectious sources of lymphadenitis are bacteria and viruses, with fungi and parasites accounting for fewer infections. Lymphadenitis in children usually is acute, with rapid onset and symptoms involving the lymph nodes of the head and neck. Lymph nodes in other sites, including the groin and on one or both sides of the body may be affected. The affected lymph node(s) may be swollen with areas of redness overlying the swelling and may be painful to touch. In some cases a "chain" of lymph nodes may be palpated. The inflammation of one or more lymph nodes may represent an infectious etiology. Evaluation by a primary care provider may be indicated to define the underlying etiology and to assess potential for transmission and need for treatment.

RATIONALE: Lymphadenitis is a common presentation of a number of infectious and non-infectious etiologies. Most types of infectious lymphadenitis may be described as acute and bilateral, acute and unilateral, and subacute or chronic (1). It is helpful to categorize lymphadenitis because certain infectious organisms are more likely to be associated with one of the three categories. It also is important to identify the infectious organism responsible for the lymphadenitis because this information has implications for management and treatment, including child care inclusion and exclusion policies. Careful hand hygiene and disinfection of surfaces and objects potentially exposed to infectious material are the best ways to prevent spread. The presence of children with lymphadenitis should be noted by caregivers/teachers, and parents/guardians of children should be notified to seek care, if indicated.

COMMENTS: Occasionally, lymphadenitis might occur in several children or staff members at the same time or within a few of days of each other.

For more information, consult the current edition of the *Red Book* from the American Academy of Pediatrics (AAP).

TYPE OF FACILITY: Center; Large Family Child Care Home; Small Family Child Care Home

REFERENCES:

1. Thorrell, E. A., P. J. Chesney. 2008. Cervical lymphadenitis and neck infections. In *Principles and practice of infectious diseases,* eds. S. S. Long, L. K. Pickering, C. G. Prober. 3rd ed. Philadelphia: Churchill Livingstone.

7.5.6 Measles

STANDARD 7.5.6.1: Immunization for Measles

All children in a child care facility should have received age-appropriate immunizations with measles, mumps, and rubella (MMR) vaccine or with measles, mumps, rubella, and varicella (MMRV) vaccine (1). If a case of measles occurs in a child care setting, interrupting subsequent spread depends on prompt immunization of people at risk of exposure or people already exposed who cannot provide documentation of measles immunity, including date of immunization. Children and adults in child care who are not immunized or not age-appropriately immunized against measles should be excluded from care immediately if the child care facility has been notified of a documented case of measles occurring in a child or adult in the center. These children should not be allowed to return to the facility until at least two weeks after the onset of rash in the last case of measles, as determined by health department officials.

Adults born before 1957 can be considered immune to measles. Adults born during or after 1957 should receive one or more doses of MMR vaccine unless they have a medical contraindication, documentation of one or more dose of vaccine, history of measles based on primary care provider diagnosis, or laboratory evidence of immunity.

RATIONALE: Measles is one of the most highly infectious of all infections transmitted by direct contact with infectious droplets or by airborne spread. Outbreaks of measles have been reported in unimmunized populations. Transmission to unimmunized people in the U.S. from importation of measles by international travelers occurs on a regular basis (2). Appropriate immunization of children and adults with MMR vaccine prevents the occurrence of measles disease. Any case of measles identified in a child or adult in a child care setting should be reported to local or state health department officials immediately.

TYPE OF FACILITY: Center; Large Family Child Care Home; Small Family Child Care Home

REFERENCES:

1. Pickering, L. K., C. J. Baker, D. W. Kimberlin, S. S. Long, eds. 2009. Measles. In *Red book: 2009 report of the Committee on Infectious Diseases*. 28th ed. Elk Grove Village, IL: American Academy of Pediatrics.

2. Centers for Disease Control and Prevention. 2008. Update: Measles – United States, January-July 2008. *MMWR* 57:893-96. http://www.cdc.gov/mmwr/preview/mmwrhtml/mm5733a1.htm.

7.5.7 Molluscum Contagiosum

STANDARD 7.5.7.1: Molluscum Contagiosum

Molluscum contagiosum is a skin disease, similar to warts, that causes one or more flesh-colored, translucent lesions with small indentations. Some lesions also have an eczema-like appearance to their outer edge. The virus that causes molluscum contagiosum is spread by person-to-person contact. It also may be transmitted by sharing towels and clothing containing residual virus acquired by contact with the lesions of an infected person. The virus may be spread to other sites by scratching and manipulating lesions. Clusters of molluscum-associated lesions commonly occur on the trunk, extremities, and face. People with eczema or who are immunocompromised may have more extensive lesions that are present for prolonged periods of time (2).

The virus causing these lesions is spread via person-to-person or person-to-object-to person; however, it is not very contagious. Despite its name, it is more likely that a person will spread the virus to a site on his or her body than to another individual. Lesions do not require covering with a dressing. Hand hygiene should be regularly practiced to reduce opportunities for transmission of the virus causing molluscum contagiosum.

Children and staff with molluscum contagiosum should not be excluded from child care.

RATIONALE: The length of time that a person with a molluscum contagiosum lesion is considered contagious varies; however, the presence of a lesion likely represents an opportunity for transmission. The time from contact to the appearance of a lesion or lesions may vary from weeks to months. In addition to hand hygiene after contact with lesions, sharing of clothing and towels should be avoided. People with molluscum contagiosum should be discouraged from touching and scratching their lesions (1).

COMMENTS: Molluscum contagiosum lesions may be pruritic (itchy), resulting in release of virus from and introduction

of bacteria into the area. The application of a bag filled with ice may reduce the urge to scratch. Treatment of lesions is a cosmetic issue and does not usually affect resolution. Over time, lesions disappear without treatment.

TYPE OF FACILITY: Center; Large Family Child Care Home; Small Family Child Care Home

RELATED STANDARDS:
Standard 7.5.3.1: Human Papillomaviruses (HPV) (Warts)

REFERENCES:

1. Aronson, S. S., T. R. Shope, eds. 2009. Molluscum contagiosum. In *Managing infectious diseases in child care and schools: A quick reference guide*. 2nd ed. Elk Grove Village, IL: American Academy of Pediatrics.
2. Pickering, L. K., C. J. Baker, D. W. Kimberlin, S. S. Long, eds. 2009. Molluscum contagiosum. In *Red book: 2009 report of the Committee on Infectious Diseases*. 28th ed. Elk Grove Village, IL: American Academy of Pediatrics.

7.5.8 Pediculosis Capitis (Head Lice)

STANDARD 7.5.8.1: Attendance of Children with Head Lice

Children should not be excluded immediately or sent home early from child care due to the presence of head lice. Parents/guardians of affected children should be notified and informed that their child must be treated before returning to the child care facility. In addition to treating the affected child with a pediculicide (an agent used to destroy lice), any items such as headgear, pillowcases, and towels that have come into contact with the affected child in the forty-eight hours prior to treatment should be laundered in hot water. Children and staff who have been in close contact with an affected child should be examined and treated if infested, defined as the presence of adult lice or nits (eggs) on a hair shaft within three to four millimeters from the scalp.

RATIONALE: Head lice infestation in children attending child care is common and is NOT a sign of poor hygiene. Transmission occurs by direct contact with hair of infested people and less commonly by direct contact with personal items of infested people. Head lice are not a health hazard because they are not responsible for spread of any disease. The institution of "no-nit" policies before permitting return of an infested child to child care or school are not effective in controlling transmission (2).

Child care programs should not institute a "no-nit" policy.

COMMENTS: Treatments for head lice generally are safe and effective when used as directed. Some treatments may cause an itching or a burning sensation of the scalp. Most products used to treat head lice are pesticides that can be absorbed through the skin. Therefore, all medicines used for treatment of lice should be used with care and only as directed. Although not medically necessary, removal of nits that are attached within one centimeter of the base of the hair shaft may be manually performed (1). Removing the nits may help in situations where outbreaks are occurring in the group to determine whether a child who has been treated became reinfested after treatment or merely has residual non-viable nits. Utilize your child care health consultant to help with this issue. In addition, the following resources may be useful to help with education and information about treatment: http://www.cdc.gov/parasites/lice/ and http://www.healthychildren.org/English/health-issues/conditions/from-insects-animals/Pages/Signs-of-Lice.aspx.

TYPE OF FACILITY: Center; Large Family Child Care Home; Small Family Child Care Home

REFERENCES:

1. Centers for Disease Control and Prevention. 2008. Head lice: Treatment FAQs. http://www.cdc.gov/parasites/lice/.
2. American Academy of Pediatrics, Committee on School Health, Committee on Infectious Diseases. 2010. Clinical report: Head lice. *Pediatrics* 126:392-403.

7.5.9 Tinea Capitis and Tinea Cruris (Ringworm)

STANDARD 7.5.9.1: Attendance of Children with Ringworm

Children with ringworm of the scalp (tinea capitis) or body (tinea corporis) should receive appropriate treatment. Children receiving treatment should not be excluded from child care.

Children and staff in close contact with an affected child should receive periodic inspections for early lesions and should receive therapy, if lesions are noted. Contact with lesions should be avoided. Dry coverings over treated lesions should be encouraged.

RATIONALE: Ringworm infections result from a fungus that is transmitted by contact with an infected person (scalp and body) and by contact with infected animals (body). Treatment of ringworm of the scalp requires oral medicine for four to six weeks (1). Treatment of ringworm of the body requires topical medicine for a minimum of four weeks (2). Oral therapy is available if lesions are extensive or unresponsive to topical therapy. Direct contact with sources of ringworm should be avoided to prevent transmission (1,2).

COMMENTS: Personal items should not be shared. The lesion resulting from the fungal infection is usually circular (hence the term "ringworm") but other non-fungal and non-infectious rashes may have a similar appearance. People receiving oral treatment for ringworm of the scalp may attend child care or school. Haircuts, shaving of the scalp, and wearing of head coverings are not indicated for treatment of tinea capitis. Using long sleeves or long pants to cover extremity lesions is sufficient to reduce the shedding of spores and transfer of topical medications from the sores to surfaces in the child care facility.

For additional information regarding ringworm, consult the current edition of the *Red Book* from the American Academy of Pediatrics (AAP).

TYPE OF FACILITY: Center; Large Family Child Care Home; Small Family Child Care Home

REFERENCES:

1. Pickering, L. K., C. J. Baker, D. W. Kimberlin, S. S. Long, eds.

2009. Tinea capitis. In *Red book: 2009 report of the Committee on Infectious Diseases*. 28th ed. Elk Grove Village, IL: American Academy of Pediatrics.
2. Pickering, L. K., C. J. Baker, D. W. Kimberlin, S. S. Long, eds. 2009. Tinea corporis. In *Red book: 2009 report of the Committee on Infectious Diseases*. 28th ed. Elk Grove Village, IL: American Academy of Pediatrics.

7.5.10 *Staphylococcus Aureus* Skin Infections Including MRSA

STANDARD 7.5.10.1: *Staphylococcus Aureus* Skin Infections Including MRSA

The following should be implemented when children or staff with lesions suspicious for *Staphylococcus aureus* infections are identified:

a) Lesions should be covered with a dressing;
b) Report the lesions to the parent/guardian with a recommendation for evaluation by a primary care provider;
c) Exclusion is not warranted unless the individual meets any of the following criteria:
    1) Care for other children would be compromised by care required for the person with the *S. aureus* infection;
    2) The individual with the *S. aureus* infection has fever or a change in behavior;
    3) The lesion(s) cannot be adequately covered by a bandage or the bandage needs frequent changing;
    4) A health care professional or health department official recommends exclusion of the person with *S. aureus* infection.

Meticulous hand hygiene following contact with lesions should be practiced. Careful hand hygiene and sanitization of surfaces and objects potentially exposed to infectious material are the best ways to prevent spread. Children and staff in close contact with an infected person should be observed for symptoms of *S. aureus* infection and referred for evaluation, if indicated.

A child may return to group child care when staff members are able to care for the child without compromising their ability to care for others, the child is able to participate in activities, appropriate therapy is being given, and the lesions can be covered.

S. aureus skin infections initially may appear as red raised areas that may become pus-filled abscesses or "boils," surrounded by areas of redness and tenderness. Fever and other symptoms including decreased activity, bone and joint pain, and difficulty breathing may occur when the infection occurs in other body systems. If any of these signs or symptoms occur, the child should be evaluated by his/her primary care provider.

RATIONALE: *S. aureus* (also known as *"Staph")* is a bacterium that commonly causes superficial skin infections (cellulitis and abscesses). It also may cause muscle, bone, lung, and blood (invasive) infections. One type of *S. aureus*, called methicillin-resistant *S. aureus* or "MRSA," is resistant to one or more classes of antibiotics. *S. aureus* and MRSA have been the source of attention due to increasing rates of infections from these bacteria associated with health care associated (HCA) infections and in healthy children and adults in the community. Transmissibility and infectivity is comparable to infections with *S. aureus* without methicillin resistance. Therefore signs and symptoms, incubation and contagion periods, control of spread, and exclusion guidelines are identical for all *S. aureus* infections, including infections with methicillin resistance or MRSA (1,2).

Most people with skin infections due to *S. aureus* do not develop invasive infections; they may experience recurrent skin infections. Infants and children who are diapered and pre-adolescents and adolescents who participate in team sports may have an increased risk for developing *S. aureus* skin infections. This is likely due to frequent breaks of skin and the sharing of towels. The incubation period for *S. aureus* skin infections is unknown. Some people may carry MRSA without having symptoms of active infection. These people are considered to be "colonized" with *S. aureus*; however, they are not considered to be infectious when they do not have active infection.

S. aureus skin infections may occur at sites of skin trauma. Pus and other material draining from skin lesions should be considered to be infectious. Treatment of *S. aureus* skin infections may be accomplished with an oral or an intravenous antibiotic or a combination of both. In some cases, incision and drainage of the lesion(s) alone may be required. In other instances, incision and drainage of smaller lesions with the use of a topical antibiotic may result in a cure. Skin lesions are considered to be infectious until they have healed; therefore, they should be kept covered and dry. Frequent hand hygiene to prevent spread of *S. aureus* should be practiced at home and in child care. Evaluation by a primary care provider in people with severe or prolonged symptoms may be indicated.

COMMENTS: *S. aureus* skin infections are common, especially among infants wearing diapers and adolescent members of sports teams. Infections may be more common among children where other family members have or have had skin lesions and during the warmer months when skin exposure to trauma may be increased. Shedding of bacteria from skin lesions may occur until the lesion has healed. Occasionally *S. aureus* infections may occur in several children at the same time or within a few of days of each other. Consultation with a health care professional and the local health department may be sought when several people have these symptoms.

For additional information for parents/guardians and caregivers/teachers, refer to information posted by the Centers for Disease Control and Prevention (CDC) at http://cdc.gov/mrsa/groups/advice-for-family-caregivers.html.

TYPE OF FACILITY: Center; Large Family Child Care Home; Small Family Child Care Home

REFERENCES:

1. Pickering, L. K., C. J. Baker, D. W. Kimberlin, S. S. Long, eds. 2009. Staphylococcal infections. In *Red book: 2009 report of the*

Committee on Infectious Diseases. 28th ed. Elk Grove Village, IL: American Academy of Pediatrics.
2. Aronson, S. S., T. R. Shope, eds. 2009. Impetigo. In *Managing infectious diseases in child care and schools: A quick reference guide*. 2nd ed. Elk Grove Village, IL: American Academy of Pediatrics.

7.5.11 Scabies

STANDARD 7.5.11.1: Attendance of Children with Scabies

Children with scabies should be removed from the child care facility until appropriate treatment has been administered. Children should be allowed to return to child care after treatment has been completed.

RATIONALE: Scabies is caused by a mite and manifests as an intensely itchy, red rash caused by burrowing of female mites into the skin. These burrows appear as gray or white thread-like crooked lines. Transmission usually occurs through prolonged close contact (1). Epidemics and localized outbreaks may require stringent and consistent measures to treat contacts. Individuals who have had prolonged skin-to-skin contact with infested people may benefit from prophylactic treatment. Bedding used and clothing worn next to the skin for three days prior to treatment should be washed in hot water and dried in a hot dryer cycle. Items that cannot be laundered should be stored in sealed plastic bags for seven days.

COMMENTS: Environmental disinfestation and cleaning with potentially toxic agents are unnecessary and are not efficacious in reducing transmission of scabies mites. Optimal control is achieved by treatment of infested people and their close contacts.

For additional information, see the Centers for Disease Control and Prevention (CDC) Website at http://www.cdc.gov/parasites/scabies/.

TYPE OF FACILITY: Center; Large Family Child Care Home; Small Family Child Care Home

REFERENCES:

1. Pickering, L. K., C. J. Baker, D. W. Kimberlin, S. S. Long, eds. 2009. Scabies. In *Red book: 2009 report of the Committee on Infectious Diseases*. 28th ed. Elk Grove Village, IL: American Academy of Pediatrics.

7.5.12 Thrush

STANDARD 7.5.12.1: Thrush (Candidiasis)

Children with thrush do not need to be excluded from group settings. Careful hand hygiene and sanitization of surfaces and objects potentially exposed to oral secretions including pacifiers and toothbrushes is the best way to prevent spread. Toothbrushes and pacifiers should be labeled individually so that children do not share toothbrushes or pacifiers, as specified in Standard 3.1.5.2. The presence of children with thrush should be noted by caregivers/teachers, and parents/guardians of the children should be notified to seek care, if indicated.

Treatment of thrush may consist of a topical or an oral medication. Most people are able to control thrush without treatment. Evaluation by a primary care provider of people with severe or prolonged symptoms may be indicated.

RATIONALE: Thrush is a common infection, especially among infants. Thrush is caused by yeast, a type of fungus called *Candida*. This fungus thrives in warm, moist areas (skin, skin under a diaper, and on mucous membranes). Thrush appears as white patches on the mucous membranes, commonly on the inner cheeks, gums, and tongue, and may cause diaper rash. The yeast that causes thrush lives on skin and mucous membranes of healthy people and is present on surfaces throughout the environment. An imbalance in the normal bacteria and fungi on the skin may cause the yeast to begin growing on the mucous membranes, appearing as white plaques that are adherent. Intermittent thrush may be normal in infants and young children. People with exposure to moisture, those receiving antibiotics, or those with an illness may develop thrush (1).

COMMENTS: Occasionally, thrush might occur in several individuals at the same time or within a couple of days of each other. Consultation with a health care professional and the local health department may be sought when several individuals have these symptoms.

TYPE OF FACILITY: Center; Large Family Child Care Home; Small Family Child Care Home

RELATED STANDARDS:
Standard 3.1.5.2: Toothbrushes and Toothpaste
Standards 3.3.0.2-3.3.0.3: Cleaning and Sanitizing Toys and Objects Intended for the Mouth

REFERENCES:

1. Pickering, L. K., C. J. Baker, D. W. Kimberlin, S. S. Long, eds. 2009. Candidiasis. In *Red book: 2009 report of the Committee on Infectious Diseases*. 28th ed. Elk Grove Village, IL: American Academy of Pediatrics.

7.6 Bloodborne Infections

7.6.1 Hepatitis B Virus (HBV)

STANDARD 7.6.1.1: Disease Recognition and Control of Hepatitis B Virus (HBV) Infection

Facilities should have written policies for inclusion and exclusion of children known to be infected with hepatitis B virus (HBV) and for immunization of all children with hepatitis B vaccine per the "Recommended Immunization Schedules" for children and adolescents. All infants should complete a three dose series of hepatitis B vaccine beginning at birth as recommended by the American Academy of Pediatrics (AAP) and Centers for Disease Control and Prevention (CDC) (1). When a child who is an HBV carrier is admitted to a facility, the facility director and primary caregivers/teachers should be informed.

Children who carry HBV chronically and who have no behavioral or medical risk factors, such as aggressive behavior (such as biting or frequent scratching), generalized dermatitis (weeping skin lesions), or bleeding problems, may be admitted to the facility without restrictions.

Testing of children for HBV should not be a prerequisite for admission to facilities.

With regard to infection control measures and handling of blood or blood-containing body fluids, every person should be assumed to be an HBV carrier with regard to blood exposure. All blood should be considered as potentially containing HBV. Child care personnel should adopt Standard Precautions, as outlined in Prevention of Exposure to Blood and Body Fluids, Standard 3.2.3.4.

Toys and objects that young children (infants and toddlers) mouth should be cleaned and sanitized, as stated in Standards 3.3.0.2-3.3.0.3.

Toothbrushes and pacifiers should be individually labeled so that the children do not share toothbrushes or pacifiers, as specified in Standard 3.1.5.2.

RATIONALE: Prior to routine hepatitis B immunization of infants, transmission in child care facilities was reported (2,3). Currently the risk of transmitting the disease in child care is theoretically small because of the low risk of transmission, implementation of infection control measures, and high immunization rates. Immunization not only will reduce the potential for transmission but also will allay anxiety about transmission from children and staff in the child care setting who may be carriers of hepatitis B (1). However, children who are HBV carriers (particularly children born in countries highly endemic for HBV) could be enrolled in child care. Thus, transmission of HBV in the child care setting is of concern to public health authorities.

The risk of disease transmission from an HBV-carrier child or staff member with no behavioral risk factors and without generalized dermatitis or bleeding problems is considered rare. This extremely low risk does not justify exclusion of an HBV-carrier child from out-of-home care, nor does it justify the routine screening of children as possible HBV carriers prior to admission to child care.

HBV transmission in a child care setting is most likely to occur through direct exposure via bites or scratches that break the skin and introduce blood or body secretions from the HBV carrier into a susceptible person. Indirect transmission via blood or saliva through environmental contamination may be possible but has not been documented. Saliva contains much less virus (1/1000) than blood; therefore, the potential infection from saliva is much lower than that of blood.

No data are available to indicate the risk of transmission if a susceptible person bites an HBV carrier. When the HBV statuses of both the biting child and the victim are unknown, the risk of HBV transmission would be extremely low because of the expected low incidence of HBV carriage by children of preschool-age and the low efficiency of disease transmission by bite exposure. Because a bite in this situation is extremely unlikely to involve an HBV-carrier child, screening is not warranted, particularly in children who are immunized appropriately against HBV (1), but each situation should be evaluated individually. In the rare circumstance that an unimmunized child bites a known HBV carrier, the hepatitis B vaccine series should be initiated (4).

COMMENTS: Parents/guardians are not required to share information about their child's HBV status, but they should be encouraged to do so. For additional information regarding HBV consult the current edition of the *Red Book* from the AAP.

TYPE OF FACILITY: Center; Large Family Child Care Home; Small Family Child Care Home

RELATED STANDARDS:

Standard 3.1.5.2: Toothbrushes and Toothpaste
Standard 3.2.3.4: Prevention of Exposure to Blood and Body Fluids
Standards 3.3.0.2-3.3.0.3: Cleaning and Sanitizing Toys and Objects Intended for the Mouth

REFERENCES:

1. Centers for Disease Control and Prevention. 2005. A comprehensive immunization strategy to eliminate transmission of hepatitis B virus infection in the United States. *MMWR* 54 (RR16). http://www.cdc.gov/mmwr/preview/mmwrhtml/rr5416a1.htm.
2. Deseda, D. D., C. N. Shapiro, K. Carroll. 1994. Hepatitis B virus transmission between a child and staff member at a day-care center. *Pediatr Infect Dis J* 13:828-30.
3. Shapiro, C. N., L. F. McCaig, K. F. Genesheimer, et al. 1989. Hepatitis B virus transmission between children in day care. *Pediatr Infect Dis J* 8:870-75.
4. Shane, A. L., L. K. Pickering. 2008. Infections associated with group child care. In *Principles and practice of pediatric infectious diseases,* eds. S. S. Long, L. K. Pickering, C. G. Prober. 3rd ed. Philadelphia: Churchill Livingstone.

STANDARD 7.6.1.2: Observation and Follow-Up of a Child Who is a Hepatitis B Virus (HBV) Carrier

The primary caregiver/teacher should observe a child who is a known hepatitis B virus (HBV) carrier and the other children in the group for development of aggressive behavior (such as biting or frequent scratching) that might facilitate transmission of HBV. If this type of behavior occurs, the child's primary care provider or the health department should evaluate the need for immediate disease prevention measures with hepatitis B immune globulin and should reevaluate the child's continuing attendance in the facility.

RATIONALE: Regular assessment of behavioral risk factors and medical conditions of enrolled children who are HBV carriers is important. It is helpful if the center director and primary caregivers/teachers are informed that a known HBV-carrier child is in care. However, parents/guardians are not required to share this information. Most children in child care facilities have been immunized against hepatitis B as part of their routine immunization schedule, minimizing the risk of transmission (1).

COMMENTS: For additional information regarding HBV infections, consult the current edition of the *Red Book* from the American Academy of Pediatrics (AAP).

TYPE OF FACILITY: Center; Large Family Child Care Home; Small Family Child Care Home

REFERENCES:

1. Centers for Disease Control and Prevention. 2005. A comprehensive immunization strategy to eliminate transmission of hepatitis B virus infection in the United States. *MMWR* 54 (RR16). http://www.cdc.gov/mmwr/preview/mmwrhtml/rr5416a1.htm.

STANDARD 7.6.1.3: Staff Education on Prevention of Bloodborne Diseases

All caregivers/teachers should receive training at employment and annually thereafter as required by the Occupational Safety and Health Administration (OSHA) on how to prevent transmission of bloodborne diseases, including hepatitis B virus (HBV), hepatitis C virus (HCV), and HIV (1).

RATIONALE: Efforts to reduce risk of transmitting diseases in child care through hygiene and environmental standards in general should focus primarily on blood precautions, limiting saliva contamination (no sharing of utensils, pacifiers, tooth brushes), and ensuring that children are appropriately immunized against HBV. People, including caregivers/teachers, who may be expected to come into contact with blood as a part of their employment, are required to be trained how to protect themselves from bloodborne diseases by their employers and be offered hepatitis B vaccine at no charge to them, within ten working days of initial assignment (1,2).

COMMENTS: If the employee initially declines hepatitis B vaccination but at a later date, while still covered under the acceptable timeline (ten working days), decides to accept the vaccination, the employer should make hepatitis B vaccination available at that time. The employer should require that employees who decline to accept the offer of hepatitis B vaccination sign the Occupational Safety and Health Administration's (OSHA) "Hepatitis B Vaccine Declination" statement (1). The "Hepatitis B Vaccine Declination" statement can be found at http://www.ecels-healthychildcarepa.org/content/Keeping Safe 07-27-10.pdf.

For additional information regarding HBV and HCV infections, consult the associated chapters in the current edition of the *Red Book* from the American Academy of Pediatrics (AAP).

TYPE OF FACILITY: Center; Large Family Child Care Home; Small Family Child Care Home

RELATED STANDARDS:

Standard 3.2.3.4: Prevention of Exposure to Blood and Body Fluids

REFERENCES:

1. Occupational Safety and Health Administration. 2008. *Bloodborne pathogens.* Title 29, pt. 1910.1030. http://www.osha.gov/pls/oshaweb/owadisp.show_document?p_table=STANDARDS&p_id=10051.

2. Centers for Disease Control and Prevention. 2005. A comprehensive immunization strategy to eliminate transmission of hepatitis B virus infection in the United States. *MMWR* 54 (RR16). http://www.cdc.gov/mmwr/preview/mmwrhtml/rr5416a1.htm.

STANDARD 7.6.1.4: Informing Public Health Authorities of Hepatitis B Virus (HBV) Cases

Staff members known to have acute or chronic hepatitis B virus (HBV) infection should not be restricted from work but should receive training on how to prevent transmission of bloodborne diseases. HBV infection is designated as a notifiable disease at the national level. Cases of acute HBV in any child or employee of a facility should be reported to the health department for determination of the need for further investigation or preventive measures (1).

RATIONALE: The risk of disease transmission from a HBV-carrier child or staff member with normal behavior and without generalized dermatitis or bleeding problems is considered to be rare. This extremely low risk does not justify exclusion of an HBV-carrier staff member from providing child care, nor does it justify the routine screening of staff as possible HBV carriers prior to admission to child care.

COMMENTS: For additional information regarding HBV infections, consult the current edition of the *Red Book* from the American Academy of Pediatrics (AAP).

TYPE OF FACILITY: Center; Large Family Child Care Home; Small Family Child Care Home

RELATED STANDARDS:

Standard 3.2.3.4: Prevention of Exposure to Blood and Bodily Fluids

Standards 3.6.4.3-3.6.4.4: Reporting Requirements for Infectious Diseases

REFERENCES:

1. Centers for Disease Control and Prevention. 2008. Recommendations for identification and public health management of persons with chronic hepatitis B virus infection. *MMWR* 57 (RR08). http://www.cdc.gov/mmwr/preview/mmwrhtml/rr5708a1.htm.

STANDARD 7.6.1.5: Handling Injuries to a Hepatitis B Virus (HBV) Carrier

Injuries that lead to bleeding by a hepatitis B virus (HBV) carrier child or adult should be handled promptly in the manner recommended for any such injury in any child or adult using Standard Precautions.

RATIONALE: Efforts to reduce the risk of transmitting diseases in child care through hygienic and environmental standards in general should focus primarily on blood precautions and ensuring appropriate immunization of children and adults against HBV (1).

COMMENTS: For additional information regarding HBV infections, consult the current edition of the *Red Book* from the American Academy of Pediatrics (AAP).

TYPE OF FACILITY: Center; Large Family Child Care Home; Small Family Child Care Home

RELATED STANDARDS:

Standard 3.2.3.4: Prevention of Exposure to Blood and Bodily Fluids

REFERENCES:
1. Centers for Disease Control and Prevention. 2008. Recommendations for identification and public health management of persons with chronic hepatitis B virus infection. *MMWR* 57 (RR08). http://www.cdc.gov/mmwr/preview/mmwrhtml/rr5708a1.htm.

7.6.2 Hepatitis C Virus (HCV)

STANDARD 7.6.2.1: Infection Control Measures with Hepatitis C Virus (HCV)

Standard Precautions, as outlined in Standard 3.2.3.4, should be followed to prevent infection with hepatitis C virus (HCV) infection. Children with HCV infection should not be excluded from out-of-home child care. Hepatitis C is designated as a notifiable disease at the national level and local and/or state public health authorities should be notified about cases of hepatitis C infections involving children or adults in the child care setting.

RATIONALE: The seroprevalence (frequency) of HCV infection in young children is less than 1% and most acute infections are asymptomatic. Transmission risks of HCV in a child care setting are unknown. The general risk of HCV infection from exposure to blood-containing body fluids entering through the skin is estimated to be ten times greater than that of HIV but lower than that of hepatitis B virus (HBV) (1). Transmission of HCV via contamination of mucous membranes (eyes, nose, mouth) or broken skin probably has an intermediate risk between that for blood infected with HIV and HBV (2).

COMMENTS: For additional information regarding HCV infections, consult the current edition of the *Red Book* from the American Academy of Pediatrics (AAP).

TYPE OF FACILITY: Center; Large Family Child Care Home; Small Family Child Care Home

RELATED STANDARDS:
Standard 3.2.3.4: Prevention of Exposure to Blood and Body Fluids

REFERENCES:
1. Centers for Disease Control and Prevention. 2009. Guidelines for prevention and treatment of opportunistic infections in HIV-infected adults and adolescents. *MMWR* 58 (RR04). http://www.cdc.gov/mmwr/pdf/rr/rr5804.pdf.
2. Centers for Disease Control and Prevention. 2008. Hepatitis C. http://www.cdc.gov/hepatitis/ChooseC.htm.

7.6.3 Human Immunodeficiency Virus (HIV)

STANDARD 7.6.3.1: Attendance of Children with HIV

Children who enter child care should not be required to be tested for HIV or to disclose their HIV status (1). There is no need to restrict placement of HIV-infected children, without risk factors for transmission of bloodborne pathogens, in child care facilities to protect other children or staff members in these settings. Because HIV-infected children whose status is unknown may attend child care, Standard Precautions should be adopted for handling of all blood and blood-containing body fluids and wound exudates from all children.

RATIONALE: The decision to admit known HIV-infected children to child care is best made on an individual basis by qualified people, including the child's primary care provider, who are able to evaluate whether the child will receive optimal care in the program and whether an HIV-infected child poses a significant risk to others (2). Specifically, admission of each HIV-infected child with one or more potential risk factors for transmission of bloodborne pathogens (e.g., biting, if the child has oral bleeding, frequent scratching, generalized dermatitis, or bleeding problems) should be assessed by the child's primary care provider and the program director. A public health authority with expertise in HIV prevention/transmission should be consulted as appropriate.

COMMENTS: For additional information regarding HIV, consult the current edition of the *Red Book* from the American Academy of Pediatrics (AAP).

TYPE OF FACILITY: Center; Large Family Child Care Home; Small Family Child Care Home

RELATED STANDARDS:
Standard 3.2.3.4: Prevention of Exposure to Blood and Body Fluids

REFERENCES:
1. American Academy of Pediatrics, Committee on Pediatric AIDS, and Committee on Infectious Disease. 1999. Issues related to human immunodeficiency virus transmission in schools, child care, medical settings, the home, and community. *Pediatrics* 104:318-24.
2. California Child Care Health Program. 2009. Illness fact sheet: HIV/AIDS. http://www.ucsfchildcarehealth.org/pdfs/illnesses/HIV_0509.pdf.

STANDARD 7.6.3.2: Protecting HIV-Infected Children and Adults in Child Care

Parents/guardians of all children, including children infected with HIV, should be notified immediately if the child has been exposed to chickenpox, tuberculosis, fifth disease (parvovirus B19), diarrheal disease, measles, or other infectious diseases through contact with other children in the facility. In particular, immune-compromised children who are exposed to measles or chickenpox should be referred immediately to their primary care provider to receive the appropriate preventive measure (immune globulin or immunization) following exposure and decision about readmission to the child care facility (1). Information regarding a child whose immune system does not function properly to prevent infection, whatever the cause, should be available to caregivers/teachers who need to know so they can reduce the likelihood of transmission of infection to the child. Accordingly, infections in other children and staff members in the facility should be brought to the prompt attention of the parent/guardian of the child whose immune system does not function properly. The parent/guardian may elect to seek medical advice regarding the child's continued participation in the facility. Injuries that lead to bleeding by a child with HIV should be handled promptly using Standard Precau-

tions in the manner recommended for any such injury to any child.

RATIONALE: The immune system of children and adults who are infected with HIV often does not function properly to prevent infections. Children and adults with immunosuppression for multiple other reasons are at greater risk for severe complications from several infections including chickenpox, cytomegalovirus (CMV), tuberculosis, *Cryptosporidium*, *Salmonella*, and measles virus (1,2). Available data indicate that infection with measles is a more serious illness in HIV-infected children than in children who are not HIV-infected. The first deaths from measles in the United States reported to the Centers for Disease Control and Prevention (CDC) after 1985 were in HIV-infected children.

Caregivers/teachers should know about a child's special health care needs so they can offer protection for that child. Standard Precautions should be adopted in caring for all adults and all children in out-of-home child care when blood or blood-containing body fluids are handled, to minimize the possibility of transmission of any bloodborne disease.

COMMENTS: Staff should have training on Standard Precautions for bloodborne pathogens, HIV and other causes of immune deficiency, confidentiality, and implications of suspicions about HIV status. Annual training on use of Standard Precautions and periodic staff monitoring may increase compliance and staff knowledge of this policy.

All caregivers/teachers should be taught the basic principles of individuals' rights to confidentiality.

For additional information regarding HIV, consult the current edition of the *Red Book* from the American Academy of Pediatrics (AAP).

TYPE OF FACILITY: Center; Large Family Child Care Home; Small Family Child Care Home

RELATED STANDARDS:
Standard 3.2.3.4: Prevention of Exposure to Blood and Body Fluids
Standards 9.4.1.3-9.4.1.6: Confidentiality and Access to Records

REFERENCES:
1. Centers for Disease Control and Prevention. 2009. Guidelines for prevention and treatment of opportunistic infections in HIV-infected adults and adolescents. *MMWR* 58 (RR04). http://www.cdc.gov/mmwr/pdf/rr/rr5804.pdf.
2. Centers for Disease Control and Prevention. 2009. Guidelines for the prevention and treatment of opportunistic infections among HIV-exposed and HIV-infected children. *MMWR* 58 (RR11). http://www.cdc.gov/mmwr/preview/mmwrhtml/rr5811a1.htm.

STANDARD 7.6.3.3: Staff Education About Preventing Transmission of HIV Infection

Caregivers/teachers should be knowledgeable about routes of transmission and about prevention of transmission of bloodborne pathogens, including HIV, and should practice measures recommended by the U.S. Public Health Service for prevention of transmission of these infections.

RATIONALE: Unwarranted fear about HIV transmission in child care should be dispelled. Studies examining transmission of HIV support the concept that HIV is not a highly infectious agent (1). The major routes of transmission are through sexual contact, through contact with blood or body fluids containing blood, and from mother to child during the birth process. Several studies have shown that HIV-infected people do not spread the HIV virus to other members of their households except through sexual contact.

HIV has been isolated in low volumes in saliva, urine, and human milk. Transmission of HIV through saliva does not occur. Cases suggest that contact with blood from an HIV-infected person is a possible mode of transmission through contact between broken skin and blood or blood-containing fluids. Theoretically, biting is a possible mode of transmission of bloodborne illness, such as HIV infection. However, the risk of such transmission is rare. If a bite results in blood exposure to either person involved, the U.S. Public Health Service recommends post-exposure follow-up, including consideration of post-exposure prophylaxis (2). Due to risks of disease transmission, as a part of Standard Precautions, no food should be given to a child (or adult) that initially was in the mouth (or pre-chewed) by someone else.

COMMENTS: For additional information regarding HIV, consult the current edition of the *Red Book* from the American Academy of Pediatrics (AAP).

TYPE OF FACILITY: Center; Large Family Child Care Home; Small Family Child Care Home

RELATED STANDARDS:
Standard 3.2.3.4: Prevention of Exposure to Blood and Body Fluids

REFERENCES:
1. Tokars, J. L., R. Marcus, D. H. Culver, et al. 1993. Surveillance of HIV infection and Zidovudine use among healthcare workers after occupational exposure to HIV-infected blood. *Ann Intern Med* 118:913-19.
2. Havens, P. L., L. M. Mofenson. 2009. Evaluation of management of the infant exposed to HIV in the U.S. *Pediatrics* 123:175-87.

STANDARD 7.6.3.4: Ability of Caregivers/ Teachers with HIV Infection to Care for Children

HIV-infected adults who do not have open and uncoverable skin lesions, other conditions that would result in contact with their body fluids, or a transmissible infectious disease may care for children in child care programs. However, immunosuppressed adults with HIV infection may be at increased risk of acquiring infectious agents from children and should consult their primary care provider about the safety of continuing to work in child care. All caregivers/teachers, especially caregivers/teachers known to be HIV-infected, should be notified immediately if they may have been exposed to varicella, fifth disease (parvovirus B19), tuberculosis, diarrheal disease, measles, or other infectious diseases through contact with children or other adults in the facility, in order to obtain appropriate therapy (1).

RATIONALE: Based on available data, there is no reason to believe that HIV-infected adults will transmit HIV in the course of their normal child care duties. Therefore, HIV-infected adults who do not: a) have open skin sores that cannot be covered, b) other conditions that would allow contact with their body fluids, or c) a transmissible infectious disease, may care for children in facilities. Immunosuppressed adults with acquired immunodeficiency syndrome (AIDS) may be more likely to acquire infectious agents from children and should consult with their own primary care providers regarding the advisability of their continuing to work in a facility.

COMMENTS: For additional information regarding HIV, consult the current edition of the *Red Book* from the American Academy of Pediatrics (AAP).

TYPE OF FACILITY: Center; Large Family Child Care Home; Small Family Child Care Home

RELATED STANDARDS:

Standard 3.2.3.4: Prevention of Exposure to Blood and Body Fluids

REFERENCES:

1. Centers for Disease Control and Prevention. 2009. Guidelines for prevention and treatment of opportunistic infections in HIV-infected adults and adolescents. *MMWR* 58 (RR04). http://www.cdc.gov/mmwr/pdf/rr/rr5804.pdf.

7.7 Herpes Viruses

7.7.1 Cytomegalovirus (CMV)

STANDARD 7.7.1.1: Staff Education and Policies on Cytomegalovirus (CMV)

Facilities that employ women of childbearing age should provide information to employees providing care to infants and children with regard to the following:

a) The increased probability of exposure to cytomegalovirus (CMV) in the child care setting;
b) The potential for fetal damage when CMV is acquired during pregnancy;
c) Hygiene measures (especially handwashing and avoiding contact with urine, saliva, and nasal secretions) aimed at reducing acquisition of CMV;
d) The availability of counseling and testing for serum antibody to CMV to determine the caregiver/teacher's immune status.

Female employees of childbearing age should be referred to their primary care provider or to the health department authority for counseling about their risk of CMV infection. This counseling may include testing for serum antibodies to CMV to determine the employee's immunity against CMV infection.

Staff should be advised not to kiss children on the lips or allow children to put their fingers or hands in another person's mouth. Additionally, since saliva can transmit CMV, cups or eating utensils should not be shared.

RATIONALE: CMV is the leading cause of congenital infection in the United States, with approximately 1% of live born infants infected prenatally (1). While most infected fetuses escape resulting illness or disability, 10% to 20% will have hearing loss, developmental delay, cerebral palsy, or vision disturbances. Although maternal immunity does not prevent congenital CMV infection, evidence indicates that acquisition of CMV during pregnancy (primary maternal infection) carries the greatest risk for resulting illness or disability of the fetus (1).

Children enrolled in child care facilities are more likely to acquire CMV than are children cared for at home. Epidemiologic data, as well as laboratory testing of viral strains, has provided evidence for child-to-child transmission of CMV in the child care setting (1). Rates of CMV excretion vary among facilities and between class groups within a facility. Children between one and three years of age have the highest rates of excretion; published studies report excretion rates between 20% and 80%. Many children excrete CMV asymptomatically and intermittently for years.

With regard to child-to-staff transmission, studies have shown increased rates of infection with CMV in caregivers/teachers ranging from 14% to 20% (1). The increased risk for exposure to CMV and high rates of acquisition of CMV in caregivers/teachers could lead to increased rates of congenital CMV infection in CMV-naive women. Pregnant women who have antibodies to CMV prior to pregnancy (previously infected with CMV) have a low risk of having an infant with a symptomatic congenital CMV infection (1). Prevention of CMV transmission with meticulous hand hygiene reduces transmission of CMV and therefore reduces rates of infection. With current knowledge on the risk of CMV infection in child care staff members and the potential consequences of gestational CMV infection, child care staff members should receive counseling in regard to the risks of acquiring CMV.

Epidemiologic data and study of CMV strains have shown that premature newborn infants who acquire CMV from other children in the nursery can transmit the virus to their parents/guardians. Moreover, parents/guardians of children who attend group child care centers have a higher rate of development of antibodies to CMV than parents/guardians with children not enrolled in group child care (1).

COMMENTS: Assays for measuring antibody to CMV are available commercially and seem to perform well when used by qualified laboratories. They are accepted for screening blood products, transfusion recipients, and organ donors and recipients.

For additional information regarding CMV, consult the CMV chapter in the current edition of the *Red Book* from the American Academy of Pediatrics (AAP).

TYPE OF FACILITY: Center; Large Family Child Care Home; Small Family Child Care Home

REFERENCES:

1. Pass, R. F. 2008. Cytomegalovirus. In *Principles and practices of pediatric infectious diseases,* eds. S. S. Long, L. K. Pickering, C. G. Prober. 3rd ed. Philadelphia: Churchill Livingstone.

STANDARD 7.7.1.2: Testing of Children with Cytomegalovirus (CMV)

Testing children to detect cytomegalovirus (CMV) excretion or excluding children known to be CMV-infected is not recommended since all infants and toddlers should be assumed to excrete CMV in their urine and saliva. Therefore, appropriate hand hygiene practices should be reinforced.

RATIONALE: Testing of urine and saliva for CMV excretion in children is expensive and is likely to be misleading, since excretion of CMV by children in child care is intermittent and common (1).

COMMENTS: For additional information regarding CMV, consult the CMV chapter in the current edition of the *Red Book* from the American Academy of Pediatrics (AAP).

TYPE OF FACILITY: Center; Large Family Child Care Home; Small Family Child Care Home

REFERENCES:

1. Pass, R. F. 2008. Cytomegalovirus. In *Principles and practices of pediatric infectious diseases,* eds. S. S. Long, L. K. Pickering, C. G. Prober. 3rd ed. Philadelphia: Churchill Livingstone.

7.7.2 Herpes Simplex

STANDARD 7.7.2.1: Disease Recognition and Control of Herpes Simplex Virus

Children with herpetic gingivostomatitis, an infection of the mouth caused by the herpes simplex virus, who do not have control of oral secretions, should be excluded from child care. In selected situations, children with mild disease who are in control of their oral secretions may not need to be excluded. The facility's child care health consultant or health department officials should be consulted.

Caregivers/teachers with herpetic gingivostomatitis, cold sores, or herpes labialis should do the following:

a) Refrain from kissing and nuzzling children;
b) Refrain from sharing food and drinks with children and other caregivers;
c) Avoid touching the lesions;
d) Wash their hands frequently;
e) Cover any skin lesion with a bandage, clothing, or an appropriate dressing if practical.

Caregivers/teachers should be instructed in the importance of and technique for hand hygiene and other measures aimed at limiting transfer of infected material, such as saliva, tissue fluid, or fluid from a skin sore.

Caregivers/teachers who work in a child care program with young infants should avoid caring for infants including neonates when the caregiver has an active "fever blister" on their lips.

RATIONALE: Initial herpes simplex virus disease in children often produces a sudden illness of short duration characterized by fever and sores around and within the mouth. Illness and viral excretion may persist for a week or more. Multiple, painful sores in the mouth and throat may prevent oral intake and necessitate hospitalization for hydration (1). Recurrent oral herpes is manifested as small, fluid-filled blisters on the lips and entails a much shorter period of virus shedding from sores. Adults and children also can shed the virus in oral secretions in the absence of identifiable sores.

Although the risk of transmission of herpes simplex virus in the child care setting has not been documented, spread of infection within families has been reported and is thought to require direct contact with infected secretions (1). Transmission of herpes simplex in child care is uncommon (2). However, neonates are at the highest risk for disseminated disease.

For additional information regarding herpes simplex, consult the herpes simplex chapter in the current edition of the *Red Book* from the American Academy of Pediatrics (AAP).

TYPE OF FACILITY: Center; Large Family Child Care Home; Small Family Child Care Home

RELATED STANDARDS:
Standards 3.2.1.1-3.2.3.4: Hygiene
Standards 3.6.1.1-3.6.1.4: Child and Staff Inclusion/Exclusion/Dismissal

REFERENCES:

1. Prober, C. G. 2008. Herpes simplex virus. In *Principles and practice of pediatric infectious diseases,* eds. S. S. Long, L. K. Pickering, C. G. Prober. 3rd ed. Philadelphia: Churchill Livingstone.
2. Schmitt, D. L., D. W. Johnson, F. W. Henderson. 1991. Herpes simplex type I infections in group care. *Pediatr Infect Dis J* 10:729-34.

7.7.3 Herpes Virus 6 and 7 (Roseola)

STANDARD 7.7.3.1: Roseola

Children with roseola (exanthema subitum) or clinical evidence of infection with human herpes virus 6 or 7 need not be excluded from child care as long as they are able to participate in normal activities comfortably and staff finds they can care for the child without jeopardizing the health or safety of other children.

RATIONALE: Roseola is a viral disease caused by human herpes virus 6 or 7 (HHV6, HHV7) that causes fever for three to seven days and then, as the fever disappears, a red, raised rash appears often on the trunk with spread to the face and extremities. A seizure may occur as a CNS (central nervous system) manifestation in patients with primary infection. Almost all children have been infected with HHV6 by two years of age. The virus is transmitted to children from healthy adults via saliva. The incubation period is reported to be nine to ten days, so a child may expose others at home and in child care before becoming ill. No antiviral therapy is recommended in otherwise healthy children. The virus, like other herpes viruses, can become latent in the body (virus DNA persists in some cells, including salivary glands) (1).

COMMENTS: Once the rash appears, the child is usually felling better.

TYPE OF FACILITY: Center; Large Family Child Care Home; Small Family Child Care Home

REFERENCES:

1. Hall, C. B. 2008. Human herpes viruses 6 and 7 (roseola, exanthem subitum). In *Principles and practices of pediatric infectious diseases,* eds. S. S. Long, L. K. Pickering, C. G. Prober. 3rd ed. Philadelphia: Churchill Livingstone.

7.7.4 Varicella-Zoster (Chickenpox) Virus

STANDARD 7.7.4.1: Staff and Parent/Guardian Notification About Varicella-Zoster (Chickenpox) Virus

The child care facility should notify all staff members and parents/guardians when a case of chickenpox occurs, informing them of the greater likelihood of serious infection in susceptible adults, the potential for fetal damage if infection occurs during pregnancy, and the risk of severe varicella in children or adults with impaired immunity for any reason including HIV infection, steroid use, cancer chemotherapy, or organ transplantation (1).

RATIONALE: Prior to introduction of varicella vaccine, about 5% to 10% of adults were susceptible to varicella-zoster virus. Within twenty-four hours after exposure is recognized, susceptible child care staff members who are pregnant and are exposed to children with chickenpox should be referred to health care professionals who are knowledgeable in the area of varicella infection during pregnancy. The Centers for Disease Control and Prevention (CDC) and the American Academy of Pediatrics (AAP) recommend use of varicella vaccine in non-pregnant susceptible people twelve months of age and older within three days but up to five days after exposure to varicella. When indicated, VariZIG, an immune globulin preparation, or intravenous immune globulin (IGIV) also can be administered following exposure (1).

COMMENTS: Outbreaks of varicella in child care have decreased since institution of the two dose varicella recommendations (2).

Sample letters of notification to parents/guardians that their child may have been exposed to an infectious disease are contained in the publication of the American Academy of Pediatrics (AAP), *Managing Infectious Diseases in Child Care and Schools, 2nd Ed*. For additional information regarding varicella, consult the current edition of the *Red Book,* also from the AAP.

TYPE OF FACILITY: Center; Large Family Child Care Home; Small Family Child Care Home

RELATED STANDARDS:
Section 2.4: Health Education

REFERENCES:

1. Centers for Disease Control and Prevention. 2007. Prevention of varicella: Recommendations of the Advisory Committee on Immunization Practices. *MMWR* 56 (RR04). http://www.cdc.gov/mmwr/preview/mmwrhtml/rr5604a1.htm.
2. Lopez, A. S., M. Marin. 2008. *Strategies for the control and investigation of a varicella outbreaks 2008*. Atlanta: Centers for Disease Control and Prevention, National Center for Immunization and Respiratory Diseases. http://www.cdc.gov/vaccines/vpd-vac/varicella/outbreaks/downloads/manual.pdf.

STANDARD 7.7.4.2: Exclusion of Children with Varicella-Zoster (Chickenpox) Virus

Children who develop chickenpox should be excluded until all sores have dried and crusted (usually six days). The need for excluding an infected person should be decided based on the recommendations of the person's primary care provider. If a conflict or question about return to the child care facility arises, the facility should consult their child care health consultant or personnel at the health department. Until the conflict is resolved, readmission should be delayed.

Varicella-zoster virus is the cause of shingles as well as of chickenpox. Staff members or children with shingles (herpes zoster) should keep sores covered by clothing or a dressing until sores have crusted. With shingles, the virus is present in small, fluid-filled blisters, and is spread by direct contact. Sores that are covered seem to pose little risk to susceptible persons. Older children and staff members with herpes zoster should be instructed to wash their hands if they touch potentially infectious lesions. If a child or staff member has zoster lesions which cannot be covered, they should be excluded until the lesions are crusted and the person is able to function normally and return.

RATIONALE: Exclusion of children infected with varicella-zoster virus may not control illness in child care, but exclusion may help control disease caused by this virus in some people (such as adults, children and adults who have a compromised immune system, and newborn infants). Children should receive two doses of a varicella containing vaccine, the first at twelve through fifteen months of age and the second at four through six years of age. The second dose may be given as early as three months after the first. If the second dose is given one month after the first, it should not be repeated.

Person-to-person transmission of this highly contagious virus occurs by direct contact with vesicular fluid from patients with varicella or by airborne spread from respiratory tract secretions. Patients are most contagious from one to two days before to shortly after onset of the rash. Contagiousness persists until crusting of all lesions.

Prior to introduction of varicella vaccine, about 5% to 10% of adults were susceptible to varicella-zoster virus. All adults without evidence of immunity to varicella should receive two doses of single-antigen varicella vaccine if not previously vaccinated or the second dose if they have received only one dose, unless they have a medical contraindication. Special consideration should be given to those who 1) have close contact with persons at high risk for severe disease (e.g., health care personnel and family contacts of people with immunocompromising conditions) or 2) are at high risk for exposure or transmission (e.g., teachers; child care employees; residents and staff members of institutional settings, including correctional institutions; college students; military personnel; adolescents and adults living in house-

holds with children; nonpregnant women of childbearing age; and international travelers).

Evidence of immunity to varicella in adults includes any of the following:

a) Documentation of two doses of varicella vaccine at least four weeks apart;
b) U.S.-born before 1980 (although for health care personnel and pregnant women, birth before 1980 should not be considered evidence of immunity);
c) History of varicella based on diagnosis or verification of varicella by a health care professional (for a patient reporting a history of or presenting with an atypical case, a mild case, or both, health care professionals should seek either an epidemiologic link to a typical varicella case or to a laboratory-confirmed case or evidence of laboratory confirmation, if performed at the time of acute disease);
d) History of herpes zoster based on health care professional diagnosis or verification of herpes zoster by a health care professional;
e) Laboratory evidence of immunity or laboratory confirmation of disease.

Pregnant women not previously immunized for varicella should be assessed for evidence of varicella immunity. Women who do not have evidence of immunity should receive the first dose of varicella vaccine upon completion or termination of pregnancy and before discharge from the health care facility. The second dose should be administered at a minimum of four weeks after the first dose. Susceptible child care staff members who are pregnant and are exposed to children with chickenpox should be referred to their primary care professional or other health care professionals who are knowledgeable in the area of varicella infection during pregnancy within twenty-four hours after the exposure is recognized.

COMMENTS: Initial viral infection with varicella-zoster virus produces an acute fever and the appearance of chickenpox blisters; reactivation of the virus results in shingles (herpes zoster).

Routine use of varicella vaccine as recommended by the American Academy of Pediatrics (AAP) and the Centers for Disease Control and Prevention (CDC) will reduce the likelihood of transmission of wild type strains of varicella virus (1,2). A zoster vaccine is available for people sixty years of age and older (3).

In mild cases with only a few sores and rapid recovery, an otherwise healthy child may be able to return to child care sooner once the lesions are crusted. Children whose immune system does not function properly and children with more severe cases of chickenpox should be excluded from child care until lesions are crusted.

For additional information regarding varicella, consult the current edition of the *Red Book* from the AAP.

TYPE OF FACILITY: Center; Large Family Child Care Home; Small Family Child Care Home

RELATED STANDARDS:
Section 2.4: Health Education
Standards 3.6.1.1-3.6.1.4: Child and Staff Inclusion/Exclusion/Dismissal
Standard 3.6.2.1: Exclusion and Alternative Care for Children Who are Ill

REFERENCES:

1. Centers for Disease Control and Prevention. 2007. Prevention of varicella: Recommendations of the Advisory Committee on Immunization Practices. *MMWR* 56 (RR04). http://www.cdc.gov/mmwr/preview/mmwrhtml/rr5604a1.htm.
2. American Academy of Pediatrics, Committee on Infectious Disease. 2007. Prevention of varicella: Recommendations for use of varicella vaccines in children, including a recommendation for a routine 2-dose varicella immunization schedule. *Pediatrics* 120:221-31.
3. Centers for Disease Control and Prevention. 2008. Prevention of herpes zoster: Recommendations of the Advisory Committee on Immunization Practices. *MMWR* 57 (RR05). http://www.cdc.gov/mmwr/pdf/rr/rr5705.pdf.

7.8 Interaction with State or Local Health Departments

Prompt reporting of infectious diseases is the foundation of public health surveillance and disease control. Diseases that are reportable in the United States at a national level are included weekly in *Morbidity and Mortality Weekly Report* (http://www.cdc.gov/mmwr/), and are summarized annually by Centers for Disease Control and Prevention (CDC) in the "Summary of Notifiable Diseases in the United States." Infectious disease reporting is regulated by individual states. Although details may differ from state to state, every state has regulations mandating that specified diseases or conditions be reported to local or state public health agencies. In general, selected infections with high mortality or large public health implications (such as meningococcal infections, measles, or smallpox) must be reported immediately; other infections (such as pertussis, varicella, or invasive group A streptococcal [GAS] infection) may in some cases be reported in a slightly less emergent fashion (e.g., one to two business days). If child care staff have any question regarding a potentially infectious illness among attendees or staff members, they should consult their local or state public health agency immediately for guidance. Child care health consultants are also very helpful. Caregivers/teachers should understand which infections are reported to local boards of health and which are reported directly to the state health department. For details about regulations for individual states, refer to local and state public health agencies.

7.9 Note to Reader on Judicious Use of Antibiotics

The spread of antimicrobial resistance is an issue of concern to patients and parents/guardians as well as to health care professionals. Children treated with antibiotics are at increased risk of becoming carriers of resistant bacteria. If

they develop an illness from resistant bacteria, they may be more difficult to treat and may be likely to fail standard antimicrobial therapy (1,2). While antibiotic therapy for a diagnosis of pharyngitis due to group A streptococci is indicated, for some conditions such as otitis media, antibiotic therapy is only occasionally recommended. For other conditions such as the common cold and nonspecific cough illness/bronchitis, antibiotic therapy is not indicated. Principles of judicious use of antimicrobial agents with detailed supporting evidence were published by the American Academy of Pediatrics (AAP), the American Academy of Family Practice (AAFP), and the Centers for Disease Control and Prevention (CDC) to identify areas where antimicrobial therapy might be curtailed without compromising patient care (1).

REFERENCES:

1. Dowell, S. F., S. M. Marcy, W. R. Phillips, et al. 1998. Principles of judicious use of antimicrobial agents for pediatric upper respiratory tract infections. *Pediatrics* 101:163-65.

2. Centers for Disease Control and Prevention. Get smart: Know when antibiotics work. http://www.cdc.gov/getsmart/.

Chapter 8

8

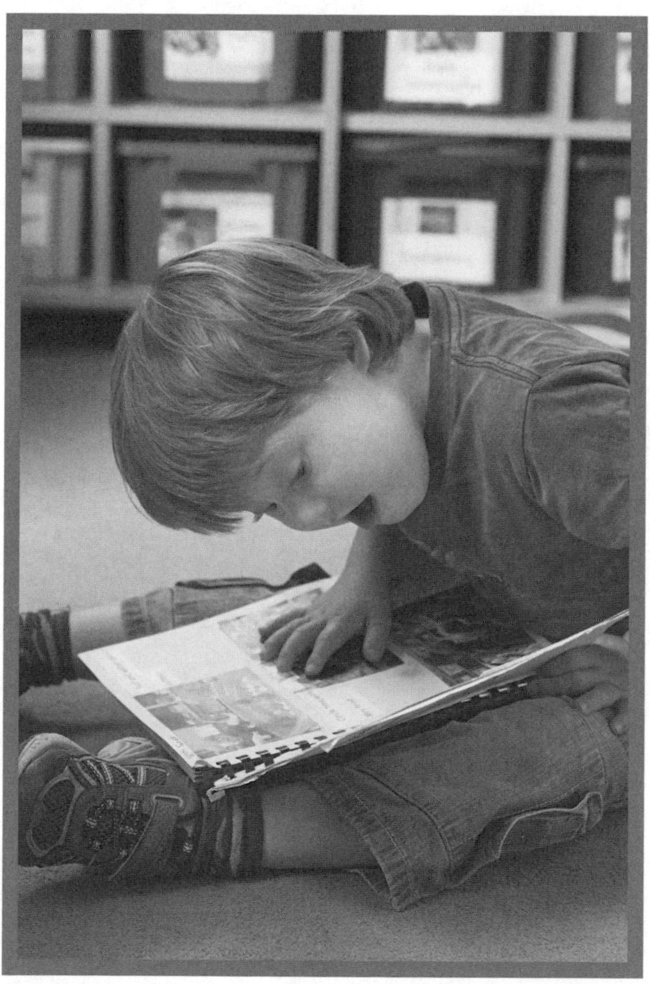

Children with Special Health Care Needs and Disabilities

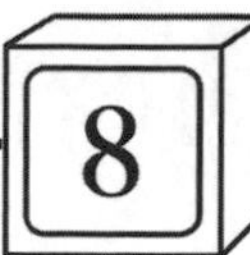

8.1 Guiding Principles for This Chapter and Introduction

The information in Chapter 8 is provided to acquaint caregivers/teachers with the care and services required and the types of programs available for both children with special health care needs as well as children with disabilities who are eligible for services under the Individuals with Disabilities Education Improvement Act (IDEA), a federal law most recently amended in 2004 (1). It also identifies what roles the caregiver/teacher has in helping these children to achieve full inclusion in the child care facility and in providing optimal developmental opportunities for children who are receiving services under IDEA. Because Chapter 8 focuses in part on children who are eligible for services under IDEA, a federal law, the reader is encouraged to review relevant state statutes and regulations which implement this statutory framework in your state, as well as state and county agency policies concerning the management of specific situations or diseases. This publication primarily focuses on national standards.

The content of this chapter was prepared with the guidance of five principles:

1) Standards that are relevant to children with special health care needs, as well as to all children, are integrated into other chapters within this document. This does not diminish the importance of making sure that children with disabilities or chronic illnesses receive the special care that typically developing children would not require to participate fully in the child care service or program.

2) Standards for children with special health care needs have been integrated throughout this book with those for all other children so as to emphasize the need to promote an inclusionary approach. Standards in this chapter are primarily those that apply to the special service needs and planning mechanisms, including those addressed in IDEA, for a child whose needs differ from those of a typically developing child. Standards addressing health, safety, nutritional, and transportation issues for care of children with special health care needs are found in other chapters. See list on page 342.

3) This chapter includes standards that enable accommodation and full inclusion of children with disabilities and special health care needs in child care facilities to achieve a level of participation as close as possible to that of typically developing children. The content of these standards will not segregate or discriminate against participation of children with disabilities and/or special health care needs, but specify the practices needed to ensure that the child with a disability or chronic illness has full, safe inclusion in the child care program.

4) To assure confidentiality and maximum family input, consent from a parent/guardian is required to obtain information about a child's special health care needs from other service providers or to share information obtained by the caregiver/teacher. However, with parent/guardian consent, the caregiver/teacher should have available important information relevant to meeting the health and safety needs of the child in the child care setting.

5) It is important that all children, especially those with special health care needs, receive their medical care in a family-centered, community-oriented health care practice, identified as a medical home. The medical home team should collaborate with other care providers, including the child care facility, in order to assure that the care for the child with special health care needs is coordinated and appropriately implemented.

Serving Children with Special Health Care Needs and Disabilities Including Children Eligible Under IDEA

The Individuals with Disabilities Education Act (IDEA), a federal law most recently amended in 2004 (1), affords caregivers/teachers a unique opportunity to support children with disabilities that might affect their educational success and to improve services for both the children and families in the child care setting. The purpose of the law is to provide "free appropriate public education" for all "eligible" children, from birth to twenty-one years, in a natural or least restrictive environment. Eligible children under IDEA include those with developmental delays or those with physical or mental conditions that may result in a developmental delay. Part B, Section 619 of this statute supports the needs of eligible preschool-age children through the local school district. Part C provides for a comprehensive system to serve the needs of eligible infants and toddlers between the ages of birth and three years and their families. Child care programs can play a significant role in supporting the developmental needs of children with special health care needs and disabilities in the child care setting.

Historical Information

The original statute of IDEA, then titled The Education for All Handicapped Children Act (2), was passed in 1975 and initially covered only children aged five through twenty-one years. This law was amended in 1986 (3) to include preschool education services to children aged three through five and early intervention services for children from birth to age two. The preschool services are included in Part B of the act. The infant and toddler portion of the act, which was Part H when initially passed, is now Part C under the 1997 reauthorized version of the act. The law is now identified as the Individuals with Disabilities Education Act. Information about IDEA can be obtained from the Office of Special Education and Rehabilitative Services (OSERS), U.S. Department of Education.

Part C Supports Collaborative Efforts

Part C of IDEA makes federal funds available for states to implement a system of early intervention services for eligible infants and toddlers and their families using evidence-based practices. The governor of each state must designate a lead agency, such as education, health or another agency, to provide the assessment, coordination of services, and the administrative functions required under Part C. The intent of Part C is to enhance the development of, and to provide

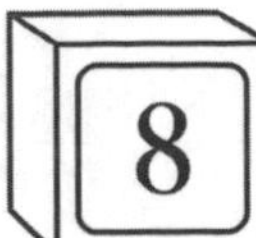

other needed services for, infants and toddlers who have developmental delays or are at risk of developing such delays and to support the capacity of families to enhance the development of their children in the home and community. A further intent is to transition children into effective and inclusionary school-age services.

Although each state must designate a lead agency for implementing this federally funded program, the program is designed to be a coordinated, collaborative effort among a variety of state agencies for screening of children, assessment, service coordination and development of an Individualized Family Service Plan (IFSP) for every eligible infant or toddler and his or her family. The IFSP describes early intervention services for an infant or toddler and the child's family, including family support and the child's educational, therapeutic, and health needs. A Service Coordinator should be appointed who is assigned to oversee the IFSP and assure that the recommended services are provided.

Among the more important aspects of this interagency model is the belief that children and their families should be viewed from the perspective of an ability model rather than a deficit model, i.e., emphasizing the strengths and capabilities of the family and child rather than the family's or child's perceived weaknesses. This means that the approach of the providers of services and supports identified in the IFSP should be that of enhancing and supporting already-existing resources, priorities, and concerns of the child and family rather than assuming that services can correct "deficiencies" of the child or family.

The focus of services and supports to the child and family under Part C is the achievement of two related goals:

a) To enhance and support the development of young children with disabilities and chronic illness and using developmentally appropriate practices, to minimize their future need for special education and related services when they enter the public school system.
b) To maximize the potential for infants and toddlers with disabilities and chronic illness to enjoy the benefits of their communities and grow into adults capable of living independently, pursuing vocations, and participating in the benefits their communities offer all citizens.

Serving Children in Natural Environments

Part C of the IDEA emphasizes the delivery of services in natural environments. These are defined generally as settings that are "natural or typical for the child's same-age peers who have no disabilities." Natural environments reflect those places that are routinely used by families and typically developing children and represent a wide variety of options such as the child's home, the neighborhood, community programs, and services such as child care centers, parks, recreation centers, stores, malls, museums, etc. By incorporating elements of the child's typical environment (e.g., furniture, toys, schedule, siblings, care providers, extended family, etc.) in the planning and delivery of services and supports, the family and caregivers/teachers can best discover the child's talents and gifts and enhance these in the normal course of routines, play relationships, and caregiving.

Learning about and understanding the child's routines and using real life opportunities and activities, such as eating, playing, interacting with others, and working on developmental skills, greatly enhances a child's ability to achieve the functional outcomes identified in the IFSP. For these reasons, it is critical to have a representative from the child care setting that the child attends or may attend at the table when the IFSP is developed or revised. The presence of the service coordinator is also essential. It is also imperative that written informed consent is obtained from parents/guardians before confidential information (written or verbal) is shared among caregivers/teachers. For these same reasons, it is very important that a caregiver/teacher become familiar with a child's IFSP and understand both the role the provider is to play and the resources available through the IFSP to support the family and caregiver/teacher.

Other federal legislation, such as the Americans with Disabilities Act (ADA) (4) and Section 504 of the Rehabilitation Act of 1973 (5), prohibit discrimination against children and adults with disabilities by requiring equal access to offered programs and services. Section 504 covers only those programs receiving federal dollars while ADA applies to public and private child care programs. The IDEA promotes inclusion of infants, toddlers, and preschoolers in the same activities as their peers by providing services within children's natural environments.

Part B - The Individualized Education Program

Three- through five-year-olds eligible for services under Part B Section 619 of the IDEA are served through a written Individualized Education Program (IEP). The IEP is also developed by a team, with the local education agency assuming responsibility for its implementation in either a public preschool program or a private preschool setting. Although federal funds are not specifically designated to support services provided by agencies outside of the public school system, local education agencies may contract with private providers for preschool services and cover educationally related services identified in the IEP, such as speech and language therapy, in the preschool setting. The IEP is often coordinated by a representative of a local school district with a team and leadership designated by the local educational authority.

Caregivers/teachers should become as familiar with a preschooler's special health care needs, as identified in the IEP, as they should with the services for an infant or toddler set forth in an IFSP. The caregiver/teacher may wish to send a representative, with prior informed written parental/guardian consent, to the child's IEP review meetings to share valuable insight and information regarding the child's special health care needs in both the educational and child care settings. Continued contact with the child's primary care provider or medical home is also desirable to assure coordinated care.

The standards in this chapter are intended to articulate those opportunities and responsibilities that child care agen-

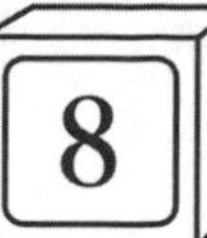

cies share with other agencies in serving a child with special health care needs, whether the child is served through an IFSP or an IEP.

8.2 Inclusion of Children with Special Needs in the Child Care Setting

STANDARD 8.2.0.1: Inclusion in All Activities

All children should be included in all activities possible unless a specific medical contraindication exists.

RATIONALE: The goal is to provide fully integrated care to the extent feasible given each child's limitations. Federal and state laws do not permit discrimination on the basis of the disability (i.e., Americans with Disabilities Act [ADA] and Section 504 of the Rehabilitation Act) (4,5).

Studies have found the following benefits of inclusive child care: Children with special needs develop increased social skills and self-esteem; families of children with special needs gain social support and develop more positive attitudes about their child; children and families without special needs become more understanding and accepting of differences and disabilities; caregivers/teachers learn from working with children, families, and service providers and develop skills in individualizing care for all children (6).

COMMENTS: Caregivers/teachers may need to seek professional guidance and obtain appropriate training in order to include children with special needs, such as children with severe disabilities and children with special health care needs such as chronic illnesses, into child care settings. These may include technology-dependent children and children with serious and severe chronic medical problems. The child care health consultant should be involved in the transition and enrollment process in order to support individual accommodations and the care of children with special health care needs. Every attempt should be made, however, to achieve inclusion if the parent/guardian so wishes.

The facility should pursue mechanisms available to supplement funding for services in the facility. These resources usually require the parents/guardians' consent and may require that the parents be actively involved in the pursuit for funding. Even so, caregivers/teachers can and should discuss options with the parents/guardian as potential sources of financial assistance for needed services. These sources might include:

a) Medicaid, including waiver funding (Title XIX);
b) Private health insurance;
c) State or federal funds for child care, education, or for Children with Special Health Care Needs (Title V);
d) IDEA (particularly Part C funding);
e) Community resources (e.g., volunteers, lending libraries, and free equipment available from community-based organizations);
f) Tax incentives (credits and deductions are available under federal law to most for-profit child care programs).

Section 504 is a civil rights law, and protects children from discrimination. It provides for supports and accommodations so a child can access the curriculum. In order to qualify for supports, a child must have a physical or mental impairment that substantially limits at least one major life activity such as walking, hearing, seeing, breathing, learning, reading, writing, etc. Section 504 requires an evaluation from multiple sources. There is no federally mandated plan, nor do parents/guardians have to be involved in the creation of the plan. We know from best practice, however, that parents/guardians should be active participants in plans to care for their children. Section 504 provides for accommodations during testing and for accessibility. It does not provide for the individual plans and protections that are provided under IDEA. For more information, go to http://www.wrightslaw.com.

Another resource for parents/guardians and caregivers/teachers are the Protection and Advocacy Centers funded by the federal government to protect rights of persons with disabilities.

TYPE OF FACILITY: Center; Large Family Child Care Home; Small Family Child Care Home

RELATED STANDARDS:
Standard 8.2.0.2: Planning for Inclusion

STANDARD 8.2.0.2: Planning for Inclusion

Inclusion and participation of children with special health care needs requires proactive planning. The facility must plan for the resources, support, and education necessary to increase the understanding and knowledge of staff, but also of parents/guardians, and the children without disabilities within the facility. Planning to include children with disabilities and with special health care needs requires time, resources, support and education. Every effort should be made to plan fully to include children with disabilities and children with special health care needs to maximize success. In planning for the inclusion of children with disabilities and children with special health care needs, safety considerations should be an additional factor considered.

RATIONALE: Inclusion without adequate preparation, understanding, training, mobilization of resources, and development of skills among all those involved, may lead to failure.

COMMENTS: Available resources include, but are not limited to: brochures, books, guest speakers, advice from parents/guardians of children with special health care needs, expert consultation from child care health consultants, and utilization of child care health consultants. Methods may vary according to need and availability and, specific to educating children without disabilities in the facility, using age-appropriate resources is particularly important. Communication between child care, parents/guardians, and primary care providers (with written parental/guardian permission) helps facilitate a smooth inclusion process. The facility should provide opportunities to discuss the similarities as well as the differences among all the children enrolled. Professionals or knowledgeable parents/guardians who facilitate such discussions should assure that caregivers and typically developing children in the facility receive presentations and participate in discussions about the special equipment that the children with special needs may require, and that they understand other differences, such as a prescribed diet or limitations of activity. Children without disabilities or special health care needs should be given the opportunity to explore and learn about these differences. Caregivers/teachers should take special care to demonstrate cultural competency, confidentiality, respect for privacy, and be generally sensitive in all communications with parents/guardians and when discussing the child and the family, particularly in discussion of an inherited condition.

TYPE OF FACILITY: Center; Large Family Child Care Home; Small Family Child Care Home

RELATED STANDARDS:
Standard 8.2.0.1: Inclusion in All Activities

8.3 Process Prior to Enrolling at a Facility

STANDARD 8.3.0.1: Initial Assessment of the Child to Determine His or Her Special Needs

Children with disabilities and children with special health care needs and their families and caregivers/teachers should have access to and be encouraged to receive a multidisciplinary, interdisciplinary, or transdisciplinary assessment by qualified health providers before the child starts in the facility. This information needs to be shared, with the parents/guardians' consent and agreement to disclose information if it is relevant to the health and safety concerns in the child care setting. If the parents/guardians consent to disclose the information and if the information is relevant to health and safety concerns in the child care setting, this evaluation should consist of the following:

a) A medical care plan developed by the child's primary care provider/medical home;
b) Results of medical and developmental examinations;
c) Assessments of the child's behavior, cognitive functioning, or current overall adaptive functioning;
d) Evaluations of the family's needs, cultural and linguistic differences, concerns, and priorities;
e) Other evaluations as needed.

The multidisciplinary, interdisciplinary, or transdisciplinary assessment should also consider a family's needs, cultural and linguistic differences, priorities, and resources as the team develops recommendations for interventions. Such recommendations should be focused on optimizing the child's development, health, and safety.

RATIONALE: The definitive characteristic of services for children and their families is the necessity of individualizing their care to meet their needs. Therefore, individual assessments must precede services.

The family's needs, values, and childrearing practices are highly relevant and respected in the provision of care to the child; however, the child's special needs continue to be the central focus of intervention.

COMMENTS: This comprehensive assessment would be done largely by an outside center, clinic, school district, or professionals who conduct evaluations of this nature. The multi-disciplinary, interdisciplinary or transdisciplinary assessment must be administered by qualified individuals using reliable and valid age and culturally and linguistically appropriate instruments and methodologies. For young children with disabilities, the designated lead agency for Part C would be responsible for conducting the initial evaluation. Under Part B (three- through five-year-olds), the school district is responsible for conducting the initial evaluation. This evaluation forms the basis of planning for the child's needs in the child care setting and for the pertinent information available to the staff. The comprehensive assessment should be used to develop a written plan for the child's caregivers/teachers that they believe they can implement. Relevant medical information will form the basis of the health care plan for the child in the program. This may need to be created with help of parents/guardians, child care health consultants, and medical providers.

The facility should pursue the many funding mechanisms available to supplement funding for services in the facility. Even so, caregivers/teachers can and should discuss these options with the parents/guardians as potential sources of financial assistance for the needed services. These sources might include:

a) Medicaid, including waiver funding (Title XIX);
b) Private health insurance and state-subsidized private health insurance under programs such as SCHIP;
c) State or federal funds for child care, education, or for Children with Special Health Care Needs (Title V);
d) Individuals with Disabilities Education Improvement Act (IDEA) (particularly Part C funding);
e) Tax incentives (credits and deductions are available under federal law to most for-profit child care programs).

TYPE OF FACILITY: Center; Large Family Child Care Home; Small Family Child Care Home

RELATED STANDARDS:
Standard 3.5.0.1: Care Plans for Children with Special Health Care Needs
Standard 10.3.4.6: Compensation for Participation in Multidisciplinary Assessments for Children with Special Health Care or Education Needs
Appendix O: Care Plan for Children with Special Health Care Needs

8.4 Developing a Service Plan for a Child with a Disability or a Child with Special Health Care Needs

STANDARD 8.4.0.1: Determining the Type and Frequency of Services

The parents/guardians of a child with a disability or a child with special health care needs, the child's primary care provider, any authorized service coordinator, any provider of intervention services, and the caregiver/teacher should discuss and determine the type and frequency of the services to be provided within the child care facility.

RATIONALE: To serve children with varying forms and severities of disabilities or special health care needs, caregivers/teachers should take a flexible approach to combine and deliver services. Parents/guardians must be involved to assure that the plan is compatible with their care and expectations for the child.

COMMENTS: In facilities that are not designed primarily to serve a population with disabilities or special health care needs, the additional therapeutic services may be obtained through consultants or arrangements with outside programs serving children with disabilities or children with special health care needs. These services may be available, as arranged, through the Individualized Family Service Plan (IFSP) or the Individualized Education Program (IEP) or through special health personnel such as RNs or LPNs under RN supervision. Most States have a case manager for Developmental Disabilities Services under a Medicaid Waiver for DD/MR children. The caregiver/teacher may become a member of the IFSP or IEP team if the parents/guardians of a child with disabilities so request.

When there is an IFSP, IDEA requires the appointment of an authorized service coordinator.

TYPE OF FACILITY: Center; Large Family Child Care Home; Small Family Child Care Home

RELATED STANDARDS:
Standard 3.5.0.1: Care Plans for Children with Special Health Care Needs
Standard 8.4.0.4: Designation and Role of Staff Person Responsible for Coordinating Care in the Child Care Facility

STANDARD 8.4.0.2: Formulation of an Action Plan

The formulation of a plan on how to best meet the child's needs should be based on the assessment process specified in Standards 8.3.0.1 and 8.4.0.1 and by the child's medical care plan which is created by the child's primary care provider in collaboration with the child care health consultant and family. Such a plan should be written, reviewed with the parents/guardians and should be maintained as part of each child's confidential record.

RATIONALE: The plan may be developed and implemented after the parents/guardians have discussed and approved it. The facility should keep the plan as a permanent part of the child's confidential record.

COMMENTS: All issues and questions should be dealt with during the discussion with families; consensus should be obtained and the plan written accordingly. Parents/guardians should provide written consent for the agreement to any plan before implementation for the child. Parents/guardians may revoke their consent at any time by written notice. This is standard procedure in the implementation of the Individuals with Disabilities Education Act (IDEA) for those child care programs involved with the Individualized Education Program (IEP) and the Individualized Family Service Plan (IFSP). All release of information must be in accordance with IDEA, as well as state regulations.

TYPE OF FACILITY: Center; Large Family Child Care Home; Small Family Child Care Home

RELATED STANDARDS:
Section 2.3: Parent/Guardian Relationships
Standard 3.5.0.1: Care Plans for Children with Special Health Care Needs
Standard 8.4.0.4: Designation and Role of Staff Person Responsible for Coordinating Care in the Child Care Facility
Appendix O: Care Plan for Children with Special Health Care Needs

STANDARD 8.4.0.3: Determination of Eligibility for Special Services

The Individualized Family Service Plan (IFSP) or Individualized Education Program (IEP) and any other plans for special services should be developed for children identified as eligible in collaboration with the family, representatives from disciplines and organizations involved with the child and family, the child's primary care provider, and the staff of the facility, depending on the family's wishes, the agency's resources, and state laws and regulations.

RATIONALE: For the IFSP, IEP, or any other needed or required special service plan to provide systematic guidance of the child's developmental achievement and to promote efficient service delivery, service providers from all of the involved disciplines/settings must be familiar with the overall multidisciplinary or interdisciplinary plans and work toward the same goals for the child. To be optimally effective, one comprehensive IFSP or IEP is developed and one service or care coordinator is designated to oversee implementation of the plan. If the parents/guardians choose to involve them, the caregivers/teachers should be partners in developing and implementing the IFSP or IEP to obtain the best possible evaluation and plan for the child with a disability within the child care facility.

COMMENTS: Development and implementation of the IFSP or IEP is a team effort. The various aspects of planning include the input of the child care program in which the child is enrolled in the evaluation for eligibility for Part B or C, the development of IFSP/IEP, and the child care program's role in implementation. Components of the IFSP or IEP may include elements developed to meet service needs developed elsewhere, when applicable in the child care setting.

TYPE OF FACILITY: Center; Large Family Child Care Home; Small Family Child Care Home

RELATED STANDARDS:
Standard 8.5.0.1: Coordinating and Documenting Services
Standards 10.3.4.5-10.3.4.6: Consultants and Technical Assistance for Children with Special Health Care Needs

STANDARD 8.4.0.4: Designation and Role of Staff Person Responsible for Coordinating Care in the Child Care Facility

If a child has an Individualized Education Program (IEP) or Individualized Family Service Plan (IFSP), or any plan for medical services, the child care facility should designate one person in the child care setting to be responsible for coordinating care within the facility and with any caregiver/teacher or coordinator in other service settings, in accordance with the written plan. The role of the designated person should include:

a) Documentation of coordination;
b) Written or electronic communication with other care or service providers for the child, including their medical home, to ensure a coordinated, coherent service plan;
c) Sharing information about the plan, staff conferences, written reports, consultations, and other services provided to the child and family (informed, written parental/guardian consent must be sought before sharing this confidential information);
d) Ensuring implementation of the components of the plan that is relevant to the facility.

When the evaluators who are to determine if the child has special health care needs or is eligible for services under the Individuals with Disabilities Education Improvement Act (IDEA) are not part of the child care staff, the lead agency should develop a formal mechanism for coordinating reevaluations and program revisions. The designated staff member from the facility should routinely be included in the evaluation process and team conferences. Any care plan should be updated whenever the child is hospitalized or has a significant change in therapy.

RATIONALE: One person being responsible for coordinating all elements of services avoids confusion and allows easier and more consistent communication with the family. When carrying out coordination duties, this person is called a child care coordinator or service coordinator. Each child should have a care coordinator/service coordinator assigned in the child care facility at the time the service plan is developed.

With more than half of all mothers in the workforce, caregivers other than the parents/guardians (such as teachers, grandparents, foster parents, or neighbors) frequently spend considerable time with the children. These caregivers/teachers need to know and understand the aims and goals of the service plan; otherwise, program approaches will not carry over into the home environment.

This requirement does not preclude outside agencies or caregivers/teachers from having their own care coordinator, service coordinator, or case manager. The intent is to ensure communication and coordination among all the child's sources of care, both in the facility and elsewhere in the community. The child's care coordinator or service coordinator does not have responsibility for directly implementing all program components but, rather, is accountable for checking to make sure the plans in the facility are being carried out, encouraging implementation of the service plan, and helping obtain or gain access to services.

A facility assuming responsibility for serving children with disabilities or children with special health care needs must develop mechanisms for identifying the needs of the children and families and obtaining appropriate services, whether or not those children have an IEP/IFSP. The child care coordinator will be responsible for coordination of health services with the program child care health consultant, as needed.

COMMENTS: Usually, the person who coordinates care or services within the child care facility will not be the person assigned to coordinate overall care or provide overall case management for the child and family. Nevertheless, the facility may assume both roles if the parents/guardians so request and state law permits. The components and the role may vary, and each facility will determine these components and roles, which may depend on the roles and responsibilities of the staff in the facility and the responsibilities assumed by the family and care providers in the community. The person who coordinates care or services within the child care facility may be the Health Advocate or someone else who is working closely with the child's family and the teaching staff in the facility.

TYPE OF FACILITY: Center; Large Family Child Care Home; Small Family Child Care Home

RELATED STANDARDS:
Standard 1.3.2.7: Qualifications and Responsibilities for Health Advocates
Standard 1.6.0.1: Child Care Health Consultants
Standards 10.3.4.5-10.3.4.6: Consultants and Technical Assistance for Children with Special Health Care Needs

STANDARD 8.4.0.5: Development of Measurable Objectives

The individualized service or treatment plan for a child with disabilities or a child with special health care needs should include services aimed at enhancing and improving the child's health and developmental functioning, based on measurable, functional outcomes agreed to by the parents/guardians. Each functional outcome objective should delineate the services, along with the designated responsibility for provision and financing. The development of the plan and its goals and objectives should not only include the child care agency staff, but all of the professionals, including various therapists and/or consultants, who will have the responsibility to assure its implementation.

With the assistance of the child's service coordinator, the caregiver/teacher should contribute to the assessment of measurable outcome objectives (service plan) within the child care setting at least every three months, or more often if the child's or family's circumstances change, and should contribute to a full, documented case review each year. Reevaluations should consider a self-assessment by the caregiver/teacher of the caregiver's competence to provide services that the child requires.

Service reviews should involve the child care staff or persons providing the intervention and supervision, the parents/guardians, and any independent observers. The results of such evaluations should be documented in a written plan given to each of the child's caregivers/teachers and the child's family. Such conferences and lists of participants should be documented in the child's health record at the facility.

Each objective should include persons responsible for its monitoring.

RATIONALE: When measurable-outcome objectives form the basis for the service plan, the family and service providers jointly formulate the expected and desired outcomes for the child and family. By using measurable-outcome objectives rather than service units, all interested parties can concentrate on how well the child is achieving the outcome objectives. Thus, for example, progress toward speech and language development assumes more importance than the number of hours of speech and language therapy provided.

Further, measurable outcome objectives constitute an individualized approach to meeting the needs of the child and family and, as such, can be integrated into, but are not solely dependent upon, the array of services available in a specific geographic area. The measurable-outcome objectives will provide the facility with a meaningful framework for enhancing the child's health and developmental status on an ongoing basis.

Regularly scheduled reassessments of the outcome objectives provide the family and service providers with a framework for anticipating changes in the kind of services that may be needed, the financial requirements for providing the services, and identification of the appropriate service provider. The changing needs of children with disabilities and/or special health care needs do not always follow a predictable course. Ad hoc reevaluations may be necessitated by changes in circumstances.

COMMENTS: The defining of measurable objectives provides a useful structure for the caregiver/teacher and aids in assessing the child's progress and the appropriateness of components of the service plan. Though this principle should apply to all children in all settings, implementation, especially in small and large family child care homes, will require ongoing assistance from and participation of specialists, including those connected with programs outside of the child care setting, to provide the needed services.

Many facilities that provide intervention services review the child's progress at least every three months. This is not a comprehensive review, but an interim analysis of the progress toward meeting objectives and to decide if any modifications are needed in the service plan and its implementation. Generally, the entire plan and the child's progress receive a comprehensive review annually. It is likely that caregivers/teachers will need training on development of goals and the means of assessing progress.

It is assumed that staff members who interact with the child will have the training described in Pre-service Qualifications and Special Training, Standards 1.3.1.1-1.3.3.1, and Training, Standards 1.4.2.1-1.4.6.2, which includes child growth and development. These topics are intended to extend caregivers'/teachers' basic knowledge and skills to help them work more effectively with children who have disabilities or children who have special health care needs and their families. Caregivers/teachers should have a basic knowledge of what constitutes a disability or special health care need, supplemented by specialized training for children with disabilities and children with special health care needs. The number of hours offered in any in-service training program should be determined by the experience and professional background of the staff.

Training and other technical assistance can be obtained from the following sources:

a) American Academy of Pediatrics (AAP);
b) American Nurses Association (ANA);
c) National Association for the Education of Young Children (NAEYC) and its local chapters;
d) National Association of Pediatric Nurse Practitioners (NAPNAP) Child Care Special Interest Group;
e) National Association of School Nurses (NASN);
f) State and community nursing associations;
g) National therapy associations (e.g., National Rehabilitation Association, Association for Behavioral and Cognitive Therapies);
h) National Association of Child Care Resource and Referral Agencies (NACCRRA) and its local resource and referral agencies;
i) Federally funded University Centers for Excellence in Developmental Disabilities Education, Research, and Service (UCEDD);
j) Local children's hospitals;
k) Other colleges and universities with expertise in training people to work with children who have special needs;
l) Community-based organizations serving people with disabilities and/or special health care needs (e.g., Autism Society of America, United Cerebral Palsy Associations, The ARC, Easter Seals, American Diabetes Association, American Lung Association, Epilepsy Foundation, etc.);
m) Zero to Three Policy Network.

The state-designated lead agency responsible for implementing IDEA may provide additional help. If the child has an IFSP, the lead agency will be responsible for coordinating the review process. If the child has an IEP, the local education agency will be responsible for seeing that the review occurs. If not, a less formal evaluation process may need to be conducted.

Assessments may be the financial responsibility of the IDEA Part C State-designated lead agency or other organizations

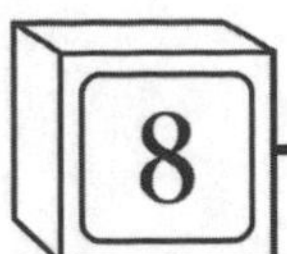

(see Standard 8.4.0.6). Funding available through implementation of IDEA Part C should provide resources to assist in implementing the IFSP.

TYPE OF FACILITY: Center; Large Family Child Care Home; Small Family Child Care Home

RELATED STANDARDS:
Section 1.3: Pre-service Qualifications
Section 1.4: Professional Development/Training
Standard 8.4.0.2: Formulation of an Action Plan
Standard 9.4.2.1: Contents of Child's Records
Standards 10.3.4.5-10.3.4.6: Consultants and Technical Assistance for Children with Special Health Care Needs

STANDARD 8.4.0.6: Contracts and Reimbursement

If a child with a disability and/or special health care needs has an Individualized Family Service Plan (IFSP), the lead agency may arrange and contract for specialized services to be conducted in the child care facility in addition to the child's home and other natural environments. If a child with disabilities or special health care needs has an Individualized Education Program (IEP), the local education agency may arrange and contract for specialized services to be conducted in the child care facility.

If the child or the specialized service or intervention is not covered by IEP/IFSP:

a) The caregiver/teacher should cover the cost when the service is reasonable and necessary for the child to participate in the program;
b) The parents/guardians or source arranged by the parents/guardians should cover the cost when the service is not a reasonable expectation of the caregiver/teacher or if it is provided while the child is in child care only for convenience and is separately billable (such as speech and language therapy).

RATIONALE: Child care facilities may have to collaborate with other service providers to meet the needs of a child and family, particularly if the number of children who require these services is too few to maintain the service onsite. To achieve maximum benefit from services, those services should be provided in the setting that is the most natural and convenient for the child and family. Whenever possible, treatment specialists (therapists) should provide these services in the facility where the child receives daytime care.

"Reasonableness" is a legal standard that looks at the impact of cost and other factors.

COMMENTS: The agency that has evaluated the child and/or is planning the entire service plan, or the facility, should make the arrangements. The specific methods by which these services will be coordinated with the child care facility is determined locally.

The facility should pursue the many funding mechanisms available to supplement funding for services in the facility. Even so, caregivers/teachers can and should discuss these options with the parents/guardians as potential sources of financial assistance for the needed accommodations. These sources might include:

a) Medicaid, including waiver funding (Title XIX);
b) Private health insurance, publicly subsidized private health insurance such as under the state child health insurance program (SCHIP);
c) State or federal funds for child care, education, or for children with special health care needs (Title V);
d) Individuals with Disabilities Education Improvement Act (IDEA) (particularly Part C funding);
e) Community resources (such as volunteers, lending libraries, and free equipment available from community-based organizations);
f) Tax incentives (credit and deductions are available under federal law to most for profit child care programs);
g) Local Community Development Block Grants (CDBG) and other community development funding.

TYPE OF FACILITY: Center

RELATED STANDARDS:
Standards 10.3.4.5-10.3.4.6: Consultants and Technical Assistance for Children with Special Health Care Needs

8.5 Coordination and Documentation

STANDARD 8.5.0.1: Coordinating and Documenting Services

Services for all children should be coordinated in a systematic manner so the facility can document all of the services the child is receiving inside of the facility and is aware of the services the child is receiving outside of the facility. If the parents/guardians of a child with disabilities or a child with special health care needs so choose, the facility should be an integral component of the child's overall service plan.

RATIONALE: Coordination of individualized services is a fundamental component in implementing a plan for care of a child with special health care needs. This is particularly true of the need to coordinate the overall child care with specialized developmental services, therapies, and child care procedures in the facility.

COMMENTS: Children with Individualized Family Service Plans (IFSP) have a service coordinator; children with Individualized Education Programs (IEP) have a primary provider or other identified service coordinator. These are the contact persons within the local education agency or lead agency. This method of service coordination is consistent throughout all of the states under the Individuals with Disabilities Education Improvement Act (IDEA). Caregivers/teachers need to become informed of how this system works and what their responsibilities are.

TYPE OF FACILITY: Center; Large Family Child Care Home; Small Family Child Care Home

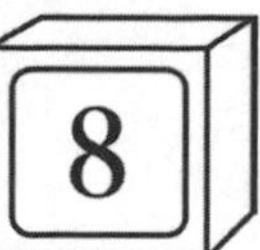

RELATED STANDARDS:
Standard 8.4.0.4: Designation and Role of Staff Person Responsible for Coordinating Care in the Child Care Facility

STANDARD 8.5.0.2: Written Reports on IFSPs/IEPs to Caregivers/Teachers

With the prior written, informed consent of the parents/guardians in the parents/guardians' native language, child care facilities may obtain written reports on Individualized Family Service Plans (IFSPs) or Individualized Education Programs (IEPs), conferences, and treatments provided.

RATIONALE: This information is confidential and parental/guardian consent for release is required if the child care facility is to gain access to it. Written documentation ensures better accountability.

TYPE OF FACILITY: Center; Large Family Child Care Home; Small Family Child Care Home

8.6 Periodic Reevaluation

STANDARD 8.6.0.1: Reevaluation Process

The facility care coordinator should ensure that formal reevaluations of the child's functioning and health care needs in the child care setting and the family's needs are conducted at least yearly, or as often as is necessary to deal with changes in the child's or family's circumstances. Medical care plans should be reviewed and revised if needed whenever there is a significant health event such as a hospitalization, or at least annually. This reevaluation should include the parents/guardians and caregiver/teacher. Such conferences and lists of participants should be documented in the child's health record at the facility.

RATIONALE: The changing needs of children with disabilities and children with special health care needs do not follow a predictable course. A periodic, thorough process of reevaluation is essential to identify appropriate goals and services for the child. The child's primary care provider or medical home and the program's child care health consultant should be involved in the development and reevaluation of the plan. A child's health is such an integral part of his or her availability to learn and to retain learned information that health- and development-related information is critical for a complete review/reevaluation process to occur.

COMMENTS: Though regular intervention services are recommended for review at three-month intervals, ad hoc reevaluations may be necessitated by changes in circumstances.

TYPE OF FACILITY: Center; Large Family Child Care Home; Small Family Child Care Home

RELATED STANDARDS:
Standard 8.4.0.5: Development of Measurable Objectives

STANDARD 8.6.0.2: Statement of Program Needs and Plans

Each reevaluation conference should result in a new statement of program needs and plans which parents/guardians have agreed to and support.

RATIONALE: Continued collaboration, participation, and coordination among all involved parties are essential.

TYPE OF FACILITY: Center; Large Family Child Care Home; Small Family Child Care Home

8.7 Assessment of Facilities for Children with Special Needs

STANDARD 8.7.0.1: Facility Self-Assessment

Facilities that serve children with special health care needs and children with disabilities eligible for services under IDEA should have a written self-assessment developed in consultation with an expert multi-disciplinary team of professionals experienced in the care and education of children with disabilities and children with special health care needs. These self-assessments should be used to create a plan for the facility to determine how it may become more accessible and ready to care for children with disabilities and children with special health care needs. The facility should review and update the plan at least every two years, unless a caregiver requests a revision at an earlier date.

RATIONALE: A self-assessment stimulates thought about the caregiver's/teacher's present capabilities and attitudes and the medical and educational particulars of a range of special health care needs and disabilities. Also, parents/guardians will have the opportunity to review the records of the written self-assessment and decide whether a facility is well-prepared to handle children with, for example, developmental delays, cognitive disabilities, or hearing impairment but is not able to offer proper care to a child with more complex medical needs.

COMMENTS: Under both the Americans with Disabilities Act (ADA) and Section 504 of the Rehabilitation Act of 1973, a program must make reasonable accommodations in order to serve a child with disabilities and/or special health care needs. Often, if architectural or other major changes are made to accommodate a particular child with physical or other disability, many other children and adults are helped by the changes. An important source of information for self-assessment is interviewing the parents/guardians of children with disabilities and/or special health care needs to see how well the program is working for their family and what could be improved. "Reasonableness" is a legal standard that looks at cost and other ADA criteria. Section 504 applies to recipients of federal funds. The ADA extends coverage to private entities that do not receive federal funds.

Parents/guardians have the right to choose which child care program will care for their child. Self-assessment should be done to evaluate what the program needs to do to be more inclusive by developing staff capability and program activities to accommodate the child's needs.

SpeciaLink: The National Centre for Child Care Inclusion, at the University of Winnipeg (http://www.specialinkcanada.org) has developed an inclusion scale much like ECERS to determine how well a program is providing inclusive care.

TYPE OF FACILITY: Center; Large Family Child Care Home; Small Family Child Care Home

STANDARD 8.7.0.2: Technical Assistance in Developing Plan

The caregiver/teacher should seek technical assistance in developing and formulating the plan for future services for children with special health care needs.

RATIONALE: Assistance is needed where caregivers/teachers lack specific capabilities.

COMMENTS: Documentation of the caregiver's/teacher's request and of the regulating agencies' responses in offering or providing assistance furnishes evidence of compliance. State regulatory agencies should be in a position to provide such assistance to facilities.

Training and other technical assistance sources can be obtained from or arranged by the following:

a) Child's primary care provider;
b) Program's child care health consultant;
c) Local children's hospital;
d) American Academy of Pediatrics (AAP);
e) National Association of Pediatric Nurse Practitioners (NAPNAP);
f) American Nurses Association (ANA);
g) National Association of School Nurses (NASN);
h) State and community nursing associations;
i) National therapy associations (e.g., National Rehabilitation Association, Association for Behavioral and Cognitive Therapies);
j) Local resource and referral agencies;
k) Federally funded University Centers for Excellence in Developmental Disabilities Education, Research, and Service (UCEDD);
l) Other colleges and universities with expertise in training others to work with children who have special health care needs;
m) Community-based organizations serving people with disabilities and/or special health care needs (e.g., Autism Society of America, United Cerebral Palsy Associations, ARC, Easter Seals, American Diabetes Association, American Lung Association, Epilepsy Foundation, etc.);
n) ADA regional technical assistance offices.

TYPE OF FACILITY: Center; Large Family Child Care Home; Small Family Child Care Home

RELATED STANDARDS:
Standards 10.3.4.5-10.3.4.6: Consultants and Technical Assistance for Children with Special Health Care Needs

STANDARD 8.7.0.3: Review of Plan for Serving Children with Disabilities or Children with Special Health Care Needs

The facility's plan for serving children with or children with special health care needs should be reviewed at least annually to see if it is in compliance with the legal requirements of the Individuals with Disabilities Education Improvement Act (IDEA) and Americans with Disabilities Act (ADA), as well as Section 504 of the Rehabilitation Act of 1973 (if it receives federal funding and is achieving the overall objectives for the agency or facility).

RATIONALE: An annual review by caregivers/teachers is a cornerstone of any quality assurance procedure.

TYPE OF FACILITY: Center; Large Family Child Care Home; Small Family Child Care Home

RELATED STANDARDS:
Section 2.3: Parent/Guardian Relationships
Standard 3.5.0.1: Care Plan for Children with Special Health Care Needs
Standards 10.3.4.5-10.3.4.6: Consultants and Technical Assistance for Children with Special Health Care Needs

8.8 Additional Standards for Providers Caring for Children with Special Health Care Needs

Standard 1.1.1.3: Ratios for Facilities Serving Children with Special Health Care Needs and Disabilities
Standard 1.3.1.1: General Qualifications of Directors
Standards 1.3.2.2 and 1.3.3.1: Qualifications for Caregiving Staff
Standards 1.4.2.1-1.4.2.3: Orientation Training
Standard 1.4.3.1: First Aid and CPR Training for Staff
Standards 1.4.4.1-1.4.4.2: Continuing Education
Standard 1.6.0.1: Child Care Health Consultants
Standard 2.1.2.5: Toilet Learning/Training
Standard 2.3.1.1: Mutual Responsibility of Parents/Guardians and Staff
Standards 2.3.1.2-2.3.3.2: Parental/Guardian Participation
Standard 3.4.3.1: Emergency Procedures
Standard 3.5.0.1: Care Plan for Children with Special Health Care Needs
Standard 3.5.0.2: Caring for Children Who Require Medical Procedures
Standards 4.2.0.8-4.2.0.9: Feeding Plans/Modifications and Menus/New Foods
Standard 4.2.0.10: Care for Children with Food Allergies
Standard 5.1.1.4: Accessibility of Facility
Standard 5.1.2.1: Space Required Per Child
Standard 5.1.4.2: Evacuation of Children with Special Health Care Needs and Children with Disabilities
Standard 5.1.4.7: Access to Exits
Standard 5.3.2.1: Therapeutic and Recreational Equipment
Standards 5.3.2.2-5.3.2.3: Special Adaptive Equipment
Standard 5.4.6.2: Space for Therapy Services
Standard 5.6.0.1: First Aid and Emergency Supplies
Standards 6.5.1.1 and 6.5.2.2: Transportation
Standard 9.2.2.1: Planning for Child's Transition to New Services
Standard 9.2.3.4: Written Policy for Obtaining Preventive Health Service Information

Standards 9.2.3.6-9.2.3.7 and 9.4.2.8: Information Exchange/Release of Records
Standard 9.4.2.1: Contents of Child's Records

REFERENCES:

1. The Individuals with Disabilities Education Act. 2004. 20 USC § 1400.
2. The Education for All Handicapped Children Act. 1975. 20 USC § 1400.
3. Dugan, S. 1986. *Education of the Handicapped Act amendments of 1986*. Alexandria, VA: Capitol Publications.
4. The Americans with Disabilities Act. 1990. 3 USC § 421.
5. The Rehabilitation Act. 1973. 29 USC § 701.
6. State of Florida Department of Education Technical Assistance and Training System. 2010. System level considerations for inclusion. *TATS eUpdate: Inclusion/Program Effectiveness* (March). http://www.tats.ucf.edu/docs/eUpdates/Inclusion-11.pdf.

Chapter 9

9

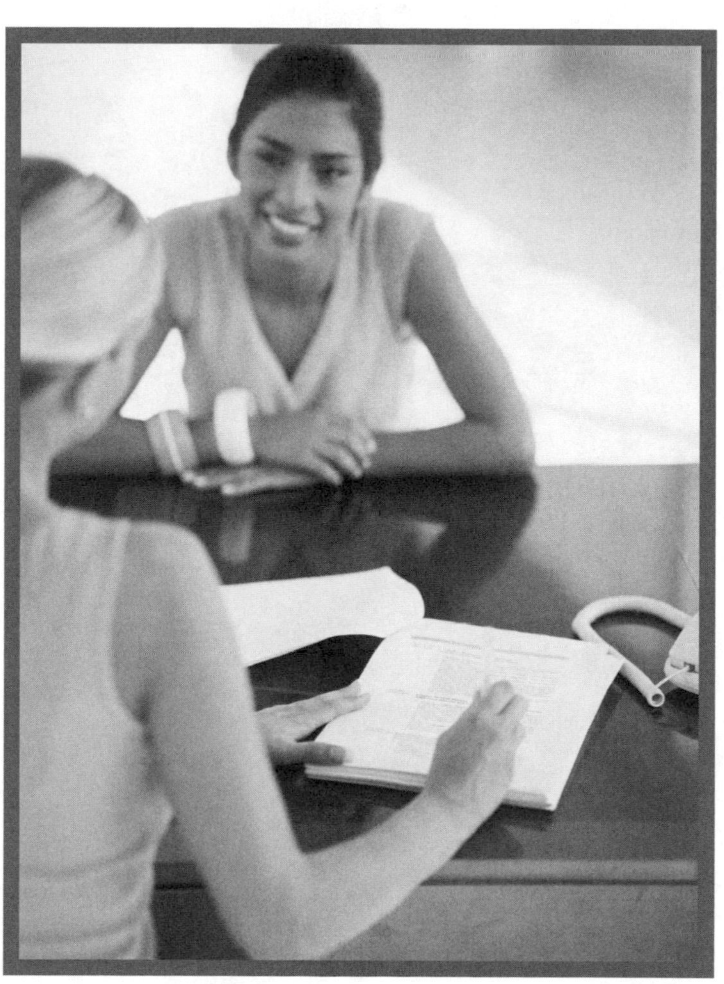

Administration

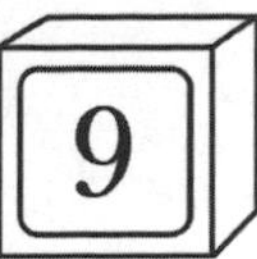

9.1 Governance

STANDARD 9.1.0.1: Governing Body of the Facility

The facility should have an identifiable governing body or person with the responsibility for and authority over the operation of the center or program. The governing body should appoint one person at the facility, or two in the case of co-directors, who is responsible for day-to-day management. The director for facilities licensed for more than thirty children should have no other assigned duties (1). Centers with fewer than thirty children may employ a director who teaches as well.

Responsibilities of the person in charge of the operation of the facility should include, but should not be limited to, the following:

a) Ensuring stable and continuing compliance with all applicable rules, regulations, and facility policies and procedures while also assuring a safe and healthy environment;
b) Developing and implementing policies that promote the achievement of quality child care;
c) Ensuring that all written policies are updated and used, as described in this chapter;
d) Assuring the reliability and integrity of staff by hiring; firing/dismissals; assigning roles, duties, and responsibilities; supervising; and evaluating personnel;
e) Providing orientation of all new parents/guardians, employees, and volunteers to the physical structure, policies, and procedures of the facility;
f) Notifying all staff, volunteers, and parents/guardians of any changes in the facility's policies and procedures;
g) Providing for continuous supervision of visitors and all non-facility personnel;
h) When problems are identified, planning for corrective action, and assigning and verifying that a specific person corrects the problem by a specified date;
i) Arranging or providing repair, maintenance, or other services at the facility;
j) Providing or arranging for in-service training and supplemental education for staff and volunteers, based on the needs of the facility and qualifications and skills of staff and volunteers;
k) Recommending an annual budget and managing the finances of the facility;
l) Maintaining required records for staff, volunteers, and children at the facility;
m) Providing for parent/guardian involvement, including parent education;
n) Reporting to the governing or advisory board on a regular basis as to the status of the facility's operation;
o) Providing oversight of research studies conducted at the facility and joint supervision of students using the facility for clinical practice.

RATIONALE: Management principles of quality improvement in any human service require identification of goals and leadership to ensure that all those involved (those with authority and experience, and those affected) participate in working toward those goals. Problem-solving approaches that are effective in other settings also work in early childhood programs. This standard describes accepted personnel management practices. For any organization to function effectively, lines of responsibility must be clearly delineated with an individual who is designated to have ultimate responsibility (1).

COMMENTS: Management should ensure policy is carried out by providing staff and parents/guardians with written handbooks, training, supervision with frequent feedback, and monitoring with checklists. A comprehensive site observation checklist is available in the print version of *Model Child Care Health Policies*, available online at http://www.ecels-healthychildcarepa.org/content/MHP4thEd Total.pdf. Copies of this publication can be purchased from the National Association for the Education of Young Children (NAEYC) at http://www.naeyc.org or from the American Academy of Pediatrics (AAP) at http://www.aap.org. It is also available on the Healthy Child Care Pennsylvania Website for download at http://www.ecels-healthychildcarepa.org.

TYPE OF FACILITY: Center; Large Family Child Care Home

RELATED STANDARDS:

Standard 1.3.1.2: Mixed Director/Teacher Role
Standards 1.4.2.1-1.4.2.3: Orientation Training
Standards 1.4.4.1-1.4.6.2: Continuing Education
Standards 2.3.1.1-2.3.3.1: Parent/Guardian Relationships

REFERENCES:

1. National Association for the Education of Young Children (NAEYC). 2004. Standard 10.A.04: NAEYC accreditation criteria for leadership and management standard. Washington, DC: NAEYC.

STANDARD 9.1.0.2: Written Delegation of Administrative Authority

There should be written delegation of administrative authority, designating the person in charge of the facility and the person(s) in charge of individual children, for all hours of operation.

RATIONALE: Caregivers/teachers are responsible for the protection of the children in their care at all times. In group care, each child must be assigned to an adult to ensure individual children are supervised and individual needs are addressed. Children should not be placed in the care of unauthorized family members or other individuals (1-8).

TYPE OF FACILITY: Center, Large Family Child Care Home

RELATED STANDARDS:

Standard 1.1.1.1: Ratios for Small Family Child Care Homes
Standard 1.1.1.2: Ratios for Large Family Child Care Homes and Centers
Standard 1.1.1.3: Ratios for Facilities Serving Children with Special Health Care Needs and Disabilities

REFERENCES:

1. Zero to Three. 2007. *The infant-toddler set-aside of the Child Care and Development Block Grant: Improving quality child care for infants and toddlers*. Washington, DC: Zero to Three. http://main.zerotothree.org/site/DocServer/Jan_07_Child_Care_Fact_Sheet.pdf.
2. National Institute of Child Health and Human Development (NICHD). 2006. *The NICHD study of early child care and youth development: Findings for children up to age 4 1/2 years*. Rockville, MD: NICHD. http://www.nichd.nih.gov/publications/pubs/upload/seccyd_051206.pdf.
3. Goldstein, A., K. Hamm, R. Schumacher. *Supporting growth and development of babies in child care: What does the research say?* Washington, DC: Center for Law and Social Policy (CLASP); Zero to Three. http://main.zerotothree.org/site/DocServer/ChildCareResearchBrief.pdf.
4. de Schipper, E. J., J. M. Riksen-Walraven, S. A. E. Geurts. 2006. Effects of child-caregiver ratio on the interactions between caregivers and children in child-care centers: An experimental study. *Child Devel* 77:861-74.
5. National Fire Protection Association (NFPA). 2009. *NFPA 101: Life safety code*. 2009 ed. Quincy, MA: NFPA.
6. Fiene, R. 2002. *13 indicators of quality child care: Research update*. Washington, DC: U.S. Department of Health and Human Services, Office of the Assistant Secretary for Planning and Evaluation. http://aspe.hhs.gov/hsp/ccquality-ind02/.
7. Zigler, E., W. S. Gilliam, S. M. Jones. 2006. *A vision for universal preschool education,* 107-29. New York: Cambridge University Press.
8. Stebbins, H. 2007. *State policies to improve the odds for the healthy development and school readiness of infants and toddlers*. Washington, DC: Zero to Three. http://main.zerotothree.org/site/DocServer/NCCP_article_for_BM_final.pdf.

9.2 Policies

9.2.1 Overview

STANDARD 9.2.1.1: Content of Policies

The facility should have policies to specify how the caregiver/teacher addresses the developmental functioning and individual or special health care needs of children of different ages and abilities who can be served by the facility, as well as other services and procedures. These policies should include, but not be limited to, the following:

a) Admissions criteria, enrollment procedures, and daily sign-in/sign-out policies, including authorized individuals for pick-up and allowing parent/guardian access whenever their child is in care;
b) Inclusion of children with special health care needs;
c) Nondiscrimination;
d) Payment of fees, deposits, and refunds;
e) Termination of enrollment and parent/guardian notification of termination;
f) Supervision;
g) Staffing, including caregivers/teachers, the use of volunteers, helpers, or substitute caregivers/teachers, and deployment of staff for different activities;
h) A written comprehensive and coordinated planned program based on a statement of principles;
i) Discipline;
j) Methods and schedules for conferences or other methods of communication between parents/guardians and staff;
k) Care of children and staff who are ill;
l) Temporary exclusion for children and staff who are ill and alternative care for children who are ill;
m) Health assessments and immunizations;
n) Handling urgent medical care or threatening incidents;
o) Medication administration;
p) Use of child care health consultants and education and mental health consultants;
q) Plan for health promotion and prevention (e.g., tracking routine child health care, health consultation, health education for children/staff/families, oral health, sun safety, safety surveillance, preventing obesity, etc.);
r) Disasters, emergency plan and drills, evacuation plan, and alternative shelter arrangements;
s) Security;
t) Confidentiality of records;
u) Transportation and field trips;
v) Physical activity (both outdoors and when children are kept indoors), play areas, screen time, and outdoor play policy;
w) Sleeping, safe sleep policy, areas used for sleeping/napping, sleep equipment, and bed linen;
x) Sanitation and hygiene;
y) Presence and care of any animals on the premises;
z) Food and nutrition including food handling, human milk, feeding and food brought from home, as well as a daily schedule of meals and snacks;
aa) Evening and night care plan;
ab) Smoking, tobacco use, alcohol, prohibited substances, and firearms;
ac) Human resource management;
ad) Staff health;
ae) Maintenance of the facility and equipment;
af) Preventing and reporting child abuse and neglect;
ag) Use of pesticides and other potentially toxic substances in or around the facility;
ah) Review and revision of policies, plans, and procedures.

The facility should have specific strategies for implementing each policy. For centers, all of these items should be written. Facility policies should vary according to the ages and abilities of the children enrolled to accommodate individual or special health care needs. Program planning should precede, not follow the enrollment and care of children at different developmental levels and abilities and with different health care needs. Policies, plans, and procedures should generally be reviewed annually or when any changes are made. A child care health consultant can be very helpful in developing and implementing model policies.

RATIONALE: Neither plans nor policies affect quality unless the program has devised a way to implement the plan or policy. Children develop special health care needs and have developmental differences recognized while they are enrolled in child care (2). Effort should be made to facilitate accommodation as quickly as possible to minimize delay or interruption of care (1). For examples of policies see *Model Child Care Health Policies* at http://www.ecels-healthy childcarepa.org/content/MHP4thEd Total.pdf and the California Childcare Health Program at http://www .ucsfchildcarehealth.org. Nutrition and physical activity policies for child care developed by the NAP SACC Program, Center for Health Promotion and Disease Prevention, University of North Carolina are available at http://www .center-trt.org.

TYPE OF FACILITY: Center; Large Family Child Care Home; Small Family Child Care Home

RELATED STANDARDS:
1.8.2.1: Staff Familiarity with Facility Policies, Plans, and Procedures
Reader's note: Chapter 9 includes many standards containing additional information on specific policies noted above.

REFERENCES:
1. Aronson, S. S., ed. 2002. *Model child care health policies.* 4th ed. Elk Grove Village, IL: American Academy of Pediatrics.
2. Child Care Law Center. 2009. *Questions and answers about the Americans with Disabilities Act: A quick reference for child care providers*. Updated Version. http://www.childcarelaw.org/docs/ ADA Q and A 2009 Final 3 09.pdf.

STANDARD 9.2.1.2: Review and Communication of Written Policies

All written policies should be reviewed and updated at least annually. The facility should provide copies of policies, which include pertinent plans and procedures, to all staff and parents/guardians at least annually, and two weeks before new policies or changes to existing policies go into effect. When a child enters a facility, when new policies are written, and when changes to existing policies have been made, parents/guardians should sign a statement that they have received a copy of the policy and read and/or understand the content of the policy.

Parents/guardians who are not able to read should have the policies presented orally to them. Parents/guardians who are not able to understand the policies because of a language barrier should have the policies presented to them in a language with which they are familiar (1).

RATIONALE: State of the art information changes. A yearly review encourages child care administrators to keep information and policies current. Current information on health and safety practices that is shared and developed cooperatively among caregivers/teachers and parents/guardians invites more participation and compliance with health and safety practices.

TYPE OF FACILITY: Center; Large Family Child Care Home; Small Family Child Care Homes

REFERENCES:
1. Gonzalez-Mena, J. 2007. *50 early childhood strategies for working and communicating with diverse families*. Upper Saddle River, NJ: Pearson Merrill Prentice Hall.

STANDARD 9.2.1.3: Enrollment Information to Parents/Guardians and Caregivers/Teachers

At enrollment, and before assumption of supervision of children by caregivers/teachers at the facility, the facility should provide parents/guardians and caregivers/teachers with a statement of services, policies, and procedures, including, but not limited, to the following:

a) The licensed capacity, child:staff ratios, ages and number of children in care. If names of children and parents/guardians are made available, parental/guardian permission for any release to others should be obtained;
b) Services offered to children including a written daily activity plan, sleep positioning policies and arrangements, napping routines, guidance and discipline policies, diaper changing and toilet learning/training methods, child handwashing, medication administration policies, oral health, physical activity, health education, and willingness for special health or therapy services delivered at the program (special requirements for a child should be clearly defined in writing before enrollment);
c) Hours and days of operation;
d) Admissions criteria, enrollment procedures, and daily sign-in/sign-out policies, including authorized individuals for pick-up and allowing parent/guardian access whenever their child is in care;
e) Payment of fees, deposits, and refunds;
f) Methods and schedules for conferences or other methods of communication between parents/guardians and staff.

Policies on:

a) Staffing, including caregivers/teachers, the use of volunteers, helpers, or substitute caregivers/teachers, and deployment of staff for different activities;
b) Inclusion of children with special health care needs;
c) Nondiscrimination;
d) Termination and parent/guardian notification of termination;
e) Supervision;
f) Discipline;
g) Care of children and caregivers/teachers who are ill;
h) Temporary exclusion and alternative care for children who are ill;
i) Health assessments and immunizations;
j) Handling urgent medical care or threatening incidents;
k) Medication administration;
l) Use of child care health consultants, education and mental health consultants;
m) Plan for health promotion and prevention (tracking routine child health care, health consultation, health education for children/staff/families, oral health, sun safety, safety surveillance, etc.);
n) Disasters, emergency plan and drills, evacuation plan, and alternative shelter arrangements;
o) Security;
p) Confidentiality of records;

q) Transportation and field trips;
r) Physical activity (both outdoors and when children are kept indoors), play areas, screen time, and outdoor play policy;
s) Sleeping, safe sleep policy, areas used for sleeping/napping, sleep equipment, and bed linen;
t) Sanitation and hygiene;
u) Presence and care of any animals on the premises;
v) Food and nutrition including food handling, human milk, feeding and food brought from home, as well as a daily schedule of meals and snacks;
w) Evening and night care plan;
x) Smoking, tobacco use, alcohol, prohibited substances, and firearms;
y) Preventing and reporting child abuse and neglect;
z) Use of pesticides and other potentially toxic substances in or around the facility.

Parents/guardians and caregivers/teachers should sign that they have reviewed and accepted this statement of services, policies, and procedures. Policies, plans and procedures should generally be reviewed annually or when any changes are made.

RATIONALE: *Model Child Care Health Policies*, available at http://www.ecels-healthychildcarepa.org/content/MHP4thEd Total.pdf, has text to comply with many of the topics covered in this standard. Each policy has a place for the facility to fill in blanks to customize the policies for a specific site. The text of the policies can be edited to match individual program operations. Starting with a template such as the one in *Model Child Care Health Policies* can be helpful.

COMMENTS: For large and small family child care homes, a written statement of services, policies, and procedures is strongly recommended and should be added to the "Parent Handbook." Conflict over policies can lead to termination of services and inconsistency in the child's care arrangements. If the statement is provided orally, parents/guardians should sign a statement attesting to their acceptance of the statement of services, policies and procedures presented to them. *Model Child Care Health Policies* can be adapted to these smaller settings.

TYPE OF FACILITY: Center; Large Family Child Care Home; Small Family Child Care Home

RELATED STANDARDS:
Standards 1.1.1.1-1.1.1.5: Child:Staff Ratio and Group Size
Standard 1.6.0.1: Child Care Health Consultants
Standards 2.1.1.1-2.1.4.6: Program of Developmental Activities
Standards 2.2.0.1-2.2.0.10: Supervision and Discipline
Standards 2.4.1.2-2.4.3.2: Health Education
Standards 3.1.1.1-3.1.1.2: Daily Health Check
Standard 3.1.2.1: Routine Health Supervision and Growth Monitoring
Standard 3.1.3.1: Active Opportunities for Physical Activity
Standard 3.1.3.2: Playing Outdoors
Standard 3.1.4.1: Safe Sleep Practices and SIDS/Suffocation Risk Reduction
Standards 3.1.5.1-3.1.5.3: Oral Health
Standards 3.2.1.1-3.2.1.5: Diapering and Changing Soiled Clothing
Standards 3.2.2.1-3.2.2.5: Handwashing
Standards 3.3.0.1-3.3.0.5: Cleaning, Sanitizing, and Disinfecting
Standard 3.4.1.1: Use of Tobacco, Alcohol, and Illegal Drugs
Standards 3.4.2.1-3.4.2.3: Animals
Standards 3.4.3.1-3.4.3.3: Emergency Procedures
Standard 3.6.1.1: Inclusion/Exclusion/Dismissal of Children
Standards 3.6.2.1-3.6.2.10: Caring for Children Who are Ill
Standards 3.6.3.1-3.6.3.3: Medications
Standards 4.2.0.1-4.2.0.12: General Requirements for Nutrition
Standards 4.3.1.1-4.3.3.1: Requirements for Special Groups or Ages of Children
Standards 4.6.0.1-4.6.0.2: Food Brought From Home
Standards 6.5.1.1-6.4.2.2: Transportation
Standards 7.2.0.1-7.2.0.3: Immunizations
Standard 9.2.1.1: Content of Policies
Standard 9.2.3.2: Content and Development of the Plan for Care of Children and Staff Who Are Ill
Standard 9.2.3.9: Written Policy on Use of Medications
Standard 9.2.3.11: Food and Nutrition Service Policies and Plans
Standard 9.2.3.12: Infant Feeding Policy
Standard 9.2.3.13: Plans for Evening and Nighttime Child Care
Standards 9.2.3.15-9.2.3.16: Policies Prohibiting Smoking, Tobacco, Alcohol, Illegal Drugs, Toxic Substances, and Firearms
Standards 9.2.4.1-9.2.4.10: Emergency/Security Policies and Plans
Standard 9.4.1.3: Written Policy on Confidentiality of Records

STANDARD 9.2.1.4: Exchange of Information Upon Enrollment

Arrangements for enrollment of children should be made in person by the parents/guardians. The facility should advise the parents/guardians of their responsibility to provide information to the facility regarding their children and inform them of the facility's confidentiality guidelines.

RATIONALE: Parents/guardians should be fully informed about the facility's services before delegating responsibility for care of the child. The facility and parents/guardians should exchange information necessary for the safety and health of the child.

TYPE OF FACILITY: Center; Large Family Child Care Home; Small Family Child Care Home

STANDARD 9.2.1.5: Nondiscriminatory Policy

The facility's written admission policy should be nondiscriminatory in regard to race, culture, sex, religion, national origin, ancestry, sexual preference, or disability. A copy of the policy and definitions of eligibility should be available for review on demand.

RATIONALE: Nondiscriminatory policies advocate for quality child care services for all children regardless of the child's citizenship, residency status, financial resources, and language differences (1).

COMMENTS: Facilities should be able to accommodate all children except those whose needs require extreme modifications beyond the capability of the facility's resources. Facilities should not have blanket policies against admitting children with disabilities. Instead, a facility should make an individual assessment of a child's needs and the facility's ability to meet those needs. Federal laws (e.g., Americans with Disabilities Act) do not permit discrimination based on disability. Inclusion of children with special health care

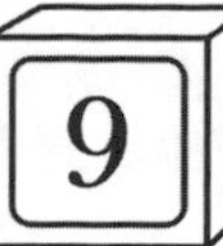

needs and disabilities in all child care and early childhood educational programs is strongly encouraged.

TYPE OF FACILITY: Center; Large Family Child Care Home; Small Family Child Care Home

RELATED STANDARDS:
Chapter 8: Children with Special Health Care Needs and Disabilities

REFERENCES:

1. U.S. Department of Justice, Civil Rights Division, Disability Rights Section. 1997. Commonly asked questions about child care centers and the Americans with Disabilities Act. http://www.ada.gov/childq%26a.htm.

STANDARD 9.2.1.6: Written Discipline Policies

Each facility should have a written discipline policy reflective of the positive methods of guidance appropriate to the ages of the children enrolled outlined in Standard 2.2.0.6 and prohibited caregiver behaviors as outlined in Standard 2.2.0.9.

The facility should have policies for dealing with biting, hitting, and other undesired behavior by children and written protocol reflective guidance outlined in Standard 2.2.0.7.

Policies should explicitly prohibit corporal punishment, psychological abuse, humiliation, abusive language, binding or tying to restrict movement, restriction of access to large motor physical activities, and the withdrawal or forcing of food and other basic needs.

All caregivers/teachers should sign an agreement to implement the facility's discipline policies. A policy explicitly stating the consequence for staff who do not follow the discipline policies should be reviewed and signed by each staff member prior to hiring.

RATIONALE: Caregivers/teachers are more likely to avoid abusive practices if they are well-informed about effective, non-abusive methods for managing children's behaviors. Positive methods of discipline create a constructive and supportive social group and reduce incidents of aggression.

Corporal punishment may be physical abuse or may become abusive very easily. Research links corporal punishment with negative effects such as later criminal behavior and impairment of learning (1-3). Primary factors supporting the prohibition of certain methods of punishment include current child development theory and practice, legal aspects (namely that a caregiver/teacher is not acting in place of parents/guardians with regard to the child), and increasing liability suits. According to the *NARA 2008 Child Care Licensing Study*, forty-eight states prohibit corporal punishment in centers; forty-three of forty-four states that license small family child care homes prohibit corporal punishment and only one state does not prohibit corporal punishment in large family child care homes (4).

COMMENTS: Parents/guardians should be encouraged to utilize similar positive discipline methods at home in order to encourage these practices and to provide a more consistent discipline approach for the child.

TYPE OF FACILITY: Center; Large Family Child Care Home; Small Family Child Care Home

RELATED STANDARDS:
Standard 2.2.0.6: Discipline Measures
Standard 2.2.0.7: Handling Physical Aggression, Biting, and Hitting
Standard 2.2.0.8: Preventing Expulsions, Suspensions, and Other Limitations in Services
Standard 2.2.0.9: Prohibited Caregiver Behaviors

REFERENCES:

1. Paintal, S. 1999. Banning corporal punishment of children: A position paper. *Child Educ* 76:36-39.
2. Education Commission of the States. 1999. *Collection of clearinghouse notes, 1998-1999*. Denver, CO: ECS.
3. American Academy of Pediatrics, Committee on School Health. 2006. Policy statement: Corporal punishment in the schools. *Pediatrics* 106:343.
4. National Child Care Information and Technical Assistance Center and the National Association for Regulatory Administration. 2010. *The 2008 child care licensing study*. http://www.naralicensing.org/displaycommon.cfm?an=1&subarticlenbr=205.

9.2.2 Transitions

STANDARD 9.2.2.1: Planning for Child's Transition to New Services

If a parent/guardian requests assistance with the transition process from the facility to a public school or another program, the designated care or service coordinator at the facility should review the child's records, including needs, learning style, supports, progress, and recommendations. The designated care or service coordinator should obtain written informed consent from the parent/guardian prior to sharing information at a transition meeting, in a written summary, or in some other verbal or written format.

The process for the child's departure should also involve sharing and the exchange of progress reports with other care providers for the child and the parents/guardians of the child within the realm of confidentiality guidelines.

Any special health care need of the child and successful strategies that have been employed while at child care should be shared. For children who are receiving services under Part C of IDEA, a transition plan is required, usually at least ninety days prior to the time that the child will leave the facility or program.

In the case of a child who may be eligible for preschool services, with approval of the family of the child, a conference should be convened among the lead agency, the family, and the local educational agency not less than ninety days (and at the discretion of all such parties, not more than nine months) before the child is eligible for the preschool services, to discuss any such services that the child may receive. In the case of a child who may not be eligible for such preschool services, with the approval of the family, reasonable efforts should be made to convene a conference among the lead agency, the family, and providers of other appropriate services, to discuss the appropriate services that the child may receive; to review the child's program options; for the period from the child's third birthday through the remainder of the school year; and to establish a transition plan, including as appropriate, steps to exit from the program. A plan also requires description of efforts to promote collaboration among Early Head Start programs under section 645A of the Head Start Act, early education and child care programs.

The facility should determine in what form and for how long archival records of transitioned children should be maintained by the facility.

RATIONALE: All children and their families will experience one or more program transitions during early childhood. One of the most common transitions is from preschool to kindergarten. Families in transition benefit when support and advocacy are available from a facility representative who is aware of their needs and of the community's resources (1). This process is essential in planning the child's departure or transition to another program. Information regarding successful behavior strategies, motivational strategies, and similar information may be helpful to staff in the setting to which the child is transitioning.

COMMENTS: Some families are capable of advocating effectively for themselves and their children; others require help negotiating the system outside of the facility. An interdisciplinary process is encouraged. Though coordinating and evaluating health and therapeutic services for children with special health care needs is primarily the responsibility of the school district or regional center, staff from the child care facility (one of many service providers) should participate, as staff members have had a unique opportunity to observe the child. In small and large family child care homes where an interdisciplinary team is not present, the caregivers/teachers should participate in the planning and preparation along with other care or treatment providers, with parent/guardian written consent.

It is important for all providers of care to coordinate their activities and referrals; otherwise the family may not be well informed. If records are shared electronically, providers should ensure that the records are encrypted for security and confidentiality.

TYPE OF FACILITY: Center; Large Family Child Care Home; Small Family Child Care Home

RELATED STANDARDS:
Standard 9.2.2.2: Format for the Transition Plan
Standards 9.4.1.3-9.4.1.6: Confidentiality and Access to Records/Documents

REFERENCES:
1. Harbin, G., B. Rous, N. Peeler, J. Schuster, K. McCormick. 2007. *Research brief: Desired family outcomes of the early childhood transition process.* http://community.fpg.unc.edu/connect/Desired-Family-Outcomes-of-the-Early-Childhood-Transition-Process-1.pdf.

STANDARD 9.2.2.2: Format for the Transition Plan

Each service agency or primary care provider should have a format and timeline for the process of developing a transition plan for children with special health care needs to be followed when each child leaves the facility. The plan should include the following components:

a) Review and final preparation of the child's records;
b) A child and family needs assessment;
c) Identification of potential child care, educational, or programmatic arrangements;
d) Summary of any special health care needs and successful strategies that were employed in child care.

RATIONALE: Many factors contribute to the success or failure of a transition. These concerns can be monitored effectively when a written plan is developed and followed to ensure that all steps in a transition are included and are undertaken in a timely, responsive manner (1).

COMMENTS: Though the child care provider can and should offer support in this process, child care is a free-market system where the parent/guardian is the consumer and decision-maker.

It is best if the process of planning begins at least nine months prior to the child turning three and an anticipated transition, since finding the proper facility for a child can be a complex and time consuming process in some communities. Each state is required to develop transition guidelines that implement the federal guidelines in respect to timelines, procedural due process expectations, and the required representation at the various meetings. Each agency can adapt the format to its own needs. However, consistent formats for planning and information exchange, requiring written parental/guardian consent, would be useful to both caregivers/teachers and families in both localities when children with special health care needs are involved. The use of outside consultants for small and large family child care homes is especially important in meeting this type of standard.

TYPE OF FACILITY: Center; Large Family Child Care Home; Small Family Child Care Home

RELATED STANDARDS:
Standard 9.2.2.1: Planning for Child's Transition to New Services

REFERENCES:
1. Harbin, G., B. Rous, N. Peeler, J. Schuster, K. McCormick. 2007. *Research brief: Desired family outcomes of the early childhood transition process.* http://community.fpg.unc.edu/connect/Desired-Family-Outcomes-of-the-Early-Childhood-Transition-Process-1.pdf.

STANDARD 9.2.2.3: Exchange of Information at Transitions

A written communication policy should be in place to describe needed communication between parents/guardians and caregivers/teachers during transitions that occur at times when children are being dropped off or picked up and other interactions with parents/guardians. When several staff shifts are involved, information about the child should be exchanged between caregivers/teachers assigned to each shift.

RATIONALE: Personal contact on a daily basis between the child care staff and parents/guardians is essential to ensure the transfer of information required to provide for the child's needs. Information about the child's experiences and health

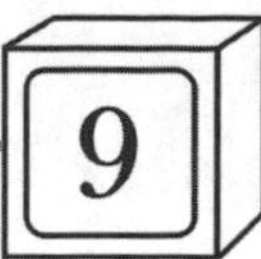

during the interval when an adult other than the parent/guardian is in charge should be provided to parents/guardians because they may need such information to understand the child's later behavior.

COMMENTS: A sample of issues that should be communicated and exchanged include change in routine at home/program, change in child's health status, recent problems sleeping/eating, or change in family routines or family health.

TYPE OF FACILITY: Center; Large Family Child Care Home; Small Family Child Care Home

RELATED STANDARDS:
Standard 2.3.1.1: Mutual Responsibility of Parents/Guardians and Staff
Standard 2.3.3.1: Parents'/Guardians' Provision of Information on Their Child's Health and Behavior

9.2.3 Health Policies

STANDARD 9.2.3.1: Policies and Practices that Promote Physical Activity

The facility should have written policies on the promotion of physical activity and the removal of potential barriers to physical activity participation. Policies should cover the following:

a) Benefits: benefits of physical activity and outdoor play;
b) Duration: children will spend sixty to one hundred and twenty minutes each day outdoors depending on their age, weather permitting. Policies will describe what will be done to ensure physical activity and provisions for gross motor activities indoors on days with more extreme conditions (i.e., very wet, very hot, or very cold);
c) Setting: provision of covered areas for shade and shelter on playgrounds, if feasible (2);
d) Clothing: clothing should permit easy movement (not too loose and not too tight) that enables children to participate fully in active play; footwear should provide support for running and climbing.

Examples of appropriate clothing/footwear include:

a) Gym shoes or sturdy gym-shoe-equivalent;
b) Clothes for the weather, including heavy coat, hat, and mittens in the winter/snow; raincoat and boots for the rain; and layered clothes for climates in which the temperature can vary dramatically on a daily basis.

Examples of inappropriate clothing/footwear include:

a) Footwear that can come off while running or that provide insufficient support for climbing (3);
b) Clothing that can catch on playground equipment (e.g., those with drawstrings or loops).

If children wear "dress clothes" or special outfits that cannot be easily laundered, caregivers/teachers should talk with the children's parents/guardians about the program's goals in providing physical activity during the program day and encourage them to provide a set of clothes that can be used during physical activities.

Facilities should discuss the importance of this policy with parents/guardians upon enrollment and periodically thereafter.

In addition to outdoor play, the facility is encouraged to incorporate movement activities or games into the standard indoor curriculum.

RATIONALE: If appropriately dressed, children can safely play outdoors in most weather conditions. Children can learn math, science, and language concepts through games involving movement (1).

COMMENTS: Lack of coat, mittens/gloves, and/or hat has been cited as a barrier to children's physical activity in early care and education (3). Caregivers/teachers can mitigate this issue by having extra clean clothing on hand. Only when weather-related health alerts are issued should restrictions be placed on outdoor activity. Children can play in the rain, snow, and in low temperatures, when wearing clothing that keeps them dry and warm. When it is very warm, children can play outdoors if they play in shady areas, wear sun-protective clothing, have water available to mist or sprinkle, and have plenty of water available for drinking.

Having a policy on outdoor physical activity that will take place on days when weather is moderately (but not severely) inclement informs all caregivers/teachers and families about the facility's expectations. The policy can make clear that outdoor activity may require special clothing in colder weather, or arrangements for cooling off when it is warm. By having such a policy, the facility encourages caregivers/teachers and families to anticipate and prepare for outdoor activity when cold, hot, or wet weather prevail. The policy also identifies when alternate large muscle activity should be held indoors so that weather conditions do not dictate lack of physical activity.

For examples of policies, see the Nemours Health and Prevention Services guide on best practices for physical activity at: http://www.nemours.org/content/dam/nemours/www/filebox/service/preventive/nhps/heguide.pdf.

TYPE OF FACILITY: Center; Large Family Child Care Home; Small Family Child Care Home

RELATED STANDARDS:
Standard 3.1.3.1: Active Opportunities for Physical Activity
Standard 3.1.3.2: Playing Outdoors
Standard 3.1.3.4: Caregivers'/Teachers' Encouragement of Physical Activity
Appendix S: Physical Activity: How Much Is Needed?

REFERENCES:
1. Trost, S. G., B. Fees, D. Dzewaltowski. 2008. Feasibility and efficacy of a "move and learn" physical activity curriculum in preschool children. *J Phys Act Health* 5:88-103.
2. McWilliams, C., S. G. Ball, S. E. Benjamin, D. Hales, A. Vaughn, D. S. Ward. 2009. Best-practice guidelines for physical activity at child care. *Pediatrics* 124:1650-59.
3. Copeland, K. A., S. N. Sherman, C. A. Kendeigh, B. E. Saelens, H. J. Kalkwarf. 2009. Flip flops, dress clothes, and no coat: Clothing barriers to children's physical activity in child-care centers identified

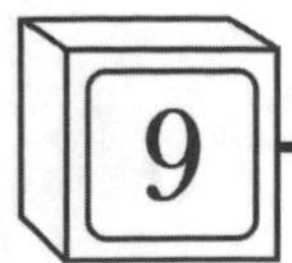

from a qualitative study. *Int J Behav Nutr and Physical Activity* 6, no. 74 (November 6). http://ijbnpa.org/content/6/1/74.

STANDARD 9.2.3.2: Content and Development of the Plan for Care of Children and Staff Who Are Ill

All child care facilities should have written policies for the management and care of children and staff who are ill. The facility's plan for the care of children and staff who are ill should be developed in consultation with the facility's child care health consultant and other health care professionals to address current understanding of the technical issues of contagion and other health risks. This plan should include:

a) Policies and procedures for urgent and emergency care;
b) Admission and inclusion/exclusion policies;
c) A description of illnesses common to children in child care, their management, and precautions to address the needs and behavior of the child who is ill, as well as to protect the health of other children and staff;
d) A procedure to obtain and maintain updated individual care plans for children and staff with special health care needs;
e) A procedure for documenting the name of person affected, date and time of illness, a description of symptoms, the response of the caregiver/teacher or other staff to these symptoms, who was notified (such as a parent/guardian, primary care provider, nurse, physician, or health department), and the response;
f) Medication policy;
g) Seasonal and pandemic influenza policy;
h) Staff illness-guidelines for exclusion and re-entry.

In group care, the facility should address the well-being of all those affected by illness: the child, the staff, parents/guardians of the child, other children in the facility and their parents/guardians, and the community. The priority of the policy should be to meet the needs of the child who is ill and the other children in the facility. The policy should address the circumstances under which separation of the affected individual (child or staff person) from the group is required; the circumstances under which the staff, parents/guardians, or other designated persons need to be informed; and the procedures to be followed in these cases. The policy should take into consideration:

a) The physical facility;
b) The number and the qualifications of the facility's personnel;
c) The fact that children do become ill frequently and at unpredictable times;
d) The fact that adults may be on staff with known health problems or may develop health problems while at work;
e) The fact that working parents/guardians often are not given leave for their children's illnesses;
f) The amount of care the child who is ill requires if the child remains in the program, can staff devote the time for caring of a child who is ill in the classroom without leaving other children unattended, and can the child participate in any of the classroom activities (1).

RATIONALE: Infectious diseases are a major concern of parents/guardians and staff. Since children, especially those in group settings, can be a reservoir for many infectious agents, and since caregivers/teachers and other staff come into close and frequent contact with children, they are at risk for developing a wide variety of infectious diseases. Following the infection control standards will help protect both children and staff from infectious disease. Recording the occurrence of illness in a facility and the response to the illness characterizes and defines the frequency of the illness, suggests whether an outbreak has occurred, may suggest an effective intervention, and provides documentation for administrative purposes.

COMMENTS: Facilities may comply by adopting a model policy and using reference materials as authoritative resources. *Managing Infectious Diseases in Child Care and Schools, 2nd Ed.,* available from the American Academy of Pediatrics (AAP), is a reference for policies and their implementation. This publication includes detailed handouts that can be used to inform parents/guardians and outline guidelines and rationale for exclusion, return to care and notification of public health authorities. Other helpful references include *Model Child Care Health Policies,* available at http://www.ecels-healthychildcarepa.org/content/MHP 4thEd Total.pdf, or the current edition of the *Red Book*. Caregivers/teachers can check for other materials provided by the licensing agency, resource and referral agency, or health department. *Curriculum for Managing Infectious Diseases,* an online training module for caregivers/teachers is available from the AAP at http://www.healthychildcare.org/ParticipantsManualID.html.

TYPE OF FACILITY: Center; Large Family Child Care Home; Small Family Child Care Home

RELATED STANDARDS:
Standard 1.6.0.1: Child Care Health Consultants
Standards 3.4.3.1-3.4.3.3: Emergency Procedures
Standard 3.6.1.1: Inclusion/Exclusion/Dismissal of Children
Standard 3.6.1.2: Staff Exclusion for Illness
Standard 3.6.3.1: Medication Administration
Chapter 7: Infectious Diseases
Standard 9.2.3.9: Written Policy on Use of Medications
Standard 9.2.4.3: Disaster Planning, Training, and Communication
Standard 9.2.4.4: Written Plan for Seasonal and Pandemic Influenza
Standard 9.4.2.1: Contents of Child's Records
Appendix A: Signs and Symptoms Chart
Appendix F: Enrollment/Attendance/Symptom Record
Appendix AA: Medication Administration Packet

REFERENCES:
1. Aronson, S. S., T. R. Shope, eds. 2009. *Managing infectious diseases in child care and schools: A quick reference guide*. 2nd ed. Elk Grove Village, IL: American Academy of Pediatrics.

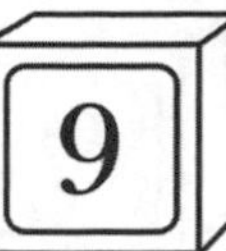

STANDARD 9.2.3.3: Written Policy for Reporting Notifiable Diseases to the Health Department

The facility should have a written policy that complies with the state's reporting requirements for children who are ill. All notifiable diseases should be reported to the health department. The facility should have the telephone number of the responsible health authority to whom confirmed or suspected cases of these diseases, or outbreaks of other infectious diseases, should be reported, and should designate a staff member as responsible for reporting the disease.

RATIONALE: Reporting to the health department provides the department with knowledge of illnesses within the community and ability to offer preventive measures to children and families exposed to the outbreak of a disease. In some states, caregivers/teachers may not be a mandatory reporter. In those states, caregivers/teachers are encouraged to report any infectious disease to the responsible health authority.

TYPE OF FACILITY: Center; Large Family Child Care Home; Small Family Child Care Home

RELATED STANDARDS:
Section 7.8: Interaction with State or Local Health Departments

STANDARD 9.2.3.4: Written Policy for Obtaining Preventive Health Service Information

Each facility should develop and follow a written policy for obtaining necessary medical information including immunizations (see Appendix G: Recommended Childhood Immunization Schedule) and periodic preventive health assessments (see Appendix I: Recommendations for Preventive Pediatric Health Care) as recommended by the American Academy of Pediatrics (AAP) in *Bright Futures Guidelines for Health Supervision of Infants, Children, and Adolescents* (1-3). Facility staff should encourage parents/guardians to schedule these preventive health services in a timely fashion.

Documentation of an age-appropriate health assessment that includes current immunizations and health screenings should be filed in the child's record at the facility. Immunization records should be provided at the time of enrollment. The health assessment should be provided within two weeks of admission or indication that an appointment has been made with the health care provider. Updates of the health record should be maintained according to the American Academy of Pediatrics' (AAP's) periodicity schedule, Appendix I: Recommendations for Preventive Pediatric Health Care. Health record information should be reviewed by the staff of the facility and information sharing between the staff, the parents/guardians, and the child's health care professional should be encouraged and facilitated in order to provide better care for the child in the child care setting.

Centers should have written procedures for the verification of compliance with recommended immunizations and periodic health assessments of children. Centers should maintain confidential records of immunizations, periodic health assessments, including Body Mass Index (BMI) for children age two and older, and any special health considerations.

RATIONALE: Health assessments are important to ensure prevention, early detection of remediable problems, and planning for adaptations needed so that all children can reach their potential. When age-appropriate health assessments and use of health insurance benefits are promoted by caregivers/teachers, children enrolled in child care will have increased access to immunizations and other preventive services (4). With the expansion of eligibility for medical assistance and the federal subsidy of state child health insurance plans (SCHIP), the numbers of children who lack insurance for routine preventive health care should lessen.

Requiring facilities to maintain a current health record encourages and supports discussion of a child's health needs between parents/guardians, caregivers/teachers, and the child's primary care provider. It also encourages parents/guardians to seek preventive and primary care services in a timely fashion for their child.

The facility should have accurate, current information regarding the medical status and treatment of each child so it will be able to determine and adjust its capability to provide needed services. This documentation should consist of more than a statement from the child's primary care provider that the child is up-to-date. Because of the administrative burden posed by requests to fill out forms, unless the specifics of services rendered are requested, the information may not reflect the child's actual receipt of services according to the nationally recommended schedule. Instead, it may only represent that the child has a current health record in the primary care provider's office. Until tracking systems become more widespread and effective in health care settings, a joint effort by the education system, family and primary care provider is required to ensure that children receive the preventive health services that ensure they are healthy and ready to learn.

COMMENTS: Assistance for caregivers/teachers and low income parents/guardians can be obtained through the Medicaid Early Periodic Screening and Diagnostic Treatment (EPSDT) program (Title XIX) and the state's version of the federal Child Health Insurance Program (SCHIP) (5).

Most states require that caregivers/teachers document that the child's health records are up-to-date to protect the child and other children whom the unimmunized child would expose to increased risk of vaccine-preventable disease. State regulations regarding immunization requirements for children may differ, but the child care facility should strive to comply with the national, annually published, "Recommended Childhood Immunization Schedule," available at http://www.cispimmunize.org from the AAP, Centers for Disease Control and Prevention (CDC), and the American Academy of Family Physicians (AAFP).

A child's entrance into the facility need not be delayed if an appointment for health supervision is scheduled. Often appointments for well-child care must be scheduled several weeks in advance. In such cases, the child care facility should obtain a health history report from the parents/guardians and documentation of an appointment for routine health supervision, as a minimum requirement for the child to attend the facility on a routine basis. The child should receive immunizations on admission or provide evidence of an immunization plan to prevent an increased exposure to vaccine-preventable diseases.

Local public health staff (such as the staff of immunization units, EPSDT programs) should provide assistance to caregivers/teachers in the form of record-keeping materials, educational materials, and on-site visits for education and help with surveillance activities. A copy of a form to use for documentation of routine health supervision services is available from *Model Child Care Health Policies* at http://www.ecels-healthychildcarepa.org/content/MHP4th Ed Total.pdf.

TYPE OF FACILITY: Center; Large Family Child Care Home; Small Family Child Care Home

RELATED STANDARDS:
Standard 2.1.1.4: Monitoring Children's Development/Obtaining Consent for Screening
Standard 9.4.1.3: Written Policy on Confidentiality of Records
Appendix G: Recommended Childhood Immunization Schedule
Appendix I: Recommendations for Preventive Pediatric Health Care
Appendix FF: Child Health Assessment

REFERENCES:
1. American Academy of Pediatrics. 2011. Recommended childhood immunization schedules. http://www.aap.org/immunization/IZSchedule.html.
2. American Academy of Pediatrics. 2008. Recommendations for preventive pediatric health care. http://practice.aap.org/content.aspx?aid=1599&nodeID=4000.
3. Hagan, J. F., J. S. Shaw, P. M. Duncan, eds. 2008. *Bright futures: Guidelines for health supervision of infants, children, and adolescents*. 3rd ed. Elk Grove Village, IL: American Academy of Pediatrics.
4. Haskins, R., J. Kotch. 1986. Day care and illness: Evidence, costs, and public policy. *Pediatrics* 77:951-82.
5. U.S. Department of Health and Human Services, Centers for Medicare and Medicaid. Children's health insurance program. http://www.cms.hhs.gov/home/chip.asp.

STANDARD 9.2.3.5: Documentation of Exemptions and Exclusion of Children Who Lack Immunizations

For children who have been exempted from required, up-to-date immunizations, these exemptions should be documented in the child's health record as a cross reference, (acceptable documentation includes a statement from the child's primary provider, a legal exemption with notarization, waiver, or other state-specific required documentation signed by the parent/guardian). See Standard 7.2.0.2 for more information.

Within two weeks of enrollment the parent/guardian should provide documentation to the child care program regarding progress in obtaining immunizations. The parent/guardian should receive written notice of exclusion if noncompliance or lack of progress is evident. If more than one immunization is needed in a series, time should be allowed for the immunizations to be obtained at the appropriate intervals. Exemptions from the requirement related to compliance with the federal McKinney-Vento Homeless Assistance Act for children experiencing homelessness are documented and include a plan for obtaining available documents within a reasonable period of time.

RATIONALE: National surveys document that child care has a positive influence on protection from vaccine-preventable illness (1). Immunizations should be required for all children in child care and early education settings. Facilities must consider the consequences if they accept responsibility for exposing a child who cannot be fully immunized (because of immaturity) to an unimmunized child who may bring disease to the facility. Although up to two weeks after the child starts to participate in child care may be allowed for the acquisition of immunizations for which the child is eligible, parents/guardians should maintain their child's immunization status according to the nationally recommended schedule to avoid potential exposure of other children in the facility to vaccine-preventable disease.

COMMENTS: An updated immunization schedule is published annually near the beginning of the calendar year in the AAP's *Pediatrics* journal and in the CDC's *MMWR* and should be consulted for current information. In addition to print versions of the recommended childhood immunization schedule, the "Recommended Immunization Schedules for Persons Aged 0 through 18 Years – United States" is posted on the Websites of the CDC at http://www.cdc.gov/vaccines/ and the AAP at http://www.aap.org/immunization/IZSchedule.html.

When a child who has a medical exemption from immunization is included in child care, reasonable accommodation of that child requires planning to exclude such a child in the event of an outbreak. Caregivers/teachers should check the Website http://www.immunize.org/laws/ for specific state-mandated immunization requirements and exemptions.

TYPE OF FACILITY: Center; Large Family Child Care Home; Small Family Child Care Home

RELATED STANDARDS:
Standard 7.2.0.2: Unimmunized Children
Appendix G: Recommended Childhood Immunization Schedule

REFERENCES:
1. Aronson, S. S. 1986. Maintaining health in child care settings. In *Group care for young children*, ed. N. Gunzenhauser, B. M. Caldwell. New Brunswick, NJ: Johnson and Johnson Baby Products Company.

STANDARD 9.2.3.6: Identification of Child's Medical Home and Parental Consent for Information Exchange

As part of the enrollment of a child, the caregiver/teacher should ask the family to identify the child's primary care provider, his or her medical home, and other specialty health care professionals. The parent/guardian should provide

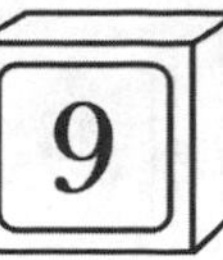

written consent to enable the caregiver/teacher to establish communication with those providers. The family should always be informed prior to the use of the permission unless it is an emergency. The providers with whom the facility should exchange information (with parental consent) should include:

a) Sources of regular medical and dental care (such as the child's primary care provider, dentist, and medical facility);
b) Special clinics the child may attend, including sessions with medical specialists and registered dietitians;
c) Special therapists for the child (e.g., occupational, physical, speech, and nutritional), along with written documentation of the services rendered provided by the special therapist;
d) Counselors, therapists, or mental health service providers for parents/guardians (e.g., social workers, psychologists, or psychiatrists);
e) Pharmacists for children who take prescription medication on a regular basis or have emergency medications for specific conditions.

RATIONALE: Primary care providers are involved not only in the medical care of the child but also involved in supporting the child's emotional and developmental needs (1-3). A major barrier to productive working relationships between child care and health care professionals is inadequate communication (1,2).

Knowing who is treating the child and coordinating services with these sources of service is vital to the ability of the caregivers/teachers to offer appropriate care to the child. Every child should have a medical home and those with special health care needs may have additional specialists and therapists (4-7). The primary care provider and needed specialists will create the Care Plan which will be the blueprint for healthy and safe inclusion into child care for the child with special health care needs.

COMMENTS: A source of health care may be a community or specialty clinic, a public health department, specialist, or a private primary care provider. Families should also know the location of the hospital emergency room departments nearest to their home and child care facility.

The California Childcare Health Program has developed a form to help facilitate the exchange of information between the health professionals and the parents/guardians and caregivers/teachers at http://ucsfchildcarehealth.org/pdfs/forms/CForm_ExchangeofInfo.pdf. They also release an information form at http://ucsfchildcarehealth.org/pdfs/forms/CF_ReferralRel.pdf. For more information on the medical home concept, see the American Academy of Pediatrics' (AAP) Medical Home Website at http://www.medicalhomeinfo.org.

TYPE OF FACILITY: Center; Large Family Child Care Home; Small Family Child Care Home

RELATED STANDARDS:

Standard 2.3.3.1: Parents'/Guardians' Provision of Information on Their Child's Health and Behavior
Standard 3.5.0.1: Care Plan for Children with Special Health Care Needs
Standards 9.4.1.3-9.4.1.6: Confidentiality and Access to Records/Documents
Appendix O: Care Plan for Children with Special Health Care Needs
Appendix AA: Medication Administration Packet
Appendix FF: Child Health Assessment

REFERENCES:

1. American Academy of Pediatrics (AAP). 2001. *The pediatrician's role in promoting health and safety in child care*. Elk Grove Village, IL: AAP.
2. Murph, J. R., S. D. Palmer, D. Glassy, eds. 2005. *Health in child care: A manual for health professionals*. 4th ed. Elk Grove Village, IL: American Academy of Pediatrics.
3. Hagan, J. F., J. S. Shaw, P. M. Duncan, eds. 2008. *Bright futures: Guidelines for health supervision of infants, children, and adolescents*. 3rd ed. Elk Grove Village, IL: American Academy of Pediatrics.
4. Starfield, B., L. Shi. 2004. The medical home, access to care, and insurance: A review of evidence. *Pediatrics* 113:1493-98.
5. Homer, C. J., K. Klatka, D. Romm, K. Kuhlthau, S. Bloom, P. Newacheck, J. Van Cleave, J. M. Perrin. 2008. A review of the evidence for the medical home for children with special health care needs. *Pediatrics* 122:e922–37.
6. Inkelas, M., M. Regolado, N. Halfon. 2005. *Stategies for integrating developmental services and promoting medical homes*. Los Angeles: National Center for Infant and Early Childhood Health Policy.
7. Nowak, A. J., P. S. Casamassimo. 2002. The dental home: A primary care concept. *JADA* 133:93-98.

STANDARD 9.2.3.7: Information Sharing on Therapies and Treatments Needed

The person at the child care facility who is responsible for planning care for the child with special therapies or treatments should obtain an individualized care plan, developed by the child's primary care provider or specialist on allergies, medications, therapies, and treatments being provided to the child that are directly relevant to the health and safety of the child in the child care facility. The written consent of the child's parents/guardians and, where appropriate, the child's primary care provider should be obtained before this confidential information is sought from outside sources. Therapies and treatments need to meet the criteria for evidenced based practices.

RATIONALE: The facility must have accurate, current information regarding the health status and treatment of the child so it will be able to determine the facility's capability to provide needed services or to obtain them elsewhere.

Medicines can be crucial to the health and wellness of children. They can also be very dangerous if the wrong type or wrong amount is given to the wrong person or at the wrong time.

Parents/guardians should always be notified in every instance when medication is used. Telephone instructions from a primary care provider are acceptable if the caregiver/teacher fully documents them and if the parent/guardian initiates the request for primary care provider or child care health consultant instruction. In the event medication for a child becomes necessary during the day or in the event of an emergency, administration instructions from a parent/guardian and the child's primary care provider are required before a caregiver/teacher may administer medication.

TYPE OF FACILITY: Center; Large Family Child Care Home; Small Family Child Care Home

RELATED STANDARDS:
Standard 3.5.0.1: Care Plan for Children with Special Health Care Needs
Standard 3.6.3.1: Medication Administration
Standards 9.4.1.3-9.4.1.6: Confidentiality and Access to Records/Documents
Appendix O: Care Plan for Children with Special Health Care Needs
Appendix AA: Medication Administration Packet

STANDARD 9.2.3.8: Information Sharing on Family Health

Families should be asked to share information about family health (such as chronic diseases) that might affect the child's health. Families should be guaranteed that all information will be kept confidential.

RATIONALE: A family history of chronic disease helps caregivers/teachers understand family stress and experiences of the child within the family.

COMMENTS: Information on family health can be gathered by asking parents/guardians to tell the caregiver/teacher about any chronic health problems that the child's parents/guardians, siblings, or household members have that might affect the child's health. This information could also be obtained from the child's primary care provider with permission from the parent/guardian.

TYPE OF FACILITY: Center; Large Family Child Care Home; Small Family Child Care Home

STANDARD 9.2.3.9: Written Policy on Use of Medications

The facility should have a written policy for the administration of any prescription or non-prescription (over-the-counter [OTC]) medication. The policy should address at least the following:

a) The use of written parental/guardian consent forms for each prescription and OTC medication to be administered at the child care facility. The consent form should include:
   1) The child's name;
   2) The name of the medication;
   3) The date(s) and times the medication is to be given;
   4) The dose or amount of medication to be given;
   5) How the medication is to be administered;
   6) The period of time the consent form is valid, which may not exceed the length of time the medication is prescribed for, the expiration date of the medication or one year, whichever is less.

b) The use of the prescribing health professional's authorization forms for each prescription and OTC medication to be administered at the child care facility.

c) The circumstances under which the facility will agree to administer medication. This may include the administration of:
   1) Topical medications such as non-medicated diaper creams, insect repellants, and sun screens;
   2) OTC medicines for fever including acetaminophen and ibuprofen;
   3) Long-term medications that are administered daily for children with chronic health conditions that are managed with medications;
   4) Controlled substances, such as psychotropic medications;
   5) Emergency medications for children with health conditions that may become life-threatening such as asthma, diabetes, and severe allergies;
   6) One-time medications to prevent conditions such as febrile seizures.

d) The circumstances under which the facility will not administer medication. This should include:
   1) No authorization from parent/guardian and/or prescribing health professional;
   2) Prohibition of administering OTC cough and cold medication;
   3) Not administering a new medication for the first time to a child while he or she is in child care;
   4) If the instructions are unclear or the supplies needed to measure doses or administer the medication are not available or not in good working condition;
   5) The medication has expired;
   6) If a staff person or his/her backup who has been trained to give that particular medication is not present (in the case of training for medications that require specific skills to administer properly, such as inhalers, injections, or feeding tubes/ports).

e) The process of accepting medication from parents/guardians. This should include:
   1) Verifying the consent form;
   2) Verifying the medication matches what is on the consent form;
   3) Accepting authorization for prescription medications from the child's prescribing health professional only if the medications are in their original container and have the child's name, the name of the medication, the dose and directions for giving the medication, the expiration date of the medication, and a list of warnings and possible side effects;
   4) Accepting authorization for OTC medications from the child's prescribing health professional only if the authorization indicates the purpose of the medication and time intervals of administration, and if the medications are in their original container and include the child's name, the name of the medication, dose and directions for use, an expiration date for the medication, and a list of warnings and possible side effects;

5) Verifying that a valid Care Plan accompanies all long-term medications (i.e., medications that are to be given routinely or available routinely for chronic conditions such as asthma, allergies, and seizures);
6) Verifying any special storage requirements and any precautions to take while the child is on the prescription or OTC medication.

f) The proper handling and storage of medications, including:
1) Emergency medications – totally inaccessible to children but readily available to supervising caregivers/teachers trained to give them;
2) Medications that require refrigeration;
3) Controlled substances;
4) Expired medications;
5) A policy to insure confidentiality;
6) Storing and preparing distribution in a quiet area completely out of access to children;
7) Keeping all medication at all times totally inaccessible to children (e.g., locked storage);
8) Whether to require even short-term medications be kept at the facility overnight.

g) The procedures to follow when administering medications. These should include:
1) Assigning administration only to an adequately trained, designated staff;
2) Checking the written consent form;
3) Adhering to the "six rights" of safe medication administration (child, medication, time/date, dose, route, and documentation) (1);
4) Documenting and reporting any medication errors;
5) Documenting and reporting and adverse effects of the medication;
6) Documenting and reporting whether the child vomited or spit up the medication.

h) The procedures to follow when returning medication to the family, including:
1) An accurate account of controlled substances being administered and the amount being returned to the family;
2) When disposing of unused medication, the remainder of a medication, including controlled substances.

i) The disposal of medications that cannot be returned to the parent/guardian.

A medication administration record should be maintained on an ongoing basis by designated staff and should include the following:

a) Specific, signed parental/guardian consent for the caregiver/teacher to administer medication including documentation of receiving controlled substances and verification of the amount received;
b) Specific, signed authorization from the child's prescribing health professional, prescribing the medication, including medical need, medication, dosage, and length of time to give medication.
c) Information about the medication including warnings and possible side effects;
d) Written documentation of administration of medication and any side effects;
e) Medication errors log.

The facility should consult with the State Board of Nursing, other interested organizations and their child care health consultant about required training and documentation for medication administration. Based on the information, the facility should develop and implement a plan regarding medication administration training (9).

RATIONALE: Administering medication requires skill, knowledge and careful attention to detail. Parents/guardians and prescribing health professionals must give a caregiver/teacher written authorization to administer medication to the child (12). Caregivers/teachers must be diligent in their adherence to the medication administration policy and procedures to prevent any inadvertent medication errors, which may be harmful to the child (11). There is always a risk that a child may have a negative reaction to a medication, and children should be monitored for serious side effects that may require an emergency response. Because children twenty-four months of age and younger are in a period of rapid development and are more vulnerable to the possible side effects of medications, extra care should be given to the circumstances under which medications will be administered to this population. A child may have a negative reaction to a medication that was given at home or to one administered while attending child care. For these reasons caregivers/teachers need to be aware of each of the medications a child received at child care as well as at home. They should know the names of the medication(s), when each was given, who prescribed them, and what the known reactions or side effects may be in the event that a child has a negative reaction to the medicine (2,10).

OTC medicines are often assumed to be safe and not afforded the proper diligence. Even common drugs such as acetaminophen and ibuprofen can result in significant toxicity for infants and small children. Inaccurate dosing from the use of inaccurate measuring tools can result in illness or even death (2,3).

Cough and cold medications (CCM) are readily available OTC in the United States and are widely used to treat upper respiratory infection. These products are not safe for infants and young children and were withdrawn by the Consumer Healthcare Products Association for children less than two years of age in 2007 (4-6,8). The Food and Drug Administration (FDA) issued a public health advisory in 2008 stating these medications should not be used in children less than two years of age. The American Academy of Pediatrics (AAP) states that CCMs are not effective for children less than six years of age and their use can result in serious, adverse effects (7).

The medication record protects the person administering medication by documenting the process. The medication errors log can be reviewed and will point out what kind of intervention, if any, will be helpful in reducing the number of medication errors. Accounting for medications administered and thrown away is important for several reasons. It may assist a health professional in determining whether the child is actually getting the medicine, especially when the child is not getting better from treatment. Some medications are "controlled substances," meaning that the medication is regulated by the federal government due to potential for abuse. Controlled substances include narcotic pain medicine, some behavior medications for ADHD, and some seizure medications. A prescribing health professional may need proper accounting for these types of medications to assure that requests for refills are because the medication was given to the patient and not used/abused by adults. Some medications, (i.e., antibiotics), can have a harmful affect on the environment if not disposed of properly.

For children with chronic health conditions or special health care needs, administering medications while the child is attending child care may be part of the child's individualized family service plan (IFSP) or individualized education plan (IEP). Child care facilities must comply with the Americans with Disabilities Act.

COMMENTS: When a child care facility cannot return unused medication to the parent/guardian, the facility needs to dispose of the medication. An example of when medication cannot be returned is when a parent/guardian has removed the child from care and the facility cannot reach the parent/guardian to return the medication. Herbal and folk medicines and home remedies are not regulated and should not be given at child cares without a prescribing health professional's order and complete pharmaceutical labeling. If they are given at home, the caregiver/teacher should be aware of their use and possible side effects.

A curriculum for child care providers on safe administration of medications in child care is available from the AAP at http://www.healthychildcare.org/HealthyFutures.html. A sample medication administration policy is located in Appendix AA: Medication Administration Packet.

TYPE OF FACILITY: Center; Large Family Child Care Home; Small Family Child Care Home

RELATED STANDARDS:

Standards 3.6.3.1-3.6.3.3: Medications
Standard 9.4.2.6: Contents of Medication Record
Appendix AA: Medication Administration Packet

REFERENCES:

1. North Carolina Child Care Health & Safety Resource Center. 2007. Steps to administering medication. http://www.healthychildcarenc.org/PDFs/steps_admin_medication.pdf.
2. American Academy of Pediatrics. 2009. Healthy futures: Medication administration in early education and child care settings. http://www.healthychildcare.org/HealthyFutures.html.
3. American Academy of Pediatrics, Council on School Health. 2009. Policy statement: Guidance for the administration of medication in school. *Pediatrics* 124:1244-51.
4. American Academy of Pediatrics, Committee on Drugs. 2009. Policy statement: Acetaminophen toxicity in children. *Pediatrics* 123:1421-22.
5. Vernacchio, L., J. Kelly, D. Kaufman, A. Mitchell. 2008. Cough and cold medication use by U.S. children, 1999-2006: Results from the Sloan Survey. *Pediatrics* 122:e323-29.
6. Schaefer, M. K., N. Shehab, A. Cohen, D. S. Budnitz. 2008. Adverse events from cough and cold medicines in children. *Pediatrics* 121:783-87.
7. Centers for Disease Control and Prevention. 2007. Infant deaths associated with cough and cold medications: Two states. *MMWR* 56:1-4.
8. U.S. Food and Drug Administration. 2007. Nonperscription cough and cold medicine use in children. http://www.fda.gov/Safety/MedWatch/SafetyInformation/SafetyAlertsforHumanMedicalProducts/ucm152691.htm.
9. Consumer Healthcare Products Association. Makers of OTC cough and cold medicines announce voluntary withdrawal of oral infant medicines. http://www.chpa-info.org/pressroom/10_11_07_OralInfantMedicines.aspx.
10. Heschel, R. T., A. A. Crowley, S. S. Cohen. 2005. State policies regarding nursing delegation and medication administration in child care setttings: A case study. *Policy, Politics, and Nurs Prac* 6:86-98.
11. Friedman, J. F., G. M. Lee, K. P. Kleinman, J. A. Finkelstein. 2004. Child care center policies and practices for management of ill children. *Ambulatory Pediatrics* 4:455-60.
12. Sinkovits, H. S., M. W. Kelly, M. E. Ernst. 2003. Medication administration in day care centers for children. *J Am Pharm Assoc* 43:379-82.

STANDARD 9.2.3.10: Sanitation Policies and Procedures

The child care facility should have written sanitation policies and procedures for the following items:

a) Maintaining equipment used for hand hygiene, toilet use, and toilet learning/training in a sanitary condition;
b) Maintaining diaper changing areas and equipment in a sanitary condition;
c) Maintaining toys in a sanitary condition;
d) Managing animals in a safe and sanitary manner;
e) Practicing proper handwashing and diapering procedures (the facility should display proper handwashing instruction signs conspicuously);
f) Practicing proper personal hygiene of caregivers/teachers and children;
g) Practicing environmental sanitation policies and procedures, such as sanitary disposal of soiled diapers;
h) Maintaining sanitation for food preparation and food service.

RATIONALE: Many infectious diseases can be prevented through appropriate hygiene and sanitation practices. Bacterial cultures of environmental surfaces in facilities, which are used to gauge the adequacy of sanitation and hygiene practices, have demonstrated evidence of fecal contamination. Contamination of hands, toys, and other equipment in the room has appeared to play a role in the transmission of diseases in child care settings (1). Regular and thorough cleaning of toys, equipment, and rooms helps to prevent transmission of illness (1).

Animals can be a source of illness for people, and people may be a source of illness for animals (1).

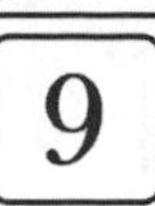

The steps involved in effective handwashing (to reduce the amount of bacterial contamination) can be easily forgotten. Posted signs provide frequent reminders to staff and orientation for new staff. Education of caregivers/teachers regarding handwashing, cleaning, and other sanitation procedures can reduce the occurrence of illness in the group of children with whom they work (2).

Illnesses may be spread by way of:

a) Human waste (such as urine and feces);
b) Body fluids (such as saliva, nasal discharge, eye discharge, open skin sores, and blood);
c) Direct skin-to-skin contact;
d) Touching a contaminated object;
e) The air (by droplets that result from sneezes and coughs).

Since many infected people carry communicable diseases without symptoms, and many are contagious before they experience a symptom, caregivers/teachers need to protect themselves and the children they serve by carrying out, on a routine basis, standard precautions and sanitation procedures that approach every potential illness-spreading condition in the same way.

Handling food in a safe and careful manner prevents the spread of bacteria, viruses, and fungi. Outbreaks of foodborne illness have occurred in many settings, including child care facilities.

COMMENTS: State health department rules and regulations may also guide the child care provider.

TYPE OF FACILITY: Center; Large Family Child Care Home; Small Family Child Care Home

RELATED STANDARDS:
Standards 3.2.1.1-3.2.1.5: Diapering and Changing Soiled Clothing
Standards 3.2.2.1-3.2.2.5: Hand Hygiene
Standards 3.3.0.2-3.3.0.3: Cleaning and Sanitizing Toys and Objects Intended for the Mouth
Standards 3.4.2.1-3.4.2.3: Animals
Standards 4.8.0.1-4.8.0.8: Kitchen and Equipment
Standards 4.9.0.1-4.9.0.7: Food Safety
Standards 4.9.0.9-4.9.0.13: Kitchen Maintenance
Standards 5.4.1.1-5.4.3.2: Toilet, Diapering, and Bath Areas
Standards 5.7.0.6-5.7.0.10: Interior Maintenance
Section 7.1: How Infections Spread
Appendix J: Selecting an Appropriate Sanitizer or Disinfectant
Appendix K: Guide for Cleaning, Sanitizing, and Disinfecting

REFERENCES:

1. Chin, J., ed. 2000. *Control of communicable diseases manual.* Washington, DC: American Public Health Association.
2. Kotch, J., P. Isbell, D. J. Weber, et al. 2007. Hand-washing and diapering equipment reduces disease among children in out-of-home child care centers. *Pediatrics* 120:e29-36.

STANDARD 9.2.3.11: Food and Nutrition Service Policies and Plans

The facility should have food handling, feeding, and nutrition policies and plans under the direction of the administration that address the following items and assigns responsibility for each:

a) Kitchen layout;
b) Food budget;
c) Food procurement and storage;
d) Menu and meal planning;
e) Food preparation and service;
f) Kitchen and meal service staffing;
g) Nutrition education for children, staff, and parents/guardians;
h) Emergency preparedness for nutrition services;
i) Food brought from home including food brought for celebrations;
j) Age-appropriate portion sizes of food to meet nutritional needs;
k) Age-appropriate eating utensils and tableware;
l) Promotion of breastfeeding and provision of community resources to support mothers.

A nutritionist/registered dietitian and a food service expert should provide input for and facilitate the development and implementation of a written nutrition plan for the early care and education facility.

RATIONALE: Having a plan that clearly assigns responsibility and that encompasses the pertinent nutrition elements will promote the optimal health of children and staff in early care and education settings.

For sample policies see the Nemours Health and Prevention Services guide on best practices for healthy eating at http://www.nemours.org/content/dam/nemours/www/filebox/service/preventive/nhps/heguide.pdf.

TYPE OF FACILITY: Center; Large Family Child Care Home; Small Family Child Care Home

RELATED STANDARDS:
Standard 4.2.0.1: Written Nutrition Plan
Standard 4.2.0.9: Written Menus and Introduction of New Foods
Standard 4.3.1.1: General Plan for Feeding Infants
Standard 4.3.1.2: Feeding Infants on Cue by a Consistent Caregiver/Teacher
Standard 4.3.1.3: Preparing, Feeding, and Storing Human Milk
Standard 4.3.2.2: Serving Size for Toddlers and Preschoolers
Standard 4.4.0.2: Use of Nutritionist/Registered Dietitian
Standards 4.6.0.1-4.6.0.2: Food Brought from Home
Standard 4.7.0.1: Nutrition Learning Experiences for Children
Standard 4.7.0.2: Nutrition Education for Parents/Guardians
Appendix C: Nutrition Specialist, Registered Dietitian, Licensed Nutritionist, Consultant, and Food Service Staff Qualifications
Appendix JJ: Our Child Care Center Supports Breastfeeding

STANDARD 9.2.3.12: Infant Feeding Policy

A policy about infant feeding should be developed with the input and approval from the nutritionist/registered dietitian and should include the following:

a) Storage and handling of expressed human milk;
b) Determination of the kind and amount of commercially prepared formula to be prepared for infants as appropriate;
c) Preparation, storage, and handling of infant formula;
d) Proper handwashing of the caregiver/teacher and the children;

e) Use and proper sanitizing of feeding chairs and of mechanical food preparation and feeding devices, including blenders, feeding bottles, and food warmers;
f) Whether expressed human milk, formula, or infant food should be provided from home, and if so, how much food preparation and use of feeding devices, including blenders, feeding bottles, and food warmers, should be the responsibility of the caregiver/teacher;
g) Holding infants during bottle-feeding or feeding them sitting up;
h) Prohibiting bottle propping during feeding or prolonging feeding;
i) Responding to infants' need for food in a flexible fashion to allow cue feedings in a manner that is consistent with the developmental abilities of the child (policy acknowledges that feeding infants on cue rather than on a schedule may help prevent obesity) (1,2);
j) Introduction and feeding of age-appropriate solid foods (complementary foods);
k) Specification of the number of children who can be fed by one adult at one time;
l) Handling of food intolerance or allergies (e.g., cow's milk, peanuts, orange juice, eggs, wheat).

Individual written infant feeding plans regarding feeding needs and feeding schedule should be developed for each infant in consultation with the infant's primary care provider and parents/guardians.

RATIONALE: Growth and development during infancy require that nourishing, wholesome, and developmentally appropriate food be provided, using safe approaches to feeding. Because individual needs must be accommodated and improper practices can have dire consequences for the child's health and safety, the policy for infant feeding should be developed with professional nutritionists/registered dietitians. The infant feeding plans should be developed with each infant's parents/guardians and, when appropriate, in collaboration with the child's primary care provider.

TYPE OF FACILITY: Center; Large Family Child Care Home; Small Family Child Care Home

RELATED STANDARDS:
Standard 4.3.1.1: General Plan for Feeding Infants
Standard 4.3.1.2: Feeding Infants on Cue by a Consistent Caregiver/Teacher
Standard 4.3.1.3: Preparing, Feeding, and Storing Human Milk
Standard 4.3.1.4: Feeding Human Milk to Another Mother's Child
Standard 4.3.1.5: Preparing, Feeding, and Storing Infant Formula
Standard 4.3.1.8: Techniques for Bottle Feeding
Standard 4.3.1.11: Introduction of Age-Appropriate Solid Foods to Infants
Standard 4.3.1.12: Feeding Age-Appropriate Solid Foods to Infants
Appendix JJ: Our Child Care Center Supports Breastfeeding

REFERENCES:
1. Birch, L., W. Dietz. 2008. *Eating behaviors of young child: Prenatal and postnatal influences on healthy eating*, 59-93. Elk Grove Village, IL: American Academy of Pediatrics.

2. Taveras, E. M., S. L. Rifas-Shiman, K. S. Scanlon, L. M. Grummer-Strawn, B. Sherry, M. W. Gillman. 2006. To what extent is the protective effect of breastfeeding on future overweight explained by decreased maternal feeding restriction? *Pediatrics* 118:2341-48.

STANDARD 9.2.3.13: Plans for Evening and Nighttime Child Care

Facilities that provide evening and nighttime care should have plans for such care that include the supervision of sleeping children and the management and maintenance of sleep equipment including their sanitation and disinfection. Evacuation drills should occur during hours children are in care. Centers should have these plans in writing.

RATIONALE: Evening child care routines are similar to those required for daytime child care with the exception of sleep routines. Evening and nighttime child care requires special attention to sleep routines, safe sleep environment, supervision of sleeping children, and personal care routines, including bathing and tooth brushing. Nighttime child care must meet the nutritional needs of the children and address morning personal care routines such as toileting/diapering, hygiene, and dressing for the day. Children and staff must be familiar with evacuation procedures in case a natural or human generated disaster occurs during evening child care and nighttime child care hours.

COMMENTS: Sleeping time is a very sensitive time for infants and young children. Attention should be paid to individual needs, transitional objects, lighting preferences, and bedtime routines.

TYPE OF FACILITY: Center; Large Family Child Care Home; Small Family Child Care Home

RELATED STANDARDS:
Standard 2.2.0.1: Methods of Supervision of Children
Standards 3.3.0.4-3.3.0.5: Cleaning Individual Bedding and Crib Surfaces
Standards 5.4.5.1-5.4.5.5: Sleep and Rest Areas
Standards 9.2.4.3-9.2.4.5: Evacuation and Emergency Plans, Drills, and Communication

STANDARD 9.2.3.14: Oral Health Policy

The program should have an oral health policy that includes the following:

a) Information about fluoride content of water at the facility;
b) Contact information for each child's dentist;
c) Resource list for children without a dentist;
d) Implementation of daily tooth brushing or rinsing the mouth with water after eating;
e) Use of sippy cups and bottles only at mealtimes during the day, not at naptimes;
f) Prohibition of serving sweetened food products;
g) Promotion of healthy foods per the USDA's Child and Adult Care Food Program (CACFP);
h) Early identification of tooth decay;
i) Age-appropriate oral health educational activities;
j) Plan for handling dental emergencies.

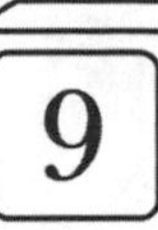

RATIONALE: Good oral hygiene is as important for a six-month-old child with one tooth as it is for a six-year-old with many teeth (1). Tooth brushing and activities at home may not suffice to develop the skill of proper tooth brushing or accomplish the necessary plaque removal, especially when children eat most of their meals and snacks during a full day in child care.

TYPE OF FACILITY: Center; Large Family Child Care Home; Small Family Child Care Home

RELATED STANDARDS:
Standard 3.1.5.1-3.1.5.3: Oral Health
Standard 5.5.0.1: Storage and Labeling of Personal Articles

REFERENCES:

1. American Academy of Pediatric Dentistry. 2009. Clinical guideline on periodicity of examination, preventive dental services, anticipatory guidance, and oral treatment for children. *Pediatric Dentistry* 30:112-18.

STANDARD 9.2.3.15: Policies Prohibiting Smoking, Tobacco, Alcohol, Illegal Drugs, and Toxic Substances

Facilities should have written policies addressing the use and possession of tobacco products, alcohol, illegal drugs, prescription medications that have not been prescribed for the user, and unauthorized potentially toxic substances. Policies should include that all of these substances are prohibited inside the facility, on facility grounds, and in any vehicles that transport children at all times. Policies should specify that smoking is prohibited at all times and in all areas used by the children in the program. Smoking is also prohibited in any vehicles that transport children.

Policies must also specify that use and possession of all substances referred to above is prohibited during all times when caregivers/teachers are responsible for the supervision of children, including times when children are transported, when playing in outdoor play areas not attached to the facility, and during field trips.

Child care centers and large family child care homes should provide information to employees about available drug, alcohol, and tobacco counseling and rehabilitation, and any available employee assistance programs.

RATIONALE: The age, defenselessness, and lack of discretion of the child under care make this prohibition an absolute requirement.

The hazards of second-hand and third-hand smoke exposure warrant the prohibition of smoking in proximity of child care areas at any time. Third-hand smoke refers to gases and particles clinging to smokers' hair and clothing, cushions, carpeting and outdoor equipment after visible tobacco smoke has dissipated (1). The residue includes heavy metals, carcinogens, and even radioactive materials that young children can get on their hands and ingest, especially if they're crawling or playing on the floor. Residual toxins from smoking at times when the children are not using the space can trigger asthma and allergies when the children do use the space (1,2).

Safe child care necessitates sober caregivers/teachers. Alcohol and illegal drug use and misuse of prescription or over-the-counter (OTC) drugs prevent caregivers/teachers from providing appropriate care to infants and children by impairing motor coordination, judgment, and response time. Off-site use prior to or during work, of alcohol, illegal drugs, OTC medications, or prescription medications that have not been prescribed for the user, is prohibited.

The use of alcoholic beverages in family child care homes after children are not in care is permissible.

COMMENTS: The policies related to smoking and use of prohibited substances should be discussed with staff and parents/guardians. Educational material such as handouts could include information on the health risks and dangers of these prohibited substances and referrals to services for counseling or rehabilitation programs.

For family child care home, it is strongly urged that, whenever possible, the caregivers/teachers be non-tobacco users because of the role model effect of tobacco users on children. The entire home should be kept smoke-free at all times to prevent exposure of the children who are cared for in these spaces.

TYPE OF FACILITY: Center; Large Family Child Care Home; Small Family Child Care Home

RELATED STANDARDS:
Standard 3.4.1.1: Use of Tobacco, Alcohol, and Illegal Drugs

REFERENCES:

1. Winickoff, J. P., J. Friebely, S. E. Tanski, C. Sherrod, G. E. Matt, M. F. Hovell, R. C. McMillen. 2009. Beliefs about the health effects of "thirdhand" smoke and home smoking bans. *Pediatrics* 123: e74-79.
2. U.S. Environmental Protection Agency. Smoke-free homes and cars program. http://www.epa.gov/smokefree/.

STANDARD 9.2.3.16: Policy Prohibiting Firearms

Centers should have a written policy prohibiting firearms, ammunition, and ammunition supplies.

Large or small family homes should have a written policy that if firearms and other weapons are present, they should:

a) Have child protective devices;
b) Be unloaded or disarmed;
c) Be kept under lock and key;
d) Be inaccessible to children.

For large and small family homes the policy should include that ammunition and ammunition supplies should be:

a) Placed in locked storage;
b) Separate from firearms;
c) Inaccessible to children.

Parents/guardians should be notified that firearms and other weapons are on the premises.

RATIONALE: The potential for injury to and death of young children due to firearms is apparent (1-3). These items should not be accessible to children in a facility (2,3).

TYPE OF FACILITY: Center; Large Family Child Care Home; Small Family Child Care Home

REFERENCES:

1. American Academy of Pediatrics, Committee on Injury and Poison Prevention. 2004. Policy statement: Firearm-related injuries affecting the pediatric population. *Pediatrics* 114:1126.
2. DiScala, C., R. Sege. 2004. Outcomes in children and young adults who are hospitalized for firearms-related injuries. *Pediatrics* 113:1306-12.
3. Grossman, D. C., B. A. Mueller, C. Riedy, et al. 2005. Gun storage practices and risk of youth suicide and unintentional firearm injuries. *JAMA* 296:707-14.

STANDARD 9.2.3.17: Child Care Health Consultant's Review of Health Policies

At least annually, after an incident or injury has occurred, or when changes are made in the health policies, the facility should obtain input and a review of the policies from a child care health consultant.

RATIONALE: Changes in health information may require changes in the health policies of a child care facility. These changes are best known to health professionals who stay in touch with sources of updated information and can suggest how the new information applies to the operation of the child care program (1,2). For example, when the information on the importance of back-positioning for putting infants down to sleep became available, it needed to be added to child care policies. Frequent changes in recommended immunization schedules offer another example of the need for review and modification of health policies.

TYPE OF FACILITY: Center; Large Family Child Care Home; Small Family Child Care Home

RELATED STANDARDS:
Standard 1.6.0.1: Child Care Health Consultants

REFERENCES:

1. Alkon, A., J. Farrer, J. Bernzweig. 2004. Child care health consultants' roles and responsibilities: Focus group findings. *Pediatric Nursing* 30:315-21.
2. Dellert, J. C, D. Gasalberti, K. Sternas, P. Lucarelli, J. Hall. 2006. Outcomes of child care health consultation services for child care providers in New Jersey: A pilot study. *Pediatric Nursing* 32:530-37.

9.2.4 Emergency/Security Policies and Plans

STANDARD 9.2.4.1: Written Plan and Training for Handling Urgent Medical Care or Threatening Incidents

The facility should have a written plan for reporting and managing what they assess to be an incident or unusual occurrence that is threatening to the health, safety, or welfare of the children, staff, or volunteers. The facility should also include procedures of staff training on this plan.

The management, documentation, and reporting of the following types of incidents, at a minimum, that occur at the child care facility should be addressed in the plan:

a) Lost or missing child;
b) Suspected maltreatment of a child (also see state's mandates for reporting);
c) Suspected sexual, physical, or emotional abuse of staff, volunteers, or family members occurring while they are on the premises of the child care facility;
d) Injuries to children requiring medical or dental care;
e) Illness or injuries requiring hospitalization or emergency treatment;
f) Mental health emergencies;
g) Health and safety emergencies involving parents/guardians and visitors to the program;
h) Death of a child or staff member, including a death that was the result of serious illness or injury that occurred on the premises of the child care facility, even if the death occurred outside of child care hours;
i) The presence of a threatening individual who attempts or succeeds in gaining entrance to the facility.

The following procedures, at a minimum, should be addressed in the plan for urgent care:

a) Provision for a caregiver/teacher to accompany a child to a source of urgent care and remain with the child until the parent/guardian assumes responsibility for the child;
b) Provision for the caregiver/teacher to provide the medical care personnel with an authorization form signed by the parent/guardian for emergency medical care and a written informed consent form signed by the parent/guardian allowing the facility to share the child's health records with other service providers;
c) Provision for a backup caregiver/teacher or substitute for large and small family child care homes to make the arrangement for urgent care feasible (child:staff ratios must be maintained at the facility during the emergency);
d) Notification of parent/guardian(s);
e) Pre-planning for the source of urgent medical and dental care (such as a hospital emergency room, medical or dental clinic, or other constantly staffed facility known to caregivers/teachers and acceptable to parents/guardians);
f) Completion of a written incident/injury report and the program's response;
g) Assurance that the first aid kits are resupplied following each first aid incident, and that required contents are maintained in a serviceable condition, by a monthly review of the contents;
h) Policy for scheduled reviews of staff members' ability to perform first aid for averting the need for emergency medical services;
i) Policy for staff supervision following an incident when a child is lost, missing, or seriously injured.

RATIONALE: Emergency situations are not conducive to calm and composed thinking. A written plan provides the opportunity to prepare and to prevent poor judgments made under the stress of an emergency.

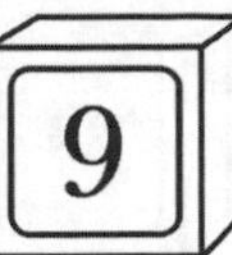

Unannounced mock situations used as drills can help ease tension and build confidence in the staff's ability to respond calmly in the event of a real incident. Discussion regarding performance and opportunities for improvement should follow the drill.

An organized, comprehensive approach to injury prevention and control is necessary to ensure that a safe environment is provided to children in child care. Such an approach requires written plans, policies, procedures, and record-keeping so that there is consistency over time and across staff and an understanding between parents/guardians and caregivers/teachers about concerns for, and attention to, the safety of children.

Routine restocking of first aid kits is necessary to ensure supplies are available at the time of an emergency. Staff should be trained in the use of standard precautions during the response to any situation in which exposure to bodily fluids could occur. Management within the first hour or so following a dental injury may save a tooth.

Intrusions by threatening individuals to child care facilities have occurred, some involved violence resulting in injury and death. These threats have come from strangers who gained access to the playground or an unsecured building, or impaired family members who had easy access to a secured building. Facilities must have a plan for what to do in such situations (1-3).

COMMENTS: The American Academy of Pediatrics' policy statement, "Medical Emergencies Occurring at School" contains information including a comprehensive list of resources that is relevant to child care facilities. The Emergency Medical Services for Children National Resource Center (http://www.childrensnational.org/emsc/) has downloadable print information for emergency medical training, particularly the brochure entitled "Emergency Guidelines for School" at http://ems.ohio.gov/EMSC web site_11_04/pdf_doc files/EMSCGuide.pdf. This site also lists internet links to emergency plans for specific health needs such as diabetes, asthma, seizures, and allergic reactions. Resources for emergency response to non-medical incidents can be found at http://www.chtc.org/dl/handouts/20061114/20061114-2.pdf and http://dcf.vermont.gov/sites/dcf/files/pdf/cdd/care/EmergencyResponse.pdf.

It is recommended that parents/guardians inform caregivers/teachers their preferred sources for medical and dental care in case of emergency. Parents/guardians should be notified, if at all possible, before dental services are rendered, but emergency care should not be delayed because the child's own dentist is not immediately available.

Facilities should develop and institute measures to control access of a threatening individual to the facility and the means of alerting others in the facility as well as summoning the police if such an event occurs.

TYPE OF FACILITY: Center; Large Family Child Care Home; Small Family Child Care Home

RELATED STANDARDS:

Standards 1.5.0.1-1.5.0.2: Substitutes
Standard 3.2.3.4: Prevention of Exposure to Blood and Bodily Fluids
Standard 3.6.4.5: Death
Standard 9.2.4.2: Review of Written Plan for Urgent Care
Standard 9.2.4.3: Disaster Planning, Training, and Communication
Standard 9.4.1.9: Records of Injury
Standard 9.4.1.10: Documentation of Parent/Guardian Notification of Injury, Illness, or Death in Program
Standard 9.4.1.11: Review and Accessibility of Injury and Illness Reports
Standard 9.4.2.1: Contents of Child's Records

REFERENCES:

1. AFP. 2009. Belgian charged over daycare killings. *Nine News,* Jan 24. http://news.ninemsn.com.au/world/.
2. Haggerty, R. 2010. Man kills self after firing shots at day care. *Journal Sentinel,* Feb 17. http://www.jsonline.com/news/crime/.
3. Guerra, C. 2010. Child care providers get lessons in Lee County on being prepared. *News-Press,* Apr 19. http://beta.news-press.com.

STANDARD 9.2.4.2: Review of Written Plan for Urgent Care

The facility's written plan for urgent medical care and threatening incidents should be reviewed and updated annually or as needed. It should be reviewed with each employee upon employment and yearly thereafter in the facility to ensure that policies and procedures are understood and followed in the event of such an occurrence. The plan and associated procedures should be reviewed with a child care health consultant once a year, signed and dated.

In the event that there is an urgent medical care or threatening incident, the facility should plan to review the process within one to two months after the incident to determine opportunities for improvement and any changes that need to be made to the plan for future incidents.

The care plan for a child with special health care needs should cover emergency care needs and be shared with and discussed between parents/guardians and caregivers/teachers prior to an emergency situation (1).

RATIONALE: Emergency situations are not conducive to calm and composed thinking. Developing a written plan and reviewing it in pre-service meetings with new employees and annually thereafter, provides the opportunity to prepare and to prevent poor judgments made under the stress of an emergency.

An organized, comprehensive approach to injury prevention and control based on current practice and evidence is necessary to ensure that a safe environment is provided to children in child care. Such an approach requires written plans, policies, procedures, and record-keeping so that there is consistency over time and across staff and an understanding between parents/guardians and caregivers/teachers about concerns for, and attention to, the safety of children.

TYPE OF FACILITY: Center; Large Family Child Care Home; Small Family Child Care Home

RELATED STANDARDS:
Standards 3.4.3.1-3.4.3.3: Emergency Procedures
Standard 3.5.0.1: Care Plan for Children with Special Health Care Needs
Standard 9.2.4.3: Disaster Planning, Training, and Communication
Appendix O: Care Plan for Children with Special Health Care Needs
Appendix CC: Incident Report Form
Appendix KK: Authorization for Emergency Medical/Dental Care

REFERENCES:

1. American Academy of Pediatrics, Committee on Pediatric Emergency Medicine. 2008. Policy statement: Emergency preparedness for children with special health care needs. *Pediatrics* 122:450.

STANDARD 9.2.4.3: Disaster Planning, Training, and Communication

Facilities should consider how to prepare for and respond to emergency or natural disaster situations and develop written plans accordingly. All programs should have procedures in place to address natural disasters that are relevant to their location (such as earthquakes, tornados, tsunamis or flash floods, storms, and volcanoes) and all hazards/disasters that could occur in any location including acts of violence, bioterrorism/terrorism, exposure to hazardous agents, facility damage, fire, missing child, power outage, and other situations that may require evacuation, lock-down, or shelter-in-place.

Written Emergency/Disaster Plan:

Facilities should develop and implement a written plan that describes the practices and procedures they use to prepare for and respond to emergency or disaster situations. This Emergency/Disaster Plan should include:

a) Information on disasters likely to occur in or near the facility, county, state, or region that require advance preparation and/or contingency planning;
b) Plans (and a schedule) to conduct regularly scheduled practice drills within the facility and in collaboration with community or other exercises;
c) Mechanisms for notifying and communicating with parents/guardians in various situations (e.g., Website postings; email notification; central telephone number, answering machine, or answering service messaging; telephone calls, use of telephone tree, or cellular phone texts; and/or posting of flyers at the facility and other community locations);
d) Mechanisms for notifying and communicating with emergency management public officials;
e) Information on crisis management (decision-making and practices) related to sheltering in place, relocating to another facility, evacuation procedures including how non-mobile children and adults will be evacuated, safe transportation of children including children with special health care needs, transporting necessary medical equipment obtaining emergency medical care, responding to an intruder, etc.;
f) Identification of primary and secondary meeting places and plans for reunification of parents/guardians with their children;
g) Details on collaborative planning with other groups and representatives (such as emergency management agencies, other child care facilities, schools, emergency personnel and first responders, pediatricians/health professionals, public health agencies, clinics, hospitals, and volunteer agencies including Red Cross and other known groups likely to provide shelter and related services);
h) Continuity of operations planning, including backing up or retrieving health and other key records/files and managing financial issues such as paying employees and bills during the aftermath of the disaster;
i) Contingency plans for various situations that address:
   1) Emergency contact information and procedures;
   2) How the facility will care for children and account for them, until the parent/guardian has accepted responsibility for their care;
   3) Acquiring, stockpiling, storing, and cycling to keep updated emergency food/water and supplies that might be needed to care for children and staff for up to one week if shelter-in-place is required and when removal to an alternate location is required;
   4) Administering medicine and implementing other instructions as described in individual special care plans;
   5) Procedures that might be implemented in the event of an outbreak, epidemic, or other infectious disease emergency (e.g., reviewing relevant immunization records, keeping symptom records, implementing tracking procedures and corrective actions, modifying exclusion and isolation guidelines, coordinating with schools, reporting or responding to notices about public health emergencies);
   6) Procedures for staff to follow in the event that they are on a field trip or are in the midst of transporting children when an emergency or disaster situation arises;
   7) Staff responsibilities and assignment of tasks (facilities should recognize that staff can and should be utilized to assist in facility preparedness and response efforts, however, they should not be hindered in addressing their own personal or family preparedness efforts, including evacuation).

Details in the Emergency/Disaster Plan should be reviewed and updated bi-annually and immediately after any relevant event to incorporate any best practices or lessons learned into the document.

Facilities should identify in advance which agency or agencies would be the primary contact for them regarding child care regulations, evacuation instructions, and other directives that might be communicated in various emergency or disaster situations.

Training:

Staff should receive training on emergency/disaster planning and response. Training should be provided by emergency management agencies, educators, child care health

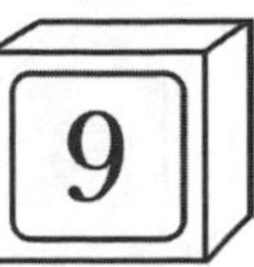

consultants, health professionals, or emergency personnel qualified and experienced in disaster preparedness and response. The training should address:

a) Why it is important for child care facilities to prepare for disasters and to have an Emergency/Disaster Plan;
b) Different types of emergency and disaster situations and when and how they may occur;
   1) Natural Disasters;
   2) Terrorism (i.e., biological, chemical, radiological, nuclear);
   3) Outbreaks, epidemics, or other infectious disease emergencies;
c) The special and unique needs of children, appropriate response to children's physical and emotional needs during and after the disaster, including information on consulting with pediatric disaster experts;
d) Providing first aid, medications, and accessing emergency health care in situations where there are not enough available resources;
e) Contingency planning including the ability to be flexible, to improvise, and to adapt to ever-changing situations;
f) Developing personal and family preparedness plans;
g) Supporting and communicating with families;
h) Floor plan safety and layout;
i) Location of emergency documents, supplies, medications, and equipment needed by children and staff with special health care needs;
j) Typical community, county, and state emergency procedures (including information on state disaster and pandemic influenza plans, emergency operation centers, and incident command structure);
k) Community resources for post-event support such as mental health consultants, safety consultants;
l) Which individuals or agency representatives have the authority to close child care programs and schools and when and why this might occur;
m) Insurance and liability issues;
n) New advances in technology, communication efforts, and disaster preparedness strategies customized to meet children's needs.

Communicating with Parents/Guardians:

Facilities should share detailed information about facility disaster planning and preparedness with parents/guardians when they enroll their children in the program, including:

a) Portions of the Emergency/Disaster Plan relevant to parents/guardians or the public;
b) Procedures and instructions for what parents/guardians can expect if something happens at the facility;
c) Description of how parents/guardians will receive information and updates during or after a potential emergency or disaster situation;
d) Situations that might require parents/guardians to have a contingency plan regarding how their children will be cared for in the unlikely event of a facility closure.

Facilities should conduct an annual drill, test, or "practice use" of the communication options/mechanisms that are selected.

RATIONALE: The only way to prepare for disasters is to consider various worst case or unique scenarios, and to develop contingency plans. By brainstorming and thinking through a variety of "what if..." situations and developing records, protocols/procedures, and checklists, facilities will be better able to respond to an unusual emergency or disaster situation.

Providing clear, accurate, and helpful information to parents/guardians as soon as possible is crucial. Sharing written policies with parents/guardians when they enroll their child, informing them of routine practices, and letting them know how they will receive information and updates, will help them understand what to expect. Notifying parents/guardians about emergencies or disaster situations without causing alarm or prompting inappropriate action is challenging. The content of such communications will depend on the situation. Sometimes, it will be necessary to provide information to parents/guardians before all details are known. In a serious situation, the federal government, the governor, or the state or county health official may announce or declare a state of emergency, a public health emergency, or a disaster. If a facility is unsure of what to do, the first point of contact in any situation should be the local health authority. The local health authority, in partnership with emergency personnel and other officials will know how to engage the appropriate public health and other professionals for the situation.

COMMENTS: Disaster planning and response protocols are unique, and they are typically customized to the type of emergency or disaster; geographical area; identified needs and available resources; applicable federal, state, and local regulations; and the incident command structure in place at the time. The U.S. Department of Homeland Security and the Federal Emergency Management Agency (FEMA) operate under a set of principles and authorities described in various laws and the National Response Framework (see http://www.fema.gov/emergency/nrf/ for details). Each state is required to maintain a state disaster preparedness plan and a separate plan for responding to a pandemic influenza. These plans may be developed by separate agencies, and the point person or the key contact for a child care facility can be the State Emergency Coordinator, a representative in the State Department of Health, an individual associated with the agency that licenses child care facilities for that state, or another official. The State Child Care Administrator is a key contact for any facility that receives federal support.

To develop an Emergency/Disaster Plan that is effective and in compliance with state requirements, the facility must identify who their key contact would be (and what the requirements for their program might be in an emergency or disaster situation) in advance of an unexpected situation. Identifying and connecting with the appropriate key contact before a disaster strikes is crucial for many reasons, but particularly because the identified official may not know how to contact or connect with individual child care facilities.

In addition, representatives within the local school system (especially school administrators and school nurses) may have effective and more direct connections to the state disaster preparedness and response system. If facilities do not communicate with the schools in their area on a regular basis, staff should consider establishing a direct link to and partnership with school representatives already involved in disaster planning and response efforts.

Certain emergency/disaster situations may result in exceptions being made regarding state or local regulations (either in existing facilities or in temporary facilities). In these situations, facilities should make every effort to meet or exceed the temporary requirements.

Early childhood professionals, child care health and safety experts, child care health consultants, health care professionals, and researchers with expertise in child development or child care may be asked to support the development of or help to implement emergency, temporary, or respite child care. These individuals may also be asked to assist with caring for children in shelters or other temporary housing situations. A "shelter-in-place" refers to "the process of staying where you are and taking shelter, rather than trying to evacuate" (2).

Early education and child care facilities and pediatricians are rarely considered or included in disaster planning or preparedness efforts, and unfortunately the needs of children are often overlooked. Children have important physical, physiological, developmental, and psychological differences from adults that can and must be anticipated in the disaster planning process. Staff, pediatricians, health care professionals, and child advocates can and should prepare to assume a primary mission of advocating for children before, during, and after a disaster (1). These professionals should be open to fulfilling this obligation in whatever manner presents, in whatever capacity is required at the moment.

For additional resources on disaster planning for child care and early education programs, see the following Websites:

http://www.aap.org/disasters/ (American Academy of Pediatrics);

http://www.naccrra.org/for_parents/coping/disaster.php (National Association of Child Care Resource and Referral Agencies);

http://nccic.acf.hhs.gov/emergency/ (National Child Care Information Center);

http://www.ecels-healthychildcarepa.org/article.cfm?contentID=27 (Healthy Child Care Pennsylvania).

A good source on business continuity or operations planning is http://www.ready.gov/business/plan/planning.html.

TYPE OF FACILITY: Center; Large Family Child Care Home; Small Family Child Care Home

RELATED STANDARDS:
Standards 3.4.3.1-3.4.3.3: Emergency Procedures
Standard 9.2.4.4: Written Plan for Seasonal and Pandemic Influenza

REFERENCES:
1. American Academy of Pediatrics, Committee on Pediatric Emergency Medicine, Task Force on Terrorism. 2006. Policy statement: The pediatrician and disaster preparedness. *Pediatrics* 117:560-65.
2. National Association of Child Care Resource and Referral and Save the Children, Domestic Emergencies Unit. 2010. *Protecting children in child care during emergencies*. http://www.naccrra.org/publications/naccrra-publications/publications/8960503_Disaster Report-SAVE_MECH.pdf.

STANDARD 9.2.4.4: Written Plan for Seasonal and Pandemic Influenza

The facility should have a written plan for seasonal and pandemic influenza (flu) to limit and contain influenza-related health hazards to the staff, children, their families and the general public. The plan should include information on:

a) Planning and coordination:
   1) Forming a committee of staff members, parents/guardians, and the child care health consultant to produce/review a plan for dealing with the flu each year including specific plans if there is a flu pandemic;
   2) Reviewing the seasonal flu plan during and after flu season so that key staff could discuss how the program would plan for a more serious outbreak or pandemic;
   3) Assigning one person to identify reliable sources of information regarding the seasonal flu strain or pandemic flu outbreak considering local, state and national resources, monitor public health department announcements and other guidance, and forward key information to staff and parents/guardians as needed (the child care health consultant can be especially helpful with this);
   4) Including the infection control policy and procedure (see below) and a communication plan (see below) in the seasonal flu plan;
   5) Including a communication plan (see below), the infection control policy and procedure (see below), and the child learning and program operations plan (see below) in the pandemic flu plan. In addition the pandemic flu plan should include:
      i) Identification of who in the program's community has legal authority to close child care programs if there is a public health emergency or pandemic;
      ii) A list of key contacts such as representatives at the local/state health departments and agencies that regulate child care and their plans to combat or address seasonal or pandemic influenza (programs can extend an invitation for consultation from these departments when formulating the plan).
      iii) Development of a plan of action for addressing key business continuity and programmatic issues relevant to pandemic flu;
      iv) Communication to parents/guardians encouraging them to have a back-up plan for

care for their children if the program must be closed;

v) Collaboration with those in charge of the community's planning to find other sources of meals for low-income children who receive subsidized meals in child care in case of a closure;

vi) Knowledge of services in the community that can help staff, children, and their families deal with stress and other problems caused by a flu pandemic;

vii) Communicate with other child care programs in the area to share information and possibly share expertise and resources.

b) Communications plan:

1) Developing a plan for keeping in touch during the flu and/or pandemic with staff members and children's families;

2) Ensuring staff and families have read and understand the flu and/or pandemic plan and understand why it's needed;

3) Communicating reliable information to staff and children's families on the issues listed below in their languages and at their reading levels:

i) How to help control the spread of flu by handwashing/cleansing and covering the mouth when coughing or sneezing (see http://www.cdc.gov/flu/school/);

ii) How to recognize a person that may have the flu, and what to do if they think they have the flu (see http://www.pandemicflu.gov);

iii) How to care for family members who are ill (see http://www.hhs.gov/pandemicflu/plan/sup5.html#box4/);

iv) How to develop a family plan for dealing with a flu pandemic (see http://pandemicflu.gov/individualfamily/).

c) Infection control policy and procedures:

1) Developing a plan for keeping children who become ill at the child care facility away from other children until the family arrives, such as a fixed place for holding children who are ill in an area of their usual caregiving room or in a separate room where interactions with unexposed children and staff will be limited;

2) Establishing and enforcing guidelines for excluding children with infectious diseases from attending the child care facility (1);

3) Teaching staff, children, and their parents/guardians how to limit the spread of infection (see http://www.cdc.gov/flu/school/ and http://www.healthykids.us/cleanliness.htm);

4) Maintaining adequate supplies of items to control the spread of infection;

5) Educating families about the influenza vaccine, including that experts recommend yearly influenza vaccine (and an influenza-specific vaccine, for example H1N1, if necessary) for everyone, however, if there is a vaccine shortage, priority should be given to children and adolescents six months through eighteen years of age, caregivers/teachers of all children younger than five years of age, and health care professionals (see http://www.cdc.gov/flu/);

6) Staff caring for all children should receive annual vaccination against influenza (and an influenza-specific vaccine such as what was used during the 2009 H1N1 pandemic, if necessary) each year, preferably before the start of the influenza season (as early as August or September) and as long as influenza is circulating in the community, immunization should continue through March or April;

7) Maintaining accurate records when children or staff are ill with details regarding their symptoms and/or the kind of illness (especially when influenza was verified through testing);

8) Practicing daily health checks of children and adults each day for illness;

9) Determining guidelines to support staff members to remain home if they think they might be ill and a mechanism to provide paid sick leave so they can stay home until completely well without losing wages.

d) Child learning and program operations:

1) Plan how to deal with program closings and staff absences;

2) Support families in continuing their child's learning if the child care program or preschool is closed;

3) Plan ways to continue basic functions (meeting payroll, maintaining communication with staff, children, and families) if modifications to program planning are necessary or the program is closed.

The facility should also include procedures for staff and parent/guardian training on this plan.

Some of the above plan components may be beyond the scope of ability in a small family child care home. In this case, the caregiver/teacher should work closely with a child care health consultant to determine what specific procedures can be implemented and/or adapted to best meet the needs of the caregiver/teacher and the families s/he serves.

RATIONALE: Yearly or seasonal influenza is a serious illness that requires specific management to keep children healthy. A pandemic flu is a flu virus that spreads much more easily and is much more deadly. The goals of planning for an influenza pandemic are to save lives and to reduce adverse personal, social, and economic consequences of a pandemic. Pandemics, while rare, are not new. In the twentieth century, three flu pandemics were responsible for more than fifty million deaths worldwide and almost a million deaths in the United States (7,8). As it is not possible to predict with certainty when the next flu pandemic will occur or how severe it will be, seasonal flu management and preparation is essential to minimize the potentially devastating effects (1-4).

COMMENTS: The Centers for Disease Control and Prevention (CDC) and the American Academy of Pediatrics (AAP) recommend annual influenza vaccination for children and caregivers/teachers in child care settings. Vaccination is the best method for preventing flu and its potentially severe complications in children (5,6). The CDC and AAP recommend children and adolescents six months through eighteen years of age, for all adults including household contacts, caregivers/teachers of all children younger than five years of age, and health care professionals get the flu vaccine. Certain groups of children are at increased risk for flu complications. Child care health consultants are very helpful with finding and coordinating the local resources for this planning. In addition most state and/or local health departments have resources for pandemic flu planning.

For additional resources, see:

- Children, the Flu and the Flu Vaccine at http://www.cdc.gov/flu/protect/children.htm;
- Protecting Against Influenza (Flu): Advice for Caregivers of Children Less Than 6 Months Old at http://www.cdc.gov/flu/protect/infantcare.htm;
- Preparing for the Flu: A Communication Toolkit for Child Care and Early Childhood Programs at http://www.cdc.gov/h1n1flu/childcare/toolkit/; and
- U.S. Health and Human Services Interagency Public Affairs Group on Influenza Preparedness and Response at http://www.flu.gov.

TYPE OF FACILITY: Center; Large Family Child Care Home; Small Family Child Care Home

RELATED STANDARDS:
Standard 3.1.1.1: Conduct of Daily Health Check
Standard 3.2.2.2: Handwashing Procedure
Standard 3.2.3.2: Cough and Sneeze Etiquette
Standard 3.6.1.1: Inclusion/Exclusion/Dismissal of Children
Standard 3.6.1.2: Staff Exclusion for Illness
Standard 3.6.1.4: Infectious Disease Outbreak Control
Standard 3.6.2.1: Exclusion and Alternative Care for Children Who Are Ill
Standard 7.3.3.1: Influenza Immunization for Children and Caregivers/Teachers
Standard 9.2.4.3: Disaster Planning, Training, and Communication
Standard 9.4.1.2: Maintenance of Records

REFERENCES:

1. Dailey, L. 2009. Excluding children due to illness. Health and Safety Notes. Berkeley, CA: California Childcare Health Program. http://www.ucsfchildcarehealth.org/pdfs/healthandsafety/excl_en0909.pdf.
2. Germann, T. C., K. Kadau, I. M. Longini, C. A. Macken. 2006. Mitigation strategies for pandemic influenza in the U.S. *PNAS* 103:5935-40.
3. American Academy of Pediatrics. 2007. *Pandemic influenza: Warning, children at risk.* Trust for America's Health. http://healthyamericans.org/reports/fluchildren/KidsPandemicFlu.pdf.
4. American Academy of Pediatrics. 2010. Children and disasters: Disaster preparedness to meet children's needs. http://www.aap.org/disasters/pandemic-flu-cc.cfm.
5. Aronson, S. S., T. R. Shope, eds. 2009. *Managing infectious diseases in child care and schools: A quick reference guide.* 2nd ed. Elk Grove Village, IL: American Academy of Pediatrics.
6. American Academy of Pediatrics, Committee on Infectious Diseases. 2010. Policy statement: Recommendation for mandatory influenza immunization of all health care personnel. *Pediatrics* 126:809-15.
7. American Academy of Pediatrics. 2010. Policy statement: Recommendations for prevention and control of influenza in children, 2010-2011. *Pediatrics* 126:816-26.
8. Centers for Disease Control and Prevention. 2010. Influenza vaccination: A summary for clinicians. http://www.cdc.gov/flu/professionals/vaccination/vax-summary.htm.

STANDARD 9.2.4.5: Emergency and Evacuation Drills/Exercises Policy

The facility should have a policy documenting that emergency drills/exercises should be regularly practiced for geographically appropriate natural disasters and human generated events such as:

a) Fire, monthly;
b) Tornadoes, on a monthly basis in tornado season;
c) Floods, before the flood season;
d) Earthquakes, every six months;
e) Hurricanes, annually;
f) Threatening person outside or inside the facility;
g) Rabid animal;
h) Toxic chemical spill;
i) Nuclear event.

All drills/exercises should be recorded. Please see Standard 9.4.1.16: Evacuation and Shelter-in-Place Drill Record for more information.

A fire evacuation procedure should be approved and certified in writing by a fire inspector for centers, and by a local fire department representative for large and small family child care homes, during an annual on-site visit when an evacuation drill is observed and the facility is inspected for fire safety hazards.

Depending on the type of disaster, the emergency drill may be within the existing facility such as in the case of earthquakes or tornadoes where the drill might be moving to a certain location within the building (basements, away from windows, etc.) Evacuation drills/exercises should be practiced at various times of the day, including nap time, during varied activities and from all exits. Children should be accounted for during the practice.

The facility should time evacuation procedures. They should aim to evacuate all persons in the specific number of minutes recommended by the local fire department for the fire evacuation, or recommended by emergency response personnel.

Cribs designed to be used as evacuation cribs, can be used to evacuate infants, if rolling is possible on the evacuation route(s).

RATIONALE: Regular emergency and evacuation drills/exercises constitute an important safety practice in areas where these natural or human generated disasters might occur. The routine practice of such drills fosters a calm, competent response to a natural or human generated disaster when it occurs (1). The extensive turnover of both staff and children, in addition to the changing developmental abilities of the

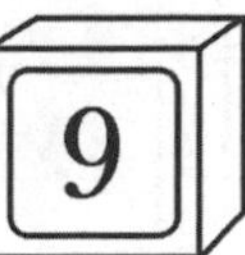

children to participant in evacuation procedures in child care, necessitates frequent practice of the exercises.

COMMENTS: Fire inspectors or local fire department representatives can contribute their expertise when observing evacuation plans and drills. They also gain familiarity with the facility and the facility's plans in the event they are called upon to respond in an emergency. In family child care homes, the possibility of infant rooms or napping areas being located on levels other than the main level makes having consideration and written approval from the fire inspector or local fire department representative of the program's evacuation plan especially important since infants require more assistance compared to other age groups during an evacuation.

TYPE OF FACILITY: Center; Large Family Child Care Home; Small Family Child Care Home

RELATED STANDARDS:
Standard 5.4.5.2: Cribs
Standard 9.2.4.3: Disaster Planning, Training, and Communication
Standard 9.2.4.6: Use of Daily Roster During Evacuation Drills
Standard 9.4.1.16: Evacuation and Shelter-in-Place Drill Record

REFERENCES:
1. Fiene, R. 2002. *13 indicators of quality child care: Research update*. Washington, DC: U.S. Department of Health and Human Services, Office of the Assistant Secretary for Planning and Evaluation. http://aspe.hhs.gov/hsp/ccquality-ind02/.

STANDARD 9.2.4.6: Use of Daily Roster During Evacuation Drills

The center director or his/her designees should use the daily class roster(s) in checking the evacuation and return to a safe space for ongoing care of all children and staff members in attendance during an evacuation drill. In centers caring for more than thirty children enrolled, the center director should assign one caregiver per classroom, the responsibility of bringing the class roster on evacuation drills and accounting for every child and classroom staff at the onset of the evacuation, at the evacuation site and upon return to a safe place. The center director or designee should account for all non-classroom staff, volunteers, and visitors during the evacuation drill process using the program's sign-in/sign-out system.

Small and large family home child caregivers/teachers should count or use a daily roster to be sure that all children and staff are safely evacuated and returned to a safe space for ongoing care during an evacuation drill.

RATIONALE: There must be a plan to account for all the children and adults in a facility at the time of an evacuation. Assigning responsibility to use a roster(s) in a center, or count the children and adults in a large or small family child care home, ensures that all children and adults are accounted for. Practice accounting for children and adults during evacuation drills makes it easier to do in an emergency situation.

TYPE OF FACILITY: Center; Large Family Child Care Home; Small Family Child Care Home

RELATED STANDARDS:
Standard 9.2.4.7: Sign-In/Sign-Out System

STANDARD 9.2.4.7: Sign-In/Sign-Out System

The facility should have a sign-in/sign-out system to track who enters and exits the facility. The system should include name, contact number, relationship to facility (e.g., parent/guardian, vendor, guest, etc.) and recorded time in and out.

RATIONALE: This system helps to maintain a secure environment for children and staff. It also provides a means to contact visitors if needed (such as a disease outbreak) or to ensure all individuals in the building are evacuated in case of an emergency.

TYPE OF FACILITY: Center; Large Family Child Care Home

RELATED STANDARDS:
Standard 9.2.4.8: Authorized Persons to Pick Up Child
Standard 9.2.4.9: Policy on Actions to be Followed When No Authorized Person Arrives to Pick Up a Child
Standard 9.2.4.10: Documentation of Drop-Off, Pick-Up, Daily Attendance of Child, and Parent/Provider Communication

STANDARD 9.2.4.8: Authorized Persons to Pick Up Child

Names, addresses, and telephone numbers of persons authorized to take a child under care out of the facility should be maintained during the enrollment process along with clarification/documentation of any custody issues/court orders. The legal guardian(s) of the child should be established and documented at this time.

If there is an extenuating circumstance (e.g., the parent/guardian or other authorized person is not able to pick up the child), another individual may pick up a child from child care if they are authorized to do so by the parent/guardian in authenticated communication such as a witnessed phone conversation in which the caller provides pre-specified identifying information or writing with pre-specified identifying information. The telephone authorization should be confirmed by a return call to the parents/guardians. The facility should establish a mechanism for identifying a person for whom the parents/guardians have given the facility prior written authorization to pick up their child, such as requiring photo ID or including a photo of each authorized person in the child's file.

If a previously unauthorized individual drops off the child, he or she will not be authorized to pick up the child without first being added to the authorization record. Policies should address how the facility will handle the situation if a parent/guardian arrives who is intoxicated or otherwise incapable of bringing the child home safely, or if a non-custodial parent attempts to claim the child without the consent of the custodial parent.

Should an unauthorized individual arrive without the facility receiving prior communication with the parent/guardian, the parent/guardian should be contacted immediately, preferably privately. If the information provided by the parent/guardian does not match the information and identification

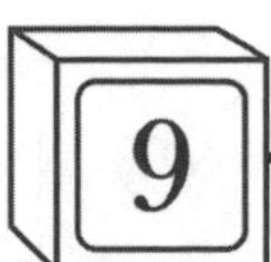

of the unauthorized individual, the child will not be permitted to leave the child care facility. If it is determined that the parent/guardian is unaware of the individual's attempt to pick-up the child, or if the parent/guardian has not or will not authorize the individual to take the child from the child care facility, information regarding the individual should be documented and the individual should be asked to leave. If the individual does not leave and his or her behavior is concerning to the child care staff or if the child is abducted by force, then the police should be contacted immediately with a detailed description of the individual and any other obtainable information such as a license plate number.

RATIONALE: Releasing a child into the care of an unauthorized person may put the child at risk. If the caregiver/teacher does not know the person, it is the caregiver's/teacher's responsibility to verify that the person picking up the child is authorized to do so. This requires checking the written authorization in the child's file and verifying the identity of the person. Caregivers/teachers must not be unwitting accomplices in schemes to gain custody of children by accepting a telephone authorization provided falsely by a person claiming to be the child's custodial parent or claiming to be authorized by the parent/guardian to pick up the child.

COMMENTS: The facility can use photo identification such as photographs supplied by the parents/guardians, photo taken with a camera by the facility, photo ID such as a driver's license, as a mechanism for verifying the identification of a new person to whom the parents/guardians have given written authorization to pick up their child. Identification methods may include passwords.

Caregivers/teachers should consider having a child car seat policy stating all authorized persons that pick-up a child have an age-appropriate car seat to transport a child from the child care program. This policy is discussed with parents/guardians during the enrollment process. Repeated failure to comply with the policy may be grounds for dismissal. Many child care facilities have extra car seats on hand to lend in case a parent/guardian forgets one (1).

Caregivers/teachers should not attempt to handle on their own an unstable (e.g., intoxicated) parent/guardian who wants to be admitted but whose behavior poses a risk to the children. Caregivers/teachers should consult local police or the local child protection agency about their recommendations for how staff can obtain support from law enforcement authorities to avoid incurring increased liability by releasing a child into an unsafe situation or by improperly refusing to release a child.

TYPE OF FACILITY: Center; Large Family Child Care Home; Small Family Child Care Home

RELATED STANDARDS:
Standard 9.2.4.9: Policy on Actions to Be Followed When No Authorized Person Arrives to Pick Up a Child

REFERENCES:
1. Public Counsel Law Center in California. 1998. Guidelines for releasing children and custody issues. http://www.publiccounsel.org/publications/release.pdf.

STANDARD 9.2.4.9: Policy on Actions to Be Followed When No Authorized Person Arrives to Pick Up a Child

Child care facilities should have a written policy identifying actions to be taken when no authorized person arrives to pick up a child. The plan should be developed in consultation with the child care health consultant and child protective services.

In the event that no authorized person arrives to pick up a child, the facility should attempt to reach each authorized contact listed in the child's record. If these efforts fail, the facility should immediately implement the written policy on actions to be followed when no authorized person arrives to pick up a child.

RATIONALE: Child care facilities are responsible for all the children in their care. If an authorized person does not come to pick up a child, and one cannot be reached, the caregiver/teacher must know what authority to call and to whom they can legally and safely release the child. This is to insure the safety of the child and to protect the caregiver/teacher.

COMMENTS: A sample pick-up and drop-off policy is provided in *Model Child Care Health Policies*, available at http://www.ecels-healthychildcarepa.org/content/MHP4th Ed Total.pdf.

TYPE OF FACILITY: Center; Large Family Child Care Home; Small Family Child Care Home

RELATED STANDARDS:
Standard 9.2.4.8: Authorized Persons to Pick Up Child

STANDARD 9.2.4.10: Documentation of Drop-Off, Pick-Up, Daily Attendance of Child, and Parent/Provider Communication

Child care programs should have policies that include:

a) A daily attendance record should be maintained, listing the times of arrival and departure of the child, as well as the person dropping off and picking up;
b) Parents/guardians are expected to communicate (confirmation required) with the caregiver/teacher/program on a daily basis by a specified time if their child will not be in attendance;
c) The caregiver/teacher/program must communicate as early as possible (within one hour) with the parent/guardian if there is no communication from the parent/guardian about a child's absence. If the caregiver/teacher/program is unable to reach the child's parent/guardian, emergency contacts will be notified;
d) A timely method of communication (phone, email, text, etc.) between the parent/guardian and the caregiver/teacher/program should be agreed upon at the time of enrollment;
e) A printed roster should be available in the event of an evacuation drill or evacuation to account for the children in care.

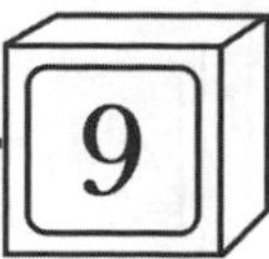

RATIONALE: Operational control to accommodate the health and safety of individual children requires basic information regarding each child in care. This standard ensures that the facility knows which children are receiving care at any given time including evacuation. It aids in the surveillance of child:staff ratios, knowledge of potentially infectious diseases (i.e., influenza), planning for staffing, and provides data for program planning. Accurate record keeping also aids in tracking the amount (and date) of service for reimbursement and allows for documentation in the event of child abuse allegations or legal action involving the facility. Furthermore, each year, twenty to forty children die from hyperthermia after being left/locked in a car or van. Some of these unfortunate deaths include children whose parents/guardians meant to drop their child off at a child care program or preschool; thus, timely communication with these parents/guardians could prevent death from hyperthermia (1,2).

COMMENTS: Time clocks and cards can serve as verification, but they should be signed by the adult who drops off and picks up the child each day. Some notification system should be used to alert the caregiver/teacher whenever the responsibility for the care of the child is being transferred to or from the caregiver/teacher to another person.

TYPE OF FACILITY: Center; Large Family Child Care Home, Small Family Child Care Home

RELATED STANDARDS:
Standard 9.2.4.7: Sign-In/Sign-Out System
Appendix F: Enrollment/Attendance/Symptom Record

REFERENCES:
1. Guard, A., S. S. Gallagher. 2005. Heat related deaths to young children in parked cars: An analysis of 171 fatalities in the United States, 1995-2002. *Injury Prevention* 11:33-37.
2. Null, J. 2010. Hyperthermia deaths of children in vehicles. San Francisco State University. http://ggweather.com/heat/.

9.2.5 Transportation Policies

STANDARD 9.2.5.1: Transportation Policy for Centers and Large Family Homes

Written policies should address the safe transport of children by vehicle to or from the facility, including field trips, home pick-ups and deliveries, and special outings. The transportation policy should include:

a) Licensing of vehicles and drivers;
b) Vehicle selection to safely transport children, based on vehicle design and condition;
c) Operation and maintenance of vehicles;
d) Driver selection, training, and supervision;
e) Child:staff ratio during transport;
f) Accessibility to first aid kit, emergency ID/contact and pertinent health information for passengers, cell phone, or two-way radio;
g) Permitted and prohibited activities during transport;
h) Backup arrangements for emergencies;
i) Use of seat belt and car safety seat, including booster seats;
j) Drop-off and pick-up plans;
k) Plan for communication between the driver and the child care facility staff;
l) Maximum travel time for children (no more than forty-five minutes in one trip);
m) Procedures to ensure that no child is left in the vehicle at the end of the trip or left unsupervised outside or inside the vehicle during loading and unloading the vehicle;
n) Use of passenger vans.

RATIONALE: Motor vehicle crashes are the leading cause of death in children two to fourteen years of age in the United States (1). It is necessary for the safety of children to require that the caregiver/teacher comply with requirements governing the transportation of children in care, in the absence of the parent/guardian. Not all vehicles are designed to safely transport children, especially young children. The National Highway Traffic Safety Administration (NHTSA) recommends that preschool and school aged children should not be transported in twelve- or fifteen-passenger vehicles due to safety concerns (2,3). Children have died because they have fallen asleep and been left in vehicles. Others have died or been injured when left outside the vehicle when thought to have been loaded into the vehicle. The process of loading and unloading children from a vehicle can distract caregivers/teachers from adequate supervision of children either inside or outside the vehicle. Policies and procedures must account for the management of these risks.

COMMENTS: Maintenance should include an inspection checklist for every trip. Vehicle maintenance service should be performed according to the manufacturer's recommendations or at least every three months.

TYPE OF FACILITY: Center; Large Family Child Care Homes

RELATED STANDARDS:
Standard 1.1.1.4: Ratios and Supervision During Transportation
Standard 6.5.1.2: Qualifications for Drivers
Standard 6.5.2.1: Drop-Off and Pick-Up
Standard 6.5.2.2: Child Passenger Safety
Standard 6.5.3.1: Passenger Vans

REFERENCES:
1. National Safety Council (NSC). 2009. *Injury facts*. 2009 ed. Chicago: NSC.
2. National Highway Traffic Safety Association. Safecar.gov. http://www.safercar.gov.
3. National Highway Traffic Safety Association. Passenger van safety. http://www.safercar.gov/Vehicle+Shoppers/Passenger+Van+Safety/.

STANDARD 9.2.5.2: Transportation Policy for Small Family Child Care Homes

Written policies should address the safe transport of children by vehicle to and from the small family child care home for any reason while the children are attending child care. Policies should include field trips or special outings. The following should be provided for:

a) Child:staff ratio during transport;
b) Backup arrangements for emergencies;

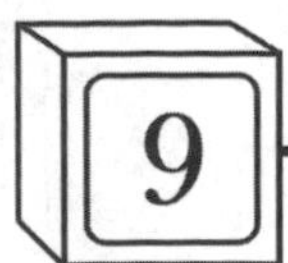

c) Use of seat belt and car safety seat, including booster seats;
d) Accessibility to first aid kit, emergency ID/contact and pertinent health information for passengers, and cell phone or two-way radio;
e) Licensing of vehicles and drivers;
f) Maintenance of the vehicles;
g) Safe use of air bags;
h) Maximum travel time for children (no more than forty-five minutes in one trip);
i) Procedures to ensure that no child is left in the vehicle at the end of the trip or left unsupervised outside or inside the vehicle during loading and unloading the vehicle;
j) Use of passenger vans.

RATIONALE: Motor vehicle crashes are the leading cause of death for children between one and fourteen years of age in the United States (1). It is necessary for the safety of children to require that the caregiver comply with minimum requirements governing the transportation of children in care, in the absence of the parent/guardian. Children have died because they have fallen asleep and left in vehicles. Others have died or been injured when left outside the vehicle when thought to have been loaded into the vehicle. The process of loading and unloading children from a vehicle can distract caregivers/teachers from adequate supervision of children either inside or outside the vehicle. Policies and procedures should account for the management of these risks.

TYPE OF FACILITY: Small Family Child Care Home

RELATED STANDARDS:

Standard 1.1.1.4: Ratios and Supervision During Transportation
Standard 6.5.2.2: Child Passenger Safety
Standard 6.5.3.1: Passenger Vans

REFERENCES:

1. Centers for Disease Control and Prevention, National Center for Injury Prevention and Control. 2008. Web-based injury statistics query and reporting system. http://www.cdc.gov/ncipc/wisqars/.

9.2.6 Play Area Policies

STANDARD 9.2.6.1: Policy on Use and Maintenance of Play Areas

Child care facilities should have a policy on the use and maintenance of play areas that address the following:

a) Safety, purpose, and use of indoor and outdoor equipment for gross motor play;
b) Selection of age-appropriate equipment;
c) Supervision of indoor and outdoor play spaces;
d) Staff training (to be addressed as employees receive training for other safety measures);
e) Recommended inspections of the facility and equipment, as follows:
   1) Inventory, once at the time of purchase, and updated when changes to equipment are made in the playground;
   2) Audits of the active (gross motor) play areas (indoors and outdoors) by an individual with specialized training in playground inspection, once a year;
   3) Monthly inspections to check for U.S. Consumer Product Safety Commission (CPSC) recalled or hazard warnings on equipment, broken equipment or equipment in poor repair that requires immediate attention;
   4) Daily safety check of the grounds for safety hazards such as broken bottles and toys, discarded cigarettes, stinging insect nests, and packed surfacing under frequently used equipment like swings and slides;
   5) Whenever injuries occur.

For centers, the policy should be written. Documentation of the recommended inspections should be maintained in a master file.

RATIONALE: Properly laid out outdoor play spaces, age-appropriate, properly designed and maintained equipment, installation of energy-absorbing surfaces, and adequate supervision of the play space by caregivers/teachers/parents/guardians help to reduce both the potential and the severity of injury (2). Indoor play spaces must also be properly laid out with care given to the location of equipment and the energy-absorbing surface under the equipment. A written policy with procedures is essential for education of staff and may be useful in situations where liability is an issue. The technical issues associated with the selection, maintenance, and use of playground equipment and surfacing are complex and specialized training is required to conduct annual inspections. Active play areas are associated with the most frequent and the most severe injuries in child care (1).

COMMENTS: Increasing awareness and understanding of issues in child safety highlight the importance of developing and maintaining safe play spaces for children in child care settings (3). Parents/guardians expect that their child will be adequately supervised and will not be exposed to hazardous play environments, yet will have the opportunity for free, creative play.

To obtain information on identifying a Certified Playground Safety Inspector (CPSI) to inspect a playground, contact the National Recreation and Park Association (NRPA) at http://www.nrpa.org/Content.aspx?id=3531.

The National Program for Playground Safety (NPPS) is another source of information on playground safety at http://www.uni.edu/playground/.

TYPE OF FACILITY: Center; Large Family Child Care Home; Small Family Child Care Home

RELATED STANDARDS:

Chapter 6: Play Areas and Equipment
Standards 9.2.6.2-9.2.6.3: Play Area and Equipment Records/Reports

REFERENCES:

1. Rivara, F. P., J. J. Sacks. 1994. Injuries in child day care: An overview. *Pediatrics* 94:1031-33.
2. U.S. Consumer Product Safety Commission. 2008. *Public playground safety handbook*. Washington, DC: CPSC. http://www.cpsc.gov/cpscpub/pubs/325.pdf.

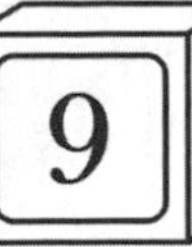

3. Quality in Outdoor Environments for Child Care. POEMS Website. http://www.poemsnc.org.

STANDARD 9.2.6.2: Reports of Annual Audits/ Monthly Maintenance Checks of Play Areas and Equipment

Report forms should be used to record the results of the annual audits of the indoor and outdoor play areas and monthly maintenance inspections of play equipment and surfaces. Corrective actions taken to eliminate hazards and reduce the risk of injury should be included in the reports. The forms should be filed in the facility's master file. The forms should be reviewed by the facility annually and should be retained for the number of years required by the state's statute of limitations.

RATIONALE: Written records of annual audits of the indoor and outdoor play areas, monthly maintenance inspections and appropriate corrective action are necessary to reduce the risk of potential injury. Annual review of such records provides a mechanism for periodic monitoring and improvement of equipment and surface type and quality (1).

COMMENTS: Individual jurisdictions may have specific regulations regarding information, records, equipment, policies, and procedures.

A sample site checklist is provided in *Model Child Care Health Policies*, available at http://www.ecels-healthychildcarepa.org/content/MHP4thEd Total.pdf.

For more information regarding facility equipment, contact ASTM International (ASTM) at http://www.astm.org, the U.S. Consumer Product Safety Commission (CPSC) at http://www.cpsc.gov, and the National Program for Playground Safety (NPPS) at http://www.uni.edu/playground/.

For information about playground safety see the *Public Playground Safety Handbook*, available at http://www.cpsc.gov/cpscpub/pubs/325.pdf and *Outdoor Home Playground Safety Handbook* available at http://www.cpsc.gov/cpscpub/pubs/324.pdf.

TYPE OF FACILITY: Center; Large Family Child Care Home

RELATED STANDARDS:
Standard 9.2.6.1: Policy on Use and Maintenance of Play Areas

REFERENCES:
1. U.S. Consumer Product Safety Commission. 2010. *Public playground safety handbook*. http://www.cpsc.gov/cpscpub/pubs/325.pdf.

STANDARD 9.2.6.3: Records of Proper Installation and Maintenance of Facility Equipment

The facility should maintain all information and records pertaining to the manufacture, installation, and regular inspection of facility equipment. Recordkeeping on play area equipment is specified in Standard 9.2.6.2. No second-hand equipment should be used in areas occupied by children, unless all pertinent data, including checking for recalls and the manufacturer's instructions, can be obtained from the previous owner or from the manufacturer. All equipment should meet ASTM International (ASTM) standards.

RATIONALE: Information regarding manufacture, installation, and maintenance of equipment is essential so that the staff can follow appropriate instructions regarding installation, repair, and maintenance procedures. Also, in the event of recalls, the information provided by the manufacturer allows the owner to identify the applicability of the recall to the equipment on hand. Products used in areas occupied by children must have these instructions for identification, maintenance, repair, and reference in case of recall.

COMMENTS: Individual jurisdictions may have specific regulations regarding information, records, equipment, policies, and procedures.

For more information regarding facility equipment requirements, contact the ASTM at http://www.astm.org and the U.S. Consumer Product Safety Commission (CPSC) at http://www.cpsc.gov.

TYPE OF FACILITY: Center; Large Family Child Care Home; Small Family Child Care Home

RELATED STANDARDS:
Standard 9.2.6.1: Policy on Use and Maintenance of Play Areas

9.3 Human Resource Management

STANDARD 9.3.0.1: Written Human Resource Management Policies for Centers and Large Family Child Care Homes

Centers and large family child care homes should have and implement written human resource management policies. All written policies should be reviewed and signed by the employee affected by them upon hiring and annually thereafter.

These policies should address:

a) A wage scale with merit increases;
b) Sick leave;
c) Vacation leave;
d) Family, parental, medical leave;
e) Personal leave;
f) Educational benefits and professional development expectations;
g) Health insurance and coverage for occupational health services;
h) Social security or other retirement plan;
i) Holidays;
j) Workers' compensation or a disability plan as required by the number of staff;
k) Maternity/paternity benefits;
l) Overtime/compensatory time policy;
m) Grievance procedures;
n) Probation period;
o) Grounds for termination;
p) Training of new caregivers/teachers and substitute staff;
q) Personal/bereavement leave;

r) Disciplinary action;
s) Periodic review of performance;
t) Exclusion policies pertaining to staff illness;
u) Staff health appraisal;
v) Professional development leave.

RATIONALE: Written human resource management provides a means of staff orientation and evaluation essential to the operation of any organization. Caregivers/teachers who are responsible for compliance with policies must have reviewed and understood the policies.

The quality and continuity of the child care workforce is a main determiner of the quality of care (3). Nurturing the nurturers is essential to prevent burnout and promote retention. Fair labor practices apply to child care settings. Caregivers/teachers should be considered as worthy of benefits as workers in other career areas.

Medical coverage should include the cost of the health appraisals and immunizations required of caregivers/teachers. Information abounds about the incidence of infectious disease for children in child care settings (4). Staff members come into close and frequent contact with children and their excretions and secretions and are vulnerable to these illnesses. In addition, many caregivers/teachers are women who are planning a pregnancy or who are pregnant, and they may be vulnerable to the potentially serious effects of infection on the outcome of pregnancy.

Sick leave is important to minimize the spread of infectious diseases and maintain the health of staff members. Sick leave may promote recovery from illness and thereby decreases the further spread or recurrence of illness.

Benefits contribute to higher morale and less staff turnover, thus promoting quality child care (2). Lack of benefits is a major reason reported for high turnover of child care staff (1).

COMMENTS: Staff benefits may be appropriately addressed in human resource management and in state and federal labor standards. Many options are available for providing leave benefits, professional development opportunities, and education reimbursements, ranging from partial to full employer contribution, based on time employed with the facility.

The Center for the Child Care Workforce (CCW) has developed model work standards for both center-based staff and family child care home caregivers/teachers with specific recommendations for these elements of human resource management. Model work standards serve as a tool to help programs assess the quality of the work environment and set goals to make improvements. More information on the CCW is available at http://www.ccw.org.

A policy of encouraging sick leave, even without pay, or of permitting a flexible schedule will allow the caregiver/teacher to take time off when needed for illness. An acknowledgment that the facility does not provide paid leave but does give time off will begin to address workers' rights to these benefits and improve quality of care. There may be other nontraditional ways to achieve these benefits.

The subsidy costs of staff benefits will need to be addressed for child care to be affordable to parents/guardians (5).

Caregivers/teachers should be encouraged to have health insurance. Health benefits can include full coverage, partial coverage (at least 75% employer paid), or merely access to group rates. Some local or state child care associations offer reduced group rates for health insurance for child care facilities and individual caregivers/teachers.

TYPE OF FACILITY: Centers; Large Family Child Care Home

RELATED STANDARDS:
Standards 1.4.2.1-1.4.5.3: Training/Development
Standards 1.5.0.1-1.5.0.2: Substitutes
Standard 1.7.0.1: Pre-Employment and Ongoing Adult Health Appraisals, Including Immunization
Standards 1.8.2.1-1.8.2.5: Evaluation
Standard 3.6.1.2: Staff Exclusion for Illness

REFERENCES:
1. Whitebook, M., D. Bellm. 1999. *Taking on turnover: An action guide for child care center teachers and directors*. Washington, DC: Center for the Child Care Workforce.
2. Klinker, J. M., D. Rile, M. A. Roach. 2005. Organizational climate as a tool for child care staff retention. *Young Children* 60:90-95.
3. Crosland, K. A., G. Dunlap, W. Sager, et al. 2008. The effects of staff training on the types of interactions observed at two group homes for foster care children. *Research on Social Work* 18:410-20.
4. Pickering, L. K., C. J. Baker, D. W. Kimberlin, S. S. Long, eds. *Red book: 2009 report of the Committee on Infectious Diseases*. 28th ed. Elk Grove Village, IL: American Academy of Pediatrics.
5. Towers Perrin. 2009. *Health care reform 2009: Leading employers weigh in—Pulse survey report.* http://www.towersperrin.com/tp/getwebcachedoc?webc=USA/2009/200909/HCR_Pulse-Survey_Sept-09_Final.pdf.

STANDARD 9.3.0.2: Written Human Resource Management Policies for Small Family Child Care Homes

Small family child care home caregivers/teachers should develop policies for themselves, which are reviewed and revised annually.

These policies should address the following items:
a) Vacation leave;
b) Holidays;
c) Professional development leave;
d) Sick Leave;
e) Scheduled increases of small family child care home fees.

If there are assistants or other employees in the home, the following should also be included in the policies:
a) Educational benefits;
b) Personal leave;
c) Family, parental, medical leave;
d) Health insurance and coverage for occupational health services;
e) Social security or other retirement plan;
f) Overtime/compensatory time policy;
g) Workers' compensation or a disability plan as required by the number of staff;

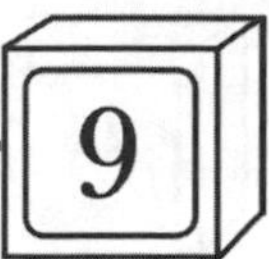

h) Minimally, breaks totaling thirty minutes over an eight-hour period of work, or as required by state labor laws;
i) Grievance procedures;
j) Probation period;
k) Grounds for termination;
l) Training of new caregivers/teachers and substitute staff;
m) Personal/bereavement leave;
n) Disciplinary action;
o) Periodic review of performance;
p) Exclusion policies pertaining to staff illness;
q) Staff health appraisal.

RATIONALE: Written human resource management provides a means of staff orientation and evaluation essential to the operation of any organization. Caregivers/teachers who are responsible for compliance with policies must have reviewed and understood the policies.

The quality and continuity of the child care workforce is a main determiner of the quality of care (3). Nurturing the nurturers is essential to prevent burnout and promote retention. Fair labor practices apply to child care settings. Caregivers/teachers should be considered as worthy of benefits as workers in other career areas.

Medical coverage should include the cost of the health appraisals and immunizations required of caregivers/teachers. Information abounds about the incidence of infectious disease for children in child care settings (4). Staff members come into close and frequent contact with children and their excretions and secretions and are vulnerable to these illnesses. In addition, many caregivers/teachers are women who are planning a pregnancy or who are pregnant, and they may be vulnerable to the potentially serious effects of infection on the outcome of pregnancy.

Sick leave is important to minimize the spread of infectious diseases and maintain the health of staff members. Sick leave may promote recovery from illness and thereby decreases the further spread or recurrence of illness.

Benefits contribute to higher morale and less staff turnover, thus promoting quality child care (2). Lack of benefits is a major reason reported for high turnover of child care staff (1).

COMMENTS: The Center for the Child Care Workforce (CCW) has developed model work standards for both center-based staff and family child care home caregivers/teachers with specific recommendations for these elements of human resource management. Model work standards serve as a tool to help programs assess the quality of the work environment and set goals to make improvements. More information on the CCW is available at http://www.ccw.org.

Caregivers/teachers should be encouraged to have health insurance. Some local or state child care associations offer reduced group rates for health insurance for individual caregivers/teachers.

TYPE OF FACILITY: Small Family Child Care Home

RELATED STANDARDS:
Standards 1.4.2.1-1.4.5.3: Training/Development/Continuing Education
Standards 1.5.0.1-1.5.0.2: Substitutes
Standard 1.7.0.1: Pre-Employment and Ongoing Adult Health Appraisals, Including Immunization
Standards 1.8.2.1-1.8.2.5: Evaluation
Standard 3.6.1.2: Staff Exclusion for Illness

REFERENCES:

1. Whitebook, M., D. Bellm. 1999. *Taking on turnover: An action guide for child care center teachers and directors*. Washington, DC: Center for the Child Care Workforce.
2. Klinker, J. M., D. Rile, M. A. Roach. 2005. Organizational climate as a tool for child care staff retention. *Young Children* 60:90-95.
3. Crosland, K. A., G. Dunlap, W. Sager, et al. 2008. The effects of staff training on the types of interactions observed at two group homes for foster care children. *Research on Social Work* 18:410-20.
4. Pickering, L. K., C. J. Baker, D. W. Kimberlin, S. S. Long, eds. *Red book: 2009 report of the Committee on Infectious Diseases*. 28th ed. Elk Grove Village, IL: American Academy of Pediatrics.

9.4 Records

9.4.1 Facility Records/Reports

STANDARD 9.4.1.1: Facility Insurance Coverage

Facilities should carry the following insurance:
a) Injury insurance on children;
b) Liability insurance;
c) Vehicle insurance on any vehicle owned or leased by the facility and used to transport children;
d) Property insurance.

Small and large family child care home caregivers/teachers should carry this insurance if available.

RATIONALE: Reasonable protection against liability action through proper insurance is essential for reasons of economic security, peace of mind, and public relations. Requiring insurance reduces risks because insurance companies stipulate compliance with health and safety regulations before issuing or continuing a policy. Property insurance is desirable since the costs of adverse events occurring at a facility can easily cause a financial disaster that can disrupt children's care. Protection, via insurance, should be secured to provide stability and protection for both the individuals and the facility. Liability insurance carried by the facility provides recourse for parents/guardians of children enrolled in the event of negligence.

COMMENTS: The liability insurance should include coverage for administration of medications, as well as for unintentional injuries and illnesses. Individual health injury coverage may be documented by evidence of personal health insurance coverage as a dependent.

TYPE OF FACILITY: Center; Large Family Child Care Home; Small Family Child Care Home

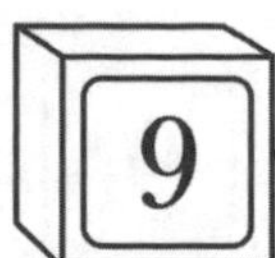

STANDARD 9.4.1.2: Maintenance of Records

The facility should maintain the following records:

a) A copy of the facility's license, insurance coverage, child care regulations or registration, all inspection reports, correction plans for deficiencies, and any legal actions;
b) Physical health records for any adult who has direct contact with children;
c) Training records of the caregiver/teacher and any assistants;
d) Criminal history records and child abuse and neglect records, as required by state licensing regulations;
e) Results of well-water tests where applicable;
f) Results of lead tests;
g) Insurance records;
h) Child health records;
i) Attendance records and sign-in/sign-out records, as well as authorization for pick-up;
j) List of reportable diseases;
k) Incident reports;
l) Fire extinguisher records and smoke detector and carbon monoxide detector battery checks;
m) Evacuation, emergency, and shelter-in-place drill records;
n) Play area and equipment warranty, maintenance, and inspection records;
o) Consultation records;
p) Medication administration logs; and
q) Nutrition and food service records.

The length of time to maintain records should follow state regulation requirements. A sample of a state regulation is below.

RATIONALE: Operational control to accommodate the health and safety of individual children requires that information regarding each child in care be kept and made available on a need-to-know basis. These records and reports are necessary to protect the health and safety of children in care.

An organized, comprehensive approach to injury prevention and control is necessary to ensure that a safe environment is provided for children in child care. Such an approach requires written plans, policies, and procedures, and record keeping so that there is consistency over time and across staff and an understanding between parents/guardians and caregivers/teachers about concerns for, and attention to, the safety of children.

COMMENTS: A file of all purchased equipment and toys with warranty information and model numbers will help identify items that have hazard warnings or are recalled by the U.S. Consumer Product Safety Commission (CPSC). A photo of the purchased items can be added to the file.

A sample of state regulations for length of time to maintain records is below.

Retention of Records

a) Documentation of the previous twelve months activity should be available for review. Records should be accessible during the hours the facility is open and operating.
b) For licensing purposes, children's information should be kept on file a minimum of one year from date of discharge from the facility.
c) For licensing purposes, personnel records should be kept on file a minimum of one year from termination of employment from the facility.
d) For licensing purposes, staff training certificates and continuing education certificates should be kept on file for a minimum of five years for currently employed staff (1).

TYPE OF FACILITY: Center; Large Family Child Care Home; Small Family Child Care Home

RELATED STANDARDS:

Standard 1.2.0.1: Staff Recruitment
Standards 1.4.2.1-1.4.5.3: Training/Development/Continuing Education
Standard 1.7.0.1: Pre-employment and Ongoing Staff Health Appraisal, Including Immunizations
Standards 3.6.4.3-3.6.4.4: Reporting Illness
Standards 5.2.6.2-5.2.6.5: Water Testing
Standard 5.2.9.13: Testing for Lead
Standards 9.2.6.2-9.2.6.3: Play Area and Equipment Warranty, Maintenance, and Inspection Records
Standard 9.4.1.1: Facility Insurance Coverage
Standard 9.4.1.6: Availability of Documents to Parents/Guardians
Standards 9.4.1.8-9.4.1.11: Incident Logs of Illness, Injury, and Other Situations That Require Documentation
Standard 9.4.1.12-9.4.1.18: Maintenance and Availability of Records
Standards 9.4.2.1-9.4.2.7: Child Records
Standard 9.4.3.2: Maintenance of Attendance Records for Staff Who Care for Children

REFERENCES:

1. Louisiana Department of Social Services, Bureau of Licensing. 2003. *Child day care center class "A" minimum standards.* Louisiana Administrative Code Title 48 – Chapter 53. http://www.daycare.com/louisiana/state-a.html.

STANDARD 9.4.1.3: Written Policy on Confidentiality of Records

The facility should establish and follow a written policy on confidentiality of the records of staff and children that ensures that the facility will not disclose material in the records (including conference reports, service plans, immunization records, and follow-up reports) without the written consent of parents/guardians for children, or of staff for themselves. Consent forms should be in the native language of the parents/guardians, whenever possible, and communicated to them in their normal mode of communication. Foreign language interpreters should be used whenever possible to inform parents/guardians about their confidentiality rights. At the time when facilities obtain prior, informed consent from parents/guardians for release of records, caregivers/teachers should inform parents/guardians who may be looking at the records (e.g., child care health consultants, mental health consultants, and specialized agencies providing services).

Written releases should be obtained from the child's parent/guardian prior to forwarding or sharing information and/or the child's records to other service providers. The content of the written procedures for protecting the confidentiality of medical and social information should be consistent with federal, state, and local guidelines and regulations and should be taught to caregivers/teachers. Confidential medical information pertinent to safe care of the child should be provided to facilities within the guidelines of state or local public health regulations. However, under all circumstances, confidentiality about the child's medical condition and the family's status should be preserved unless such information is released at the written request of the family, except in cases where child maltreatment is a concern or to determine compliance with licensing regulations. In such cases, state laws and regulations apply.

The director of the facility should decide who among the staff may have confidential information shared with them. Clearly, this decision must be made selectively, and all caregivers/teachers should be taught the basic principles of all individuals' rights to confidentiality. Caregivers/teachers should not disclose or discuss personal information regarding children and their families with any unauthorized person. Confidential information should be seen by and discussed only with staff members who need the information in order to provide services. Caregivers/teachers should not discuss confidential information about families in the presence of others in the facility.

Procedures should be developed and a method established to ensure accountability and to ensure that the exchange is being carried out. The child's record should be available to the parents/guardians for inspection at all times.

If other children are mentioned in a child's record that is authorized for release, the confidentiality of those children should be maintained. The record should be edited to remove any information that could identify another child.

Caregivers/teachers should not disclose or discuss personal information regarding children and their families with any unauthorized person. Confidential information should be seen by and discussed only with staff members who need the information in order to provide services. Caregivers/teachers should not discuss confidential information about families in the presence of others in the facility.

RATIONALE: Confidentiality must be maintained to protect the child and family and is defined by law (1). Serving children and families involves significant facility responsibilities in obtaining, maintaining, and sharing confidential information. Each caregiver/teacher must respect the confidentiality of information pertaining to all families, staff, and volunteers served (2).

Someone in each facility must be authorized to make decisions about the sharing of confidential information, and the director is the logical choice. The decision about sharing information must also involve the parent/guardian(s). Sharing of confidential information should be selective and should be based on a need-to-know and on the parent's/guardian's authorization for disclosure of such information (3).

Requiring written releases ensures confidentiality. Continuity of care and information is invaluable during childhood when growth and development are rapidly changing. Providing consent forms in the native language of the parents/guardians and providing an interpreter to explain the confidentiality policy and procedures helps to insure that the signed consent is informed consent.

The California Childcare Health Program developed with the Child Care Law Center, "Consent for Exchange of Information Form" that can be viewed at: http://ucsfchildcarehealth.org/pdfs/forms/CForm_ExchangeofInfo.pdf.

COMMENTS: Parental trust in the caregiver is the key to the caregiver's ability to work toward health promotion and to obtain needed information to use in decision making and planning for the child's best interest. Assurance of confidentiality fosters this trust. When custody has been awarded to only one parent, access to records must be limited to the custodial parent. In cases of disputed access, the facility may need to request that the parents/guardians supply a copy of the court document that defines parental rights. Operational control to accommodate the health and safety of individual children requires basic information regarding each child in care.

Release formats may vary from state to state and within facilities. User friendly forms furnished for all caregivers/teachers may facilitate the exchange of information.

TYPE OF FACILITY: Center

RELATED STANDARDS:

Standard 9.4.2.8: Release of Child's Records

REFERENCES:

1. U.S. Congress. 1974. Family Educational Rights and Privacy Act (FERPA). 20 USC Sec 1232.
2. U.S. Department of Health and Human Services (DHHS), Office for Civil Rights. HIPAA administrative simplification statute and rules. Washington, DC: DHHS. http://www.hhs.gov/ocr/privacy/hipaa/administrative/index.html.
3. U.S. Department of Education. FERPA regulations. http://www2.ed.gov/policy/gen/reg/ferpa/.

STANDARD 9.4.1.4: Access to Facility Records

The designated person in charge should have access to the records necessary to manage the facility and should allow regulatory staff access to the facility and records.

RATIONALE: Those with responsibility must have access to the information required to carry out their duties and make reasonable decisions.

TYPE OF FACILITY: Center

RELATED STANDARDS:

Standard 9.4.1.5: Availability of Records to Licensing Agency
Standard 9.4.1.11: Review and Accessibility of Injury and Illness Reports

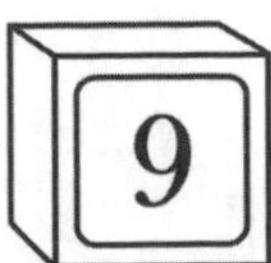

STANDARD 9.4.1.5: Availability of Records to Licensing Agency

Where these standards require the facility to have written policies, reports, and records, these documents should be available to the licensing agency for inspection. In addition, the facility should make available any other policies, reports, or records that are required by the licensing agency that are not specified in these standards.

RATIONALE: The licensing agency monitors policies, reports, and records required to determine the facility's compliance with licensing regulations. Inspection of the policies, reports, and records required by licensing regulations may also include inspection of those addressed by the standards.

TYPE OF FACILITY: Center; Large Family Child Care Home; Small Family Child Care Home

RELATED STANDARDS:
Standard 9.4.1.4: Access to Facility Records

STANDARD 9.4.1.6: Availability of Documents to Parents/Guardians

In an easily available space that parents/guardians are made aware of and able to access, facilities should make available the following items:

a) The facility's license, child care regulations, or registration, which also includes information on how to file a complaint and the telephone number for filing complaints with the regulatory agency;
b) A statement informing parents/guardians about how they may obtain a copy of the licensing or registration requirements from the regulatory agency;
c) Inspection certificates;
d) Reports of any legal sanctions and documentation that all required corrections have been completed;
e) A notice that inspection reports/certificates, legal actions, and compliance letters are available for inspection in the facility;
f) Accreditation certificates;
g) Quality rating score, if applicable;
h) Evacuation route;
i) Emergency evacuation procedures, including fire evacuation and weather related evacuation procedures, to be posted in each room of the center;
j) Procedures for the reporting of child abuse and neglect consistent with state law and local law enforcement and child protective service contacts;
k) Notice announcing the "open-door policy" (parents/guardians may visit at any time and will be admitted without delay);
l) The action the facility will take to handle a visitor's request for access if the caregiver/teacher is concerned about the safety of the children;
m) A current weekly menu of any food or beverage served in the facility to the children for parents/guardians and caregivers/teachers including changes in the menus as they are served; the facility should provide copies of menus to parents/guardians, if requested, and copies of menus served should be kept on file for six months;
n) A statement of nondiscrimination for programs participating in the U.S. Department of Agriculture (USDA) Child and Adult Care Food Program (CACFP) and for programs who receive Child Care Assistance Child Care Development Block Grant (CCDBG) funds;
o) Policy manual (health and safety policies, nutrition and oral health policies, etc.);
p) A copy of the policy and procedures for discipline, including the prohibition of corporal punishment;
q) Legible safety rules for the use of swimming and built-in wading pools if the facility has such pools (safety rules should be posted conspicuously on the pool enclosure);
r) Phone numbers and instructions for contacting the fire department, police, emergency medical services, physicians, dentists, rescue and ambulance services, and the poison center, child abuse reporting hotline; the address of the facility; and directions to the facility from major routes north, south, east, and west (this information should be conspicuously posted adjacent to the telephone);
s) A list of reportable infectious diseases as required by the state and local health authorities;
t) Employee rights and safety standards as required by the Occupational Safety and Health Administration (OSHA) and/or state agencies;
u) Breastfeeding policy that includes information and guidance for mothers on how to store and transport human milk;
v) A notice of what, where and when pesticides have been applied within or around the program's property (this notice should be put up forty-eight hours in advance of any pesticide use);
w) Reports of lead concentration and water quality.

RATIONALE: Each local and/or state regulatory agency gives official permission to certain persons to operate child care programs by virtue of their compliance with regulations. Therefore, documents relating to investigations, inspections, and approval to operate should be made available to consumers, caregivers/teachers, concerned persons, and the community. Posting other documents listed in this standard increases access to parents/guardians over having the policies filed in a less accessible location.

Awareness of the child abuse and neglect reporting requirements and procedures is essential to the prevention of child abuse. State requirements may differ, but those for whom the reporting of child abuse and neglect is mandatory usually include child care personnel. Information on how to call and how to report should be readily available to parents/guardians and caregivers/teachers.

The open-door policy may be the single most important method for preventing maltreatment of children in child care (1). When access is restricted, areas observable by the parents/guardians may not reflect the care the children actually receive.

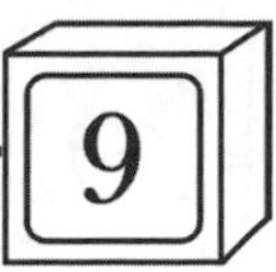

A roster helps parents/guardians see how facility responsibility is assigned and know which children receive care in their child's group.

Primary caregiver assignments foster and channel meaningful communication between parents/guardians and caregivers/teachers.

Children are offered nutritious foods that help assure that children can meet the minimum daily requirements of nutrients. A child care facility is not responsible for the children receiving all of their nutrients. Parents/guardians need to know what food and beverages their children receive while in child care. Menus filed should reflect last-minute changes so that parents/guardians and any nutritionist/registered dietitian who reviews these documents can get an accurate picture of what was actually served. Food allergies should be posted for caregivers/teachers to view easily while still maintaining confidentiality from the public.

Parents/guardians and caregivers/teachers must have a common basis of understanding about what disciplinary measures are to be used to avoid conflict and promote consistency in approach between caregivers/teachers and parents/guardians. Corporal punishment may be physical abuse or become abusive very easily.

Parents/guardians have a right to see any reports and notices of any legal actions taken against the facility that have been sustained by the court. Since unfounded suits may be filed, knowledge of which could undermine parent/guardian confidence, only actions that result in corrections or judgment needs to be made accessible.

Pool safety requires reminders to users of pool rules. Making pool rules available serves as reminder that all pool rules must be strictly adhered to for the safety of the children.

In an emergency, phone numbers must be immediately accessible.

COMMENTS: Compliance can be measured by asking for the location of documents and how accessible they are.

A sample telephone emergency list is provided in *Healthy Young Children* from the National Association for the Education of Young Children (NAEYC) at http://www.naeyc.org.

When it is possible to translate documents into the native language of the parents/guardians of children in care, it increases the level of communication between facility and parents/guardians.

TYPE OF FACILITY: Center; Large Family Child Care Home; Small Family Child Care Home

RELATED STANDARDS:
Standards 2.2.0.4-2.2.0.5: Water Safety
Standards 3.6.4.3-3.6.4.4: Reporting Illness
Standards 4.3.1.1-4.3.1.12: Nutrition for Infants
Standard 5.2.8.1: Integrated Pest Management
Standard 6.3.1.7: Pool Safety Rules
Standard 9.2.1.6: Written Discipline Policies
Standard 9.2.4.3: Disaster Planning, Training, and Communication
Standard 9.4.1.2: Maintenance of Records
Standard 9.4.1.12: Record of Valid License, Certificate, or Registration of Facility
Standard 9.4.1.13: Maintenance and Display of Inspection Reports
Standard 9.4.1.14: Written Plan/Record to Resolve Deficiencies
Standard 9.4.1.18: Records of Nutrition Service
Standards 10.4.3.1-10.4.3.2: Procedures for Complaints and Reporting

REFERENCES:
1. Murph, J. R., S. D. Palmer, D. Glassy, eds. 2005. *Health in child care: A manual for health professionals*. 4th ed. Elk Grove Village, IL: American Academy of Pediatrics.

STANDARD 9.4.1.7: Requirements for Compliance of Contract Services

The facility should assure that any contracted services will comply with all applicable standards and state regulations.

RATIONALE: Whether the director or family child care provider contracts for a service directly or hires an agency to provide the services to be performed, children's safety must be protected and their growth and development supported by strict adherence to applicable standards and state regulations.

COMMENTS: The contract language should not only specify the requirement for compliance, but should also define methods for monitoring and for redress. An example of such a contract is a food service contract or a temporary service agency contract that provides substitute caregivers/teachers.

TYPE OF FACILITY: Center; Large Family Child Care Home; Small Family Child Care Home

STANDARD 9.4.1.8: Records of Illness

In situations where illnesses are reported by a parent/guardian or become evident while a child or staff member is at the facility and may potentially require exclusion, the facility should record the following:

a) Date and time of the illness;
b) Person(s) affected;
c) Description of the symptoms;
d) Response of the staff to these symptoms;
e) Persons notified (such as a parent/guardian, primary care provider, or the local health department representative, if applicable), and their response;
f) Name of person completing the form.

RATIONALE: Recording the occurrence of illness in a facility and the response to the illness, as well as reviewing the daily patterns, characterizes and defines the frequency of the illness, suggests whether an outbreak has occurred, may suggest an effective intervention (improved sanitation and handwashing best practices initially), and provides documentation for administrative purposes.

COMMENTS: Surveillance for symptoms can be accomplished easily by using a combined attendance and symptom records. Any symptoms can be noted when the child is signed in and the daily health check is performed, with added notations made during the day when additional symptoms appear. Simple forms, for a weekly or monthly period, that record data for the entire group help caregivers/

teachers spot patterns of illness for an individual child or among the children in the group or center.

TYPE OF FACILITY: Center; Large Family Child Care Home; Small Family Child Care Home

RELATED STANDARDS:
Standard 3.1.1.1: Conduct of Daily Health Check
Standard 3.6.1.1: Inclusion/Exclusion/Dismissal of Children
Standard 9.4.1.2: Maintenance of Records
Standard 9.4.1.10: Documentation of Parent/Guardian Notification of Injury, Illness, or Death in Program
Appendix F: Enrollment/Attendance/Symptom Record

STANDARD 9.4.1.9: Records of Injury

When an injury occurs in the facility that results in first aid or medical attention for a child or adult, the facility should complete a report form that provides the following information:

a) Name, sex, and age of the injured person;
b) Date and time of injury;
c) Location where injury took place;
d) Description of how the injury occurred, including who (name, address, and phone number) saw the incident and what they reported, as well as what was reported by the child;
e) Body part(s) involved;
f) Description of any consumer product involved;
g) Name and location of the staff member responsible for supervising the child at the time of the injury;
h) Actions taken by staff members on behalf of the injured following the injury as well as specifically whether emergency medical services and/or professional dental/medical care was required;
i) Recommendations of preventive strategies that could be taken to avoid future occurrences of this type of injury;
j) Name of person who completed the report;
k) Name, address, and phone number of the facility;
l) Signature of the parent/guardian of the child injured or signature of the adult injured and the date signature obtained (recommended that the signature be obtained the same day as the injury);
m) If parent/guardian of child was notified at time of injury;
n) Documentation that written report was sent home the day of the injury, regardless of parental signature.

Examples of injuries that should be documented include:

a) Child maltreatment (physical, sexual, emotional, and neglect abuse);
b) Bites that are continuous in nature, break the skin, left a mark, and cause significant pain;
c) Falls, burns, broken limbs, tooth loss, other injury;
d) Motor vehicle injury;
e) Aggressive/unusual behavior;
f) Ingestion of non-food substances;
g) Medication error;
h) Blows to the head;
i) Death.

Three copies of the injury report form should be completed. One copy should be given to the child's parent/guardian (or to the injured adult). The second copy should be kept in the child's (or adult's) folder at the facility. A third copy should be kept in a chronologically filed injury log that is analyzed periodically to determine any patterns regarding time of day, equipment, location or supervision issues. This last copy should be kept in the facility for the period required by the state's statute of limitations. If required by state regulations, a copy of an injury report for each injury that required medical attention should be sent to the state licensing agency.

Based on the logs, the facility should plan to take corrective action. Examples of corrective action include: adjusting schedules, removing or limiting the use of equipment, relocating equipment or furnishings, and/or increasing supervision.

RATIONALE: Injury patterns and child abuse and neglect can be discerned from such records and can be used to prevent future problems (1,2). Known data on typical injuries (scanning for hazards, providing direct supervision, etc.) can also how to prevent them. A report form is also necessary for providing information to the child's parents/guardians and primary care provider and other appropriate health or state agencies.

COMMENTS: Caregivers/teachers should report specific products that may have played a role in the injury to the U.S. Consumer Product Safety Commission (CPSC) via their toll-free consumer hotline: 800-638-2772 (TTY 800-638-8270) or online at http://www.cpsc.gov/talk.html. This data helps CPSC respond with needed recalls. Multi-copy forms can be used to make copies of an injury report simultaneously for the child's record, for the parent/guardian, for the folder that logs all injuries at the facility, and for the regulatory agency.

Facilities should secure the parent's/guardian's signature on the form at the time it is presented to the parent/guardian.

TYPE OF FACILITY: Center; Large Family Child Care Home; Small Family Child Care Home

RELATED STANDARDS:
Standard 9.2.4.1: Written Plan and Training for Handling Urgent Medical Care or Threatening Incidents
Standard 9.4.1.10: Documentation of Parent/Guardian Notification of Injury, Illness, or Death in Program
Standard 9.4.1.11: Review and Accessibility of Injury and Illness Reports
Appendix CC: Incident Report Form
Appendix DD: Injury Report Form for Indoor and Outdoor Injuries
Appendix EE: America's Playgrounds Safety Report Card

REFERENCES:
1. Murph, J. R., S. D. Palmer, D. Glassy, eds. 2005. *Health in child care: A manual for health professionals*. 4th ed. Elk Grove Village, IL: American Academy of Pediatrics.
2. ChildCare.net. Incident reports. http://www.childcare.net/library/incidentreports.shtml.

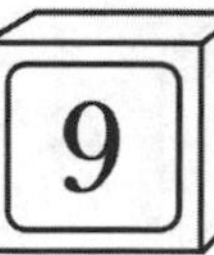

STANDARD 9.4.1.10: Documentation of Parent/Guardian Notification of Injury, Illness, or Death in Program

The facility should document that a child's parent/guardian was notified immediately in the event of a death of their child, of an injury or illness of their child that required professional medical attention, or if their child was lost/missing.

Documentation should also occur noting when law enforcement was notified (immediately) in the event of a death of a child or a lost/missing child.

The facility should document in accordance with state regulations, its response to any of the following events:

a) Death;
b) Serious injury or illness that required medical attention;
c) Reportable infectious disease;
d) Any other significant event relating to the health and safety of a child (such as a lost child, a fire or other structural damage, work stoppage, or closure of the facility).

The caregiver/teacher should call 9-1-1 to insure immediate emergency medical support for a death or serious injury or illness. They should follow state regulations with regard to when they should notify state agencies such as the licensing agency and the local or state health department about any of the above events.

RATIONALE: The licensing agency should be notified according to state regulations regarding any of the events listed above because each involves special action by the licensing agency to protect children, their families, and/or the community. If death, serious injury, or illness or any of the events in item d) occur due to negligence by the caregiver/teacher, immediate suspension of the license may be necessary. Public health staff can assist in stopping the spread of the infectious disease if they are notified quickly by the licensing agency or the facility (1,2). The action by the facility in response to an illness requiring medical attention is subject to licensing review.

A report form that records death, maltreatment, serious injury or illness is also necessary for providing information to the child's parents/guardians and primary care provider, other appropriate health agencies, law enforcement agency, and the insurance companies covering the parents/guardians and the facility.

COMMENTS: Guidance on policies for parental notification of child maltreatment reports should be sought from child care health consultants or local child abuse prevention agencies. Surveillance for symptoms can be accomplished easily by using a combined attendance and symptom record. Any symptoms can be noted when the child is signed in, with added notations made during the day when additional symptoms appear. Simple forms, for a weekly or monthly period, that record data for the entire group help caregivers/teachers spot patterns of illness for an individual child or among the children in the group or center.

Multi-copy forms can be used to make copies of an injury report simultaneously for the child's record, for the parent/guardian, for the folder that logs all injuries at the facility, and for the licensing agency. Facilities should secure the parent/guardian's signature on the form at the time it is presented to the parent/guardian.

TYPE OF FACILITY: Center; Large Family Child Care Home; Small Family Child Care Home

RELATED STANDARDS:

Standard 7.3.5.1: Recommended Control Measures for Invasive Meningococcal Infection In Child Care
Standard 7.3.5.2: Informing Public Health Authorities of Meningococcal Infections
Standard 7.3.7.1: Informing Public Health Authorities of Pertussis Cases
Standard 7.3.10.1: Measures for Detection, Control, and Reporting of Tuberculosis
Standard 7.4.0.1: Control of Enteric (Diarrheal) and Hepatitis A Virus (HAV) Infections
Standard 7.4.0.3: Disease Surveillance of Enteric (Diarrheal) and Hepatitis A Virus (HAV) Infections
Standard 7.4.0.4: Maintenance of Records on Incidents of Diarrhea
Standard 7.6.1.4: Informing Public Health Authorities of Hepatitis B Virus (HBV) Cases
Section 7.8: Interaction with State or Local Health Departments
Standard 9.2.4.1: Written Plan and Training for Handling Urgent Medical Care or Threatening Incidents
Standard 9.4.1.9: Records of Injury
Standard 9.4.1.11: Review and Accessibility of Injury and Illness Reports
Appendix F: Enrollment/Attendance/Symptom Record
Appendix CC: Incident Report Form
Appendix DD: Injury Report Form for Indoor and Outdoor Injuries
Appendix EE: America's Playgrounds Safety Report Card

REFERENCES:

1. Aguero, J., M. Ortega-Mendi, M. Eliecer Cano, A. Gonzalez de Aledo, J. Calvo, L. Viloria, P. Mellado, T. Pelayo, A. Fernandez-Rodriguez, L. Martinez-Martinez. 2008. Outbreak of invasive group A streptococcal disease among children attending a day-care center. *Pediatr Infect Dis J* 27:602-4.
2. Galil, K., B. Lee, T. Strine, C. Carraher, A. L. Baughman, M. Eaton, J. Montero, J. Seward. 2002. Outbreak of varicella at a day-care center despite vaccination. *N Engl J Med* 347:1909-15.

STANDARD 9.4.1.11: Review and Accessibility of Injury and Illness Reports

The injury and illness log should be reviewed by caregivers/teachers at least semi-annually and inspected by licensing staff and child care health consultants at least annually. In addition to maintaining a record for documentation of liability, forms should be used to identify patterns of injury and illness occurring in child care that are amenable to prevention.

RATIONALE: Injury patterns and child abuse and neglect can be detected from such records and can be used to prevent future problems (1). A report form is also necessary for providing information to the child's parents/guardians, primary care provider and other appropriate health agencies.

COMMENTS: Surveillance for symptoms can be accomplished easily by using a combined attendance and symptom record. Any symptoms can be noted when the child is signed in, with added notations made during the day when additional symptoms appear. Simple forms, for a weekly or monthly period, that record data for the entire group help caregivers/teachers spot patterns of illness for an individual child or among the children in the group or center. Child care health consultants can be especially helpful in helping to spot patterns of illness or injury.

TYPE OF FACILITY: Center; Large Family Child Care Home; Small Family Child Care Home

RELATED STANDARDS:
Standard 1.6.0.1: Child Care Health Consultants
Standard 9.2.4.1: Written Plan and Training for Handling Urgent Medical Care or Threatening Incidents
Standard 9.4.1.9: Records of Injury
Standard 9.4.1.10: Documentation of Parent/Guardian Notification of Injury, Illness, or Death in Program
Standards 10.4.2.2-10.4.2.3: Inspections
Appendix F: Enrollment/Attendance/Symptom Record

REFERENCES:
1. Murph, J. R., S. D. Palmer, D. Glassy, eds. 2005. *Health in child care: A manual for health professionals*. 4th ed. Elk Grove Village, IL: American Academy of Pediatrics.

STANDARD 9.4.1.12: Record of Valid License, Certificate, or Registration of Facility

Every facility should hold a valid license or certificate, or documentation of, registration prior to operation as required by the local and/or state statute.

RATIONALE: Licensing registration provides recognition that the facility meets regulatory requirements which are written to insure that children are cared for by qualified staff in a safe environment that supports the children's development and protects them from maltreatment while they are in child care programs.

TYPE OF FACILITY: Center; Large Family Child Care Home; Small Family Child Care Home

STANDARD 9.4.1.13: Maintenance and Display of Inspection Reports

The facility should maintain and display, in one central area within the facility, current copies of inspection reports required by the state licensing office. These reports and documentation may include the following:

a) Licensing/registration reports;
b) Fire inspection reports;
c) Sanitation inspection reports;
d) Building code inspection reports;
e) Plumbing, gas, and electrical inspection reports;
f) Termite and other insect inspection report;
g) Zoning approval;
h) Results of all water tests;
i) Evacuation and shelter-in-place drill records;
j) Any accreditation certificates and/or quality rating score, if applicable;
k) Reports of any legal actions and documentation that all required corrections have been completed;
l) Results of lead tests;
m) Insurance records;
n) Playground inspection report, equipment inspection/maintenance records and reports,
o) Child care health consultant's assessment reports that do not pertain to any specific children.

RATIONALE: Facility safeguarding is not achieved by one agency carrying out a single regulatory program. Total safeguarding is achieved through a multiplicity of regulatory programs and agencies (1). Licensing staff, consumers, and concerned individuals benefit from having documents of regulatory approval and legal action in one central location. Parents/guardians, staff, consultants, and visitors should be able to assess the extent of evaluation and compliance of the facility with regulatory and voluntary requirements. Accreditation documentation provides additional information about surveillance and quality improvement efforts of the facility (2).

TYPE OF FACILITY: Center; Large Family Child Care Home; Small Family Child Care Home

RELATED STANDARDS:
Standards 5.2.6.2-5.2.6.5: Water Testing
Standard 5.2.9.13: Testing for Lead
Standards 9.2.4.3-9.2.4.5: Emergency and Evacuation Plans, Drills, and Communication
Standard 9.2.6.2: Reports of Annual Audits/Monthly Maintenance Checks of Play Areas and Equipment
Standard 9.4.1.1: Facility Insurance Coverage
Standard 9.4.1.16: Evacuation and Shelter-in-Place Drill Record

REFERENCES:
1. National Association for Regulatory Administration (NARA). 2009. *Recommended best practices for human care and regulatory agencies.* The NARA Vision Series Part 1. http://www.naralicensing.org/associations/4734/files/Recommended Best Practices.pdf.
2. National Association for Regulatory Administration (NARA). 2010. *Strong licensing: The foundation for a quality early care and education system; NARA's call to action.* http://www.naralicensing.org/associations/4734/files/NARA_Call_to_Action.pdf.

STANDARD 9.4.1.14: Written Plan/Record to Resolve Deficiencies

When deficiencies are identified during annual policy and performance reviews by the licensing department, funding agency, or accreditation organization, the director or small or large family child care home caregiver/teacher should follow a written plan for resolution, developed with the regulatory agency.

This plan should include the following:

a) Description of the problem;
b) Proposed timeline for resolution;
c) Designation of responsibility for correcting the deficiency;
d) Description of the successful resolution of the problem.

RATIONALE: A written plan or contract for change may be required and is more likely to achieve the desired change (1).

COMMENTS: Simple problems amenable to immediate correction do not require extensive documentation. For these,

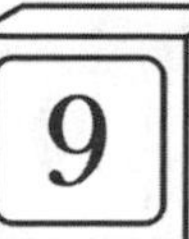

a simple notation of the problem and that the problem was immediately corrected will suffice. However, a notation of the problem is necessary so that recurring problems of the same type can be addressed by a more lasting solution.

TYPE OF FACILITY: Center; Large Family Child Care Home; Small Family Child Care Home

REFERENCES:

1. National Association for Regulatory Administration (NARA). 2000. *The NARA licensing curriculum.* Lexington, KY: NARA.

STANDARD 9.4.1.15: Availability of Reports on Inspections of Fire Protection Devices

A report of the inspection and maintenance of fire extinguishers, smoke detectors, carbon monoxide detectors, or other fire prevention mechanisms should be available for review. The report should include the following information:

a) Location of the fire extinguishers, smoke detectors, carbon monoxide detectors, or other equipment;
b) Date the inspection was performed and by whom;
c) Condition of the equipment;
d) Description of any service provided for the equipment.

Fire extinguishers should be inspected semi-annually. Smoke detectors should be inspected monthly. Carbon monoxide detectors should be checked monthly.

Inspections should be performed in compliance with local and/or state regulations.

RATIONALE: A fire extinguisher may lose its effectiveness over time. It should work properly at any time in case it is needed to put out a small fire or to clear an escape path (1). Since chemicals tend to separate within the canister, maintenance instructions should be followed.

Smoke detectors are often powered by batteries and will need to be checked monthly to ensure they are in operating condition.

COMMENTS: Caregivers/teachers can do the inspection themselves, since many fire extinguishers are equipped with gauges that can be read easily.

TYPE OF FACILITY: Center; Large Family Child Care Home; Small Family Child Care Home

RELATED STANDARDS:

Standard 3.4.3.2: Use of Fire Extinguishers
Standard 5.1.1.3: Compliance with Fire Prevention Code
Standard 5.2.9.5: Carbon Monoxide Detectors

REFERENCES:

1. U.S. Fire Administration. Home fire prevention. http://www.usfa.dhs.gov/citizens/all_citizens/home_fire_prev/index.shtm.

STANDARD 9.4.1.16: Evacuation and Shelter-In-Place Drill Record

A record of evacuation drills, shelter-in-place drills, lock down drills, and of facility participation in community evacuation drills should be kept on file. Type of drill, date and time should be recorded.

RATIONALE: Routine practice of emergency evacuation plans fosters calm, competent use of the plans in an emergency.

COMMENTS: Suggested timing for specific drills:

a) Fire: monthly;
b) Geographically appropriate natural disasters:
    1) Tornadoes: on a monthly basis in tornado season;
    2) Floods: before the flood season;
    3) Earthquakes: every six months;
    4) Hurricanes: annually.

A "shelter-in-place" refers to "the process of staying where you are and taking shelter, rather than trying to evacuate" (1).

TYPE OF FACILITY: Center; Large Family Child Care Home; Small Family Child Care Home

RELATED STANDARDS:

Standards 9.2.4.3-9.2.4.5: Emergency and Evacuation Plans, Drills, and Communication

REFERENCES:

1. National Association of Child Care Resource and Referral and Save the Children, Domestic Emergencies Unit. 2010. Protecting children in child care during emergencies. http://www.naccrra.org/publications/naccrra-publications/publications/8960503_DisasterReport-SAVE_MECH.pdf.

STANDARD 9.4.1.17: Documentation of Child Care Health Consultation/Training Visits

Documentation of child care health/early childhood mental health consultation visits should be maintained in the facility's files. Documentation should include at least the following:

a) Name of child care health/early childhood mental health consultant;
b) Date and time of visit;
c) Recipient(s) of service;
d) Reason for the visit/phone/internet consultation;
e) Type of service provided;
f) Recommendations;
g) Follow-up, if any.

All training or education provided by child care health consultants for early care and education professionals should be documented in a manner that can be used to meet professional development requirements or documentation. Recommendations and improvement plans should be provided to the staff.

RATIONALE: Child care health consultants, including mental health consultants, licensing agents, health departments, and fellow caregivers/teachers should reinforce the importance of appropriate health behavior. Documentation of health consultation by a child care health consultant or other health professional provides a record of the assessed need in a facility, the strategies to make improvements, and the barriers that result from implementing strategies. The documentation can also be useful in evaluating the effectiveness of the services provided (1).

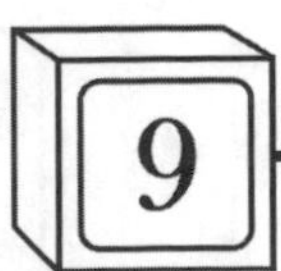

The documentation from the child care health consultant should take the form of a quality improvement plan that includes goals, objectives, timeline, and financial considerations. All encounters should be documented by the child care health consultant. The child care health consultant should use the same standards as would be used to document "patient care" the patient or client in this case is the child care business.

TYPE OF FACILITY: Center; Large Family Child Care Home; Small Family Child Care Home

RELATED STANDARDS:
Standard 1.6.0.1: Child Care Health Consultants
Standard 1.6.0.3: Early Childhood Mental Health Consultants
Standard 1.6.0.4: Early Childhood Education Consultants

REFERENCES:

1. Norwood, S. L. 2003. *Nursing consultation: A Framework for working with communities.* 2nd ed. Upper Saddle River, NJ: Prentice Hall.

STANDARD 9.4.1.18: Records of Nutrition Service

The facility should maintain records covering the nutrition services budget, expenditures for food, menus, numbers and types of meals served daily with separate recordings for children and adults, inspection reports made by health authorities, nutrition education and recipes. Copies should be maintained in the facility files for six months or according to state/local regulations.

RATIONALE: Food service records permit efficient and effective management of the facility's nutrition component and provide data from which a nutritionist/registered dietitian can develop recommendations for program improvement. If a facility is large enough to employ a supervisor for food service who holds certification equivalent to the Food Service Manager's Protection (Sanitation) Certificate, records of this certification should be maintained (1).

COMMENTS: For information on the USDA's Child and Adult Care Food Program (CACFP) and resources for child care, including feeding infants, see the Child Care Providers page on USDA's Food and Nutrition Website http://www.fns.usda.gov/tn/childcare.html and MyPlate for Preschoolers Website http://www.choosemyplate.gov/specificaudiences.html.

TYPE OF FACILITY: Center; Large Family Child Care Home; Small Family Child Care Home

RELATED STANDARDS:
Appendix C: Nutrition Specialist, Registered Dietitian, Licensed Nutritionist, Consultant, and Food Service Staff Qualifications
Appendix Q: Getting Started with MyPlate
Appendix R: Choose MyPlate: 10 Tips to a Great Plate
Appendix S: Physical Activity: How Much Is Needed?

REFERENCES:

1. U.S. Department of Agriculture. 2000. Child and Adult Care Food Program; Improving management and program integrity; Proposed rule. 7 CFR 226. http://www.fns.usda.gov/cnd/Care/Regs-Policy/policymemo/2000-2003/2000-09-12.pdf.

STANDARD 9.4.1.19: Community Resource Information

The facility should obtain or have access to a community resource file that is updated at least annually. This resource file should be made available to parents/guardians as needed. For families who do not speak English, community resource information should be provided in the parents'/guardians' native language or through the use of interpreters (1).

RATIONALE: Posting resources in a public place is a service to the community.

COMMENTS: In many communities, community agencies (such as resource and referral agencies) offer community resource files and may be able to supply updated information or service directories to local caregivers/teachers. Even small family child care home caregivers/teachers will be able to maintain a list of telephone numbers of human services, such as that published in the telephone directory. If a resource file is maintained, it must be updated regularly and should be used by a caregiver/teacher knowledgeable about health and the community (i.e., Health Advocate).

Local resource and referral agencies, mental health services, WIC (Women, Infants, and Children), Child Find, Legal Aid, specialty clinics serving the developmentally disabled, poison centers, social services, community health centers, hospitals, private physicians, state child health insurance programs (SCHIP), medical homes, food banks and pantries, energy/housing assistance, churches, child care payment assistance, public health nurses, Head Start, the American Red Cross, public schools, early intervention programs, and county extension services, faith-based organizations, local government agencies are examples of potential resources.

For locating community resources, see the Maternal and Child Health Library Community Services Locator at http://www.mchlibrary.info/KnowledgePaths/kp_community.html. American Academy of Pediatrics' State Chapter Child Care Contacts are available at http://www.healthychildcare.org.

TYPE OF FACILITY: Center

RELATED STANDARDS:
Standard 2.3.2.3: Support Services for Parents/Guardians
Standard 10.3.4.5: Resources for Parents/Guardians of Children with Special Health Care Needs

REFERENCES:

1. Gonzalez-Mena, J. 2007. *50 early childhood strategies for working and communicating with diverse families.* Upper Saddle River, NJ: Pearson Merrill Prentice Hall.

9.4.2 Child Records

STANDARD 9.4.2.1: Contents of Child's Records

The facility should maintain a file for each child in one central location within the facility. This file should be kept in a confidential manner but should be immediately available to the child's caregivers/teachers (who should have parental/

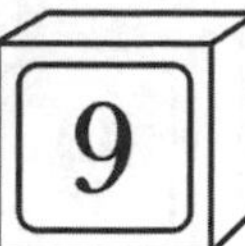

guardian consent for access to records), the child's parents/guardians, and the licensing authority upon request.

The file for each child should include the following:

a) Pre-admission enrollment information;
b) Admission agreement signed by the parent/guardian at enrollment;
c) Initial health care professional assessment, completed and signed by the child's primary care provider and based on the child's most recent well care visit and containing a complete immunization record as recommended at http://www.aap.org/immunization/ and a statement of any special needs with a care plan for how the program should accommodate these special needs (this should be on file preferably at enrollment or a two week written plan should be provided upon admission);
d) Updated health care professional assessments should be completed from the initial assessment filed except that such assessments should be at the recommended intervals by the American Academy of Pediatrics (AAP) until the age of two years and annually thereafter;
e) Health history to be completed by the parent/guardian at admission, preferably with staff involvement;
f) Medication record, maintained on an ongoing basis by designated staff;
g) Authorization form for emergency medical care (see Appendix KK: Authorization for Emergency Medical/Dental Care for an example; this form should not be used for routine problems or when the parent can be reached);
h) Any written informed consent forms signed by the parent/guardian allowing the facility to share the child's health records with other service providers.

RATIONALE: The health and safety of individual children requires that information regarding each child in care be kept and made available on a need-to-know basis. Prior informed, written consent of the parent/guardian is required for the release of records/information (verbal and written) to other service providers, including process for secondary release of records. Consent forms should be in the native language of the parents/guardians, whenever possible, and communicated to them in their normal mode of communication. Foreign language interpreters should be used whenever possible to inform parents/guardians about their confidentiality rights (1).

TYPE OF FACILITY: Center; Large Family Child Care Home; Small Family Child Care Home

RELATED STANDARDS:

Standard 9.4.2.4: Contents of Child's Primary Care Provider's Assessment
Standard 9.4.1.3: Written Policy on Confidentiality of Records
Appendix I: Recommendations for Preventive Pediatric Health Care
Appendix KK: Authorization for Emergency Medical/Dental Care

REFERENCES:

1. American Academy of Pediatrics, Committee on Pediatric Emergency Medicine. 2007. Policy statement: Consent for emergency medical services for children and adolescents. *Pediatrics* 120:683-84.

STANDARD 9.4.2.2: Pre-Admission Enrollment Information for Each Child

The file for each child should include the following pre-admission enrollment information (pre-admission requirements may be waived to comply with the federal McKinney-Vento Homeless Assistance Act regarding health and health records):

a) The child's name, address, sex, and date of birth;
b) The full names of the child's parents/guardians, and their home and work addresses and telephone numbers, which should be updated quarterly (telephone contact numbers should be confirmed by a call placed to the contact number during the facility's hours of operation);
c) The names, addresses, and telephone numbers of at least two additional persons to be notified in the event that the parents/guardians cannot be located (telephone information should be confirmed and updated as specified in item b) above);
d) The names and telephone numbers of the child's medical home provider and main sources of specialty medical care (if any), emergency medical care, and dental care;
e) The child's health payment resource or health insurance;
f) Written instructions (in the form of a care plan) of the parent/guardian and the child's primary care provider for any special dietary needs or special needs due to a health condition or allergy; or any other special instructions from the parent/guardian;
g) Scheduled days and hours of attendance;
h) In the event that a custody or guardianship order has been issued regarding the child, legal documentation evidencing the child's custodian or guardian;
i) Enrollment date, reason for entry in child care, and fee arrangements;
j) Signed permission to act on parent/guardian's behalf for emergency treatment;
k) Authorization to release child to designated individuals other than the custodial parent/guardian.

The emergency information in items a) through e) above should be obtained in duplicate with original parent/guardian signatures on both copies. One copy should be in the child's confidential record and one copy should be easily accessible at all times. This information should be updated quarterly and as necessary. A copy of the emergency information must accompany the child to all offsite excursions.

RATIONALE: These records and reports are necessary to protect the health and safety of children in care. An organized, comprehensive approach to illness and injury prevention and control is necessary to ensure that a healthy and safe environment is provided for children in child care. Such an approach requires written plans, policies, procedures, and record-keeping so that there is consistency over time and across staff and an understanding between parents/guardians and caregivers/teachers about concerns for, and attention to, the safety of children.

Emergency information is the key to obtaining needed care in emergency situations (1). Caregivers/teachers must have written parental permission to allow them access to information they and emergency medical services personnel may need to care for the child in an emergency (1). Contact information must be verified for accuracy. Health payment resource information is usually required before any non-life-threatening emergency care is provided.

COMMENTS: Duplicate records are easily made by scanning copies or making photocopies.

TYPE OF FACILITY: Center; Large Family Child Care Home; Small Family Child Care Home

RELATED STANDARDS:
Standards 9.2.4.8-9.2.4.10: Child Pick-up/Drop-off Policies and Procedures
Appendix BB: Emergency Information for Children with Special Health Care Needs
Appendix KK: Authorization for Emergency Medical/Dental Care

REFERENCES:
1. Murph, J. R., S. D. Palmer, D. Glassy, eds. 2005. *Health in child care: A manual for health professionals*. 4th ed. Elk Grove Village, IL: American Academy of Pediatrics.

STANDARD 9.4.2.3: Contents of Admission Agreement Between Child Care Program and Parent/Guardian

The file for each child should include an admission agreement signed by the parent/guardian at enrollment. The admission agreement should contain the following topics and documentation of consent:

- a) General topics:
  - 1) Operating days and hours;
  - 2) Holiday closure dates;
  - 3) Payment for services;
  - 4) Drop-off and pick-up procedures;
  - 5) Family access (visiting site at any time when their child is there and admitted immediately under normal circumstances) and involvement in child care activities;
  - 6) Name and contact information of any primary staff person designation, especially primary caregivers/teachers designated for infants and toddlers, to make parent/guardian contact of a caregiver/teacher more comfortable.
- b) Health topics:
  - 1) Immunization record;
  - 2) Breast feeding policy;
  - 3) For infants, statement that parent/guardian(s) has received and discussed a copy of the program's infant safe sleep policy;
  - 4) Documentation of written consent signed and dated by the parent/guardian for:
    - i) Any health service obtained for the child by the facility on behalf of the parent/guardian. Such consent should be specific for the type of care provided to meet the tests for "informed consent" to cover on-site screenings or other services provided;
    - ii) Administration of medication for prescriptions and non-prescription medications (over-the-counter [OTC]) including records and special care plans (if needed).
- c) Safety topics:
  - 1) Prohibition of corporal punishment in the child care facility;
  - 2) Statement that parent/guardian has received and discussed a copy of the state child abuse and neglect reporting requirements;
  - 3) Documentation of written consent signed and dated by the parent/guardian for:
    - i) Emergency transportation;
    - ii) All other transportation provided by the facility;
    - iii) Planned or unplanned activities off-premises (such consent should give specific information about where, when, and how such activities should take place, including specific information about walking to and from activities away from the facility);
    - iv) Swimming, if the child will be participating;
    - v) Release of any information to agencies, schools, or providers of services;
    - vi) Written authorization to release the child to designated individuals other than the parent/guardian.

RATIONALE: These records and reports are necessary to protect the health and safety of children in care.

These consents are needed by the person delivering the medical care. Advance consent for emergency medical or surgical service is not legally valid, since the nature and extent of injury, proposed medical treatment, risks, and benefits cannot be known until after the injury occurs, but it does allow the parent/guardian to guide the caregiver/teacher in emergency situations when the parent/guardian cannot be reached (1). See Appendix KK: Authorization for Emergency Medical/Dental Care for an example.

The parent/guardian/child care partnership is vital.

TYPE OF FACILITY: Center; Large Family Child Care Home; Small Family Child Care Home

RELATED STANDARDS:
Appendix KK: Authorization for Emergency Medical/Dental Care

REFERENCES:
1. American Academy of Pediatrics, Committee on Pediatric Emergency Medicine. 2007. Policy statement: Consent for emergency medical services for children and adolescents. *Pediatrics* 120:683-84.

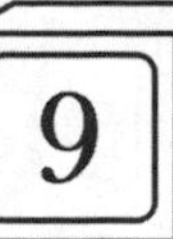

STANDARD 9.4.2.4: Contents of Child's Primary Care Provider's Assessment

The file for each child should include an initial health assessment completed and signed by the child's primary care provider. This should be on file preferably at enrollment and no later than within six weeks of admission. (Requirements may be waived to comply with the federal McKinney-Vento Homeless Assistance Act regarding health and health records.) It should include:

a) Immunization Records;
b) Growth Assessment – may include percentiles of weight, height, and head circumference (under age of two); recording body mass index (BMI) and percentile for age is especially helpful in those children age two years and older who are over or underweight;
c) Health Assessment – includes descriptions of any current acute and/or chronic health issues and should also include any findings from an exam or screening that may need follow-up, e.g., vision, hearing, dental, obesity, or nutritional screens or tests for lead, anemia, or tuberculosis (these health concerns may require a care plan and possibly a medication plan [see h) below]);
d) Developmental Issues – includes descriptions of concerns and the child's special needs in a child care setting, (for example, a vision or hearing deficit, a developmental variation, prematurity, or an emotional or behavioral disturbance);
e) Significant physical findings so that caregivers/teachers can note if there are changes from baseline and report those findings;
f) Dates of Significant Illnesses and/or Injuries;
g) Allergies;
h) Medication(s) List – includes dosage, time and frequency of administration of any ongoing prescription or non-prescription (over-the-counter [OTC]) medication that the person with prescriptive authority recommends for the child. This list would also include information on recognizing side-effects and responding to them appropriately and it may also contain the same information for intermittent use of a fever reducer medication;
i) Dietary modifications;
j) Emergency plans;
k) Other special instructions for the caregiver/teacher;
l) Care Plan – (if the child has a special health need as indicated by c) or d) above) includes routine and emergency management plans that might be required by the child while in child care. This plan also includes specific instructions for caregiver/teacher observations, activities or services that differ from those required by typically developing children and should include specific instructions to caregivers/teachers on how to provide medications, procedures, or implement modifications required by children with asthma, severe allergic reactions, diabetes, medically-indicated special feedings, seizures, hearing impairments, vision problems, or any other condition that requires accommodation in child care;
m) Parent's/Guardian's assessment and concerns (4).

For children up the age of three years, health care professional assessments should be at the recommended intervals indicated by the American Academy of Pediatrics (AAP) (3). For all other children, the Health Care Professional Assessment updates should be obtained annually. It should include any significant health status changes, any new medications, any hospitalizations, and any new immunizations given since the previous health assessment. This health report will be supplemented by the health history obtained from the parents/guardians by the child care provider at enrollment.

RATIONALE: The requirement of a health report for each child reflecting completion of health assessments and immunizations is a valid way to ensure timely preventive care for children who might not otherwise receive it and can be used in decision-making at the time of admission and during ongoing care (2). This requirement encourages families to have a primary care provider (medical home) for each child where timely and periodic well-child evaluations are done. The objective of timely and periodic evaluations is to permit detection and treatment for improved oral, physical, mental, and emotional/social health (1,3). The reports of such evaluations provide a conduit for communication of information that helps the primary care provider and the caregiver/teacher determine appropriate services for the child. When the parent/guardian carries the request for the report to the primary care provider, concerns of the caregiver/teacher can be delivered by the parent/guardian to the child's primary care provider and consent for communication is thereby given. The parent/guardian can give written consent for direct communication between the primary care provider and the caregiver/teacher so that the forms can be faxed or mailed.

Quality child care requires information about the child's health status and need for accommodations in child care (2).

COMMENTS: The purpose of a health care professional assessment is to:

a) Give information about a child's health history, special health care needs, and current health status to allow the caregiver/teacher to provide a safe setting and healthy experience for each child;
b) Promote individual and collective health by fostering compliance with approved standards for health care assessments and immunizations;
c) Document compliance with licensing standards;
d) Serve as a means to ensure early detection of health problems and a guide to steps for remediation;
e) Serve as a means to facilitate and encourage communication and learning about the child's needs among caregivers/teachers, primary care providers, and parents/guardians.

This approach is usually the most efficient, effective and least costly since the primary care provider has the child, the family member, and the record in hand, to provide the information that the child care facility should have. When the data are requested separate from the visit to the primary care provider for the health assessment, the record must be pulled from the file and the information retrieved from the notes in the file. Some health care facilities charge families for the cost of the additional work to complete forms either at the time of a health care visit or later. Collaborating in reducing the burden of form completion by writing in as much information as is known before giving the forms to the primary care provider helps foster effective communication. Many primary care providers appreciate having identifying information filled in on the form about the child care facility, the child, the family and a note about any concerns to be addressed.

Caregivers/teachers may offer a four-week grace period during which the parent/guardian can arrange to get this assessment. The health history can serve as an interim health assessment during this grace period.

Health data should be presented in a form usable for caregivers/teachers to help identify any special needs for care. Local Early Periodic Screening and Diagnostic Treatment (EPSDT) program contractor, if available, should be called upon to help with liaison and education activities. In some situations, screenings may be performed at the facilities, but it is always preferable that the child have a medical home and primary care provider who screens the child and provides the information. When clinicians do not fill out forms completely enough to assist the caregiver/teacher in understanding the significance of health assessment findings or the unique characteristics of a child, the caregiver/teacher should obtain parental consent to contact the child's primary care provider to explain why the information is needed and to request clarification.

Health assessments should be in a format easily usable by caregivers/teachers to identify any special needs for care.

A child's primary care provider is a key resource to families when racial, ethnic, socioeconomic, or educational disparities create barriers to the child receiving regular dental care. He or she can perform an oral examination and conduct an oral health risk assessment and triage for infants and young children. Children with suspected oral problems should see a dentist immediately, regardless of age or interval.

The American Academy of Pediatrics (AAP) and Bright Futures recommend vision/hearing and dental screenings are:

a) Vision/hearing at every well care visit (with objective measures of visual acuity by four years and audiometry measures of hearing by five years of age); and
b) Dental exam at one year (or sooner if there are suspected oral problems) (3).

TYPE OF FACILITY: Center; Large Family Child Care Home; Small Family Child Care Home

RELATED STANDARDS:
Standard 9.4.2.1: Contents of Child's Records
Standard 9.4.2.5: Health History
Appendix O: Care Plan for Children with Special Health Care Needs
Appendix FF: Child Health Assessment

REFERENCES:
1. Hagan, J. F., J. S. Shaw, P. M. Duncan, eds. 2008. *Bright Futures: Guidelines for health supervision of infants, children, and adolescents*. 3rd ed. Elk Grove Village, IL: American Academy of Pediatrics.
2. Murph, J. R., S. D. Palmer, D. Glassy, eds. 2005. *Health in child care: A manual for health professionals*. 4th ed. Elk Grove Village, IL: American Academy of Pediatrics.
3. American Academy of Pediatrics, Committee on Practice and Ambulatory Medicine, Bright Futures Steering Committee. 2007. Policy statement: Recommendations for preventive pediatric health care. *Pediatrics* 120:1376.
4. Crowley A. A., G. C. Whitney. 2005. Connecticut's new comprehensive and universal early childhood health assessment form. *J School Health* 75:281-85.

STANDARD 9.4.2.5: Health History

The file for each child should include a health history completed by the parent/guardian at admission, preferably with staff involvement. This history should include the following:

a) Identification of the child's medical home/primary care provider and dental home;
b) Permission to contact these professionals in case of emergency;
c) Chronic diseases/health issues currently under treatment;
d) Developmental variations, sensory impairment, serious behavior problems or disabilities that may need consideration in the child care setting;
e) Description of current physical, social, and language developmental levels;
f) Current medications, medical treatments and other therapeutic interventions;
g) Special concerns (such as allergies, chronic illness, pediatric first aid information needs);
h) Specific diet restrictions, if the child is on a special diet;
i) Individual characteristics or personality factors relevant to child care;
j) Special family considerations;
k) Dates of infectious diseases;
l) Plans for medical emergencies;
m) Any special equipment that might be needed;
n) Special transportation adaptations.

RATIONALE: A health history is the basis for meeting the child's medical and psychosocial needs in the child care setting. This information must be obtained and reviewed at admission by the significant caregiver/teacher. This information may be the only health information on file for up to the first four weeks following enrollment.

COMMENTS: This history will complement the child's health history which is completed by the primary care provider.

TYPE OF FACILITY: Center; Large Family Child Care Home; Small Family Child Care Home

RELATED STANDARDS:
Standard 9.4.2.1: Contents of Child's Records

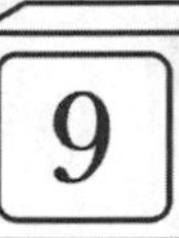

STANDARD 9.4.2.6: Contents of Medication Record

The file for each child should include a medication record maintained on an ongoing basis by designated staff for all prescription and non-prescription (over-the-counter [OTC]) medications. State requirements should be checked and followed. The medication record for prescription and non-prescription medications should include the following:

a) A separate consent signed by the parent/guardian for each medication the caregiver/teacher has permission to administer to the child; each consent should include the child's name, medication, time, dose, how to give the medication, and start and end dates when it should be given;
b) Authorization from the prescribing health professional for each prescription and non-prescription medication; this authorization should also include potential side effects and other warnings about the medication (exception: non-prescription sunscreen and insect repellent always require parental/guardian consent but do not require instructions from each child's individual medical provider);
c) Administration log which includes the child's name, the medication that was given, the dose, the route of administration, the time and date, and the signature or initials of the person administering the medication. For medications given "as needed," record the reason the medication was given. Space should be available for notations of any side-effects noted after the medication was given or if the dose was not retained because of the child vomiting or spitting out the medication. Documentation should also be made of attempts to give medications that were refused by the child;
d) Information about prescription medication brought to the facility by the parents/guardians in the original, labeled container with a label that includes the child's name, date filled, prescribing clinician's name, pharmacy name and phone number, dosage/ instructions, and relevant warnings. Potential side effects and other warnings about the medication should be listed on the authorization form;
e) Non prescription medications should be brought to the facility in the original container, labeled with the child's complete name and administered according to the authorization completed by the person with prescriptive authority;
f) For medications that are to be given or available to be given for the entire year, a Care Plan should also be in place (for instance, inhalers for asthma or epinephrine for possible allergy);
g) Side effects.

RATIONALE: Before assuming responsibility for administration of prescription or non-prescription medicine, facilities must have written confirmation of orders from the prescribing health professional that includes clear, accurate instructions and medical confirmation of the child's need for medication while in the facility. Caregivers/teachers should not administer medication based solely on a parent's/guardian's request. Proper labeling of medications is crucial for safety (1). Both the child's name and the name and dose of the medication should be clear. Medications should never be removed from their original container. All containers should have child resistant packaging. Potential side-effects are usually included on prescription and OTC medications if the packaging is left intact (2).

Medications may have side-effects, and parents/guardians might not be aware that their child is experiencing those symptoms unless they are recorded and reported. Serious medication side-effects might require emergency care. Adjustments or additional medications might help those symptoms if the prescribing health professional is made aware of them. Children who do not tolerate medications may vomit or spit up the medication. Notation should be made if any of the medication was retained in those cases. Children may also vigorously refuse medications, and plans to deal with this should be made (1,2).

The Medication Log is a legal document and should be kept in the child's file for as long as required by state licensing requires.

COMMENTS: A curriculum for child care providers on safe administration of medications in child care is available from the American Academy of Pediatrics at: http://www.healthychildcare.org/HealthyFutures.html.

TYPE OF FACILITY: Center; Large Family Child Care Home; Small Family Child Care Home

RELATED STANDARDS:
Standards 3.6.3.1-3.6.3.3: Medication
Standard 9.2.3.9: Written Policy on Use of Medications
Standard 9.4.2.1: Contents of Child's Records
Appendix AA: Medication Administration Packet

REFERENCES:
1. Healthy Child Care America. 2010. Healthy futures: Medication administration in early education and child care settings. American Academy of Pediatrics. http://www.healthychildcare.org/ HealthyFutures.html.
2. American Academy of Pediatrics, Council on School Health. 2009. Policy statement: Guidance for the administration of medication in school. *Pediatrics* 124:1244-51.

STANDARD 9.4.2.7: Contents of Facility Health Log for Each Child

The file for each child should include a facility health log maintained on an ongoing basis by designated staff. The facility health log should include:

a) Staff and parent/guardian observations of the child's health status, behavior, and physical condition;
b) Response to any treatment provided while the child is in child care, and any observable side effects;
c) Notations of health-related referrals and follow-up action;
d) Notations of health-related communications with parents/guardians or the child's primary care provider;

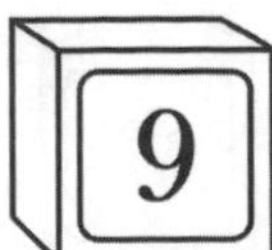

e) Staff observations of changes in and assessments of the child's learning and social activity;
f) Documentation of planned communication with parents/guardians and a list of participants involved;
g) Documentation of parent/guardian participation in health education.

RATIONALE: A facility health log maintained by caregivers/teachers can document staff's observations and concerns that may lead to intervention decisions.

COMMENTS: The facility health log is a confidential, chronologically-oriented location for the recording of staff observations, patterns of illness, and parent/guardian concerns. It can be followed and can become guidelines for intervention, if needed.

Facility observation logs provide useful information over time on each child's unique characteristics. Parents/guardians and caregivers/teachers can use these logs in planning for the child's needs. On occasion, the child's primary care provider can use them as an aid in diagnosing health conditions.

"Hands-on" opportunities for parents/guardians to work with their own child or others in the company of caregivers/teachers should be encouraged and documented.

Staff notations on communication with parents/guardians can be in a parent/guardian log separate from the child's health record.

TYPE OF FACILITY: Center; Large Family Child Care Home; Small Family Child Care Home

RELATED STANDARDS:
Standard 2.3.2.1: Parent/Guardian Conferences
Standard 2.3.2.3: Support Services for Parents/Guardians
Standards 2.4.3.1-2.4.3.2: Health Education for Parents/Guardians
Standard 9.4.1.6: Availability of Documents to Parents/Guardians
Appendix F: Enrollment/Attendance/Symptom Record
Appendix AA: Medication Administration Packet

STANDARD 9.4.2.8: Release of Child's Records

The parents'/guardians' written requests to release their child's records must be specific about to whom the record is being released, for what purpose, and what parts of the record are being copied and sent. Upon parent/guardian request, designated portions or all of the child's records should be copied and released to specific individuals named and authorized in writing by the parents/guardians to receive this information. The original records and the written requests should be retained by the facility.

RATIONALE: The facility must retain the original records in case legal defense is required, but parents/guardians have the right to know and have the full contents of the records. Sending the record to another source of service for the child may enhance the ability of other service providers to provide appropriate care for the child and family.

COMMENTS: Parents/guardians may want a copy of the record themselves or may want the record sent to another source of care for the child. An effective way to educate parents/guardians on the value of maintaining the child's developmental and health information is to have them focus on their own child's records. Such records should be used as a mutual education tool by parents/guardians and caregivers/teachers. Facilities may charge a reasonable fee for making a copy.

TYPE OF FACILITY: Center

RELATED STANDARDS:
Standard 9.4.1.3: Written Policy on Confidentiality of Records

9.4.3 Staff Records

STANDARD 9.4.3.1: Maintenance and Content of Staff and Volunteer Records

Individual files for all staff members and volunteers, should be maintained in a central location within the facility and should contain the following:

a) The individual's name, birth date, address, and telephone number;
b) The position application, which includes a record of work experience and work references; verification of reference information, education, and training; and records of any checking for background screenings, driving records, criminal records, and/or listing in child abuse registry;
c) The health assessment record, a copy of which, having been dated and signed by the employee's primary care provider, should be kept in a confidential file in the facility; this record should be updated by another health appraisal when recommended by the staff member's primary care provider or supervisory or regulatory/certifying personnel;
d) The name and telephone number of the person, primary care provider, or health facility to be notified in case of emergency;
e) The job description or the job expectations for staff and substitutes;
f) Required licenses, certificates, and transcripts;
g) The date of employment or volunteer assignment;
h) A signed statement of agreement that the employee understands and will abide by the following:
    1) Regulations and statutes governing child care;
    2) Human resource management and procedures;
    3) Health policies and procedures;
    4) Discipline policy;
    5) Guidelines for reporting suspected child abuse, neglect, and sexual abuse;
    6) Confidentiality policy.
i) The date and content of staff and volunteer orientation(s);
j) A daily record of hours worked, including paid planning time and parent/guardian conference time;
k) A record of professional development completed by each staff member and volunteer, including dates and clock or credit hours;
l) Written performance evaluations.

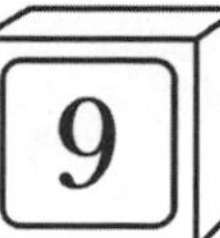

RATIONALE: Complete identification of staff, paid or volunteer, is an essential step in safeguarding children in child care. Maintaining complete records on each staff person employed at the facility is a sound administrative practice. Employment history, a daily record of days worked, performance evaluations, a record of benefits, and who to notify in case of emergency provide important information for the employer. Licensors will check the records to assure that applicable licensing requirements are met (such as identifying information, educational qualifications, health assessment on file, record of continuing education, signed statement of agreement to observe the discipline policy, and guidelines for reporting suspected child abuse, neglect, and sexual abuse).

Emergency contact information for staff, paid or volunteer is needed in child care in the event that an adult becomes ill or injured at the facility.

The signature of the employee confirms the employee's notification of responsibilities that might otherwise by overlooked by the employee.

COMMENTS: If a small family child care home has employees, this standard would apply.

TYPE OF FACILITY: Center; Large Family Child Care Home

RELATED STANDARDS:
Standards 1.3.1.1-1.3.3.2: Pre-Service Qualifications
Standards 1.4.2.1-1.5.0.2: Training/Development
Standard 1.7.0.1: Pre-Employment and Ongoing Adult Health Appraisals, Including Immunization
Standards 1.8.2.2-1.8.2.3: Performance Evaluations
Standards 2.2.0.6-2.2.0.10: Discipline
Standard 9.2.1.1: Content of Policies
Standard 9.2.1.3: Enrollment Information to Parents/Guardians and Caregivers/Teachers
Standard 9.2.1.6: Written Discipline Policies
Standard 9.3.0.1: Written Human Resource Management Policies for Centers and Large Family Child Care Homes
Standard 9.4.1.3: Written Policy on Confidentiality of Records

STANDARD 9.4.3.2: Maintenance of Attendance Records for Staff Who Care for Children

Centers and large family child care homes should keep daily attendance records listing the names of each caregiver/teacher and/or substitute in attendance, the hours each individual worked, and the names of the children in their care. When a caregiver/teacher, substitute provider and/or volunteer cares for more than one group of children during their hours worked, daily attendance records will reflect the names of the children cared for during each block of time.

RATIONALE: Promoting the health and safety of individual children requires keeping records regarding supervision of each child in care. This standard ensures that the facility knows which children are receiving care at any given time and who is responsible for directly supervising each child. It also aids in the surveillance of child:staff ratios and provides data for program planning. Past attendance records are essential in conducting complaint investigations including child abuse.

TYPE OF FACILITY: Center; Large Family Child Care Home

RELATED STANDARDS:
Standard 9.4.3.1: Maintenance and Content of Staff and Volunteer Records

STANDARD 9.4.3.3: Training Record

The director of a center or a large or small family child care home should provide and maintain documentation or participate in the state's training/professional development registry of training/professional development received by, or provided for, staff. For centers, the date of the training, the number of hours, the names of staff participants, the name(s) and qualification(s) of the trainer(s), and the content of the training (both orientation and continuing education) should be recorded in each staff person's file or in a separate training file. If the state has a training/professional development registry, the director should provide training documentation to the registry.

Small family child care home caregivers/teachers should keep a written record of training acquired and certificates containing the same information as the documentation recommended for centers and large homes.

RATIONALE: The training record should be used to assess each employee's need for additional training and to provide regulators with a tool to monitor compliance. Continuing education with course credit should be recorded and the records made available to staff members to document their applications for licenses/certificates or for license upgrading. All accrediting bodies for child care facilities, homes and centers, require documentation of training.

In many states, small family child care home caregivers/teachers are required to keep records of training.

COMMENTS: Colleges issue transcripts, workshops can issue certificates, and facility administrators can maintain individual training logs.

TYPE OF FACILITY: Center; Large Family Child Care Home; Small Family Child Care Home

RELATED STANDARDS:
Standard 9.4.3.1: Maintenance and Content of Staff and Volunteer Records

Chapter 10

10

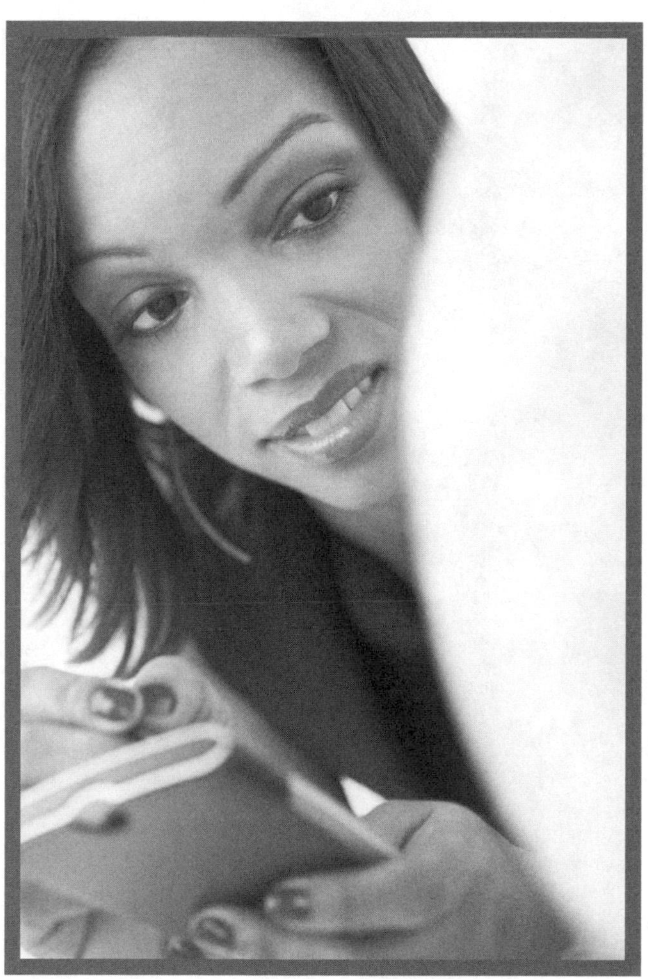

Licensing and Community Action

10.1 Introduction

This chapter contains standards for the responsibilities of agencies, organizations, and society, not for the individual caregiver/teacher or child care facility. These standards provide the support systems for implementation of the standards in the preceding chapters. Although many of these standards are directed to state administrative activity, they define necessary actions to assure the health and safety of children in out-of-home settings. The chapter addresses standards for the licensing of child care facilities, a process by which states grant official permission to operate an activity which would otherwise be prohibited by law. Licensing can also be known as "permission," "certification," "registration," or "approval." For the purposes of simplicity, licensing will be used to convey these other terms in this chapter. The term "license" can also be known as "permit," "certificate," "registration," or "approval" and will be used to convey these other terms.

10.2 Regulatory Policy

STANDARD 10.2.0.1: Regulation of All Out-of-Home Child Care

Every state should have a statute that identifies the licensing agency and mandates the licensing and regulation of all full-time and part-time out-of-home care of children, regardless of setting, except care provided by parents or legal guardians, grandparents, siblings, aunts, or uncles (sometimes called relative, friend, and neighbor care) or when a family engages an individual in the family's home to care solely for their children (1,2).

RATIONALE: A state statute gives government the authority to protect children as vulnerable and dependent citizens and to protect families as consumers of child care service. Licensing must have a statutory basis, because it is unknown to the common law. The statute must address the administration and location of the responsibility. Fifty states have child care regulatory statutes. The laws of some states exempt part-day centers, school-age child care, care provided by religious organizations, drop-in care, summer camps, or care provided in small or large family child care homes (3). In some states the threshold for family child care homes being regulated leaves many children unprotected (4). These exclusions and gaps in coverage expose children to unacceptable risks.

REFERENCES:

1. National Association for the Education of Young Children (NAEYC). 1997. *Licensing and public regulation of early childhood programs: A position statement*. Washington, DC: NAEYC.
2. U.S. Department of Health and Human Services, Administration for Children and Families, National Child Care Information and Technical Assistance Center. 2010. Understanding and supporting family, friend, and neighbor child care. http://nccic.acf.hhs.gov/resource/understanding-and-supporting-family-friend-and-neighbor-child-care/.
3. Child Care and Early Education Research Connections. 2010. *Child care licensing and regulation: A key topic resource list. 2nd ed.* http://www.researchconnections.org/files/childcare/keytopics/licensing.pdf.
4. National Association of Child Care Resource and Referral Agencies (NACCRRA). 2010. *Leaving children to chance: NACCRRA's ranking of state standards and oversight of small family child care homes, 2010 update.* Arlington, VA: NACCRRA. http://www.naccrra.org/publications/naccrra-publications/publications/854-0000_Lvng Children 2 Chance_rev_031510.pdf.

STANDARD 10.2.0.2: Adequacy of Staff and Funding for Regulatory Enforcement

All phases of regulatory administration should have authorization, funding, and enough qualified staff to monitor and enforce the law and regulations of the state.

RATIONALE: For regulations to be effective, the regulatory body must formulate, implement, and enforce licensing requirements and assure that licensing inspectors are both sufficient in numbers and capable of fairly and effectively developing and applying the regulations. Funds for all phases of the licensing process should be provided, or faulty administrative operations may result; such as inadequate protection of children, formulation of irresponsible standards, inadequate investigations, and insufficient and unfair enforcement (1).

REFERENCES:

1. National Association for Regulatory Administration (NARA). 2009. *Recommended best practices for human care licensing agencies.* The NARA Vision Series Part I. Lexington, KY: NARA. http://www.naralicensing.org/associations/4734/files/Recommended Best Practices.pdf.

STANDARD 10.2.0.3: State Statute Support of Regulatory Enforcement

The state statute should authorize the suppression of illegal operations and enforcement of child care regulations and statutory provisions. Reports of unlicensed care should be promptly investigated and illegally operating providers either brought into the regulated system or forced to terminate offering care. Fines for continuing to provide unlicensed care should be substantial enough to serve as an effective deterrent.

RATIONALE: Without proper enforcement, especially the suppression of illegal operations, licensing could become a ritual and lose its safeguarding intent. Some state laws lack adequate provisions for enforcement. Without effective enforcement, licensing fails to meet its responsibility to protect children from harm (1).

REFERENCES:

1. National Association for Regulatory Administration (NARA). 2000. Suppressing illegal operations. In *NARA licensing curriculum*. 2000 ed. Lexington, KY: NARA.

10.3 Licensing Agency

10.3.1 The Regulation Setting Process

STANDARD 10.3.1.1: Operation Permits

The licensing agency should issue permits of operation to all facilities that comply with the state's licensing regulations and rules.

RATIONALE: Every child has a right to protective care that meets the regulations and rules, regardless of the child care setting in which the child is enrolled. Public and private schools, nurseries, preschools, centers, child development programs, babysitting centers, early childhood observation centers, small and large family child care homes, drop-in care, and all other settings where young children receive care by individuals who are not close relatives should be regulated. Facilities have been able to circumvent rules and regulations in some states by claiming to be specialized facilities. Nothing in the educational philosophy, religious orientation, or setting of an early childhood program inherently protects children from health and safety risks or provides assurance of quality of child care.

Any exemptions for care provided outside the family may place children at risk. In addition to the basic protection afforded by stipulating requirements and inspecting for licensing, facilities should be required to be authorized for operation. Authorization for operation gives states a mechanism to identify facilities and individuals that are providing child care and authority to monitor compliance. These facilities and individuals may be identified as potential customers for training, technical assistance, and consultation services. Currently, many church run nurseries, nursery schools, group play centers, and home based programs operate incognito in the community because they are not required to notify any centralized agency that they care for children (2).

The lead agency for licensing of child care in most states is the human services agency. However, the state public health agency can be an appropriate licensing authority for safeguarding children in some states. The education system is increasingly involved in providing services to children in early childhood. The standards should be equally stringent no matter what agency assumes the responsibility for regulating child care.

In-home care, which is the care of a child in his/her own home by someone whom the parent has employed, not a family child care home, should not be licensed as a child care facility. The relationship between the parent and caregiver/teacher is that of employer and employee rather than that of purchaser and provider of care, thus licensing or certification of the individual who provides such care, rather than of the service itself, is desirable and recommended.

COMMENTS: A good resource on licensing, regulatory, and enforcement issues is the National Association for Regulatory Administration (NARA) at http://www.naralicensing.org, an international professional organization for licensors, dedicated to promoting excellence in human care regulation and licensing through leadership, education, collaboration, and services. In addition, the "Licensing and Public Regulation of Early Childhood Programs" document published by the National Association for the Education of Young Children (NAEYC) includes rationale for policy decisions related to licensing and regulation (1). In addition, the National Association for Child Care Resource and Referral Agencies (NACCRRA) publishes periodic reports comparing the licensing regulations of the states against standards formulated by NACCRRA; these reports are available at http://www.naccrra.org.

RELATED STANDARDS:

Appendix GG: Licensing and Public Regulation of Early Childhood Programs

REFERENCES:

1. National Association for the Education of Young Children (NAEYC). 1997. *Licensing and public regulation of early childhood programs: A position statement.* Revised ed. Washington, DC: NAEYC.

2. National Association for Regulatory Administration (NARA), National Child Care Association (NCCA). 2004. License exempt early care and education programs: Equal protection and quality education for every child. Joint position paper. http://nara.affiniscape.com/associations/4734/files/JointPP.pdf.

STANDARD 10.3.1.2: Rational Basis of Regulations

The state child care licensing agency should formulate, implement, and enforce regulations that reduce risks to children in out-of-home child care (1,2).

RATIONALE: Regulations describe the minimum performance required of a facility. Regulations must be:

a) Understandable to any reasonable citizen;
b) Specific enough that any person knows what is to be done and what is not to be done;
c) Enforceable, in that they are capable of measurement;
d) Consistent with new technical knowledge, current research findings and changes in public views to offer necessary protection and to avoid unacceptable risk;
e) Easily available in both print and electronic media.

REFERENCES:

1. National Association for Regulatory Administration (NARA). 2000. Formulation of rules. In *NARA licensing curriculum*. 2000 ed. Lexington, KY: NARA.

2. Class, N. E., J. English. 1983. Formulating operationally valid standards. The administrative regulation of community care facilities with special reference to child care. A compilation of papers by Norris E. Class, Professor Emeritus, School of Social Work, University of Southern California.

STANDARD 10.3.1.3: Community Participation in Development of Licensing Rules

State licensing rules should be developed with active community participation by all interested parties including parents/guardians, service providers, advocates, professionals in medical and child development fields, funding and training sources (1,2).

Regulations formulated through a representative citizen process should come before the public at well-publicized public hearings held at convenient times and places in different parts of the state. The licensing rules should be re-examined and revised at least every five years, to assure that the rules can be informed by new relevant research findings and significant social data. The regulatory development process should include many opportunities for public debate and discussion as well as the ability to provide written input.

RATIONALE: The legal principle of broad interest representation has long been applied to the formulation of regulations for child care. Changes in regulation can be implemented only with broad support from the different interests affected. State administrative laws and constitutional principles require public review. The interests of the child must take precedence over all other interests. The system should allow for more frequent changes when required to protect children's health or safety, e.g., updates on Sudden Infant Death Syndrome (SIDS) risk reduction measures.

REFERENCES:

1. National Association for Regulatory Administration (NARA). 2000. Formulation of rules. In *NARA licensing curriculum.* 2000 ed. Lexington, KY: NARA.
2. Class, N. E., J. English. 1985. Formulating valid standards for licensing. *J Am Public Welfare Assoc* 43:32-35.

10.3.2 Advisory Groups

STANDARD 10.3.2.1: Child Care Licensing Advisory Board

States should have an official child care licensing advisory body for regulatory and related policy issues. A child care advisory board should:

a) Review proposed rules and regulations prior to adoption;
b) Recommend administrative policy;
c) Recommend changes in legislation; and
d) Guide enforcement, if granted this authority via the legislative process.

The advisory group should include representatives from the following agencies and groups:

a) State agencies with regulatory responsibility or an interest in child care (human services, public health, fire marshal, emergency medical services, education, human resources, attorney general, safety council);
b) Organizations with a child care emphasis;
c) Operators, directors, owners, and caregivers/teachers reflecting various types of child care programs including for-profit and non-profit;
d) Professionals with expertise related to the rules; may include pediatrics, physical activity, nutrition, mental health, oral health, injury prevention, resource and referral, early childhood education, and early childhood professional development;
e) Parents/guardians who reflect the diversity of the families that are consumers of licensed child care programs.

This advisory board should be linked to the State Early Childhood Advisory Council (see Standard 10.3.2.2) as required by the Head Start Act of 2007 (1).

RATIONALE: The advisory group should actively seek citizen participation in the development of child care policy, including parents/guardians, child care administrators, and caregivers/teachers. The licensing advisory board should report directly to the agency having administrative authority over licensing.

RELATED STANDARDS:

Standard 10.3.2.2: State Early Childhood Advisory Council

REFERENCES:

1. U.S. Congress. 2007. Head Start Act. 42 USC 9801. http://eclkc.ohs.acf.hhs.gov/hslc/Head Start Program/Program Design and Management/Head Start Requirements/Head Start Act/.

STANDARD 10.3.2.2: State Early Childhood Advisory Council

Each state should establish a state early childhood advisory council or charge an existing commission with the responsibility for developing a early childhood plan and facilitating cooperation among government public health, human service, and education departments; institutions of higher education; early childhood professional development systems; early childhood professional organizations; as well as community-based human services agencies. Schools, employers, parents/guardians, and caregivers/teachers should also be involved to ensure that the health, safety, and child development needs of children are met by the child care services provided in the state. The council should be mandated by law, and should report to the legislature and to the governor at least annually. Larger communities should have a network of local councils to advise the state council. The state child care licensing advisory board (see Standard 10.3.2.1) should have representation on the council.

RATIONALE: Coordination among public and private sources of health, social service, and education services is essential, especially when young children are in care. Some states have separate groups that advise the health agency, the social service agency, the education agency, the licensing agency, the governor, and the legislature (1). Other states have some, but not all, of these advisory bodies; each of which has some relevance to child care, but often with a different focus. National initiatives such as the Early Childhood Comprehensive Systems (ECCS) Initiative and the Healthy Child Care America (HCCA) program have done much to encourage effective collaboration among agencies and organizations with the ability to impact child care within states (2).

Time limited task forces could be created for specific purposes, but there is a need for one standing council that addresses early childhood as its primary responsibility. Mandating the council by law will reduce the likelihood that the council will be rendered ineffective by changes in political leadership or dissolved when its recommendations are not in agreement with a current administration.

Large municipalities with a similarly diverse group of agencies, authorities, and public and private resources should also have a council to coordinate early childhood activity. Participation of parent/guardian representatives in planning and implementing early childhood initiatives at the state and local levels promotes effective partnerships between parents/guardians and caregivers/teachers (1).

RELATED STANDARDS:
Standard 10.3.2.1: Child Care Licensing Advisory Board

REFERENCES:
1. U.S. Congress. 2007. Head Start Act. 42 USC 9801. http://eclkc.ohs.acf.hhs.gov/hslc/Head Start Program/Program Design and Management/Head Start Requirements/Head Start Act/.
2. Healthy Child Care America (HCCA). 2010. About us. American Academy of Pediatrics. http://www.healthychildcare.org/about.html.

STANDARD 10.3.2.3: Collaborative Development of Child Care Requirements and Guidelines for Children Who Are Ill

Local and state health departments, child care licensing agencies, education and health professionals, attorneys, caregivers/teachers, parents/guardians, and representatives of the business community, including employers, should work together to develop child care licensing requirements and guidelines for children who are ill.

RATIONALE: Local and state health departments have the legal responsibility to control infectious diseases in their jurisdictions (1). To meet this responsibility, health departments generally have the expertise to provide leadership and technical assistance to licensing authorities, caregivers/teachers, parents/guardians, and health professionals in the development of licensing requirements and guidelines for the management of children who are ill. The heavy reliance on the expertise of local and state health departments in the establishment of facilities to care for children who are ill has fostered a partnership in many states among health departments, licensing authorities, caregivers/teachers, and parents/guardians for the adequate care of children who are ill in child care settings. Early care and education professionals can provide the information required to ensure child care settings support children's social-emotional, language and cognitive development. In addition, the business community has a vested interest in assuring that parents/guardians have facilities that provide quality care for children who are ill so parents/guardians can be productive in the workplace. This vested interest is likely to produce meaningful contributions from the business community to creative solutions and innovative ideas about how to approach the regulation of facilities for children who are ill. All stakeholders in the care of children who are ill should be involved for the solutions that are developed in regulations to be most successful.

RELATED STANDARDS:
Standards 3.6.2.1-3.6.2.10: Caring for Children Who Are Ill

REFERENCES:
1. Grad, F. P. 2004. *The public health law manual*. 3rd ed. Washington, DC: American Public Health Association.

STANDARD 10.3.2.4: Public-Private Collaboration on Care of Children Who Are Ill

State and regional agencies should collaborate with employers to facilitate arrangements for the care of children who are ill in the following settings:

f) The child's own home, under the supervision of an adult known to the parents/guardians and the child;
g) A separate area in the child's own facility or in a specialized center, where both the caregiver/teacher and the facility are familiar to the child;
h) A child's own small family child care home;
i) A space within the small family child care home network's central place that serves children from participating small family child care homes, where both the caregiver and the facility are familiar to the child.

RATIONALE: The most appropriate care of a child who is ill is at the child's own home by a parent/guardian. This is in the best interests of the child, family, and community. Businesses should be encouraged to allow the use of paid sick leave for this purpose. However, when parent care puts the family income or parent employment at risk, the child should receive care that is appropriate for the child. Often, when faced with the pressures of the workplace, parents/guardians take children who are ill to work, leave them in places where either or both the caregiver/teacher and place are unfamiliar, or leave them alone. Under the stress of illness, children need familiar caregivers/teachers and familiar places where their illnesses and their emotional needs can be managed competently.

RELATED STANDARDS:
Standards 3.6.2.1-3.6.2.10: Caring for Children Who Are Ill

10.3.3 Licensing Role with Staff Credentials, Child Abuse Prevention, and ADA Compliance

STANDARD 10.3.3.1: Credentialing of Individual Child Care Providers

The state licensing agency or a credentialing body recognized by the state child care regulatory agency should credential or license all persons who provide child care or who may be responsible for children or who may be alone with children in a facility. The credential should be granted to individuals who meet age, education, and experience qualifications, whose health status facilitates providing safe and nurturing care, and who have no record of conviction for criminal offenses against persons, especially children, or confirmed act of child abuse. The state should establish qualifications for differentiated roles in child care and a procedure for verifying that the individual who is authorized to perform a specified role meets the qualifications and is credentialed for that role.

RATIONALE: Individual credentialing will enhance child health and development and protect children by ensuring that the staff who care for children are healthy and are quali-

fied for their roles. The current system, in which the details of staff qualifications and ongoing training are checked as part of facility inspection, is cumbersome for child care administrators and licensing inspectors alike. If staff qualifications were established as part of a separate, more central process, the licensing agency staff could check center records of character references and whether staff members have licenses for the roles for which they are employed.

Centralizing individual credentialing, qualifying, or licensing (whichever term is consistent with the state's approach to authorizing legal professional activity) will improve control over quality, encourage a career ladder with increasing qualifications, and reduce the risk of abuse. It will help consumers know that individuals who are caring for their children have met basic requirements for consumer protection. Such a process is analogous to that provided for other education professionals (teachers), and even those service providers with less potential for harm than is involved in caring for children (such as beauticians, barbers, taxi drivers).

The cost of individual certification, credentialing, or licensure will be offset by the benefits to consumers of reliable and consistent qualifications of child care personnel. Program administrators, licensors, and child care personnel, who do not have to undertake the tedious process of verification of each portion of an individual's credentials during all site visits, when sites are licensed, or when individuals change jobs, will experience cost savings and assurance of compliance. Public and private policymakers should use financial and other incentives to help caregivers/teachers meet credentialing requirements. They should encourage community colleges to offer courses appropriate for provider training at times convenient for child care workers to attend and for other agencies to offer online courses available to providers from their homes or places of employment.

Periodic renewal of the credential should be required, and should be related to requirements for continuing education and the absence of founded claims of child abuse or criminal convictions. The requirement for renewable certification is likely to deter people from applying for work in child care as a way of gaining access to children for sexual purposes since the process would include a background screening that includes a check of the sex offender registry and child abuse registry (1).

COMMENTS: In a centralized individual credentialing system, successful completion of education should be verified by requiring the individual to submit evidence of completion of credit-bearing courses that have been previously approved as meeting the state's requirements to a central verification office where this transcript should be continually updated. Background screening records should be checked by state licensing agency staff for evidence of behavior that would disqualify an individual for work in specified child care roles. Evidence of a recent health examination indicating ability to care for children can be submitted at the same time. The center director then knows whether job applicants who have been working in the field previously are qualified at the time they apply for the job, without lengthy waiting for background checks of a prospective employee and without having to hire before background checks have been completed. By this means, children are not exposed to health and safety risks from understaffing, or to care by unqualified or even dangerous individuals employed provisionally because the results of a check are not yet available to the director.

RELATED STANDARDS:
Section 1.3: Pre-service Qualifications

REFERENCES:
1. Finkelhor, D., L. M. William, N. Burns. 1988. *Nursery crimes: Sexual abuse in day care*. Beverly Hills, CA: Sage Publications.

STANDARD 10.3.3.2: Background Screening

Every state should have a statute which mandates the licensing agency or other authority to obtain a background screening that includes a criminal records check, a sex offender registry check, and a child abuse registry check on every prospective child care staff person, volunteer, or on a family child care home provider's family member who is over ten years of age and who comes in contact with children. The expense of background screenings should be a public responsibility. No staff (paid or volunteer) or family member should be unsupervised with the children until all background screenings have been completed and found to be acceptable.

RATIONALE: Some states do not regulate family child care providers who care for just a few children. Caregivers/teachers who care for more children are required to comply with legal requirements in most states. In nearly all States, regulations require background screenings for all child care center staff. This screening requirement may protect children from abuse and reduce liability risks (1). Some local governments regulate family child care caregivers/teachers who are not covered by State regulations or have regulations that exceed the state requirements.

COMMENTS: The cost of background screenings, where they have been implemented, has become an additional financial burden on programs, which are forced to pass on the expense to parents/guardians or staff. Placing the burden on potential new staff, volunteers, and substitute caregivers/teachers themselves proves to be another disincentive to enter this field of work. A solution to this problem should be sought in addressing the overall need to support development of a well educated and competent early education workforce. For workers who enter the field as a first work experience, previous child abuse histories may be unknown. In many cases juvenile records are sealed and cannot be used for the purposes of background screenings. Juvenile offender records begin at age ten. Most state regulations are not clear on whether sex offender registries are to be checked (2).

Some states have established definitions for regular volunteers (for whom criminal record and child abuse registry checks should be required) and for short-term visitors, such as entertainers and others, who will not be unsupervised with the children.

REFERENCES:
1. U.S. Department of Labor, Bureau of Labor Statistics. 2010. Career guide to industries, 2010-11 edition: Child day care services. http://www.bls.gov/oco/cg/cgs032.htm.
2. National Association of Child Care Resource and Referral Agencies. 2009. *Comprehensive background checks.* http://www.naccrra.org/policy/docs/Background-Checks-Sept22.pdf.

STANDARD 10.3.3.3: Licensing Agency Role in Communicating the Importance of Reporting Suspected Child Abuse

Licensing agencies should consistently make known the requirements for reporting and methods of reporting suspected child abuse.

RATIONALE: Child care staff and parents/guardians should be aware of the reporting requirements and the procedures for handling reports of child abuse (1,2). State requirements may differ, but those for whom reporting suspected abuse is mandatory usually include child care personnel. Information on how to call and how to report should be posted in licensed facilities so it is readily available to parents/guardians and staff. Emotional abuse can be extremely harmful to children, but unlike physical or sexual abuse, it is not adequately defined in most state child abuse reporting laws. State licensing agencies need to report suspected abuse or neglect which they become aware of to the State Child Protective Agency for appropriate follow-up.

Procedures for evaluating allegations of physical and emotional abuse may or may not be the purview of the licensing agency. This responsibility may fall to another agency to which the licensing agency refers child abuse allegations.

RELATED STANDARDS:
Standards 3.4.4.1-3.4.4.5: Child Abuse and Neglect

REFERENCES:
1. Child Welfare Information Gateway. Reporting. http://www.childwelfare.gov/responding/reporting.cfm.
2. Child Help. Prevention and treatment of child abuse. http://www.childhelp.org.

STANDARD 10.3.3.4: Licensing Agency Provision of Child Abuse Prevention Materials

The licensing agency should be a resource for or have knowledge of sources of child abuse prevention materials for child care facilities and parents/guardians. Guidance and technical assistance should also be provided related to their state's child abuse/neglect statute and procedures including the facility's responsibilities of reporting suspected child abuse and neglect.

RATIONALE: Centers and small and large family child care homes are good locations to distribute materials for the prevention of abuse and host community training events (1).

COMMENTS: State Child Welfare Agencies are a good source of information and materials and resources on prevention and may have designated staff who provide training in the community, including to early care and education program staff and parents/guardians.

Additional resources for licensing agencies can be found at: http://www.childwelfare.gov/preventing/ and http://www.childwelfare.gov/pubs/res_packet_2008/.

REFERENCES:
1. Center for the Study of Social Policy. Strengthening families. http://www.strengtheningfamilies.net.

STANDARD 10.3.3.5: Licensing Agency Role in Communicating the Importance of Compliance with Americans with Disabilities Act

Licensing agencies should consistently make known the requirements under the Americans with Disabilities Act that child care programs must follow.

RATIONALE: Child care programs must comply with the requirements of the Americans with Disabilities Act.

COMMENTS: Procedures for evaluating allegations of physical and emotional abuse may or may not be the purview of the licensing agency. This responsibility may fall to another agency to which the licensing agency refers child abuse allegations.

10.3.4 Technical Assistance from the Licensing Agency

STANDARD 10.3.4.1: Sources of Technical Assistance to Support Quality of Child Care

Public authorities (such as licensing agencies) and private agencies (such as resource and referral agencies), should develop systems for technical assistance to states, localities, child care agencies, and caregivers/teachers that address the following:

a) Meeting licensing requirements;
b) Establishing programs that meet the developmental needs of children;
c) Educating parents/guardians on specific health and safety issues through the production and distribution of related material.

RATIONALE: The administrative practice of developing systems for technical assistance is designed to enhance the overall quality of child care that meets the social and developmental needs of children. The chief sources of technical assistance are:

a) Licensing agencies (on ways to meet the regulations);
b) Health departments (on health related matters);
c) Resource and referral agencies (on ways to achieve quality, how to start a new facility, supply and demand data, how to get licensed, and what parents/guardians want);
d) Child care health, education, mental health consultant networks; American Academy of Pediatrics (AAP) state chapters and child care contacts; and state Early Childhood Comprehensive Systems (ECCS) grants are examples of partners providing technical assistance on health and related child care matters.

The state agency has a continuing responsibility to assist an applicant in qualifying for a license and to help licensees improve and maintain the quality of their facility. Regulations should be available to parents/guardians and interested citizens upon request and should be translated if needed. Licensing inspectors throughout the state should be required to offer assistance and consultation as a regular part of their duties and to coordinate consultation with other technical assistance providers as this is an integral part of the licensing process.

The Maternal and Child Health Bureau (MCHB) of the Health Resources and Services Administration (HRSA) and the Office of Child Care (OCC) of the Administration for Children and Families (ACF) continue to develop initiatives that provide funding to support technical assistance to early care and education. States should check with their State Child Care Administrators, Maternal and Child Health Directors, and Head Start State Collaboration Directors, for more information.

Providing centers and networks of small or large family child care homes with guidelines and information on establishing a program of care is intended to promote appropriate programs of activities. Child care staff is rarely trained health professionals. Since staff and time are often limited, caregivers/teachers should have access to consultation on available resources in a variety of fields (such as physical and mental health care; nutrition; safety, including fire safety; oral health care; developmental disabilities; and cultural sensitivity) (1,2).

The public agencies can facilitate access to children and their families by providing useful materials to child care providers.

RELATED STANDARDS:

Standards 2.4.3.1-2.4.3.2: Health Education for Parents/Guardians
Standard 10.3.3.1: Credentialing of Individual Health Care Providers
Standard 10.4.1.3: Licensing Agency Procedures Prior to Issuing a License

REFERENCES:

1. American Academy of Pediatrics. 2001. *The pediatrician's role in promoting health and safety in child care*. Elk Grove Village, IL: AAP.
2. Alkon, A., J. Bernzweig, K. To, M. Wolff, J. F. Mackie. 2009. Child care health consultation improves health and safety policies and practices. *Acad Pediatr* 9:366-70.

STANDARD 10.3.4.2: Licensing Agency Provision of Written Agreements for Parents/Guardians and Caregivers/Teachers

The licensing agency or a resource and referral agency should provide guidance, technical assistance, and training to support caregivers/teachers in developing written agreements between the child care facility and parents/guardians, as required by licensing regulations. The written agreement should be available at the time of an inspection visit.

RATIONALE: The licensing agency and the resource and referral agency can develop sample agreement forms or be a resource to parents/guardians and caregivers/teachers in locating the appropriate materials and tools.

STANDARD 10.3.4.3: Support for Consultants to Provide Technical Assistance to Facilities

State agencies should encourage the arrangement and coordination of and the fiscal support for consultants from the local community to provide technical assistance for program development and maintenance. Consultants should have training and experience in early childhood education, early childhood growth and development, issues of health and safety in child care settings, business practices, ability to establish collegial relationships with child care providers, adult learning techniques, and ability to help establish links between facilities and community resources. There should be collaboration among all parts of the early care and education community to provide technical assistance and consultation to improve the quality of care. The licensing agency should be an integral part of the quality rating and improvement system (QRIS) in the state; all parts of the system must collaborate to assure the most effective and efficient use of resources to encourage quality improvement. *See Glossary for definition of QRIS.*

The state regulatory agency with the Title V or State Child Care Resource and Referral Agency should provide or arrange for other public agencies, private organizations or technical assistance agencies (such as a resource and referral agency) to make the following consultants available to the community of child care providers of all types:

a) Program consultant, to provide technical assistance for program development and maintenance and business practices. Consultants should be chosen on the basis of training and experience in early childhood education and ability to help establish links between the facility and community resources;
b) Child care health consultant (CCHC), who has knowledge and expertise in child health and child development, is knowledgeable about the special needs of children in out-of-home care settings, and knows the child care licensing requirements and available health resources. A regional plan to make consultants accessible to facilities for ongoing relationships should be developed;
c) Nutritionist/registered dietitian, who also has the knowledge of infant and child development, food service, nutrition and nutrition education methods, to be responsible for the development of policies and procedures and for the implementation of nutrition standards to provide high quality meals, nutrition education programs and appropriately trained personnel, and to provide consultation to agency personnel, including collaborating with licensing inspectors;
d) Early childhood education consultant, to assist centers, large family child care homes, and networks of small family child care homes in partnering with families in meeting the individual development and learning needs of children, including any special developmental and educational needs that a child may have. Early Childhood Education Consultants can assist providers n early detection and referral for

identifying and addressing special learning needs, especially infants and toddlers;

e) Early childhood mental health consultant (ECMHC), to assist centers, large family child care homes, and networks of small family child care homes in meeting the emotional needs of children and families. The state mental health agency should promote funding through community mental health agencies and child guidance clinics for these services. At the least, such consultants should be available when caregivers/ teachers identify children whose behaviors are more difficult to manage than typically developing children;

f) Dental health consultant, to assist centers, large family child care homes and networks small family child care homes in meeting the oral health needs of children. The dental health consultant should have knowledge of pediatric oral health and be able to help with policy and procedure development in this area;

g) Physical activity consultant, who has knowledge in infant and child motor development (developmental biomechanics), locomotion, ballistic, and manipulative skills, sensory-perceptual development, social, psychosocial, and cultural constraints in motor development, and development of cardio-respiratory endurance, strength and flexibility, and body composition, to be responsible for the development of policies and procedures for the implementation of age and developmentally appropriate physical activity standards to provide children with the movement experiences needed for optimal growth and development, physical education/movement programs, and appropriately trained personnel, and to provide consultation to agency personnel, including collaborating with licensing inspectors.

A plan should be in place that supports the interdisciplinary collaboration of consultant support to programs to ensure coordinated support, avoid duplication and stress on programs and families, and promote efficient use of consultant resources.

Additionally, a plan should be in place that outlines how the state identifies, trains, and supports consultants who, in turn, support programs. Minimum qualifications required of consultants may be specified in state regulations. There are resources for training consultants, e.g., The National Training Institute for Child Care Health Consultants (NTI) that can be integrated into state plans for supporting health and other early childhood consultants. States will ideally take advantage of opportunities to partner with Head Start, child welfare, Part C and Part B, and others to maintain an ongoing system of supporting consultants and fostering partnerships that support children, families and programs and help improve the overall quality of services provided in the community.

RATIONALE: Securing expertise is acceptable by whatever method is most workable at the state or local level (for example, consultation could be provided from a resource and referral agency). Providers, not the regulatory agency, are responsible for securing the type of consultation that is required by their individual facilities. Ongoing relationships with CCHCs, nutritionists/registered dietitians, and ECMHCs are effective in promoting healthy and safe environments (3-5).

COMMENTS: Several states now have mental health consultants specifically serving the child care community. There are different models of mental health consultation. Some models are programmatic and only include the staff, others work with individual children with behavioral and emotional problems and the third model integrates both approaches. MHCs are usually social workers or professionals with a child development or psychology background who are trained to work in child care settings (2). There is no formal or standardized training for ECMHCs nationally. Developmental and behavioral pediatricians, child and adolescent psychiatrists, and child psychologists are resources for the behavioral and mental health needs of young children (1). Some, but not all, adolescent and child psychiatrists and psychologists, social workers and child counselors have the necessary skills to work with behavior problems of this youngest age group. To find such specialists, contact the Department of Pediatrics at academic centers or the State Department of Mental Health. The faculty at such centers can usually refer child care facilities to individuals with the necessary skills in their area.

The administrative practice of developing systems for technical assistance is designed to enhance the overall quality of child care that meets the social and developmental needs of children. The chief sources of technical assistance are:

a) AAP Chapter Child Care Contact (contact information can be found at http://www.healthychildcare.org);
b) Licensing agencies (on ways to meet the regulations and make quality improvements);
c) Health departments (on health related matters);
d) Resource and referral agencies (on ways to achieve quality, how to start a new facility, supply and demand data, how to get licensed, and what parents/ guardians want);
e) Community action programs or non-profit organizations (on health related matters including physical education, for health education and/or quality improvement issues);
f) Local university kinesiology departments (on early childhood motor development and physical activity issues);
g) Small business administration (on financial issues related to program operations);
h) Subsidy agencies may fund a variety of consultants to programs through the Child Care and Development Fund (CCDF) quality dollars;
i) Education departments often administer the food program dollars and may have technical assistance related to the Individuals with Disabilities Education Act (IDEA).

REFERENCES:

1. American Academy of Pediatrics (AAP). 2001. *The pediatrician's role in promoting health and safety in child care*. Elk Grove Village, IL: AAP.

2. Healthy Child Care America. 2006. *The influence of child care health consultants in promoting children's health and well-being: A status report*. Rockville, MD: Maternal and Child Health Bureau.
3. Crowley, A. A., J. M. Kulikowich. Impact of training on child care health consultant knowledge and practice. *Ped Nurs* 35:93-100.
4. Dellert, J. C., D. Gasalberti, K. Sternas, P. Lucarelli, J. Hall. 2006. Outcomes of child care health consultation services for child care providers in New Jersey: A pilot study. *Pediatric Nursing* 32:530-37.
5. Alkon, A., J. Bernzweig, K. To, M. Wolff, J. F. Mackie. 2009. Child care health consultation improves health and safety policies and practices. *Acad Pediatr* 9:366-70.

STANDARD 10.3.4.4: Development of List of Providers of Services to Facilities

The local regulatory agency or resource and referral agency should assist centers and small and large family child care homes to formulate and maintain a list of community professionals and agencies available to provide needed health, dental, and social services to families.

RATIONALE: Families depend on their child care facilities to provide information about obtaining health and dental care and other community services. A number of communities have Family Resource Centers, which are central points for information. It is important that regulatory agencies and resource and referral agencies have knowledge of family resource centers or can provide a directory of community services to child care facilities.

Partnerships among health care professionals and community agencies are necessary to provide a medical home for all children. The American Academy of Pediatrics (AAP) defines the medical home as care that is accessible, family-centered, continuous, comprehensive, coordinated, compassionate, and culturally competent. The medical home is not a building, house, or hospital, but an approach to providing health care services in a high-quality and cost-effective manner (1,2). Health care professionals and other community service agencies are beginning to recognize that child care facilities are a logical opportunity to provide information or referral of children to a medical home. Child care programs also provide opportunities for education in health promotion and disease prevention for children and families (3).

REFERENCES:

1. Kempe, A., B. Beaty, B. P. Englund, R. J. Roark, N. Hester, J. F. Steiner. 2000. Quality of care and use of the medical home in a state-funded capitated primary care plan for low-income children. *Pediatrics* 105:1020-28.
2. American Academy of Pediatrics. 2008. Policy statement: The medical home. *Pediatrics* 122:450.
3. Gupta, R. S., S. Shuman, E. M. Taveras, M. Kulldorff, J. A. Finkelstein. 2005. Opportunities for health promotion education in child care. *Pediatrics* 116: e499-e505.

STANDARD 10.3.4.5: Resources for Parents/ Guardians of Children with Special Health Care Needs

The state agency or council of agencies responsible for child care services for children with special health care needs should aid parents/guardians in their assessment of facilities for care of children with special health care needs. Agencies should provide printed and audiovisual information about assessment of specialized health care to the parents/ guardians.

In addition, the regulatory agency should refer parents/ guardians of children with special health care needs to a medical home for assistance in development and formulation of a written care plan to be used within a child care program.

RATIONALE: Parents/guardians of children with special health care needs require support to enable their identification and evaluation of facilities where their children can receive quality child care.

Parents/guardians should participate in the facility evaluation, both formally and informally. Unless the Interagency Coordinating Council (ICC) or some similar body provides information to parents/guardians, they are unlikely to be able to find and evaluate options for child care for children with special health care needs. While the professionals involved with the family may do this on behalf of the family, the parents/guardians should have every opportunity to play a significant role in the process.

The state licensing agency as well as the state agencies responsible for implementation of the Individuals with Disabilities Education Act (IDEA) should assist child care caregivers/teachers to recognize the opportunity they have to participate in the child's overall care planning and to obtain training on effective inclusion in order to provide care to the children (1).

RELATED STANDARDS:
Section 1.6: Consultants

REFERENCES:

1. U.S. Department of Health and Human Services, Health Resources and Services Administration, Maternal and Child Health Bureau. State Title V contacts. https://perfdata.hrsa.gov/mchb/mchreports/link/state_links.asp.

STANDARD 10.3.4.6: Compensation for Participation in Multidisciplinary Assessments for Children with Special Health Care or Education Needs

The agency (or a council of such agencies) within the state responsible for overseeing child care for children with special health care or educational needs should assure that the Individualized Family Service Plan (IFSP) or the Individualized Education Program (IEP) includes compensation for the hours of time spent by members of the multidisciplinary team and the staff from the child care program in developing the assessment defined in Standards 8.7.0.1-8.7.0.3.

RATIONALE: Unless there is a source of compensation for the time spent in planning and completing assessments, these requirements cannot be implemented.

Funding under Individuals with Disabilities Education Act (IDEA) makes it possible for the resources and funding for service to follow the child. Traditionally, these funds have paid for individual therapists only, and not for others who participate in formulating the IFSP or IEP. This tradition of restrained spending inhibits effective service delivery for children and families (1).

COMMENTS: For more information and resources, contact the State Children with Special Health Care Needs Program Director. Contact information for each state can be found at: https://perfdata.hrsa.gov/mchb/mchreports/link/state_links.asp.

RELATED STANDARDS:

Standards 8.7.0.1-8.7.0.3: Assessment of Facilities for Children with Special Needs

REFERENCES:

1. U.S. Department of Health and Human Services, Health Resources and Services Administration, Maternal and Child Health Bureau. State Title V contacts. https://perfdata.hrsa.gov/mchb/mchreports/link/state_links.asp.

STANDARD 10.3.4.7: Technical Assistance to Facilities to Address Diversity in the Community

Technical assistance and incentives should be provided by state, municipal, public, and private agencies to encourage facilities to address within their programs, the cultural and socioeconomic diversity in the broader community, not just in the neighborhood where the child care facility is located.

RATIONALE: Children who are exposed to cultural and socioeconomic diversity in early childhood are more likely to value and accept differences between their own backgrounds and those of others as they move through life (1,2). This attitude results in improved self-esteem and mental health in children from all backgrounds. Facilities may be able to attract participants from different income and cultural groups by paying attention to the location of the facility and available subsidies for low income families.

REFERENCES:

1. National Childcare Accreditation Council. 2005. *Diversity in programming: Family day care quality assurance - Factsheet #4*. http://www.ncac.gov.au/factsheets/factsheet4.pdf.
2. Biles, B. Activities that promote racial and cultural awareness. http://www.pbs.org/kcts/preciouschildren/diversity/read_activities.html.

10.3.5 Licensing Staff Training

STANDARD 10.3.5.1: Education, Experience and Training of Licensing Inspectors

Licensing inspectors, and others in licensing positions, should be pre-qualified by education and experience to be knowledgeable about the form of child care they are assigned to inspect. Prior to employment or within the first six months of employment, licensing inspectors should receive training in regulatory administration based on the concepts and principles found in the National Association for Regulatory Administration (NARA) Licensing Curriculum through onsite platform training or online coursework (1). In addition, they should receive no less than forty clock hours of orientation training upon employment (1). In addition, they should receive no less than twenty-four clock hours of continuing education each year (1), covering the following topics and other such topics as necessary based on competency needs:

a) The licensing statutes and rules for child care;
b) Other applicable state and federal statutes and regulations;
c) The historical, conceptual, and theoretical basis for licensing, investigation, and enforcement;
d) Technical skills related to the person's duties and responsibilities, such as investigative techniques, interviewing, rule-writing, due process, and data management;
e) Child development, early childhood education principles, child care programming, scheduling, and design of space;
f) Law enforcement and the rights of licensees;
g) Center and large or small family child care home management;
h) Child and staff health in child care;
i) Detection, prevention, and management of child abuse;
j) Practical techniques and ADA requirements for inclusion of children with special needs;
k) Exclusion/inclusion of children who are ill;
l) Health, safety, physical activity, and nutrition;
m) Recognition of hazards.

RATIONALE: Licensing inspectors are a point of contact and linkage for caregivers/teachers and sources of technical information needed to improve the quality of child care. This is particularly true for areas not usually within the network of early childhood professionals, such as health and safety expertise. Unless the licensing inspector is competent and able to recognize areas where facilities need to improve their health and safety provisions (for example prevention of infectious disease), the opportunity for such linkages will be lost. To effectively carry out their responsibilities to license and monitor child care facilities, it is critical that licensing inspectors have appropriate, conceptually based professional development in the principles, concepts and practices of child care licensing as well as in the principles and practices of the form or child care to which they are assigned. When developed, it will be important for licensing inspectors to secure NARA Licensing Credentials.

REFERENCES:

1. National Association for Regulatory Administration (NARA). 2000. Phases of licensing. In *NARA licensing curriculum.* 2000 ed. Lexington, KY: NARA.

STANDARD 10.3.5.2: Performance Monitoring of Licensing Inspectors

Licensing inspectors should receive initial and periodic competency-based training on the principles and practices of conducting licensing and monitoring inspections for compliance with licensing standards. Competency should be initially and periodically assessed by simultaneous,

independent monitoring by a skilled licensing inspector until the trainee attains the necessary skills. Consistency in interpretation of licensing rules is essential for effective and equitable enforcement of the rules. Achieving consistency across inspectors throughout the state is difficult to achieve and maintain. Examples of effective techniques to achieve consistency are: development of interpretive guidelines which are designed to provide the intent of each rule, the means to achieve compliance, and the criteria to be used to measure compliance.

RATIONALE: Objective assessment of compliance is a learned skill that can be fostered by classroom and self teaching methods but should be mastered through direct practice and apprenticeship. To ensure consistent protection of children, licensing inspectors should undergo periodic retraining and reevaluation to assess their ability to recognize sound and unsound practices. In addition, all staff involved in licensing such as agency directors, attorneys, policy staff, managers, clerical/support personnel, and information system staff need periodic training updates. Training for licensors/inspectors should include best practice programming, child development theory, and law enforcement. The National Association for Regulatory Administration (NARA) professional development system is the primary source for training in the principles and practices of child care licensing (1).

Interpretive guidelines (also known as indicator manuals or field guides) assist staff in consistent interpretation and also assist providers to better understand the intent of the rules and how to achieve compliance. States are beginning to put interpretive guidelines on their Websites for ready use by providers. Licensing staff must be trained on the interpretive guidelines and treat it as a living document which is frequently reviewed and revised as interpretation is refined. Another practice used by some states is to hold periodic case reviews by a licensing office with one individual presenting the case(s) which are critiqued by others. Procedure manuals, consisting of well developed and currendly used procedures to be used in the enforcement of licensing rules and regulatinos are also effective in achieving consistency when there is frequent training and revision as needed. Documents used by the agency for achieving consistency should be conveniently accessible to caregivers/teachers (1).

REFERENCES:

1. Stevens, C. 2008. *Achieving the vision: A workbook for human care regulatory agencies.* Lexington, KY: National Association for Regulatory Administration.

STANDARD 10.3.5.3: Training of Licensing Agency Personnel about Child Abuse

Staff and administrators in licensing agencies and state supported resource and referral agencies should receive sixteen hours of training about child abuse with an emphasis on how child abuse occurs in child care.

RATIONALE: Licensing and resource and referral persons should be at least as well informed about child abuse issues as caregivers/teachers. States should establish procedures to ensure compliance of the training requirement by agency personnel.

10.4 Facility Licensing

10.4.1 Initial Considerations for Licensing

STANDARD 10.4.1.1: Uniform Categories and Definitions

Each state should adopt uniform categories and definitions for its own licensing requirements. Every state should have individual standards that are applied to the following types of facilities:

a) Family child care home: A facility providing care and education of children, including the caregiver/teacher's own children in the home of the caregiver/teacher:
   1) Small family child care home – one to six children;
   2) Large family child care home – seven to twelve children, with one or more qualified adult assistants to meet child: staff ratio requirements;
b) Center: A facility providing care and education of any number of children in a nonresidential setting, or thirteen or more children in any setting if the facility is open on a regular basis (for instance, if it is not a drop-in facility);
c) Drop-in facility: A child care program where children are cared for over short periods of time on a one-time, intermittent, unscheduled and/or occasional basis. Drop-in care is often operated in connection with a business (e.g., health club, hotel, shopping center, or recreation centers);
d) School-age child care facility: A facility offering activities to school-age children before and after school, during vacations, and non-school days set aside for such activities as caregivers'/teachers' in-service programs;
e) Facility for children who are mildly ill: A facility providing care of one or more children who are mildly ill, children who are temporarily excluded from care in their regular child care setting;
f) Integrated or small group care for children who are mildly ill: A facility that has been approved by the licensing agency to care for well children and to include up to six children who are mildly ill;
g) Special facility for children who are mildly ill: A facility that cares only for children who are mildly ill, or a facility that cares for more than six children who are mildly ill at a time.

RATIONALE: Lack of standard terminology hampers the ability of citizens and professionals to compare rules from state to state or to apply national guidance material to upgrade the quality of care (1). For example, child care for seven to twelve children in the residence of the caregiver/teacher may be referred to as family day care, a group day care home, or a mini-center in different states. While it is not essential that each state use the same terms and some variability in definitions of types of care may occur, terminology should be consistent within the state and as consistent as possible from state to state in the way different types of settings are classified. Child care facilities should be differentiated from community facilities that primarily care for those with developmental disabilities, the elderly, and other adults and teenagers who need supervised care (2).

RELATED STANDARDS:

Standards 3.6.2.1-3.6.2.10: Caring for Children Who Are Ill

REFERENCES:

1. National Association for the Education of Young Children (NAEYC). 1997. *Licensing and public regulation of early childhood programs: A position statement*. Washington, DC: NAEYC.
2. Newacheck, P. W., B. Strickland, J. P. Shonkoff, et al. 1998. An epidemiologic profile of children with special health care needs. *Pediatrics* 102:117-23.

STANDARD 10.4.1.2: Quality Rating and Improvement Systems

States should develop a quality rating and improvement system (QRIS) to provide incentives to improve the quality of child care based on or using the licensing system as its foundation.

RATIONALE: A highly functioning licensing system has to be the foundation for a quality rating and improvement system in order to work properly (3). It is important to recognize the relevance of health and safety in the quality criteria (1,2).

COMMENTS: Quality rating and improvement systems (QRIS) are initiatives in states to provide incentives for improved child care in licensed child care centers and small and large family child care homes. It is important for the QRIS system to work closely with all parts of the early care and education system and the health care system. Examples include ensuring health and safety measures are part of the ratings and access to a child care health consultant is required.

REFERENCES:

1. Friedman, D. E. 2007. Quality rating systems: The experiences of center directors. *Child Care Exchange* 173:6-12.
2. U.S. Department of Health and Human Services, Administration for Children and Families, National Child Care Information and Technical Assistance Center. Quality improvement systems. http://nccic.acf.hhs.gov/topics/quality-improvement-systems.
3. Mitchell, A. W. 2005. *Stair steps to quality: A guide for states and communities developing quality rating systems for early care and education*. Alexandria, VA: United Way of America, Success By 6.

STANDARD 10.4.1.3: Licensing Agency Procedures Prior to Issuing a License

Before granting a license to a facility, the licensing agency should check as specified below for a record of a physical examination and for educational qualifications, and should check background screening records for all adults who are permitted to be alone with children in a facility. The licensing agency should also check background screening records for all persons over ten years of age who live in a small or large family child care home where child care is provided.

a) Staff health appraisals, as specified in Standard 1.7.0.1;
b) Educational requirements, as specified in Sections 1.3 and 1.4;
c) Criminal record files, for crimes of violence against persons, especially children, within the state of residence, and for personnel who have moved into the state within the past five years, federal or out of state criminal records of the other state(s) where the individual has resided in the past five years;
d) The child abuse registry, for a known history of child abuse or neglect in the state of residence and for personnel who have moved into the state within the past five years, the other state(s) where the individual has resided in the past five years (1);
e) The sex offender registry, for a known history of sex-related crimes in the state of residence and for personnel who have moved into the state within the past five years, the other state(s) where the individual has resided in the past five years.

RATIONALE: Requiring a check of both criminal records and the sex offender registry provides additional protection against individuals avoiding detection by using other names or files not being forwarded to the applicable agencies.

COMMENTS: In many cases juvenile records are sealed and cannot be used for the purposes of background checks. To determine the policy in your state or local jurisdiction contact the State Attorney General's Office or the local County Prosecutor.

RELATED STANDARDS:

Section 1.3: Pre-service Qualifications
Section 1.4: Professional Development/Training
Standard 1.7.0.1: Pre-Employment and Ongoing Adult Health Appraisals, Including Immunization

REFERENCES:

1. National Association for Regulatory Administration (NARA). 2000. Phases of licensing. In *NARA licensing curriculum.* 2000 ed. Lexington, KY: NARA.

STANDARD 10.4.1.4: Alternative Means of Compliance

Alternative means of compliance should be granted from state licensing requirements when the intent of the requirement is being met by equivalent means and does not compromise the health, safety or protection of children (1).

RATIONALE: The ability to grant alternative means of compliance recognizes the variety of settings and services that can effectively and safely meet children's needs. Flexibility in applying licensing regulations should be permitted to the extent that children's need for protection is met.

REFERENCES:

1. National Association for Regulatory Administration (NARA). 2000. Phases of licensing. In *NARA licensing curriculum.* 2000 ed. Lexington, KY: NARA.

10.4.2 Facility Inspections and Monitoring

STANDARD 10.4.2.1: Frequency of Inspections for Child Care Centers, Large Family Child Care Homes, and Small Family Child Care Homes

The licensing inspector should make an onsite inspection to measure compliance with licensing rules prior to issuing an initial license and at least two inspections each year to each center and large and small family child care home thereafter. At least one of the inspections should be unannounced and more if needed for the facility to achieve satisfactory compliance or is closed at any time (1). Sufficient numbers of licensing inspectors should be hired to provide adequate time visiting and inspecting facilities to insure compliance with regulations

The number of inspections should not include those inspections conducted for the purpose of investigating complaints. Complaints should be investigated promptly, based on severity of the complaint. States are encouraged to post the results of licensing inspections, including complaints, on the Internet for parent and public review. Parents/guardians should be provided easy access to the licensing rules and made aware of how to report complaints to the licensing agency.

RATIONALE: Licensing inspections are important to assist facilities to achieve and maintain full compliance with licensing rules. Supervision and monitoring of child care facilities are critical to facilitate continued compliance with the rules in order to prevent or correct problems before they become serious (2). Technical assistance and consultation provided by licensing inspectors on an on-going basis are essential to help programs achieve compliance with the rules and go beyond the basic level of quality. These positive strategies are most effective when they are coupled with the non-regulatory methods used by other parts of the early care and education community to promote quality (such as professional development, quality and improvement rating systems, accreditation, peer support, and consumer education) (3). All of these methods are most effective when they work together within a coordinated early care and education system. Research has demonstrated that posting of licensing information on the Internet has a positive effect on compliance with licensing rules (3).

REFERENCES:

1. National Association for Regulatory Administration (NARA). 2010. *Strong licensing: The foundation for a quality early care and education system: NARA's call to action.* http://www.naralicensing.org/associations/4734/files/NARA_Call_to_Action.pdf.
2. National Association for Regulatory Administration (NARA). 1999. *Licensing workload assessment*. Technical assistance bulletin #99-01. Lexington, KY: NARA.
3. Witte, A. D., M. Queralt. 2004. What happens when child care inspections and complaints are made available on the internet? Faculty Working Paper 10227, Wellesley College Department of Economics and National Bureau of Economic Research, Wellesley Child Care Research Partnership.
3. National Association for Regulatory Administration (NARA). 2000. Phases of licensing. In *NARA licensing curriculum.* 2000 ed. Lexington, KY: NARA.

STANDARD 10.4.2.2: Statutory Authorization of On-Site Inspections

The state statute should authorize the state regulatory agency to conduct on-site inspections of child care/early care and education facilities.

RATIONALE: The National Association for the Education of Young Children (NAEYC) Position Statement says, "Effective enforcement requires periodic on-site inspections on both an announced and unannounced basis with meaningful sanctions for noncompliance" (1). When unannounced inspections are used, they should be conducted at any hour the facility is in operation, i.e., evenings and nights included if the facility operates at those times (2). NAEYC recommends that all centers and large and small family child care homes receive at least one site visit per year. Unannounced inspections have been shown to be especially effective when targeted to providers with a history of low compliance (1).

REFERENCES:

1. National Association for the Education of Young Children (NAEYC). 1997. *Licensing and public regulation of early childhood programs: A position statement*. Washington, DC: NAEYC.
2. U.S. Department of Health, Education, and Welfare (DHEW), Office of Child Development (OCD). 1973. *Guides for day care licensing*. DHEW Publication no. OCD 73-1053. Washington, DC: DHEW, OCD.

STANDARD 10.4.2.3: Monitoring Strategies

The licensing agency should adopt monitoring strategies that ensure compliance with licensing requirements. These strategies should include the provision of technical assistance, advice and guidance to help providers achieve and maintain compliance with licensing requirements and consultation, advice and guidance to encourage upgrading the quality of care to exceed licensing requirements (1). When these strategies do not include a total annual review of all licensing requirements, the agency should review selected policies and performance indicators and/or conduct a random sampling of licensing requirements at least annually. The licensing agency should have procedures and staffing in place to increase the level of compliance monitoring for any facility found in significant noncompliance.

RATIONALE: Due to an insufficient number of inspectors in licensing agencies across the country, it is important to use various methods in the licensing process to insure quality (2). Monitoring with a focus on teaching, encouraging, upgrading and safeguarding, can be very successful in assisting programs and providers to achieve and maintain compliance with licensing requirements (2).

REFERENCES:

1. National Association for Regulatory Administration (NARA). 2000. Phases of licensing. In *NARA licensing curriculum.* 2000 ed. Lexington, KY: NARA.

2. Fiene, R. 2002. *13 indicators of quality child care: Research update*. Washington, DC: U.S. Department of Health and Human Services, Office of the Assistant Secretary for Planning and Evaluation. http://aspe.hhs.gov/hsp/ccquality-ind02/.

STANDARD 10.4.2.4: Agency Collaboration to Safeguard Children in Child Care

The child care licensing, building, fire safety, and health authorities, as well as any other regulators (e.g., environmental, sanitation, and food safety), should work together as a team to safeguard children in child care. The team should eliminate duplication of inspections to create more efficient regulatory efforts. Examples of activities to be coordinated include:

a) Inspection of child care facility;
b) Reporting and surveillance systems;
c) Guidance in managing outbreaks of infectious diseases;
d) Preventing exposure of children to hazards;
e) Reporting child abuse;
f) Training and technical consultation;
g) Disaster preparedness and response planning (1).

Regulatory agents should collaborate to educate caregivers/teachers, parents/guardians, health care providers, public health workers, licensors, and employers about their roles in ensuring health and safety in child care settings.

RATIONALE: Frequently, caregivers/teachers are burdened by complicated procedures and conflicting requirements to obtain clearance from various authorities to operate. To use limited resources, agencies must avoid contradictions in regulatory codes, simplify inspection procedures, and reduce bureaucratic disincentives to the provision of safe and healthy care for children. When regulatory authorities work as a team, collaboration should focus on establishing the role of each agency in ensuring that necessary services and systems exist to prevent and control health and safety problems in facilities. Each member of the team gains opportunities to learn about the responsibilities of other team members so that close working relationships can be established, conflicts can be resolved, and decisions can be reached. In small states, a state level task force may be sufficient. In larger or more populous states, local task forces may be needed to promote effective use of resources.

COMMENTS: The licensing agency can facilitate communication and collaboration between the child care facility and the state health department, Emergency Medical Services (EMS) agencies, other regulatory agencies, funding agencies, child protection agencies, law enforcement agencies, community service agencies, school districts and school personnel, including school nurses, and local government to safeguard children in child care.

RELATED STANDARDS:

Standard 3.4.4.1: Recognizing and Reporting Suspected Child Abuse, Neglect, and Exploitation
Standard 6.2.5.1: Inspection of Indoor and Outdoor Play Areas and Equipment
Chapter 7: Infectious Disease
Standards 9.2.4.1-9.2.4.10: Emergency/Security Policies and Plans

REFERENCES:

1. American Academy of Pediatrics. Children and disasters. http://www.aap.org/disasters/.

10.4.3 Procedures for Complaints, Reporting, and Data Collecting

STANDARD 10.4.3.1: Procedure for Receiving Complaints

Each licensing agency should have a procedure for receiving complaints regarding violation of the regulations. Such complaints should be recorded, investigated, and appropriate action, if indicated, should be taken.

RATIONALE: The telephone number, email address, or other contact method for filing complaints should be listed on material about licensing that is given to parents/guardians by the state licensing agency and the resource and referral agency. At a minimum, the licensing agency has responsibility for consumer protection. Complaints serve as an early warning before more serious adverse events occur. A fair and equitable process for handling complaints is essential to protect both the person complaining and the target of the complaint from harassment. In most cases complaint investigation should include an unannounced inspection.

STANDARD 10.4.3.2: Whistle-Blower Protection under State Law

State law should ensure that caregivers/teachers and child care staff who report violation of licensing requirements in the settings where they work are immune from discharge, retaliation, or other disciplinary action for that reason alone, unless it is proven that the report was malicious.

RATIONALE: Staff in child care facilities are in an excellent position to note areas of noncompliance with licensing requirements in the setting where they work. However, so that they feel safe about reporting these deficiencies, they must be assured immunity from retaliation by the child care facility unless the report is malicious. This immunity is best provided when a state statute mandates it. Individuals who report problems in their own workplace may be known as "whistle-blowers" (1).

Retaliatory complaints against a caregiver/teacher by disgruntled staff or parents/guardians at times serve only to harass the provider and expend valuable licensing resources or unnecessary work. States should recognize and develop a system to deal with these nuisance complaints.

REFERENCES:

1. U.S. Department of Labor, Northern Hudson Valley Job Services Employer Committee. 2010. Whistleblower protection laws. http://eclkc.ohs.acf.hhs.gov/hslc/tta-system/operations/Management and Administration/Human Resources/Personnel Policies/WhistleblowerPro.htm.

STANDARD 10.4.3.3: Collection of Data on Illness or Harm to Children in Facilities

The state regulatory agency should have access to an information system for collecting data relative to the incidence of illness and injuries, confirmed child abuse and neglect, and death of children in facilities. This data should be shared with appropriate agencies and the child care health consultant for analysis.

RATIONALE: Sound public policy planning in respect to health and safety in facilities starts with the collection of epidemiological data. When outbreaks or emergencies occur, quick identification of, and appropriate response to, an unusual circumstance is critical. Conducting daily health checks and keeping symptom records is a good way to identify the potential for an infectious disease emergency or outbreak. When children in a group seem to have similar symptoms that suggest a contagious disease is spreading, the program should consult with its child care health consultant or medical advisor (1). Licensing agencies can make appropriate and preventive changes to licensing regulations and program monitoring if they have accurate data on which to base those changes (2).

RELATED STANDARDS:
Standard 3.1.1.1: Conduct of Daily Health Check
Standards 3.4.4.1-3.4.4.5: Child Abuse and Neglect
Standard 3.6.4.5: Death

REFERENCES:
1. Aronson, S. S., T. R. Shope, eds. 2009. *Managing infectious diseases in child care and schools: A quick reference guide.* 2nd ed. Elk Grove Village, IL: American Academy of Pediatrics.
2. Wrigley, J., J. Derby. 2005. Fatalities and the organization of child care in the United States. *Am Socio Rev* 70:729-57.

10.5 Health Department Responsibilities and Role

STANDARD 10.5.0.1: State and Local Health Department Role

State and local health departments should play an important role in the identification, prevention and control of injuries, injury risk, and infectious disease in child care settings as well as in using the child care setting to promote health and safety. This role includes the following activities to be conducted in collaboration with the child care licensing agency:

a) Assisting in the planning of a comprehensive health and safety program for children and child care providers, including promoting and ensuring maintenance of a system of child care health consultation;
b) Monitoring the occurrence of serious injury events and outbreaks involving children or providers;
c) Alerting the responsible child care administrators about identified or potential injury hazards and infectious disease risks in the child care setting;
d) Controlling outbreaks, identifying and reporting infectious diseases in child care settings including:
    1) Methods for notifying parents/guardians, caregivers/teachers, and health care providers of the problem;
    2) Providing appropriate actions for the child care provider to take;
    3) Providing policies for exclusion or isolation of infected children;
    4) Arranging a source and method for the administration of needed medication;
    5) Providing a list of reportable diseases, including descriptions of these diseases. The list should specify where diseases are to be reported and what information is to be provided by the child care provider to the health department and to parents/guardians;
    6) Requiring that all facilities, regardless of licensure status, and all health care providers report certain infectious diseases to the responsible local or state public health authority. The child care licensing authority should require such reporting under its regulatory jurisdiction and should collaborate fully with the health department when the latter is engaged in an enforcement action with a licensed facility;
    7) Determining whether a disease represents a potential health risk to children in out-of-home child care;
    8) Conducting the epidemiological investigation necessary to initiate public health and safety interventions;
    9) Recommending a disease prevention or control strategy that is based on sound public health and clinical practices (such as the use of vaccine, immunoglobulin, or antibiotics taken to prevent an infection);
    10) Verifying reports of infectious diseases received from facilities with the assessment and diagnosis of the disease made by a health care provider and, or the local or state health department;
e) Designing systems and forms for use by facilities for the care of children who are ill to document the surveillance of cared for illnesses and problems that arise in the care of children in such child care settings;
f) Assisting in the development of orientation and annual training programs for caregivers/teachers. Such training should include specialized education for staff of facilities that include child who are ill, as well as those in special facilities that serve only children who are ill. Specialized training for staff who care for children who are ill should focus on the recognition and management of childhood illnesses, as well as the care of children with infectious diseases;
g) Assisting the licensing authority in the periodic review of facility performance related to caring for children who are ill by:
    1) Reviewing written policies developed by facilities regarding inclusion, exclusion, dismissal criteria

and plans for health care, urgent and emergency care, and reporting and managing children with infectious disease;

2) Assisting with periodic compliance reviews for those rules relating to inclusion, exclusion, dismissal, daily health care, urgent and emergency care, and reporting and management of children with infectious disease;

h) Collaborating in the planning and implementation of appropriate training and educational programs related to health and safety in child care facilities. Such training should include education of parents/guardians, primary care providers, public health and safety workers, licensing inspectors, and employers about how to prevent injury and disease as well as promote health and safety of children and their caregivers/teachers;

i) Promoting that health care personnel, such as qualified public health nurses, pediatric and family nurse practitioners, and pediatricians serve as child care health consultants;

j) Ensuring child care programs are included and represented in local and state disaster preparedness and pandemic flu planning.

RATIONALE: A number of studies have described the incidence of injuries in the child care setting (7-10). Although the injuries described have not been serious, these occur frequently, and may require medical or emergency attention. Child care programs need the assistance of local and state health agencies in planning of the safety program that will minimize the risk for serious injury (11). This would include planning for such significant emergencies as fire, flood, tornado, or earthquake (11-13). A community health agency can collect information that can promptly identify an injury risk or hazard and provide an early notice about the risk or hazard (14). An example is the recent identification of unpowered scooters as a significant injury risk for preschool children (15). Once the injury risk is identified, appropriate channels of communication are required to alert the child care administrators and to provide training and educational activities.

Effective control and prevention of infectious diseases in child care settings depends on affirmative relationships among parents/guardians, caregivers/teachers, public health authorities, regulatory agencies, and primary health care providers. The major barriers to productive working relationships between caregivers/teachers and health care providers are inadequate channels of communication and uncertainty of role definition (4). Public health authorities can play a major role in improving the relationship between caregivers/teachers and primary care providers by disseminating information regarding disease reporting laws, prescribed measures for control and prevention of diseases and injuries, and resources that are available for these activities (11). Child care health consultant networks have proven to be effective in improving the health and safety of children in child care settings (16-18).

State and local health departments are legally required to control certain infectious diseases within their jurisdictions (20). All states have laws that grant extraordinary powers to public health departments during outbreaks of infectious diseases (1,11,12). Since infectious disease is likely to occur in child care settings, a plan for the control of infectious diseases in these settings is essential and often legally required. Early recognition and prompt intervention will reduce the spread of infection. Outbreaks of infectious disease in child care settings can have great implications for the general community (2). Programs administered by local health departments have been more successful in controlling outbreaks of hepatitis A than those that rely primarily on private physicians. Programs coordinated by the local health department also provide reassurance to caregivers/teachers, staff, and parents/guardians, and thereby promote cooperation with other disease control policies (3). Infectious diseases in child care settings pose new epidemiological considerations. Only in recent decades has it been so common for very young children to spend most of their days together in groups. Public health authorities should expand their role in studying this situation and designing new preventive health measures (4,5).

Collaboration is necessary to use limited resources most effectively. In small states, a state level task force that includes the Department of Health might be sufficient. In larger or more populous states, local task forces in addition to coordination at the state level may be needed. The collaboration should focus on establishing the role of each agency in ensuring that necessary services and systems exist to prevent and control injuries and infectious diseases in facilities (6,19).

Health departments generally have or should develop the expertise to provide leadership and technical assistance to licensing authorities, caregivers/teachers, parents/guardians, and primary care providers in the development of licensing requirements and guidelines for the management of children who are ill. The heavy reliance on the expertise of local and state health departments in the establishment of facilities to care for children who are ill has fostered a partnership in many states among health departments, licensing authorities, caregivers/teachers, and parents/guardians for the adequate care of children who are ill in child care settings (16-18).

RELATED STANDARDS:
Section 1.6: Consultants
Standard 3.6.2.5: Caregiver Qualifications for Facilities that Care for Children Who Are Ill
Standard 3.6.2.7: Child Care Health Consultants for Facilities that Care for Children Who Are Ill
Standards 3.6.4.3-3.6.4.4: Reporting Policies

REFERENCES:
1. Grad, F. P. 2004. *The public health law manual*. 3rd ed. Washington, DC: American Public Health Association.
2. Brady, M. T. 2005. Infectious disease in pediatric out-of-home child care. *Am J Infect Control* 33:276-85.
3. Heymann, D. L. 2008. *Control of communicable diseases manual*. 19th ed. Washington, DC: American Public Health Association.

4. Ginter, P. M., Wingate, M. S., A. C. Rucks, R. D. Vasconez, L. C. McCormick, S. Baldwin, C. A. Fargason. 2006. Creating a regional pediatric medical disaster preparedness network: Imperative and issues. *Maternal Child Health J* 10:391-96.
5. Buttross, S. 2006. Caring for children of caretakers during a disaster. *Pediatrics* 117: S446-47.
6. Wilson, S. A., B. J. Temple, M. E. Milliron, C. Vazquez, M. D. Packard, B. S. Rudy. 2008. The lack of disaster preparedness by the public and it's affect on communities. *Internet J Rescue Disaster Med* 7 (2): 1.
7. Murray, J. S. 2009. Disaster care: Public health emergencies and children. *Am J Nursing* 109: 28-29, 31.
8. Vollman, D., R. Witsaman, D. R. Comstock, G. A. Smith. 2009. Epidemiology of playground equipment-related injuries to children in the United States, 1996-2005. *Clinical Pediatrics* 48:66-71.
9. Gordon, R. A., R. Kaestner, S. Korenman. 2007. The effects of maternal employment on child injuries and infectious disease. *Demography* 44:307-33.
10. Jansson, B., A. P. De Leon, N. Ahmed, V. Jansson. 2006. Why does Sweden have the lowest childhood mortality in the world? The role of architecture and public pre-school services. *J Public Health Policy* 27:146-65.
11. Gaines, S. K., J. M. Leary. 2004. Public health emergency preparedness in the setting of child care. *Family and Comm Health* 27:260-65.
12. American Academy of Pediatrics, Committee on Pediatric Emergency Medicine, Task Force on Terrorism. 2006. Policy statement: The pediatrician and disaster preparedness. *Pediatrics* 117:560-65.
13. National Association of Child Care Resource and Referral Agencies. Helping families and children cope with trauma in the aftermath of disaster. http://www.naccrra.org/for_parents/coping/trauma.php.
14. Samet, J. M. 2004. Risk assessment and child health. *Pediatrics* 113:952-56.
15. Kubiak, R., T. Slongo. 2003. Unpowered scooter injuries in children. *Acta Paediatrics* 92:50-54.
16. Crowley, A. A. and Kulikowich, J. M. 2009. Impact of training on child care health consultant knowledge and practice. *Pediatric Nurs* 35:93-100.
17. Dellert, J. C., D. Gasalberti, K. Sternas, P. Lucarelli, J. Hall. 2006. Outcomes of child care health consultation services for child care providers in New Jersey: A pilot study. *Pediatric Nursing* 32:530-37.
18. Alkon, A., J. Bernzweig, K. To, M. Wolff, J. F. Mackie. 2009. Child care health consultation improves health and safety policies and practices. *Academic Pediatrics* 9:366-70.
19. Garrett, A. L., R. Grant, P. Madrid, A. Brito, D. Abramson, I. Redlener. 2007. Children and megadisasters: Lessons learned in the new millennium. *Advances Pediatrics* 54:189-214.
20. National Child Care Information and Technical Assistance Center. State and territory emergency preparedness plans. http://nccic.acf.hhs.gov/poptopics/disasterprep.html.

STANDARD 10.5.0.2: Written Plans for the Health Department Role

The health department's role defined in Standard 10.5.0.1 should be described in written plans that assign the responsibilities of community agencies and organizations involved in the prevention and control of injury, injury risk, and infectious disease in facilities. The plan should identify child care related risks and diseases as well as provide guidance for risk reduction, disease prevention and control. The health department should develop these written plans in collaboration with the licensing agency (if other than the health department), health care providers, caregivers/teachers, and parents/guardians to ensure the availability of sufficient community resources for successful implementation. In addition, the health department should provide assistance to the licensing agency (if other than the health department) for the promulgation and enforcement of child care facility standards. These services should be in addition to the health agency's assigned responsibilities for enforcement of the state's immunization and other health laws and regulations.

In addition to *Caring for Our Children (CFOC)* and *Stepping Stones*, the following resources should be consulted in the development of the health department plan:

a) Guidelines from the American Academy of Pediatrics (AAP), including current editions of *Red Book, Managing Infectious Diseases in Child Care and Schools, Managing Chronic Health Needs in Child Care and Schools*, and the many other relevant technical manuals on such topics as environment and nutrition;
b) Guidelines from the American Public Health Association (APHA), including *Control of Communicable Diseases Manual;*
c) Guidelines provided by the Centers for Disease Control and Prevention (CDC);
d) Guidelines from the U.S. Public Health Service's Advisory Committee on Immunization Practices, as reported periodically in *Morbidity and Mortality Weekly Report (MMWR);*
e) State and local regulations and guidelines regarding infectious diseases in facilities;
f) *Bright Futures - Guidelines for Health Supervision of Infants, Children, and Adolescents;*
g) Current early childhood nutrition guidelines such as *Preventing Childhood Obesity and Making Food Healthy and Safe for Children.*
h) Current early childhood physical activity resources, such as *Active Start: A Statement of Physical Activity Guidelines for Children From Birth to Age 5, 2nd Edition; Moving with a Purpose: Developing Programs for Preschoolers of All Abilities;* and *Purposeful Play: Early Childhood Movement Activities on a Budget.*

RATIONALE: Written plans help define delegation and accountability, providing the continuity of purpose that helps to institutionalize performance.

RELATED STANDARDS:
Standard 10.5.0.4: Use of Fact Sheets on Common Illnesses Associated with Child Care

STANDARD 10.5.0.3: Requirements for Facilities to Report to Health Department

The child care licensing authority should require all facilities under its regulatory jurisdiction to report outbreaks to the health department and comply with state and local rules and regulations intended to prevent infectious disease that apply to child care facilities.

RATIONALE: State and local health departments are legally required to control certain infectious diseases within their jurisdictions. All states have laws that grant extraordinary powers to public health departments during outbreaks or epidemics of infectious disease or bioterrorism attacks. Since infectious disease is likely to occur in child care settings, a plan for the control of infectious diseases in these settings is essential and often legally required. Early recognition and prompt intervention will reduce the spread of infection.

Outbreaks of infectious disease in child care settings can have great implications for the general community (1,4). Programs administered by local health departments have been more successful in controlling outbreaks of hepatitis A than those that rely primarily on private physicians. Programs coordinated by the local health department also provide reassurance to caregivers/teachers, staff, and parents/guardians, and thereby promote cooperation with other disease and safety control policies (2). Infectious diseases in child care settings pose epidemiological considerations. Public health authorities should expand their role in studying this situation and designing new preventive health and safety measures (3).

REFERENCES:

1. Churchill, R. B., L. K. Pickering. 1997. Infection control challenges in child-care centers. *Infect Dis Clin North Am* 11:347-65.
2. Heymann, D. L. 2008. *Control of communicable diseases manual*. 19th ed. Washington, DC: American Public Health Association.
3. Reves, R. R., L. K. Pickering. 1992. Impact of child day care on infectious diseases in adults. *Infect Dis Clin North Am* 6:239-50.
4. Aronson, S. S., T. R. Shope, eds. 2009. *Managing infectious diseases in child care and schools: A quick reference guide.* 2nd ed. Elk Grove Village, IL: American Academy of Pediatrics.

STANDARD 10.5.0.4: Use of Fact Sheets on Common Illnesses Associated with Child Care

Health departments should help child care providers use prepared prototype parent and staff fact sheets on common illnesses associated with child care. These fact sheets should:

a) Be provided to parents/guardians when their child is first admitted to the facility, to staff at the time of employment and to both parents/guardians and staff when infectious disease notification is recommended;
b) Contain the following information:
c) Disease (case or outbreak) to which the child was exposed;
d) Signs and symptoms of the disease that the parents/guardians and caregivers/teachers should watch for in the child;
e) Mode of transmission of the disease;
f) Period of communicability;
g) Disease prevention measures recommended by the public health department (if appropriate);
h) Emphasize modes of transmission of respiratory disease and infections of the intestines (often with diarrhea) and liver, common methods of infection control (such as hand hygiene).

RATIONALE: Education is a primary method for providing information to primary care providers and parents/guardians about the incidence of infectious diseases in child care settings (1). Education of child care staff and parents/guardians on the recognition and transmission of various infectious diseases is important to any infection control policy (1). Training of child care staff has improved the quality of their health related behaviors and practices. Training should be available to all parties involved, including caregivers/teachers, public health workers, health care providers, parents/guardians, and children. Good quality training, with imaginative and accessible methods of presentation supported by well-designed materials, will facilitate learning. The number of studies evaluating the importance of education of child care staff in the prevention of disease is limited. However, data from numerous studies in hospitals illustrate the important role of continuing education in preventing and minimizing the transmission of infectious disease (1). The provision of fact sheets on infectious childhood diseases at the time their child is admitted to a facility helps educate parents/guardians as to the early signs and symptoms of these illnesses and the need to inform caregivers/teachers of their existence. Illness information sheets can be assembled in a convenient booklet for this purpose. Health departments may consult or use nationally accepted fact sheets on common illnesses available from such agencies as the American Academy of Pediatrics (AAP) in its *Managing Infectious Diseases in Child Care and Schools, 2nd ed*. and the Centers for Disease Control and Prevention (CDC).

RELATED STANDARDS:

Standards 3.2.1.1-3.2.3.4: Hygiene
Chapter 7: Infectious Disease

REFERENCES:

1. Pickering, L. K., C. J. Baker, D. W. Kimberlin, S. S. Long, eds. 2009. *Red book: 2009 report of the Committee on Infectious Diseases*. 28th ed. Elk Grove Village, IL: American Academy of Pediatrics.

10.6 Caregiver/Teacher Support

10.6.1 Caregiver/Teacher Training

STANDARD 10.6.1.1: Regulatory Agency Provision of Caregiver/Teacher and Consumer Training and Support Services

The licensing agency should promote participation in a variety of caregiver/teacher and consumer training and support services as an integral component of its mission to reduce risks to children in out-of-home child care. Such training should emphasize the importance of conducting regular safety checks and providing direct supervision of children at all times. Training plans should include mechanisms for training of prospective child care staff prior to their assuming responsibility for the care of children and for ongoing/continuing education. The higher education institutions providing early education degree programs should be coordinated with training provided at the community level to

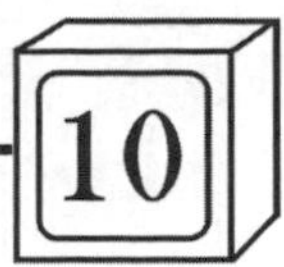

encourage continuing education and availability of appropriate content in the coursework provide by these institutions of higher education.

Persons wanting to enter the child care field should be able to learn from the regulatory agency about training opportunities offered by public and private agencies. Discussions of these trainings can emphasize critical child care health and safety messages. Some training can be provided online to reinforce classroom education.

Training programs should address the following:

a) Child growth and development including social-emotional, cognitive, language, and physical development;
b) Child care programming and activities;
c) Discipline and behavior management;
d) Mandated child abuse and neglect reporting;
e) Health and safety practices including injury prevention, basic first aid and CPR, reporting, preventing and controlling infectious diseases, children's environmental health and health promotion, and reducing the risk of SIDS and use of safe sleep practices;
f) Cultural diversity;
g) Nutrition and eating habits including the importance of breastfeeding and the prevention of obesity and related chronic diseases;
h) Parent/guardian education;
i) Design, use and safe cleaning of physical space;
j) Care and education of children with special health care needs;
k) Oral health care;
l) Reporting requirements for infectious disease outbreaks;
m) Caregiver/teacher health;
n) Age-appropriate physical activity.

RATIONALE: Training enhances staff competence (1,2,4). In addition to low child:staff ratio, group size, age mix of children, and continuity of caregiver/teacher, the training/education of caregivers/teachers is a specific indicator of child care quality (1,2). Most states require limited training for child care staff depending on their functions and responsibilities. Some states do not require completion of a high school degree or GED for various levels of teacher positions (5). Staff members who are better trained are more able to prevent, recognize, and correct health and safety problems. Decisions about management of illness are facilitated by the caregiver's/teacher's increased skill in assessing a child's behavior that suggests illness (2,3). Training should promote increased opportunity in the field and openings to advance through further degree-credentialed education.

RELATED STANDARDS:

Standards 1.4.2.1-1.4.2.3: Orientation Training
Standard 10.6.2.1: Development of Child Care Provider Organizations and Networks

REFERENCES:

1. U.S. General Accounting Office (USGAO); Health, Education, and Human Services Division. 1994. Child care: Promoting quality in family child care. Report to the chairman, subcommittee on regulation, business opportunities, and technology, committee on small business, House of Representatives. Publication no. GAO-HEHS-95-36. Washington, DC: USGAO.
2. Galinsky, E., C. Howes, S. Kontos, M. Shinn. 1994. *The study of children in family child care and relative care*. New York: Families and Work Institute.
19. Aronson, S. S., L. S. Aiken. 1980. Compliance of child care programs with health and safety standards: Impact of program evaluation and advocate training. *Pediatrics* 65:318-25.
3. Kendrick, A. S. 1994. Training to ensure healthy child day-care programs. *Pediatrics* 94:1108-10.
4. Moon, R. Y., R. P. Oden. 2003. Back to sleep: Can we influence child care providers? *Pediatrics* 112:878-82.
5. National Child Care Information and Technical Assistance Center, National Association for Regulatory Administration (NARA). 2010. *The 2008 child care licensing study: Final report*. Lexington, KY: NARA. http://www.naralicensing.org/associations/4734/files/1005_2008_Child Care Licensing Study_Full_Report.pdf.

STANDARD 10.6.1.2: Provision of Training to Facilities by Health Agencies

Public health departments, other state departments charged with professional development for out of home child care providers, and Emergency Medical Services (EMS) agencies should provide training, written information, consultation in at least the following subject areas or referral to other community resources (e.g., child care health consultants, licensing personnel, health care professionals, including school nurses) who can provide such training in:

a) Immunization;
b) Reporting, preventing, and managing of infectious diseases;
c) Techniques for the prevention and control of infectious diseases;
d) Exclusion and inclusion guidelines and care of children who are acutely ill;
e) General hygiene and sanitation;
f) Food service, nutrition, and infant and child-feeding;
g) Care of children with special health care needs (chronic illnesses, physical and developmental disabilities, and behavior problems);
h) Prevention and management of injury;
i) Managing emergencies;
j) Oral health;
k) Environmental health;
l) Health promotion, including routine health supervision and the importance of a medical or health home for children and adults;
m) Health insurance, including Medicaid and the Children's Health Insurance Program (CHIP);
n) Strategies for preparing for and responding to infectious disease outbreaks, such as a pandemic influenza;
o) Age-appropriate physical activity;
p) Sudden Infant Death Syndrome (SIDS) and Shaken Baby Syndrome/Abusive Head Trauma.

RATIONALE: Training of child care staff has improved the quality of their health related behaviors and practices. Training should be available to all parties involved, includ-

ing caregivers/teachers, public health workers, health care providers, parents/guardians, and children. Good quality training, with imaginative and accessible methods of presentation supported by well-designed materials, will facilitate learning.

RELATED STANDARDS:
Standards 1.4.4.1-1.4.6.2: Continuing Education
Standard 10.5.0.1: State and Local Health Department Role

10.6.2 Caregiver/Teacher Networking and Collaboration

STANDARD 10.6.2.1: Development of Child Care Provider Organizations and Networks

State-level agencies and resource and referral agencies should encourage the development of child care provider organizations or networks, to attract, train, support, and encourage participation in facility quality ratings and accreditation, for those caregivers/teachers who would like to be part of an organization or system. National professional organizations should encourage the development of local child care provider organizations and networks.

When possible, these networks should include a central facility for enrichment activities for groups of children and support in-service programs for caregivers/teachers.

RATIONALE: To enhance staff qualifications and a nurturing environment, child care providers need support (1,3). This especially applies to family child care home providers who tend to be more isolated than those employed in centers. In studies of the quality of care in family child care homes, the caregivers/teachers who provided better care were those who viewed their role as a profession and acted accordingly, participating in continuous improvement activities (2).

COMMENTS: Professional networking organizations offer professional encouragement, support, and training to promote rigorous professional standards (3). This should include the promotion of quality ratings, accreditation, credentialing, and other quality improvement initiatives that are based on implementing best practices in early childhood education.

RELATED STANDARDS:
Standard 10.3.3.1: Credentialing of Individual Child Care Providers

REFERENCES:

1. Pickering, L. K., C. J. Baker, D. W. Kimberlin, S. S. Long, eds. 2009. *Red book: 2009 report of the Committee on Infectious Diseases*. 28th ed. Elk Grove Village, IL: American Academy of Pediatrics.
2. Galinsky, E., C. Howes, S. Kontos, M. Shinn. 1994. *The study of children in family child care and relative care*. New York: Families and Work Institute.
3. Bromer, J. 2009. *The Family Child Care Network impact study: Promising strategies for improving family child care quality.* http://www.erikson.edu/hrc/researchdetail.aspx?c=1296.

STANDARD 10.6.2.2: Fostering Collaboration to Establish Programs for School-Age Children

Public and private agencies should foster collaboration among the schools, child care facilities, and resource and referral agencies to establish programs for school-age children, ages five to twelve and older. Such care should be designed to meet the social and developmental needs of children who receive care in any setting.

RATIONALE: More than fifteen million children in the United States are left alone after school each day (1). School-age children who are under-supervised ("latchkey children") are exposed to considerable health and safety risks. Bringing these children into supervised, quality child care is a societal responsibility. In addition to providing protection for children, these programs can offer homework assistance, tutoring and other support for school achievement.

REFERENCES:

1. Afterschool Alliance. Facts and research: America after 3pm. http://www.afterschoolalliance.org/AA3PM.cfm.

10.7 Public Policy Issues and Resource Development

STANDARD 10.7.0.1: Development of Resource and Referral Agencies

States should encourage the use of public and private resources in local communities to develop resource and referral agencies. The functions of these agencies should include the following:

a) Helping parents/guardians find developmentally appropriate child care that protects the health and safety of children;
b) Giving parents/guardians consumer information to enable them to know about, evaluate, and choose among available child care options;
c) Helping parents/guardians maintain a dialogue with their caregivers/teachers;
d) Recruiting new potential caregivers/teachers;
e) Providing training, technical assistance, and consultation, including health and safety, to new facilities and to all caregivers/teachers;
f) Compiling data on supply and demand to identify community needs for child care;
g) Providing information to employers on options for their involvement in meeting community child care needs;
h) Participating in and/or supporting the state's Quality Rating Improvement System (QRIS) and/or similar quality improvements;
i) Assisting programs in achieving accreditation and providers in achieving credentials.

RATIONALE: Resource and referral agencies provide a locus in the community to assist parents/guardians in fulfilling their childrearing responsibilities, a mechanism to coordinate and provide the resources and services that supplement and facilitate the functions of the family, and a mechanism for the coordination of services that helps keep children safe and healthy (1).

REFERENCES:

1. National Association of Child Care Resource and Referral Agencies (NACCRRA). 2008. *Covering the map: Child care resource and referral agencies providing vital services to parents throughout the United States.* Arlington, VA: NACCRRA. http://www.naccrra.org/publications/naccrra-publications/publications/Parent Svc Report_MECH_screen.pdf.

STANDARD 10.7.0.2: Coordination of Public and Private Resources to Ensure Families' Access to Quality Child Care

National and state agencies should coordinate public and private resources to ensure that all families have access to affordable, safe, and healthy child care for their children. To the extent possible, communities should coordinate multiple funding streams to support child care. Strengthening the child care workforce through professional development opportunities and commensurate compensation should be a major goal in improving available child care.

RATIONALE: Research provides clear evidence that a well qualified and consistent staff is essential to the provision of good care for children (4). Quality cannot be attained by merely applying standards to caregivers/teachers; resources are necessary to meet the cost of quality care at a price that parents/guardians can afford. Quality care requires not only lower child:staff ratios and smaller group sizes, but also well trained staff to reduce the spread of infectious diseases, provide for safe evacuation and management of emergency situations, and to offer developmentally appropriate program activities (1). Currently, the low wages and benefits earned by child care staff result in high staff turnover, which adversely affects the health and safety of children. Staff wages make up the largest cost in providing care, and caregiver/teacher wages in the United States are currently too low to attract and retain qualified staff (4). Facilities cannot benefit from training provided to staff if the staff members leave their jobs before the training is implemented (1).

See The Child Care Bureau's Case Studies of Public-Private Partnerships for Child Care (2) and Head Start State Collaboration Annual Profiles (3) for examples of successful state-wide collaborative projects.

REFERENCES:

1. Kendrick, A. S. 1994. Training to ensure healthy child day-care programs. *Pediatrics* 94:1108-10.
2. U.S. Department of Health and Human Services (HHS), Administration for Children and Families, Child Care Bureau. 1998. *The child care partnership project: Case studies of public-private partnerships for child care.* Fairfax, VA: National Child Care Information and Technical Assistance Center.
3. U.S. Department of Health and Human Services, Administration for Children and Families, Office of Head Start. Head Start collaboration offices. http://eclkc.ohs.acf.hhs.gov/hslc/hsd/SCO/.
4. Gable, S., T. C. Rothrauff, K. R. Thornburg, D. Mauzy. Cash incentives and turnover in center-based child care staff. *Early Childhood Res Quarter* 22:363-78.

Appendices

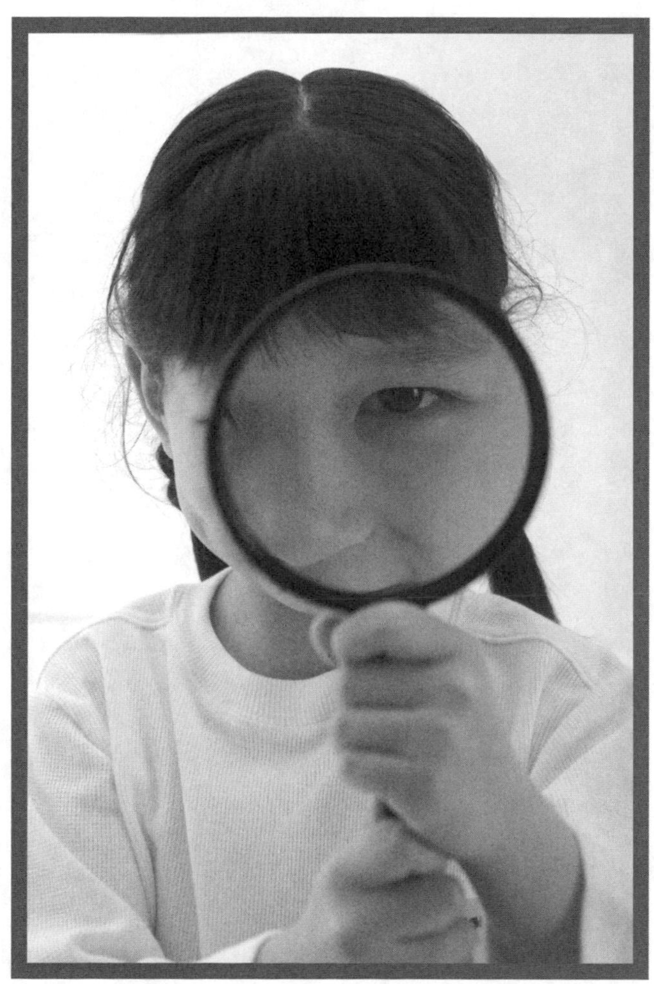

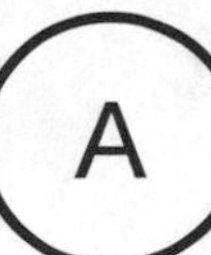

Signs and Symptoms Chart

Symptom	Common Causes	Complaints or What Might Be Seen	Notify Health Consultant	Notify Parent	Temporarily Exclude?	If Excluded, Readmit When
Cold Symptoms	*Viruses* (early stage of many viruses) • Adenovirus • Coxsackievirus • Enterovirus • Parainfluenza virus • Respiratory syncytial virus • Rhinovirus • Coronavirus • Influenza *Bacteria* • Mycoplasma	• Runny or stuffy nose • Scratchy throat • Coughing • Sneezing • Watery eyes • Fever	Not necessary	Yes	No, unless • Fever accompanied by behavior change. • Child looks or acts very ill. • Child has difficulty breathing. • Child has blood red or purple rash not associated with injury. • Child meets other exclusion criteria	• Exclusion criteria are resolved.
Cough (May come from congestion any where from ears to lungs. Cough is a body response to something that is irritating tissues in the airway.)	• Common cold • Lower respiratory infection (eg, pneumonia, bronchiolitis) • Croup • Asthma • Sinus infection • Bronchitis	• Dry or wet cough • Runny nose (clear, white, or yellow-green) • Sore throat • Throat irritation • Hoarse voice, barking cough	Not necessary	Yes	No, unless • Severe cough • Rapid and/or difficult breathing • Wheezing if not already evaluated and treated • Cyanosis (ie, blue color of skin and mucous membranes)	• Exclusion criteria are resolved.
Diaper Rash	• Irritation by rubbing of diaper material against skin wet with urine or stool • Infection with yeast or bacteria	• Redness • Scaling • Red bumps • Sores • Cracking of skin indiaper region	Not necessary	Yes	No, unless • Oozing sores that leak body fluids outside the diaper	• Exclusion criteria are resolved.
Diarrhea	Usually viral, less commonly bacterial or parasitic	• Frequent loose or watery stools compared to child's normal pattern. (Note that exclusively breastfed infants normally have frequent unformed and somewhat watery stools, or may have several days with no stools.) • Abdominal cramps. • Fever. • Generally not feeling well. • Sometimes accompanied by vomiting.	For one or more cases of bloody diarrhea or 2 or more children with diarrhea in group within a week	Yes	Yes, if • Stool is not contained in the diaper for diapered children. • Diarrhea is causing "accidents" for toilet-trained children. • Stool frequency exceeds 2 or more stools above normal for that child, because this may cause too much work for the teacher/caregivers and make it difficult to maintain good sanitation. • Blood/mucus in stool. • Abnormal color of stool for child (eg, all black or very pale). • No urine output in 8 hours. • Jaundice (ie, yellow skin or eyes). • Fever with behavior change. • Looks or acts very ill.	• Cleared to return by health professional for all cases of bloody diarrhea and diarrhea caused by *Shigella*, *Salmonella*, or *Giardia*. • Diapered children have their stool contained by the diaper (even if the stools remain loose) and toilet-trained children do not have toileting accidents. • Able to participate.

American Academy of Pediatrics. *Managing Infectious Diseases in Child Care and Schools: A Quick Reference Guide*. Aronson SS, Shope TR, eds. 2nd ed. Elk Grove Village, IL: American Academy of Pediatrics; 2009. Used with permission of the American Academy of Pediatrics, 2009.

Symptom	Common Causes	Complaints or What Might Be Seen	Notify Health Consultant	Notify Parent	Temporarily Exclude?	If Excluded, Readmit When
Difficult or Noisy Breathing	1. Common cold 2. Croup 3. Epiglottitis 4. Bronchiolitis 5. Asthma 6. Pneumonia 7. Object stuck in airway	1. Common cold: Stuffy nose, sore throat, cough, and/or mild fever. 2. Croup: Barking cough, hoarseness, fever, possible chest discomfort (symptoms worse at night), and/or very noisy breathing, especially when breathing in. 3. Epiglottitis: Gasping noisily for breath with mouth wide open, chin pulled down, high fever, and/or bluish (cyanotic) nails and skin; drooling, unwilling to lie down. 4 and 5. Bronchiolitis and Asthma: Child is working hard to breathe; rapid breathing; space between ribs looks like it is sucked in with each breath (retractions); wheezing; whistling sound with breathing; cold/cough; irritable and unwell. Takes longer to breathe out than to breathe in. 6. Pneumonia: Deep cough, fever, rapid breathing, or space between ribs looks like it is sucked in with each breath (retractions). 7. Object stuck in airway: Symptoms similar to croup (2 above).	Not necessary	Yes	Yes, if • Fever accompanied by behavior change. • Child looks or acts very ill. • Child has difficulty breathing. • Child has blood red or purple rash not associated with injury. • The child meets other exclusion criteria	• Exclusion criteria are resolved.
Earache	• Bacteria or viruses • Often occurs in context of common cold	• Fever • Pain or irritability • Difficulty hearing • "Blocked ears" • Drainage • Swelling around ear	Not necessary	Yes	No, unless • Unable to participate. • Care would compromise staff's ability to care for other children. • Fever with behavior change.	• Exclusion criteria are resolved.
Eye Irritation, Pinkeye	1. Bacterial infection of the membrane covering the eye and eyelid (bacterial conjunctivitis) 2. Viral infection of the membrane covering the eye and eyelid (viral conjunctivitis) 3. Allergic irritation of the membrane covering the eye and eyelid (allergic conjunctivitis) 4. Chemical irritation of the membrane covering the eye and eyelid (irritant conjunctivitis) (eg, swimming in heavily chlorinated water, air pollution)	1. Bacterial infection: Pink color instead of whites of eyes and thick yellow/green discharge. May be irritated, swollen, or crusted in the morning. 2. Viral infection: Pinkish/red, irritated, swollen eyes; watery discharge; possible upper respiratory infection. 3 and 4. Allergic and chemical irritation: Red, tearing, itchy eyes; runny nose, sneezing; watery discharge.	Yes, if 2 or more children have red eyes with watery discharge	Yes	*For bacterial conjunctivitis* No. Exclusion is no longer required for this condition. Health professionals may vary on whether to treat this condition with antibiotic medication. The role of antibiotics in treatment and preventing spread is unclear. Most children with pinkeye get better after 5 or 6 days without antibiotics. *For other forms* **No, unless** • The child meets other exclusion criteria Note: One type of viral conjunctivitis spreads rapidly and requires exclusion. If 2 or more children in the group have watery red eyes without any known chemical irritant exposure, exclusion may be required and health authorities should be notified.	• *For bacterial conjunctivitis*, once parent has discussed with health professional. Antibiotics may or may not be prescribed. • Exclusion criteria are resolved.

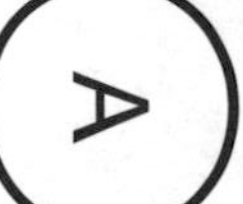

Symptom	Common Causes	Complaints or What Might Be Seen	Notify Health Consultant	Notify Parent	Temporarily Exclude?	If Excluded, Readmit When
Fever	• Any viral, bacterial, or parasitic infection • Overheating • Reaction to medication (eg, vaccine, oral) • Other noninfectious illnesses (eg, rheumatoid arthritis, malignancy)	Flushing, tired, irritable, decreased activity Notes • Fever alone is not harmful. When a child has an infection, raising the body temperature is part of the body's normal defense against outside attacks. • Rapid elevation of body temperature sometimes triggers a febrile seizure in young children; this usually is outgrown by age 6 years. The first time a febrile seizure happens, the child requires evaluation. These seizures are frightening, but do not cause the child any long-term harm. Parents should inform their child's health professional every time the child has a seizure, even if the child is known to have febrile seizures. Warning: *Do not* give aspirin. It has been linked to an increased risk of Reye syndrome (a rare and serious disease affecting the brain and liver).	Not necessary	Yes	No, unless • Behavior change. • Unable to participate. • Care would compromise staff's ability to care for other children. Note: Temperatures considered meaningfully elevated above normal, although not necessarily an indication of a significant health problem, for children older than 4 months are • 100°F (37.8°C) axillary (armpit) • 101°F (38.3°C) orally • 102°F (38.9°C) rectally • Aural (ear) temperature equal to oral or rectal temperature **Get immediate medical attention when** infant younger than 4 months has unexplained temperature of 101°F (38.3°C) rectally or 100°F (37.8°C) axillary. Any infant younger than 2 months with fever should get medical attention within an hour.	• Able to participate • Exclusion criteria are resolved.
Headache	• Any bacterial/viral infection • Other noninfectious causes	• Tired and irritable • Can occur with or without other symptoms	Not necessary	Yes	**No, unless** • Child is unable to participate Note: **Notify health professional** in case of sudden, severe headache with vomiting or stiff neck that might signal meningitis. The stiff neck of concern is reluctance and unusual discomfort when the child is asked to look at his or her "belly button" (putting chin to chest)—different from soreness in the side of the neck.	• Able to participate

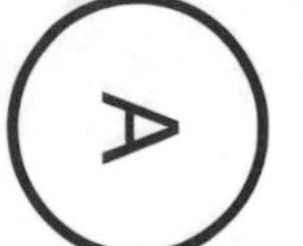

Symptom	Common Causes	Complaints or What Might Be Seen	Notify Health Consultant	Notify Parent	Temporarily Exclude?	If Excluded, Readmit When
Itching	1. Ringworm 2. Chickenpox 3. Pinworm 4. Head lice 5. Scabies 6. Allergic or irritant reaction (eg, poison ivy) 7. Dry skin or eczema 8. Impetigo	1. Ringworm: Itchy ring-shaped patches on skin or bald patches on scalp. 2. Chickenpox: Blister-like spots surrounded by red halos on scalp, face, and body; fever; irritable. 3. Pinworm: Anal itching. 4. Head lice: Small insects or white egg sheaths (nits) in hair. 5. Scabies: Severely itchy red bumps on warm areas of body, especially between fingers or toes. 6. Allergic or irritant reaction: Raised, circular, mobile rash; reddening of the skin; blisters occur with local reactions (poison ivy, contact reaction). 7. Dry skin or eczema: Dry areas on body. More often worse on cheeks, in front of elbows, and behind knees. In infants, may be dry areas on fronts of legs and anywhere else on body, but not usually in diaper area. If swollen, red, or oozing, think about infection. 8. Impetigo: Areas of crusted yellow, oozing sores. Often around mouth or nasal openings.	For infestations such as lice and scabies; if more than one child in group has impetigo or ringworm; for chickenpox	**Yes**	For chickenpox, scabies, and impetigo **Yes** For ringworm and head lice **Yes, at the end of the day** • Children should be referred to a health professional at the end of the day for treatment. For pinworm, allergic or irritant reactions, and eczema **No, unless** • Appears infected as a weeping or crusty sore Note: Exclusion for hives is only necessary to obtain medical advice for care, if there is no previously made assessment and care plan for the hives.	• Exclusion criteria are resolved. • On medication or treated as recommended by a health professional if indicated for the condition and for the time required to be readmitted. For conditions that require application of antibiotics to lesions or taking of antibiotics by mouth, the period of treatment to reduce the risk of spread to others is usually 24 hours. For most children with insect infestations or parasites, readmission as soon as the treatment has been given is acceptable.
Mouth Sores	1. Oral thrush (yeast infection) 2. Herpes or coxsackievirus infection 3. Canker sores	1. Oral thrush: White patches on tongue and along cheeks 2. Herpes or coxsackievirus infection: Pain on swallowing; fever; painful, yellowish spots in mouth; swollen neck glands; fever blister, cold sore; reddened, swollen, painful lips 3. Canker sores: Painful ulcers on cheeks or gums	Not necessary	**Yes**	**No, unless** • Drooling steadily related to mouth sores. • Unable to participate. • Care would compromise staff's ability to care for other children.	• Able to participate. • Exclusion criteria are resolved.
Rash	Many causes 1. Viral: roseola infantum, fifth disease, chickenpox, herpesvirus, molluscum contagiosum, warts, cold sores, shingles (herpes zoster), and others 2. Skin infections and infestations: ringworm (fungus), scabies (parasite), impetigo, abscesses, and cellulitis (bacteria) 3. Severe bacterial infections: meningococcus, pneumococcus, *Staphylococcus aureus* (MSSA, MRSA).	• Skin may show similar findings with many different causes. Determining cause of rash requires a competent health professional evaluation that takes into account information other than just how rash looks. 1. Viral: Usually signs of general illness such as runny nose, cough, and fever (except for warts or molluscum). Each viral rash may have a distinctive appearance. 2. Minor skin infections and infestations: See "Itching." More serious skin infections: redness, pain, fever, pus. 3. Severe bacterial infections: Rare. These children have fever with rash and may be very ill.	For outbreaks	**Yes**	**No, unless** • Rash with behavior change or fever • Has oozing/open wound • Has bruising not associated with injury • Has joint pain and rash • Unable to participate • Tender, red area of skin, especially if it is increasing in size or tenderness	• Able to participate in daily activities. • On antibiotic medication at least 24 hours (if indicated). • Exclusion criteria are resolved.

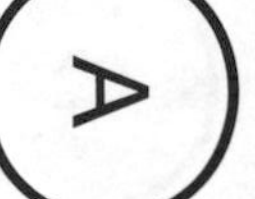

Symptom	Common Causes	Complaints or What Might Be Seen	Notify Health Consultant	Notify Parent	Temporarily Exclude?	If Excluded, Readmit When
Sore Throat (pharyngitis)	1. Viral—common cold viruses that cause upper respiratory infections 2. Strep throat	1. Viral: Verbal children will complain of sore throat; younger children may be irritable with decreased appetite and increased drooling (refusal to swallow). May see symptoms associated with upper respiratory illness, such as runny nose, cough, and congestion. 2. Strep throat: Strep infection usually does not result in cough or runny nose. Signs of the body's fight against infection include red tissue with white patches on sides of throat, at back of tongue (tonsil area), and at back wall of throat. Tonsils may be large, even touching each other. Swollen lymph nodes (sometimes incorrectly called "swollen glands") occur as body fights off the infection.	Not necessary	**Yes**	**No, unless** • Inability to swallow. • Excessive drooling with breathing difficulty. • Fever with behavior change. • The child meets other exclusion criteria	• Able to swallow. • Able to participate. • On medication at least 24 hours (if strep). • Exclusion criteria are resolved.
Stomachache	1. Viral gastroenteritis or strep throat 2. Problems with internal organs of the abdomen such as intestine, colon, liver, bladder	1. Viral gastroenteritis or strep throat: Vomiting and diarrhea and/or cramping are signs of a viral infection of stomach and/or intestine. Strep throat may cause stomachache with sore throat, headache, and possible fever. If cough or runny nose is present, strep is very unlikely. 2. Problems with internal organs of the abdomen: Persistent severe pain in abdomen.	Not unless multiple cases in same group within 1 week.	**Yes**	**No, unless** • Severe pain causing child to double over or scream • Abdominal pain after injury • Bloody/black stools • No urine output for 8 hours • Diarrhea • Vomiting • Yellow skin/eyes • Fever with behavior change • Looks or acts very ill	• Pain resolves. • Able to participate. • Exclusion criteria are resolved.
Swollen Glands (properly called swollen lymph nodes)	1. Normal body defense response to viral or bacterial infection in the area where lymph nodes are located (ie, in the neck for any upper respiratory infection) 2. Bacterial infection of lymph nodes that become overcome and infected by bacteria they are responding to as part of the body's defense system	1. Normal lymph node response: Swelling at front, sides, and back of the neck and ear, in the armpit or groin, or anywhere else near an area of an infection. 2. Bacterial infection of lymph nodes: Swollen, warm lymph nodes with overlying pink skin, tender to the touch, usually located near an area of the body that has been infected.	Not necessary	**Yes**	**No, unless** • Difficulty breathing or swallowing • Red, tender, warm glands • Fever with behavior change	• Child is on antibiotics (if indicated). • Able to participate. • Exclusion criteria are resolved.
Vomiting	• Viral infection of the stomach or intestine (gastroenteritis) • Coughing strongly • Other viral illness with fever	Diarrhea, vomiting, and/or cramping for viral gastroenteritis	For outbreak	**Yes**	**Yes, if** • Vomited more than 2 times in 24 hours • Vomiting and fever • Vomit that appears green/bloody • No urine output in 8 hours • Recent history of head injury • Looks or acts very ill • Vomit that appears green/bloody	• Vomiting ends.

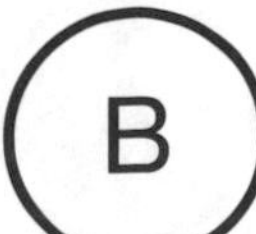

MAJOR OCCUPATIONAL HEALTH HAZARDS

Infectious Diseases and Organisms

General Types of Infectious Diseases
Diarrhea (infectious)
Respiratory tract infection

Specific Infectious Diseases and Organisms
Adenovirus
Astrovirus
Caliciviruses
Campylobacter jejuni/coli
Chickenpox (varicella)
Clostridium parvum
Cytomegalovirus (CMV)
Escherichia coli 0157:H7
Giardia lamblia
Hepatitis A
Hepatitis B
Hepatitis C
Herpes 6
Herpes 7
Herpes simplex
Herpes zoster
Human Immunodeficiency Virus (HIV)
Impetigo
Influenza and H1N1
Lice
Measles
Meningitis (bacterial, viral)
Meningococcus (Neisseria meningitidis)
Mumps
Parvovirus B19
Pertussis
Pinworm
Ringworm
Rotavirus
Rubella
Salmonella organisms
Scabies
Shigella organisms
Staphylococcus aureus
Streptococcus, Group A
Tuberculosis

Injuries and Noninfectious Diseases
Back injuries
Bites
Dermatitis
Falls

Environmental exposure
Art materials
Cleaning, sanitizing and disinfecting solutions
Indoor air pollution
Outdoor air pollution
Noise
Odor

Stress
Fear of liability
Inadequate break time, sick time, and personal days
Inadequate facilities
Inadequate pay
Inadequate recognition
Inadequate training
Insufficient professional recognition
Lack of adequate medical/dental health insurance
Responsibility for children's welfare
Undervaluing of work
Working alone/Isolation

Reference: American Academy of Pediatrics, Committee on Infectious Diseases. *Red book 2009: Report of the Committee on Infectious Diseases.* Elk Grove Village, IL: AAP.

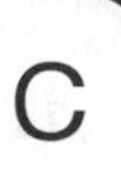

Nutrition Specialist, Registered Dietitian, Licensed Nutritionist, Consultant, and Food Service Staff Qualifications

TITLE	LEVEL OF PROFESSIONAL RESPONSIBILITY	EDUCATION AND EXPERIENCE
Nutrition Specialist/ Registered Dietician/Licensed Nutritionist/Child Care Nutrition Consultant (state level)	Develops policies and procedures for implementation of nutrition food standards statewide and provides consultation to state agency personnel, including staff involved with licensure.	Current registration with the Commission on Dietetic Registration of the American Dietetic Association or eligibility for registration with a Bachelor's and Master's degree in nutrition (including or supplemented by course(s) in child growth and development), plus at least two years of related experience as a nutritionist or dietitian in a health program including services to infants and children is preferred. A Master's degree from an approved program in public health nutrition may be substituted for registration with the Commission on Dietetic Registration. Current state licensure or certification as a nutritionist or dietitian is acceptable.
Nutrition Specialist/ Registered Dietitian (local level)	Provides expertise to child care center director and provides ongoing guidance, consultation, and inservice training to facility's nutrition component. The number of sites and facilities for one child care Nutrition Specialist will vary according to size and complexity of local facilities.	Registered Dietitian, as above. At least one year of experience as described above.
Food Service Manager	Has overall supervisory responsibility for the food service unit at one or more facility sites.	High school diploma or GED. Successful completion of a food handler food protection class. Coursework in basic menu-planning skills, basic foods, introduction to child feeding programs for managers, and/or other relevant courses (offered at community colleges). Two years of food service experience.
Food Service Worker (Cook)	Under the supervision of the Food Service Manager, carries out food service operations including menu planning, food preparation and service, and related duties in a designated area.	High school diploma or GED. Successful completion of a food handler food protection class. Coursework in basic menu-planning skills and basic foods (offered through adult education or a community college). One year of food service experience.
Food Service Aide	Works no more than four hours a day, under the supervision of an employee at a higher level in food service unit.	High school diploma or GED. Must pass the food handler test within one to two months of employment. No prior experience is required for semi-skilled persons who perform assigned tasks in designated areas.

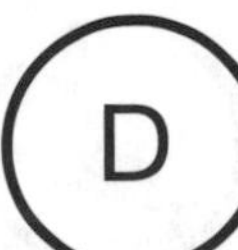

Gloving

Wash hands prior to using gloves if hands are visibly soiled.

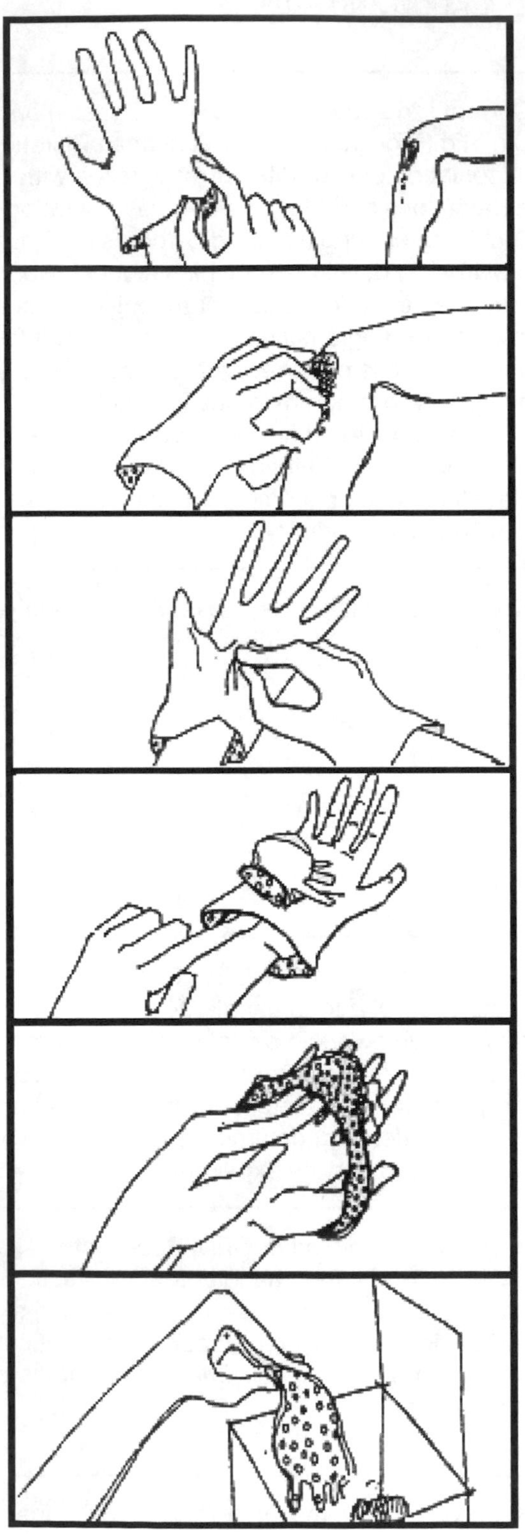

Put on a clean pair of gloves.

Provide the appropriate care.

Remove each glove carefully. Grab the first glove at the palm and strip the glove off. Touch dirty surfaces only to dirty surfaces.

Ball-up the dirty glove in the palm of the other gloved hand.

With the clean hand strip the glove off from underneath at the wrist, turning the glove inside out. Touch dirty surfaces only to dirty surfaces.

Discard the dirty gloves immediately in a step can. Wash your hands.

Note that sensitivity to latex is a growing problem. If caregivers/teachers or children who are sensitive to latex are present in the facility, non-latex gloves should be used.

Adapted with permission from: California Department of Education. *Keeping Kids Healthy Preventing and Managing Communicable Disease in Child Care.* Sacramento CA:California Department of Education, 1995.

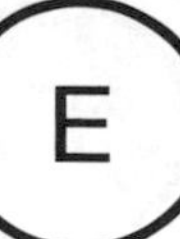

Child Care Staff Health Assessment

********* Employer should complete this section. ********

Name of person to be examined: ____________________

Employer for whom examination is being done: ____________________

Employer's Location: ____________________ Phone number: ____________________

Purpose of examination: ☐pre-employment (with conditional offer of employment) ☐annual re-examination

Type of activity on the job: ☐lifting, carrying children ☐close contact with children ☐food preparation ☐desk work ☐driver of vehicles ☐facility maintenance

****** Part I and Part II below must be completed and signed by a licensed physician or CRNP. ******

Based on a review of the medical record, health history, and examination, does this person have any of the following conditions or problems that might affect job performance or require accommodation?

Date of exam: ____________________

Part I:Health Problems

(circle)

Visual acuity less than 20/40 (combined, obtained with lenses if needed)?..........yes .... no

Decreased hearing or difficulty functioning in a noisy environment (less than 20 db at 500, 1000, 2000, 4000 Hz)? .yes .... no

Respiratory problems (asthma, emphysema, airway allergies, current smoker, other)?..........yes .... no

Heart, blood pressure, or other cardiovascular problems?..........yes .... no

Gastrointestinal problems (ulcer, colitis, special dietary requirements, obesity, other)?..........yes .... no

Endocrine problems (diabetes, thyroid, other)?..........yes .... no

Emotional disorders or addiction (depression, substance dependency, difficulty handling stress, other)?..........yes .... no

Neurologic problems (epilepsy, Parkinsonism, other)?..........yes .... no

Musculoskeletal problems (low back pain or susceptibility to back injury, neck problems, arthritis, limitations on activity)?..........yes .... no

Skin problems (eczema, rashes, conditions incompatible with frequent handwashing, other)?..........yes .... no

Immune system problems (from medication, inherent susceptibility to infection, illness, allergies)?..........yes .... no

Need for more frequent health visits or sick days than the average person?..........yes .... no

Other special medical problem or chronic disease that requires work restrictions or accommodation?..........yes .... no

Part II: Infectious Disease Status

Female of childbearing age susceptible to CMV or parvovirus?..........yes .... no

Immunizations now due/overdue for:

- Tdap*..........yes .... no
- MMR (2 doses for persons born after 1989; 1 dose for those born in or after 1957)..........yes .... no
- polio (OPV or IPV in childhood)..........yes .... no
- hepatitis B (3 dose series)..........yes .... no
- varicella (2 doses or had the disease)..........yes .... no
- influenza..........yes .... no
- pneumococcal vaccine..........yes .... no

*Reference: Centers for Disease Control and Prevention. 2006. Preventing Tetanus, Diphtheria, and Pertussis Among Adults: Use of Tetanus Toxoid, Reduced Diphtheria Toxoid and Acellular Pertussis Vaccine. *MMWR* 55(RR17): 1-33.

Evaluation of tuberculosis status shows a risk for communicable TB?..........yes** .... no

☐ Tuberculin Skin Test (TST) ☐ Interferon-Gamma Release Assay (IGRA) Test Date: ____________ Result: ____________
(Check Test Used)

Transmission of tuberculosis infection should be controlled by requiring all adolescents and adults who are present while children are in care to have their tuberculosis status assessed with a tuberculin skin test (TST) or interferon-gamma release assay (IGRA) blood test before caregiving activities are initiated.
In people with a reactive TST or positive IGRA, chest radiography without evidence of active pulmonary disease and/or documentation of completion of therapy for latent tuberculosis infection (LTBI) or completion of therapy for active disease should be required.

**Health professions should consult the current edition of *Red Book: Report of the Committee on Infectious Diseases* (www.aapredbook.org) for guidance on TB screening.
For current adult immunization requirements see: www.cispimmunize.org; www.aapredbook.org; and www.cdc.ogv/vaccines/recs/schedules/default.htm.

Please attach additional sheets to explain all "yes" answers above. Include the plan for follow up.

______ ____________________ ____________________ MD DO CRNP
(Date) (Signature) (Printed last name) (Title)

Phone number of physician or CRNP: ____________________

I have read and understand the above information.

______ ____________________
(Date) (Patient's Signature)

Reference: Pennsylvania Chapter, American Academy of Pediatrics. 2002. *Model Child Care Health Policies*. 4th ed. Washington, DC: National Association for the Education of Young Children.
This form was adapted from *Model Child Care Health Policies*, 2002, by the Early Childhood Education Linkage System (ECELS), a program funded by the Pennsylvania Depts. of Health & Public Welfare and contractually administered by the PA Chapter, American Academy of Pediatrics.

Enrollment / Attendance / Symptom Record

Classroom ______________

MONTH 20

NAME	AGE IN MONTHS	DAILY HOURS IN CARE	FOR EACH CHILD, EACH DAY CODE TOP BOX "+" = PRESENT or "O" = ABSENT, N = NOT SCHEDULED CODE BOTTOM BOX "O" = WELL or " " SYMPTOM CODE FROM BOTTOM OF PAGE.																														
			1	2	3	4	5	6	7	8	9	10	11	12	13	14	15	16	17	18	19	20	21	22	23	24	25	26	27	28	29	30	31

TOTAL PLACED ON REGISTER		NUMBER OF DAYS FACILITY WAS OPEN	

Symptom Codes: 1 = ASTHMA, WHEEZING, 2 = BEHAVIOR CHANGE WITH NO OTHER SYMPTOM, 3 = DIARRHEA, 4 = FEVER, 5 = HEADACHE, 6 = RASH, 7 = RESPIRATORY (COLD, COUGH, RUNNY NOSE, EARACHE, SORE THROAT, PINK EYE), 8 = STOMACHACHE, 9 = URINE PROBLEM, 10 = VOMITING, 11 = OTHER (SPECIFY ON BACK OF FORM)

This form was adapted from Pennsylvania Chapter, American Academy of Pediatrics. *Model Child Care Health Policies*. 4th ed. Washington, DC: National Association for the Education of Young Children, 2002.

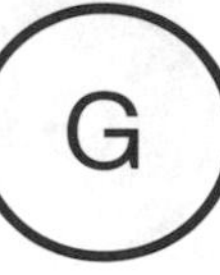

This schedule was current at time of Caring for Our Children printing in 2011.
To check for latest edition, go to http://www.cdc.gov/vaccines/recs/schedules/default.htm

Recommended Immunization Schedule for Persons Aged 0 Through 6 Years—United States • 2011

For those who fall behind or start late, see the catch-up schedule

Vaccine ▼ Age ▶	Birth	1 month	2 months	4 months	6 months	12 months	15 months	18 months	19–23 months	2–3 years	4–6 years
Hepatitis B[1]	HepB	HepB	HepB		HepB	HepB	HepB	HepB			
Rotavirus[2]			RV	RV	RV[2]						
Diphtheria, Tetanus, Pertussis[3]			DTaP	DTaP	DTaP	see footnote[3]	DTaP	DTaP			DTaP
Haemophilus influenzae type b[4]			Hib	Hib	Hib[4]	Hib	Hib				
Pneumococcal[5]			PCV	PCV	PCV	PCV	PCV			PPSV	PPSV
Inactivated Poliovirus[6]			IPV	IPV	IPV	IPV	IPV	IPV			IPV
Influenza[7]					Influenza (Yearly)	Influenza (Yearly)	Influenza (Yearly)	Influenza (Yearly)	Influenza (Yearly)	Influenza (Yearly)	Influenza (Yearly)
Measles, Mumps, Rubella[8]						MMR	MMR	see footnote[8]			MMR
Varicella[9]						Varicella	Varicella	see footnote[9]			Varicella
Hepatitis A[10]						HepA (2 doses)	HepA (2 doses)	HepA (2 doses)	HepA (2 doses)	HepA Series	HepA Series
Meningococcal[11]										MCV4	MCV4

Range of recommended ages for all children

Range of recommended ages for certain high-risk groups

This schedule includes recommendations in effect as of December 21, 2010. Any dose not administered at the recommended age should be administered at a subsequent visit, when indicated and feasible. The use of a combination vaccine generally is preferred over separate injections of its equivalent component vaccines. Considerations should include provider assessment, patient preference, and the potential for adverse events. Providers should consult the relevant Advisory Committee on Immunization Practices statement for detailed recommendations: **http://www.cdc.gov/vaccines/pubs/acip-list.htm**. Clinically significant adverse events that follow immunization should be reported to the Vaccine Adverse Event Reporting System (VAERS) at **http://www.vaers.hhs.gov** or by telephone, **800-822-7967**.

1. **Hepatitis B vaccine (HepB).** (Minimum age: birth)
   At birth:
   - Administer monovalent HepB to all newborns before hospital discharge.
   - If mother is hepatitis B surface antigen (HBsAg)-positive, administer HepB and 0.5 mL of hepatitis B immune globulin (HBIG) within 12 hours of birth.
   - If mother's HBsAg status is unknown, administer HepB within 12 hours of birth. Determine mother's HBsAg status as soon as possible and, if HBsAg-positive, administer HBIG (no later than age 1 week).

   Doses following the birth dose:
   - The second dose should be administered at age 1 or 2 months. Monovalent HepB should be used for doses administered before age 6 weeks.
   - Infants born to HBsAg-positive mothers should be tested for HBsAg and antibody to HBsAg 1 to 2 months after completion of at least 3 doses of the HepB series, at age 9 through 18 months (generally at the next well-child visit).
   - Administration of 4 doses of HepB to infants is permissible when a combination vaccine containing HepB is administered after the birth dose.
   - Infants who did not receive a birth dose should receive 3 doses of HepB on a schedule of 0, 1, and 6 months.
   - The final (3rd or 4th) dose in the HepB series should be administered no earlier than age 24 weeks.
2. **Rotavirus vaccine (RV).** (Minimum age: 6 weeks)
   - Administer the first dose at age 6 through 14 weeks (maximum age: 14 weeks 6 days). Vaccination should not be initiated for infants aged 15 weeks 0 days or older.
   - The maximum age for the final dose in the series is 8 months 0 days
   - If Rotarix is administered at ages 2 and 4 months, a dose at 6 months is not indicated.
3. **Diphtheria and tetanus toxoids and acellular pertussis vaccine (DTaP).** (Minimum age: 6 weeks)
   - The fourth dose may be administered as early as age 12 months, provided at least 6 months have elapsed since the third dose.
4. Haemophilus influenzae **type b conjugate vaccine (Hib).** (Minimum age: 6 weeks)
   - If PRP-OMP (PedvaxHIB or Comvax [HepB-Hib]) is administered at ages 2 and 4 months, a dose at age 6 months is not indicated.
   - Hiberix should not be used for doses at ages 2, 4, or 6 months for the primary series but can be used as the final dose in children aged 12 months through 4 years.
5. **Pneumococcal vaccine.** (Minimum age: 6 weeks for pneumococcal conjugate vaccine [PCV]; 2 years for pneumococcal polysaccharide vaccine [PPSV])
   - PCV is recommended for all children aged younger than 5 years. Administer 1 dose of PCV to all healthy children aged 24 through 59 months who are not completely vaccinated for their age.
   - A PCV series begun with 7-valent PCV (PCV7) should be completed with 13-valent PCV (PCV13).
   - A single supplemental dose of PCV13 is recommended for all children aged 14 through 59 months who have received an age-appropriate series of PCV7.
   - A single supplemental dose of PCV13 is recommended for all children aged 60 through 71 months with underlying medical conditions who have received an age-appropriate series of PCV7.
   - The supplemental dose of PCV13 should be administered at least 8 weeks after the previous dose of PCV7. See *MMWR* 2010:59(No. RR-11).
   - Administer PPSV at least 8 weeks after last dose of PCV to children aged 2 years or older with certain underlying medical conditions, including a cochlear implant.
6. **Inactivated poliovirus vaccine (IPV).** (Minimum age: 6 weeks)
   - If 4 or more doses are administered prior to age 4 years an additional dose should be administered at age 4 through 6 years.
   - The final dose in the series should be administered on or after the fourth birthday and at least 6 months following the previous dose.
7. **Influenza vaccine (seasonal).** (Minimum age: 6 months for trivalent inactivated influenza vaccine [TIV]; 2 years for live, attenuated influenza vaccine [LAIV])
   - For healthy children aged 2 years and older (i.e., those who do not have underlying medical conditions that predispose them to influenza complications), either LAIV or TIV may be used, except LAIV should not be given to children aged 2 through 4 years who have had wheezing in the past 12 months.
   - Administer 2 doses (separated by at least 4 weeks) to children aged 6 months through 8 years who are receiving seasonal influenza vaccine for the first time or who were vaccinated for the first time during the previous influenza season but only received 1 dose.
   - Children aged 6 months through 8 years who received no doses of monovalent 2009 H1N1 vaccine should receive 2 doses of 2010–2011 seasonal influenza vaccine. See *MMWR* 2010;59(No. RR-8):33–34.
8. **Measles, mumps, and rubella vaccine (MMR).** (Minimum age: 12 months)
   - The second dose may be administered before age 4 years, provided at least 4 weeks have elapsed since the first dose.
9. **Varicella vaccine.** (Minimum age: 12 months)
   - The second dose may be administered before age 4 years, provided at least 3 months have elapsed since the first dose.
   - For children aged 12 months through 12 years the recommended minimum interval between doses is 3 months. However, if the second dose was administered at least 4 weeks after the first dose, it can be accepted as valid.
10. **Hepatitis A vaccine (HepA).** (Minimum age: 12 months)
    - Administer 2 doses at least 6 months apart.
    - HepA is recommended for children aged older than 23 months who live in areas where vaccination programs target older children, who are at increased risk for infection, or for whom immunity against hepatitis A is desired.
11. **Meningococcal conjugate vaccine, quadrivalent (MCV4).** (Minimum age: 2 years)
    - Administer 2 doses of MCV4 at least 8 weeks apart to children aged 2 through 10 years with persistent complement component deficiency and anatomic or functional asplenia, and 1 dose every 5 years thereafter.
    - Persons with human immunodeficiency virus (HIV) infection who are vaccinated with MCV4 should receive 2 doses at least 8 weeks apart.
    - Administer 1 dose of MCV4 to children aged 2 through 10 years who travel to countries with highly endemic or epidemic disease and during outbreaks caused by a vaccine serogroup.
    - Administer MCV4 to children at continued risk for meningococcal disease who were previously vaccinated with MCV4 or meningococcal polysaccharide vaccine after 3 years if the first dose was administered at age 2 through 6 years.

The Recommended Immunization Schedules for Persons Aged 0 Through 18 Years are approved by the Advisory Committee on Immunization Practices (**http://www.cdc.gov/vaccines/recs/acip**), the American Academy of Pediatrics (**http://www.aap.org**), and the American Academy of Family Physicians (**http://www.aafp.org**).

Department of Health and Human Services • Centers for Disease Control and Prevention

This schedule was current at time of Caring for Our Children printing in 2011.
To check for latest edition, go to http://www.cdc.gov/vaccines/recs/schedules/default.htm

Recommended Immunization Schedule for Persons Aged 7 Through 18 Years—United States • 2011

For those who fall behind or start late, see the schedule below and the catch-up schedule

Vaccine ▼ Age ▶	7–10 years	11–12 years	13–18 years
Tetanus, Diphtheria, Pertussis[1]		Tdap	Tdap
Human Papillomavirus[2]	*see footnote* 2	HPV (3 doses)(females)	HPV series
Meningococcal[3]	MCV4	MCV4	MCV4
Influenza[4]	Influenza (Yearly)		
Pneumococcal[5]	Pneumococcal		
Hepatitis A[6]	HepA Series		
Hepatitis B[7]	Hep B Series		
Inactivated Poliovirus[8]	IPV Series		
Measles, Mumps, Rubella[9]	MMR Series		
Varicella[10]	Varicella Series		

Range of recommended ages for all children

Range of recommended ages for catch-up immunization

Range of recommended ages for certain high-risk groups

This schedule includes recommendations in effect as of December 21, 2010. Any dose not administered at the recommended age should be administered at a subsequent visit, when indicated and feasible. The use of a combination vaccine generally is preferred over separate injections of its equivalent component vaccines. Considerations should include provider assessment, patient preference, and the potential for adverse events. Providers should consult the relevant Advisory Committee on Immunization Practices statement for detailed recommendations: **http://www.cdc.gov/vaccines/pubs/acip-list.htm.** Clinically significant adverse events that follow immunization should be reported to the Vaccine Adverse Event Reporting System (VAERS) at **http://www.vaers.hhs.gov** or by telephone, **800-822-7967.**

1. **Tetanus and diphtheria toxoids and acellular pertussis vaccine (Tdap).** (Minimum age: 10 years for Boostrix and 11 years for Adacel))
   - Persons aged 11 through 18 years who have not received Tdap should receive a dose followed by Td booster doses every 10 years thereafter.
   - Persons aged 7 through 10 years who are not fully immunized against pertussis (including those never vaccinated or with unknown pertussis vaccination status) should receive a single dose of Tdap. Refer to the catch-up schedule if additional doses of tetanus and diphtheria toxoid–containing vaccine are needed.
   - Tdap can be administered regardless of the interval since the last tetanus and diphtheria toxoid–containing vaccine.
2. **Human papillomavirus vaccine (HPV).** (Minimum age: 9 years)
   - Quadrivalent HPV vaccine (HPV4) or bivalent HPV vaccine (HPV2) is recommended for the prevention of cervical precancers and cancers in females.
   - HPV4 is recommended for prevention of cervical precancers, cancers, and genital warts in females.
   - HPV4 may be administered in a 3-dose series to males aged 9 through 18 years to reduce their likelihood of genital warts.
   - Administer the second dose 1 to 2 months after the first dose and the third dose 6 months after the first dose (at least 24 weeks after the first dose).
3. **Meningococcal conjugate vaccine, quadrivalent (MCV4).** (Minimum age: 2 years)
   - Administer MCV4 at age 11 through 12 years with a booster dose at age 16 years.
   - Administer 1 dose at age 13 through 18 years if not previously vaccinated.
   - Persons who received their first dose at age 13 through 15 years should receive a booster dose at age 16 through 18 years.
   - Administer 1 dose to previously unvaccinated college freshmen living in a dormitory.
   - Administer 2 doses at least 8 weeks apart to children aged 2 through 10 years with persistent complement component deficiency and anatomic or functional asplenia, and 1 dose every 5 years thereafter.
   - Persons with HIV infection who are vaccinated with MCV4 should receive 2 doses at least 8 weeks apart.
   - Administer 1 dose of MCV4 to children aged 2 through 10 years who travel to countries with highly endemic or epidemic disease and during outbreaks caused by a vaccine serogroup.
   - Administer MCV4 to children at continued risk for meningococcal disease who were previously vaccinated with MCV4 or meningococcal polysaccharide vaccine after 3 years (if first dose administered at age 2 through 6 years) or after 5 years (if first dose administered at age 7 years or older).
4. **Influenza vaccine (seasonal).**
   - For healthy nonpregnant persons aged 7 through 18 years (i.e., those who do not have underlying medical conditions that predispose them to influenza complications), either LAIV or TIV may be used.
   - Administer 2 doses (separated by at least 4 weeks) to children aged 6 months through 8 years who are receiving seasonal influenza vaccine for the first time or who were vaccinated for the first time during the previous influenza season but only received 1 dose.
   - Children 6 months through 8 years of age who received no doses of monovalent 2009 H1N1 vaccine should receive 2 doses of 2010-2011 seasonal influenza vaccine. See *MMWR* 2010;59(No. RR-8):33–34.
5. **Pneumococcal vaccines.**
   - A single dose of 13-valent pneumococcal conjugate vaccine (PCV13) may be administered to children aged 6 through 18 years who have functional or anatomic asplenia, HIV infection or other immunocompromising condition, cochlear implant or CSF leak. See *MMWR* 2010;59(No. RR-11).
   - The dose of PCV13 should be administered at least 8 weeks after the previous dose of PCV7.
   - Administer pneumococcal polysaccharide vaccine at least 8 weeks after the last dose of PCV to children aged 2 years or older with certain underlying medical conditions, including a cochlear implant. A single revaccination should be administered after 5 years to children with functional or anatomic asplenia or an immunocompromising condition.
6. **Hepatitis A vaccine (HepA).**
   - Administer 2 doses at least 6 months apart.
   - HepA is recommended for children aged older than 23 months who live in areas where vaccination programs target older children, or who are at increased risk for infection, or for whom immunity against hepatitis A is desired.
7. **Hepatitis B vaccine (HepB).**
   - Administer the 3-dose series to those not previously vaccinated. For those with incomplete vaccination, follow the catch-up schedule.
   - A 2-dose series (separated by at least 4 months) of adult formulation Recombivax HB is licensed for children aged 11 through 15 years.
8. **Inactivated poliovirus vaccine (IPV).**
   - The final dose in the series should be administered on or after the fourth birthday and at least 6 months following the previous dose.
   - If both OPV and IPV were administered as part of a series, a total of 4 doses should be administered, regardless of the child's current age.
9. **Measles, mumps, and rubella vaccine (MMR).**
   - The minimum interval between the 2 doses of MMR is 4 weeks.
10. **Varicella vaccine.**
    - For persons aged 7 through 18 years without evidence of immunity (see *MMWR* 2007;56[No. RR-4]), administer 2 doses if not previously vaccinated or the second dose if only 1 dose has been administered.
    - For persons aged 7 through 12 years, the recommended minimum interval between doses is 3 months. However, if the second dose was administered at least 4 weeks after the first dose, it can be accepted as valid.
    - For persons aged 13 years and older, the minimum interval between doses is 4 weeks.

The Recommended Immunization Schedules for Persons Aged 0 Through 18 Years are approved by the Advisory Committee on Immunization Practices (**http://www.cdc.gov/vaccines/recs/acip**), the American Academy of Pediatrics (**http://www.aap.org**), and the American Academy of Family Physicians (**http://www.aafp.org**).
Department of Health and Human Services • Centers for Disease Control and Prevention

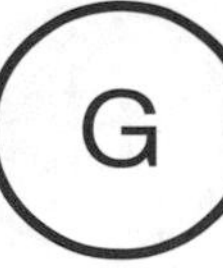

This schedule was current at time of Caring for Our Children printing in 2011.
To check for latest edition, go to http://www.cdc.gov/vaccines/recs/schedules/default.htm

Catch-up Immunization Schedule for Persons Aged 4 Months Through 18 Years Who Start Late or Who Are More Than 1 Month Behind—United States • 2011

The table below provides catch-up schedules and minimum intervals between doses for children whose vaccinations have been delayed. A vaccine series does not need to be restarted, regardless of the time that has elapsed between doses. Use the section appropriate for the child's age

Vaccine	Minimum Age for Dose 1	Minimum Interval Between Doses			
		Dose 1 to Dose 2	Dose 2 to Dose 3	Dose 3 to Dose 4	Dose 4 to Dose 5
PERSONS AGED 4 MONTHS THROUGH 6 YEARS					
Hepatitis B[1]	Birth	4 weeks	8 weeks (and at least 16 weeks after first dose)		
Rotavirus[2]	6 wks	4 weeks	4 weeks[2]		
Diphtheria, Tetanus, Pertussis[3]	6 wks	4 weeks	4 weeks	6 months	6 months[3]
Haemophilus influenzae type b[4]	6 wks	**4 weeks** if first dose administered at younger than age 12 months **8 weeks (as final dose)** if first dose administered at age 12–14 months **No further doses needed** if first dose administered at age 15 months or older	**4 weeks[4]** if current age is younger than 12 months **8 weeks (as final dose)[4]** if current age is 12 months or older and first dose administered at younger than age 12 months and second dose administered at younger than 15 months **No further doses needed** if previous dose administered at age 15 months or older	**8 weeks (as final dose)** This dose only necessary for children aged 12 months through 59 months who received 3 doses before age 12 months	
Pneumococcal[5]	6 wks	**4 weeks** if first dose administered at younger than age 12 months **8 weeks (as final dose for healthy children)** if first dose administered at age 12 months or older or current age 24 through 59 months **No further doses needed** for healthy children if first dose administered at age 24 months or older	**4 weeks** if current age is younger than 12 months **8 weeks (as final dose for healthy children)** if current age is 12 months or older **No further doses needed** for healthy children if previous dose administered at age 24 months or older	**8 weeks (as final dose)** This dose only necessary for children aged 12 months through 59 months who received 3 doses before age 12 months or for children at high risk who received 3 doses at any age	
Inactivated Poliovirus[6]	6 wks	4 weeks	4 weeks	6 months[6]	
Measles, Mumps, Rubella[7]	12 mos	4 weeks			
Varicella[8]	12 mos	3 months			
Hepatitis A[9]	12 mos	6 months			
PERSONS AGED 7 THROUGH 18 YEARS					
Tetanus, Diphtheria/ Tetanus, Diphtheria, Pertussis[10]	7 yrs[10]	4 weeks	**4 weeks** if first dose administered at younger than age 12 months **6 months** if first dose administered at 12 months or older	**6 months** if first dose administered at younger than age 12 months	
Human Papillomavirus[11]	9 yrs	Routine dosing intervals are recommended (females)[11]			
Hepatitis A[9]	12 mos	6 months			
Hepatitis B[1]	Birth	4 weeks	8 weeks (and at least 16 weeks after first dose)		
Inactivated Poliovirus[6]	6 wks	4 weeks	4 weeks[6]	6 months[6]	
Measles, Mumps, Rubella[7]	12 mos	4 weeks			
Varicella[8]	12 mos	**3 months** if person is younger than age 13 years **4 weeks** if person is aged 13 years or older			

1. **Hepatitis B vaccine (HepB).**
   - Administer the 3-dose series to those not previously vaccinated.
   - The minimum age for the third dose of HepB is 24 weeks.
   - A 2-dose series (separated by at least 4 months) of adult formulation Recombivax HB is licensed for children aged 11 through 15 years.
2. **Rotavirus vaccine (RV).**
   - The maximum age for the first dose is 14 weeks 6 days. Vaccination should not be initiated for infants aged 15 weeks 0 days or older.
   - The maximum age for the final dose in the series is 8 months 0 days.
   - If Rotarix was administered for the first and second doses, a third dose is not indicated.
3. **Diphtheria and tetanus toxoids and acellular pertussis vaccine (DTaP).**
   - The fifth dose is not necessary if the fourth dose was administered at age 4 years or older.
4. ***Haemophilus influenzae* type b conjugate vaccine (Hib).**
   - 1 dose of Hib vaccine should be considered for unvaccinated persons aged 5 years or older who have sickle cell disease, leukemia, or HIV infection, or who have had a splenectomy.
   - If the first 2 doses were PRP-OMP (PedvaxHIB or Comvax), and administered at age 11 months or younger, the third (and final) dose should be administered at age 12 through 15 months and at least 8 weeks after the second dose.
   - If the first dose was administered at age 7 through 11 months, administer the second dose at least 4 weeks later and a final dose at age 12 through 15 months.
5. **Pneumococcal vaccine.**
   - Administer 1 dose of 13-valent pneumococcal conjugate vaccine (PCV13) to all healthy children aged 24 through 59 months with any incomplete PCV schedule (PCV7 or PCV13).
   - For children aged 24 through 71 months with underlying medical conditions, administer 1 dose of PCV13 if 3 doses of PCV were received previously or administer 2 doses of PCV13 at least 8 weeks apart if fewer than 3 doses of PCV were received previously.
   - A single dose of PCV13 is recommended for certain children with underlying medical conditions through 18 years of age. See age-specific schedules for details.
   - Administer pneumococcal polysaccharide vaccine (PPSV) to children aged 2 years or older with certain underlying medical conditions, including a cochlear implant, at least 8 weeks after the last dose of PCV. A single revaccination should be administered after 5 years to children with functional or anatomic asplenia or an immunocompromising condition. See *MMWR* 2010;59(No. RR-11).
6. **Inactivated poliovirus vaccine (IPV).**
   - The final dose in the series should be administered on or after the fourth birthday and at least 6 months following the previous dose.
   - A fourth dose is not necessary if the third dose was administered at age 4 years or older and at least 6 months following the previous dose.
   - In the first 6 months of life, minimum age and minimum intervals are only recommended if the person is at risk for imminent exposure to circulating poliovirus (i.e., travel to a polio-endemic region or during an outbreak).
7. **Measles, mumps, and rubella vaccine (MMR).**
   - Administer the second dose routinely at age 4 through 6 years. The minimum interval between the 2 doses of MMR is 4 weeks.
8. **Varicella vaccine.**
   - Administer the second dose routinely at age 4 through 6 years.
   - If the second dose was administered at least 4 weeks after the first dose, it can be accepted as valid.
9. **Hepatitis A vaccine (HepA).**
   - HepA is recommended for children aged older than age 23 months who live in areas where vaccination programs target older children, or who are at increased risk for infection, or for whom immunity against hepatitis A is desired.
10. **Tetanus and diphtheria toxoids (Td) and tetanus and diphtheria toxoids and acellular pertussis vaccine (Tdap).**
    - Doses of DTaP are counted as part of the Td/Tdap series.
    - Tdap should be substituted for a single dose of Td in the catch-up series for children aged 7 through 10 years or as a booster for children aged 11 through 18 years; use Td for other doses.
11. **Human papillomavirus vaccine (HPV).**
    - Administer the series to females at age 13 through 18 years if not previously vaccinated or have not completed the vaccine series.
    - Quadrivalent HPV vaccine (HPV4) may be administered in a 3-dose series to males aged 9 through 18 years to reduce their likelihood of genital warts.
    - Use recommended routine dosing intervals for series catch-up (i.e., the second and third doses should be administered at 1 to 2 and 6 months after the first dose). The minimum interval between the first and second doses is 4 weeks. The minimum interval between the second and third doses is 12 weeks, and the third dose should be administered at least 24 weeks after the first dose.

Information about reporting reactions after immunization is available online at **http://www.vaers.hhs.gov** or by telephone, **800-822-7967**. Suspected cases of vaccine-preventable diseases should be reported to the state or local health department. Additional information, including precautions and contraindications for immunization, is available from the National Center for Immunization and Respiratory Diseases at **http://www.cdc.gov/vaccines** or telephone, **800-CDC-INFO** (800-232-4636).
Department of Health and Human Services • Centers for Disease Control and Prevention

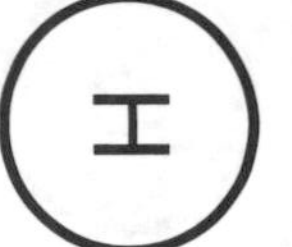

This schedule was current at time of Caring for Our Children printing in 2011.
To check for latest edition, go to http://www.cdc.gov/vaccines/recs/schedules/default.htm

Recommended Adult Immunization Schedule

UNITED STATES - 2011

Note: These recommendations *must* be read with the footnotes that follow containing number of doses, intervals between doses, and other important information.

Figure 1. Recommended adult immunization schedule, by vaccine and age group

<table>
<tr><th>VACCINE ▼ AGE GROUP▶</th><th>19–26 years</th><th>27–49 years</th><th>50–59 years</th><th>60–64 years</th><th>≥65 years</th></tr>
<tr><td>Influenza[1,*]</td><td colspan="5">1 dose annually</td></tr>
<tr><td>Tetanus, diphtheria, pertussis (Td/Tdap)[2,*]</td><td colspan="4">Substitute 1-time dose of Tdap for Td booster; then boost with Td every 10 yrs</td><td>Td booster every 10 yrs</td></tr>
<tr><td>Varicella[3,*]</td><td colspan="5">2 doses</td></tr>
<tr><td>Human papillomavirus (HPV)[4,*]</td><td>3 doses (females)</td><td></td><td></td><td></td><td></td></tr>
<tr><td>Zoster[5]</td><td></td><td></td><td></td><td colspan="2">1 dose</td></tr>
<tr><td>Measles, mumps, rubella (MMR)[6,*]</td><td colspan="2">1 or 2 doses</td><td colspan="3">1 dose</td></tr>
<tr><td>Pneumococcal (polysaccharide)[7,8]</td><td colspan="4">1 or 2 doses</td><td>1 dose</td></tr>
<tr><td>Meningococcal[9,*]</td><td colspan="5">1 or more doses</td></tr>
<tr><td>Hepatitis A[10,*]</td><td colspan="5">2 doses</td></tr>
<tr><td>Hepatitis B[11,*]</td><td colspan="5">3 doses</td></tr>
</table>

*Covered by the Vaccine Injury Compensation Program.

For all persons in this category who meet the age requirements and who lack evidence of immunity (e.g., lack documentation of vaccination or have no evidence of previous infection)

Recommended if some other risk factor is present (e.g., based on medical, occupational, lifestyle, or other indications)

No recommendation

Report all clinically significant postvaccination reactions to the Vaccine Adverse Event Reporting System (VAERS). Reporting forms and instructions on filing a VAERS report are available at http://www.vaers.hhs.gov or by telephone, 800-822-7967.

Information on how to file a Vaccine Injury Compensation Program claim is available at http://www.hrsa.gov/vaccinecompensation or by telephone, 800-338-2382. Information about filing a claim for vaccine injury is available through the U.S. Court of Federal Claims, 717 Madison Place, N.W., Washington, D.C. 20005; telephone, 202-357-6400.

Additional information about the vaccines in this schedule, extent of available data, and contraindications for vaccination also is available at http://www.cdc.gov/vaccines or from the CDC-INFO Contact Center at 800-CDC-INFO (800-232-4636) in English and Spanish, 24 hours a day, 7 days a week.

This schedule was current at time of Caring for Our Children printing in 2011.
To check for latest edition, go to http://www.cdc.gov/vaccines/recs/schedules/default.htm

Figure 2. Vaccines that might be indicated for adults based on medical and other indications

VACCINE ▼ / INDICATION ▶	Pregnancy	Immuno-compromising conditions (excluding human immunodeficiency virus [HIV])[3,5,6,13]	HIV infection[3,6,12,13] CD4+ T lymphocyte count <200 cells/µL	HIV infection[3,6,12,13] CD4+ T lymphocyte count ≥200 cells/µL	Diabetes, heart disease, chronic lung disease, chronic alcoholism	Asplenia[12] (including elective splenectomy) and persistent complement component deficiencies	Chronic liver disease	Kidney failure, end-stage renal disease, receipt of hemodialysis	Healthcare personnel
Influenza[1,*]	1 dose TIV annually								1 dose TIV or LAIV annually
Tetanus, diphtheria, pertussis (Td/Tdap)[2,*]	Td	Substitute 1-time dose of Tdap for Td booster; then boost with Td every 10 yrs							
Varicella[3,*]	Contraindicated			2 doses					
Human papillomavirus (HPV)[4,*]		3 doses through age 26 yrs							
Zoster[5]	Contraindicated				1 dose				
Measles, mumps, rubella (MMR)[6,*]	Contraindicated			1 or 2 doses					
Pneumococcal (polysaccharide)[7,8]		1 or 2 doses							
Meningococcal[9,*]	1 or more doses								
Hepatitis A[10,*]	2 doses								
Hepatitis B[11,*]					3 doses				

*Covered by the Vaccine Injury Compensation Program.

For all persons in this category who meet the age requirements and who lack evidence of immunity (e.g., lack documentation of vaccination or have no evidence of previous infection)

Recommended if some other risk factor is present (e.g., on the basis of medical, occupational, lifestyle, or other indications)

No recommendation

These schedules indicate the recommended age groups and medical indications for which administration of currently licensed vaccines is commonly indicated for adults ages 19 years and older, as of February 4, 2011. For all vaccines being recommended on the adult immunization schedule, a vaccine series does not need to be restarted, regardless of the time that has elapsed between doses. Licensed combination vaccines may be used whenever any components of the combination are indicated and when the vaccine's other components are not contraindicated. For detailed recommendations on all vaccines, including those used primarily for travelers or that are issued during the year, consult the manufacturers' package inserts and the complete statements from the Advisory Committee on Immunization Practices (http:// www.cdc.gov/vaccines/pubs/acip-list.htm).

The recommendations in this schedule were approved by the Centers for Disease Control and Prevention's (CDC) Advisory Committee on Immunization Practices (ACIP), the American Academy of Family Physicians (AAFP), the American College of Obstetricians and Gynecologists (ACOG), and the American College of Physicians (ACP).

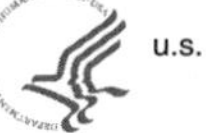

u.s. department of health and human services
centers for disease control and prevention

CDC

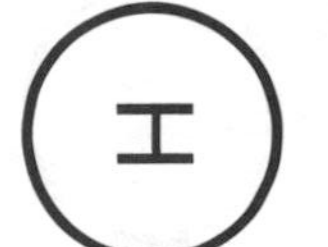

This schedule was current at time of Caring for Our Children printing in 2011.
To check for latest edition, go to http://www.cdc.gov/vaccines/recs/schedules/default.htm

Footnotes

Recommended Adult Immunization Schedule—UNITED STATES - 2011

For complete statements by the Advisory Committee on Immunization Practices (ACIP), visit www.cdc.gov/vaccines/pubs/ACIP-list.htm.

1. Influenza vaccination

Annual vaccination against influenza is recommended for all persons aged 6 months and older, including all adults. Healthy, nonpregnant adults aged less than 50 years without high-risk medical conditions can receive either intranasally administered live, attenuated influenza vaccine (FluMist), or inactivated vaccine. Other persons should receive the inactivated vaccine. Adults aged 65 years and older can receive the standard influenza vaccine or the high-dose (Fluzone) influenza vaccine. Additional information about influenza vaccination is available at http://www.cdc.gov/vaccines/vpd-vac/flu/default.htm.

2. Tetanus, diphtheria, and acellular pertussis (Td/Tdap) vaccination

Administer a one-time dose of Tdap to adults aged less than 65 years who have not received Tdap previously or for whom vaccine status is unknown to replace one of the 10-year Td boosters, and as soon as feasible to all 1) postpartum women, 2) close contacts of infants younger than age 12 months (e.g., grandparents and child-care providers), and 3) healthcare personnel with direct patient contact. Adults aged 65 years and older who have not previously received Tdap and who have close contact with an infant aged less than 12 months also should be vaccinated. Other adults aged 65 years and older may receive Tdap. Tdap can be administered regardless of interval since the most recent tetanus or diphtheria-containing vaccine.

Adults with uncertain or incomplete history of completing a 3-dose primary vaccination series with Td-containing vaccines should begin or complete a primary vaccination series. For unvaccinated adults, administer the first 2 doses at least 4 weeks apart and the third dose 6–12 months after the second. If incompletely vaccinated (i.e., less than 3 doses), administer remaining doses. Substitute a one-time dose of Tdap for one of the doses of Td, either in the primary series or for the routine booster, whichever comes first.

If a woman is pregnant and received the most recent Td vaccination 10 or more years previously, administer Td during the second or third trimester. If the woman received the most recent Td vaccination less than 10 years previously, administer Tdap during the immediate postpartum period. At the clinician's discretion, Td may be deferred during pregnancy and Tdap substituted in the immediate postpartum period, or Tdap may be administered instead of Td to a pregnant woman after an informed discussion with the woman.

The ACIP statement for recommendations for administering Td as prophylaxis in wound management is available at http://www.cdc.gov/vaccines/pubs/acip-list.htm.

3. Varicella vaccination

All adults without evidence of immunity to varicella should receive 2 doses of single-antigen varicella vaccine if not previously vaccinated or a second dose if they have received only 1 dose, unless they have a medical contraindication. Special consideration should be given to those who 1) have close contact with persons at high risk for severe disease (e.g., healthcare personnel and family contacts of persons with immunocompromising conditions) or 2) are at high risk for exposure or transmission (e.g., teachers; child-care employees; residents and staff members of institutional settings, including correctional institutions; college students; military personnel; adolescents and adults living in households with children; nonpregnant women of childbearing age; and international travelers).

Evidence of immunity to varicella in adults includes any of the following: 1) documentation of 2 doses of varicella vaccine at least 4 weeks apart; 2) U.S.-born before 1980 (although for healthcare personnel and pregnant women, birth before 1980 should not be considered evidence of immunity); 3) history of varicella based on diagnosis or verification of varicella by a healthcare provider (for a patient reporting a history of or having an atypical case, a mild case, or both, healthcare providers should seek either an epidemiologic link with a typical varicella case or to a laboratory-confirmed case or evidence of laboratory confirmation, if it was performed at the time of acute disease); 4) history of herpes zoster based on diagnosis or verification of herpes zoster by a healthcare provider; or 5) laboratory evidence of immunity or laboratory confirmation of disease.

Pregnant women should be assessed for evidence of varicella immunity. Women who do not have evidence of immunity should receive the first dose of varicella vaccine upon completion or termination of pregnancy and before discharge from the healthcare facility. The second dose should be administered 4–8 weeks after the first dose.

4. Human papillomavirus (HPV) vaccination

HPV vaccination with either quadrivalent (HPV4) vaccine or bivalent vaccine (HPV2) is recommended for females at age 11 or 12 years and catch-up vaccination for females aged 13 through 26 years.

Ideally, vaccine should be administered before potential exposure to HPV through sexual activity; however, females who are sexually active should still be vaccinated consistent with age-based recommendations. Sexually active females who have not been infected with any of the four HPV vaccine types (types 6, 11, 16, and 18, all of which HPV4 prevents) or any of the two HPV vaccine types (types 16 and 18, both of which HPV2 prevents) receive the full benefit of the vaccination. Vaccination is less beneficial for females who have already been infected with one or more of the HPV vaccine types. HPV4 or HPV2 can be administered to persons with a history of genital warts, abnormal Papanicolaou test, or positive HPV DNA test, because these conditions are not evidence of previous infection with all vaccine HPV types.

HPV4 may be administered to males aged 9 through 26 years to reduce their likelihood of genital warts. HPV4 would be most effective when administered before exposure to HPV through sexual contact.

A complete series for either HPV4 or HPV2 consists of 3 doses. The second dose should be administered 1–2 months after the first dose; the third dose should be administered 6 months after the first dose.

Although HPV vaccination is not specifically recommended for persons with the medical indications described in Figure 2, "Vaccines that might be indicated for adults based on medical and other indications," it may be administered to these persons because the HPV vaccine is not a live-virus vaccine. However, the immune response and vaccine efficacy might be less for persons with the medical indications described in Figure 2 than in persons who do not have the medical indications described or who are immunocompetent.

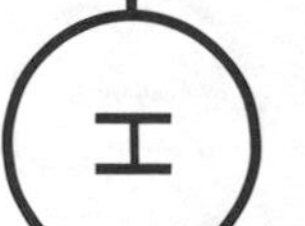

This schedule was current at time of Caring for Our Children printing in 2011.
To check for latest edition, go to http://www.cdc.gov/vaccines/recs/schedules/default.htm

5. Herpes zoster vaccination

A single dose of zoster vaccine is recommended for adults aged 60 years and older regardless of whether they report a previous episode of herpes zoster. Persons with chronic medical conditions may be vaccinated unless their condition constitutes a contraindication.

6. Measles, mumps, rubella (MMR) vaccination

Adults born before 1957 generally are considered immune to measles and mumps. All adults born in 1957 or later should have documentation of 1 or more doses of MMR vaccine unless they have a medical contraindication to the vaccine, laboratory evidence of immunity to each of the three diseases, or documentation of provider-diagnosed measles or mumps disease. For rubella, documentation of provider-diagnosed disease is not considered acceptable evidence of immunity.

Measles component: A second dose of MMR vaccine, administered a minimum of 28 days after the first dose, is recommended for adults who 1) have been recently exposed to measles or are in an outbreak setting; 2) are students in postsecondary educational institutions; 3) work in a healthcare facility; or 4) plan to travel internationally. Persons who received inactivated (killed) measles vaccine or measles vaccine of unknown type during 1963–1967 should be revaccinated with 2 doses of MMR vaccine.

Mumps component: A second dose of MMR vaccine, administered a minimum of 28 days after the first dose, is recommended for adults who 1) live in a community experiencing a mumps outbreak and are in an affected age group; 2) are students in postsecondary educational institutions; 3) work in a healthcare facility; or 4) plan to travel internationally. Persons vaccinated before 1979 with either killed mumps vaccine or mumps vaccine of unknown type who are at high risk for mumps infection (e.g. persons who are working in a healthcare facility) should be revaccinated with 2 doses of MMR vaccine.

Rubella component: For women of childbearing age, regardless of birth year, rubella immunity should be determined. If there is no evidence of immunity, women who are not pregnant should be vaccinated. Pregnant women who do not have evidence of immunity should receive MMR vaccine upon completion or termination of pregnancy and before discharge from the healthcare facility.

Healthcare personnel born before 1957: For unvaccinated healthcare personnel born before 1957 who lack laboratory evidence of measles, mumps, and/or rubella immunity or laboratory confirmation of disease, healthcare facilities should 1) consider routinely vaccinating personnel with 2 doses of MMR vaccine at the appropriate interval (for measles and mumps) and 1 dose of MMR vaccine (for rubella), and 2) recommend 2 doses of MMR vaccine at the appropriate interval during an outbreak of measles or mumps, and 1 dose during an outbreak of rubella. Complete information about evidence of immunity is available at http://www.cdc.gov/vaccines/recs/provisional/default.htm.

7. Pneumococcal polysaccharide (PPSV) vaccination

Vaccinate all persons with the following indications:

Medical: Chronic lung disease (including asthma); chronic cardiovascular diseases; diabetes mellitus; chronic liver diseases; cirrhosis; chronic alcoholism; functional or anatomic asplenia (e.g., sickle cell disease or splenectomy [if elective splenectomy is planned, vaccinate at least 2 weeks before surgery]); immunocompromising conditions (including chronic renal failure or nephrotic syndrome); and cochlear implants and cerebrospinal fluid leaks. Vaccinate as close to HIV diagnosis as possible.

Other: Residents of nursing homes or long-term care facilities and persons who smoke cigarettes. Routine use of PPSV is not recommended for American Indians/Alaska Natives or persons aged less than 65 years unless they have underlying medical conditions that are PPSV indications. However, public health authorities may consider recommending PPSV for American Indians/Alaska Natives and persons aged 50 through 64 years who are living in areas where the risk for invasive pneumococcal disease is increased

8. Revaccination with PPSV

One-time revaccination after 5 years is recommended for persons aged 19 through 64 years with chronic renal failure or nephrotic syndrome; functional or anatomic asplenia (e.g., sickle cell disease or splenectomy); and for persons with immunocompromising conditions. For persons aged 65 years and older, one-time revaccination is recommended if they were vaccinated 5 or more years previously and were aged less than 65 years at the time of primary vaccination.

9. Meningococcal vaccination

Meningococcal vaccine should be administered to persons with the following indications:

Medical: A 2-dose series of meningococcal conjugate vaccine is recommended for adults with anatomic or functional asplenia, or persistent complement component deficiencies. Adults with HIV infection who are vaccinated should also receive a routine 2-dose series. The 2 doses should be administered at 0 and 2 months.

Other: A single dose of meningococcal vaccine is recommended for unvaccinated first-year college students living in dormitories; microbiologists routinely exposed to isolates of *Neisseria meningitidis*; military recruits; and persons who travel to or live in countries in which meningococcal disease is hyperendemic or epidemic (e.g., the "meningitis belt" of sub-Saharan Africa during the dry season [December through June]), particularly if their contact with local populations will be prolonged. Vaccination is required by the government of Saudi Arabia for all travelers to Mecca during the annual Hajj.

Meningococcal conjugate vaccine, quadrivalent (MCV4) is preferred for adults with any of the preceding indications who are aged 55 years and younger; meningococcal polysaccharide vaccine (MPSV4) is preferred for adults aged 56 years and older. Revaccination with MCV4 every 5 years is recommended for adults previously vaccinated with MCV4 or MPSV4 who remain at increased risk for infection (e.g., adults with anatomic or functional asplenia, or persistent complement component deficiencies).

This schedule was current at time of Caring for Our Children printing in 2011.
To check for latest edition, go to http://www.cdc.gov/vaccines/recs/schedules/default.htm

10. Hepatitis A vaccination

Vaccinate persons with any of the following indications and any person seeking protection from hepatitis A virus (HAV) infection:

Behavioral: Men who have sex with men and persons who use injection drugs.

Occupational: Persons working with HAV-infected primates or with HAV in a research laboratory setting.

Medical: Persons with chronic liver disease and persons who receive clotting factor concentrates.

Other: Persons traveling to or working in countries that have high or intermediate endemicity of hepatitis A (a list of countries is available at http://wwwn.cdc.gov/travel/contentdiseases.aspx).

Unvaccinated persons who anticipate close personal contact (e.g., household or regular babysitting) with an international adoptee during the first 60 days after arrival in the United States from a country with high or intermediate endemicity should be vaccinated. The first dose of the 2-dose hepatitis A vaccine series should be administered as soon as adoption is planned, ideally 2 or more weeks before the arrival of the adoptee.

Single-antigen vaccine formulations should be administered in a 2-dose schedule at either 0 and 6–12 months (Havrix), or 0 and 6–18 months (Vaqta). If the combined hepatitis A and hepatitis B vaccine (Twinrix) is used, administer 3 doses at 0, 1, and 6 months; alternatively, a 4-dose schedule may be used, administered on days 0, 7, and 21–30, followed by a booster dose at month 12.

11. Hepatitis B vaccination

Vaccinate persons with any of the following indications and any person seeking protection from hepatitis B virus (HBV) infection:

Behavioral: Sexually active persons who are not in a long-term, mutually monogamous relationship (e.g., persons with more than one sex partner during the previous 6 months); persons seeking evaluation or treatment for a sexually transmitted disease (STD); current or recent injection-drug users; and men who have sex with men.

Occupational: Healthcare personnel and public-safety workers who are exposed to blood or other potentially infectious body fluids.

Medical: Persons with end-stage renal disease, including patients receiving hemodialysis; persons with HIV infection; and persons with chronic liver disease.

Other: Household contacts and sex partners of persons with chronic HBV infection; clients and staff members of institutions for persons with developmental disabilities; and international travelers to countries with high or intermediate prevalence of chronic HBV infection (a list of countries is available at http://wwwn.cdc.gov/travel/contentdiseases.aspx).

Hepatitis B vaccination is recommended for all adults in the following settings: STD treatment facilities; HIV testing and treatment facilities; facilities providing drug-abuse treatment and prevention services; healthcare settings targeting services to injection-drug users or men who have sex with men; correctional facilities; end-stage renal disease programs and facilities for chronic hemodialysis patients; and institutions and nonresidential day-care facilities for persons with developmental disabilities.

Administer missing doses to complete a 3-dose series of hepatitis B vaccine to those persons not vaccinated or not completely vaccinated. The second dose should be administered 1 month after the first dose; the third dose should be given at least 2 months after the second dose (and at least 4 months after the first dose). If the combined hepatitis A and hepatitis B vaccine (Twinrix) is used, administer 3 doses at 0, 1, and 6 months; alternatively, a 4-dose Twinrix schedule, administered on days 0, 7, and 21 to 30, followed by a booster dose at month 12 may be used.

Adult patients receiving hemodialysis or with other immunocompromising conditions should receive 1 dose of 40 µg/mL (Recombivax HB) administered on a 3-dose schedule or 2 doses of 20 µg/mL (Engerix-B) administered simultaneously on a 4-dose schedule at 0, 1, 2, and 6 months.

12. Selected conditions for which Haemophilus influenzae type b (Hib) vaccine may be used

1 dose of Hib vaccine should be considered for persons who have sickle cell disease, leukemia, or HIV infection, or who have had a splenectomy, if they have not previously received Hib vaccine.

13. Immunocompromising conditions

Inactivated vaccines generally are acceptable (e.g., pneumococcal, meningococcal, influenza [inactivated influenza vaccine]) and live vaccines generally are avoided in persons with immune deficiencies or immunocompromising conditions. Information on specific conditions is available at http://www.cdc.gov/vaccines/pubs/acip-list.htm.

American Academy of Pediatrics
DEDICATED TO THE HEALTH OF ALL CHILDREN™

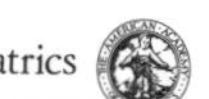

Recommendations for Preventive Pediatric Health Care

Bright Futures/American Academy of Pediatrics

Bright Futures. prevention and health promotion for infants, children, adolescents, and their families™

These recommendations were current at the time of *Caring for Our Children* printing in 2011. To check for the latest edition, go to Http://www.aap.org.

Each child and family is unique; therefore, these **Recommendations for Preventive Pediatric Health Care** are designed for the care of children who are receiving competent parenting, have no manifestations of any important health problems, and are growing and developing in satisfactory fashion. **Additional visits may become necessary** if circumstances suggest variations from normal.

Developmental, psychosocial, and chronic disease issues for children and adolescents may require frequent counseling and treatment visits separate from preventive care visits.

These guidelines represent a consensus by the American Academy of Pediatrics (AAP) and Bright Futures. The AAP continues to emphasize the great importance of **continuity of care** in comprehensive health supervision and the need to avoid **fragmentation of care.**

The recommendations in this statement do not indicate an exclusive course of treatment or standard of medical care. Variations, taking into account individual circumstances, may be appropriate.

	INFANCY								EARLY CHILDHOOD							MIDDLE CHILDHOOD						ADOLESCENCE										
AGE[1]	PRENATAL[2]	NEWBORN[3]	3–5 d[4]	By 1 mo	2 mo	4 mo	6 mo	9 mo	12 m	15 mo	18 mo	24 mo	30 mo	3 y	4 y	5 y	6 y	7 y	8 y	9 y	10 y	11 y	12 y	13 y	14 y	15 y	16 y	17 y	18 y	19 y	20 y	21 y
HISTORY																																
Initial/Interval	●	●	●	●	●	●	●	●	●	●	●	●	●	●	●	●	●	●	●	●	●	●	●	●	●	●	●	●	●	●	●	●
MEASUREMENTS																																
Length/Height and Weight		●	●	●	●	●	●	●	●	●	●	●	●	●	●	●	●	●	●	●	●	●	●	●	●	●	●	●	●	●	●	●
Head Circumference		●	●	●	●	●	●	●	●	●	●	●																				
Weight for Length		●	●	●	●	●	●	●	●	●	●																					
Body Mass Index												●	●	●	●	●	●	●	●	●	●	●	●	●	●	●	●	●	●	●	●	●
Blood Pressure[5]		★	★	★	★	★	★	★	★	★	★	★	★	●	●	●	●	●	●	●	●	●	●	●	●	●	●	●	●	●	●	●
SENSORY SCREENING																																
Vision		★	★	★	★	★	★	★	★	★	★	★	★	●[6]	●	●	●	★	●	★	●	★	●	★	★	●	★	★	●	★	★	★
Hearing		●[7]	★	★	★	★	★	★	★	★	★	★	★	★	●	●	●	★	●	★	●	★	★	★	★	★	★	★	★	★	★	★
DEVELOPMENTAL/BEHAVIORAL ASSESSMENT																																
Developmental Screening[8]								●			●		●																			
Autism Screening[9]											●	●																				
Developmental Surveillance[8]		●	●	●	●	●	●		●	●		●		●	●	●	●	●	●	●	●	●	●	●	●	●	●	●	●	●	●	●
Psychosocial/Behavioral Assessment		●	●	●	●	●	●	●	●	●	●	●	●	●	●	●	●	●	●	●	●	●	●	●	●	●	●	●	●	●	●	●
Alcohol and Drug Use Assessment																						★	★	★	★	★	★	★	★	★	★	★
PHYSICAL EXAMINATION[10]		●	●	●	●	●	●	●	●	●	●	●	●	●	●	●	●	●	●	●	●	●	●	●	●	●	●	●	●	●	●	●
PROCEDURES[11]																																
Newborn Metabolic/Hemoglobin Screening[12]		←	●	—	→																											
Immunization[13]		●	●	●	●	●	●	●	●	●	●	●	●	●	●	●	●	●	●	●	●	●	●	●	●	●	●	●	●	●	●	●
Hematocrit or Hemoglobin[14]						★			●		★	★		★	★	★	★	★	★	★	★	★	★	★	★	★	★	★	★	★	★	★
Lead Screening[15]							★	★	● or ★[16]		★	● or ★[16]		★	★	★	★															
Tuberculin Test[17]				★			★		★		★	★		★	★	★	★	★	★	★	★	★	★	★	★	★	★	★	★	★	★	★
Dyslipidemia Screening[18]												★			★		★		★		★	★	★	★	★	★	★	★	←	—	●	→
STI Screening[19]																						★	★	★	★	★	★	★	★	★	★	★
Cervical Dysplasia Screening[20]																						★	★	★	★	★	★	★	★	★	★	★
ORAL HEALTH[21]							★	★	● or ★[21]		● or ★[21]	● or ★[21]	● or ★[21]	●[22]			●[22]															
ANTICIPATORY GUIDANCE[23]	●	●	●	●	●	●	●	●	●	●	●	●	●	●	●	●	●	●	●	●	●	●	●	●	●	●	●	●	●	●	●	●

1. If a child comes under care for the first time at any point on the schedule, or if any items are not accomplished at the suggested age, the schedule should be brought up to date at the earliest possible time.
2. A prenatal visit is recommended for parents who are at high risk, for first-time parents, and for those who request a conference. The prenatal visit should include anticipatory guidance, pertinent medical history, and a discussion of benefits of breastfeeding and planned method of feeding per AAP statement "The Prenatal Visit" (2001) [URL: http://aappolicy.aappublications.org/cgi/content/full/pediatrics;107/6/1456].
3. Every infant should have a newborn evaluation after birth, breastfeeding encouraged, and instruction and support offered.
4. Every infant should have an evaluation within 3 to 5 days of birth and within 48 to 72 hours after discharge from the hospital, to include evaluation for feeding and jaundice. Breastfeeding infants should receive formal breastfeeding evaluation, encouragement, and instruction as recommended in AAP statement "Breastfeeding and the Use of Human Milk" (2005) [URL: http://aappolicy.aappublications.org/cgi/content/full/pediatrics;115/2/496]. For newborns discharged in less than 48 hours after delivery, the infant must be examined within 48 hours of discharge per AAP statement "Hospital Stay for Healthy Term Newborns" (2004) [URL: http://aappolicy.aappublications.org/cgi/content/full/pediatrics;113/5/1434].
5. Blood pressure measurement in infants and children with specific risk conditions should be performed at visits before age 3 years.
6. If the patient is uncooperative, rescreen within 6 months per the AAP statement "Eye Examination in Infants, Children, and Young Adults by Pediatricians" (2007) [URL: http://aappolicy.aappublications.org/cgi/content/full/pediatrics;111/4/902].
7. All newborns should be screened per AAP statement "Year 2000 Position Statement: Principles and Guidelines for Early Hearing Detection and Intervention Programs " (2000) [URL: http://aappolicy.aappublications.org/cgi/content/full/pediatrics;106/4/798]. Joint Committee on Infant Hearing. Year 2007 position statement: principles and guidelines for early hearing detection and intervention programs. *Pediatrics.* 2007;120:898–921.
8. AAP Council on Children With Disabilities, AAP Section on Developmental Behavioral Pediatrics, AAP Bright Futures Steering Committee, AAP Medical Home Initiatives for Children With Special Needs Project Advisory Committee. Identifying infants and young children with developmental disorders in the medical home: an algorithm for developmental surveillance and screening. *Pediatrics.* 2006;118:405–420 [URL: http://aappolicy.aappublications.org/cgi/content/full/pediatrics;118/1/405].
9. Gupta VB, Hyman SL, Johnson CP, et al. Identifying children with autism early? *Pediatrics.* 2007;119:152–153 [URL: http://pediatrics.aappublications.org/cgi/content/full/119/1/152].
10. At each visit, age-appropriate physical examination is essential, with infant totally unclothed, older child undressed and suitably draped.
11. These may be modified, depending on entry point into schedule and individual need.
12. Newborn metabolic and hemoglobinopathy screening should be done according to state law. Results should be reviewed at visits and appropriate retesting or referral done as needed.
13. Schedules per the Committee on Infectious Diseases, published annually in the January issue of *Pediatrics.* Every visit should be an opportunity to update and complete a child's immunizations.
14. See AAP *Pediatric Nutrition Handbook*, 5th Edition (2003) for a discussion of universal and selective screening options. See also Recommendations to prevent and control iron deficiency in the United States. *MMWR.* 1998;47(RR-3):1–36.
15. For children at risk of lead exposure, consult the AAP statement "Lead Exposure in Children: Prevention, Detection, and Management" (2005) [URL: http://aappolicy.aappublications.org/cgi/content/full/pediatrics;116/4/1036]. Additionally, screening should be done in accordance with state law where applicable.
16. Perform risk assessments or screens as appropriate, based on universal screening requirements for patients with Medicaid or high prevalence areas.
17. Tuberculosis testing per recommendations of the Committee on Infectious Diseases, published in the current edition of *Red Book: Report of the Committee on Infectious Diseases.* Testing should be done on recognition of high-risk factors.
18. "Third Report of the National Cholesterol Education Program (NCEP) Expert Panel on Detection, Evaluation, and Treatment of High Blood Cholesterol in Adults (Adult Treatment Panel III) Final Report" (2002) [URL: http://circ.ahajournals.org/cgi/content/full/106/25/3143] and "The Expert Committee Recommendations on the Assessment, Prevention, and Treatment of Child and Adolescent Overweight and Obesity." Supplement to *Pediatrics.* In press.
19. All sexually active patients should be screened for sexually transmitted infections (STIs).
20. All sexually active girls should have screening for cervical dysplasia as part of a pelvic examination beginning within 3 years of onset of sexual activity or age 21 (whichever comes first).
21. Referral to dental home, if available. Otherwise, administer oral health risk assessment. If the primary water source is deficient in fluoride, consider oral fluoride supplementation.
22. At the visits for 3 years and 6 years of age, it should be determined whether the patient has a dental home. If the patient does not have a dental home, a referral should be made to one. If the primary water source is deficient in fluoride, consider oral fluoride supplementation.
23. Refer to the specific guidance by age as listed in Bright Futures Guidelines. (Hagan JF, Shaw JS, Duncan PM, eds. *Bright Futures: Guidelines for Health Supervision of Infants, Children, and Adolescents.* 3rd ed. Elk Grove Village, IL: American Academy of Pediatrics; 2008.)

KEY

● = to be performed ★ = risk assessment to be performed, with appropriate action to follow, if positive ←●→ = range during which a service may be provided, with the symbol indicating the preferred age

Reference: American Academy of Pediatrics, Committee on Practice and Ambulatory Medicine, Bright Futures Steering Committee. 2007. Recommendations for preventive pediatric health care. Pediatrics 120:1376. Used with permission of the American Academy of Pediatrics, 2009.
Also available at http://brightfutures.aap.org/pdfs/AAP%20Bright%20Futures%20Periodicity%20Sched%20101107.pdf.

Selecting an Appropriate Sanitizer or Disinfectant

One of the most important steps in reducing the spread of infectious diseases in child care settings is cleaning, sanitizing, and disinfecting surfaces that could possibly pose a risk to children or staff. Routine cleaning with detergent and water is the most useful method for removing germs from surfaces in the child care setting. However, some items and surfaces require an additional step after cleaning to further reduce the number of germs on a surface to a level that is unlikely to transmit disease.

What is the difference between sanitizing and disinfecting?

Sometimes these terms are used as if they mean the same thing, but they are not the same.

Sanitizer is a product that reduces germs on inanimate surfaces to levels considered safe by public health codes or regulations. A sanitizer may be appropriate to use on food contact surfaces (dishes, utensils, cutting boards, high chair trays), toys that children may place in their mouths, and pacifiers.

Disinfectant is a product that destroys or inactivates germs on an inanimate object. A disinfectant may be appropriate to use on non-porous surfaces such as diaper change tables, counter tops, door and cabinet handles, and toilets and other bathroom surfaces.

The U.S. Environmental Protection Agency (EPA) recommends that EPA-registered products be used whenever possible. Only a sanitizer or disinfectant product with an EPA registration number on the label can make public health claims that they are effective in inactivating germs. Major manufacturers of chlorine bleach and hydrogen peroxide products offer products that are EPA-registered and sold either in retail stores or commercial janitorial supply stores.

Always follow the manufacturer's instructions when using EPA-registered products described as sanitizers or disinfectants. This includes pre-cleaning, how long the product needs to remain wet on the surface or item, whether or not the product should be diluted or used as is, and if rinsing is needed. Please note that the label instructions on most disinfectants indicate that the surface must be pre-cleaned before applying the disinfectant.

Are there alternatives to chlorine bleach?

If a product that is not chlorine bleach is registered with the EPA and described as a sanitizer or as a disinfectant and is used according to the manufacturer's instructions, it can be used in child care settings. Check the label to see how long you need to leave the sanitizer or disinfectant in contact with the surface you are treating, whether you need to rinse it off before contact by children, and for any precautions when handling.

Some child care settings are using products with hydrogen peroxide as the active ingredient instead of chlorine bleach. Hydrogen peroxide breaks down into water and oxygen. Check to see if the product has an EPA registration number and follow the manufacturer's instructions for use and safe handling. Remember that EPA-registered products will also have available a Material Safety Data Sheet (MSDS) that will provide instructions for the safe use of the product and guidance for first aid response to inadvertent exposure to the chemical.

If you are looking for environmentally friendly products, one EPA-registered product is a botanical-based disinfectant whose active ingredient is thymol which requires a ten minute contact time and, if applied to toys or food contact surfaces, a water rinse is required before use.

In addition, some manufacturers of sanitizer and disinfectant products are working towards developing "green cleaning products" that can attain EPA registration. As new environmentally friendly cleaning products appear in the market, check to see if they are EPA-registered.

Household Bleach and Water

If purchasing an EPA-registered product for sanitizing or disinfecting is not an option, then household bleach diluted with water is a practical alternative. It is economical, convenient, and readily available. It is effective if the proportional amount of bleach to water is appropriate for the task. Using too little bleach may make the mixture ineffective. However, using too much bleach may create a potential health hazard.

When purchasing chlorine bleach, make sure that the bleach concentration is for household use, and not for industrial applications. Household chlorine bleach is typically sold in retail stores as 5-10% hypochlorite solution (regular strength). Use only unscented bleach.

Some chlorine bleach products sold in retail stores may be EPA-registered and described as a sanitizer or disinfectant. Check the label to see if the product has an EPA registration number and follow the manufacturer's instructions

If the chlorine bleach product is for household use and does not have an EPA registration number, here are two recipes that you can use. Which recipe you choose will depend on whether you need to sanitize or disinfect a surface.

To safely prepare bleach solutions:

- Dilute bleach with cool water and do not use more than the recommended amount of bleach.
- Select a bottle made of opaque material.
- Make a fresh bleach dilution daily; label the bottle with contents and the date mixed.
- Wear gloves and eye protection when diluting bleach.
- Use a funnel.
- Add bleach to the water rather than the water to bleach to reduce fumes.
- Make sure the room is well ventilated.
- Never mix or store ammonia with bleach or products that contain bleach.

Purpose	Recipe
Sanitizer For food contact surface sanitizing (dishes, utensils, cutting boards, high chair trays), toys that children may place in their mouths, and pacifiers.	1 tablespoon of bleach + 1 gallon of cool water Let stand for 2 minutes or air dry.
Disinfectant For use on non-porous surfaces such as diaper change tables, counter tops, door and cabinet handles, toilets.	¼**- ¾ cup of bleach + 1 gallon of cool water (or 1 to 3 tablespoons of bleach + 1 quart of cool water) applied as a spray or poured fresh solution, not by dipping into a container with a cloth that has been in contact with a contaminated surface Let stand for 2 minutes or air dry.

To safely use bleach solutions:

- Apply the bleach dilution after cleaning the surface with soap or detergent and rinsing with water.
- If using a spray bottle, adjust the setting to produce a heavy spray instead of a fine mist.
- Allow for a two minute contact time or air dry.
- Apply when children are not present in the area.
- Ventilate the area by allowing fresh air to circulate and allow the surfaces to completely air dry or wipe dry after two minutes of contact with the surface before allowing children back into the area.
- Store all chemicals securely, out of reach of children and in a way that they will not tip and spill.

Adapted from: California Childcare Health Program. 2009. Sanitize safely and effectively: Bleach and alternatives in child care programs. *Health and Safety Notes* (July).

A Final Note

Remember that any cleaning, sanitizing, or disinfecting product must always be safely stored and out of reach of children. Always follow the manufacturer's instruction for safe handling to protect yourselves and those in your care.

References:

1. California Childcare Health Program. 2009. Sanitize safely and effectively: Bleach and alternatives in child care programs. *Health and Safety Notes* (July). http://www.ucsfchildcarehealth.org/pdfs/healthandsafety/SanitizeSafely_En0709.pdf.
2. U.S. Environmental Protection Agency. 2008. What are antimicrobial pesticides? Pesticides Website. http://www.epa.gov/oppad001/ad_info.htm.
3. U.S. Environmental Protection Agency. 2009. Selected EPA-registered disinfectants. Pesticides Website. www.epa.gov/oppad001/chemregindex.htm.
4. Grenier, D., D. Leduc, eds. 2008. *Well beings: A guide to health in child care.* 3rd ed. Ottawa: Canadian Paediatric Society.
5. Rutala, W. A., D. J. Weber, the Healthcare Infection Control Practices Advisory Committee (HICPAC). 2008. *Guideline for disinfection and sterilization in healthcare facilities, 2008*. Atlanta, GA: Centers for Disease Control and Prevention, National Center for Preparedness, Detection, and Control of Infectious Diseases, Division of Healthcare Quality Promotion. http://www.cdc.gov/hicpac/pdf/guidelines/Disinfection_Nov_2008.pdf.
6. U.S. Department of Health and Human Services, Public Health Service, Food and Drug Administration. 2009. Food code. College Park, MD: Food and Drug Administration. http://www.fda.gov/Food/FoodSafety/RetailFoodProtection/FoodCode/FoodCode2009/default.htm.

** Corrected to "1/4" from "1/2" in second printing, August 2011.

Routine Schedule** for Cleaning, Sanitizing, and Disinfecting

Areas	Before Each Use	After Each Use	Daily (At the End of the Day)	Weekly	Monthly	Comments
Food Areas						
• Food preparation surfaces	Clean, Sanitize	Clean, Sanitize				Use a sanitizer safe for food contact
• Eating utensils & dishes		Clean, Sanitize				If washing the dishes and utensils by hand, use a sanitizer safe for food contact as the final step in the process; Use of an automated dishwasher will sanitize
• Tables & highchair trays	Clean, Sanitize	Clean, Sanitize				
• Countertops		Clean	Clean, Sanitize			Use a sanitizer safe for food contact
• Food preparation appliances		Clean	Clean, Sanitize			
• Mixed use tables	Clean, Sanitize					Before serving food
• Refrigerator					Clean	
Child Care Areas						
• Plastic mouthed toys		Clean	Clean, Sanitize			
• Pacifiers		Clean	Clean, Sanitize			Reserve for use by only one child; Use dishwasher or boil for one minute
• Hats			Clean			Clean after each use if head lice present
• Door & cabinet handles			Clean, Disinfect			

**Corrected to "Routine Schedule" from "Guide" in second printing, August 2011.

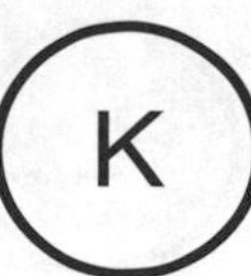

• Floors			Clean			Sweep or vacuum, then damp mop, (consider micro fiber damp mop to pick up most particles)
• Machine washable cloth toys				Clean		Launder
• Dress-up clothes				Clean		Launder
• Play activity centers				Clean		
• Drinking Fountains			Clean, Disinfect			
• Computer keyboards		Clean, Sanitize				Use sanitizing wipes, do not use spray
• Phone receivers			Clean			
Toilet & Diapering Areas						
• Changing tables		Clean, Disinfect				Clean with detergent, rinse, disinfect
• Potty chairs		Clean, Disinfect				
• Handwashing sinks & faucets			Clean, Disinfect			
• Countertops			Clean, Disinfect			
• Toilets			Clean, Disinfect			
• Diaper pails			Clean, Disinfect			
• Floors			Clean, Disinfect			Damp mop with a floor cleaner/ disinfectant
Sleeping Areas						
• Bed sheets & pillow cases				Clean		Clean before use by another child
• Cribs, cots, & mats				Clean		Clean before use by another child
• Blankets					Clean	

Cleaning Up Body Fluids

Treat urine, stool, vomit, blood, and body fluids, except for human milk, as potentially infectious. Spills of body fluid should be cleaned up and surfaces disinfected immediately.

a) For small amounts of urine and stool on smooth surfaces, wipe off and clean away visible soil with a little detergent solution. Then rinse the surface with clean water.

b) Apply a disinfectant following the manufacturer's instructions. See Appendix J.

For larger spills on floors, or any spills on rugs or carpets:

c) Wear gloves while cleaning. While disposable gloves can be used, household rubber gloves are adequate for all spills except blood and bloody body fluids. Disposable gloves should be used when blood may be present in the spill;

d) Take care to avoid splashing any contaminated material onto the mucous membranes of your eyes, nose or mouth, or into any open sores you may have;

e) Wipe up as much of the visible material as possible with disposable paper towels and carefully place the soiled paper towels and other soiled disposable material in a leak-proof, plastic bag that has been securely tied or sealed. Use a wet/dry vacuum on carpets, if such equipment is available;

f) Immediately use a detergent, or a combination detergent/disinfectant to clean the spill area. Then rinse the area with clean water. Additional cleaning by shampooing or steam cleaning the contaminated surface may be necessary;

g) For blood and body fluid spills on carpeting, blot to remove body fluids from the fabric as quickly as possible. Then disinfect by spot-cleaning with a combination detergent/disinfectant, and shampooing, or steam-cleaning the contaminated surface;

h) If directed by the manufacturer's instructions, dry the surface;

i) Clean and rinse reusable household rubber gloves, then apply disinfectant. Remove, dry and store these gloves away from food or food surfaces. Discard disposable gloves;

j) Mops and other equipment used to clean up body fluids should be:

   1) Cleaned with detergent and rinsed with water;

   2) Rinsed with a fresh disinfectant solution;

   3) Wrung as dry as possible;

   4) Air-dried.

k) Wash your hands afterward, even though you wore gloves;

l) Remove and bag clothing (yours and those worn by children) soiled by body fluids;

m) Put on fresh clothes after washing the soiled skin and hands of everyone involved.

For guidance on sanitizers and disinfectants, please refer to Appendix J, Selecting an Appropriate Sanitizer or Disinfectant.

References:

1. Grenier, D., D. Leduc, eds. 2008. *Well beings: A guide to health in child care*. 3rd ed. Ottawa: Canadian Paediatric Society.
2. Centers for Disease Control and Prevention, National Institute for Occupational Safety and Health. 2010. *Preventing exposures to bloodborne pathogens among paramedics*. http://www.cdc.gov/niosh/docs/wp-solutions/2010-139/pdfs/2010-139.pdf.
3. Centers for Disease Control and Prevention. 2010. Bloodborne infectious diseases: HIV/AIDS, hepatitis B, hepatitis C. http://www.cdc.gov/niosh/topics/bbp/.
4. Pickering, L. K., C. J. Baker, D. W. Kimberlin, S. S. Long, eds. 2009. Infections spread by blood and body fluids. In *Red book: 2009 report of the Committee on Infectious Diseases.* 28th ed. Elk Grove Village, IL: American Academy of Pediatrics.
5. Occupational Safety and Health Administration (OSHA). 2008. Bloodborne pathogens. 29 CFR 1910.1030. http://www.osha.gov/pls/oshaweb/owadisp.show_document?p_table=standards&p_id=10051.
6. Clark, Roger A. 1992. Standard interpretations: 1910.1030, written at the request of Marjorie P. Alloy. Occupational Safety and Health Administration (OSHA). http://www.osha.gov/pls/oshaweb/owadisp.show_document?p_table=INTERPRETATIONS&p_id=20952.

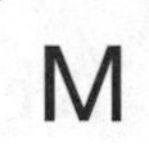

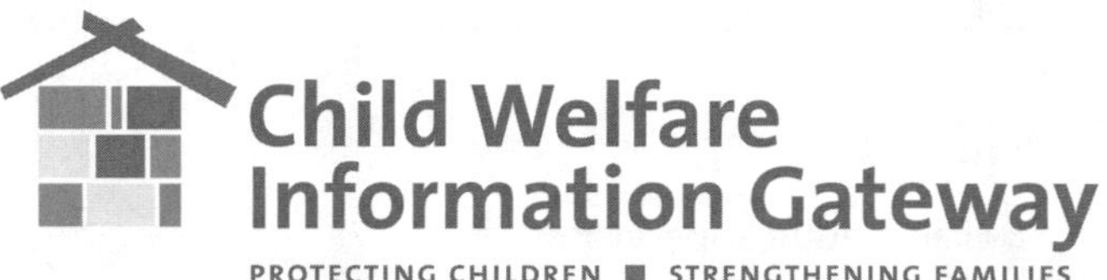

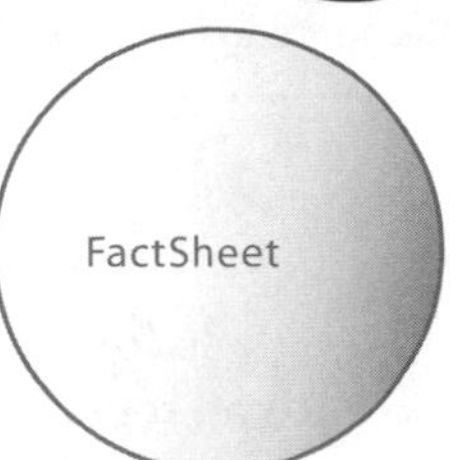

June 2007

Disponible en español
www.childwelfare.gov/pubs/
factsheets/sp_signs.cfm

Recognizing Child Abuse and Neglect: Signs and Symptoms

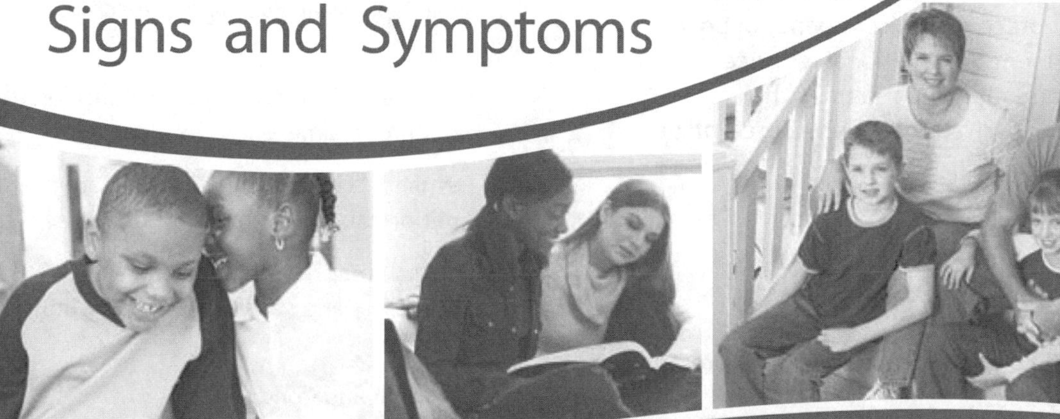

The first step in helping abused or neglected children is learning to recognize the signs of child abuse and neglect. The presence of a single sign does not prove child abuse is occurring in a family, but a closer look at the situation may be warranted when these signs appear repeatedly or in combination.

If you do suspect a child is being harmed, reporting your suspicions may protect the child and get

What's Inside:

U.S. Department of Health and Human Services
Administration for Children and Families
Administration on Children, Youth and Families
Children's Bureau

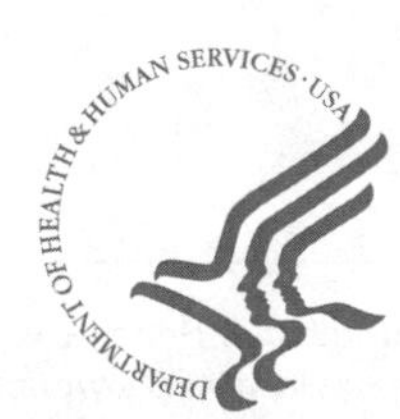

Child Welfare Information Gateway
Children's Bureau/ACYF
1250 Maryland Avenue, SW
Eighth Floor
Washington, DC 20024
703.385.7565 or 800.394.3366
Email: info@childwelfare.gov
www.childwelfare.gov

help for the family. Any concerned person can report suspicions of child abuse and neglect. Some people (typically certain types of professionals) are required by law to make a report of child maltreatment under specific circumstances—these are called mandatory reporters. For more information, see the Child Welfare Information Gateway publication, Mandatory Reporters of Child Abuse and Neglect: www.childwelfare.gov/systemwide/laws_policies/statutes/manda.cfm

For more information about where and how to file a report, contact your local child protective services agency or police department. An additional resource for information and referral is the Childhelp ® National Child Abuse Hotline (800.4.A.CHILD).

Recognizing child abuse

The following signs may signal the presence of child abuse or neglect.

The Child:

- Shows sudden changes in behavior or school performance
- Has not received help for physical or medical problems brought to the parents' attention
- Has learning problems (or difficulty concentrating) that cannot be attributed to specific physical or psychological causes
- Is always watchful, as though preparing for something bad to happen
- Lacks adult supervision
- Is overly compliant, passive, or withdrawn
- Comes to school or other activities early, stays late, and does not want to go home

The Parent:

- Shows little concern for the child
- Denies the existence of—or blames the child for—the child's problems in school or at home
- Asks teachers or other caregivers to use harsh physical discipline if the child misbehaves
- Sees the child as entirely bad, worthless, or burdensome
- Demands a level of physical or academic performance the child cannot achieve
- Looks primarily to the child for care, attention, and satisfaction of emotional needs

The Parent and Child:

- Rarely touch or look at each other
- Consider their relationship entirely negative
- State that they do not like each other

types of abuse

The following are some signs often associated with particular types of child abuse and neglect: physical abuse, neglect, sexual abuse, and emotional abuse. It is important to note, however, that these types of abuse are more typically found in combination than alone. A physically abused child, for example, is often emotionally abused as well, and a sexually abused child also may be neglected.

Signs of Physical abuse

Consider the possibility of physical abuse when the child:

- Has unexplained burns, bites, bruises, broken bones, or black eyes
- Has fading bruises or other marks noticeable after an absence from school
- Seems frightened of the parents and protests or cries when it is time to go home
- Shrinks at the approach of adults
- Reports injury by a parent or another adult caregiver

Consider the possibility of physical abuse when the parent or other adult caregiver:

- Offers conflicting, unconvincing, or no explanation for the child's injury
- Describes the child as "evil," or in some other very negative way
- Uses harsh physical discipline with the child
- Has a history of abuse as a child

Signs of Neglect

Consider the possibility of neglect when the child:

- Is frequently absent from school
- Begs or steals food or money
- Lacks needed medical or dental care, immunizations, or glasses
- Is consistently dirty and has severe body odor
- Lacks sufficient clothing for the weather
- Abuses alcohol or other drugs
- States that there is no one at home to provide care

Consider the possibility of neglect when the parent or other adult caregiver:

- Appears to be indifferent to the child
- Seems apathetic or depressed
- Behaves irrationally or in a bizarre manner
- Is abusing alcohol or other drugs

Signs of Sexual abuse

Consider the possibility of sexual abuse when the child:

- Has difficulty walking or sitting
- Suddenly refuses to change for gym or to participate in physical activities
- Reports nightmares or bedwetting

- Experiences a sudden change in appetite
- Demonstrates bizarre, sophisticated, or unusual sexual knowledge or behavior
- Becomes pregnant or contracts a venereal disease, particularly if under age 14
- Runs away
- Reports sexual abuse by a parent or another adult caregiver

Consider the possibility of sexual abuse when the parent or other adult caregiver:

- Is unduly protective of the child or severely limits the child's contact with other children, especially of the opposite sex
- Is secretive and isolated
- Is jealous or controlling with family members

Signs of emotional Maltreatment

Consider the possibility of emotional maltreatment when the child:

- Shows extremes in behavior, such as overly compliant or demanding behavior, extreme passivity, or aggression
- Is either inappropriately adult (parenting other children, for example) or inappropriately infantile (frequently rocking or head-banging, for example)
- Is delayed in physical or emotional development
- Has attempted suicide
- Reports a lack of attachment to the parent

Consider the possibility of emotional maltreatment when the parent or other adult caregiver:

- Constantly blames, belittles, or berates the child
- Is unconcerned about the child and refuses to consider offers of help for the child's problems
- Overtly rejects the child

Resources on the Child Welfare Information Gateway Website

Child Abuse and Neglect
www.childwelfare.gov/can/index.cfm

Defining Child Abuse and Neglect
www.childwelfare.gov/can/defining/

Preventing Child Abuse and Neglect
www.childwelfare.gov/preventing/

Reporting Child Abuse and Neglect
www.childwelfare.gov/responding/reporting.cfm

This factsheet was adapted, with permission, from Recognizing Child Abuse: What Parents Should Know. Prevent Child Abuse America. © 2003.

Protective Factors Regarding Child Abuse and Neglect

Protective factors that quality child care can enhance:

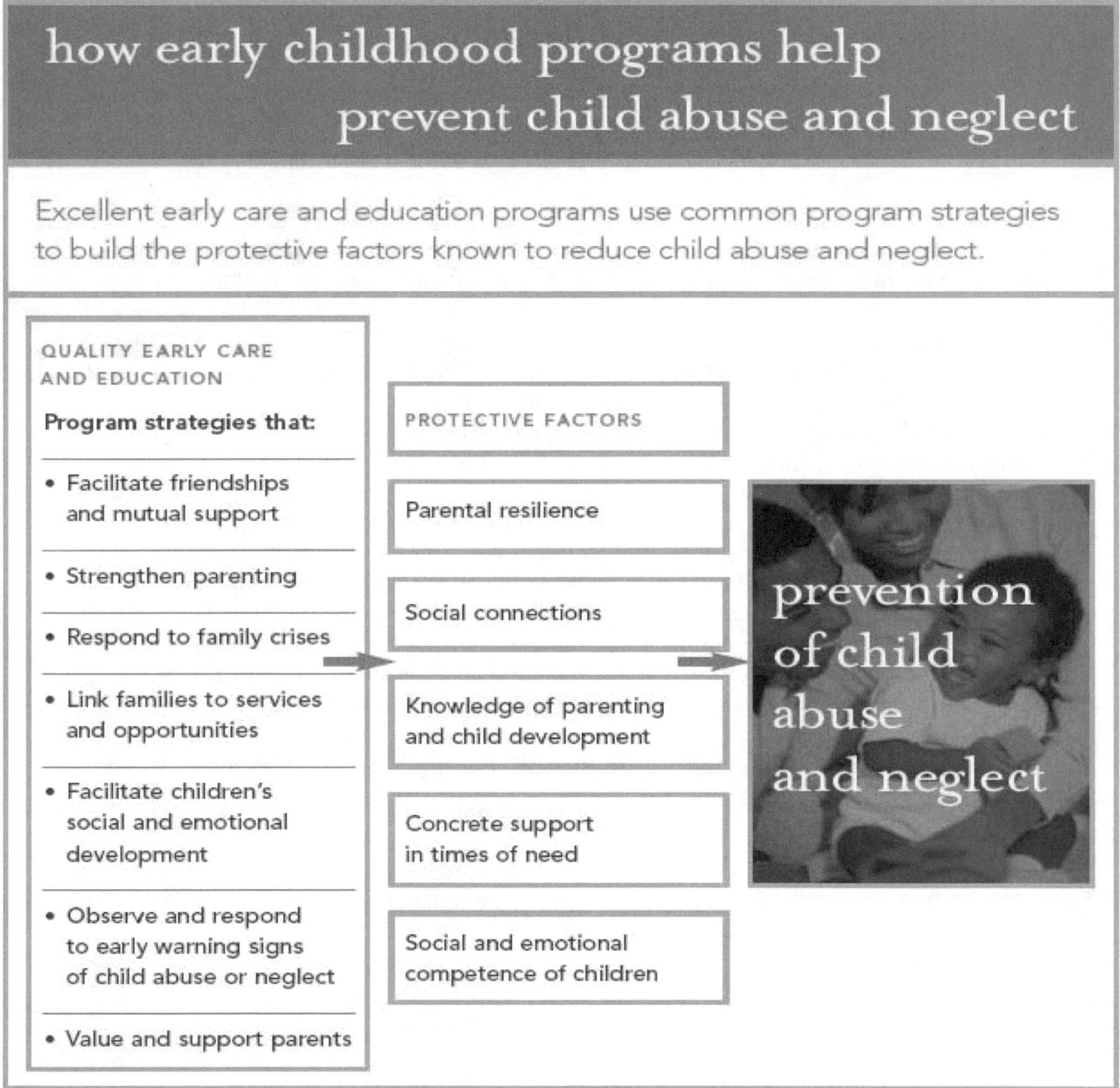

Reproduced with permission from: Strengthening Families – Center for Study of Social Policy http://www.strengtheningFamilies.net.

1. Parental resilience
    - value and support parents/guardians, assist development of parental self-efficacy, link to community resources including mental health professionals when needed
2. Social connections

   - provide a place where parents/guardians may develop positive social interactions in a child-friendly environment
3. Parenting skills and knowledge about normal child development
   - model and teach positive, effective parenting/discipline techniques, educate parents/guardians about child development and appropriate expectations
4. Support structures in place during times of need
   - identify needs and connect families stressed or in crisis with center and/or community resources
5. Children's social and emotional competence
   - provide children with a healthy, nurturing environment that encourages trust and attachment

References/Resources:

The Child Welfare Information Gateway. Stay connected! U.S. Department of Health and Human Services, Administration for Children and Families, Children's Bureau. www.childwelfare.gov.

Additional resources

1. The Child Welfare Information Gateway. Enhancing protective factors. U.S. Department of Health and Human Services, Administration for Children and Families, Children's Bureau. http://www.childwelfare.gov/preventing/promoting/protectfactors/.
2. Strengthening Families. Strengthening families Website. Center for the Study of Social Policy. http://www.strengtheningfamilies.net/index.php/about.
3. American Academy of Pediatrics. Connected kids Website. www.aap.org/connectedkids.
4. American Academy of Pediatrics. 2010. What to know about child abuse. Healthy Children. http://www.healthychildren.org/English/safety-prevention/at-home/Pages/What-to-Know-about-Child-Abuse.aspx?nfstatus=401&nftoken=00000000-0000-0000-0000-000000000000&nfstatusdescription=ERROR:+No+local+token.
5. American Academy of Pediatrics. 2010. What to know about child abuse. Healthy Children. http://www.healthychildren.org/english/safety-prevention/at-home/Pages/What-to-Know-about-Child-Abuse.aspx.
6. American Academy of Pediatrics. 2007. Policy statement: Assessment of maltreatment of children with disabilities. *Pediatrics* 108:508-12.

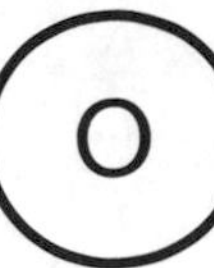

CARE PLAN FOR CHILDREN WITH SPECIAL HEALTH NEEDS

-To be completed by a Health Care Provider-

	Today's Date
Child's Full Name	Date of Birth
Parent's/Guardian's Name	Telephone No. ( )
Primary Health Care Provider	Telephone No. ( )
Specialty Provider	Telephone No. ( )
Specialty Provider	Telephone No. ( )
Diagnosis(es)	
Allergies	

ROUTINE CARE

Medication To Be Given at Child Care	Schedule/Dose (When and How Much?)	Route (How?)	Reason Prescribed	Possible Side Effects

List medications given at home:

NEEDED ACCOMMODATION(S)

Describe any needed accommodation(s) the child needs in daily activities and why:

Diet or Feeding: ____________________

Classroom Activities: ____________________

Naptime/Sleeping: ____________________

Toileting: ____________________

Outdoor or Field Trips: ____________________

Transportation: ____________________

Other: ____________________

Additional comments: ____________________

____

CH-15
MAR 05

Page 1 of 2 Pages.

Source: New Jersey Department of Health and Senior Services, 2005.

CARE PLAN FOR CHILDREN WITH SPECIAL HEALTH NEEDS
Continued

SPECIAL EQUIPMENT / MEDICAL SUPPLIES

1. ______________________________
2. ______________________________
3. ______________________________

EMERGENCY CARE

CALL PARENTS/GUARDIANS if the following symptoms are present:

____

____

CALL 911 (EMERGENCY MEDICAL SERVICES) if the following symptoms are present, as well as contacting the parents/guardians:

____

____

TAKE THESE MEASURES while waiting for parents or medical help to arrive:

____

____

____

SUGGESTED SPECIAL TRAINING FOR STAFF

____

____

____

Health Care Provider Signature	Date

PARENT NOTES (OPTIONAL)

____

____

____

I hereby give consent for my child's health care provider or specialist to communicate with my child's child care provider or school nurse to discuss any of the information contained in this care plan.

Parent/Guardian Signature	Date

Important: In order to ensure the health and safety of your child, it is vital that any person involved in the care of your child be aware of your child's special health needs, medication your child is taking, or needs in case of a health care emergency, and the specific actions to take regarding your child's special health needs.

CH-15
MAR 05
New Jersey Department of Health and Senior Services

Page 2 of 2 Pages.

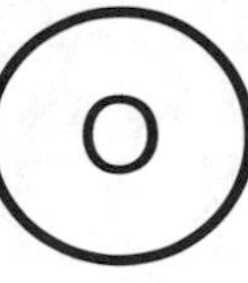

Special Health Care Plan

The special health care plan defines all members of the care team, communication guidelines (how, when, and how often), and all information on appropriately accommodating the special health concerns and needs of this child while in child care.

Name of Child: ______________________ **Date:** ______________

Facility Name: ______________________

Description of condition(s): (include description of difficulties associated with each condition) ______________________

Team Member Names and Titles (parents of the child are to be included)

Care Coordinator (responsible for developing and administering the Special Health Care Plan): ______________________

ⓘ If training is necessary, then all team members will be trained.

☐ Individualized Family Service Plan **(IFSP)** attached ☐ Individualized Education Plan **(IEP)** attached

Outside Professionals Involved	**Telephone**
Health Care Provider (MD, NP, etc.):	
Speech & Language Therapist:	
Occupational Therapist:	
Physical Therapist:	
Psychologist/Mental Health Consultant:	
Social Worker:	
Family-Child Advocate:	
Other:	

Communication

How the team will communicate (notes, communication log, phone calls, meetings, etc.):

How often will team communication occur: ☐ **Daily** ☐ **Weekly** ☐ **Monthly** ☐ **Bi-monthly** ☐ **Other** ______________

Date and time specifics: ______________________

Page 1 of 3 California Childcare Health Program www.ucsfchildcarehealth.org rev. 08/04

Specific Medical Information

* Medical documentation provided and attached: ☐ Yes ☐ No

☐ **Information Exchange Form** completed by health care provider is in child's file on site.

* Medication to be administered: ☐ Yes ☐ No

☐ **Medication Administration Form** completed by health care provider and parents are in child's file on site (including: type of medications, method, amount, time schedule, potential side effects, etc.)

Any known allergies to foods and/or medications: ______

Specific health-related needs: ______

Planned strategies to support the child's needs and any safety issues while in child care: (diapering/toileting, outdoor play, circle time, nap/sleeping, etc.) ______

Plan for absences of personnel trained and responsible for health-related procedure(s): ______

Other (i.e., transportation, field trips, etc.): ______

Special Staff Training Needs

Training monitored by: ______

1) Type (be specific): ______

Training done by: ______ Date of Training: ______

2) Type (be specific): ______

Training done by: ______ Date of Training: ______

3) Type (be specific): ______

Training done by: ______ Date of Training: ______

Equipment/Positioning

* Physical Therapist (PT) and/or Occupational Therapist (OT) consult provided: ☐ Yes ☐ No ☐ Not Needed

Special equipment needed/to be used: ______

Positioning requirements (attach additional documentation as necessary): ______

Equipment care/maintenance notes: ______

Page 2 of 3 California Childcare Health Program www.ucsfchildcarehealth.org rev. 08/04

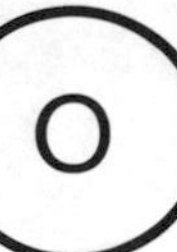

Nutrition and Feeding Needs

☐ **Nutrition and Feeding Care Plan Form** completed by team is in child's file on-site.(See for detailed requirements/needs.)

Behavior Changes

(be specific when listing changes in behavior that arise as a result of the health-related condition/concerns)

____

____

____

Additional Information

(include any unusual episodes that might arise while in care and how the situation should be handled)

____

____

____

Support Programs the Child Is Involved with Outside of Child Care

1. Name of program: ______________________ Contact person: ______________________

   Address and telephone: ______________________

   Frequency of attendance: ______________________

2. Name of program: ______________________ Contact person: ______________________

   Address and telephone: ______________________

   Frequency of attendance: ______________________

   ☐

3. Name of program: ______________________ Contact person: ______________________

   Address and telephone: ______________________

   Frequency of attendance: ______________________

Emergency Procedures

☐ Special emergency and/or medical procedure required (additional documentation attached)

Emergency instructions: ______________________

____

____

Emergency contact: ______________________ Telephone: ______________________

Follow-up: Updates/Revisions

This Special Health Care Plan is to be updated/revised whenever child's health status changes or at least every __________ months as a result of the collective input from team members.

Due date for revision and team meeting: ______________________

Page 3 of 3

California Childcare Health Program www.ucsfchildcarehealth.org rev. 08/04

Nutrition and Feeding Care Plan

The nutrition and feeding care plan defines all members of the care team, communication guidelines (how, when, and how often), and all information on a child's diet and feeding needs for this child while in child care.

Name of Child: ______________________________ **Date:** ____________________

Facility Name: ______________________________

Team Member Names and Titles (parents of the child are to be included)

Care Coordinator (responsible for developing and administering *Nutrition and Feeding Care Plan*): ______________________________

____

____

ⓘ If training is necessary, then all team members will be trained.

☐ Individualized Family Service Plan **(IFSP)** attached ☐ Individualized Education Plan **(IEP)** attached

Communication

What is the team's communication goal and how will it be achieved (notes, communication log, phone calls, meetings, etc.):

____

____

How often will team communication occur: ☐ **Daily** ☐ **Weekly** ☐ **Monthly** ☐ **Bi-monthly** ☐ **Other** __________

Date and time specifics: ______________________________

Specific Diet Information

* Medical documentation provided and attached: ☐ Yes ☐ No ☐ Not Needed

Specific nutrition/feeding-related needs and any safety issues: ______________________________

____

____

____

* **Foods to avoid (*allergies* and/or *intolerances*):** ______________________________

Planned strategies to support the child's needs: ______________________________

____

____

____

Plan for absences of personnel trained and responsible for nutrition/feeding-related procedure(s): __________

____

____

* Food texture/consistency needs: ______________________________

* Special dietary needs: ______________________________

* Other: ______________________________

Eating Equipment/Positioning

* Physical Therapist (PT) and/or Occupational Therapist (OT) consult provided ☐ Yes ☐ No ☐ Not Needed

Special equipment needed: ______________________________

Specific body positioning for feeding (attach additional documentation as necessary): ______________________________

____

Page 1 of 2 California Childcare Health Program www.ucsfchildcarehealth.org rev. 05/03

Behavior Changes (be specific when listing changes in behavior that arise before, during, or after feeding/eating)

____

____

Medical Information

☐ **Information Exchange Form** completed by Health Care Provider is in child's file onsite.

* Medication to be administered as part of feeding routine: ☐ Yes ☐ No

☐ **Medication Administration Form** completed by health care provider and parents is in child's file on-site (including type of medication, who administers, when administered, potential side effects, etc.)

Tube Feeding Information

Primary person responsible for daily feeding: ______________________________

Additional person to support feeding: ______________________________

☐ Breast Milk ☐ Formula (list brand information): ______________________________

Time(s) of day: ______________________________

Volume (how much to feed): ______________ Rate of flow: ______________ Length of feeding: ______________

Position of child: ______________________________

☐ Oral feeding and/or stimulation (attach detailed instructions as necessary): ______________________________

Special Training Needed by Staff

Training monitored by: ______________________________

1) Type (be specific): ______________________________

Training done by: ______________________ Date of Training: ______________________

2) Type (be specific): ______________________________

Training done by: ______________________ Date of Training: ______________________

Additional Information (include any unusual episodes that might arise while in care and how the situation should be handled)

____

____

____

Emergency Procedures

☐ Special emergency and/or medical procedure required (additional documentation attached)

Emergency instructions: ______________________________

____

Emergency contact: ______________________ Telephone: ______________________

Follow-up: Updates/Revisions

This Nutrition and Feeding Care Plan is to be updated/revised whenever child's health status changes or at least every ___ months as a result of the collective input from team members.

Due date for revision and team meeting: ______________

Page 2 of 2 California Childcare Health Program www.ucsfchildcarehealth.org rev. 05/03

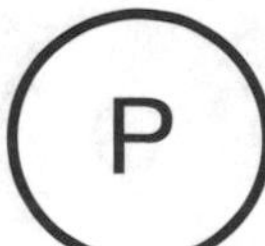

Situations that Require Medical Attention Right Away

In the two boxes below, you will find lists of common medical emergencies or urgent situations you may encounter as a child care provider. To prepare for such situations:

1) Know how to access Emergency Medical Services (EMS) in your area. See Glossary for definition of EMS.
2) Know how to reach your Poison Center right away, nationally call 1-800-222-1222.
3) Educate staff on the recognition of an emergency, and when in doubt, call EMS.
4) Know how to contact each child's guardian and primary health care provider. Obtain permission from parents/guardians to speak directly to each child's health care professional.
5) Develop plans for children with special medical needs together with their family and primary care provider.
6) Compile information on when and how to contact public health authorities.

Call Emergency Medical Services (EMS) immediately if:

- You believe the child's life is at risk or there is a risk of permanent injury.
- The child is acting strangely, much less alert, or much more withdrawn than usual.
- The child has difficulty breathing, is having an asthma exacerbation, or is unable to speak.
- The child's skin or lips look blue, purple, or gray.
- The child has rhythmic jerking of arms and legs and a loss of consciousness (seizure).
- The child is unconscious.
- The child is less and less responsive.
- The child has any of the following after a head injury: decrease in level of alertness, confusion, headache, vomiting, irritability, or difficulty walking.
- The child has increasing or severe pain anywhere.
- The child has a cut or burn that is large, deep, and/or won't stop bleeding.
- The child is vomiting blood.
- The child has a severe stiff neck, headache, and fever.
- The child is significantly dehydrated: sunken eyes, lethargic, not making tears, not urinating.
- Multiple children affected by injury or serious illness at the same time.
- When in doubt, call EMS.
- After you have called EMS, remember to contact the child's legal guardian.

At any time you believe the child's life may be at risk, or you believe there is a risk of permanent injury, seek immediate medical treatment. Do not hesitate, when in doubt, call EMS.

Determine contingency plans for times when there may be power outages, transportation issues etc.

Document what happened and what actions were taken; share verbally and in writing with parents/guardians.

Some children may have urgent situations that do not necessarily require ambulance transport but still need medical attention. The box below lists some of these more common situations. The legal guardian should be informed of the following conditions. If you or the guardian cannot reach the physician within one hour, the child should be brought to a hospital.

Get medical attention within one hour for:

- Fever* in any age child who looks more than mildly ill.
- Fever * in a child less than two months (eight weeks) of age.
- A quickly spreading purple or red rash.
- A large volume of blood in the stools.
- A cut that may require stitches.
- Any medical condition specifically outlined in a child's care plan requiring parental notification.

**Fever is defined as a temperature above 101°F (38.3°C) orally, above 102°F (38.9°C) rectally, or 100°F (37.8°C) or higher taken axillary (armpit) or measured by an equivalent method.*

References:

1. Aronson, S., ed. 2005. *Pediatric first aid for caregivers and teachers.* Elk Grove Village, IL: American Academy of Pediatrics.

2. Aronson, S., T. R. Shope, eds. 2008. Managing infectious diseases in child care and schools: A quick reference guide. Elk Grove Village, IL: American Academy of Pediatrics.

Approved by the AAP Committee on Pediatric Emergency Medicine, January 2009.

Getting Started with *MyPlate*

- MyPlate is part of a larger communications initiative based on *2010 Dietary Guidelines for Americans* to help consumers make better food choices.
- MyPlate is designed to remind Americans to eat healthfully; it is not intended to change consumer behavior alone.
- MyPlate illustrates the five food groups using a familiar mealtime visual, a place setting.

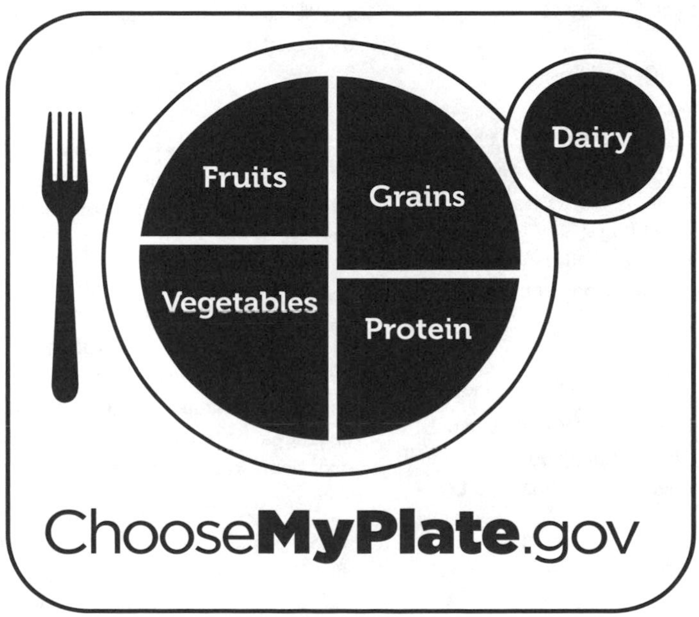

ChooseMyPlate.gov features practical information and tips to help Americans build healthier diets. It features selected messages to help consumers focus on key behaviors. Selected messages include:

o Enjoy your food, but eat less.

o Avoid oversized portions.

o Make half your plate fruits and vegetables.

o Switch to fat-free or low-fat (1%) milk.

o Make at least half your grains whole grains.

o Compare sodium in foods like soup, bread, and frozenmeals - and choose foods with lower numbers.

o Drink water instead of sugary drinks.

Source: U.S. Department of Agriculture. 2011. MyPlate. http://www.choosemyplate.gov.

10 tips
Nutrition Education Series

choose MyPlate

10 tips to a great plate

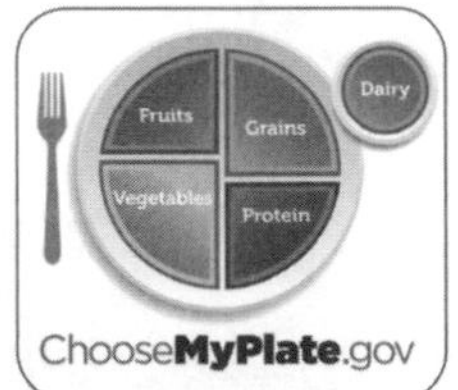

Making food choices for a healthy lifestyle can be as simple as using these 10 Tips.
Use the ideas in this list to *balance your calories*, to choose foods to *eat more often*, and to cut back on foods to *eat less often*.

1 balance calories

Find out how many calories YOU need for a day as a first step in managing your weight. Go to www.ChooseMyPlate.gov to find your calorie level. Being physically active also helps you balance calories.

2 enjoy your food, but eat less

Take the time to fully enjoy your food as you eat it. Eating too fast or when your attention is elsewhere may lead to eating too many calories. Pay attention to hunger and fullness cues before, during, and after meals. Use them to recognize when to eat and when you've had enough.

3 avoid oversized portions

Use a smaller plate, bowl, and glass. Portion out foods before you eat. When eating out, choose a smaller size option, share a dish, or take home part of your meal.

4 foods to eat more often

Eat more vegetables, fruits, whole grains, and fat-free or 1% milk and dairy products. These foods have the nutrients you need for health—including potassium, calcium, vitamin D, and fiber. Make them the basis for meals and snacks.

5 make half your plate fruits and vegetables

Choose red, orange, and dark-green vegetables like tomatoes, sweet potatoes, and broccoli, along with other vegetables for your meals. Add fruit to meals as part of main or side dishes or as dessert.

6 switch to fat-free or low-fat (1%) milk

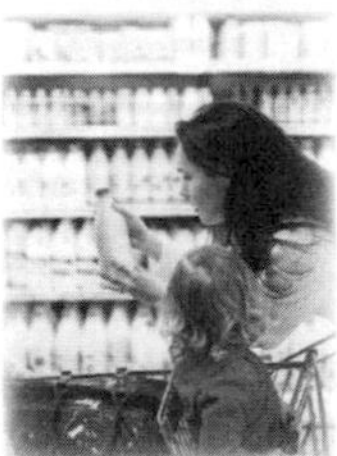

They have the same amount of calcium and other essential nutrients as whole milk, but fewer calories and less saturated fat.

7 make half your grains whole grains

To eat more whole grains, substitute a whole-grain product for a refined product—such as eating whole-wheat bread instead of white bread or brown rice instead of white rice.

8 foods to eat less often

Cut back on foods high in solid fats, added sugars, and salt. They include cakes, cookies, ice cream, candies, sweetened drinks, pizza, and fatty meats like ribs, sausages, bacon, and hot dogs. Use these foods as occasional treats, not everyday foods.

9 compare sodium in foods

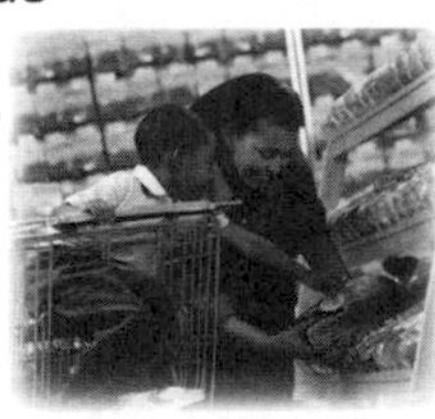

Use the Nutrition Facts label to choose lower sodium versions of foods like soup, bread, and frozen meals. Select canned foods labeled "low sodium," "reduced sodium," or "no salt added."

10 drink water instead of sugary drinks

Cut calories by drinking water or unsweetened beverages. Soda, energy drinks, and sports drinks are a major source of added sugar, and calories, in American diets.

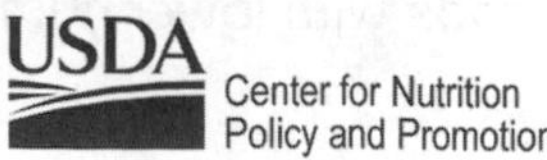

Center for Nutrition Policy and Promotion

Go to www.ChooseMyPlate.gov for more information.

DG TipSheet No. 1
June 2011
USDA is an equal opportunity provider and employer.

Physical Acitvity: How Much Is Needed?

Young Children (2 to 5 years)

Children ages two to five years should play actively several times each day. Their activity may happen in short bursts of time and not be all at once. Physical activities for young children should be developmentally-appropriate, fun, and offer variety.

Children and Adolescents (6 to 17 years)

Children and adolescents should do sixty minutes or more of physical activity each day. Most of the sixty minutes should be either moderate- or vigorous-intensity aerobic physical activity, and should include vigorous-intensity physical activity at least three days a week. As part of their sixty or more minutes of daily physical activity, children and adolescents should include muscle-strengthening activities, like climbing, at least three days a week and bone-strengthening activities, like jumping, at least three days a week. Children and adolescents are often active in short bursts of time rather than for sustained periods of time, and these short bursts can add up to meet physical activity needs. Physical activities for children and adolescents should be developmentally-appropriate, fun, and offer variety.

What is Meant by "Age-Appropriate" Physical Activities

Some physical activity is better-suited for children than adolescents. For example, children do not usually need formal muscle-strengthening programs, such as lifting weights. Younger children usually strengthen their muscles when they do gymnastics, play outside, or climb on playground structures. Also, the skill and coordination needed for complex physical activities may not allow for younger children to participate safely. It is important for child care facilities to promote a variety of physical activities that are structured and unstructured so children of all ages can enjoy physical activity and increase their likelihood of life-long adherence.

Many physical activities fall into several categories (moderate- and vigorous-intensity and muscle- and bone-strengthening), making it possible for children to gain multiple benefits with each type of activity.

Sources: U.S. Department of Agriculture. 2011. How much physical activity is needed? http://www.choosemyplate.gov/foodgroups/physicalactivity_amount.html.

Centers for Disease Control and Prevention. 2011. Physical activity for everyone: Aerobic, muscle-, and bone-strengthening: What counts? http://www.cdc.gov/physicalactivity/everyone/guidelines/what_counts.html.

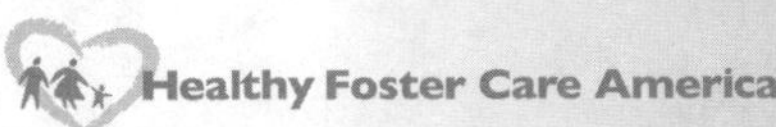

Children in foster care have special health care needs. Before foster care, most of these children lived with families that suffered from drug abuse, mental health problems, poor education, unemployment, violence, poor parenting skills, and/or involvement with the criminal justice system. The experience of living in out-of-home placement usually brings with it feelings of confusion, worry, fear, sadness, and loss of control. While it is impossible to predict all of the health concerns that these children might have, we know they have many more physical, mental, dental, and developmental health concerns than children who are not in foster care.

Ideally, when children enter foster care, they will remain with their familiar child care provider. However, this may not be possible. Sometimes, children enter child care for the first time when they enter foster care. Also, foster parents or kin may have to enroll children in child care almost immediately after placement.

Common issues for a child transitioning (changing) into child care include:

- Increased difficulty transitioning into child care due to the child also having to adjust to foster care placement and being away from the birth parent(s)
- Lack of knowledge by early education and child care professionals about how to help a child with a history of trauma
- Difficulty enrolling a child in child care because a lack of health information, sometimes resulting in a change of placement or use of unlicensed child care providers
- Behavior problems resulting in the child not being allowed to go back to child care

Behavior issues that often lead to suspension or expulsion from child care are based on childhood trauma and include acting out toward staff or other children; stealing; ruining property; and very often not following rules or listening to the child care provider.

Advice for Foster Parents or Kin

Here are some steps foster parents or kin can take to help the child make a successful transition into the child care program:

- ☐ Visit the program with the child, before she begins attending.
- ☐ Inform early education and child care professionals about the need for extra support because the child is getting used to both your home and to child care.
- ☐ Send a transitional object, such as a blanket or stuffed animal, with the child to child care every day; you can even let the child pick what to bring by offering a few choices. Note: To reduce the risk of Sudden Infant Death Syndrome, children under 1-year should not have any soft bedding or objects in the crib. Visit http://aap.org/fostercare/PDFs/HFCA_SIDS.pdf for more information on reducing the risk of SIDS.
- ☐ Let the child know who will be there to pick him up at end of the day.
- ☐ Let the child know that she will be returning to your home at the end of the day.

www.aap.org/fostercare

American Academy of Pediatrics

DEDICATED TO THE HEALTH OF ALL CHILDREN™

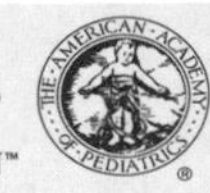

Advice for Early Education and Child Care Providers

Here are some steps early education and child care professionals can take to help the child make a successful transition into the child care program:

- ☐ Ensure that appropriate permission is in place, each time, when a child is picked up for a visit with the birth parent(s). Often the person picking up the child changes week to week, or the birth parent(s) drops in for a visit. The child care program needs to ensure that the child is only being visited or taken by permission.
- ☐ Ensure confidentiality about the fact that a particular child is in foster care. Early education and child care professionals should not reference that a child is in foster care in front of other parents or other children.
- ☐ Encourage awareness that children in foster care are often very sensitive to transitions and separation. In addition, the times right before and/or after visits can be very stressful for the child.

  Tips for easing the transition:

  - Have a consistent caregiver each day.
  - Allow the child to have pictures of key people in his life handy.
  - Prepare the child for visits with family (some happen during the day and when the child is picked up and/or returned to the child care program). Assist in the transition when the child is being picked up for a visit, especially if the person is unknown to the child (eg, a driver).
  - After a visit, allow the child to spend time with a familiar and caring adult to transition back to the child care setting.
  - Be aware that behaviors may increase before and/or after a visit and/or if the visit is canceled or the parent does not show up.
- ☐ Encourage awareness that severe tantrums or other behavior issues also need to be handled sensitively. Isolating a child (eg, using a "time out") who already feels "abandoned" can be very damaging.
- ☐ Encourage awareness about common mental health issues for children in foster care (and how to respond to them) such as:
  - Reactive attachment disorder
  - Developmental delays/disorders
  - Post Traumatic Stress Disorder
  - Drug and/or alcohol exposure (eg, Fetal Alcohol Spectrum Disorders)
- ☐ Engage the assistance of a mental health consultant if the child's behaviors are problematic and/or if the child is having chronic difficulty with transitions and/or separations.
- ☐ Encourage sensitivity regarding things like Mother's and Father's Day projects (eg, make 2 sets of gifts, one for the foster parent and one for the birth parent).

www.aap.org/fostercare

American Academy of Pediatrics

DEDICATED TO THE HEALTH OF ALL CHILDREN™

Recommended Safe Minimum Internal Cooking Temperatures

Food	**Degrees Fahrenheit (°F)**
Ground meat and meat mixtures	
Beef, pork, veal, lamb	160
Turkey, chicken	165
Fresh beef, veal, lamb	
Steaks, roasts, chops	145
Poultry	
Chicken and turkey, whole	165
Poultry breasts, roasts	165
Poultry thighs, wings	165
Duck and goose	165
Stuffing (cooked alone or in bird)	165
Fresh pork	160
Ham	
Fresh (raw)	160
Pre-cooked (to reheat)	140
Eggs and egg dishes	
Eggs	Cook until yolk and white are firm.
Egg dishes	160
Seafood	
Fish	145
	Cook fish until it is opaque (milky white) and flakes with a fork.
Shellfish	
Shrimp, lobster, scallops	Cook until the flesh of shrimp and lobster are an opaque color. Scallops should be opaque and firm.
Clams, mussels, oysters	Cook until their shells open. This means that they are done. Throw away any that were already open before cooking as well as ones that did not open after cooking.
Casseroles and reheated leftovers	165

**Consumers should use a food thermometer to determine internal temperatures of foods.

Source: U.S. Department of Agriculture and U.S. Department of Health and Human Services. 2010. *Dietary guidelines for Americans, 2010.* 7th ed. Washington, DC: U.S. GPO. http://www.health.gov/dietaryguidelines/dga2010/DietaryGuidelines2010.pdf.

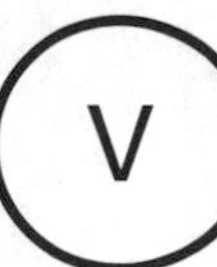

Food Storage Chart

This chart has information about keeping foods safely in the refrigerator or freezer. It does not include foods that can be stored safely in the cupboard or on the shelves where quality may be more of an issue than safety. Remember this is a guide and you should always follow any "best before" dates that are on the product.		
FOOD	**IN REFRIGERATOR**	**IN FREEZER**
Eggs		
Fresh, in shell	3 weeks	Don't freeze
Raw yolks, whites	2-4 days	1 year
Hard-cooked (boiled)	1 week	Don't freeze
Liquid pasteurized eggs or egg substitutes, opened	3 days	Don't freeze
Liquid pasteurized eggs or egg substitutes, unopened	10 days	1 year
Mayonnaise		
Commercial, refrigerate after opening	2 months	Don't freeze
TV Dinners, Frozen Casseroles		
Keep frozen until ready to heat and serve		3-4 months
Deli and Vacuum-Packed Products		
Store-prepared or homemade egg, chicken, tuna, ham, macaroni salads	3-4 days	Don't freeze
Pre-stuffed pork and lamb chops, stuffed chicken breasts	1 day	Don't freeze
Store-cooked convenience meals	1-2 days	Don't freeze
Commercial brand vacuum-packed dinners with USDA seal	2 weeks, unopened	Don't freeze
Hamburger, Ground, and Stew Meats (Raw)		
Hamburger and stew meats	1-2 days	3-4 months
Ground turkey, chicken, veal pork, lamb, and mixtures of them	1-2 days	3-4 months
Hotdogs and Lunch Meats*		
Hotdogs, opened package	1 week	
Hotdogs, unopened package	2 weeks	In freezer wrap, 1-2 months
Lunch Meats, opened	3-5 days	
Lunch Meats, unopened	2 weeks	In freezer wrap, 1-2 months
Deli sliced ham, turkey, lunch meats	2-3 days	1-2 months

Bacon and Sausage		
Bacon	1 week	1 month
Sausage, raw from pork, beef, turkey	1-2 days	1-2 months
Smoked breakfast links or patties	1 week	1-2 months
Hard Sausage-Pepperoni, Jerky Sticks	2-3 weeks	1-2 months
FOOD	**IN REFRIGERATOR**	**IN FREEZER**
Ham		
Canned, unopened, label says keep refrigerated	6-9 months	Don't freeze
Fully cooked - whole	7 days	1-2 months
Fully cooked - half	3-5 days	1-2 months
Fully cooked - slices	3-4 days	1-2 months
Fresh Meat		
Steaks, beef	3-5 days	6-12 months
Chops, pork	3-5 days	4-6 months
Chops, lamb	3-5 days	6-9 months
Roasts, beef	3-5 days	6-12 months
Roasts, lamb	3-5 days	6-9 months
Roasts, pork and veal	3-5 days	4-6 months
Fresh Poultry		
Chicken or turkey, whole	1-2 days	1 year
Chicken or turkey pieces	1-2 days	9 months
Giblets	1-2 days	3-4 months
Fresh Seafood		
Fish and shellfish	2 days	2-4 months

*Uncooked salami is not recommended because recent studies have found that the processing does not always kill the *E. coli* bacteria. Look for the label to say "Fully Cooked."

Benjamin, S. E., ed. 2007. *Making food healthy and safe for children.* 2nd ed. Chapel Hill, NC: National Training Institute for Child Care Health Consultants. http://nti.unc.edu/course_files/curriculum/nutrition/making_food_healthy_and_safe.pdf.

Sample Food Service Cleaning Schedule

TASK	HOW OFTEN?					COMMENTS
	After each use	Before & after each use	Daily	Weekly	As necessary	
RANGE						
Clean grill and grease pans	√					
Clean burners	√					
Clean outside			√			
Wipe out oven				√		
Clean edges around hood				√		
Clean hood screening and grease trap				√		
REFRIGERATOR AND FREEZER						Or when more than 1/4-inch frost develops or temperature exceeds 0°F.
Defrost freezer and clean shelves					√	
Wipe outside			√			
Dust top				√		
Clean inside shelves in order				√		
MIXER AND CAN OPENER						
Clean mixer base and attachments	√					
Clean and wipe can opener blade	√					
WORK SURFACES						
Clean and sanitize		√				
Organize for neatness			√			
WALLS AND WINDOWS						
Wipe if splattered or greasy					√	
Wipe window sills					√	
Wipe window screens					√	
SINKS						
Keep clean	√					
Scrub			√			
CARTS *(if applicable)*						
Wipe down	√					
Sanitize			√			
GARBAGE						Or more often, as needed.
Take out			√			
Clean can					√	
TABLES AND CHAIRS						
Clean and sanitize		√				
LINENS						
Wash cloth napkins	√					
Wash tablecloths and placemats	√ if plastic		√ if cloth			
Wash dishcloths			√			
Wash potholders				√		
STORAGE AREAS						
Wipe shelves, cabinets, and drawers					√	

Benjamin, S. E., ed. 2007. *Making food healthy and safe for children.* 2nd Ed. Chapel Hill, NC: National Training Institute for Child Care Health Consultants.

Adaptive Equipment for Children with Special Health Care Needs

Children on a gluten-free diet and those with latex allergies must be protected from ingesting or coming in contact with equipment/materials that may contain these substances. Check manufacturer's specifications and/or labels of all equipment, feeding materials, and toys including art supplies.

Physical Therapy/Occupational Therapy Equipment

Infants, Ages Birth to Two

Equipment

Floor mats, 2 to 3 inches of varying firmness
Therapy balls of varying sizes
Wedges: 4, 6, 8, and 12 inch
Inflatable mattress
Air compressor (for inflatables)
Therapy rolls and half rolls of varying sizes
Nesting benches, varying heights
Wooden weighted pushcart
Toddler swing
Floor mirror
Dycem non-slip matting

Feeding

Bottle straws
Cut-out cups
Bottle holders
Built-up handled utensils
Scoop bowls
Coated spoons

Toys

Books
Mirror
Ring stack
Container toys
Pegboard
Rattles
Squeeze toys
Tracking toys
Toys for pushing, swiping, cause and effect
Adapted switches
Form boards
Large beads
Large crayons

Pre-K, Ages Two to Five

Equipment

Floor mats, 2 to 3 inches of varying firmness
Therapy balls: 16, 20, 24, and 37 inch diameter
Nesting benches
Therapy rolls: 8, 10, and 12 inch diameter
Steps
Floor mirrors
Climbing equipment
Small chair and table
Scooter board
Dycem non-slip matting
Suspended equipment (see also Adaptive Physical Education Equipment, Balance/Gross Motor Coordination)
Walkers, sidelyers, proneboards, adapted chairs
Adapted tricycles

Toys

Easel
Tricycles
Ride-on scooters
Wagon
Wooden push cart
Manipulative toys (puzzles, beads, pegs and pegboard, nesting toys, etc.)
Fastening boards (zippers, snaps, laces, etc.)
Paper, crayons, chalk, markers
Sand/water table
Playdough or clay (consider gluten free and latex free alternatives)
Target activities (beanbags, ring toss)
Playground balls (see under Adaptive Physical Education Equipment, Eye-Hand Coordination)

Speech and Language Development

Infants, Ages Birth to Two

Equipment

Mirrors, wall and hand-held
Assorted spoons, cups, bowls, plates
Mats and sheets
Preston feeding chairs
High chair

Toys

Dolls (soft with large features and feeding bathing and daily living equipment)
Rattles (noisemakers and easy to grasp)
Manipulative toys (for pulling, pushing, shaking, cause and effect)
Assorted picture books (large pictures, one-a-page, photographs, simple plot)
Building blocks
Balls/belts
Telephone
Stacking rings
Shape sorters
Xylophone, Drum

Assessments and Books

Small Wonder Activity Kit

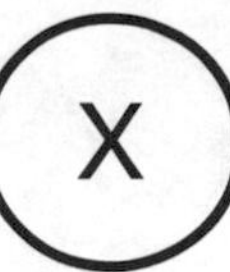

Pre-Feeding Skills by Suzanne Morris
Parent-Infant Communication
Bayley Scales of Infant Development
Communication and Symbolic Behavior Scale
Movement Assessment in Infants by S. Harris and L. Chandler
RIDES
HAWAII HELP
Early Learning Accomplishments
Profile and Kit (Kaplan)
Receptive Expressive Emergent Language Test 3
Rosetti Infant/Toddler Language Scale

Pre-K, Ages Two to Five

Equipment

Mirrors, wall and hand-held
Tongue depressors
Penlight
Stopwatch
Tape recorder and tapes
Toothettes
Horns and Whistles

Toys

Dolls (with movable parts and removable clothing)
Manipulative toys (cars and toys for pushing, stacking, cause and effect)
Building blocks
Dollhouse
Pretend play items (dress-up clothes, dishes, sink, food, telephone)
Playdough or clay (consider gluten free and latex free alternatives)
Puzzles (individual pieces or minimal interlocking parts)
Picture cards (nouns, actions, etc.)
Puppets
Animals
Storybooks with simple plot lines (large pictures and few, if any, words)

Assessments and books

Clinical evaluation of Language Fundamentals - Pre-School
Sequenced Inventory of Communication
Test of Auditory Comprehension of Language
Goldman Fristore Test of Articulation
Pre-School Language Assessment Inventory
Assessment of Phonological Processes
Expressive Vocabulary Test-2
Peabody Picture Vocabulary Test-4

Adaptive Physical Education Equipment

Pre-K, Ages Two to Five

Balance/Gross Motor Coordination

Incline mat
Balance beams, 4 and 12 inch wide
Floor mats, 2 inch
Bolsters
Rocking platforms
Scooters (sit-on type)
Tunnel (accordion style)
Training stairs
Hurdles, adjustable height
Pediatric climbing wall

Eye-Hand Coordination

Balls (to hit, throw, and catch)
Beanbags and Target
Hula hoops
Lightweight paddles/rackets
Lightweight bats
Traffic cones
Batting tees
Beachballs

Eye-Foot Coordination

Balls for kicking
Foot placement ladder
Footprints or “stepping stones”
Horizontal ladder

Even Plants Can Be Poisonous

Learn the names of your plants and label them. Below is a list of some of the more common indoor and outdoor plants that you may have in your home. This list is not a complete list. If you have a plant around your home that is not on the list, you may call thePoison Center at 1-800-2221222 to find out how poisonous it may be. You must know either the common name or the botanical name in order for the Poison Center to determine if it is poisonous. It is not possible to do plant or berry identifications over the phone, so check with a nursery for identification of all unknown plants. Carefully supervise children playing near poisonous plants. Call 1-800-222-1222 immediately if a child samples a mushroom or possibly poisonous plant.

Non-Poisonous Plants

Common Name	Botanical Name
African violet	*Saintpaulia ionantha*
Begonia	*Begonia*
Christmas cactus	*Schlumbergera bridgesii*
Coleus	*Coleus*
Dandelion	*Taraxacum officinale*
Dracaena	*Dracaena*
Forsythia	*Forsythia*
Impatiens	*Impatiens*
Jade	*Crassula argentea*
Marigold Calendula	*Tagetes*
Petunia	*Petunia*
Poinsettia	*Euphorbia pulcherrima (may cause irritation only)*
Rose	*Rosa*
Spider plant	*Chlorophytum comosum*
Swedish ivy	*Plectranthus australia*
Wandering Jew	*Tradescantia fluminesis*
Wild strawberry	*Fragaria virginiensis*

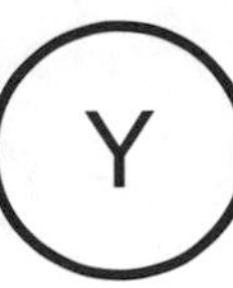

Poisonous Plants

Common Name	Botanical Name
Azalea, rhododendron	*Rhododendron*
Caladium	*Caladium*
Castor bean	*Ricinis communis*
Daffodil	*Narcissus*
Deadly nightshade	*Atropa belladonna*
Dumbcane	*Dieffenbachia*
Elephant Ear	*Colocasia esculenta*
Foxglove	*Digitalis purpurea*
Fruit pits and seeds	contain cyanogenic glycosides
Holly	*Ilex*
Iris	*Iris*
Jerusalem cherry	*Solanum pseudocapsicum*
Jimson weed	*Datura stramonium*
Lantana	*Lantana camara*
Lily-of-the-valley	*Convalleria majalis*
Mayapple	*Podophyllum peltatum*
Mistletoe	*Viscum album*
Morning glory	*Ipomoea*
Mountain laurel	*Kalmia iatifolia*
Nightshade	*Salanum spp.*
Oleander	*Nerium oleander*
Peace lily	*Spathiphyllum*
Philodendron	*Philodendron*
Pokeweed	*Phytolacca americana*
Pothos	*Epipremnum aureum*
Yew	*Taxus*

Source: National Capital Poison Center (www.poison.org). Photos of selected plants in this appendix are available at http://www.poison.org/prevent/plants.asp.

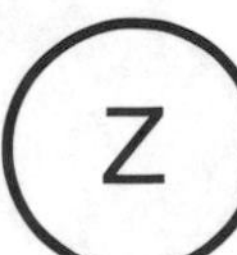

Depth Required for Shock-Absorbing Surfacing Materials for Use Under Play Equipment

The following fall heights and depth of loose-fill, impact-attenuating surfacing materials have been shown to reduce the risk of life-threatening head injuries. The depths shown assume the materials have been compressed due to use and weathering and are properly maintained to the given level.

Inches	(Loose-Fill Material)	Protects to Fall Height (feet)
6*	Shredded/recycled rubber	10
9	Sand	4
9	Pea Gravel	5
9	Wood mulch (non-CCA)	7
9	Wood chips	10

* Shredded/recycled rubber loose-fill surfacing does not compress in the same manner as other loose-fill materials. However, care should be taken to maintain a constant depth as displacement may still occur.

Reproduced from: U.S. Consumer Product Safety Commission (CPSC). 2010. *Public playground safety handbook.* http://www.cpsc.gov/cpscpub/pubs/325.pdf.

Nine important tips to consider when choosing to use loose-fill materials under play equipment:

1. Loose-fill materials will compress at least 25% over time due to use and weathering (e.g., if the playground will require nine inches of wood chips, then the initial fill level should be twelve inches). Provide a margin of safety when selecting a type and depth of material.
2. Loose-fill surfacing requires frequent maintenance to ensure levels never drop below the minimum depth. Wear mats can be installed to reduce displacement.
3. Provide a method for containing loose-fill materials within the playground.
4. Consider marking equipment supports with the minimum fill level to help with maintaining the required depth of material.
5. Ensure that drainage from the playground is effective. Standing water reduces the effectiveness of the surfacing material by compaction and decomposition.
6. Keep in mind that as the ground freezes in colder months, the safe fall height may be reduced.
7. Never use less than nine inches of loose-fill material except for shredded/recycled rubber (six inches is recommended).
8. Some loose-fill materials may not meet Americans with Disabilities Act accessibility guidelines. Contact the Access Board at http://www.access-board.gov, or refer to ASTM F1951.
9. Wood mulch containing chromated copper arsenate (CCA)-treated wood should not be used. Also, consider the possible toxicity of recycled rubber.

Note:

The fall height is the maximum height of the structure or any part of the structure for all stationary and mobile equipment except swings. For swings, the fall height is the height above the surface of the pivot point where the swing's suspending elements connect to the supporting structure.

Unitary surfacing materials (such as rubber mats, tiles, or a combination of unitary/loose-fill category materials) and loose-fill surfacing materials should be tested and comply with the ASTM International (ASTM) standard F1292 for impact-attenuation of playground surfacing materials.

The manufacturer of unitary surfacing materials should provide test data to show a match between the fall height of the equipment to be used and the critical height shock-absorbing characteristics of the surfacing materials.

References:
U.S. Consumer Product Safety Commission (CPSC). 2010. *Public playground safety handbook.* http://www.cpsc.gov/cpscpub/pubs/325.pdf.
ASTM International (ASTM). 2009. F1292 – 09: Standard specification for impact attenuation of surfacing materials within the use zone of playground equipment. West Conshohocken, PA: ASTM.

Medication Administration Packet

Authorization to Give Medicine
PAGE 1

CHILD'S INFORMATION

Name of Facility/School ____________________ Today's Date ___/___/___

Name of Child (First and Last) ____________________ Date of Birth ___/___/___

Name of Medicine ____________________

Reason medicine is needed during school hours ____________________

Dose ____________________ Route ____________________

Time to give medicine ____________________

Additional instructions ____________________

Date to start medicine ____/____/____ Stop date ____/____/____

Known side effects of medicine ____________________

Plan of management of side effects ____________________

Child allergies ____________________

PRESCRIBER'S INFORMATION

Prescribing Health Professional's Name and Signature ____________________

Phone Number ____________________

PERMISSION TO GIVE MEDICINE

I hereby give permission for the facility/school to administer medicine as prescribed above. **I also give permission for the caregiver/teacher to contact the prescribing health professional about the administration of this medicine. I have administered at least one dose of medicine to my child without adverse effects.**

Parent or Guardian Name (Print) ____________________

Parent or Guardian Signature ____________________

Address ____________________

Home Phone Number ____________ Work Phone Number ____________ Cell Phone Number ____________

Adapted with permission from the NC Division of Child Development to the Department of Maternal and Child Health at the University of North Carolina at Chapel Hill, Connecticut Department of Public Health, and Healthy Child Care Pennsylvania.

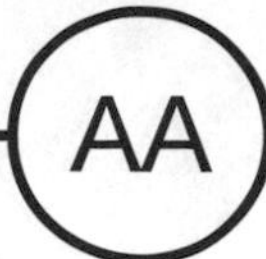

Receiving Medication

PAGE 2—TO BE COMPLETED BY CAREGIVER/TEACHER

Name of child ____

Name of medicine ____

Date medicine was received _____/_____/_____

Safety Check

☐ 1. Child-resistant container.

☐ 2. Original prescription or manufacturer's label with the name and strength of the medicine.

☐ 3. Name of child on container is correct (first and last names).

☐ 4. Current date on prescription/expiration label covers period when medicine is to be given.

☐ 5. Name and phone number of licensed health care professional who ordered medicine is on container and licensed health care professional's signature and parent signature are on Authorization form.

☐ 6. Copy of Child Health Record is on file.

☐ 7. Instructions are clear for dose, route, and time to give medicine.

☐ 8. Instructions are clear for storage (eg, temperature) and medicine has been safely stored.

☐ 9. Child has had a previous trial dose.

Y ☐ N ☐ 10. Is this a controlled substance? If yes, special storage and log may be needed.

____
Caregiver/Teacher Name (Print)

____
Caregiver/Teacher Signature

Medication Log

PAGE 3—TO BE COMPLETED BY CAREGIVER/TEACHER

Name of child ____________________ Weight of child ____________

	Monday	Tuesday	Wednesday	Thursday	Friday
Medicine					
Date	/ /	/ /	/ /	/ /	/ /
Actual time given	AM ______ PM ______	AM ______ PM ______	AM ______ PM ______	AM ______ PM ______	AM ______ PM ______
Dosage/amount					
Route					
Staff signature					

	Monday	Tuesday	Wednesday	Thursday	Friday
Medicine					
Date	/ /	/ /	/ /	/ /	/ /
Actual time given	AM ______ PM ______	AM ______ PM ______	AM ______ PM ______	AM ______ PM ______	AM ______ PM ______
Dosage/amount					
Route					
Staff signature					

Describe error/problem in detail in a Medical Incident Form. Observations can be noted here.

Date/time	Error/problem/reaction to medication	Action taken	Name of parent/guardian notified and time/date	Caregiver/teacher signature

RETURNED to parent/guardian	Date	Parent/guardian signature	Caregiver/teacher signature
	/ /		
DISPOSED of medicine	Date	Caregiver/teacher signature	Witness signature
	/ /		

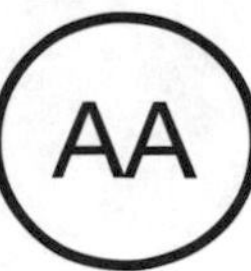

Medication Incident Report

Date of report ______________________ School/center ______________________

Name of person completing this report ______________________

Signature of person completing this report ______________________

Child's name ______________________

Date of birth ______________________ Classroom/grade ______________________

Date incident occurred ______________________ Time noted ______________________

Person administering medication ______________________

Prescribing health care provider ______________________

Name of medication ______________________

Dose ______________________ Scheduled time ______________________

Describe the incident and how it occurred (wrong child, medication, dose, time, or route?)

____

____

____

Action taken/intervention ______________________

Parent/guardian notified? Yes __________ No __________ Date __________ Time __________

Name of the parent/guardian that was notified ______________________

Follow-up and outcome ______________________

Administrator's signature ______________________

Adapted with permission from Healthy Child Care Colorado.

Preparing to Give Medication

This is a checklist to use at your child care facility/school to make sure that your program is ready to give medication. There is also a Receiving Medication checklist (page 146) with more detail to use whenever a parent drops off medication.

1. Paperwork

- ☐ Parent authorization to give medications is signed.
- ☐ Health care professional authorization or instructions are on file.
- ☐ Child Health Record is on file.

2. Medication checked when received

- ☐ Properly labeled.
- ☐ Proper container.
- ☐ Stored correctly.
- ☐ Instructions are clear.
- ☐ Disposal plan is developed.

3. Administering medication

- ☐ Area is clean and quiet.
- ☐ Staff is trained.
- ☐ Hands are washed.
- ☐ The 5 rights are followed—right child, medication, dose, time, and route.
- ☐ Child is observed for side effects.

4. Documentation

- ☐ Medication log is completed fully and in ink.

Documents in Appendix AA adopted with permission from the NC Division of Child Development to the Department of Maternal and Child Health at the University of North Carolina at Chapel Hill, American Academy of Pediatrics, Connecticut Department of Public, Healthy Child Care Pennsylvania and Healthy Child Care Colorado, 2011.

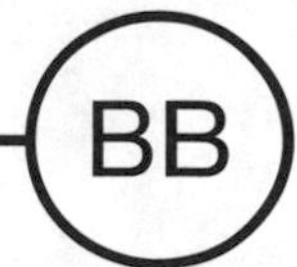

Emergency Information Form for Children With Special Needs

American College of Emergency Physicians®

American Academy of Pediatrics
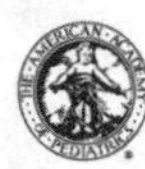

Date form completed	Revised	Initials
By Whom	Revised	Initials

Last Name:

Name:	Birth date:	Nickname:
Home Address:	Home/Work Phone:	
Parent/Guardian:	Emergency Contact Names & Relationship:	
Signature/Consent*:		
Primary Language:	Phone Number(s):	

Physicians:	
Primary care physician:	Emergency Phone:
	Fax:
Current Specialty physician:	Emergency Phone:
Specialty:	Fax:
Current Specialty physician:	Emergency Phone:
Specialty:	Fax:
Anticipated Primary ED:	Pharmacy:
Anticipated Tertiary Care Center:	

Diagnoses/Past Procedures/Physical Exam:

1.	Baseline physical findings:
2.	
3.	Baseline vital signs:
4.	
Synopsis:	
	Baseline neurological status:

*Consent for release of this form to health care providers

Last Name:

Diagnoses/Past Procedures/Physical Exam continued:

Medications:

1.
2.
3.
4.
5.
6.

Significant baseline ancillary findings (lab, x-ray, ECG):

Prostheses/Appliances/Advanced Technology Devices:

Management Data:

Allergies: Medications/Foods to be avoided **and why:**

1.
2.
3.

Procedures to be avoided **and why:**

1.
2.
3.

Immunizations (mm/yy)

Dates						**Dates**					
DPT						Hep B					
OPV						Varicella					
MMR						TB status					
HIB						Other					

Antibiotic prophylaxis: Indication: Medication and dose:

Common Presenting Problems/Findings With Specific Suggested Managements

Problem	Suggested Diagnostic Studies	Treatment Considerations

Comments on child, family, or other specific medical issues:

Physician/Provider Signature: **Print Name:**

Reference: American College of Emergency Physicians and the American Academy of Pediatrics. ©2001. Emergency Information Form for Children with Special Needs. Used with Permission, 2011.

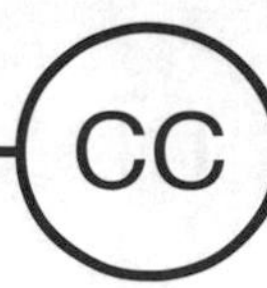

Incident Report Form

Fill in all blanks and boxes that apply.

Name of Program: ______________________________ Phone: ____________________

Address of Facility: ____

Child's Name: ______________________ Sex: M F Birthdate: ___/___/___ Incident Date: ___/___/___

Time of Incident: ___:___am/pm Witnesses:____

Name of Legal Guardian/Parent Notified: ____________ Notified by: ____________ Time Notified: ___:___am/pm

EMS (911) or other medical professional ☐Not notified ☐Notified Time Notified: ___:___am/pm

Location where incident occurred: ☐Playground ☐Classroom ☐Bathroom ☐Hall ☐Kitchen ☐Doorway ☐Gym ☐Office ☐Dining Room ☐Stairway ☐Unknown ☐Other (specify)____________

Equipment / Product involved: ☐Climber ☐Slide ☐Swing ☐Playground Surface ☐Sandbox ☐Trike/Bike ☐Handtoy (specify): ______________________________ ☐Other Equipment (specify):______________________________

Cause of Injury (describe): ____

☐Fall to surface; Estimated height of fall ___feet; Type of surface: ____________________
☐Fall from running or tripping ☐Bitten by child ☐Motor vehicle ☐Hit or pushed by child
☐Injured by object ☐Eating or choking ☐Insect sting/bite ☐Animal bite ☐Exposure to cold
☐Other (specify):____

Parts of body injured: ☐Eye ☐Ear ☐Nose ☐Mouth ☐Tooth ☐Part of face ☐Part of head ☐Neck ☐Arm/Wrist/Hand ☐Leg/Ankle/Foot ☐Trunk ☐Other (specify): ____________

First aid given at the facility (e.g. comfort, pressure, elevation, cold pack, washing, bandage): ____________________
____

Treatment provided by: ____

☐No doctor's or dentist's treatment required
☐Treated as an outpatient (e.g. office or emergency room)
☐Hospitalized (overnight) # of days: _________

Number of days of limited activity from this incident: _________ Follow-up plan for care of the child: ____________
____

Corrective action needed to prevent reoccurrence:
____

Name of Official/Agency notified: ____

Signature of Staff Member: ______________________________ Date: ____________

Signature of Legal Guardian/Parent:______________________________ Date: ____________

Reference: American Academy of Pediatrics, Pennsylvania Chapter. 2002. *Model child care health policies*. 4th ed. Washhington, DC: national Association for the Education of Young Children.
This form was developed for *Model Child Care Health Policies*, 2002, by the Early Chhildhood Education Linkage System (ECELS), a program funded by the Pennsylvania Depts. of Health & Public Welfare and contractually administered by the PA Chapter, American Academy of Pediatrics.

Child Injury Report Form for Indoor and Outdoor Injuries

1. Child's name______________________ 3. Grade ____________ 5. ( ) Male ( ) Female
2. School name ______________________ 4. Date of injury __________ 6. Time of injury ______
7. Days absent: ___Less than ½ ___1/2 ___1 ___1 ½ - 2 ___2 ½ - 3 ___Other: ______________________
8. First Aid given: _____ Ice _____Washed wound _____Kept immobile _____Observed _____ Stopped bleeding _____Applied splint _____Applied dressing _____Other
   Explain: ______________________
9. Body part injured:

Head	Trunk	Extremities		Other
___Ear	___Abdomen	___Ankle	___Lower arm	
___Eye	___Back	___Elbow	___Lower leg	____________
___Face	___Chest	___Finger	___Thumb	
___Head	___Groin	___Foot	___Toes	____________
___Neck	___Shoulder	___Hand	___Upper arm	
___Scalp	___Trunk	___Hip	___Upper leg	____________
		___Knee	___Wrist	

10. Type of injury suspected:
    _____Laceration/Abrasion _____Bruise/Contusion
    _____Sprain/Strain _____Dislocation
    _____Fracture _____Concussion
    _____Surface cut/Scratch _____Burn
    _____Other : ______________________
11. Action taken: ______Parent took home ______Transfer to hospital _______Parent took to doctor
    ______Returned to class ______Called 911 _______Parent took to ER
    ______Other : ______________________ _______Time spent in nurse's office
12. Explanation of accident:
    _____Collision with person _____Collision with obstacle
    _____Hit with object _____Injury to self
    _____Fall ________Height of fall _____Other ______________________
13. Accident location: _____ Classroom _____Playground _____Gym _____Assembly
    _____Stairs _____Hallway _____ Bus _____P.E. class
    _____Before School _____After school _____ Other ______________________
14. Surface: _____Blacktop ____Dirt ____Grass ____Synthetic surface
    _____Carpet ____Pea gravel ____Mats ____Rubber tile
    _____Concrete ____Ice/Snow ____Sand ____Wood products
    _____Other: ______________________
    _____Depth of loose fill material
15. Activity: ☐

1. Baseball/Softball	6. Fighting	11. Playing on bars	16. Soccer	20. Volleyball
2. Basketball	7. Flag/Touch football	12. Running	17. Swinging	21. Walking
3. Bicycling	8. Jumping	13. Rough housing	18. Throwing rocks or snowballs	22. Other: ________
4. Climbing	9. Kickball	14. Sliding		________
5. Dodge ball	10. Playground equipment	15. Sliding on ice	19. Track/Field	________

16. Equipment: Was playground equipment involved in injury? ___Yes ___No
    IF YES, (a) Did equipment appear to be used appropriately? ___Yes ___No
    (b) Was there any apparent malfunction of equipment? ___Yes ___No

    Check which piece → ___Arch climber ___Slide ___Cargo net ___Sliding pole ___Chinning bar ___Track ride ___Horizontal ladder ___Swing ___See Saw ___Other______
17. Describe: Describe specifically how the injury happened. ______________________

____

____

____

____

____

Signed: ______________________ (Person filing report) **Signed:** ______________________ (Director)

Adapted from National Program for Playground Safety. 2005. Student Injury Report Form.

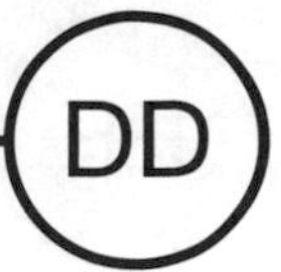

CHILD INJURY REPORT FORM INSTRUCTIONS

This form is to be completed immediately following the occurrence of any injury that is severe enough to:

a. Cause the loss of one-half day or more of school
b. Warrant medical attention and treatment (i.e., school nurse, M.D., E.R., etc.), and/or
c. Require reporting according to School District policy.

Number	Description of Each Number
1- 6	Self explanatory.
7	Do not file a form until you have filled in days missed. If student is going to be absent for an extended period of time, use parent's estimate. If no school is missed, check less than ½.
8 -11	Self explanatory. Record the amount of time child was in the nurse's office. Please include H or M. H= hours: M=minutes (i.e., 1h:40m).
12	*Collision with person* includes injuries which result from interactions between players from incidental or intended contact. *Hit with object* includes that the student got hit by an object (ball, backpacks, etc.) *Fall* injuries are those when the student falls from equipment or falls while running. *Collision with obstacle* includes contact when the child collides into an object (playground equipment, fence, etc.) *Injury to self* occurs when a child got injured because of an action s/he carried out.
	Height of fall – Report the height from where the child fell.
13	Self explanatory.
14	Describe surface over which injury occurred.
15	In the small box indicate the number of the activity that the child was doing when s/he got injured.
16	Self explanatory. See attached document with pictures of each piece of equipment.
17	Briefly describe specifically how the incident happened. Make sure to include all names of witnesses present. If additional space is needed, continue on another sheet of paper and attach.

National Program for Playground Safety
School of HPELS
University of Northern Iowa
Cedar Falls, IA 50614-0618
www.playgroundsafety.org
(800) 554 –PLAY : (319) 273-7308 (fax)

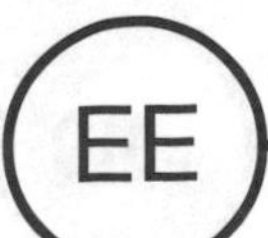

America's Playgrounds

Safety Report Card

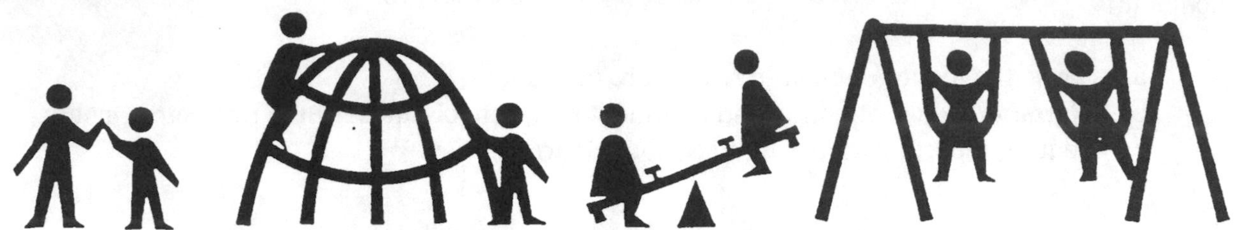

DOES YOUR PLAYGROUND MAKE THE GRADE?
Evaluate your playground using the following criteria.
A full explanation of the criteria is on the following page.

	Yes	No
SUPERVISION		
Adults present when children are on equipment		
Children can be easily viewed on equipment		
Children can be viewed in crawl spaces		
Rules posted regarding expected behavior		
AGE-APPROPRIATE DESIGN		
Playgrounds have separate areas for ages 2-5 and 5-12		
Platforms have appropriate guardrails		
Platforms allow change of directions to get on/off structure		
Signage indicating age group for equipment provided		
Equipment design prevents climbing outside the structure		
Supporting structure prevents climbing on it		
FALL SURFACING		
Suitable surfacing materials provided		
Height of all equipment is 8 feet or lower		
Appropriate depth of loose fill provided		
Six foot use zone has appropriate surfacing		
Concrete footings are covered		
Surface free of foreign objects		
EQUIPMENT MAINTENANCE		
Equipment is free of noticeable gaps		
Equipment is free of head entrapments		
Equipment is free of broken parts		
Equipment is free of missing parts		
Equipment is free of protruding bolts		
Equipment is free of rust		
Equipment is free of splinters		
Equipment is free of cracks/holes		
TOTAL POINTS		

SCORING SYSTEM

Total the number of "Yes" answers in the "Total Points" box in the table.

24 – 20 = A
Congratulations on having a SAFE playground. Please continue to maintain this excellence.

19 – 17 = B
Your playground is on its way to providing a safe environment for children. Work on the areas checked 'No'.

16 – 13 = C
Your playground is potentially hazardous for children. Take corrective measures.

12 – 8 = D
Children are at risk on this playground. Start to make improvements.

7 & = F
Do not allow children on this playground. Make changes immediately.

****If any of the gray boxes are marked 'NO', the potential of a life-threatening injury is significantly increased. Contact the owner of the playground.**

For Additional Resources and Information Contact:
National Program for Playground Safety: 1-800-554-PLAY (7529) ~ www.playgroundsafety.org
Reference: National Program for Playground Safety, 2006.

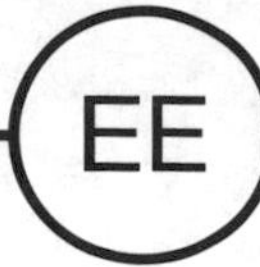

Explanation of Risk Factor Criteria

SUPERVISION

*1. Since equipment can't supervise children, it is important that adult supervision is present when children are playing on the playground.
2. In order to properly supervise, children need to be seen. This question is asking if there are any blind spots where children can hide out of the sight of the supervisor.
3. Many crawl spaces, tunnels, and boxed areas have plexiglas or some type of transparent material present to allow the supervisor to see that a child is inside the space. When blind tunnels are present, children cannot be properly supervised.
4. Rules help reinforce expected behavior. Therefore, the posting of playground rules is recommended. For children, ages 2-5, no more than three rules should be posted. Children over the age of five will remember five rules. These rules should be general in nature, such as "respect each other and take turns."

AGE APPROPRIATE DESIGN

*1. It is recommended that playgrounds have separate areas with appropriately sized equipment and materials to serve ages 2-5 and ages 5-12. Further, the intended user group should be obvious from the design and scale of equipment. In playgrounds designed to serve children of all ages, the layout of pathways and the landscaping of the playground should show the distinct areas for the different age groups. The areas should be separated at least by a buffer zone, which could be an area with shrubs or benches.
*2. Either guardrails or protective barriers may be used to prevent inadvertent or unintentional falls off elevated platforms. However, to provide greater protection, protective barriers should be designed to prevent intentional attempts by children.
3. Platforms over six feet in height should provide an intermediate standing surface where a decision can be made to halt the ascent or to pursue an alternative means of descent.
4. Signs posted in the playground area can be used to give some guidance to adults as to the age appropriateness of equipment.
5. Children use equipment in creative ways which are not necessarily what the manufacturer intended when designing the piece. Certain equipment pieces, like high tube slides, can put the child at risk if they can easily climb on the outside of the piece. The answer to this question is a judgment on your part as to whether the piece was designed to minimize risk to the child for injury from a fall.
6. Support structures such as long poles, bars, swing frames, etc. become the play activity. The problem is that many times these structures have no safe surfacing underneath and children fall from dangerous heights to hard surfaces.

FALL SURFACING

*1. Appropriate surfaces are either loose fill (engineered wood fiber, sand, pea gravel, or shredded tires) or unitary surfaces (rubber tiles, rubber mats, and poured in place rubber). Inappropriate surface materials are asphalt, concrete, dirt, and grass. It should be noted that falls from 1 ft. onto concrete could cause a concussion. Falls from a height of eight feet onto dirt is the same as a child hitting a brick wall traveling 30 mph.
*2. Research has shown that equipment heights can double the probability of a child getting injured. We recommend that the height of equipment for pre-school age children be no higher than 6 feet and the height of equipment for school age children be limited to 8 feet.
*3. Proper loose fill surfacing must be at the appropriate depth to cushion falls. An inch of sand upon hard packed dirt will not provide any protection. We recommend 12 inches of loose fill material under and around playground equipment.
*4. Appropriate surfacing should be located directly underneath equipment and extend six feet in all directions with the exception of slides and swings, which have a longer use zone.
*5. You should not be able to see concrete footings around any of the equipment. Deaths or permanent disabilities have occurred from children falling off equipment and striking their heads on exposed footings.
6. Glass, bottle caps, needles, trash, etc. can also cause injury if present on playground surfaces.

EQUIPMENT MAINTENANCE

*1. Strangulation is the leading cause of playground fatalities. Some of these deaths occur when drawstrings on sweatshirts, coats, and other clothing get caught in gaps in the equipment. The area on top of slides is one potential trouble spot.
*2. Entrapment places include between guardrails and underneath merry-go-rounds. Head entrapment occurs when the body fits through a space but the child's head cannot pass through the same space. This occurs because generally, young children's heads are larger than their bodies. If the space between two parts (usually guardrails) is more than three and a half inches then it must be greater than nine inches to avoid potential entrapment.
*3. Broken equipment pieces are accidents waiting to happen. If a piece of equipment is broken, measures need to be taken to repair the piece. In the meantime, children should be kept off the equipment.
*4. Missing parts also create a playground hazard. A rung missing from a ladder, which is the major access point onto a piece of equipment, poses an unnecessary injury hazard for the child.
5. Protruding bolts or fixtures can cause problems with children running into equipment or catching clothing. Therefore, they pose a potential safety hazard.
6. Exposed metal will rust. This weakens the equipment and will eventually create a serious playground hazard.
7. Wood structures must be treated on a regular basis to avoid weather related problems such as splinters. Splintering can cause serious injuries to children.
8. Plastic equipment may crack or develop holes due to temperature extremes and/or vandalism. This is a playground hazard.

***If these risk factors are missing, the potential for a life-threatening injury is significantly increased.**

2006 National Program for Playground Safety

Playground Safety Report Card Follow-up

For any item checked NO on the Playground Safety (PS) Report card, indicate how the item will be remedied and the date of completion.

Highlight any item checked NO from the PS Report Card	How item will be fixed	Date completed
SUPERVISION		
Adults present when children are on equipment		
Children can be easily viewed on equipment		
Children can be viewed in crawl spaces		
Rules posted regarding expected behavior		
AGE-APPROPRIATE DESIGN		
Playgrounds have separate areas for ages 2-5 and 5-12		
Platforms have appropriate guardrails		
Platforms allow change of directions to get on/off structure		
Signage indicating age group for equipment provided		
Equipment design prevents climbing outside the structure		
Supporting structure prevents climbing on it		
FALL SURFACING		
Suitable surfacing materials provided		
Height of all equipment is 8 feet or lower		
Appropriate depth of loose fill provided		
Six foot use zone has appropriate surfacing		
Concrete footings are covered		
Surface free of foreign objects		
EQUIPMENT MAINTENANCE		
Equipment is free of noticeable gaps		
Equipment is free of head entrapments		
Equipment is free of broken parts		
Equipment is free of missing parts		
Equipment is free of protruding bolts		
Equipment is free of rust		
Equipment is free of splinters		
Equipment is free of cracks/holes		

Adapted from National Playground Safety Program. 2006. America's Playgrounds Safety Report Card.

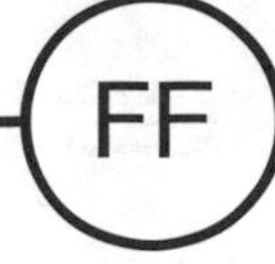

CHILD HEALTH ASSESSMENT

Parents & Child Care Providers fill-in this part.

CHILD'S NAME: (LAST)	(FIRST)	PARENT/GUARDIAN:
DATE OF BIRTH:	HOME PHONE:	ADDRESS:
CHILD CARE FACILITY NAME:		
FACILITY PHONE:	COUNTY:	WORK PHONE:

In lieu of completing this form, parent/guardian and primary healthcare provider may attach a copy of current physical exam and immunizations.

To Parents: Submission of this form to the child care provider implies consent for the child care provider to discuss the child's health with the child's clinician.
Child care providers should document that enrolled children have received age appropriate health services and immunizations that meet the current schedule of the American Academy of Pediatrics 141 Northwest Point Blvd., Elk Grove Village, IL 60007. The schedule is available at <www.aap.org>.

Health history and medical information pertinent to routine child care and emergencies (describe, if any): ☐ NONE	Date of most recent well-child exam:
Allergies to food or medicine (describe, if any): ☐ NONE	Do not omit any information. This form may be updated by health professional. (Initial and date new data.) Child care facility needs 2 copies.

ATTACH CARE PLAN FOR CHILDREN WITH SPECIAL HEALTH CARE NEEDS (Appendix O) IF NECESSARY

Parents may write immunization dates, health professionals should verify and complete all data.

LENGTH/HEIGHT	WEIGHT	HEAD CIRCUMFERENCE	BLOOD PRESSURE
________IN/CM % ILE ________	________LB/KG % ILE ________	________IN/CM % ILE ________	(BEGINNING AT AGE 3) ________/________

PHYSICAL EXAMINATION	✓= NORMAL	IF ABNORMAL - COMMENTS
HEAD/EARS/EYES/THROAT		
TEETH		
CARDIORESPIRATORY		
ABDOMEN/GI		
GENITALIA/BREATS		
EXTREMITIES/JOINTS/BACK/CHEST		
SKIN/LYMPH NODES		
NEUROLOGIC & DEVELOPMENTAL		

IMMUNIZATIONS	DATE	DATE	DATE	DATE	DATE	COMMENTS
DTaP/DTP/Td						
POLIO						
HIB						
HEP B						
MMR						
VARICELLA						
PNEUMOCOCCAL						
ROTOVIRUS						
HEP A						
MENINGOCOCCAL						
INFLUENZA						
OTHER						

SCREENING TESTS	DATE TEST DONE	NOTE HERE IF RESULTS ARE PENDING OR ABNORMAL
LEAD		
ANEMIA (HGB/HCT)		
URINALYSIS (UA) (at age 5)		
HEARING (subjective until age 4)		
VISION (subjective until age 3)		
PROFESSIONAL DENTAL EXAM		

HEALTH PROBLEMS OR SPECIAL NEEDS, RECOMMENDED TREATMENT/MEDICATIONS/SPECIAL CARE (ATTACH ADDITIONAL SHEETS IF NECESSARY)

☐ NONE **NEXT APPOINTMENT – MONTH/YEAR:**

MEDICAL CARE PROVIDER: NAME OF PHYSICIAN OR CPNP:		SIGNATURE OF PHYSICIAN OR CPNP:	
ADDRESS:			
	PHONE:	LICENSE NUMBER:	DATE FORM SIGNED:

Adapted from the Pennsylvania Department of Public Welfare, 2001, form.

Licensing and Public Regulation of Early Childhood Programs

A position statement of the National Association for the Education of Young Children

Adopted 1983; revised 1992 and 1997

One of the most dramatic changes in American family life in recent years has been the increased participation of young children in nonparental child care and early education settings. Between 1970 and 1993 the percentage of children regularly attending these types of arrangements soared from 30 to 70% (Department of Health and Human Services n.d.). Much of the demand comes from the need for child care that has accompanied the rapid rise in maternal labor force participation. Increased demand for early childhood care and education services also comes from families who—regardless of parents' employment status—want their children to experience the social and educational enrichment provided by good early childhood programs.

Background

Families seeking nonparental arrangements choose among a variety of options: *centers* (for groups of children in a nonresidential setting), *small family child care homes* (for 6 or fewer children in the home of the care provider), *large family or group child care homes* (typically for 7 to 12 children in the home of a care provider who employs a full-time assistant), *in-home* care (by a nonrelative in the family home), and *kith and kin* care (provided by a relative, neighbor, or friend to children of one family only).

The responsibility to ensure that any and all of these settings protect and nurture the children in their care is shared among many groups. Families are ultimately responsible for making informed choices about the specific programs that are most appropriate for their own children. Early childhood professionals and others engaged in providing or supporting early childhood services have an ethical obligation to uphold high standards of practice. Others within the community, including employers and community organizations, who benefit when children and families have access to high-quality early childhood programs also share in the responsibility to improve the quality and availability of early childhood services. Government serves a number of important roles, including

- **licensing** and otherwise regulating so as to define and enforce minimum requirements for the legal operation of programs available to the public;
- **funding programs and supporting infrastructure,** including professional development and supply-building activities;
- **providing financial assistance** to help families with program costs;
- **supporting research and development** related to child development and learning and early childhood programs as well as data gathering for community planning; and
- **disseminating information** to inform consumers, service providers, and the public about ways to promote children's healthy development and learning, both at home and in out-of-family settings.

While many of these functions can and should occur at multiple levels of government, the licensing function is established by laws passed by state legislatures, creating offices that traditionally play the primary role in regulating the child care market by defining requirements for legal operation. States vary considerably in the methods and scope of regulation, using processes that may be called licensing, registration, or certification. These terms can have different meanings from state to state.

The importance of an effective system of public regulation

The primary benefit from public regulation of the child care and early education market is its help in ensuring children's rights to care settings that protect them from harm and promote their healthy development. The importance of these rights is underscored by a growing body of research evidence that emphasizes the importance of children's earliest experiences to their development and later learning (Center for the Future of Children 1995; Hart & Risley 1995; Bredekamp & Copple 1997; Kagan & Cohen 1997). Emerging research on brain development indicates that the degree of responsive caregiving that children receive as infants and toddlers positively affects the connections between neurons in the brain, the architecture of the brain itself (Newberger 1997; Shore 1997). Given the proportion of children who spend significant portions of their day in settings outside their family, ensuring that these environments promote healthy development becomes increasingly important.

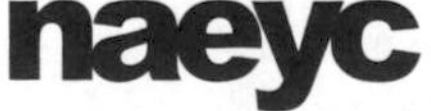

1509 16th Street, N.W., Washington, DC 20036-1426 • 202-232-8777 • 800-424-2460 • FAX: 202-328-1846

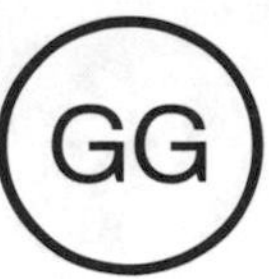

Research documents that those states with more effective regulatory structures have a greater supply of higher quality programs (Phillips, Howes, & Whitebook 1992; Helburn 1995). Additionally, in such states differences in quality are minimized between service sectors (e.g., nonprofit and proprietary programs) (Kagan & Newton 1989).

Children who attend higher quality programs consistently demonstrate better outcomes. These differences are apparent in many areas: *cognitive functioning and intellectual development* (Lazar et al. 1982; Clarke-Stewart & Gruber 1984; Goelman & Pence 1987; Burchinal, Lee, & Ramey 1989; Epstein 1993; Helburn 1995; Peisner-Feinberg & Burchinal 1997); *language development* (McCartney 1984; Whitebook, Howes, & Phillips 1989; Peisner-Feinberg & Burchinal 1997); and *social development* (McCartney et al. 1982; Clarke-Stewart 1987; Howes 1988; Whitebook, Howes, & Phillips 1989; Peisner-Feinberg & Burchinal 1997). The demonstrated outcomes appear in cross-sectional studies conducted at a specific point in time as well as in longitudinal studies over time (Carew 1980; Howes1988; Vandell, Henderson, & Wilson 1988; Howes 1990; Schweinhart et al. 1993; Barnett 1995). The differences in outcomes occur even when other family variables are controlled for, including maternal education and family income level (Helburn 1995; NICHD 1997).

Research is also consistent in identifying the structural factors most related to high quality in early childhood programs:

- small groups of children with a sufficient number of adults to provide sensitive, responsive caregiving;
- higher levels of general education and specialized preparation for caregivers or teachers as well as program administrators; and
- higher rates of compensation and lower rates of turnover for program personnel (Whitebook, Howes, & Phillips 1989; Hayes, Palmer, & Zaslow 1990; Galinsky et al. 1994; Helburn 1995; Kagan & Cohen 1997; Whitebook, Sakai, & Howes 1997). Many of these factors can be regulated directly or influenced by regulatory policy.

Despite widespread knowledge of what is needed to provide good quality in early childhood programs, many programs fail to do so. Two large-scale studies of licensed centers and family child care homes found that only about 10 to 15% of the settings offered care that promoted children's healthy development and learning. For infants and toddlers, the situation is grave: as many as 35 to 40% of the settings were found to be inadequate and potentially harmful to children's healthy development (Galinsky et al. 1994; Helburn 1995).

Support for an effective licensing system falls short

An effective licensing system minimizes the potential for harmful care, but regulatory systems in many states receive inadequate support to fully protect children's healthy development and learning. The lack of support can be seen in five broad areas: (1) some states set their basic floor for protection too low, failing to reflect research findings about the factors that create risk of harm; (2) a large number of settings in some states are exempt from regulation; (3) the licensing office in some states is not empowered to adequately enforce the rules; (4) multiple regulatory systems may apply to individual programs, resulting sometimes in overlapping or even contradictory requirements; and (5) policymakers may view licensing as unnecessary because they believe it seeks the ideal or imposes an elitist definition of quality rather than establishing a baseline of protection. Each of these issues is discussed briefly below.

1. Some states set their basic floor for protection too low, with licensing rules that fail to reflect research findings about the factors that promote or hinder children's healthy development. Clear links exist between the quality of early childhood programs in child care centers and homes and the quality of the public regulatory systems governing these services. Not only is the overall quality level of services provided to children higher in states with more stringent licensing systems (Phillips, Howes, & Whitebook 1992; Helburn 1995), but also demonstrable improvements can be seen in program quality in states that have worked to improve aspects of their licensing processes (Howes, Smith, & Galinsky 1995). Despite such compelling evidence as to the importance of strong licensing systems, a 1997 study looking at grouping, staff qualifications, and program requirements found that "the majority of states' child care regulations do not meet basic standards of acceptable/appropriate practice that assure the safe and healthy development of very young children" (Young, Marsland, & Zigler in press). Similar findings also have been reported on licensing standards for the care of four-year-olds (Snow, Teleki, & Reguero-de-Atiles 1996).

2. A large number of settings in some states are exempt from regulation. Many children are unprotected because they receive care outside their families in programs that are legally exempt from regulation. Exemptions affect both centers and family child care homes. Among centers the most common licensing exemptions are for part-day programs (roughly half of the states) and programs operated by religious institutions (nine states) (Children's Foundation

1509 16th Street, N.W., Washington, DC 20036-1426 • 202-232-8777 • 800-424-2460 • FAX: 202-328-1846

1997). Programs operated by or in public schools are sometimes exempt from licensing, although in some cases public school programs must meet comparable regulatory standards. Many states exempt family child care providers from regulation if they care for fewer children than stipulated as the threshold for regulation. About half of the states set such a threshold, ranging from 4 to 13 children (Child Care Law Center 1996).

3. States do not always provide the licensing office with sufficient funding and power to effectively enforce licensing rules. A 1992 report found that "many states face difficulties protecting children from care that does not meet minimum safety and health standards" (General Accounting Office 1992, 3). According to the report, staffing and budget cuts forced many states to reduce on-site monitoring, a key oversight activity for effective enforcement. These cutbacks occurred during a time of tremendous growth in the number of centers and family child care homes. The number of centers is estimated to have tripled between the mid 1970s and early 1990s, while the number of children enrolled quadrupled (Willer et al. 1991). An indicator of the growth in the number of regulated family child care providers is found in the recorded increase in the number of home-based participants in the USDA Child and Adult Care Food Program (regulation being a requirement of participation) from 82,000 in 1986 to nearly 200,000 in 1996 (Morawetz 1997).

Lack of meaningful sanctions makes enforcement of existing regulations difficult (Gormley 1997). Licensing offices in all states have the power to revoke licenses, but some states have a much broader range of enforcement tools. Others lack funding to adequately train licensing personnel and fail to receive appropriate legal backup for effective enforcement.

Although most states require that a facility license be prominently posted, many states do not require prominent posting or public printing of violation notices when facilities fail inspections. Information about licensing violations is only available in some states by checking the files in the state licensing office (Scurria 1994). The high demand for child care and early education services can exert pressures to keep even inadequate facilities open (Gormley 1995).

4. Multiple regulatory layers exist, sometimes with overlapping or even contradictory requirements. Different laws have created different inspection systems for different reasons, all affecting child care programs. Programs typically must comply with local zoning, building and fire safety, and health and sanitation codes in addition to licensing. A lack of coordination of requirements can frustrate new and existing providers and undermine the overall effectiveness of the regulatory system. For example, state and local regulatory structures sometimes impose contradictory requirements on family child care providers (Gormley 1995). If providers react by "going underground," children suffer.

5. Policymakers may view licensing as unnecessary because they believe it seeks the ideal or imposes an elitist definition of quality rather than establishing a baseline of protection. By definition, licensing rules represent the most basic level of protection for children. Licensing constitutes official permission to operate a center or family child care home; without this permission, the facility is operating illegally. Licensing rules combined with other regulatory requirements, such as environmental health codes, zoning provisions, and building and fire safety codes, define the floor for acceptable care that all child care programs must meet. In the current deregulatory climate, efforts to improve licensing rules and provide better basic protections for children's healthy development have sometimes been misrepresented as attempts to impose a "Cadillac" or ideal of quality child care that is too costly and unrealistic for all programs to achieve. When such misrepresentations succeed, the floor or safety net that licensing provides to protect children in out-of-family care is weakened.

Drawing upon a conceptual framework first espoused by Norris Class (1969), Morgan (1996) distinguishes multiple levels of standards needed to achieve quality in early childhood programs. As the strongest of governmental interventions, licensing must rest on a basis of the prevention of harm. Other regulatory methods, including approval of publicly operated programs, fiscal control and rate setting, and credentialing and accreditation, provide additional mechanisms that, building upon the basic floor of licensing, can encourage programs to achieve higher standards.

Nonregulatory methods can also promote higher quality services: for example, public and consumer awareness and engagement, professional development of teachers/caregivers and administrators, networking and information sharing among professionals, and dissemination of information regarding best practices. These standards can interact and be dynamic. For example, licensing rules can reference credentialing standards, or fiscal regulation can reflect higher rates for accredited programs. Also, greater knowledge of the importance of various factors in preventing harm to children's healthy development and learning can result in changes in licensing rules so as to raise the level of basic protection over time.

1509 16th Street, N.W., Washington, DC 20036-1426 ● 202-232-8777 ● 800-424-2460 ● FAX: 202-328-1846

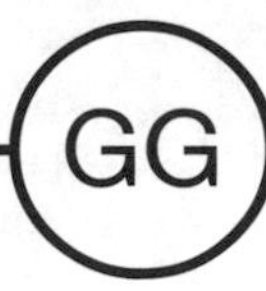

NAEYC's position

The National Association for the Education of Young Children (NAEYC) affirms the responsibility of states to license and regulate the early care and education market by regulating centers, schools, and family and group child care homes. The fundamental purpose of public regulation is to protect children from harm, not only threats to their immediate physical health and safety but also threats of long-term developmental impairment.

NAEYC recommends that states continue to adopt and improve requirements that establish a basic floor of protection below which no center, school, or family child care or group home may legally operate. Basic protections should, at a minimum, protect children by striving to prevent the risk of the spread of disease, fire in buildings as well as other structural safety hazards, pesonal injury, child abuse or neglect, and developmental impairment.

Licensing rules should be coordinated statewide and streamlined to focus on those aspects that research and practice most clearly demonstrate as reducing these types of harm. Licensing rules and procedures should be developed in a context that recognizes other strategies and policies that encourage all programs to strive continuously for higher standards of quality. Such strategies and policies include application of levels of funding standards and rates for the public purchase or operation of services; maintenance of broadly accessible registries of programs or providers who meet nationally recognized standards of quality (such as NAEYC accreditation); provision of a broad array of training and technical assistance programs to meet the varied needs of different types of providers; and development and dissemination of model standards or best practices.

Public regulation of early childhood program facilities, including licensing, represents a basic level of protection afforded to all children in settings outside their family. Additional strategies and policies along with licensing are needed to support the provision of high-quality services for all families who want or need them. These strategies and policies, however, cannot substitute for licensing in providing basic protection.

NAEYC's principles for effective regulation

NAEYC offers the following 10 principles for implementing an effective regulatory system.

1. Any program providing care and education to children from two or more unrelated families should be regulated; there should be no exemptions from this principle.

NAEYC believes that all types of care and education programs within the child care market should be regulated to provide basic protections to children. These protections must apply to all programs, without limiting definitions, exemptions, or exceptions. Whenever programs are exempted, not covered, or given special treatment, children are vulnerable and the entire regulatory system is weakened. NAEYC believes that programs should be regulated regardless of sponsorship, regardless of the length of program day, and regardless of the age of children served. NAEYC explicitly opposes exemption of part-day programs or programs sponsored by religious organizations because such exemption does not provide an equal level of health and safety protection for all children.

NAEYC's definition of licensed care specifically excludes care by kith and kin when a family engages an individual to care solely for their children. A family support/education model that provides helpful information and support to individuals caring for children is likely to be more effective and meaningful in reaching kith-and-kin providers than a formal licensing model. Programs targeted to parents of young children to help them in their role as their child's first teacher should also be accessible to kith-and-kin caregivers. If kith-and-kin providers are paid with public funds, NAEYC supports the application of funding standards to these arrangements.

2. States should license all facilities that provide services to the public, including all centers, large family or group child care homes, and small family child care homes (i.e., grant permission to operate).

NAEYC recommends that all centers or schools (serving 10 or more children in a nonresidential setting) be licensed facilities. Facility licensure should include an on-site visit prior to licensure and periodic inspections to monitor continued compliance. Licensing rules should focus on the aspects deemed most critical to maintaining children's safety and their healthy development, both in terms of their immediate physical health and well-being and their long-term well-being in all areas of development. NAEYC supports the use of *Stepping Stones to Using "Caring for Our Children"* (National Resource Center for Health and Safety in Child Care 1997) to identify those requirements in the National Health and Safety Performance Standards (APHA & AAP 1992) most needed for prevention of injury, morbidity, and mortality in child care settings.

Licenses are typically granted to privately administered programs rather than publicly operated programs, although some states do require publicly operated programs (such as those administered by the state department of education) to be licensed. If licensure is not required of publicly operated

1509 16th Street, N.W., Washington, DC 20036-1426 • 202-232-8777 • 800-424-2460 • FAX: 202-328-1846

programs, the administering agency should ensure that the program's regulatory standards and enforcement procedures are at least equivalent to those applied to licensed facilities. Such language should be written into law to empower the administering agency to develop statewide policies for implementation.

States currently vary widely in their definitions and procedures for regulating family child care homes. NAEYC recommends the adoption of consistent definitions of *small family child care homes* as care of no more than 6 children by a single caregiver in her home, including the caregiver's children age 12 or younger; and of *large family child care homes* as care in the caregiver's residence employing a full-time assistant and serving 7 to 12 children, including the caregiver's children age 12 or younger. When infants and toddlers are present in a small family child care home, no more than three children should be younger than age three, unless only infants and toddlers are in the group and the total group size does not exceed four. Large family child care homes should meet the same ratios and group sizes recommended for use in centers.

For small family child care homes, NAEYC supports licensing methods that are designed to achieve full regulatory coverage of all home-based care providers in a state. These methods sometimes do not require an on-site inspection prior to operation. NAEYC believes that such methods—whether called registration, certification, or another form of licensing—are viable ways to license small family child care homes provided that (1) standards are developed and applied; (2) permission to operate may be removed from homes that refuse to comply with the rules; (3) parents are well informed about the standards and the process; and (4) an effective monitoring process, including on-site inspections, is in place. NAEYC believes that large family child care homes should be licensed in the same way as centers, with an inspection prior to licensure.

3. In addition to licensing facilities, states should establish complementary processes for professional licensing of individuals as teachers, caregivers, or program administrators (i.e., grant permission to practice).

The skills and qualifications of the individuals working in an early childhood program are critically essential to creating environments that promote children's healthy development and learning. Establishing licenses for the various roles included in early childhood centers and family child care homes not only protects children's healthy development by requiring the demonstration of key competencies but also enhances early childhood professionalism and career development. In addition, individual licensure holds promise for increasing the compensation of staff (Kagan & Cohen 1997). Licensing of individuals is also a more cost-effective way of regulating qualifications centrally rather than through a licensing visit.

A number of states are implementing career or personnel registries (Azer, Capraro, & Elliott 1997); individual licensure can build upon and complement these efforts. Personnel licensure should provide for multiple levels and roles, such as teacher/caregiver, master or lead teacher/caregiver, family child care provider, master family child care provider, and early childhood administrator. Attaining a license should require demonstration of the skills, knowledge, and competencies needed for the specific role. (For further information, see NAEYC's *Guidelines for Preparation of Early Childhood Professionals* [NAEYC 1996] and "A Conceptual Framework for Early Childhood Professional Development" [Willer 1994]).

Multiple licenses are needed because of the diversity of roles and functions fulfilled by program personnel; multiple levels help to establish a career ladder with meaningful opportunities for career advancement, with higher levels of compensation linked to higher levels of qualification and demonstrated competence. In states in which early childhood teacher licensure or certification already exists for public school personnel, early childhood personnel licensing should be coordinated with these efforts. Individual licensure efforts may also be used to provide a form of consumer protection for families using in-home care by enabling them to check the credentials of a potential employee.

4. Licensing standards should be clear and reasonable and reflect current research findings related to regulative aspects that reduce the risk of harm.

Licensing rules reflect public policy, not program specifications. Highly detailed descriptions of program implementation are inappropriate for inclusion in licensing rules. Such areas are better addressed through consumer education and professional development. For example, requiring programs to establish a planned program of activities to enhance children's development and learning would be an appropriate licensing rule; specifying the number of blocks to be available in a classroom would not.

NAEYC recommends that the licensing standards address health and safety aspects, group size, adult-child ratios, and preservice qualifications and inservice requirements for staff (referencing individual licensing standards). Periodic review and revision (every five years) are needed to ensure that rules reflect current issues as well as the latest knowledge and practice. Licensing rules should be widely publicized to parents and the public; these groups, along with service providers, should also participate in the review and revision of the rules.

1509 16th Street, N.W., Washington, DC 20036-1426 • 202-232-8777 • 800-424-2460 • FAX: 202-328-1846

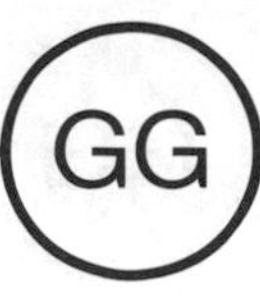

5. Regulations should be vigorously and equitably enforced.

Enforcement is critical to effective regulation. Effective enforcement requires periodic on-site inspections on both an announced and unannounced basis, with meaningful sanctions for noncompliance. NAEYC recommends that all centers and large and small family child care homes receive at least one site visit per year. Additional inspections should be completed if there are reasons (such as newness of the facility, sanction history, recent staff turnover, history of violations, complaint history) to suspect regulatory violations. Unannounced visits have been shown to be especially effective when targeted to providers with a history of low compliance (Fiene 1996).

Clear, well-publicized processes should be established for reporting, investigating, and appealing complaints against programs. Parents and consumers especially should be informed of these processes. Staff should be encouraged to report program violations of licensing rules. If whistle-blowing laws do not exist or do not cover early care and education workers, such legislation should be enacted. Substantiated violations should be well publicized at the program site as well as in other venues (such as resource-and-referral agencies, newspapers, public libraries, online, etc.) easily accessible to parents and consumers. Lists of programs with exemplary compliance records alsoshould be widely publicized along with lists of programs that meet the requirements of recognized systems of quality approval, such as NAEYC accreditation.

Sanctions should be included in the regulatory system to give binding force to its requirements. Enforcement provisions should provide an array of enforcement options such as the ability to impose fines; to revoke, suspend, or limit licenses; to restrict enrollment oradmissions; and to take emergency action to close programs in circumstances that are dangerous to children. When threats to children's health and safety are discovered, sanctions should be promptly imposed without a delayed administrative hearing process. Thevulnerability of children mandates the highest level of official scrutiny of out-of-family care and education environments.

6. Licensing agencies should have sufficient staff and resources to effectively implement the regulatory process.

Staffing to handle licensing must be adequate not only to provide for timely processing of applications but also to implement periodic monitoring inspections and to follow up complaints against programs. Licensing agencies must consider a number of factors in determining reasonable caseloads, for example, program size and travel time between programs. NAEYC believes that, on the average, regulators' caseloads should be no more than 75 centers and large family child care homes or the equivalent; NAEYC recommends 50 as a more desirable number. States that do not make on-site inspections prior to licensing small family child care homes may assume larger caseloads, but allow for timely processing of licenses, periodic on-site inspections, and prompt follow-ups to complaints.

Regulatory personnel responsible for inspecting and monitoring programs should have preparation and demonstrated competence in early childhood education and child development, program administration, and regulatory enforcement, including the use of sanctions. These criteria should be included in civil service requirements for licensing staff.

7. Regulatory processes should be coordinated and streamlined to promote greater effectiveness and efficiency.

Rules and inspections should be coordinated between the licensing agency and those agencies responsible for building and fire safety and health and sanitation codes so that any overlap is reduced to a minimum and contradictions resolved. In many cases coordination will require reform at a statewide level, as different requirements derive from different laws, are implemented by different agencies, and respond to different constituencies (Center for Career Development 1995). Coordination with funding agencies is also crucial. Licensing personnel can provide program monitoring for the funding agency, thus eliminating duplicate visits; funding possibly can be withheld in cases of substantiated violations.

Other methods for consideration in streamlining the regulatory process include (1) establishing permanent rather than annual licenses for centers, allowing for the revocation of the license for cause at any time, and conducting inspection visits at least annually to determine continued compliance; (2) coordinating local teams that monitor and inspect for licensing and regulation of health, fire, and building safety codes; and (3) removing zoning barriers. NAEYC believes that centers and family child care homes should be regarded as a needed community service rather than as commercial development and should be permitted in any residential zone. Planning officials should take into account the need for these services as communities develop new housing and commercial uses.

8. Incentive mechanisms should encourage the achievement of a higher quality of service beyond the basic floor.

In addition to mandated licensing rules that establish a floor for quality below which no program is allowed to operate, governments can use incentive mechanisms to encourage programs to achieve higher levels of quality. Examples of incentive mechanisms include funding stan-

1509 16th Street, N.W., Washington, DC 20036-1426 ● 202-232-8777 ● 800-424-2460 ● FAX: 202-328-1846

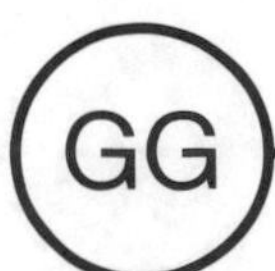

dards, higher payment rates tied to demonstrated compliance with higher levels of quality, and active publicity on programs achieving higher quality. Given the nature of the early childhood field as severely underfunded, these mechanisms should be implemented in conjunction with funding targeted to help programs achieve and maintain higher levels of quality, or else the strategy simply enlarges the gulf between the *haves* and *have-nots* Differential monitoring strategies, whereby programs maintaining strong track records and experiencing low turnover in pesonnel receive shortened inspections or are eligible for longer-term licenses, also may serve as incentives to programs for providing higher quality care.

9. Consumer and public education should inform families, providers, and the public of the importance of the early years and of ways to create environments that promote children's learning and development.

Actively promoting messages about what constitutes good settings for young children not only encourages parents to be better consumers of services in the marketplace but also, because these messages will reach providers outside the scope of regulation (family members and in-home providers), may help improve the quality of other settings. Public service announcements, the development and dissemination of brochures and flyers that describe state/local standards, open workshops, and ongoing communication with organized parent groups and well-care programs are all excellent ways for the regulatory agency to raise the child-caring consciousness of a community. A highly visible regulatory system also helps to inform potential and existing providers of the existence of standards and the need to comply with the law.

10. States should invest sufficient levels of resources to ensure that children's healthy development and learning are not harmed in early care and education settings.

NAEYC believes that public regulation is a basic and necessary component of government's responsibility for protecting all children in all programs from the risk of harm and for promoting the conditions that are essential for children's healthy development and learning and must be adequately funded. Additionally, government at every level can and should support early childhood programs by ensuring sufficient funding for high-quality services, opportunities for professional development and technical assistance to service providers, consumer education to families and the general public, and child care resource-and-referral services to families.

Early childhood regulation in context

An effective system of public regulation is the cornerstone of an effective system of early childhood care and education services, because it alone reaches all programs in the market. But for the regulatory system to be most effective, other pieces of the early childhood care and education services system also must be in place, including (1) a holistic approach to addressing the needs of children and families that stresses collaborative planning and service integration across traditional boundaries of child care, education, health, employment, and social services; (2) systems that recognize and promote quality; (3) an effective system of professional development that provides meaningful opportunities for career advancement to ensure a stable, well-qualified workforce; (4) equitable financing that ensures access for all children and families to high-quality services; and (5) active involvement of all stakeholders—providers, practitioners, parents, and community leaders from both public and private sectors—in all aspects of program planning and delivery. NAEYC is committed to ensuring that each of these elements is in place. As early childhood educators, we believe that nothing less than the future of our nation—the well-being of its children—is at stake.

References

APHA & AAP (American Public Health Association & American Academy of Pediatrics). 1992. *Caring for our children—National health and safety performance: Guidelines for out-of-home child care programs.* Washington, DC: APHA.

Azer, S.L., L. Capraro, & K. Elliott. 1997. Working *toward making a career of it: A profile of career development initiatives in 1996.* Boston: Center for Career Development in Early Care and Education, Wheelock College.

Barnett, W.S. 1995. Long-term effects of early childhood programs on cognitive and social outcomes. *Center for the Future of Children* 5 (3): 25–50.

Bredekamp, S., & C. Copple, eds. 1997. *Developmentally appropriate practice in early childhood programs.* Rev. ed. Washington, DC: NAEYC.

Burchinal, M., M.W. Lee, & C.T. Ramey. 1989. Type of day care and preschool intellectual development in disadvantaged children. *Child Development* 60: 128–37.

Carew, J. 1980. *Experience and development of intelligence in young children at home and in day care.* Monographs of the Society for Research in Child Development, vol. 45, nos. 6–7, ser. no. 187.

Center for Career Development in Early Care and Education at Wheelock College. 1995. *Regulation and the prevention of harm.* Boston: Author.

Center for the Future of Children. 1995. Long-term outcomes of early childhood programs. *The Future of Children* 5 (3).

Child Care Law Center. 1996. *Regulation-exempt family child care in the context of publicly subsidized child care: An exploratory study.* San Francisco: Author.

Children's Foundation. 1997. *1997 Child care licensing study.* Washington, DC: Author.

Clarke-Stewart, K.A. 1987. Predicting child development from child care forms and features: The Chicago Study. In *Quality in child care: What does research tell us?* ed. D.A. Phillips. Washington, DC: NAEYC.

1509 16th Street, N.W., Washington, DC 20036-1426 ● 202-232-8777 ● 800-424-2460 ● FAX: 202-328-1846

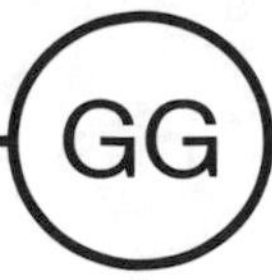

Clarke-Stewart, K.A., & C. Gruber. 1984. Daycare forms and features. In *Quality variations in daycare,* ed. R.C. Ainslie, 35–62. New York: Praeger.

Class, N.E. 1969. Safeguarding day care through regulatory programs: The need for a multiple approach. Paper presented at the NAEYC Annual Conference, Seattle, Washington.

Epstein, A. 1993. *Training for quality: Improving early childhood programs through systematic inservice training*Ypsilanti, MI: High/Scope Press.

Fiene, R. 1996. Unannounced versus announced licensing inspections in monitoring child care programs. Paper developed for the Cross-systems licensing project, Pennsylvania State University at Harrisburg and Pennsylvania Department of Public Welfare.

Galinsky, E., C. Howes, S. Kontos, & M. Shinn. 1994. *The study of children in family child care and relative care. Highlights and findings.* New York: Families and Work Institute.

Goelman, H., & A. Pence. 1987. Effects of child care, family and individual characteristics on children's language development: The Victoria day care research project. In *Quality in child care: What does research tell us?* ed. D.A. Phillips, 89–104. Washington, DC: NAEYC.

Gormley, W.T., Jr. 1995. *Everybody's children: Child care as a public problem.* Washington, DC: Brookings Institution.

Gormley, W.T., Jr. 1997. Regulatory enforcement: Accommodation and conflict in four states. *Public Administration Review* 57 (4): 285–93.

Hart, B., & T. Risley. 1995. *Meaningful differences in the everyday experiences of young American children*Baltimore: Paul H. Brookes.

Hayes, C.D., J.L. Palmer, & M.J. Zaslow, eds. 1990. *Who cares for America's children? Child care policy in the 1990s.*Washington, DC: National Academy Press.

Helburn, S., ed. 1995. *Cost, quality, and child outcomes in child care centers.* Technical report. Denver: University of Colorado at Denver.

Howes, C. 1988. Relations between early child care and schooling. *Developmental Psychology*24: 53–57.

Howes, C. 1990. Can the age of entry into child care and the quality of child care predict adjustment in kindergarten? *Developmental Psychology* 26 (2): 292–303.

Howes, C., E. Smith, & E. Galinsky. 1995. *The Florida child care quality improvement study. Interim report.* New York: Families and Work Institute.

Kagan, S.L., & N. Cohen. 1997. *Not by chance: Creating an early care and education system*New Haven, CT: Bush Center for Child Development and Social Policy, Yale University.

Kagan, S.L., & J.W. Newton. 1989. Public policy report. For-profit and nonprofit child care: Similarities and differences. *Young Children* 45 (1): 4–10.

Lazar, I., R. Darlington, H. Murray, J. Royce, & A. Snipper. 1982. *Lasting effects of early education: A report from the Consortium for Longitudinal Studies.* Monographs of the Society for Research in Child Development, vol. 47, ser. no. 201.

McCartney, K. 1984. The effect of quality of day care environment upon children's language development. *Developmental Psychology* 20: 224–60.

McCartney, K., S. Scarr, D. Phillips, S. Grajek, & C. Schwarz. 1982. Environmental differences among day care centers and their effects on children's development. In *Day care: Scientific and social policy issues,* eds. E.G. Zigler & E.W. Gordon. Boston: Auburn House.

Morawetz, E. 1997. Personal communication in July. Unpublished data, Child and Adult Care Food Program, U.S. Department of Agriculture, Food and Consumer Service, Child Nutrition Division, Alexandria, VA.

Morgan, G. 1996. Licensing and accreditation: How much quality is *quality*? In *NAEYC accreditation: A decade of learning and the years ahead* , eds. S. Bredekamp & B.A. Willer, 129–38.Washington, DC: NAEYC.

NAEYC. 1996. *Guidelines for preparation of early childhood professionals.* Washington, DC: Author.

National Resource Center for Health and Safety in Child Care. 1997. *Stepping stones to using "Caring for our children: National health and safety performance standards guidelines for out-of-home child care programs."* Denver: Author.

Newberger, J.J. 1997. New brain development research—A wonderful window of opportunity to build public support for early childhood education. *Young Children* 52 (4): 4–9.

NICHD Early Child Care Research Network. 1997. Mother-child interaction and cognitive outcomes associated with early child care: Results of the NICHD study. Paper presented at the 1997 Biennial Conference of the Society for Research in Child Development, Washington, DC.

Peisner-Feinberg, E.S., & M.R. Burchinal. 1997. Relations between preschool children's child-care experiences and concurrent development: The Cost, Quality, and Outcomes Study. *Merrill-Palmer Quarterly* 43 (3): 451–77.

Phillips, D., C. Howes, & M. Whitebook. 1992. The social policy context of child care: Effects on quality. *American Journal of Community Psychology* 20 (1): 25–51.

Schweinhart, L.J., H.V. Barnes, & D.P. Weikart with W.S. Barnett & A.S. Epstein. 1993. *Significant benefits: The High/Scope Perry Preschool Study through age 27.* High/Scope Educational Research Foundation Monograph, no. 10. Ypsilanti, MI: High/Scope Press.

Scurria, K.L. 1994. Alternative approaches to regulation of child care: Lessons from other fields. Working paper prepared for the Quality 2000: Advancing Early Care and Education Initiative.

Shore, R. 1997. *Rethinking the brain: New insights into early development.* New York: Families and Work Institute.

Snow, C.W., J.K. Teleki, & J.T. Reguero-de-Atiles. 1996. Child care center licensing standards in the United States: 1981 to 1995. *Young Children* 51 (6): 36–41.

U.S. Department of Health and Human Services. n.d. *Blueprint for action. Healthy Child Care America campaign.* Washington, DC: Author.

U.S. General Accounting Office. 1992. *Child care: States face difficulties enforcing standards and promoting quality*GAO/HRD-93-13. Washington, DC: GPO.

Vandell, D.L., V.K. Henderson, & K.S. Wilson. 1988. A longitudinal study of children with day-care experiences of varying quality. *Child Development* 59: 1286–92.

Whitebook, M., C. Howes, & D.A. Phillips. 1989. *Who cares? Child care teachers and the quality of care in America. The National Child Care Staffing Study.* Oakland, CA: Child Care Employee Project.

Whitebook, M., L. Sakai, & C. Howes. 1997. *NAEYC accreditation as a strategy for improving child care quality, executive summary.* Washington, DC: National Center for the Early Childhood Work Force.

Willer, B. ed. 1994. A conceptual framework for early childhood professional development: NAEYC position statement. In *The early childhood career lattice: Perspectives on professional development,* eds. J. Johnson & J.B. McCracken, 4–23. Washington, DC: NAEYC.

Willer, B., S.L. Hofferth, E.E. Kisker, P. Divine-Hawkins, E. Farquhar, & F.B. Glantz. 1991. *The demand and supply of child care in 1990.* Washington, DC: NAEYC.

Young, K., K.W. Marsland, & E.G. Zigler. In press. *American Journal of Orthopsychiatry.*

1509 16th Street, N.W., Washington, DC 20036-1426 • 202-232-8777 • 800-424-2460 • FAX: 202-328-1846

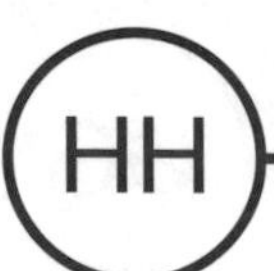

Use Zones and Clearance Dimensions for Single- and Multi-Axis Swings

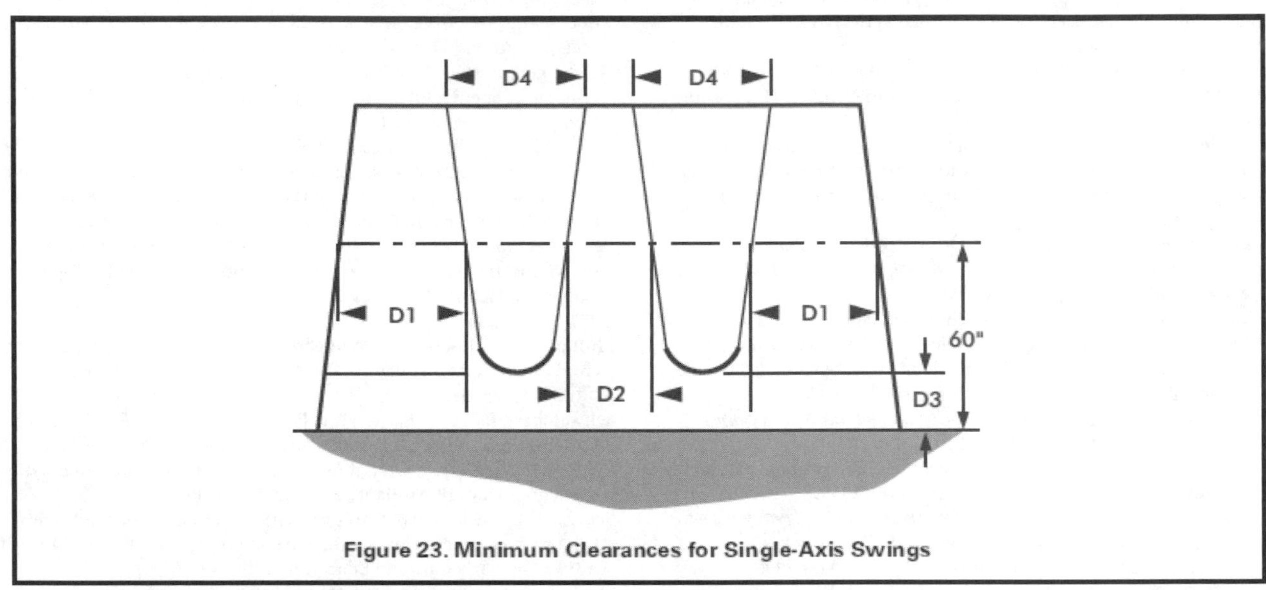

Figure 23. Minimum Clearances for Single-Axis Swings

Table 7. Clearance dimensions for swings

Reason	Dimension	Toddler Full bucket	Preschool-age Belt	School-age Belt
Minimizes collisions between a swing and the supporting structure	D1	20 inches	30 inches	30 inches
Minimizes collisions between swings	D2	20 inches	24 inches	24 inches
Allows access	D3	24 inches	12 inches	12 inches
Reduces side-to-side motion	D4	20 inches	20 inches	20 inches

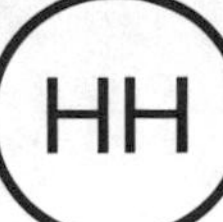

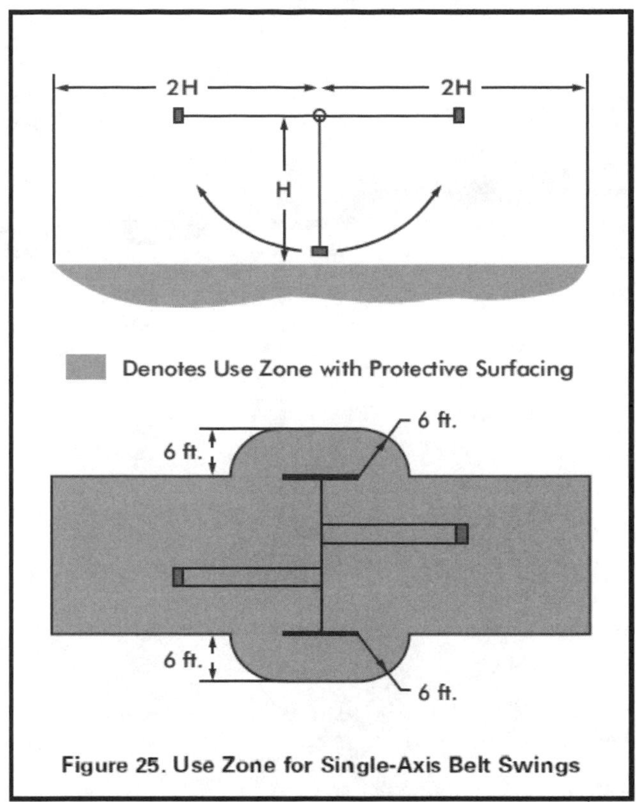

Figure 25. Use Zone for Single-Axis Belt Swings

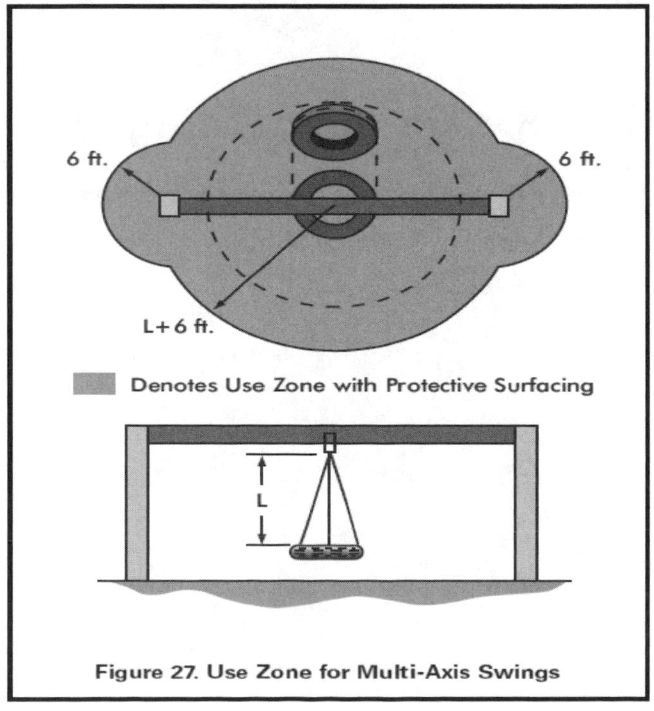

Figure 27. Use Zone for Multi-Axis Swings

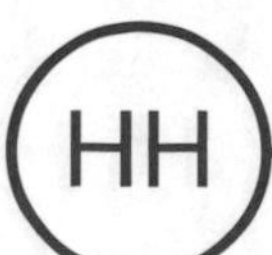

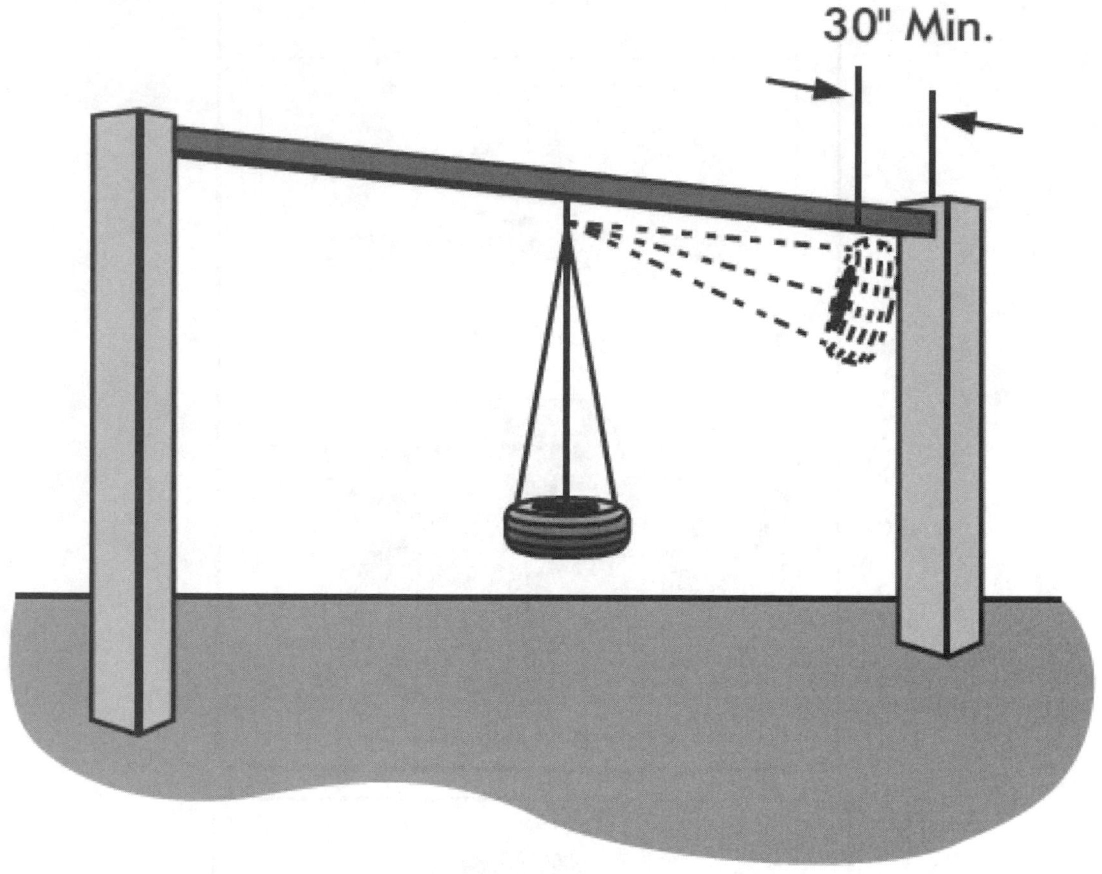

30" Min.

Figure 26. Multi-Axis Swing Clearance

Reference: U.S. Consumer Product Safety Commission. 2010. *Public playground safety handbook.* http://www.cpsc.gov/cpscpub/pubs/325.pdf.

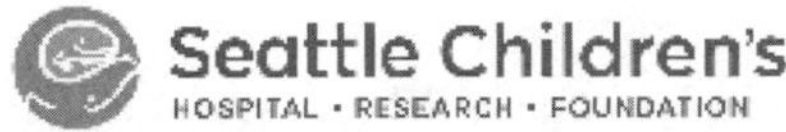

Community Education

Bike Helmets: Quick-Fit Check

Use this easy, three-point check to test for a proper helmet fit

1. Eyes

Helmet sits level on your child's head and rests low on the forehead, one to two finger widths above the eyebrows. Your child should be able to see the very edge of their helmet by looking up with their eyes only, while keeping their head still. A helmet pushed up too high will not protect the face or head well in a fall or crash.

2. Ears

The straps are even and form a "Y" under each earlobe. The straps are snug against the head.

3. Mouth

The buckled chin strap is loose enough so that your child can breathe. There should be enough room so you can insert a finger between the buckle and chin, but it should be tight enough that if your child opens their mouth, you can feel the helmet pull down on top.

Why are bike helmets needed?

Helmets provide the best protection against injury, whether your child is riding a bike, scooter or on skates. Wearing a helmet can prevent about 85 percent of head injuries from bike crashes. However, a helmet will only protect when it fits well.

Help your child get in the habit of wearing a helmet by starting when they're young. Be a good role model and wear a helmet yourself.

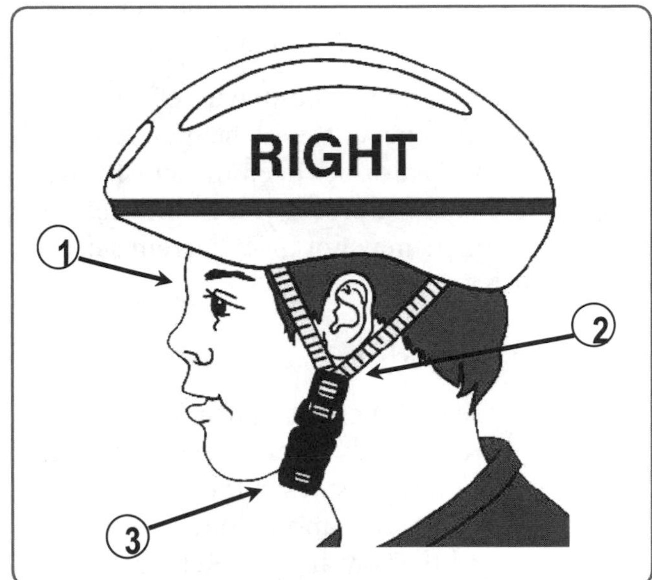

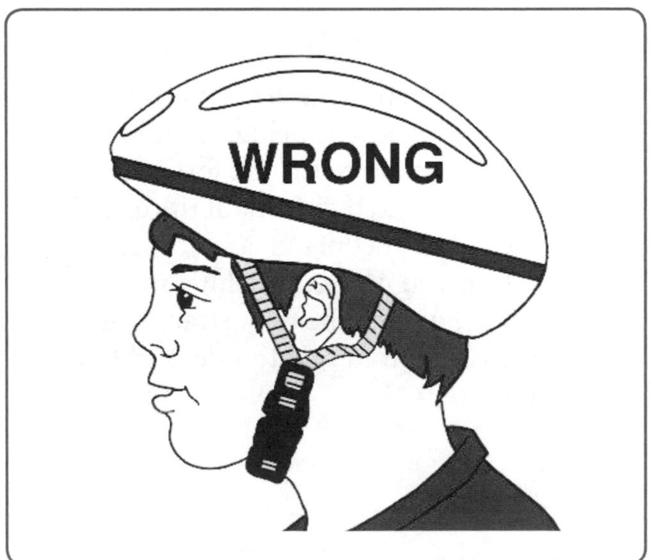

The "Eyes, Ears, Mouth Test" is courtesy of the Bicycle Coalition of Maine.

Used with Permission of the Seattle Children's Hospital, 2010.

How do I choose a helmet?

- Choose a helmet that meets safety standards. Look for a CPSC (U.S. Consumer Product Safety Commission) or Snell sticker inside the helmet.
- Helmet costs vary. Expensive helmets are not always better. Choose one that your child likes and will wear. Let your child help choose a helmet that fits well and looks good.
- Check used or hand-me-down helmets with care, and never wear a helmet that is cracked, broken or has been in a crash. Used helmets may have cracks you cannot see. Older helmets may not meet current safety standards.

What are the pads for?

Helmets come with fit pads to help ensure a proper fit. Use the pads where there is space at the front, back and/or sides of the helmet to get a snug fit. Move pads around to touch your child's head evenly all the way around. Replace thick pads with thinner ones as your child grows.

How do I check the fit?

With one hand, gently lift the front of the helmet up and back. The helmet should not move up and back to reveal the forehead. If it does, tighten the strap in front of the ear. Now lift the back of the helmet up and forward from the back. Can you move the helmet more than an inch? If so, tighten the back strap. If you can move the helmet from side to side, add thicker pads at the side.

When done, the helmet should feel level, fit solidly on your child's head and be comfortable. If it doesn't fit, keep working with the fit pads and straps or try another helmet.

Safety tips

- Teach your child to take their helmet off before playing at the playground or climbing on equipment or trees. The straps can get caught on poles or branches and prevent your child from breathing.
- Leave hair loose or tie it back at the base of the neck.
- Bike helmets can be worn with inline roller skates or scooters. For skateboarding or snowboarding, you will need another type of helmet.
- If your child does aggressive, trick or extreme skating or skateboarding, look for a true multi-impact helmet that has a sticker inside saying it meets ASTM F1492.
- Helmets are good for only one crash. Replace the helmet after a crash.

To Learn More

- www.bhsi.org, Bicycle Helmet Safety Institute
- www.cbcef.org, Cascade Bicycle Club Education Foundation
- www.seattlechildrens.org
- Seattle Children's Resource Line 206-987-2500 or 866-987-2500 toll-free Washington, Alaska, Montana, Idaho
- Your child's healthcare provider

Seattle Children's will make this information available in alternate formats upon request. Call Marketing Communications at 206-987-5205 or 206-987-2280 (TTY).

This handout has been reviewed by clinical staff at Seattle Children's. However, your child's needs are unique. Before you act or rely upon this information, please talk with your child's healthcare provider.

6/09
CE222

Our Child Care Center Supports Breastfeeding

Because we are committed to healthy mothers and children,

Our Child Care Center Supports Breastfeeding

In order to support families who are breastfeeding or who are considering breastfeeding, we strive to do the following:

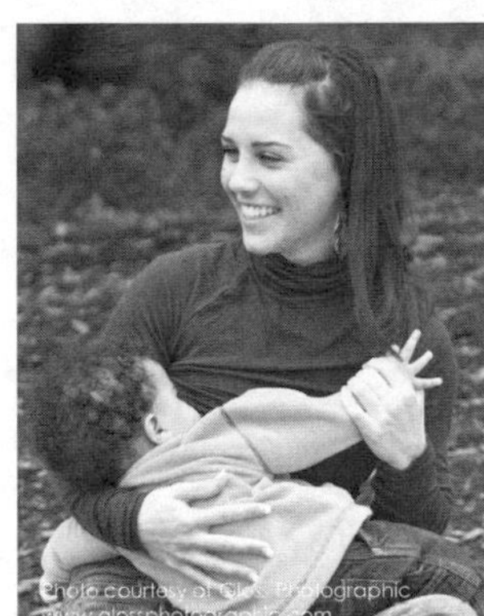

- Make a commitment to the importance of breastfeeding, especially exclusive breastfeeding, and proudly share this commitment with our staff and clients.
- Train all staff in supporting the best infant and young child feeding.
- Inform families about the importance of breastfeeding.
- Develop a breastfeeding-friendly feeding plan with each family.
- Train all staff to handle, store, and feed mother's milk properly.
- Teach our clients to properly store and label their milk for child care center use.

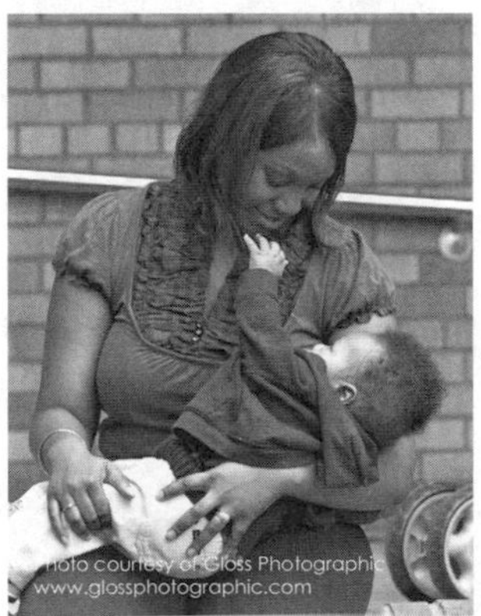

- Provide a breastfeeding-friendly environment, welcoming mothers to nurse their babies at our center.
- Display posters and brochures that support breastfeeding and show best practices.
- Contact and coordinate with local skilled breastfeeding support and actively refer.
- Continually update our information and learning about breastfeeding support.

Breastfeeding Families Welcome Here!

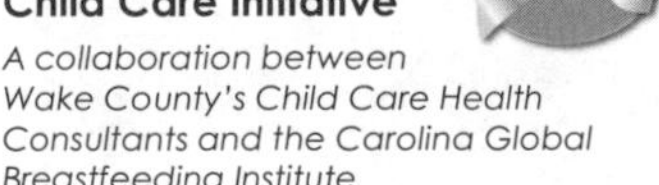

A collaboration between Wake County's Child Care Health Consultants and the Carolina Global Breastfeeding Institute

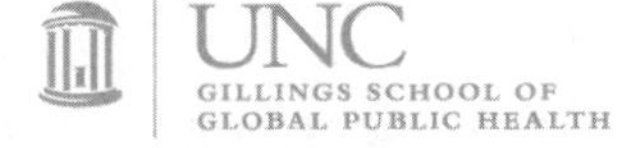

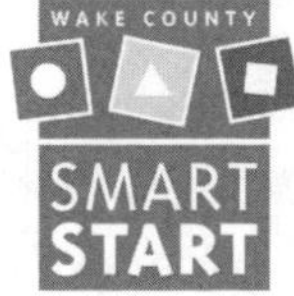

Child Care Health Consultant Program is funded by Wake County SmartStart, working to ensure children, ages 0 to 5, are prepared for success in school and in life.

AUTHORIZATION FOR EMERGENCY MEDICAL/DENTAL CARE

In cases of illness or injury requiring medical attention and when the parents/guardians cannot be reached, the undersigned authorizes _________________ (*caregiver/teacher*) to call the preferred primary/dental care provider or to take my child _________________ (*child's name*) to the nearest hospital or preferred primary/dental care provider; and it is understood that if possible, his/her services will be obtained. If the preferred primary/dental care provider cannot be contacted, the caregiver/teacher is authorized to contact another primary/dental care provider.

It is also understood that this agreement covers only those situations which, in the best judgment of the caregiver/teacher, are true emergencies.

NOTE: Every effort will be made to notify parents/guardians immediately in case of emergency.

Child's Full Name_________________________ Child's Date of Birth___/___/_____
Child's Address____

PARENT/GUARDIAN #1

Name_________________ Relationship to Child ____________

Home Ph.______________ Work Ph.______________ Cell Ph.______________

PARENT/GUARDIAN #2

Name_________________ Relationship to Child ____________

Home Ph.______________ Work Ph.______________ Cell Ph.______________

EMERGENCY CONTACT

Name_________________ Relationship to Child ____________

Home Ph.______________ Work Ph.______________ Cell Ph.______________

Any known allergies or medical conditions of child:
____
____

MEDICAL INSURANCE INFORMATION
Name of Company__________________________ Phone____________________
Name of Member___________________________ Policy #__________________
Group Number____________________________

My preferred primary care provider is:
Name:
Address:

Phone:

My preferred hospital is:
Name:
Address:

Phone:

DENTAL INSURANCE INFORMATION
Name of Company__________________________ Phone____________________
Name of Member___________________________ Policy #__________________
Group Number____________________________

My preferred dental care provider is:
Name:
Address:

Phone:

I agree to be responsible for the cost of such emergency medical care.
Signature of Parent/Guardian #1: ____________________________
Signature of Parent/Guardian #2:____________________________

Adapted from the N.C. Department of Health and Human Services, Division of Child Development. 2004. Child's Health and Emergency Information for Family Child Care Homes. http://ncchildcare.dhhs.state.nc.us/pdf_forms/DCD-0377.pdf.

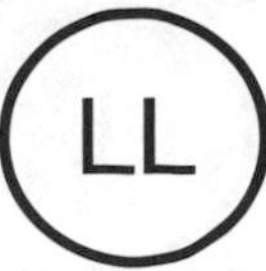

Conversion Table - Second Edition Standard Numbering to Third Edition Standard Numbering

The numbering system for the standards was changed in the 3rd Edition to facilitate recognition of standards by their placement and content grouping in each chapter. Each standard is represented by four numbers separated by a period (#.#.#.#). The first number represents the chapter, the second number represents a major chapter division, the third number represents a subdivision below a major division, and finally, the standard within that subdivision.

Numbering Example: **Numbering Scheme Explanation:**

1	**#**	**Chapter**
1.3	**#.#**	**Major chapter division**
1.3.3	**#.#.#**	**Chapter subdivision**
1.3.3.1	**#.#.#.#**	**Standard**

The conversion table below lists the 2nd Edition number side-by-side with its new 3rd Edition number and the 3rd Edition Standard Title. If a standard has been deleted from the 2nd Edition, it is indicated under the column for the 3rd Edition number. At the end of the Standard Table, there is a separate section for new standards.

Chapter 1 - Staffing		
2nd Ed. #	**3rd Ed. #**	**3rd Ed. Standard Title**
1.001	1.1.1.1	Ratios for Small Family Child Care Homes
1.002	1.1.1.2	Ratios for Large Family Child Care Homes and Centers
1.003	1.1.1.3	Ratios for Facilities Serving Children with Special Health Care Needs and Disabilities
1.004	1.1.1.4	Ratios and Supervision During Transportation
1.005	1.1.1.5	Ratios and Supervision for Swimming, Wading, and Water Play
1.006	1.4.1.1	Pre-Service Training
1.007	1.2.0.1	Staff Recruitment
1.008	1.2.0.2	Background Screening
1.009 split	1.4.1.1	Pre-Service Training
1.009 split	1.4.4.1	Continuing Education for Directors and Caregivers/Teachers in Centers and Large Family Child Care Homes
1.010	1.3.2.4	Additional Qualifications for Caregivers/Teachers Serving Children Three to Thirty-Five Months of Age
1.011	1.3.2.5	Additional Qualifications for Caregivers/Teachers Serving Children Three to Five Years of Age
1.012	1.3.2.6	Additional Qualifications for Caregivers/Teachers Serving School-Age Children
1.013	1.4.5.4	Diversity Education of Center Staff
1.014	1.3.1.1	General Qualifications of Directors
1.015	1.3.1.2	Mixed Director/Teacher Role
1.016	1.3.2.1	Differentiated Roles
1.017	1.3.2.2	Qualifications of Lead Teachers and Teachers
1.018	1.3.2.3	Qualifications for Assistant Teachers, Teacher Aides, and Volunteers
1.019	1.3.3.1	General Qualifications of Family Child Care Caregivers/Teachers to Operate a Family Child Care Home
1.020	1.3.3.2	Support Networks for Family Child Care
1.021	1.3.2.7	Qualifications and Responsibilities for Health Advocates
1.022	1.3.2.7	Qualifications and Responsibilities for Health Advocates
1.023	1.4.2.1	Initial Orientation of All Staff
1.024	1.4.2.2	Orientation for Care of Children with Special Health Care Needs
1.025	1.4.2.3	Additional Orientation Topics
1.026	1.4.3.1	First Aid and CPR Training for Staff

Chapter 1 - Staffing		
2nd Ed. #	**3rd Ed. #**	**3rd Ed. Standard Title**
1.027	1.4.3.2	Topics Covered in First Aid Training
1.028	1.4.3.3	CPR Training for Swimming and Water Play
1.029	1.4.4.1	Continuing Education for Directors and Caregivers/Teachers in Centers and Large Family Child Care Homes
1.030	1.4.4.2	Continuing Education for Small Family Child Care Home Caregivers/Teachers
1.031	1.4.5.1	Training of Staff Who Handle Food
1.032	1.4.5.2	Child Abuse and Neglect Education
1.033	1.4.5.3	Training on Occupational Risk Related to Handling Body Fluids
1.034	9.4.3.3	Training Record
1.035	1.4.6.1	Training Time and Professional Development Leave
1.036	1.4.6.2	Payment for Continuing Education
1.037	1.5.0.1	Employment of Substitutes
1.038	1.5.0.2	Orientation of Substitutes
1.039	1.5.0.2	Orientation of Substitutes
1.040	1.6.0.1	Child Care Health Consultants
1.041	1.6.0.1	Child Care Health Consultants
1.042	1.6.0.5	Specialized Consultation for Facilities Serving Children with Disabilities
1.043	1.6.0.2	Frequency of Child Care Health Consultation Visits
1.044	3.5.0.2	Caring for Children Who Require Medical Procedures
1.045	1.7.0.1	Pre-Employment and Ongoing Adult Health Appraisals, Including Immunization
1.046	1.7.0.2	Daily Staff Health Check
1.047	1.7.0.3	Health Limitations of Staff
1.048	1.7.0.4	Occupational Hazards
1.049	1.7.0.5	Stress
1.050	1.8.1.1	Basic Benefits
1.051	1.8.2.1	Staff Familiarity with Facility Policies, Plans and Procedures
1.052	1.8.2.2	Annual Staff Competency Evaluation
1.053	9.2.1.6	Written Discipline Policies
1.054	1.8.2.4	Observation of Staff
1.055	1.8.2.2	Annual Staff Competency Evaluation
1.056	1.8.2.3	Staff Improvement Plan
1.057	1.8.2.5	Handling Complaints About Caregivers/Teachers

Chapter 2 - Program: Activities for Healthy Development		
2nd Ed. #	**3rd Ed. #**	**3rd Ed. Standard Title**
2.001	2.1.1.1	Written Daily Activity Plan and Statement of Principles
2.002	2.1.1.1	Written Daily Activity Plan and Statement of Principles
2.003	2.1.1.1	Written Daily Activity Plan and Statement of Principles
2.004	2.1.1.5	Helping Families Cope with Separation
2.005	2.1.2.5	Toilet Learning/Training
2.006	2.1.1.7	Communication in Native Language Other Than English
2.007	2.1.1.8	Diversity in Enrollment and Curriculum
2.008	2.1.1.9	Verbal Interaction
2.009	3.1.3.2	Playing Outdoors
2.010	2.1.2.1	Personal Caregiver/Teacher Relationships for Infants and Toddlers

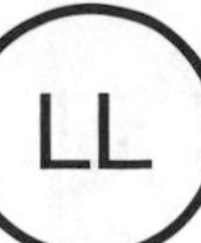

Chapter 2 - Program: Activities for Healthy Development		
2nd Ed. #	**3rd Ed. #**	**3rd Ed. Standard Title**
2.011	2.1.2.2	Interactions with Infants and Toddlers
2.012	2.1.2.3	Space and Activity to Support Learning of Infants and Toddlers
2.013	2.1.2.4	Separation of Infants and Toddlers From Older Children
2.014	2.1.3.1	Personal Caregiver/Teacher Relationships for Three- to 5-Year-Olds
2.015	2.1.3.2	Opportunities for Learning for Three- to Five-Year-Olds
2.016	2.1.3.3	Selection of Equipment for Three- to Five-Year-Olds
2.017	2.1.3.4	Expressive Activities For Three- To Five-Year-Olds
2.018	2.1.3.5	Fostering Cooperation Of Three- To Five-Year-Olds
2.019	2.1.3.6	Fostering Language Development of Three- to Five-Year-Olds
2.020	2.1.3.7	Body Mastery for Three- to Five-Year-Olds
2.021	2.1.1.2	Health, Nutrition, Physical Activity, and Safety Awareness
2.022	2.1.4.1	Supervised School-Age Activities
2.023	2.1.4.2	Space for School-Age Activity
2.024	2.1.4.3	Developing Relationships for School-Age Children
2.025	2.1.4.4	Planning Activities for School-Age Children
2.026	2.1.4.5	Community Outreach for School-Age Children
2.027	2.1.4.6	Communication Between Child Care and School
2.028	2.2.0.1	Methods of Supervision of Children
2.029	6.5.1.1	Competence and Training of Transportation Staff
2.030	6.5.1.2	Qualifications for Drivers
2.031	6.5.2.6	Route to Emergency Medical Services
2.032	6.5.2.1	Drop-Off and Pick-Up
2.033	6.5.2.2	Child Passenger Safety
2.034 split	9.2.5.1	Transportation Policy for Centers and Large Family Homes
2.034 split	9.2.5.2	Transportation Policy for Small Family Child Care Homes
2.035 split	3.4.1.1	Use of Tobacco, Alcohol, and Illegal Drugs
2.035 split	9.2.3.15	Policies Prohibiting Smoking, Tobacco, Alcohol, Illegal Drugs, and Toxic Substances
2.036	6.5.2.5	Distractions While Driving
2.037	6.5.2.3	Child Behavior During Transportation
2.038 split	5.6.0.1	First Aid and Emergency Supplies
2.038 split	5.3.1.12	Availability and Use of a Telephone or Wireless Communication Device
2.039	2.2.0.6	Discipline Measures
2.040	2.2.0.7	Handling Physical Aggression, Biting and Hitting
2.041	9.2.1.6	Written Discipline Policies
2.042	2.2.0.9	Prohibited Caregiver/Teacher Behaviors
2.043	2.2.0.10	Using Physical Restraint
2.044	2.3.1.1	Mutual Responsibility of Parents/Guardians and Staff
2.045	2.3.2.3	Support Services for Parents/Guardians
2.046	2.3.1.2	Parent/Guardian Visits
2.047	2.3.2.1	Parent/Guardian Conferences
2.048	9.4.2.3	Contents of Admission Agreement Between Child Care Program and Parent/Guardian
2.049	9.4.2.7	Contents of Facility Health Log for Each Child
2.050	2.3.2.2	Seeking Parent/Guardian Input
2.051	2.3.2.3	Support Services for Parents/Guardians

Chapter 2 - Program: Activities for Healthy Development		
2nd Ed. #	**3rd Ed. #**	**3rd Ed. Standard Title**
2.052	2.3.2.4	Parent/Guardian Complaint Procedures
2.053 split	2.1.1.4	Monitoring Children's Development/ Obtaining Consent for Screening
2.053 split	9.2.3.6	Identification of Child's Medical Home and Parental/Guardian Consent for Information Exchange
2.054	2.3.3.1	Parents'/Guardians' Provision of Information on their Child's Health and Behavior
2.055	9.4.1.19	Community Resource Information
2.056	9.4.1.19	Community Resource Information
2.057	2.4.3.2	Parent/Guardian Education Plan
2.058	8.5.0.1	Coordinating and Documenting Services
2.059	2.3.3.2	Communication From Specialists
2.060	2.4.1.2	Staff Modeling of Healthy and Safe Behavior and Health and Safety Education Activities
2.061	2.4.1.1	Health and Safety Education Topics for Children
2.062	2.4.1.3	Gender and Body Awareness
2.063	2.4.1.2	Staff Modeling of Healthy and Safe Behavior and Health and Safety Education Activities
2.064	2.4.2.1	Health and Safety Education Topics for Staff
2.065	2.4.3.1	Opportunities for Communication and Modeling of Health and Safety Education for Parents/ Guardians
2.066 split	2.4.3.1	Opportunities for Communication and Modeling of Health and Safety Education for Parents/ Guardians
2.066 split	2.4.3.2	Parent/Guardian Education Plan
2.067	2.4.3.2	Parent/Guardian Education Plan
Chapter 3 - Health Promotion and Protection in Child Care		
2nd Ed. #	**3rd Ed. #**	**3rd Ed. Standard Title**
3.001	3.1.1.1	Conduct of Daily Health Check
3.002	3.1.1.2	Documentation of the Daily Health Check
3.003	3.1.2.1	Routine Health Supervision and Growth Monitoring
3.004	4.2.0.2	Assessment and Planning of Nutrition for Individual Children
3.005	7.2.0.1	Immunization Documentation
3.006	7.2.0.2	Unimmunized Children
3.007	7.2.0.3	Immunization of Caregivers/Teachers
3.008	3.1.4.4	Scheduled Rest Periods and Sleep Arrangements
3.009	3.1.4.5	Unscheduled Access to Rest Areas
3.010	3.1.5.1	Routine Oral Hygiene Activities
3.011	3.1.5.3	Oral Health Education
3.012	3.2.1.1	Type of Diapers Worn
3.013	3.2.1.3	Checking for the Need to Change Diapers
3.014	3.2.1.4	Diaper Changing Procedure
3.015	5.4.2.4	Use, Location, and Setup of Diaper Changing Areas
3.016	5.4.2.4	Use, Location, and Setup of Diaper Changing Areas
3.017	5.4.2.4	Use, Location, and Setup of Diaper Changing Areas
3.018	3.2.1.2	Handling Cloth Diapers
3.019	5.4.2.6	Maintenance of Changing Tables
3.020	3.2.2.1	Situations that Require Hand Hygiene
3.021	3.2.2.2	Handwashing Procedure
3.022	3.2.2.3	Assisting Children with Hand Hygiene
3.023	3.2.2.4	Training and Monitoring for Hand Hygiene

Chapter 3 - Health Promotion and Protection in Child Care		
2nd Ed. #	**3rd Ed. #**	**3rd Ed. Standard Title**
3.024	3.2.3.1	Procedure for Nasal Secretions and Use of Nasal Bulb Syringes
3.025	3.2.3.3	Cuts and Scrapes
3.026	3.2.3.4	Prevention of Exposure to Blood and Body Fluids
3.027	4.3.1.4	Feeding Human Milk to Another Mother's Child
3.028 split	3.3.0.1	Routine Cleaning, Sanitizing, and Disinfecting
3.028 split	Appx K	Routine Schedule for Cleaning, Sanitizing, and Disinfecting
3.029	5.4.1.7	Toilet Learning/Training Equipment
3.030	5.4.1.8	Equipment Used for Cleaning and Disinfecting Toileting Equipment
3.031	5.6.0.4	Microfiber Cloths, Rags, and Disposable Towels and Mops Used for Cleaning
3.032	5.2.1.6	Ventilation to Control Odors
3.033	5.4.1.9	Waste Receptacles in the Child Care Facility and in Child Care Facility Toilet Room(s)
3.034	5.3.1.4	Surfaces of Equipment, Furniture, Toys, and Play Materials
3.035	5.2.9.14	Shoes in Infant Play Areas
3.036	3.3.0.2	Cleaning and Sanitizing Toys
3.037	3.3.0.3	Cleaning and Sanitizing Objects Intended for the Mouth
3.038	6.2.5.1	Inspection of Indoor and Outdoor Play Areas and Equipment
3.039	3.3.0.4	Cleaning Individual Bedding
3.040	3.3.0.5	Cleaning Crib Surfaces
3.041	3.4.1.1	Use of Tobacco, Alcohol, and Illegal Drugs
3.042	3.4.2.1	Animals that Might Have Contact with Children and Adults
3.043	3.4.2.2	Prohibited Animals
3.044	3.4.2.3	Care for Animals
3.045	2.2.0.4	Supervision Near Bodies of Water
3.046	2.2.0.5	Behavior Around a Pool
3.047	6.4.1.1	Pool Toys
3.048	3.4.3.1	Emergency Procedures
3.049	3.5.0.1	Care Plan for Children with Special Health Care Needs
3.050	Deleted	Syrup of Ipecac
3.051	3.4.3.2	Use of Fire Extinguishers
3.052	3.4.3.3	Response to Fire and Burns
3.053	3.4.4.1	Recognizing and Reporting Suspected Child Abuse, Neglect, and Exploitation
3.054	3.4.4.1	Recognizing and Reporting Suspected Child Abuse, Neglect, and Exploitation
3.055	3.4.4.2	Immunity for Reporters of Child Abuse and Neglect
3.056	3.4.4.1	Recognizing and Reporting Suspected Child Abuse, Neglect, and Exploitation
3.057	3.4.4.4	Care for Children Who Have Been Abused/Neglected
3.058	1.7.0.5	Stress
3.059	3.4.4.5	Facility Layout to Reduce Risk of Child Abuse and Neglect
3.060	Deleted	Seizure Care Plan
3.061	Deleted	Training for Staff to Handle Seizures
3.062	Deleted	Management of Children with Asthma
3.063	3.5.0.2	Caring for Children Who Require Medical Procedures
3.064	3.6.2.8	Licensing of Facilities that Care for Children Who Are Ill
3.065	3.6.1.1	Inclusion/Exclusion/Dismissal of Children
3.066	3.5.0.2	Caring for Children Who Require Medical Procedures
3.067	3.6.1.4	Infectious Disease Outbreak Control

Chapter 3 - Health Promotion and Protection in Child Care		
2nd Ed. #	**3rd Ed. #**	**3rd Ed. Standard Title**
3.068	3.6.1.1	Inclusion/Exclusion/Dismissal of Children
3.069	3.6.1.2	Staff Exclusion for Illness
3.070	3.6.2.2	Space Requirements for Care of Children Who Are Ill
3.071	3.6.2.3	Qualifications of Directors of Facilities that Care for Children Who Are Ill
3.072	3.6.2.4	Program Requirements for Facilities that Care for Children Who Are Ill
3.073	3.6.2.5	Caregiver/Teacher Qualifications for Facilities that Care for Children Who Are Ill
3.074	3.6.2.6	Child-Staff Ratios for Facilities that Care for Children Who Are Ill
3.075	3.6.2.7	Child Care Health Consultants for Facilities that Care for Children Who Are Ill
3.076	3.6.2.8	Licensing of Facilities that Care for Children Who Are Ill
3.077	3.6.2.9	Information Required for Children Who Are Ill
3.078	3.6.2.10	Inclusion and Exclusion of Children From Facilities that Serve Children Who Are Ill
3.079 split	3.6.2.1	Exclusion and Alternative Care for Children Who Are Ill
3.079 split	10.3.2.3	Collaborative Development of Child Care Requirements and Guidelines for Children Who Are Ill
3.080	3.6.2.2	Space Requirements for Care of Children Who Are Ill
3.081	3.6.3.1	Medication Administration
3.082	3.6.3.2	Labeling, Storage, and Disposal of Medications
3.083	3.6.3.3	Training of Caregivers/Teachers to Administer Medication
3.084	3.6.4.1	Procedure for Parent/Guardian Notification About Exposure of Children to Infectious Disease
3.085	3.6.4.2	Infectious Diseases that Require Parent/Guardian Notification
3.086	3.6.4.3	Notification of the Facility About Infectious Disease or Other Problems by Parents/Guardian
3.087	3.6.4.4	List of Excludable and Reportable Conditions for Parents/Guardians
3.088	9.2.3.3	Written Policy for Reporting Notifiable Diseases to the Health Department
3.089	3.6.4.5	Death
Chapter 4 - Nutrition and Food Service		
2nd Ed. #	**3rd Ed. #**	**3rd Ed. Standard Title**
4.001	4.2.0.1	Written Nutrition Plan
4.002	4.2.0.3	Use of USDA - CACFP Guidelines
4.003	4.2.0.5	Meal and Snack Patterns
4.004	4.2.0.4	Categories of Foods
4.005	4.2.0.7	100% Fruit Juice
4.006	4.2.0.6	Availability of Drinking Water
4.007	4.2.0.8	Feeding Plans and Dietary Modifications
4.008	4.2.0.9	Written Menus and Introduction of New Foods
4.009	4.2.0.8	Feeding Plans and Dietary Modifications
4.010	4.2.0.10	Care for Children with Food Allergies
4.011	4.3.1.1	General Plan for Feeding Infants
4.012	4.3.1.11	Introduction of Age-Appropriate Solid Foods to Infants
4.013	4.3.1.2	Feeding Infants on Cue by a Consistent Caregiver/Teacher
4.014	4.3.1.8	Techniques for Bottle Feeding
4.015	4.3.1.3	Preparing, Feeding, and Storing Human Milk
4.016	4.3.1.5	Preparing, Feeding, and Storing Infant Formula
4.017	4.3.1.5	Preparing, Feeding, and Storing Infant Formula
4.018	4.3.1.9	Warming Bottles and Infant Foods
4.019	4.3.1.10	Cleaning and Sanitizing Equipment Used for Bottle Feeding

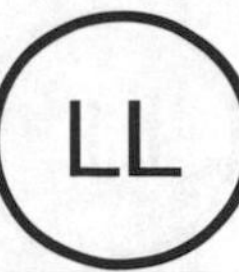

Chapter 4 - Nutrition and Food Service		
2nd Ed. #	**3rd Ed. #**	**3rd Ed. Standard Title**
4.020	4.3.1.7	Feeding Cow's Milk
4.021	4.3.1.12	Feeding Age-Appropriate Solid Foods to Infants
4.022	4.3.2.1	Meal and Snack Patterns for Toddlers and Preschoolers
4.023	4.3.2.2	Serving Size for Toddlers and Preschoolers
4.024	4.3.2.3	Encouraging Self-Feeding by Older Infants and Toddlers
4.025	4.3.3.1	Meal and Snack Patterns for School-Age Children
4.026	4.4.0.1	Food Service Staff by Type of Facility and Food Service
4.027	4.4.0.2	Use of Nutritionist/Registered Dietitian
4.028	4.5.0.1	Developmentally Appropriate Seating and Utensils for Meals
4.029	4.5.0.2	Tableware and Feeding Utensils
4.030	4.5.0.3	Activities that Are Incompatible with Eating
4.031	4.5.0.4	Socialization During Meals
4.032	4.5.0.7	Participation of Older Children and Staff in Mealtime Activities
4.033	4.5.0.8	Experience with Familiar and New Foods
4.034	4.5.0.9	Hot Liquids and Foods
4.035	4.5.0.5	Numbers of Children Fed Simultaneously by One Adult
4.036	4.5.0.6	Adult Supervision of Children Who Are Learning to Feed themselves
4.037	4.5.0.10	Foods that Are Choking Hazards
4.038	4.3.1.1	General Plan for Feeding Infants
4.039	4.5.0.11	Prohibited Uses of Food
4.040	4.6.0.1	Selection and Preparation of Food Brought From Home
4.041	4.6.0.2	Nutritional Quality of Food Brought From Home
4.042	4.8.0.1	Food Preparation Area
4.043	4.8.0.2	Design of Food Service Equipment
4.044	4.8.0.3	Maintenance of Food Service Surfaces and Equipment
4.045	4.8.0.4	Food Preparation Sinks
4.046	4.8.0.5	Handwashing Sink Separate From Food Zones
4.047	4.8.0.6	Maintaining Safe Food Temperatures
4.048	4.8.0.7	Ventilation Over Cooking Surfaces
4.049	4.8.0.8	Microwave Ovens
4.050	4.9.0.1	Compliance with U.S. Food and Drug Administration Food Sanitation Standards, State and Local Rules
4.051	4.9.0.2	Staff Restricted From Food Preparation and Handling
4.052	4.9.0.3	Precautions for a Safe Food Supply
4.053	4.9.0.4	Leftovers
4.054	4.9.0.5	Preparation for and Storage of Food in the Refrigerator
4.055	4.9.0.9	Cleaning Food Areas and Equipment
4.056	4.9.0.6	Storage of Foods Not Requiring Refrigeration
4.057	4.9.0.7	Storage of Dry Bulk Foods
4.058	4.9.0.8	Supply of Food and Water for Disasters
4.059	5.2.7.3	Containment of Garbage
4.060	5.2.9.1	Use and Storage of Toxic Substances
4.061	4.9.0.9	Cleaning Food Areas and Equipment
4.062	4.9.0.10	Cutting Boards

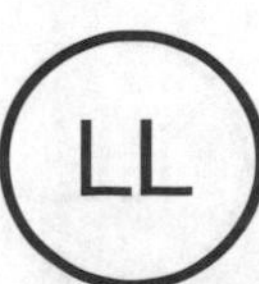

Chapter 4 - Nutrition and Food Service		
2nd Ed. #	**3rd Ed. #**	**3rd Ed. Standard Title**
4.063	4.9.0.11	Dishwashing in Centers
4.064	4.9.0.12	Dishwashing in Small and Large Family Child Care Homes
4.065	4.9.0.13	Method for Washing Dishes by Hand
4.066	4.10.0.1	Approved Off-Site Food Services
4.067	4.10.0.2	Food Safety During Transport
4.068	4.10.0.3	Holding of Food Prepared At Off-Site Food Service Facilities
4.069	4.7.0.1	Nutrition Learning Experiences for Children
4.070	4.7.0.2	Nutrition Education for Parents/Guardians
Chapter 5 - Facilities, Supplies, Equipment, and Transportation		
2nd Ed. #	**3rd Ed. #**	**3rd Ed. Standard Title**
5.001	5.1.1.1	Location of Center
5.002	5.1.1.2	Inspection of Buildings
5.003	5.1.1.3	Compliance with Fire Prevention Code
5.004	5.1.1.4	Accessibility of Facility
5.005	5.1.1.5	Environmental Audit of Site Location
5.006	5.1.1.6	Structurally Sound Facility
5.007	5.1.1.7	Use of Basements and Below Grade Areas
5.008	5.1.1.8	Buildings of Wood Frame Construction
5.009	5.1.1.9	Unrelated Business in a Child Care Area
5.010	5.1.1.10	Office Space
5.011	5.1.1.11	Separation of Operations From Child Care Areas
5.012	5.1.1.12	Multiple Use of Rooms
5.013	5.1.3.1	Weather-Tightness and Water-Tightness of Openings
5.014	5.1.3.2	Possibility of Exit From Windows
5.015	5.1.3.3	Screens for Ventilation Openings
5.016	5.1.3.4	Safety Guards for Glass Windows/Doors
5.017	5.1.3.5	Finger-Pinch Protection Devices
5.018	5.1.3.6	Directional Swing of Indoor Doors
5.019	5.1.4.3	Path of Egress
5.020	5.1.4.1	Alternate Exits and Emergency Shelter
5.021	5.1.4.2	Evacuation of Children with Special Health Care Needs and Children with Disabilities
5.022	5.1.4.3	Path of Egress
5.023	5.1.4.4	Locks
5.024	5.1.4.6	Labeled Emergency Exits
5.025	5.1.4.7	Access to Exits
5.026	5.3.1.6	Floors, Walls, and Ceilings
5.027	5.2.1.1	Fresh Air
5.028	5.2.1.2	Indoor Temperature
5.029	5.2.1.4	Ventilation When Using Art Materials
5.030	5.2.1.7	Electric Fans
5.031	5.2.1.8	Maintenance of Air Filters
5.032	5.2.1.3	Heating and Ventilation Equipment Inspection and Maintenance
5.033	5.2.1.9	Type and Placement of Room Thermometers
5.034	5.2.1.10	Gas, Oil, or Kerosene Heaters, Generators, Portable Gas Stoves, and Charcoal and Gas Grills

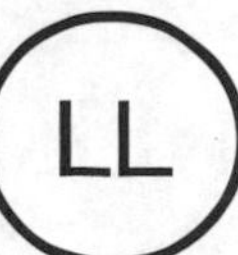

Chapter 5 - Facilities, Supplies, Equipment, and Transportation		
2nd Ed. #	**3rd Ed. #**	**3rd Ed. Standard Title**
5.035	5.2.1.11	Portable Electric Space Heaters
5.036	5.2.1.3	Heating and Ventilation Equipment Inspection and Maintenance
5.037	5.2.1.13	Barriers/Guards for Heating Equipment and Units
5.038	5.2.1.12	Fireplaces, Fireplace Inserts, and Wood/Corn Pellet Stoves
5.039	5.2.1.13	Barriers/Guards for Heating Equipment and Units
5.040	5.2.1.14	Water Heating Devices and Temperatures Allowed
5.041	5.2.1.15	Maintenance of Humidifiers and Dehumidifiers
5.042	5.2.2.1	Levels of Illumination
5.043	5.2.2.2	Light Fixtures Including Halogen Lamps
5.044	5.2.2.3	High Intensity Discharge Lamps, Multi-Vapor, and Mercury Lamps
5.045	5.2.2.4	Emergency Lighting
5.046	5.2.3.1	Noise Levels
5.047	5.2.4.1	Electrical Service
5.048	5.2.4.2	Safety Covers and Shock Protection Devices for Electrical Outlets
5.049	5.2.4.3	Ground-Fault Circuit-Interrupter for Outlets Near Water
5.050	5.2.4.4	Location of Electrical Devices Near Water
5.051	5.2.4.5	Extension Cords
5.052	5.2.4.6	Electrical Cords
5.053	5.2.5.1	Smoke Detection Systems and Smoke Alarms
5.054	5.2.5.2	Portable Fire Extinguishers
5.055	5.2.6.1	Water Supply
5.056	5.2.6.6	Water Handling and Treatment Equipment
5.057	5.2.6.7	Cross-Connections
5.058	5.2.6.8	Installation of Pipes and Plumbing Fixtures
5.059	5.2.6.2	Testing of Drinking Water Not From Public System
5.060	5.2.6.9	Handwashing Sink Using Portable Water Supply
5.061	5.2.6.3	Testing for Lead and Copper Levels in Drinking Water
5.062	5.2.6.4	Water Test Results
5.063	5.2.6.5	Emergency Safe Drinking Water and Bottled Water
5.064	5.2.7.1	On-Site Sewage Systems
5.065	5.2.7.2	Removal of Garbage
5.066	5.2.7.3	Containment of Garbage
5.067	5.2.7.4	Containment of Soiled Diapers
5.068	5.2.7.5	Labeling, Cleaning, and Disposal of Waste and Diaper Containers
5.069	5.2.7.6	Storage and Disposal of Infectious and Toxic Wastes
5.070	5.2.8.1	Integrated Pest Management
5.071	5.2.8.1	Integrated Pest Management
5.072	5.2.8.1	Integrated Pest Management
5.073	5.2.8.1	Integrated Pest Management
5.074	See toxic substance	Testing for Unsafe Levels of Toxic Chemicals
5.075	5.3.1.1	Safety of Equipment, Materials, and Furnishings
5.076	5.3.1.3	Size of Furniture
5.077	5.3.1.4	Surfaces of Equipment, Furniture, Toys, and Play Materials

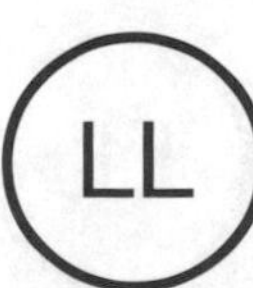

Chapter 5 - Facilities, Supplies, Equipment, and Transportation		
2nd Ed. #	**3rd Ed. #**	**3rd Ed. Standard Title**
5.078	5.3.1.5	Placement of Equipment and Furnishings
5.079	5.3.1.6	Floors, Walls, and Ceilings
5.080	5.3.1.7	Facility Arrangements to Minimize Back Injuries
5.081	5.3.1.8	High Chair Requirements
5.082	5.3.1.9	Carriage, Stroller, Gate, Enclosure, and Play Yard Requirements
5.083	5.3.1.10	Restrictive Infant Equipment Requirements
5.084	5.3.1.12	Availability and Use of a Telephone or Wireless Communication Device
5.085	6.2.1.1	Play Equipment Requirements
5.086	5.7.0.4	Inaccessibility of Hazardous Equipment
5.087	6.4.1.2	Inaccessibility of Toys or Objects to Children Under Three Years of Age
5.088	6.4.1.3	Crib Toys
5.089	6.4.1.5	Balloons
5.090	6.4.1.4	Projectile Toys
5.091	6.2.4.2	Water Play Tables
5.092	6.4.2.1	Riding Toys with Wheels and Wheeled Equipment
5.093	5.6.0.1	First Aid and Emergency Supplies
5.094	3.6.1.5	Sharing of Personal Articles Prohibited
5.095	3.1.5.2	Toothbrushes and Toothpaste
5.096	5.6.0.3	Supplies for Bathrooms and Handwashing Sinks
5.097	5.3.2.1	Therapeutic and Recreational Equipment
5.098	5.3.2.2	Special Adaptive Equipment
5.099	5.3.2.4	Orthotic and Prosthetic Devices
5.100	5.2.9.1	Use and Storage of Toxic Substances
5.101	5.2.9.2	Use of a Poison Center
5.102	5.2.9.3	Informing Staff Regarding Presence of Toxic Substances
5.103	5.2.9.4	Radon Concentrations
5.104	5.2.9.6	Preventing Exposure to Asbestos or Other Friable Materials
5.105	5.2.9.7	Proper Use of Art and Craft Materials
5.106	5.2.9.10	Prohibition of Poisonous Plants
5.107	5.2.9.11	Chemicals Used to Control Odors
5.108	5.2.1.5	Ventilation of Recently Carpeted or Paneled Areas
5.109 split	5.1.1.5	Environmental Audit of Site Location
5.109 split	5.2.9.6	Preventing Exposure to Asbestos and Other Friable Materials
5.110	5.2.9.13	Testing for Lead
5.111	5.2.9.15	Construction and Remodeling During Hours of Operation
5.112	5.1.2.1	Space Required Per Child
5.113	5.1.2.2	Floor Space Beneath Low Ceiling Heights
5.114	2.1.2.4	Separation of Infants and Toddlers From Older Children
5.115	5.1.2.3	Areas for School-Age Children
5.116	5.4.1.1	General Requirements for Toilet and Handwashing Areas
5.117	5.4.1.2	Location of Toilets and Privacy Issues
5.118	5.4.1.3	Ability to Open Toilet Room Doors
5.119	5.4.1.4	Preventing Entry to Toilet Rooms by Infants and Toddlers
5.120	5.4.1.2	Location of Toilets and Privacy Issues

Chapter 5 - Facilities, Supplies, Equipment, and Transportation		
2nd Ed. #	**3rd Ed. #**	**3rd Ed. Standard Title**
5.121	5.4.1.5	Chemical Toilets
5.122	5.4.1.6	Ratios of Toilets, Urinals, and Hand Sinks to Children
5.123	5.4.1.6	Ratios of Toilets, Urinals, and Hand Sinks to Children
5.124	5.4.1.7	Toilet Learning/Training Equipment
5.125	5.4.1.9	Waste Receptacles in the Child Care Facility and Child Care Facility Toilet Room(s)
5.126	5.4.1.10	Handwashing Sinks
5.127	5.4.1.11	Prohibited Uses of Handwashing Sinks
5.128	5.4.1.12	Mop Sinks
5.129	5.4.2.1	Diaper Changing Tables
5.130	5.4.2.2	Handwashing Sinks for Diaper Changing Areas in Centers
5.131	5.4.2.3	Handwashing Sinks for Diaper Changing Areas in Homes
5.132	5.4.2.4	Use, Location, and Setup of Diaper Changing Areas
5.133	5.4.2.5	Changing Table Requirements
5.134	5.4.3.1	Ratio and Location of Bathtubs and Showers
5.135	5.4.3.2	Safety of Bathtubs and Showers
5.136	4.2.0.6	Availability of Drinking Water
5.137	5.2.6.10	Drinking Fountains
5.138	5.2.6.3	Testing for Lead and Copper Levels in Drinking Water
5.139	5.6.0.2	Single Service Cups
5.140	5.4.4.1	Laundry Service and Equipment
5.141	5.4.4.2	Location of Laundry Equipment and Water Temperature for Laundering
5.142	5.1.1.12	Multiple Use of Rooms
5.143	3.1.4.1	Safe Sleep Practices and SIDS/Suffocation Risk Reduction
5.144	5.4.5.1	Sleeping Equipment and Supplies
5.145	5.4.5.2	Cribs
5.146	3.1.4.1	Safe Sleep Practices and SIDS Risk Reduction
5.147	5.4.5.4	Futons
5.148	5.4.5.5	Bunk Beds
5.149	5.4.6.1	Space for Children Who Are Ill
5.150	5.4.6.2	Space for therapy Services
5.151	5.5.0.1	Storage and Labeling of Personal Articles
5.152	5.3.2.3	Storage for Adaptive Equipment
5.153	5.5.0.2	Coat Hooks/Cubicles
5.154	5.5.0.3	Storage of Play and Teaching Equipment and Supplies
5.155	5.5.0.4	Storage for Soiled and Clean Linens
5.156	5.1.4.5	Closet Door Latches
5.157	5.5.0.6	Inaccessibility to Matches, Candles and Lighters
5.158	5.5.0.5	Storage of Flammable Materials
5.159	5.5.0.7	Storage of Plastic Bags
5.160	3.4.6.1	Strangulation Hazards
5.161	5.5.0.8	Firearms
5.162	6.1.0.1	Size and Location of Outdoor Play Area
5.163	6.1.0.2	Size and Requirements of Indoor Play Area
5.164	Deleted	Capacity of Outdoor Play Area

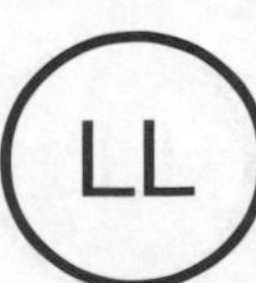

Chapter 5 - Facilities, Supplies, Equipment, and Transportation		
2nd Ed. #	**3rd Ed. #**	**3rd Ed. Standard Title**
5.165	6.1.0.3	Rooftops an Play Areas
5.166	6.1.0.4	Elevated Play Areas
5.167	5.1.6.7	Location of Satellite Dishes
5.168	6.1.0.5	Visibility of Outdoor Play Area
5.169	5.1.1.5	Environmental Audit of Site Location
5.170	6.2.2.4	Clearance Requirements of Playground Areas
5.171	6.2.2.5	Clearance Space for Swings
5.172	6.2.2.1	Use Zone for Fixed Play Equipment
5.173	6.1.0.7	Shading of Play Area
5.174	6.2.2.2	Arrangement of Play Equipment
5.175	6.2.2.3	Location of Moving Play Equipment
5.176	6.1.0.6	Location of Play Areas Near Bodies of Water
5.177	6.1.0.7	Shading of Play Area
5.178	6.1.0.8	Enclosures for Outdoor Play Areas
5.179	5.1.1.5	Environmental Audit of Site Location
5.180	6.2.4.1	Sandboxes
5.181	6.2.1.3	Design of Play Equipment
5.182	6.2.1.4	Installation of Play Equipment
5.183	6.2.3.1	Prohibited Surfaces for Placing Climbing Equipment
5.184	6.2.1.7	Enclosure of Moving Parts on Play Equipment
5.185	6.2.1.8	Material Defects and Edges on Play Equipment
5.186	6.2.1.9	Entrapment Hazards of Play Equipment
5.187	6.2.1.2	Play Equipment and Surfaces Meet Ada Requirements
5.188	6.2.1.5	Play Equipment Connecting and Linking Devices
5.189	6.2.1.6	Size and Anchoring of Crawl Spaces
5.190	5.1.6.3	Drainage of Paved Surfaces
5.191	5.1.6.4	Walking Surfaces
5.192	5.1.6.4	Walking Surfaces
5.193	5.1.6.5	Areas Used by Children for Wheeled Vehicles
5.194	5.7.0.2	Removal of Hazards From Outdoor Areas
5.195 split	5.3.1.4	Surfaces of Equipment, Furniture, Toys, and Play Materials
5.195 split	6.2.1.1	Play Equipment Requirements
5.196	6.2.5.1	Inspection of Indoor and Outdoor Play Areas and Equipment
5.197	6.2.5.2	Inspection of Play Area Surfacing
5.198	6.3.1.1	Enclosure of Bodies of Water
5.199	6.3.1.2	Accessibility to Above-Ground Pools
5.200	6.3.1.3	Sensors or Remote Monitors
5.201	6.3.1.4	Safety Covers for Swimming Pools
5.202	5.2.8.2	Insect Breeding Hazard
5.203	6.3.1.5	Deck Surface
5.204	6.3.3.1	Pool Performance Requirements
5.205	6.3.1.6	Pool Drain Covers
5.206	6.3.1.8	Supervision of Pool Pump
5.207	6.3.3.3	Electrical Safety for Pool Areas

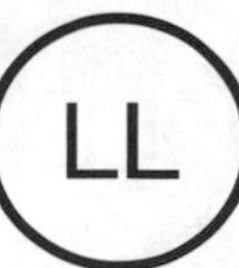

Chapter 5 - Facilities, Supplies, Equipment, and Transportation		
2nd Ed. #	**3rd Ed. #**	**3rd Ed. Standard Title**
5.208	6.3.2.1	Lifesaving Equipment
5.209	6.3.2.2	Lifeline in Pool
5.210	6.3.2.3	Pool Equipment and Chemical Storage Rooms
5.211	6.3.5.1	Hot Tubs, Spas, and Saunas
5.212	6.3.5.2	Water in Containers
5.213	6.3.5.3	Portable Wading Pools
5.214	6.3.3.2	Construction, Maintenance, and Inspection of Pools
5.215	6.3.1.7	Pool Safety Rules
5.216	6.3.4.1	Pool Water Quality
5.217	6.3.4.2	Chlorine Pucks
5.218	6.3.3.4	Pool Water Temperature
5.219	5.1.6.1	Designated Walkways, Bike Routes, and Drop-Off and Pick-Up Points
5.220	5.1.6.2	Construction and Maintenance of Walkways
5.221	5.1.6.6	Guardrails and Protective Barriers
5.222	5.1.5.1	Balusters
5.223	5.1.5.2	Handrails
5.224	5.1.5.3	Landings
5.225	5.1.5.4	Guards At Stairway Access Openings
5.226	5.7.0.1	Maintenance of Exterior Surfaces
5.227	5.7.0.3	Removal of Allergen Triggering Materials From Outdoor Areas
5.228	5.7.0.5	Cleaning Schedule for Exterior Areas
5.229	5.2.1.3	Heating and Ventilation Equipment Inspection and Maintenance
5.230	5.7.0.6	Storage Area Maintenance and Ventilation
5.231	5.7.0.7	Structure Maintenance
5.232	5.7.0.8	Electrical Fixtures and Outlets Maintenance
5.233	5.7.0.9	Plumbing and Gas Maintenance
5.234	5.7.0.10	Cleaning of Humidifiers and Related Equipment
5.235 split	9.2.5.1	Transportation Policy for Centers and Large Family Homes
5.235 split	9.2.5.2	Transportation Policy for Small Family Child Care Homes
5.236	6.5.2.2	Child Passenger Safety
5.237	5.6.0.1	First Aid and Emergency Supplies
5.238	6.5.2.4	Interior Temperature of Vehicles
5.239 split	9.2.5.1	Transportation Policy for Centers and Large Family Homes
5.239 split	9.2.5.2	Transportation Policy for Small Family Child Care Homes
5.240 split	9.2.5.1	Transportation Policy for Centers and Large Family Homes
5.240 split	9.2.5.2	Transportation Policy for Small Family Child Care Homes
5.241	6.4.2.3	Bike Routes
5.242	6.4.2.2	Helmets
Chapter 6 - Infectious Diseases		
2nd Ed. #	**3rd Ed. #**	**3rd Ed. Standard Title**
6.001	7.3.2.1	Immunization for *Haemophilus Influenzae* Type B (Hib)
6.002	7.3.2.2	Informing Parents/Guardians of *Haemophilus Influenzae* Type B (Hib) Exposure
6.003	7.3.2.3	Informing Public Health Authorities of Invasive *Haemophilus Influenzae* Type B Cases
6.004	7.3.9.1	Immunization with *Streptococcus Pneumoniae* Conjugate Vaccine (PCV13)

Chapter 6 - Infectious Diseases		
2nd Ed. #	**3rd Ed. #**	**3rd Ed. Standard Title**
6.005	7.3.9.2	Informing Public Health Authorities of Invasive *Streptococcus Pneumoniae*
6.006	7.3.5.2	Informing Public Health Authorities of Meningococcal Infections
6.007	7.3.5.1	Recommended Control Measures for Invasive Meningococcal Infection in Child Care
6.008	7.3.5.1	Recommended Control Measures for Invasive Meningococcal Infection in a Child Care Center
6.009	7.3.7.1	Informing Public Health Authorities of Pertussis Cases
6.010	7.3.7.2	Prophylactic Treatment for Pertussis
6.011	7.3.7.3	Exclusion for Pertussis
6.012	7.3.1.1	Exclusion for Group a Streptococcal (Gas) Infections
6.013	7.3.1.2	Informing Caregivers/Teachers of Group a Streptococcal (Gas) Infection
6.014	7.3.10.1	Measures for Detection, Control, and Reporting of Tuberculosis
6.015	7.3.10.2	Attendance of Children with Latent Tuberculosis Infection or Active Tuberculosis Disease
6.016	7.3.6.1	Attendance of Children with Erythema Infectiosum (EI) (Parvovirus B19)
6.017	7.3.11.1	Attendance of Children with Unspecified Respiratory Tract Infection
6.018	7.7.2.1	Disease Recognition and Control of Herpes Simplex Virus
6.019	7.7.4.1	Staff and Parent/Guardian Notification About Varicella-Zoster (Chickenpox) Virus
6.020	7.7.4.2	Exclusion of Children with Varicella-Zoster (Chickenpox) Virus
6.021	7.7.1.1	Staff Education and Policies on Cytomegalovirus (CMV)
6.022	7.7.1.2	Testing of Children with Cytomegalovirus (CMV)
6.023	7.4.0.1	Control of Enteric (Diarrheal) and Hepatitis a Virus (HAV) Infections
6.024	7.4.0.2	Staff Education and Policies on Enteric (Diarrheal) and Hepatitis a Virus (Hav) Infections
6.025	7.4.0.3	Disease Surveillance of Enteric (Diarrheal) and Hepatitis a Virus (HAV) Infections
6.026	7.4.0.4	Maintenance of Records on Incidents of Diarrhea
6.027	7.6.1.1	Disease Recognition and Control of Hepatitis B Virus (HBV) Infection
6.028	7.6.1.2	Observation and Follow-Up of a Child Who Is an Hepatitis B Virus (HBV) Carrier
6.029	7.6.1.3	Staff Education on Prevention of Bloodborne Diseases
6.030	7.6.1.4	Informing Public Health Authorities of Hepatitis B Virus (HBV) Cases
6.031	7.6.1.5	Handling Injuries to a Hepatitis B Virus (HBV) Carrier
6.032	7.6.2.1	Infection Control Measures with Hepatitis C Virus (HCV)
6.033	7.6.3.1	Attendance of Children with HIV
6.034	7.6.3.2	Protecting HIV-Infected Children and Adults in Child Care
6.035	7.6.3.3	Staff Education About Preventing Transmission of HIV Infection
6.036	7.6.3.4	Ability of Caregivers/Teachers with HIV Infection to Care for Children
6.037	7.5.11.1	Attendance of Children with Scabies
6.038	7.5.8.1	Attendance of Children with Head Lice
6.039	7.5.9.1	Attendance of Children with Ringworm
Reader's Note	7.9	Note to Reader on Judicious Use of Antibiotics
Chapter 7 - Children Who are Eligible for Services Under IDEA		
2nd Ed. #	**3rd Ed. #**	**3rd Ed. Standard Title**
7.001	8.2.0.1	Inclusion in All Activities
7.002	8.2.0.2	Planning for Inclusion
7.003	8.3.0.1	Initial Assessment of the Child to Determine His or Her Special Needs
7.004	8.4.0.1	Determining the Type and Frequency of Services
7.005	8.4.0.2	Formulation of an Action Plan

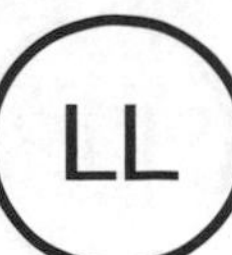

Chapter 7 - Children Who are Eligible for Services Under IDEA		
2nd Ed. #	**3rd Ed. #**	**3rd Ed. Standard Title**
7.006	8.4.0.3	Determination of Eligibility for Special Services
7.007	8.4.0.4	Designation and Role of Staff Person Responsible for Coordinating Care in the Child Care Facility
7.008	8.4.0.5	Development of Measurable Objectives
7.009	8.4.0.6	Contracts and Reimbursement
7.010	8.5.0.1	Coordinating and Documenting Services
7.011	8.5.0.2	Written Reports on IFSPs/IEPs to Caregivers/Teachers
7.012	8.6.0.1	Reevaluation Process
7.013	8.6.0.2	Statement of Program Needs and Plans
7.014	8.7.0.1	Facility Self-Assessment
7.015	8.7.0.2	Technical Assistance in Developing Plan
7.016	8.7.0.3	Review of Plan for Serving Children with Disabilities or Children with Special Health Care Needs

Chapter 8 - Administration		
2nd Ed. #	**3rd Ed. #**	**3rd Ed. Standard Title**
8.001	9.1.0.1	Governing Body of the Facility
8.002	9.1.0.2	Written Delegation of Administrative Authority
8.003	9.4.1.4	Access to Facility Records
8.004	9.2.1.1	Content of Policies
8.005	9.2.1.3	Enrollment Information to Parents/Guardians and Caregivers/Teachers
8.006	9.2.1.5	Nondiscriminatory Policy
8.007	9.2.1.4	Exchange of Information Upon Enrollment
8.008	9.2.1.6	Written Discipline Policies
8.009	2.2.0.6	Discipline Measures
8.010 split	9.2.1.6	Written Discipline Policies
8.010 split	2.2.0.7	Handling Physical Aggression, Biting and Hitting
8.011	9.2.3.2	Content and Development of the Plan for Care of Children and Staff Who Are Ill
8.012	3.6.2.1	Exclusion and Alternative Care for Children Who Are Ill
8.013	9.2.3.4	Written Policy for Obtaining Preventive Health Service Information
8.014	9.2.3.5	Documentation of Exemptions and Exclusion of Children Who Lack Immunizations
8.015	9.2.3.6	Identification of Child's Medical Home and Parental/Guardian Consent for Information Exchange
8.016	9.2.3.7	Information Sharing on therapies and Treatments Needed
8.017	9.2.3.8	Information Sharing on Family Health
8.018	9.2.2.1	Planning for Child's Transition to New Services
8.019	9.2.2.2	Format for the Transition Plan
8.020	1.6.0.1	Child Care Health Consultants
8.021	9.2.3.9	Written Policy on Use of Medications
8.022	9.2.4.1	Written Plan and Training for Handling Urgent Medical Care or Threatening Incidents
8.023	9.2.4.2	Review of Written Plan for Urgent Care
8.024	9.2.4.3	Disaster Planning, Training and Communication
8.025	9.2.4.5	Emergency and Evacuation Drills/Exercises Policy
8.026	9.2.4.6	Use of Daily Roster During Evacuation Drills
8.027	9.2.4.5	Emergency and Evacuation Drills/Exercises Policy
8.028	9.2.4.8	Authorized Persons to Pick Up Child
8.029	9.2.4.9	Policy on Actions to Be Followed When No Authorized Person Arrives to Pick Up a Child
8.030	9.2.4.10	Documentation of Drop-Off, Pick-Up, and Daily Attendance of Child, and Parent/Guardian/ Provider Communication

Chapter 8 - Administration		
2nd Ed. #	**3rd Ed. #**	**3rd Ed. Standard Title**
8.031	9.2.5.1	Transportation Policy for Centers and Large Family Homes
8.032	9.2.5.2	Transportation Policy for Small Family Child Care Homes
8.033	9.2.6.1	Policy on Use and Maintenance of Play Areas
8.034	9.2.3.10	Sanitation Policies and Procedures
8.035	9.2.3.11	Food and Nutrition Service Policies and Plans
8.036	9.2.3.12	Infant Feeding Policy
8.037	9.2.3.13	Plans for Evening and Nighttime Child Care
8.038	9.2.3.15	Policies Prohibiting Smoking, Tobacco, Alcohol, Illegal Drugs, and Toxic Substances
8.039	9.2.3.16	Policy Prohibiting Firearms
8.040	9.2.1.2	Review and Communication of Written Policies
8.041	9.2.3.17	Child Care Health Consultant's Review of Health Policies
8.042	2.1.1.1	Written Daily Activity Plan and Statement of Principles
8.043	9.2.2.3	Exchange of Information at Transitions
8.044	9.3.0.1	Written Human Resource Management Policies for Centers and Large Family Child Care Homes
8.045	Deleted	Written Statement of Services
8.046	9.4.2.1	Contents of Child's Records
8.047	9.4.2.2	Pre-Admission Enrollment Information for Each Child
8.048	9.4.2.4	Contents of Child's Primary Care Provider's Assessment
8.049	9.4.2.3	Contents of Admission Agreement Between Child Care Program and Parent/Guardian
8.050	9.4.2.5	Health History
8.051	9.4.2.6	Contents of Medication Record
8.052	9.4.2.7	Contents of Facility Health Log for Each Child
8.053	9.2.3.6	Identification of Child's Medical Home and Parental/Guardian Consent for Information Exchange
8.054	9.4.1.3	Written Policy on Confidentiality of Records
8.055	9.2.3.6	Identification of Child's Medical Home and Parental/Guardian Consent for Information Exchange
8.056	9.4.2.8	Release of Child's Records
8.057	9.4.1.5	Availability of Records to Licensing Agency
8.058	9.4.3.1	Maintenance and Content of Staff and Volunteer Records
8.059	9.2.4.10	Documentation of Drop-Off, Pick-Up, and Daily Attendance of Child, and Parent/Guardian/ Provider Communication
8.060	9.4.3.2	Maintenance of Attendance Records for Staff Who Care for Children
8.061	9.4.1.8	Records of Illness
8.062	9.4.1.9	Records of Injury
8.063	9.4.1.10	Documentation of Parent/Guardian Notification of Injury, Illness or Death in Program
8.064	9.4.1.11	Review and Accessibility of Injury and Illness Reports
8.065	9.4.1.12	Record of Valid License, Certificate or Registration of Facility
8.066	9.4.1.13	Maintenance and Display of Inspection Reports
8.067	9.4.1.14	Written Plan/Record to Resolve Deficiencies
8.068	9.4.1.15	Availability of Reports on Inspections of Fire Protection Devices
8.069	9.4.1.16	Evacuation and Shelter-In-Place Drill Record
8.070	9.4.1.1	Facility Insurance Coverage
8.071	9.2.6.3	Records of Proper Installation and Maintenance of Facility Equipment
8.072	9.2.6.2	Reports of Annual Audits/Monthly Maintenance Checks of Play Areas and Equipment
8.073	9.4.1.17	Documentation of Child Care Health Consultation/Training Visits

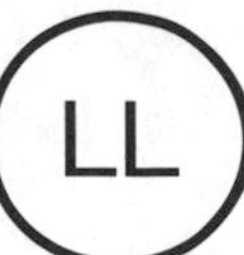

Chapter 8 - Administration		
2nd Ed. #	**3rd Ed. #**	**3rd Ed. Standard Title**
8.074	9.4.1.18	Records of Nutrition Service
8.075	9.4.1.19	Community Resource Information
8.076	9.4.1.2	Maintenance of Records
8.077	9.4.1.6	Availability of Documents to Parents/Guardians
8.078	9.4.1.7	Requirements for Compliance of Contract Services
8.079	10.4.1.1	Uniform Categories and Definitions
Chapter 9 - Licensing and Community Action		
2nd Ed. #	**3rd Ed. #**	**3rd Ed. Standard Title**
9.001	10.2.0.1	Regulation of All Out-Of-Home Child Care
9.002	10.3.1.1	Operation Permits
9.003	10.3.3.2	Background Screening
9.004	10.4.1.1	Uniform Categories and Definitions
9.005	3.6.2.8	Licensing of Facilities that Care for Children Who Are Ill
9.006	10.3.3.1	Credentialing of Individual Child Care Providers
9.007	10.4.1.3	Licensing Agency Procedures Prior to Issuing a License
9.008	10.4.1.4	Alternative Means of Compliance
9.009	10.3.1.2	Rational Basis of Regulations
9.010	10.3.1.3	Community Participation in Development of Licensing Rules
9.011	10.3.2.3	Collaborative Development of Child Care Requirements and Guidelines for Children Who are Ill
9.012	10.2.0.2	Adequacy of Staff and Funding for Regulatory Enforcement
9.013	10.3.5.2	Performance Monitoring of Licensing Inspectors
9.014	10.4.2.1	Frequency of Inspections for Child Care Centers, Large Family Child Care Homes, and Small Family Child Care Homes
9.015	10.3.5.1	Education, Experience and Training of Licensing Inspectors
9.016	10.3.5.3	Training of Licensing Agency Personnel About Child Abuse
9.017	10.4.2.2	Statutory Authorization of On-Site Inspections
9.018	10.4.2.1	Frequency of Inspections for Child Care Centers, Large Family Child Care Homes, and Small Family Child Care Homes
9.019	10.4.2.3	Monitoring Strategies
9.020	10.4.3.1	Procedure for Receiving Complaints
9.021	10.4.3.2	Whistle-Blower Protection Under State Law
9.022	10.3.3.3	Licensing Agency Role in Communicating the Importance of Reporting Suspected Child Abuse
9.023	10.2.0.3	State Statute Support of Regulatory Enforcement
9.024	10.3.2.1	Child Care Licensing Advisory Board
9.025	10.5.0.1	State and Local Health Department Role
9.026	10.5.0.2	Written Plans for the Health Department Role
9.027	10.5.0.3	Requirements for Facilities to Report to Health Department
9.028	10.5.0.4	Use of Fact Sheets on Common Illnesses Associated with Child Care
9.029	10.3.4.1	Sources of Technical Assistance to Support Quality of Child Care
9.030	10.3.3.4	Licensing Agency Provision of Child Abuse Prevention Materials
9.031	10.3.4.2	Licensing Agency Provision of Written Agreements for Parents/Guardians and Caregivers/Teachers
9.032	10.4.3.3	Collection of Data on Illness or Harm to Children in Facilities
9.033	10.3.4.3	Support for Consultants to Provide Technical Assistance to Facilities
9.034	10.3.4.4	Development of List of Providers of Services to Facilities

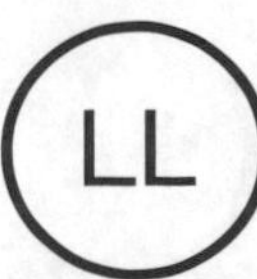

Chapter 9 - Licensing and Community Action		
2nd Ed. #	**3rd Ed. #**	**3rd Ed. Standard Title**
9.035	10.3.4.5	Resources for Parents/Guardians of Children with Special Health Care Needs
9.036	10.3.4.6	Compensation for Participation in Multidisciplinary Assessments for Children with Special Health Care or Education Needs
9.037	10.6.2.1	Development of Child Care Provider Organizations and Networks
9.038	10.6.1.1	Regulatory Agency Provision of Caregiver/Teacher and Consumer Training and Support Services
9.039	Deleted	Child Development Associate Training
9.040	10.6.1.2	Provision of Training to Facilities by Health Agencies
9.041	10.3.4.7	Technical Assistance to Facilities to Address Diversity in the Community
9.042	10.6.2.2	Fostering Collaboration to Establish Programs for School-Age Children
9.043	10.3.2.4	Public-Private Collaboration on Care of Children Who Are Ill
9.044	10.4.2.4	Agency Collaboration to Safeguard Children in Child Care
9.045	10.3.2.2	State Early Childhood Advisory Council
9.046	10.7.0.1	Development of Resource and Referral Agencies
9.047	10.7.0.2	Coordination of Public and Private Resources to Ensure Families' Access to Quality Child Care
9.048	Deleted	Arrangements for Parental/Guardian Leave
New Standards		
2nd Ed. #	**3rd Ed. #**	**Standard Title**
New	1.1.2.1	Minimum Age to Enter Child Care
New	1.6.0.3	Early Childhood Mental Health Consultants
New	1.6.0.4	Early Childhood Education Consultants
New	2.1.1.3	Coordinated Child Care Health Program Model
New	2.1.1.6	Transitioning within Programs and Indoor and Outdoor Learning/Play Environments
New	2.2.0.2	Limiting Infant/Toddler Time in Crib, High Chair, Car Seat, Etc
New	2.2.0.3	Limiting Screen Time – Media, Computer Time
New	2.2.0.8	Preventing Expulsions, Suspensions, and Other Limitations in Services
New	3.1.3.1	Active Opportunities for Physical Activity
New	3.1.3.3	Protection From Air Pollution While Children Are Outside
New	3.1.3.4	Caregivers'/Teachers' Encouragement of Physical Activity
New	3.1.4.2	Swaddling
New	3.1.4.3	Pacifier Use
New	3.2.1.5	Procedure for Changing Children's Soiled Underwear/Pull-Ups and Clothing
New	3.2.2.5	Hand Sanitizers
New	3.2.3.2	Cough and Sneeze Etiquette
New	3.4.4.3	Preventing and Identifying Shaken Baby Syndrome/Abusive Head Trauma
New	3.4.5.1	Sun Safety Including Sunscreen
New	3.4.5.2	Insect Repellent - Protection From Vector Borne Diseases
New	3.6.1.3	Thermometers for Taking Human Temperatures
New	4.2.0.11	Ingestion of Substances that Do Not Provide Nutrition
New	4.2.0.12	Vegetarian/Vegan Diets
New	4.3.1.6	Use of Soy-Based Formula and Soy Milk
New	5.2.9.5	Carbon Monoxide Detectors
New	5.2.9.8	Use of Play Dough and Other Manipulative Art or Sensory Materials
New	5.2.9.9	Plastic Containers and Toys
New	5.2.9.12	Treatment of CCA Pressure-Treated Wood

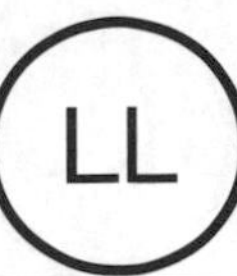

New Standards		
2nd Ed. #	**3rd Ed. #**	**Standard Title**
New	5.3.1.2	Product Recall Monitoring
New	5.3.1.11	Exercise Equipment
New	5.4.5.3	Stackable Cribs
New	6.2.4.3	Sensory Table Materials
New	6.2.4.4	Trampolines
New	6.2.4.5	Ball Pits
New	6.5.3.1	Passenger Vans
New	7.3.3.1	Influenza Immunizations for Children and Caregivers/Teachers
New	7.3.3.2	Influenza Control
New	7.3.3.3	Influenza Prevention Education
New	7.3.4.1	Mumps
New	7.3.8.1	Attendance of Children with Respiratory Syncytial Virus (RSV) Respiratory Tract Infection
New	7.5.1.1	Conjunctivitis
New	7.5.2.1	Enterovirus Infections
New	7.5.3.1	Human Papillomaviruses (HPV) (Warts)
New	7.5.4.1	Impetigo
New	7.5.5.1	Lymphadenitis
New	7.5.6.1	Immunization for Measles
New	7.5.7.1	Molluscum Contagiosum
New	7.5.10.1	*Staphylococcus Aureus* Skin Infections Including MRSA
New	7.5.12.1	Thrush (Candidiasis)
New	7.7.3.1	Roseola
New	7.8	Interaction with State or Local Health Departments
New	9.2.3.1	Policies and Practices that Promote Physical Activity
New	9.2.3.14	Oral Health Policy
New	9.2.4.4	Written Plan for Seasonal and Pandemic Influenza
New	9.2.4.7	Sign-In/Sign-Out System
New	9.3.0.2	Written Human Resource Management Policies for Small Family Child Care Homes
New	10.3.3.5	Licensing Agency Role in Communicating the Importance of Compliance with Americans with Disabilities Act
New	10.4.1.2	Quality Rating and Improvement Systems
Appendices		
2nd Ed.	**3rd Ed.**	**Appendix Title**
A	Front Matter	Guiding Principles for the Standards
B	B	Major Occupational Health Hazards
C	C	Nutrition Specialist, Registered Dietician, Licensed Nutritionist, Consultant, and Food Service Staff Qualifications
D	D	Gloving
E	E	Child Care Staff Health Assessment
F	F	Enrollment/Attendance/Symptom Record
G	G	Recommended Childhood Immunization Schedule
H	I	Recommendations for Preventive Pediatric Health Care
I	J	Selecting an Appropriate Sanitizer or Disinfectant
J	L	Cleaning Up Body Fluids

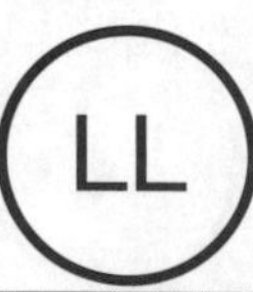

Appendices		
2nd Ed.	**3rd Ed.**	**Appendix Title**
K	M	Clues to Child Abuse and Neglect
L	Deleted	Risk Factors for Abuse and/or Neglect
M	Deleted	Special Care Plan for a Child with Asthma
N	P	Situations that Require Medical Attention Right Away
O	Deleted	Food Guide Pyramid for Young Children
P	Deleted	Child and Adult Care Food Program Child Care Infant Meal Pattern
Q	Deleted	Child and Adult Care Food Program Child Care Meal Pattern Requirements for Children Ages 1 through 12 Years
R	V	Food Storage Chart
S	W	Sample Food Service Cleaning Schedule
T	X	Adaptive Equipment for Children with Special Health Care Needs
U	Y	Non Poisonous and Poisonous Plants
V	Z	Depth of Surface Materials
W	Deleted	Permission for Medical Condition Treatment
X	BB	Emergency Information for Children with Special Health Care Needs
Y	CC	Incident Report Form
Z	FF	Child Health Assessment
AA	GG	Licensing and Public Regulation of Early Childhood Programs – NAEYC Position Statement
BB	Deleted	Contact Information
CC	Deleted	Conversion Table - 1st Edition to 2nd Edition
DD	Deleted	Conversion Table - 2nd Edition to 1st Edition
New	A	Signs and Symptoms Chart
New	H	Recommended Adult Immunization Schedule
New	K	Routine Schedule for Cleaning, Sanitizing, and Disinfecting
New	N	Protective Factors Regarding Child Abuse and Neglect
New	O	Care Plan for Children with Special Health Care Needs
New	Q	Getting Started with MyPlate
New	R	Choose MyPlate: 10 Tips to a Great Plate
New	S	Physical Activity: How Much Is Needed?
New	T	Foster Care
New	U	Recommended Safe Minimum Internal Cooking Temperatures
New	AA	Medication Administration Packet
New	DD	Injury Report Form for Indoor and Outdoor Injuries
New	EE	America's Playgrounds Safety Report Card
New	HH	Use Zones for Clearance Dimensions for Single- and Multi-Axis Swings
New	II	Bicycle Helmets: Quick- Fit Check
New	JJ	Our Child Care Center Supports Breastfeeding
New	KK	Authorization for Emergency Medical/Dental Care
New	LL	Conversion Table - 2nd Edition to 3rd Edition
New	MM	Conversion Table - 3rd Edition to 2nd Edition

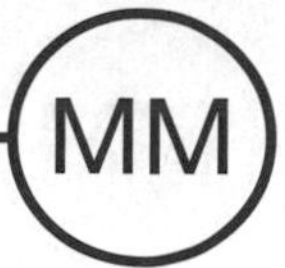

Appendix MM: Conversion Table - Third Edition Standard Numbering to Second Edition Standard Numbering

The numbering system for the standards was changed in the 3rd Edition to facilitate recognition of standards by their placement and content grouping in each chapter. Each standard is represented by four numbers separated by a period (#.#.#.#). The first number represents the chapter, the second number represents a major chapter division, the third number represents a subdivision below a major division, and finally, the standard within that subdivision.

Numbering Example:		Numbering Scheme Explanation:
1	#	Chapter
1.3	#.#	Major chapter division
1.3.3	#.#.#	Chapter subdivision
1.3.3.1	#.#.#.#	Standard

The conversion table below lists the 3rd Edition number first followed by its old 2nd Edition number, followed by the 3rd Edition Standard Title. If a standard has been deleted from the 2nd Edition, it is indicated under the column for the 3rd Edition number and is listed in a separate section at the end of the table. If standards were merged from multiple 2nd Edition standards, the merged 2nd Edition numbers are listed in the 2nd Edition column.

Chapter 1		
3rd Ed. #	**2nd Ed. #**	**3rd Ed. Standard Title**
1.1.1.1	1.001	Ratios for Small Family Child Care Homes
1.1.1.2	1.002	Ratios for Large Family Child Care Homes and Centers
1.1.1.3	1.003	Ratios for Facilities Serving Children with Special Health Care Needs and Disabilities
1.1.1.4	1.004	Ratios and Supervision During Transportation
1.1.1.5	1.005	Ratios and Supervision for Swimming, Wading, and Water Play
1.1.2.1	New	Minimum Age to Enter Child Care
1.2.0.1	1.007	Staff Recruitment
1.2.0.2	1.008	Background Screening
1.3.1.1	1.014	General Qualifications of Directors
1.3.1.2	1.015	Mixed Director/Teacher Role
1.3.2.1	1.016	Differentiated Roles
1.3.2.2	1.017	Qualifications of Lead Teachers and Teachers
1.3.2.3	1.018	Qualifications for Assistant Teachers, Teacher Aides, and Volunteers
1.3.2.4	1.010	Additional Qualifications for Caregivers/Teachers Serving Children Three to Thirty-Five Months of Age
1.3.2.5	1.011	Additional Qualifications for Caregivers/Teachers Serving Children Three to Five Years of Age
1.3.2.6	1.012	Additional Qualifications for Caregivers/Teachers Serving School-Age Children
1.3.2.7	1.021/1.022	Qualifications and Responsibilities for Health Advocates
1.3.3.1	1.019	General Qualifications of Family Child Care Caregivers/Teachers to Operate a Family Child Care Home
1.3.3.2	1.020	Support Networks for Family Child Care
1.4.1.1	1.006/1.009	Pre-Service Training
1.4.2.1	1.023	Initial Orientation of All Staff
1.4.2.2	1.024	Orientation for Care of Children with Special Health Care Needs
1.4.2.3	1.025	Additional Orientation Topics
1.4.3.1	1.026	First Aid and CPR Training for Staff
1.4.3.2	1.027	Topics Covered in First Aid Training
1.4.3.3	1.028	CPR Training for Swimming and Water Play
1.4.4.1	1.009/1.029	Continuing Education for Directors and Caregivers/Teachers in Centers and Large Family Child Care Homes

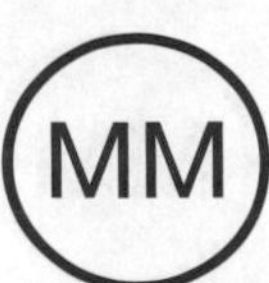

Chapter 1		
3rd Ed. #	**2nd Ed. #**	**3rd Ed. Standard Title**
1.4.4.2	1.030	Continuing Education for Small Family Child Care Home Caregivers/Teachers
1.4.5.1	1.031	Training of Staff Who Handle Food
1.4.5.2	1.032	Child Abuse and Neglect Education
1.4.5.3	1.033	Training on Occupational Risk Related to Handling Body Fluids
1.4.5.4	1.013	Diversity Education of Center Staff
1.4.6.1	1.035	Training Time and Professional Development Leave
1.4.6.2	1.036	Payment for Continuing Education
1.5.0.1	1.037	Employment of Substitutes
1.5.0.2	1.038/1.039	Orientation of Substitutes
1.6.0.1	1.040/1.041/8.020	Child Care Health Consultants
1.6.0.2	1.043	Frequency of Child Care Health Consultation Visits
1.6.0.3	New	Early Childhood Mental Health Consultants
1.6.0.4	New	Early Childhood Education Consultants
1.6.0.5	1.042	Specialized Consultation for Facilities Serving Children with Disabilities
1.7.0.1	1.045	Pre-Employment and Ongoing Adult Health Appraisals, Including Immunization
1.7.0.2	1.046	Daily Staff Health Check
1.7.0.3	1.047	Health Limitations of Staff
1.7.0.4	1.048	Occupational Hazards
1.7.0.5	1.049/3.058	Stress
1.8.1.1	1.050	Basic Benefits
1.8.2.1	1.051	Staff Familiarity with Facility Policies, Plans and Procedures
1.8.2.2	1.052/1.055	Annual Staff Competency Evaluation
1.8.2.3	1.056	Staff Improvement Plan
1.8.2.4	1.054	Observation of Staff
1.8.2.5	1.057	Handling Complaints About Caregivers/Teachers

Chapter 2		
3rd Ed. #	**2nd Ed. #**	**3rd Ed. Standard Title**
2.1.1.1	2.001/2.002/ 2.003/8.042	Written Daily Activity Plan and Statement of Principles
2.1.1.2	2.021	Health, Nutrition, Physical Activity, and Safety Awareness
2.1.1.3	New	Coordinated Child Care Health Program Model
2.1.1.4	2.053	Monitoring Children's Development/ Obtaining Consent for Screening
2.1.1.5	2.004	Helping Families Cope with Separation
2.1.1.6	New	Transitioning within Programs and Indoor and Outdoor Learning/Play Environments
2.1.1.7	2.006	Communication in Native Language Other Than English
2.1.1.8	2.007	Diversity in Enrollment and Curriculum
2.1.1.9	2.008	Verbal Interaction
2.1.2.1	2.010	Personal Caregiver/Teacher Relationships for Infants and Toddlers
2.1.2.2	2.011	Interactions with Infants and Toddlers
2.1.2.3	2.012	Space and Activity to Support Learning of Infants and Toddlers
2.1.2.4	2.013/5.114	Separation of Infants and Toddlers From Older Children
2.1.2.5	2.005	Toilet Learning/Training
2.1.3.1	2.014	Personal Caregiver/Teacher Relationships for Three- to 5-Year-Olds
2.1.3.2	2.015	Opportunities for Learning for Three- to Five-Year-Olds
2.1.3.3	2.016	Selection of Equipment for Three- to Five-Year-Olds

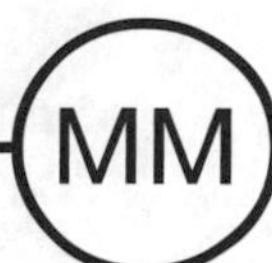

Chapter 2		
3rd Ed. #	**2nd Ed. #**	**3rd Ed. Standard Title**
2.1.3.4	2.017	Expressive Activities for Three- to Five-Year-Olds
2.1.3.5	2.018	Fostering Cooperation of Three- to Five-Year-Olds
2.1.3.6	2.019	Fostering Language Development of Three- to Five-Year-Olds
2.1.3.7	2.020	Body Mastery for Three- to Five-Year-Olds
2.1.4.1	2.022	Supervised School-Age Activities
2.1.4.2	2.023	Space for School-Age Activity
2.1.4.3	2.024	Developing Relationships for School-Age Children
2.1.4.4	2.025	Planning Activities for School-Age Children
2.1.4.5	2.026	Community Outreach for School-Age Children
2.1.4.6	2.027	Communication Between Child Care and School
2.2.0.1	2.028	Methods of Supervision of Children
2.2.0.2	New	Limiting Infant/Toddler Time in Crib, High Chair, Car Seat, Etc.
2.2.0.3	New	Limiting Screen Time – Media, Computer Time
2.2.0.4	3.045	Supervision Near Bodies of Water
2.2.0.5	3.046	Behavior Around a Pool
2.2.0.6	2.039/8.009	Discipline Measures
2.2.0.7	2.040/8.010	Handling Physical Aggression, Biting and Hitting
2.2.0.8	New	Preventing Expulsions, Suspensions, and Other Limitations in Services
2.2.0.9	2.042	Prohibited Caregiver/Teacher Behaviors
2.2.0.10	2.043	Using Physical Restraint
2.3.1.1	2.044	Mutual Responsibility of Parents/Guardians and Staff
2.3.1.2	2.046	Parent/Guardian Visits
2.3.2.1	2.047	Parent/Guardian Conferences
2.3.2.2	2.050	Seeking Parent/Guardian Input
2.3.2.3	2.045/2.051	Support Services for Parents/Guardians
2.3.2.4	2.052	Parent/Guardian Complaint Procedures
2.3.3.1	2.054	Parents'/Guardians' Provision of Information on their Child's Health and Behavior
2.3.3.2	2.059	Communication From Specialists
2.4.1.1	2.061	Health and Safety Education Topics for Children
2.4.1.2	2.060/2.063	Staff Modeling of Healthy and Safe Behavior and Health and Safety Education Activities
2.4.1.3	2.062	Gender and Body Awareness
2.4.2.1	2.064	Health and Safety Education Topics for Staff
2.4.3.1	2.065/2.066	Opportunities for Communication and Modeling of Health and Safety Education for Parents/Guardians
2.4.3.2	2.057/2.066/2.067	Parent/Guardian Education Plan

Chapter 3		
3rd Ed. #	**2nd Ed. #**	**3rd Ed. Standard Title**
3.1.1.1	3.001	Conduct of Daily Health Check
3.1.1.2	3.002	Documentation of the Daily Health Check
3.1.2.1	3.003	Routine Health Supervision and Growth Monitoring
3.1.3.1	New	Active Opportunities for Physical Activity
3.1.3.2	2.009	Playing Outdoors
3.1.3.3	New	Protection From Air Pollution While Children Are Outside
3.1.3.4	New	Caregivers'/Teachers' Encouragement of Physical Activity
3.1.4.1	5.143/5.146	Safe Sleep Practices and SIDS/Suffocation Risk Reduction

Chapter 3		
3rd Ed. #	**2nd Ed. #**	**3rd Ed. Standard Title**
3.1.4.2	New	Swaddling
3.1.4.3	New	Pacifier Use
3.1.4.4	3.008	Scheduled Rest Periods and Sleep Arrangements
3.1.4.5	3.009	Unscheduled Access to Rest Areas
3.1.5.1	3.010	Routine Oral Hygiene Activities
3.1.5.2	5.095	Toothbrushes and Toothpaste
3.1.5.3	3.011	Oral Health Education
3.2.1.1	3.012	Type of Diapers Worn
3.2.1.2	3.018	Handling Cloth Diapers
3.2.1.3	3.013	Checking for the Need to Change Diapers
3.2.1.4	3.014	Diaper Changing Procedure
3.2.1.5	New	Procedure for Changing Children's Soiled Underwear/Pull-Ups and Clothing
3.2.2.1	3.020	Situations that Require Hand Hygiene
3.2.2.2	3.021	Handwashing Procedure
3.2.2.3	3.022	Assisting Children with Hand Hygiene
3.2.2.4	3.023	Training and Monitoring for Hand Hygiene
3.2.2.5	New	Hand Sanitizers
3.2.3.1	3.024	Procedure for Nasal Secretions and Use of Nasal Bulb Syringes
3.2.3.2	New	Cough and Sneeze Etiquette
3.2.3.3	3.025	Cuts and Scrapes
3.2.3.4	3.026	Prevention of Exposure to Blood and Body Fluids
3.3.0.1	3.028	Routine Cleaning, Sanitizing, and Disinfecting
3.3.0.2	3.036	Cleaning and Sanitizing Toys
3.3.0.3	3.037	Cleaning and Sanitizing Objects Intended for the Mouth
3.3.0.4	3.039	Cleaning Individual Bedding
3.3.0.5	3.040	Cleaning Crib Surfaces
3.4.1.1	2.035/3.041	Use of Tobacco, Alcohol, and Illegal Drugs
3.4.2.1	3.042	Animals that Might Have Contact with Children and Adults
3.4.2.2	3.043	Prohibited Animals
3.4.2.3	3.044	Care for Animals
3.4.3.1	3.048	Emergency Procedures
3.4.3.2	3.051	Use of Fire Extinguishers
3.4.3.3	3.052	Response to Fire and Burns
3.4.4.1	3.053/3.054/3.056	Recognizing and Reporting Suspected Child Abuse, Neglect, and Exploitation
3.4.4.2	3.055	Immunity for Reporters of Child Abuse and Neglect
3.4.4.3	New	Preventing and Identifying Shaken Baby Syndrome/Abusive Head Trauma
3.4.4.4	3.057	Care for Children Who Have Been Abused/Neglected
3.4.4.5	3.059	Facility Layout to Reduce Risk of Child Abuse and Neglect
3.4.5.1	New	Sun Safety Including Sunscreen
3.4.5.2	New	Insect Repellent - Protection From Vector Borne Diseases
3.4.6.1	5.160	Strangulation Hazards
3.5.0.1	3.049	Care Plan for Children with Special Health Care Needs
3.5.0.2	1.044/3.063/3.066	Caring for Children Who Require Medical Procedures
3.6.1.1	3.065/3.068	Inclusion/Exclusion/Dismissal of Children

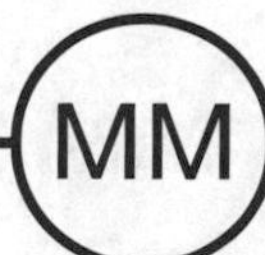

Chapter 3		
3rd Ed. #	**2nd Ed. #**	**3rd Ed. Standard Title**
3.6.1.2	3.069	Staff Exclusion for Illness
3.6.1.3	New	Thermometers for Taking Human Temperatures
3.6.1.4	3.067	Infectious Disease Outbreak Control
3.6.1.5	5.094	Sharing of Personal Articles Prohibited
3.6.2.1	3.079/8.012	Exclusion and Alternative Care for Children Who Are Ill
3.6.2.2	3.070/3.080	Space Requirements for Care of Children Who Are Ill
3.6.2.3	3.071	Qualifications of Directors of Facilities that Care for Children Who Are Ill
3.6.2.4	3.072	Program Requirements for Facilities that Care for Children Who Are Ill
3.6.2.5	3.073	Caregiver/Teacher Qualifications for Facilities that Care for Children Who Are Ill
3.6.2.6	3.074	Child-Staff Ratios for Facilities that Care for Children Who Are Ill
3.6.2.7	3.075	Child Care Health Consultants for Facilities that Care for Children Who Are Ill
3.6.2.8	3.076/3.064/9.005	Licensing of Facilities that Care for Children Who Are Ill
3.6.2.9	3.077	Information Required for Children Who Are Ill
3.6.2.10	3.078	Inclusion and Exclusion of Children From Facilities that Serve Children Who Are Ill
3.6.3.1	3.081	Medication Administration
3.6.3.2	3.082	Labeling, Storage, and Disposal of Medications
3.6.3.3	3.083	Training of Caregivers/Teachers to Administer Medication
3.6.4.1	3.084	Procedure for Parent/Guardian Notification About Exposure of Children to Infectious Disease
3.6.4.2	3.085	Infectious Diseases that Require Parent/Guardian Notification
3.6.4.3	3.086	Notification of the Facility About Infectious Disease or Other Problems by Parents
3.6.4.4	3.087	List of Excludable and Reportable Conditions for Parents
3.6.4.5	3.089	Death
Chapter 4		
3rd Ed. #	**2nd Ed. #**	**3rd Ed. Standard Title**
4.1	4.1	Introduction
4.2.0.1	4.001	Written Nutrition Plan
4.2.0.2	3.004	Assessment and Planning of Nutrition for Individual Children
4.2.0.3	4.002	Use of USDA - CACFP Guidelines
4.2.0.4	4.004	Categories of Foods
4.2.0.5	4.003	Meal and Snack Patterns
4.2.0.6	4.006/5.136	Availability of Drinking Water
4.2.0.7	4.005	100% Fruit Juice
4.2.0.8	4.007/4.009	Feeding Plans and Dietary Modifications
4.2.0.9	4.008	Written Menus and Introduction of New Foods
4.2.0.10	4.010	Care for Children with Food Allergies
4.2.0.11	New	Ingestion of Substances that Do Not Provide Nutrition
4.2.0.12	New	Vegetarian/Vegan Diets
4.3.1.1	4.011/4.038	General Plan for Feeding Infants
4.3.1.2	4.013	Feeding Infants on Cue by a Consistent Caregiver/Teacher
4.3.1.3	4.015	Preparing, Feeding, and Storing Human Milk
4.3.1.4	3.027	Feeding Human Milk to Another Mother's Child
4.3.1.5	4.016/4.017	Preparing, Feeding, and Storing Infant Formula
4.3.1.6	New	Use of Soy-Based Formula and Soy Milk

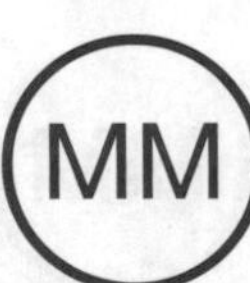

Chapter 4		
3rd Ed. #	**2nd Ed. #**	**3rd Ed. Standard Title**
4.3.1.7	4.020	Feeding Cow's Milk
4.3.1.8	4.014	Techniques for Bottle Feeding
4.3.1.9	4.018	Warming Bottles and Infant Foods
4.3.1.10	4.019	Cleaning and Sanitizing Equipment Used for Bottle Feeding
4.3.1.11	4.012	Introduction of Age-Appropriate Solid Foods to Infants
4.3.1.12	4.021	Feeding Age-Appropriate Solid Foods to Infants
4.3.2.1	4.022	Meal and Snack Patterns for Toddlers and Preschoolers
4.3.2.2	4.023	Serving Size for Toddlers and Preschoolers
4.3.2.3	4.024	Encouraging Self-Feeding by Older Infants and Toddlers
4.3.3.1	4.025	Meal and Snack Patterns for School-Age Children
4.4.0.1	4.026	Food Service Staff by Type of Facility and Food Service
4.4.0.2	4.027	Use of Nutritionist/Registered Dietitian
4.5.0.1	4.028	Developmentally Appropriate Seating and Utensils for Meals
4.5.0.2	4.029	Tableware and Feeding Utensils
4.5.0.3	4.030	Activities that Are Incompatible with Eating
4.5.0.4	4.031	Socialization During Meals
4.5.0.5	4.035	Numbers of Children Fed Simultaneously by One Adult
4.5.0.6	4.036	Adult Supervision of Children Who Are Learning to Feed themselves
4.5.0.7	4.032	Participation of Older Children and Staff in Mealtime Activities
4.5.0.8	4.033	Experience with Familiar and New Foods
4.5.0.9	4.034	Hot Liquids and Foods
4.5.0.10	4.037	Foods that Are Choking Hazards
4.5.0.11	4.039	Prohibited Uses of Food
4.6.0.1	4.040	Selection and Preparation of Food Brought From Home
4.6.0.2	4.041	Nutritional Quality of Food Brought From Home
4.7.0.1	4.069	Nutrition Learning Experiences for Children
4.7.0.2	4.070	Nutrition Education for Parents/Guardians
4.8.0.1	4.042	Food Preparation Area
4.8.0.2	4.043	Design of Food Service Equipment
4.8.0.3	4.044	Maintenance of Food Service Surfaces and Equipment
4.8.0.4	4.045	Food Preparation Sinks
4.8.0.5	4.046	Handwashing Sink Separate From Food Zones
4.8.0.6	4.047	Maintaining Safe Food Temperatures
4.8.0.7	4.048	Ventilation Over Cooking Surfaces
4.8.0.8	4.049	Microwave Ovens
4.9.0.1	4.050	Compliance with U.S. Food and Drug Administration Food Sanitation Standards, State and Local Rules
4.9.0.2	4.051	Staff Restricted From Food Preparation and Handling
4.9.0.3	4.052	Precautions for a Safe Food Supply
4.9.0.4	4.053	Leftovers
4.9.0.5	4.054	Preparation for and Storage of Food in the Refrigerator
4.9.0.6	4.056	Storage of Foods Not Requiring Refrigeration
4.9.0.7	4.057	Storage of Dry Bulk Foods
4.9.0.8	4.058	Supply of Food and Water for Disasters

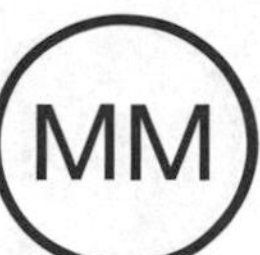

Chapter 4		
3rd Ed. #	**2nd Ed. #**	**3rd Ed. Standard Title**
4.9.0.9	4.055/4.061	Cleaning Food Areas and Equipment
4.9.0.10	4.062	Cutting Boards
4.9.0.11	4.063	Dishwashing in Centers
4.9.0.12	4.064	Dishwashing in Small and Large Family Child Care Homes
4.9.0.13	4.065	Method for Washing Dishes by Hand
4.10.0.1	4.066	Approved Off-Site Food Services
4.10.0.2	4.067	Food Safety During Transport
4.10.0.3	4.068	Holding of Food Prepared At Off-Site Food Service Facilities
Chapter 5		
3rd Ed. #	**2nd Ed. #**	**3rd Ed. Standard Title**
5.1.1.1	5.001	Location of Center
5.1.1.2	5.002	Inspection of Buildings
5.1.1.3	5.003	Compliance with Fire Prevention Code
5.1.1.4	5.004	Accessibility of Facility
5.1.1.5	5.005/5.109/ 5.169/5.179	Environmental Audit of Site Location
5.1.1.6	5.006	Structurally Sound Facility
5.1.1.7	5.007	Use of Basements and Below Grade Areas
5.1.1.8	5.008	Buildings of Wood Frame Construction
5.1.1.9	5.009	Unrelated Business in a Child Care Area
5.1.1.10	5.010	Office Space
5.1.1.11	5.011	Separation of Operations From Child Care Areas
5.1.1.12	5.012/5.142	Multiple Use of Rooms
5.1.2.1	5.112	Space Required Per Child
5.1.2.2	5.113	Floor Space Beneath Low Ceiling Heights
5.1.2.3	5.115	Areas for School-Age Children
5.1.3.1	5.013	Weather-Tightness and Water-Tightness of Openings
5.1.3.2	5.014	Possibility of Exit From Windows
5.1.3.3	5.015	Screens for Ventilation Openings
5.1.3.4	5.016	Safety Guards for Glass Windows/Doors
5.1.3.5	5.017	Finger-Pinch Protection Devices
5.1.3.6	5.018	Directional Swing of Indoor Doors
5.1.4.1	5.020	Alternate Exits and Emergency Shelter
5.1.4.2	5.021	Evacuation of Children with Special Health Care Needs and Children with Disabilities
5.1.4.3	5.022/5.019	Path of Egress
5.1.4.4	5.023	Locks
5.1.4.5	5.156	Closet Door Latches
5.1.4.6	5.024	Labeled Emergency Exits
5.1.4.7	5.025	Access to Exits
5.1.5.1	5.222	Balusters
5.1.5.2	5.223	Handrails
5.1.5.3	5.224	Landings
5.1.5.4	5.225	Guards At Stairway Access Openings
5.1.6.1	5.219	Designated Walkways, Bike Routes, and Drop-Off and Pick-Up Points

Chapter 5		
3rd Ed. #	**2nd Ed. #**	**3rd Ed. Standard Title**
5.1.6.2	5.220	Construction and Maintenance of Walkways
5.1.6.3	5.190	Drainage of Paved Surfaces
5.1.6.4	5.191/5.192	Walking Surfaces
5.1.6.5	5.193	Areas Used by Children for Wheeled Vehicles
5.1.6.6	5.221	Guardrails and Protective Barriers
5.1.6.7	5.167	Location of Satellite Dishes
5.2.1.1	5.027	Fresh Air
5.2.1.2	5.028	Indoor Temperature
5.2.1.3	5.032/5.036/5.229	Heating and Ventilation Equipment Inspection and Maintenance
5.2.1.4	5.029	Ventilation When Using Art Materials
5.2.1.5	5.108	Ventilation of Recently Carpeted or Paneled Areas
5.2.1.6	3.032	Ventilation to Control Odors
5.2.1.7	5.030	Electric Fans
5.2.1.8	5.031	Maintenance of Air Filters
5.2.1.9	5.033	Type and Placement of Room thermometers
5.2.1.10	5.034	Gas, Oil or Kerosene Heaters, Generators, Portable Gas Stoves, and Charcoal and Gas Grills
5.2.1.11	5.035	Portable Electric Space Heaters
5.2.1.12	5.038	Fireplaces, Fireplace Inserts, and Wood/Corn Pellet Stoves
5.2.1.13	5.037/5.039	Barriers/Guards for Heating Equipment and Units
5.2.1.14	5.040	Water Heating Devices and Temperatures Allowed
5.2.1.15	5.041	Maintenance of Humidifiers and Dehumidifiers
5.2.2.1	5.042	Levels of Illumination
5.2.2.2	5.043	Light Fixtures Including Halogen Lamps
5.2.2.3	5.044	High Intensity Discharge Lamps, Multi-Vapor, and Mercury Lamps
5.2.2.4	5.045	Emergency Lighting
5.2.3.1	5.046	Noise Levels
5.2.4.1	5.047	Electrical Service
5.2.4.2	5.048	Safety Covers and Shock Protection Devices for Electrical Outlets
5.2.4.3	5.049	Ground-Fault Circuit-Interrupter for Outlets Near Water
5.2.4.4	5.050	Location of Electrical Devices Near Water
5.2.4.5	5.051	Extension Cords
5.2.4.6	5.052	Electrical Cords
5.2.5.1	5.053	Smoke Detection Systems and Smoke Alarms
5.2.5.2	5.054	Portable Fire Extinguishers
5.2.6.1	5.055	Water Supply
5.2.6.2	5.059	Testing of Drinking Water Not From Public System
5.2.6.3	5.061/5.138	Testing for Lead and Copper Levels in Drinking Water
5.2.6.4	5.062	Water Test Results
5.2.6.5	5.063	Emergency Safe Drinking Water and Bottled Water
5.2.6.6	5.056	Water Handling and Treatment Equipment
5.2.6.7	5.057	Cross-Connections
5.2.6.8	5.058	Installation of Pipes and Plumbing Fixtures
5.2.6.9	5.060	Handwashing Sink Using Portable Water Supply

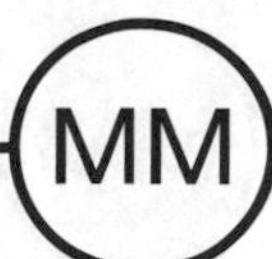

Chapter 5		
3rd Ed. #	**2nd Ed. #**	**3rd Ed. Standard Title**
5.2.6.10	5.137	Drinking Fountains
5.2.7.1	5.064	On-Site Sewage Systems
5.2.7.2	5.065	Removal of Garbage
5.2.7.3	4.059/5.066	Containment of Garbage
5.2.7.4	5.067	Containment of Soiled Diapers
5.2.7.5	5.068	Labeling, Cleaning, and Disposal of Waste and Diaper Containers
5.2.7.6	5.069	Storage and Disposal of Infectious and Toxic Wastes
5.2.8.1	5.070/5.071/ 5.072/5.073	Integrated Pest Management
5.2.8.2	5.202	Insect Breeding Hazard
5.2.9.1	4.060/5.100	Use and Storage of Toxic Substances
5.2.9.2	5.101	Use of a Poison Center
5.2.9.3	5.102	Informing Staff Regarding Presence of Toxic Substances
5.2.9.4	5.103	Radon Concentrations
5.2.9.5	New	Carbon Monoxide Detectors
5.2.9.6	5.104/5.109	Preventing Exposure to Asbestos or Other Friable Materials
5.2.9.7	5.105	Proper Use of Art and Craft Materials
5.2.9.8	New	Use of Play Dough and Other Manipulative Art or Sensory Materials
5.2.9.9	New	Plastic Containers and Toys
5.2.9.10	5.106	Prohibition of Poisonous Plants
5.2.9.11	5.107	Chemicals Used to Control Odors
5.2.9.12	New	Treatment of CCA Pressure-Treated Wood
5.2.9.13	5.110	Testing for Lead
5.2.9.14	3.035	Shoes in Infant Play Areas
5.2.9.15	5.111	Construction and Remodeling During Hours of Operation
5.3.1.1	5.075	Safety of Equipment, Materials, and Furnishings
5.3.1.2	New	Product Recall Monitoring
5.3.1.3	5.076	Size of Furniture
5.3.1.4	3.034/5.077/5.195	Surfaces of Equipment, Furniture, Toys, and Play Materials
5.3.1.5	5.078	Placement of Equipment and Furnishings
5.3.1.6	5.079/5.026	Floors, Walls, and Ceilings
5.3.1.7	5.080	Facility Arrangements to Minimize Back Injuries
5.3.1.8	5.081	High Chair Requirements
5.3.1.9	5.082	Carriage, Stroller, Gate, Enclosure, and Play Yard Requirements
5.3.1.10	5.083	Restrictive Infant Equipment Requirements
5.3.1.11	New	Exercise Equipment
5.3.1.12	2.038/5.084	Availability and Use of a Telephone or Wireless Communication Device
5.3.2.1	5.097	Therapeutic and Recreational Equipment
5.3.2.2	5.098	Special Adaptive Equipment
5.3.2.3	5.152	Storage for Adaptive Equipment
5.3.2.4	5.099	Orthotic and Prosthetic Devices
5.4.1.1	5.116	General Requirements for Toilet and Handwashing Areas
5.4.1.2	5.117/5.120	Location of Toilets and Privacy Issues
5.4.1.3	5.118	Ability to Open Toilet Room Doors

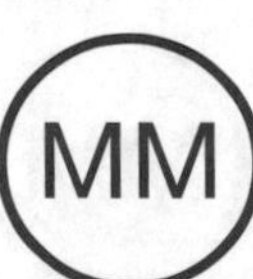

Chapter 5		
3rd Ed. #	**2nd Ed. #**	**3rd Ed. Standard Title**
5.4.1.4	5.119	Preventing Entry to Toilet Rooms by Infants and Toddlers
5.4.1.5	5.121	Chemical Toilets
5.4.1.6	5.122/5.123	Ratios of Toilets, Urinals, and Hand Sinks to Children
5.4.1.7	3.029/5.124	Toilet Learning/Training Equipment
5.4.1.8	3.030	Equipment Used for Cleaning and Disinfecting Toileting Equipment
5.4.1.9	5.125/3.033	Waste Receptacles in the Child Care Facility and Child Care Facility Toilet Room(s)
5.4.1.10	5.126	Handwashing Sinks
5.4.1.11	5.127	Prohibited Uses of Handwashing Sinks
5.4.1.12	5.128	Mop Sinks
5.4.2.1	5.129	Diaper Changing Tables
5.4.2.2	5.130	Handwashing Sinks for Diaper Changing Areas in Centers
5.4.2.3	5.131	Handwashing Sinks for Diaper Changing Areas in Homes
5.4.2.4	3.015/3.016/ 3.017/5.132	Use, Location, and Setup of Diaper Changing Areas
5.4.2.5	5.133	Changing Table Requirements
5.4.2.6	3.019	Maintenance of Changing Tables
5.4.3.1	5.134	Ratio and Location of Bathtubs and Showers
5.4.3.2	5.135	Safety of Bathtubs and Showers
5.4.4.1	5.140	Laundry Service and Equipment
5.4.4.2	5.141	Location of Laundry Equipment and Water Temperature for Laundering
5.4.5.1	5.144	Sleeping Equipment and Supplies
5.4.5.2	5.145	Cribs
5.4.5.3	New	Stackable Cribs
5.4.5.4	5.147	Futons
5.4.5.5	5.148	Bunk Beds
5.4.6.1	5.149	Space for Children Who Are Ill
5.4.6.2	5.150	Space for therapy Services
5.5.0.1	5.151	Storage and Labeling of Personal Articles
5.5.0.2	5.153	Coat Hooks/Cubicles
5.5.0.3	5.154	Storage of Play and Teaching Equipment and Supplies
5.5.0.4	5.155	Storage for Soiled and Clean Linens
5.5.0.5	5.158	Storage of Flammable Materials
5.5.0.6	5.157	Inaccessibility to Matches, Candles and Lighters
5.5.0.7	5.159	Storage of Plastic Bags
5.5.0.8	5.161	Firearms
5.6.0.1	2.038/5.093/5.237	First Aid and Emergency Supplies
5.6.0.2	5.139	Single Service Cups
5.6.0.3	5.096	Supplies for Bathrooms and Handwashing Sinks
5.6.0.4	3.031	Microfiber Cloths, Rags, and Disposable Towels and Mops Used for Cleaning
5.7.0.1	5.226	Maintenance of Exterior Surfaces
5.7.0.2	5.194	Removal of Hazards From Outdoor Areas
5.7.0.3	5.227	Removal of Allergen Triggering Materials From Outdoor Areas
5.7.0.4	5.086	Inaccessibility of Hazardous Equipment
5.7.0.5	5.228	Cleaning Schedule for Exterior Areas

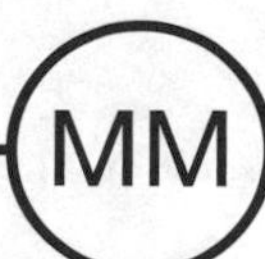

Chapter 5		
3rd Ed. #	**2nd Ed. #**	**3rd Ed. Standard Title**
5.7.0.6	5.230	Storage Area Maintenance and Ventilation
5.7.0.7	5.231	Structure Maintenance
5.7.0.8	5.232	Electrical Fixtures and Outlets Maintenance
5.7.0.9	5.233	Plumbing and Gas Maintenance
5.7.0.10	5.234	Cleaning of Humidifiers and Related Equipment
Chapter 6		
3rd Ed. #	**2nd Ed. #**	**3rd Ed. Standard Title**
6.1.0.1	5.162	Size and Location of Outdoor Play Area
6.1.0.2	5.163	Size and Requirements of Indoor Play Area
6.1.0.3	5.165	Rooftops an Play Areas
6.1.0.4	5.166	Elevated Play Areas
6.1.0.5	5.168	Visibility of Outdoor Play Area
6.1.0.6	5.176	Location of Play Areas Near Bodies of Water
6.1.0.7	5.173/5.177	Shading of Play Area
6.1.0.8	5.178	Enclosures for Outdoor Play Areas
6.2.1.1	5.085/5.195	Play Equipment Requirements
6.2.1.2	5.187	Play Equipment and Surfaces Meet Ada Requirements
6.2.1.3	5.181	Design of Play Equipment
6.2.1.4	5.182	Installation of Play Equipment
6.2.1.5	5.188	Play Equipment Connecting and Linking Devices
6.2.1.6	5.189	Size and Anchoring of Crawl Spaces
6.2.1.7	5.184	Enclosure of Moving Parts on Play Equipment
6.2.1.8	5.185	Material Defects and Edges on Play Equipment
6.2.1.9	5.186	Entrapment Hazards of Play Equipment
6.2.2.1	5.172	Use Zone for Fixed Play Equipment
6.2.2.2	5.174	Arrangement of Play Equipment
6.2.2.3	5.175	Location of Moving Play Equipment
6.2.2.4	5.170	Clearance Requirements of Playground Areas
6.2.2.5	5.171	Clearance Space for Swings
6.2.3.1	5.183	Prohibited Surfaces for Placing Climbing Equipment
6.2.4.1	5.180	Sandboxes
6.2.4.2	5.091	Water Play Tables
6.2.4.3	New	Sensory Table Materials
6.2.4.4	New	Trampolines
6.2.4.5	New	Ball Pits
6.2.5.1	3.038/5.196/5.160	Inspection of Indoor and Outdoor Play Areas and Equipment
6.2.5.2	5.197	Inspection of Play Area Surfacing
6.3.1.1	5.198	Enclosure of Bodies of Water
6.3.1.2	5.199	Accessibility to Above-Ground Pools
6.3.1.3	5.200	Sensors or Remote Monitors
6.3.1.4	5.201	Safety Covers for Swimming Pools
6.3.1.5	5.203	Deck Surface
6.3.1.6	5.205	Pool Drain Covers
6.3.1.7	5.215	Pool Safety Rules

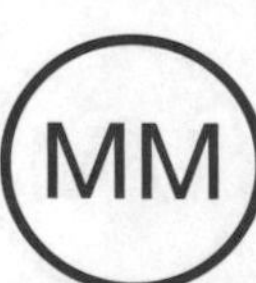

Chapter 6		
3rd Ed. #	**2nd Ed. #**	**3rd Ed. Standard Title**
6.3.1.8	5.206	Supervision of Pool Pump
6.3.2.1	5.208	Lifesaving Equipment
6.3.2.2	5.209	Lifeline in Pool
6.3.2.3	5.210	Pool Equipment and Chemical Storage Rooms
6.3.3.1	5.204	Pool Performance Requirements
6.3.3.2	5.214	Construction, Maintenance, and Inspection of Pools
6.3.3.3	5.207	Electrical Safety for Pool Areas
6.3.3.4	5.218	Pool Water Temperature
6.3.4.1	5.216	Pool Water Quality
6.3.4.2	5.217	Chlorine Pucks
6.3.5.1	5.211	Hot Tubs, Spas, and Saunas
6.3.5.2	5.212	Water in Containers
6.3.5.3	5.213	Portable Wading Pools
6.4.1.1	3.047	Pool Toys
6.4.1.2	5.087	Inaccessibility of Toys or Objects to Children Under Three Years of Age
6.4.1.3	5.088	Crib Toys
6.4.1.4	5.090	Projectile Toys
6.4.1.5	5.089	Balloons
6.4.2.1	5.092	Riding Toys with Wheels and Wheeled Equipment
6.4.2.2	5.242	Helmets
6.4.2.3	5.241	Bike Routes
6.5.1.1	2.029	Competence and Training of Transportation Staff
6.5.1.2	2.030	Qualifications for Drivers
6.5.2.1	2.032	Drop-Off and Pick-Up
6.5.2.2	2.033/5.236	Child Passenger Safety
6.5.2.3	2.037	Child Behavior During Transportation
6.5.2.4	5.238	Interior Temperature of Vehicles
6.5.2.5	2.036	Distractions While Driving
6.5.2.6	2.031	Route to Emergency Medical Services
6.5.3.1	New	Passenger Vans
Chapter 7		
3rd Ed. #	**2nd Ed. #**	**3rd Ed. Standard Title**
7.1	New	Introduction
7.2.0.1	3.005	Immunization Documentation
7.2.0.2	3.006	Unimmunized Children
7.2.0.3	3.007	Immunization of Caregivers/Teachers
7.3.1.1	6.012	Exclusion for Group a Streptococcal (Gas) Infections
7.3.1.2	6.013	Informing Caregivers/Teachers of Group a Streptococcal (Gas) Infection
7.3.2.1	6.001	Immunization for *Haemophilus Influenzae* Type B (Hib)
7.3.2.2	6.002	Informing Parents/Guardians of *Haemophilus Influenzae* Type B (Hib) Exposure
7.3.2.3	6.003	Informing Public Health Authorities of Invasive *Haemophilus Influenzae* Type B Cases
7.3.3.1	New	Influenza Immunizations for Children and Caregivers/Teachers
7.3.3.2	New	Influenza Control
7.3.3.3	New	Influenza Prevention Education

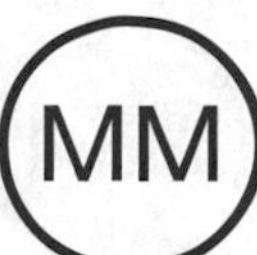

Chapter 7		
3rd Ed. #	**2nd Ed. #**	**3rd Ed. Standard Title**
7.3.4.1	New	Mumps
7.3.5.1	6.007/6.008	Recommended Control Measures for Invasive Meningococcal Infection in Child Care
7.3.5.2	6.006	Informing Public Health Authorities of Meningococcal Infections
7.3.6.1	6.016	Attendance of Children with Erythema Infectiosum (EI) (Parvovirus B19)
7.3.7.1	6.009	Informing Public Health Authorities of Pertussis Cases
7.3.7.2	6.010	Prophylactic Treatment for Pertussis
7.3.7.3	6.011	Exclusion for Pertussis
7.3.8.1	New	Attendance of Children with Respiratory Syncytial Virus (RSV) Respiratory Tract Infection
7.3.9.1	6.004	Immunization with *Streptococcus Pneumoniae* Conjugate Vaccine (PCV13)
7.3.9.2	6.005	Informing Public Health Authorities of Invasive *Streptococcus Pneumoniae*
7.3.10.1	6.014	Measures for Detection, Control, and Reporting of Tuberculosis
7.3.10.2	6.015	Attendance of Children with Latent Tuberculosis Infection or Active Tuberculosis Disease
7.3.11.1	6.017	Attendance of Children with Unspecified Respiratory Tract Infection
7.4.0.1	6.023	Control of Enteric (Diarrheal) and Hepatitis a Virus (HAV) Infections
7.4.0.2	6.024	Staff Education and Policies on Enteric (Diarrheal) and Hepatitis a Virus (Hav) Infections
7.4.0.3	6.025	Disease Surveillance of Enteric (Diarrheal) and Hepatitis a Virus (HAV) Infections
7.4.0.4	6.026	Maintenance of Records on Incidents of Diarrhea
7.5.1.1	New	Conjunctivitis
7.5.2.1	New	Enterovirus Infections
7.5.3.1	New	Human Papillomaviruses (HPV) (Warts)
7.5.4.1	New	Impetigo
7.5.5.1	New	Lymphadenitis
7.5.6.1	New	Immunization for Measles
7.5.7.1	New	Molluscum Contagiosum
7.5.8.1	6.038	Attendance of Children with Head Lice
7.5.9.1	6.039	Attendance of Children with Ringworm
7.5.10.1	New	*Staphylococcus Aureus* Skin Infections Including MRSA
7.5.11.1	6.037	Attendance of Children with Scabies
7.5.12.1	New	Thrush (Candidiasis)
7.6.1.1	6.027	Disease Recognition and Control of Hepatitis B Virus (HBV) Infection
7.6.1.2	6.028	Observation and Follow-Up of a Child Who Is an Hepatitis B Virus (HBV) Carrier
7.6.1.3	6.029	Staff Education on Prevention of Bloodborne Diseases
7.6.1.4	6.030	Informing Public Health Authorities of Hepatitis B Virus (HBV) Cases
7.6.1.5	6.031	Handling Injuries to a Hepatitis B Virus (HBV) Carrier
7.6.2.1	6.032	Infection Control Measures with Hepatitis C Virus (HCV)
7.6.3.1	6.033	Attendance of Children with HIV
7.6.3.2	6.034	Protecting HIV-Infected Children and Adults in Child Care
7.6.3.3	6.035	Staff Education About Preventing Transmission of HIV Infection
7.6.3.4	6.036	Ability of Caregivers/Teachers with HIV Infection to Care for Children
7.7.1.1	6.021	Staff Education and Policies on Cytomegalovirus (CMV)
7.7.1.2	6.022	Testing of Children with Cytomegalovirus (CMV)
7.7.2.1	6.018	Disease Recognition and Control of Herpes Simplex Virus
7.7.3.1	New	Roseola
7.7.4.1	6.019	Staff and Parent/Guardian Notification About Varicella-Zoster (Chickenpox) Virus

Chapter 7		
3rd Ed. #	**2nd Ed. #**	**3rd Ed. Standard Title**
7.7.4.2	6.020	Exclusion of Children with Varicella-Zoster (Chickenpox) Virus
7.8	New	Interaction with State or Local Health Departments
7.9	Reader's Note	Note to Reader on Judicious Use of Antibiotics
Chapter 8		
3rd Ed. #	**2nd Ed. #**	**3rd Ed. Standard Title**
8.1	8.1	Introduction
8.2.0.1	7.001	Inclusion in All Activities
8.2.0.2	7.002	Planning for Inclusion
8.3.0.1	7.003	Initial Assessment of the Child to Determine His or Her Special Needs
8.4.0.1	7.004	Determining the Type and Frequency of Services
8.4.0.2	7.005	Formulation of an Action Plan
8.4.0.3	7.006	Determination of Eligibility for Special Services
8.4.0.4	7.007	Designation and Role of Staff Person Responsible for Coordinating Care in the Child Care Facility
8.4.0.5	7.008	Development of Measurable Objectives
8.4.0.6	7.009	Contracts and Reimbursement
8.5.0.1	2.058/7.010	Coordinating and Documenting Services
8.5.0.2	7.011	Written Reports on IFSPs/IEPs to Caregivers/Teachers
8.6.0.1	7.012	Reevaluation Process
8.6.0.2	7.013	Statement of Program Needs and Plans
8.7.0.1	7.014	Facility Self-Assessment
8.7.0.2	7.015	Technical Assistance in Developing Plan
8.7.0.3	7.016	Review of Plan for Serving Children with Disabilities or Children with Special Health Care Needs
Chapter 9		
3rd Ed. #	**2nd Ed. #**	**3rd Ed. Standard Title**
9.1.0.1	8.001	Governing Body of the Facility
9.1.0.2	8.002	Written Delegation of Administrative Authority
9.2.1.1	8.004	Content of Policies
9.2.1.2	8.040	Review and Communication of Written Policies
9.2.1.3	8.005	Enrollment Information to Parents/Guardians and Caregivers/Teachers
9.2.1.4	8.007	Exchange of Information Upon Enrollment
9.2.1.5	8.006	Nondiscriminatory Policy
9.2.1.6	1.053/2.041/ 8.008/8.010	Written Discipline Policies
9.2.2.1	8.018	Planning for Child's Transition to New Services
9.2.2.2	8.019	Format for the Transition Plan
9.2.2.3	8.043	Exchange of Information At Transitions
9.2.3.1	New	Policies and Practices that Promote Physical Activity
9.2.3.2	8.011	Content and Development of the Plan for Care of Children and Staff Who Are Ill
9.2.3.3	3.088	Written Policy for Reporting Notifiable Diseases to the Health Department
9.2.3.4	8.013	Written Policy for Obtaining Preventive Health Service Information
9.2.3.5	8.014	Documentation of Exemptions and Exclusion of Children Who Lack Immunizations
9.2.3.6	2.053/8.015/ 8.053/8.055	Identification of Child's Medical Home and Parental Consent for Information Exchange
9.2.3.7	8.016	Information Sharing on therapies and Treatments Needed

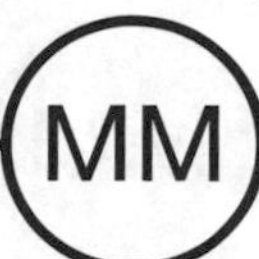

Chapter 9		
3rd Ed. #	**2nd Ed. #**	**3rd Ed. Standard Title**
9.2.3.8	8.017	Information Sharing on Family Health
9.2.3.9	8.021	Written Policy on Use of Medications
9.2.3.10	8.034	Sanitation Policies and Procedures
9.2.3.11	8.035	Food and Nutrition Service Policies and Plans
9.2.3.12	8.036	Infant Feeding Policy
9.2.3.13	8.037	Plans for Evening and Nighttime Child Care
9.2.3.14	New	Oral Health Policy
9.2.3.15	2.035/8.038	Policies Prohibiting Smoking, Tobacco, Alcohol, Illegal Drugs, and Toxic Substances
9.2.3.16	8.039	Policy Prohibiting Firearms
9.2.3.17	8.041	Child Care Health Consultant's Review of Health Policies
9.2.4.1	8.022	Written Plan and Training for Handling Urgent Medical Care or Threatening Incidents
9.2.4.2	8.023	Review of Written Plan for Urgent Care
9.2.4.3	8.024	Disaster Planning, Training and Communication
9.2.4.4	New	Written Plan for Seasonal and Pandemic Influenza
9.2.4.5	8.025/ 8.027	Emergency and Evacuation Drills/Exercises Policy
9.2.4.6	8.026	Use of Daily Roster During Evacuation Drills
9.2.4.7	New	Sign-In/Sign-Out System
9.2.4.8	8.028	Authorized Persons to Pick Up Child
9.2.4.9	8.029	Policy on Actions to Be Followed When No Authorized Person Arrives to Pick Up a Child
9.2.4.10	8.030/8.059	Documentation of Drop-Off, Pick-Up, and Daily Attendance of Child, and Parent/Provider Communication
9.2.5.1	2.034/5.235/5.239/ 5.240/8.031	Transportation Policy for Centers and Large Family Homes
9.2.5.2	2.034/5.235/5.239/ 5.240/8.032	Transportation Policy for Small Family Child Care Homes
9.2.6.1	8.033	Policy on Use and Maintenance of Play Areas
9.2.6.2	8.072	Reports of Annual Audits/Monthly Maintenance Checks of Play Areas and Equipment
9.2.6.3	8.071	Records of Proper Installation and Maintenance of Facility Equipment
9.3.0.1	8.044	Written Human Resource Management Policies for Centers and Large Family Child Care Homes
9.3.0.2	New	Written Human Resource Management Policies for Small Family Child Care Homes
9.4.1.1	8.070	Facility Insurance Coverage
9.4.1.2	8.076	Maintenance of Records
9.4.1.3	8.054	Written Policy on Confidentiality of Records
9.4.1.4	8.003	Access to Facility Records
9.4.1.5	8.057	Availability of Records to Licensing Agency
9.4.1.6	8.077	Availability of Documents to Parents/Guardians
9.4.1.7	8.078	Requirements for Compliance of Contract Services
9.4.1.8	8.061	Records of Illness
9.4.1.9	8.062	Records of Injury
9.4.1.10	8.063	Documentation of Parent/Guardian Notification of Injury, Illness or Death in Program
9.4.1.11	8.064	Review and Accessibility of Injury and Illness Reports
9.4.1.12	8.065	Record of Valid License, Certificate or Registration of Facility
9.4.1.13	8.066	Maintenance and Display of Inspection Reports
9.4.1.14	8.067	Written Plan/Record to Resolve Deficiencies
9.4.1.15	8.068	Availability of Reports on Inspections of Fire Protection Devices

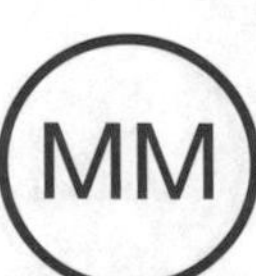

Chapter 9		
3rd Ed. #	**2nd Ed. #**	**3rd Ed. Standard Title**
9.4.1.16	8.069	Evacuation and Shelter-In-Place Drill Record
9.4.1.17	8.073	Documentation of Child Care Health Consultation/Training Visits
9.4.1.18	8.074	Records of Nutrition Service
9.4.1.19	2.055/2.056/8.075	Community Resource Information
9.4.2.1	8.046	Contents of Child's Records
9.4.2.2	8.047	Pre-Admission Enrollment Information for Each Child
9.4.2.3	2.048/8.049	Contents of Admission Agreement Between Child Care Program and Parent/Guardian
9.4.2.4	8.048	Contents of Child's Primary Care Provider's Assessment
9.4.2.5	8.050	Health History
9.4.2.6	8.051	Contents of Medication Record
9.4.2.7	2.049/8.052	Contents of Facility Health Log for Each Child
9.4.2.8	8.056	Release of Child's Records
9.4.3.1	8.058	Maintenance and Content of Staff and Volunteer Records
9.4.3.2	8.060	Maintenance of Attendance Records for Staff Who Care for Children
9.4.3.3	1.034	Training Record
Chapter 10		
3rd Ed. #	**2nd Ed. #**	**3rd Ed. Standard Title**
10.1	New	Introduction
10.2.0.1	9.001	Regulation of All Out-Of-Home Child Care
10.2.0.2	9.012	Adequacy of Staff and Funding for Regulatory Enforcement
10.2.0.3	9.023	State Statute Support of Regulatory Enforcement
10.3.1.1	9.002	Operation Permits
10.3.1.2	9.009	Rational Basis of Regulations
10.3.1.3	9.010	Community Participation in Development of Licensing Rules
10.3.2.1	9.024	Child Care Licensing Advisory Board
10.3.2.2	9.045	State Early Childhood Advisory Council
10.3.2.3	3.079/9.011	Collaborative Development of Child Care Requirements and Guidelines for Children Who Are Ill
10.3.2.4	9.043	Public-Private Collaboration on Care of Children Who Are Ill
10.3.3.1	9.006	Credentialing of Individual Child Care Providers
10.3.3.2	9.003	Background Screening
10.3.3.3	9.022	Licensing Agency Role in Communicating the Importance of Reporting Suspected Child Abuse
10.3.3.4	9.030	Licensing Agency Provision of Child Abuse Prevention Materials
10.3.3.5	New	Licensing Agency Role in Communicating the Importance of Compliance with Americans with Disabilities Act
10.3.4.1	9.029	Sources of Technical Assistance to Support Quality of Child Care
10.3.4.2	9.031	Licensing Agency Provision of Written Agreements for Parents/Guardians and Caregivers/Teachers
10.3.4.3	9.033	Support for Consultants to Provide Technical Assistance to Facilities
10.3.4.4	9.034	Development of List of Providers of Services to Facilities
10.3.4.5	9.035	Resources for Parents/Guardians of Children with Special Health Care Needs
10.3.4.6	9.036	Compensation for Participation in Multidisciplinary Assessments for Children with Special Health Care or Education Needs
10.3.4.7	9.041	Technical Assistance to Facilities to Address Diversity in the Community
10.3.5.1	9.015	Education, Experience and Training of Licensing Inspectors

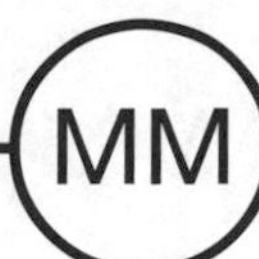

Chapter 10		
3rd Ed. #	**2nd Ed. #**	**3rd Ed. Standard Title**
10.3.5.2	9.013	Performance Monitoring of Licensing Inspectors
10.3.5.3	9.016	Training of Licensing Agency Personnel About Child Abuse
10.4.1.1	9.004	Uniform Categories and Definitions
10.4.1.2	New	Quality Rating and Improvement Systems
10.4.1.3	9.007	Licensing Agency Procedures Prior to Issuing a License
10.4.1.4	9.008	Alternative Means of Compliance
10.4.2.1	9.014/9.018	Frequency of Inspections for Child Care Centers, Large Family Child Care Homes, and Small Family Child Care Homes
10.4.2.2	9.017	Statutory Authorization of On-Site Inspections
10.4.2.3	9.019	Monitoring Strategies
10.4.2.4	9.044	Agency Collaboration to Safeguard Children in Child Care
10.4.3.1	9.020	Procedure for Receiving Complaints
10.4.3.2	9.021	Whistle-Blower Protection Under State Law
10.4.3.3	9.032	Collection of Data on Illness or Harm to Children in Facilities
10.5.0.1	9.025	State and Local Health Department Role
10.5.0.2	9.026	Written Plans for the Health Department Role
10.5.0.3	9.027	Requirements for Facilities to Report to Health Department
10.5.0.4	9.028	Use of Fact Sheets on Common Illnesses Associated with Child Care
10.6.1.1	9.038	Regulatory Agency Provision of Caregiver/Teacher and Consumer Training and Support Services
10.6.1.2	9.040	Provision of Training to Facilities by Health Agencies
10.6.2.1	9.037	Development of Child Care Provider Organizations and Networks
10.6.2.2	9.042	Fostering Collaboration to Establish Programs for School-Age Children
10.7.0.1	9.046	Development of Resource and Referral Agencies
10.7.0.2	9.047	Coordination of Public and Private Resources to Ensure Families' Access to Quality Child Care
Deleted		
3rd Ed.	**2nd Ed. #**	**Standard Title**
Deleted	3.050	Syrup of Ipecac
Deleted	3.060	Seizure Care Plan
Deleted	3.061	Training for Staff to Handle Seizures
Deleted	3.062	Management of Children with Asthma
Deleted	5.164	Capacity of Outdoor Play Area
Deleted	8.045	Written Statement of Services
Deleted	9.039	Child Development Associate Training
Deleted	9.048	Arrangements for Parental Leave
Appendices		
3rd Ed.	**2nd Ed.**	**Appendix Title**
A	New	Signs and Symptoms Chart
B	B	Major Occupational Health Hazards
C	C	Nutrition Specialist, Registered Dietician, Licensed Nutritionist, Consultant, and Food Service Staff Qualifications
D	D	Gloving
E	E	Child Care Staff Health Assessment
F	F	Enrollment/Attendance/Symptom Record

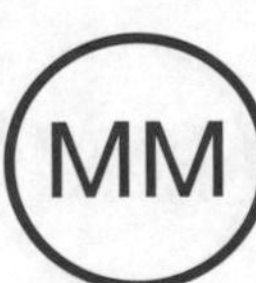

Appendices		
3rd Ed.	**2nd Ed.**	**Appendix Title**
G	G	Recommended Childhood Immunization Schedule
H	New	Recommended Adult Immunization Schedule
I	H	Recommendations for Preventive Pediatric Health Care
J	I	Selecting an Appropriate Sanitizer or Disinfectant
K	3.028	Routine Schedule for Cleaning, Sanitizing, and Disinfecting
L	J	Cleaning Up Body Fluids
M	K	Clues to Child Abuse and Neglect
N	New	Protective Factors Regarding Child Abuse and Neglect
O	New	Care Plan for Children with Special Health Care Needs
P	N	Situations that Require Medical Attention Right Away
Q	New	Getting Started with MyPlate
R	New	Choose MyPlate: 10 Tips to a Great Plate
S	New	Physical Activity: How Much Is Needed?
T	New	Foster Care
U	New	Recommended Safe Minimum Internal Cooking Temperatures
V	R	Food Storage Chart
W	S	Sample Food Service Cleaning Schedule
X	T	Adaptive Equipment for Children with Special Health Care Needs
Y	U	Non Poisonous and Poisonous Plants
Z	V	Depth of Surface Materials
AA	New	Medication Administration Packet
BB	X	Emergency Information for Children with Special Health Care Needs
CC	Y	Incident Report Form
DD	New	Injury Report Form for Indoor and Outdoor Injuries
EE	New	America's Playgrounds Safety Report Card
GG	AA	Licensing and Public Regulation of Early Childhood Programs–NAEYC Position Statement
FF	Z	Child Health Assessment
HH	New	Use Zones for Clearance Dimensions for Single- and Multi-Axis Swings
II	New	Bicycle Helmets: Quick- Fit Check
JJ	New	Our Child Care Center Supports Breastfeeding
KK	New	Authorization for Emergency Medical/Dental Care
LL	New	Conversion Table - 2nd Edition to 3rd Edition
MM	New	Conversion Table - 3rd Edition to 2nd Edition
Deleted		
3rd Ed.	**2nd Ed.**	**Standard Title**
Deleted	BB	Contact Information
Deleted	CC	Conversion Table - 1st Edition to 2nd Edition
Deleted	DD	Conversion Table - 2nd Edition to 1st Edition
Deleted	L	Risk Factors for Abuse and/or Neglect
Deleted	M	Special Care Plan for a Child with Asthma
Deleted	O	Food Guide Pyramid for Young Children
Deleted	P	Child and Adult Care Food Program Child Care Infant Meal Pattern
Deleted	Q	Child and Adult Care Food Program Child Care Meal Pattern Requirements for Children Ages 1 through 12 Years
Deleted	W	Permission for Medical Condition Treatment

ACRONYMS/ABBREVIATIONS

AAA – American Automobile Association

AAFP – American Academy of Family Physicians

AAHE – American Association for Health Education

AAOS – American Academy of Orthopedic Surgeons

AAP – American Academy of Pediatrics

AAPD – American Academy of Pediatric Dentistry

AARST – American Association of Radon Scientists and Technologists

ABCT – Association for Behavioral and Cognitive Therapies

ABT – Abusive Head Trauma

ACE – Adverse Childhood Experiences

ACEI – Association for Childhood Education International

ACIP – U.S. Public Health Service Advisory Committee on Immunization Practices

ACMI – Art and Creative Materials Institute

ADA – American Dietetic Association

ADA – Americans with Disabilities Act

ADAAG – Americans with Disabilities Act Accessibility Guidelines

ADHD – Attention-deficit Hyper-activity Disorder

AFMA – American Furniture Manufacturers Association

AGA – American Gas Association

AHA – American Heart Association

AHAM – Association of Home Appliance Manufacturers

AIDS – Acquired Immunodeficiency Syndrome

ALA – American Lung Association

ANA – American Nurses Association

ANSI – American National Standards Institute

APHA – American Public Health Association

APRN – Advanced Practice Registered Nurse

APSP – Association of Pool and Spa Professionals

AQI – Air Quality Index

ASHRAE – American Society of Heating, Refrigerating, and Air-conditioning Engineers

ASQ – Ages and Stages Questionnaire

ASME – American Society of Mechanical Engineers

ASTM – ASTM International, formerly named American Society for Testing and Materials

BPA – Bisphenol A

CPR – Cardiopulmonary Resuscitation

CACFP – Child and Adult Care Food Program

CCA – Chromated copper arsenate

CCDF – Child Care Development Fund

CCHC – Child Care Health Consultant

CCM – Cough and Cold Medication

CCSIG – Child Care Special Interest Group

CCW – Child Care Workforce

CDA – Child Development Associate

CDBG – Community Development Block Grant

CDC – Centers for Disease Control and Prevention

CFL – Compact Fluorescent Light

CFOC – Caring for Our Children: National Health and Safety Standards; Guidelines for Early Care and Education Programs

CFR – Code of Federal Regulations

CGMP – Current Good Manufacturing Practices

CHEJ – Center for Health Environment and Justice

CHES – Certified Health Education Specialist

CHIP – Children's Health Insurance Program

CISP – Childhood Immunization Support Program

CMV – Cytomegalovirus

CPSC – U.S. Consumer Product Safety Commission

CSA – Canadian Standards Association

CSHCN – Children with Special Health Care Needs

CSHP – Coordinated School Health Program

CSN – Children with Special Needs

CVD – Cardiovascular Disease

DASH – Division of Adolescent and School Health

db – Decibel

DEET – N,N-diethyl-meta-toluamide

DEHA – Diethylhexyladepate

ECE/CD – Early Childhood Education/Child Development

ECERS – Early Childhood Environment Rating Scale

ECMHC – Early Childhood Mental Health Consultant

EEI – Edison Electric Institute

EMS – Emergency Medical Services

EMSC – Emergency Medical Services for Children

EPA – U.S. Environmental Protection Agency

EPSDT – Early Periodic Screening, Diagnosis, and Treatment

FDA – U.S. Food and Drug Administration

FEMA – Federal Emergency Management Agency

FERPA – Family Educational Rights and Privacy Act

GED – General Educational Development

GFCI – Ground-fault Circuit-interrupter

GIS – Geographic Information System

HAV – Hepatitis A Virus

HBV – Hepatitis B Virus

HCV – Hepatitis C Virus

HDPE – High-density Polyethylene

HEPA – High-efficiency Particulate Air

HHS – U.S. Department of Health and Human Services

HHV-6 – Human Herpesvirus Six

HIC – Head Injury Criterion

HIV – Human Immunodeficiency Virus

HRSA – Health Resources and Services Administration

HUD – Housing and Urban Development

HVAC – Heating, Ventilation, Air-conditioning, and Cooling

ICC – Interagency Coordinating Council

IDEA – Individuals with Disabilities Education Act

IEEE – Institute of Electrical and Electronics Engineers

IEP – Individualized Education Program

IFSP – Individual Family Service Plan

IGRA – Interferon-gamma Release Assay

IPM – Integrated Pest Management

ITERS – Infant/Toddler Environment Rating Scale

IVIG – Intravenous Immune Globulin

JPMA – Juvenile Products Manufacturers Association

LCR – Lead and Copper Rule

LDPE – Low-density polyethylene

LED – Light Emitting Diode

LPN – Licensed Practical Nurse

LTBI – Latent Tuberculosis Infection

MCH – Maternal and Child Health

MHC – Mental Health Consultant

MMR – Measles, Mumps, and Rubella

MMRV – MMR Vaccine

MRSA – Methicillin-resistant Staphylococcus aureus

MSDS – Material Safety Data Sheet

MSW – Municipal Solid Waste

NAA – National AfterSchool Association

NACCRRA – National Association of Child Care Resource and Referral Agencies

NAEYC – National Association for the Education of Young Children

NAFCC – National Association for Family Child Care

NAPNAP – National Association of Pediatric Nurse Practitioners

NAP-SACC – Nutrition and Physical Activity Self-assessment for Child Care

NASCD – National Association for Sick Child Daycare

NASN – National Association of School Nurses

NASPE – National Association for Sport and Physical Education

NCCA – National Child Care Association

NCHEC – National Commission for Health Education Credentialing

NCPS – National Center for Playground Safety

NEC – National Electrical Code

NEC – Necrotizing enterocolitis

NECPA – National Early Childhood Program Accreditation

NEISS – National Electronic Injury Surveillance System

NHTSA – National Highway Traffic Safety Association

NNii – National Network for Immunization Information

NOAA – National Oceanic and Atmospheric Administration

NOWRA – National On-site Wastewater Recycling Association

NPPS – National Program for Playground Safety

NRA – National Rehabilitation Association

NRC – National Resource Center for Health and Safety in Child Care and Early Education

NRPA – National Recreation and Parks Association

NSF – National Sanitation Foundation

NTI – National Training Institute for Child Care Health Consultants

NTNCWS – Non-transient, Non-community Water System

NWR – NOAA Weather Radio

NWS – National Weather Service

OPIM – Other Potential Infectious Materials

OSERS – Office of Special Education and Rehabilitative Services

OSG – Office of the Surgeon General

OSHA – Occupational Safety and Health Administration

OTC – Over-the-counter

PBDE – Polybrominated diphenyl ethers

PC – Polycarbonate

PDCB – Para-dichlorobenzene

PedFACTS – Pediatric First Aid for Caregivers and Teachers

PETE – Polyethylene terephthalate

PP – Polypropylene

PS – Polystyrene

PVC – Polyvinyl chloride

QRIS – Quality Rating and Improvement Systems

QRS – Quality Rating Systems

RN – Registered Nurse

SBA – Safe Building Alliance

SBS – Shaken baby syndrome

SCHIP – State Children's Health Insurance Program

SIDS – Sudden infant death syndrome

SPF – Sun Protection Factor

SPMTA – Swimming Pool Manufacturers Trade Association

STIPDA – State and Territorial Injury Prevention Directors' Association

SVRS – Safety Vacuum Release System

TANF – Temporary Assistance for Needy Families

TCA – Tricyclic Antidepressants

TST – Tuberculin Skin Test

UCHR – Universal Child Health Record

UF – Urea-formaldehyde

UL – Underwriters Laboratories

USDA – U.S. Department of Agriculture

UV – Ultra-violet

WIC – Women, Infants, and Children

VNA – Visiting Nurse Association

VOC – Volatile Organic Compound

GLOSSARY

See Also Acronyms/Abbreviations** (pages 541-543)*

Note: Some of these definitions were contained in the first edition in which they were reprinted with permission from Infectious Diseases in Child Care Settings and Schools, a manual with information for directors, caregivers/teachers, and parents/guardians, by the Epidemiology Departments of Hennepin County Community Health, St. Paul Division of Public Health, Minnesota Department of Health, Washington County Public Health, and Bloomington Division of Health. Other definitions are from the resources referenced at the end of the definition. Others were supplied by our Technical Panels. Please see the Acknowledgments section for a list of the Technical Panels' members.

Abrasion – An injury (such as a scrape) that occurs when the top layer of skin is removed, with little blood loss.
Ref: American Academy of Pediatrics (AAP). 2005. *Pediatric first aid for caregivers and teachers*. Ed. S. S. Aronson. Boston: Jones and Bartlett; Elk Grove Village, IL: AAP. http://www.pedfactsonline.com.

Acute – Adjective describing an illness that has a sudden onset and is of short duration.
Ref: Donoghue, E. A., C. A. Kraft, eds. 2010. *Managing chronic health needs in child care and schools: A quick reference guide.* Elk Grove Village, IL: American Academy of Pediatrics.

Acrocyanosis – Blueness or pallor of the extremities usually associated with pain and numbness and caused by vasomotor disturbances.

Adaptive equipment – Equipment (such as eye glasses, hearing aids, wheelchairs, crutches, prostheses, oxygen tanks) that helps children with special health care needs adapt to and function within their surroundings. See also Appendix X.

Aflatoxin – A naturally occurring mycotoxin (fungus). This toxic metabolite occurs in soil, decaying vegetation, hay, and grains undergoing microbiological deterioration. Favorable conditions include high moisture content and high temperature.
Ref: Cornell University Department of Animal Science. 2009. Aflatoxins: Occurrence and health risks. http://www.ansci.cornell.edu/plants/toxicagents/aflatoxin/aflatoxin.html.

Age-appropriate physical activity – See Physical activity

Age-appropriate solid foods – Also known as complementary foods, foods introduced at the correct age to infants. Examples are iron-fortified infant cereals and pureed meats for infants.

AIDS – See Human Immunodeficiency virus (HIV)

Air Quality Index (AQI) – A tool used by EPA and other agencies to describe how clean the air is and whether or not the public should be concerned for their health. The AQI is focused on health effects that can happen within a few hours or days after breathing polluted air.
Ref: Agency for Toxic Substances and Disease Registry. 2009. The air quality index. http://www.atsdr.cdc.gov/general/theair.html#indic.

Allergens – A substance (food, pollen, pets, mold, medication, etc.) that causes an allergic reaction.

Ambient measurements – Measurements that help assess the amount of air pollutants, noise, or lighting within a specific area.

Anaphylaxis – An allergic reaction to a specific substance (food, pollen, pets, mold, medication, etc.) that causes dangerous and possibly fatal complications, including the swelling and closure of the airway that can lead to an inability to breathe.

Anemia – Having too little hemoglobin (hemoglobin carries oxygen from the lungs throughout the body). The terms anemia, iron deficiency, and iron deficiency anemia often are used interchangeably but are equivalent.
Ref: Centers for Disease Control and Prevention. 2011. Iron and iron deficiency. http://www.cdc.gov/nutrition/everyone/basics/vitamins/iron.html.

Antibiotic prophylaxis – Medicine that is prescribed to prevent infections in infants and children in situations associated with an increased risk of serious infection with a specific disease.
Ref: Pickering, L. K., C. J. Baker, D. W. Kimberlin, S. S. Long, eds. 2009. *Red book: 2009 report of the Committee on Infectious Diseases*. 28th ed. Elk Grove Village, IL: American Academy of Pediatrics.

Antibody – A protein substance produced by the body's immune defense system in response to something foreign. Antibodies help protect against infections.

Antiseptic – Antimicrobial substances that are applied to the skin or surfaces to reduce the number of microbial flora. Examples include alcohols, chlorhexidine, chlorine, hexachlorophene, iodine, chloroxylenol (PCMX), quaternary ammonium compounds, and triclosan.
Ref: Boyce, J. M., D. Pittet. 2002. Guideline for hand hygiene in healthcare settings: Recommendations of the Healthcare Infection Control Practices Advisory Committee and the HICPAC/SHEA/APIC/IDSA Hand Hygiene Task Force. *MMWR* 51(RR16): 1-44. http://www.cdc.gov/mmwr/preview/mmwrhtml/rr5116a1.htm.

Antigen – Any substance that is foreign to the body. An antigen is capable of causing a response from the immune system.

Antisiphon ballcock – An automatic valve in the toilet tank, the opening and closing of which is controlled by a spherical float at the end of a lever. The antisiphon ballcock does not allow dirty water to be admixed with clean water.

Asbestos – A mineral fiber that can pollute air or water and cause cancer or asbestosis when inhaled.

Friable asbestos – Any material containing more than one-percent asbestos, and that can be crumbled or reduced to powder by hand pressure. (May include previously non-friable material which becomes broken or damaged by mechanical force.)
Ref: U.S. Environmental Protection Agency. 2009. Terms of environment: Glossary, abbreviations and acronyms. http://www.epa.gov/glossary/.

Asphyxial crib death – Death attributed to an item within the crib that caused deprivation of oxygen or obstruction to normal breathing of an infant.

Asphyxiation – Death or unconsciousness due to inadequate oxygenation, the presence of noxious agents, or other obstructions to normal breathing.

Aspiration – The inhalation of food, liquid, or a foreign body into a person's airway which results in choking/respiratory distress.

Assessment – An in-depth appraisal conducted to diagnose a condition or determine the importance or value of a procedure.

Asymptomatic – Without symptoms. For example, a child may not have symptoms of hepatitis infection, but may still shed hepatitis A virus in the stool and may be able to infect others.

Autism spectrum disorders – A group of developmental disabilities associated with problems in the brain. Children with ASDs have trouble in three core areas of their development: language difficulties, especially no apparent desire to communicate, social interac-

*Corrected page number in second printing, August 2011
**Corrected to "Acronyms/Abbreviations" from "Acronyms" in second printing, August 2011

tion, restricted interests and behaviors that are repeated over and over again.
Ref: Donoghue, E. A., C. A. Kraft, eds. 2010. *Managing chronic health needs in child care and schools: A quick reference guide.* Elk Grove Village, IL: American Academy of Pediatrics.

Automous behavior – Behavior that is independent, free, and self-directing.
Ref: Merriam-Webster. 2009. Autonomy. Medline Plus Medical Dictionary. http://www2.merriam-webster.com/cgi-bin/mwmednlm?book=Medical&va=autonomy.

Axillary – Pertaining to the area under the arm (armpit).
Ref: American Academy of Pediatrics. 2009. How to take a child's temperature. Healthy Children. http://www.healthychildren.org/English/health-issues/conditions/fever/pages/How-to-Take-a-Childs-Temperature.aspx.

Background screenings – The process of checking the history of adults before they are allowed to care for children. See Standard 1.2.0.2 for detail on what should be included in a background screening.

Bacteria (Plural of bacterium) – Organisms that may be responsible for localized or generalized diseases and can survive in and out of the body. They are much larger than viruses and can usually be treated effectively with antibiotics.

Balusters – Vertical stair railings that support a horizontal handrail.

Bleach solution – See Appendix J: Selecting an Appropriate Sanitizer or Disinfectant.

Bloodborne pathogens – Infectious microorganisms present in blood that can cause disease in humans. These pathogens include, but are not limited to, hepatitis B virus (HBV), hepatitis C virus (HCV), and human immunodeficiency virus (HIV), the virus that causes AIDS.
Ref: Occupational Safety and Health Administration. 2011. OSHA factsheet: OSHA's bloodborne pathogens standard. http://www.osha.gov/OshDoc/data_BloodborneFacts/bbfact01.pdf.

BMI – See Body Mass Index (BMI)

Body fluids – Urine, feces, saliva, blood, nasal discharge, eye discharge, and injury or tissue discharge.

Body Mass Index (BMI) – Measurement of weight in kilograms divided by height in meters squared. Overweight and obesity can be defined by the BMI for age measurement.
Ref: Hagan, J. F., J. S. Shaw, P. M. Duncan, eds. 2008. *Bright futures: Guidelines for health supervision of infants, children and adolescents*. 3rd ed. Elk Grove Village, IL: American Academy of Pediatrics.

Bottle propping – Bottle-feeding an infant by leaning the bottle against the infant's mouth and leaving the infant alone rather than holding the bottle by hand.

Botulism – A severe illness of the nervous system. Three distinct, naturally occurring forms of human botulism exist: foodborne, wound, and infant.
Ref: Pickering, L. K., C. J. Baker, D. W. Kimberlin, S. S. Long, eds. 2009. *Red book: 2009 report of the Committee on Infectious Diseases*. 28th ed. Elk Grove Village, IL: American Academy of Pediatrics.

BPA (BISPHENOL A) – An organic compound used to manufacture polycarbonate plastics. This type of plastic is used to make some types of beverage containers, compact disks, plastic dinnerware, impact-resistant safety equipment, automobile parts, and toys. BPA epoxy resins are used in the protective linings of food cans, in dental sealants, and in other products.
Ref: Centers for Disease Control and Prevention. 2009. National report on human exposure to environmental chemicals. Fact sheet: Bisphenol A. http://www.cdc.gov/exposurereport/BisphenolA_FactSheet.html.

Bronchitis – A bacterial or viral infection that leads to swelling of the tubes (bronchioles) leading to the lungs.

Cadmium – An extremely toxic metal commonly found in industrial workplaces, particularly where any ore is being processed or smelted.
Ref: Occupational Safety and Health Administration. 2009. Safety and health topics: Cadmium. http://www.osha.gov/SLTC/cadmium/.

Campylobacter – A bacterium that causes diarrhea.

Campylobacteriosis – A diarrheal infection caused by the *Campylobacter* bacterium.

Capture velocity – Airflow that will collect the pollutant (such as dust or fumes) that you want removed.

Cardiopulmonary resuscitation (CPR) – Emergency measures performed by a person on another person whose breathing or heart activity has stopped. Measures include closed chest cardiac compressions in a regular sequence.

Care coordinator – An individual assigned to work with the child's family or alternative caretaker to assist in coordinating services, either internally within an agency directly providing services or with other service providers for the child and family. This term is also used by some agencies or caregivers in place of, or in association with, the term case manager

Care Plan – A document that provides specific health care information, including any medications, procedures, precautions, or adaptations to diet or environment that may be needed to care for a child with chronic medical conditions or special health care needs. Care Plans also describe signs and symptoms of impending illness and outline the response needed to those signs and symptoms. A Care Plan is completed by a health care professional and should be updated on a regular basis.
Ref: Donoghue, E. A., C. A. Kraft, eds. 2010. *Managing chronic health needs in child care and schools: A quick reference guide*. Elk Grove Village, IL: American Academy of Pediatrics.

Caregiver/Teacher – The primary person who works directly with the children in the center and in small and large family child care homes.

Carrier – A person or animal who carries within his/her body a specific disease causing organism, who has no symptoms of disease, and who can spread the disease to others. For example, some children may be carriers of Haemophilus influenzae or giardia and have no symptoms.

Case manager – See Care coordinator

Catheterization – The process of inserting a hollow tube into an organ of the body, either for an investigative purpose or to give some form of treatment (such as to remove urine from the bladder of a child with neurologic disease).

CCA (chromated copper arsenate) – A chemical wood preservative containing chromium, copper, and arsenic. CCA is used in pressure treated wood to protect wood from rotting due to insects and microbial agents.
Ref: U.S. Environmental Protection Agency. 2008. Pesticides: Regulating pesticides. Chromated Copper Arsenate (CCA). http://www.epa.gov/oppad001/reregistration/cca/.

Ceftriaxone – An antibiotic often prescribed for those exposed to an infection caused by *Haemophilus influenzae* type b (Hib) or *Neisseria meningitidis* (meningococcus).

Celiac disease – A digestive disease that damages the small intestine and interferes with absorption of nutrients from food. People who have celiac disease cannot tolerate gluten, a protein in wheat, rye, and barley. Gluten is found mainly in foods but may also be found in everyday products such as medicines, vitamins, and lip balms.
Ref: National Digestive Diseases Information Clearinghouse. 2008. Celiac disease. http://digestive.niddk.nih.gov/ddiseases/pubs/celiac/#what/.

Center – A facility that provides care and education of any number of children in a nonresidential setting, or thirteen or more children in any setting if the facility is open on a regular basis.

Certification (as it relates to a form of licensing) – Designation as having met the requirements to operate or practice in a specific sector.
Ref: Merriam-Webster. 2009. Certify. Medline Plus Medical Dictionary. http://www.merriam-webster.com/medlineplus/certify.

Certified playground safety inspector (CPSI) – Individuals who have attained a measured level of competency to inspect playgrounds for safety hazards and to ensure compliance with national standards set by ASTM International (ASTM) and the U.S. Consumer Product Safety Commission (CPSC).
Ref: National Recreation and Park Association. 2009. Certified Playground Safety Inspector (CPSI) certification. http://www.nrpa.org/Content.aspx?id=413.

Child abuse and neglect – See Appendix M for definitions of types of abuse and neglect.

Child and Adult Care Food Program (CACFP) – The U.S. Department of Agriculture's sponsored program whose child care component provides nutritious meals to children enrolled in centers and family child care homes throughout the country.

Child care health consultant (CCHC) – A licensed health professional with education and experience in child and community health and early care and education, preferably specialized training in child care health consultation.

Child Development Associate (CDA) – A credential awarded to those who have completed a list of requirements, including 120 hours of training, set forth by the Council for Professional Recognition.

Child:staff ratio – The amount of staff required, based on the number of children present and the ages of these children. See also Group size.

Children with special health care needs – Children who have or are at increased risk for chronic physical, developmental, behavioral, or emotional conditions who require health and related services of a type or amount beyond that required by children generally.
Ref: Maternal and Child Health Bureau. Achieving and measuring success: A national agenda for children with special health care needs. http://mchb.hrsa.gov/programs/specialneeds/measuresuccess.htm.

Children's Health Insurance Program (CHIP) – A program that provides free or low-cost health coverage for children up to age nineteen. CHIP covers U.S. citizens and eligible immigrants.

Chronic – Describing a disease or illness of long duration or frequent recurrence, often having a slow progressive course of indefinite duration.
Ref: Merriam-Webster. 2010. Chronic. Medline Plus Medical Dictionary. http://www.merriam-webster.com/medlineplus/chronic/.

Ciprofloxacin – An antibiotic often prescribed for those exposed to an infection caused by *Haemophilus influenzae* type b (Hib) or *Neisseria meningitidis* (meningococcus).

Clean – To remove dirt and debris by scrubbing and washing with a detergent solution and rinsing with water.

CMV – See Cytomegalovirus

Communicable disease – See Infectious disease

Complementary foods – Solid foods that are age-appropriate for infants such as iron-fortified infant cereals and pureed meats.

Compliance – The act of carrying out a recommendation, policy, regulation, or procedure.

Congenital – Existing from the time of birth.

Conjunctivitis – Also known as "Pink eye," inflammation (redness and swelling) of thin tissue covering the white part of the eye and the inside of the eyelids.
Ref: Aronson, S. S., T. R. Shope, eds. 2009. *Managing infectious diseases in child care and schools: A quick reference guide*. 2nd ed. Elk Grove Village, IL: American Academy of Pediatrics.

Contact dermatitis – A skin inflammation that results when the skin comes in direct contact with substances that can cause an allergic or inflammatory reaction.

Contamination – The presence of infectious microorganisms in or on the body, on environmental surfaces, on articles of clothing, or in food or water.

Contraindication – Something (as a symptom or condition) that makes a particular treatment or procedure inadvisable.

Contractual relationship – A relationship based on a signed and written contract between parents/guardians and caregivers/teachers that documents child care agreements involving policies and procedures and educational programming goals.

Corporal punishment – Physical harm inflicted on the body (such as spanking).

CPR – See Cardiopulmonary resuscitation

Croup – Spasms of the airway that cause difficult breathing and a cough sounding like a seal's bark. Croup can be caused by various bacteria and viruses.

Cryptosporidium – A parasite that causes cryptosporidiosis, a diarrheal illness.

"Cue" feeding – Feeding an infant based on their "cues" such as opening the mouth, making suckling sounds and moving the hands at random, as well as discontinuing feeding by observing cues that they are full.

Cytomegalovirus (CMV) – A viral infection common to children. In most cases, CMV causes no symptoms. When symptoms are experienced, they typically consist of fever, swollen glands, and fatigue. CMV can infect a pregnant woman who is not immune and damage the fetus, leading to mental retardation, hearing loss, and other nervous system problems in the unborn child.

Daily health check – Assessment of a child's health each day through observation of the child, talking with the parent/guardian, and if applicable, with the child. See Standard 3.1.1.1 for details.

Decibel (db) – The unit of measure of the loudness of sounds; one decibel is the lowest intensity of sound at which a given note can be heard. The decibel level is the number of decibels of noise perceived or measured in a given place.

DEET (N,N-Diethyl-meta-toluamide) – An ingredient in many insect repellents. See Standard 3.4.5.2 for instructions on use.

Delegation of medication administration – Delegation is a tool that may be used by the health professional to allow unlicensed assistive personnel to administer medication under the supervision of the health professional's guidance and assessment of the unique needs of the individual and the suitability of delegation of specific tasks.
Ref: American Academy of Pediatrics, Council on School Health. 2009. Policy statement: Guidance for the administration of medication on school. *Pediatrics* 124:1244-51.

Demand feeding – The feeding of infants whenever they indicate that they need to be fed, rather than feeding according to a clock schedule. See also "Cue" feeding.

Dental caries – A disease process that leads to holes in the teeth (commonly called dental cavities).
Ref: Aronson, S. S., T. R. Shope, eds. 2009. *Managing infectious diseases in child care and schools: A quick reference guide*. 2nd ed. Elk Grove Village, IL: American Academy of Pediatrics.

Dental Home – The ongoing relationship between the dentist and the patient, inclusive of all aspects of oral health care delivered in a comprehensive, continuously accessible, coordinated and family-centered way.
Ref: American Academy of Pediatrics, Section on Pediatric Dentistry. 2003. Policy statement: Oral health risk assessment timing and establishment of the dental home. *Pediatrics* 111:1113-16.

Dental sealants – Clear protective coatings that cover tooth surfaces and prevent bacteria and food particles from settling into the pits and grooves. Dental sealants are usually applied after a child reaches the age of six when the first permanent molars come in. Dental sealants last for four to five years and can be reapplied when they wear off.

Dermatitis – An inflammation of the skin.
Ref: Merriam-Webster. 2011. Dermatitis. Medical Dictionary. http://www.merriam-webster.com/medlineplus/dermatitis/.

Developmental screening – The use of standardized tools to identify a child at risk of a developmental delay or disorder.
Ref: American Academy of Pediatrics, Healthy Child Care America. 2009. Developmental screening in early childhood systems: Summary report. http://www.healthychildcare.org/pdf/DSECSreport.pdf.

Diabetes – A disorder that affects the way the body uses or converts food for energy and growth. Type 1 diabetes is a disease in which the immune system destroys the cells in the pancreas that make insulin. Children with type 1 diabetes need to take insulin injections to live. Type 2 diabetes is a condition in which the pancreas produces insulin, but the body cannot use it, often because of obesity; this is known as insulin resistance.
Ref: Donoghue, E. A., C. A. Kraft, eds. 2010. *Managing chronic health needs in child care and schools: A quick reference guide*. Elk Grove Village, IL: American Academy of Pediatrics.

Diarrhea – An illness in which an individual develops more watery and more frequent stools than is typical for that person.
Ref: Aronson, S. S., T. R. Shope, eds. 2009. *Managing infectious diseases in child care and schools: A quick reference guide*. 2nd ed. Elk Grove Village, IL: American Academy of Pediatrics.

Disease surveillance – Close observation for the occurrence of a disease or infection. Surveillance is performed to discover a disease problem early, to understand a disease problem better, and to evaluate the methods used to control the disease.

Disinfect – See Appendix J: Selecting an Appropriate Sanitizer or Disinfectant

Drop-in care facility – Program where children are cared for over short periods of time on a one-time, intermittent, unscheduled and/or occasional basis. It is often operated in connection with a business (e.g., health club, hotel, shopping center, or recreation centers).

Dyslipidemia – A condition marked by abnormal concentrations of lipids or lipoproteins in the blood, consisting of one or a combination of high LDL, low HDL, and high triglycerides.

E. coli – See Shiga toxin-producing *E. coli* (STEC)

Early childhood education consultant (ECEC) – Education professionals within the early childhood community who are trained in literacy, child development, curriculum development, instruction, and coaching.
Ref: Chester County Intermediate Unit. Training and consultation (TaC). http://www.cciu.org/22251042710361673/site/default.asp.

Egress – A place or means of going out. An exit.
Ref: Merriam-Webster. 2010. Egress. Merriam-Webster Online. http://www.merriam-webster.com/dictionary/egress/.

Electret test device – Equipment used to measure the short-term and long-term concentrations of radon in the air.
Ref: U.S. Environmental Protection Agency, Indoor Environments Division. 2009. A citizen's guide to radon: The guide to protecting yourself and your family from radon. http://www.epa.gov/radon/pdfs/citizensguide.pdf.

Emergency/Disaster plan – An action plan that lets affected individuals know what to do in particular disaster situations and how to be prepared in advance. See Standard 9.2.4.3 for specific components.
Ref: American Red Cross. 2007. Family disaster plan. http://www.redcross.org/images/pdfs/code/family_disaster_plan.pdf.

Emergency medical services (EMS) – A system of care for victims of sudden and serious injury or illness.
Ref: Rural Assistance Center. 2008 Emergency medical services. http://www.raconline.org/info_guides/ems/.

Emergency response plan – Procedures used to call for emergency medical assistance, to reach parents/guardians or emergency contacts, to arrange for transfer to medical assistance, and to render first aid to the injured person. See also Emergency/Disaster plan.

Emphysema – A lung disease that causes breathing-related problems by destroying the air sacs in the lungs (alveoli).
Ref: Centers for Disease Control and Prevention. 2009. Chronic obstructive pulmonary disease. http://www.cdc.gov/copd/.

Encephalitis – Inflammation (redness and swelling) of the brain, which can be caused by a number of viruses, including mumps, measles, and varicella.

Endotracheal suctioning – The mechanical aspiration and removal of mucous from a person's airway through a tracheostomy (an artificial opening in the trachea).

Enteric – Describes the location of infections affecting the intestines (often with diarrhea) or the liver.

Enterovirus – A common virus infection spread by fecal-oral and respiratory routes. A common enterovirus infection in young children is "hand-foot-and-mouth disease" in which fever and blister-

like eruptions in the mouth and/or a rash (usually on the palms and soles) may occur.
Ref: American Academy of Pediatrics (AAP). 2009. Enterovirus (non-poliovirus) infections. In *Red book: 2009 report of the Committee on Infectious Diseases*. 28th ed. Elk Grove Village, IL: AAP.

Environmental audit – Evaluation of a location site and buildings to determine if healthy and safe for humans to occupy. Assessments include: Potential air, soil, and water contamination on facility sites and outdoor play spaces; potential toxic or hazardous materials in building construction; and potential safety hazards in the community surrounding the site.

Epidemic – Affecting or tending to affect an atypically large number of individuals within a population, community, or region at the same time.
Ref: Merriam-Webster. 2010. Epidemic. Medline Plus Medical Dictionary. http://www.merriam-webster.com/medlineplus/epidemic/.

Epidemiology – The scientific study of the occurrence and distribution of diseases.

EpiPen – A registered trade name for an automatic epinephrine injector. Ephinephrine is administered in response to some allergic reactions.
Ref: Donoghue, E. A., C. A. Kraft, eds. 2010. *Managing chronic health needs in child care and schools: A quick reference guide*. Elk Grove Village, IL: American Academy of Pediatrics.

EPSDT – Abbreviation for Medicaid's Early Periodic Screening and Diagnostic Treatment program, which provides health assessments and follow up services to income-eligible children.

Ergot – A toxic fungus found as a parasite on grains of rye and other grains. Consumption of food contaminated with ergots may cause vomiting, diarrhea and may lead to gangrene in serious cases.

Erythromycin – An antibiotic medication used to treat many upper respiratory illnesses. It is often prescribed for people exposed to pertussis.

Evaluation – Impressions and recommendations formed after a careful appraisal and study.

Exclusion – Denying admission of a child or staff member to a facility (e.g., child or staff who is ill).

Excretion – A process whereby the body rids itself of waste material, such as feces and urine.

Expulsion – Expulsion is the permanent removal of the child from the child care facility.
Ref: American Academy of Pediatrics, Committee on School Health. 2008. Policy statement: Out-of-school suspension and expulsion. *Pediatrics* 122:450.

Facilitated play – Appropriate play experiences which are set-up by, but do not involve interaction from the caregiver/teacher, that facilitate development in all domains and promote autonomy, competency and a sense of joy in discovery and learning.
Ref: Liske, V., L. Bell. Play and the impaired child. Playworks. http://www.playworks.net/article-play-and-impaired-child.html.

Facility – The buildings, the grounds, the equipment, and the people involved in providing child care of any type.

Facility for children who are mildly ill – A facility providing care of one or more children who are mildly ill, children who are temporarily excluded from care in their regular child care setting; 1) Integrated or small group care for children who are mildly ill: A facility that has been approved by the licensing agency to care for well children and to include up to six children who are mildly ill; 2) Special facility for children who are mildly ill: A facility that cares only for children who are mildly ill, or a facility that cares for more than six children who are mildly ill at a time.

Failure to Thrive – Failure of a child to develop physically.

Family child care – The setting where early care and education is provided in the home of the caregiver/teacher.

Small family child care provides care and education for one to six children, including the caregiver's/teacher's own children. Family members or other helpers may be involved in assisting the caregiver/teacher, but often, there is only one caregiver/teacher present at any one time.

Large family child care provides care and education for seven to twelve children, including the caregiver/teacher's own children. One or more qualified adult assistants are present to meet child:staff ratio requirements.

Fecal coliform – Bacteria in stool that normally inhabit the gastrointestinal tract and are used as indicators of fecal pollution. They denote the presence of intestinal pathogens in water or food.

Fever – An elevation of body temperature. Temperature above 101°F (38.3°C) orally, above 102°F (38.9°C) rectally, or 100°F (37.8°C) or higher taken axillary (armpit) or measured by an equivalent method.

Fifth disease – A common viral infection with rash occurring one to three weeks after infection, also known as Parvovirus B19.
Ref: Aronson, S. S., T. R. Shope, eds. 2009. *Managing infectious diseases in child care and schools: A quick reference guide*. 2nd ed. Elk Grove Village, IL: American Academy of Pediatrics.

First aid – See Pediatric first aid

Foodborne illness/disease – An illness or disease transmitted through food products.

Foot-candles – The amount of illumination produced by a standard candle at a distance of one foot.

Formaldehyde – A colorless, flammable gas at room temperature that has a pungent, distinct odor and may cause a burning sensation to the eyes, nose, and lungs at high concentrations.
Ref: Agency for Toxic Substances and Disease Registry. 2009. Public health statement for formaldehyde. http://www.atsdr.cdc.gov/phs/phs.asp?id=218&tid=39/.

Free play – See Unstructured physical activity.

Friable asbestos – See Asbestos

Functional outcomes – Health status measures that go beyond traditional physiological assessments. By incorporating a multidimensional definition of health that encompasses physical, psychological and social aspects, functional outcome measures can capture the broader impact of disease and treatment on life from a child's (or parent's/guardian's) own perspective. Such tools enable children and parents/guardians to offer input on their quality of life and their capacity to function in normal social roles.

Fungi (singular fungus) – Plantlike organisms, such as yeasts, molds, mildews, and mushrooms, which get their nutrition from other living organisms or from dead organic matter.

Galactosemia – A condition in which the body is unable to use (metabolize) the simple sugar galactose.
Ref: Medline Plus. 2009. Galactosemia. Medical Encyclopedia. http://www.nlm.nih.gov/medlineplus/ency/article/000366.htm.

G-MAX – The measure of the maximum acceleration (shock) produced by an impact.
Ref: ASTM International (ASTM). 2009. ASTM F1292-09: Standard specification for impact attenuation of surfacing materials within the use zone of playground equipment. West Conshohocken, PA: ASTM.

Gastric tube feeding – The administration of nourishment through a tube that has been surgically inserted directly into the stomach.

Gastrointestinal (GI) tract – The human digestive tract that breaks down and absorbs food. Organs that make up the GI tract) are the mouth, esophagus, stomach, small intestine, large intestine, rectum, and anus.
Ref: National Digestive Diseases Information Clearinghouse. 2008. Your digestive system and how it works. http://digestive.niddk.nih.gov/ddiseases/pubs/yrdd/.

Gestational – Occurring during or related to pregnancy.

Giardia intestinalis – A parasite that causes giardiasis, an intestinal infection commonly referred to as "Giardia."
Ref: Aronson, S. S., T. R. Shope, eds. 2009. *Managing infectious diseases in child care and schools: A quick reference guide*. 2nd ed. Elk Grove Village, IL: American Academy of Pediatrics.

Glomerulonephritis – A type of kidney disease in which the part of the kidneys that helps filter waste and fluids from the blood is damaged.
Ref: Medline Plus. 2009. Glomerulonephritis. Medical Encyclopedia. http://www.nlm.nih.gov/medlineplus/ency/article/000484.htm.

Gross motor skills – Large movements involving the arms, legs, feet, or the entire body (such as crawling, running, and jumping).

Ground-fault circuit-interrupter (GFCI) – A piece of equipment in an electrical line that offers protection against electrocution if the line comes into contact with water.

Group A Streptococcus (GAS) – A bacterium commonly found in the throat and on the skin that can cause a range of infections, from relatively mild sore throats "strep throat" and skin infections (e.g., "scarlet fever") to life-threatening disease.

Group size – The number of children assigned to a caregiver/teacher or team of caregivers/teachers occupying an individual classroom or well defined space within a larger room. See also Child:staff ratio.

***Haemophilus influenzae* type b (Hib)** – A group of bacterial infections that can infect ears, eyes, sinuses, epiglottis (i.e., the flap that covers the windpipe), skin, lungs, blood, joints, and coverings of the brain (meningitis). Hib should not be confused with "the flu" which is a disease caused by a virus. Hib infection is a vaccine preventable disease.
Ref: Aronson, S. S., T. R. Shope, eds. 2009. *Managing infectious diseases in child care and schools: A quick reference guide*. 2nd ed. Elk Grove Village, IL: American Academy of Pediatrics.

HBV – An abbreviation for hepatitis B virus. See also Hepatitis.

Head Injury Criterion (HIC) – An empirical measure of impact severity based on published research describing the relationship between the magnitude and duration of impact accelerations and the risk of head trauma.
Ref: ASTM International (ASTM). 2009. ASTM F1292-09: Standard specification for impact attenuation of surfacing materials within the use zone of playground equipment. West Conshohocken, PA: ASTM.

Health advocate – A staff person in an early care and education setting responsible for policies and day-to-day issues related to health, development, and safety of individual children, children as a group, staff, and parents/guardians. The health advocate does not fill the same role as the child care health consultant. See also Child care health consultant.

Health care professional – Someone who practices medicine with or without supervision, and who is licensed by an established licensing body The most common types of health care professionals include physicians, nurse practitioners, nurses, and physician assistants.
Ref: Donoghue, E. A., C. A. Kraft, eds. 2010. *Managing chronic health needs in child care and schools: A quick reference guide*. Elk Grove Village, IL: American Academy of Pediatrics.

Health consultant – See Child Care Health Consultant

Health history – A compilation of health information about an individual See Standard 9.4.2.5 for list of information to be included in such a history.

Health plan – See Care Plan

Health supervision – Routine screening tests, immunizations, and chronic or acute illness monitoring. For children younger than twenty-four months of age, health supervision includes documentation and plotting of charts on standard sex-specific length, weight, weight for length, and head circumference and assessing diet and activity. For children twenty-four months of age and older, sex-specific height and weight graphs should be plotted by the primary care provider in addition to body mass index (BMI).

Hepatitis – Inflammation of the liver caused by viral infection. There are six types of infectious hepatitis: type A; type B; nonA, nonB; type C; and type D.

Herpes simplex virus – A viral organism that causes a recurrent disease which is marked by blister-like sores on mucous membranes (such as the mouth, lips, or genitals) that weep clear fluid and slowly crust over.

Herpetic gingivostomatitis – Inflammation of the mouth and lips caused by the herpes simplex virus.

Hib – See *Haemophilus influenzae* type b

HIPPA – Health Insurance Portability and Accountability Act – Federal act that provides protections for personal health information held by covered entities and gives patients an array of rights with respect to that information.

HIV – See Human Immunodeficiency Virus (HIV)

HPV (human papillomaviruses) – Viruses that cause a number of skin and mucous membrane infections; the most common infection is the skin wart

Human Immunodeficiency Virus (HIV) – A virus that affects the body in a variety of ways. In the most severe infections, the virus progressively destroys the body's immune system, causing a condition called acquired immune deficiency syndrome, or AIDS.
Ref: Aronson, S. S., T. R. Shope, eds. 2009. Managing infectious diseases in child care and schools: A quick reference guide. 2nd ed. Elk Grove Village, IL: American Academy of Pediatrics.

Hypercholesterolemia – Having elevated cholesterol levels. High levels of cholesterol increase the risk for cardiovascular disease and stroke.

IEP – See Individualized Education Program

IFSP – See Individualized Family Service Plan

Immune globulin (Gamma globulin, immunoglobulin)– An antibody preparation made from human plasma. It provides temporary protection against diseases such as hepatitis A.

Immunity – The body's ability to fight a particular infection. For example, a child acquires immunity to diseases such as measles, mumps, rubella, and pertussis after natural infection or by immunization.

Immunizations – Vaccines that are given to children and adults to help them develop protection (antibodies) against specific infections. Vaccines may contain an inactivated or killed agent or a weakened live organism.

Immunocompromised – The state of not having normal body defenses (immune responses) against diseases caused by microorganisms.

Immunosuppression – Inhibition of the body's natural immune response, used especially to describe the action of drugs that allow the surgical transplantation of a foreign organ or tissue by inhibiting its biological rejection.

Impervious – Adjective describing a smooth surface that does not become wet or retain particles.

Impetigo – A common skin infection caused by streptococcal infection or staphylococcal bacteria.
Ref: Aronson, S. S., T. R. Shope, eds. 2009. *Managing infectious diseases in child care and schools: A quick reference guide*. 2nd ed. Elk Grove Village, IL: American Academy of Pediatrics.

Incubation period – Time between exposure to an infectious microorganism and beginning of symptoms.

Individualized Education Program (IEP) – A written document, derived from Part B of IDEA (Individuals with Disabilities Education Act), that is designed to meet a child's individual educational program needs. The main purposes for an IEP are to set reasonable learning goals and to state the services that the school district will provide for a child with special educational needs. Every child who is qualified for special educational services provided by the school is required to have an IEP.

Individualized Family Service Plan (IFSP) – A written document, derived from Part C of IDEA (Individuals with Disabilities Education Act), that is formulated in collaboration with the family to meet the needs of a child with a developmental disability or delay, to assist the family in its care for a child's educational, therapeutic, and health needs, and to deal with the family's needs to the extent to which the family wishes assistance.

Infant – A child between the time of birth and the age of ambulation (usually the ages from birth through twelve months).

Infant walkers – Equipment consisting of a wheeled base supporting a rigid frame that holds a fabric seat with leg openings and usually a plastic feeding/play tray. Also known as baby walkers.

Infectious disease – A disease caused by a microorganism (bacterium, virus, fungus, or parasite) that can be transmitted from person to person via infected body fluids or respiratory spray, with or without an intermediary agent (such as a louse, mosquito) or environmental object (such as a table surface). Many infectious diseases are reportable to the local health authority.

Infested – Common usage of this term refers to parasites (such as lice or scabies) living on the outside of the body.

Influenza ("flu") – An acute viral infection of the respiratory tract. Symptoms usually include fever, chills, headache, muscle aches, dry cough, and sore throat. Influenza should not be confused with *Haemophilus influenzae* infection caused by bacteria, or with "stomach flu," which is usually an infection caused by a different type of virus.

Ingestion – The act of taking material (whether food or other substances) into the body through the mouth.

Injury, unintentional – Physical damage to a human being resulting from an unintentional event (one not done by design) involving a transfer of energy (physical, chemical, or heat energy).

Integrated pest management (IPM) – A common-sense approach to eliminating the root causes of pest problems, providing safe and effective control of insects, weeds, rodents, and other pests while minimizing risks to human health and the environment.

Intradermal – Relating to areas between the layers of the skin (as in intradermal injections).

Isolation – The physical separation of a person who is ill from other persons in order to prevent or lessen contact between other persons and the body fluids of the person who is ill.

Jaundice – Yellowish discoloration of the whites of the eyes, skin, and mucous membranes caused by deposition of bile salts in these tissues.

Kinesiology – The study of the principles of mechanics and anatomy in relation to human movement.
Ref: Merriam-Webster. 2010. Kinesiology. Merriam-Webster Online. http://www.merriam-webster.com/dictionary/kinesiology/.

Laceration – A cut, which can be jagged or smooth and may be superficial or deep, large or small.
Ref: American Academy of Pediatrics (AAP). 2005. *Pediatric first aid for caregivers and teachers.* Ed. S. S. Aronson. Boston: Jones and Bartlett; Elk Grove Village, IL: AAP. http://www.pedfactsonline.com.

Large family child care home – See Family child care

Lead – A highly toxic metal. Common sources of lead exposure are lead-based paint in older homes, contaminated soil, household dust, drinking water, lead crystal, and lead-glazed pottery.
Ref: National Institute of Environmental Health Sciences. Lead. National Institutes of Health. http://www.niehs.nih.gov/health/topics/agents/lead/.

Lead agency – An individual state's choice for the agency that will receive and allocate the federal and state funding for children with special educational needs. The federal funding is allocated to individual states in accordance with the Individuals with Disabilities Educational Act (IDEA).

Lecithin – Any of several waxy lipids which are widely distributed in animals and plants, and have emulsifying, wetting, and antioxidant properties.

Lethargy – Unusual sleepiness or low activity level.
Ref: Donoghue, E. A., C. A. Kraft, eds. 2010. *Managing chronic health needs in child care and schools: A quick reference guide*. Elk Grove Village, IL: American Academy of Pediatrics.

Lice – Parasites that live on the surface of the human body (in head, body, or pubic hair).

Light emitting diode (LED) – Small light sources that become illuminated by the movement of electrons through a semiconductor material.
Ref: U.S. Environmental Protection Agency, U.S. Department of Energy. LED light bulbs: Energy Star. http://www.energystar.gov/index.cfm?fuseaction=find_a_product.showProductGroup&pgw_code=ILB/.

Listeriosis – Diseases caused by the *Listeria* bacterium. Can cause meningitis, blood infections, heart problems, and abscesses, and can cause a pregnant woman to miscarry.

Longitudinal study – A research study in which patients are followed and examined over a period of time.

Lyme disease – An infection caused by a type of bacteria known as spirochetes, that is transmitted when particular ticks attach to a person's skin and feed on that person's blood.
Ref: Aronson, S. S., T. R. Shope, eds. 2009. *Managing infectious diseases in child care and schools: A quick reference guide*. 2nd ed. Elk Grove Village, IL: American Academy of Pediatrics.

Lymphadenitis – An acute infection of one or more lymph nodes.
Ref: Beers, M. H., R. S. Porter, T. V. Jones, J. L. Kaplan, M. Berkwits, eds. 2006. *The Merck manual of diagnosis and therapy*. 18th ed. Whitehouse Station, NJ: Merck Research Laboratories.

Lymphoma – A general term for a group of cancers that originate in the lymph system. The two primary types of lymphoma are Hodgkin lymphoma, which spreads in an orderly manner from one group of lymph nodes to another; and non-Hodgkin lymphoma, which spreads through the lymphatic system in a non-orderly manner.
Ref: Centers for Disease Control and Prevention. 2009. Hematologic (blood) cancers: Lymphoma. http://www.cdc.gov/cancer/hematologic/lymphoma/.

Mandatory reporters – Individuals required by their state laws to report concerns of child abuse and neglect.
Ref: Child Welfare Information Gateway. 2010. Mandatory reporters of child abuse and neglect: Summary. http://www.childwelfare.gov/systemwide/laws_policies/statutes/manda.pdf.

Mantoux intradermal skin test – A test to assess the likelihood of infection with tuberculosis.

Material safety data sheet (MSDS) – Information regarding the proper procedures for handling, storing, and disposing of chemical substances. Federal law dictates that employers must provide information to their employees about hazardous materials and chemicals that employees may be exposed to in the workplace. The vehicle for that information is the MSDS.
Ref: Occupational Safety and Health Administration. Occupational safety and health standards: Hazard communication. 29 CFR 1910.1200. http://www.osha.gov/pls/oshaweb/owadisp.show_document?p_table=STANDARDS&p_id=10099/.

Measles (red measles, rubeola, hard measles, 8 to 10 day measles) – A serious viral illness characterized by a red rash, high fever, lightsensitive eyes, cough, and cold symptoms.

Medicaid – A program which provides medical assistance for individuals and families with low incomes and resources. The program became law in 1965 as a jointly funded cooperative venture between the Federal and State governments to assist states in the provision of adequate medical care to eligible needy persons.

Medical home – Primary care that is accessible, continuous, comprehensive, family centered, coordinated, compassionate, and culturally effective. The child health care professional works in partnership with the family and patient to ensure that all the medical and non-medical needs of the patient are met.
Ref: Hagan, J. F., J. S. Shaw, P. M. Duncan, eds. 2008. *Bright futures: Guidelines for health supervision of infants, children and adolescents*. 3rd ed. Elk Grove Village, IL: American Academy of Pediatrics.

Medications – Any substance that is intended to diagnose, cure, treat, or prevent disease or is intended to affect the structure or function of the body of humans or other animals.

Meningitis – A swelling or inflammation of the tissue covering the spinal cord and brain. Meningitis is usually caused by a bacterial or viral infection.

Meningococcal disease – Pneumonia, arthritis, meningitis, or blood infection caused by the bacterium *Neisseria meningitides*.

Mercury – A naturally occurring metal which has several forms. Exposure to high levels of metallic, inorganic, or organic mercury can permanently damage the brain, kidneys, and developing fetus.
Ref: Agency for Toxic Substances and Disease Registry. 1999. ToxFAQs for mercury. http://www.atsdr.cdc.gov/toxfaqs/tf.asp?id=113&tid=24/.

Methemoglobinemia – Also known as blue baby syndrome, is a blood disorder caused when nitrite interacts with the hemoglobin in red blood cells and is characterized by the inability of the blood to carry sufficient oxygen to the body's cells and tissues. Although methemoglobinemia is rare among adults, it may affect infants, when nitrate-contaminated well water is used to prepare formula and other infant foods.

Methicillin-resistant Staphylococcus aureus (MRSA) – A potentially dangerous type of staph bacteria that is resistant to certain antibiotics and may cause skin and other infections.
Ref: Centers for Disease Control and Prevention. 2008. National MRSA education initiative: Preventing MRSA skin infections. http://www.cdc.gov/mrsa/.

Methionine – A sulfur containing essential amino acid that is important in many body functions.
Ref: PubChem Compound. 2004. Methionine – compound summary. National Center for Biotechnology Information. http://pubchem.ncbi.nlm.nih.gov/summary/summary.cgi?cid=6137/.

MMR – Abbreviation for the vaccine against measles, mumps, and rubella.

Mold – Fungi that are found virtually everywhere, indoors and outdoors. Mold can cause or worsen certain illnesses (e.g., some allergic and occupation-related diseases and infections in health care settings).
Ref: Centers for Disease Control and Prevention. Mold. http://www.cdc.gov/mold/.

Molluscum contagiosum – A common skin disease that is caused by a virus. Molluscum infection causes small white, pink, or flesh-colored bumps or growths with a dimple or pit in the center.
Ref: Centers for Disease Control and Prevention. 2006. Molluscum (molluscum contagiosum). http://www.cdc.gov/ncidod/dvrd/molluscum/overview.htm.

Morbidity – The incidence of a disease within a population.
Ref: Aronson, S. S., T. R. Shope, eds. 2009. *Managing infectious diseases in child care and schools: A quick reference guide*. 2nd ed. Elk Grove Village, IL: American Academy of Pediatrics.

Motor skills – Coordinated muscle movements involved in movement, object control, and postural control perceived as occurring after a stage (or stages) involving birth reflexes, with the idea that fundamental motor skills must be mastered before development of more sport-specific skills.
Ref: Barnett, L. M., E. van Beurden, P. J. Morgan, L. O. Brooks, J. R. Beard. 2009. Childhood motor skill proficiency as a predictor of adolescent physical activity. *J Adolescent Health* 44:252-59.

MRSA – See Methicillin-resistant *Staphylococcus aureus*

Mucous membranes – Membranes that line body passages and cavities which communicate directly or indirectly with the exterior (as the alimentary, respiratory, and genitourinary tracts), that func-

tions in protection, support, nutrient absorption, and secretion of mucus, enzymes, and salts.
Ref: Merriam-Webster. 2009. Mucous membrane. Medline Plus Medical Dictionary. http://www2.merriam-webster.com/cgi-bin/mwmednlm?book=medical&va=mucous+membrane/.

Mumps – A viral infection with symptoms of fever, headache, and swelling and tenderness of the salivary glands, causing the cheeks to swell.

Nasogastric tube feeding – The administration of nourishment using a plastic tube that stretches from the nose to the stomach.

Necrotizing enterocolitis – A condition when the lining of the intestinal wall dies and the tissue falls off. This disorder usually develops in an infant that is already ill or premature, and most often develops while the infant is still in the hospital.
Ref: Medline Plus. 2009. Necrotizing enterocolitis. Medical Encyclopedia. http://www.nlm.nih.gov/medlineplus/ency/article/001148.htm.

***Neisseria meningitidis* (meningococcus)** – A bacterium that can cause meningitis, blood infections, pneumonia, and arthritis.

NOAA Weather Radio All Hazards (NWR) – A nationwide network of radio stations broadcasting continuous weather information directly from the nearest National Weather Service office. NWR broadcasts official Weather Service warnings, watches, forecasts and other hazard information twenty-four hours a day, seven days a week.
Ref: National Weather Service. 2008. NOAA weather radio now numbers 1000 transmitters! http://www.nws.noaa.gov/nwr/.

Non-prescription medications – Drugs that are available without a prescription, also known as “over-the-counter” (OTC) medications.

Non-transient, non-community water supply – A non-community water system in a location that serves the same non-resident users daily. Schools, colleges, hospitals, and factories with their own water supplies are examples.
Ref: Colorado Department of Public Health and Environment, Water Quality Control Division. 2008. Safe drinking water: A Colorado guide for non-transient non-community public water systems that use surface water. http://www.cdphe.state.co.us/wq/DrinkingWater/pdf/NTNCSurWtr_Guide.pdf.

Norovirus – Virus that causes an illness in humans called gastroenteritis. Noroviruses are very contagious. They usually are found in contaminated food or drinks, but they also can live on surfaces or be spread through contact with an infected person.
Ref: National Institute of Allergy and Infectious Diseases. 2007. Norovirus infection. http://www3.niaid.nih.gov/topics/norovirus/.

Nutritionist/Registered Dietitian – A professional with current registration with the Commission on Dietetic Registration of the American Dietetic Association or eligibility for registration with a Bachelor's and Master's degree in nutrition; a Master's degree from an approved program in public health nutrition may be substituted for registration with the Commission on Dietetic Registration. Current state licensure or certification as a nutritionist or dietitian is acceptable. See also Appendix C.

Obesity – An excess percentage of body weight (Body Mass Index equal or greater than 95%) due to fat that puts people at risk for many health problems. In children older than two years of age, obesity is assessed by a measure called the Body Mass Index (BMI).
Ref: American Academy of Pediatrics. About childhood obesity. http://www.aap.org/obesity/about.html.

Occupational therapy – Treatment based on the utilization of occupational activities of a typical child (such as play, feeding, toileting, and dressing). Child specific exercises are developed in order to encourage a child with mental or physical disabilities to contribute to their own recovery and development.

Organisms – Living things. Often used as a general term for germs (such as bacteria, viruses, fungi, or parasites) that can cause disease.

Otitis media – Inflammation or infection of the middle part of the ear. Ear infections are commonly caused by *Streptococcus pneumoniae* or *Haemophilus influenzae*.

Outbreak – A sudden rise in the incidence of a disease.
Ref: Merriam-Webster. 2010. Outbreak. Medline Plus Medical Dictionary. http://www.merriam-webster.com/medlineplus/outbreak/.

Outdoor learning environment – The physical outdoor space used during the planned program of daily activities. It encompasses the objects (natural and manufactured) within the space, the specific play and learning settings, and the interactions that occur between the caregivers/teachers and children.

Over-the-counter medication (OTC) – Medicine that can be bought without a prescription.
Ref: Food and Drug Administration. 2010. Over-the-counter medicines. Medline Plus. http://www.nlm.nih.gov/medlineplus/overthe countermedicines.html.

Overweight – Children and adolescents with a Body Mass Index (BMI) equal to or over the 85th percentile for age but less than the 95th percentile for age are considered overweight.
Ref: American Academy of Pediatrics. About childhood obesity. http://www.aap.org/obesity/about.html.

Oxygen saturation – A relative measure of the amount of oxygen that is dissolved or carried in a given medium.

Paradichlorobenzene – A white crystalline compound C6H4Cl2 made by chlorinating benzene and used chiefly as a moth repellent and deodorizer (also called PDB).
Ref: Merriam-Webster. 2011. Paradichlorobenzene. Medical Dictionary. http://www.merriam-webster.com/medical/paradichloro benzene/.

Parasite – An organism that lives on or in another living organism (such as ticks, lice, mites, etc.)

Parent/Guardian – The child's natural or adoptive mother or father, guardian, or other legally responsible person.

Pasteurized – The partial sterilization of a food substance and especially a liquid (as milk) at a temperature and for a period of exposure that destroys objectionable organisms without major chemical alteration of the substance.
Ref: Merriam-Webster. 2010. Pasteurization. Merriam-Webster Online. http://www.merriam-webster.com/dictionary/pasteurization.

Pediatric first aid – The immediate care given to a suddenly ill or injured child until a medical professional or a parent or legal guardian assumes responsibility for the medical condition from becoming worse and does not take the place of proper medical treatment.
Ref: American Academy of Pediatrics (AAP). 2005. *Pediatric first aid for caregivers and teachers*. Ed. S. S. Aronson. Boston: Jones and Bartlett; Elk Grove Village, IL: AAP. http://www.pedfactsonline.com.

Pentachlorophenol – A manufactured chemical which is a restricted use pesticide and is used industrially as a wood preservative for utility poles, railroad ties, and wharf pilings. Exposure to high levels of pentachlorophenol can have negetive effects on the body.
Ref: Agency for Toxic Substances and Disease Registry. 2001. ToxFAQs for pentachlorophenol. http://www.atsdr.cdc.gov/toxfaqs/tf.asp?id=401&tid=70/.

Perishable foods – Foods (such as fruit, vegetables, meat, milk and dairy, and eggs) that are liable to spoil or decay.
Ref: Merriam-Webster. 2010. Perishable. Merriam-Webster Online. http://www.merriam-webster.com/dictionary/perishable/.

Pertussis – A highly contagious bacterial respiratory infection, which begins with cold-like symptoms and cough and becomes progressively more severe, so that the person may experience vomiting, sweating, and exhaustion with the cough, also known as whooping cough.

Pesticides – A chemical used to kill pests, particularly insects.

Phenylketonuria (PKU) – A genetic disorder in which the body can't process part of a protein called phenylalanine (Phe).
Ref: National Institute of Child Health and Human Development. 2009. Phenylketonuria. Medline Plus. http://www.nlm.nih.gov/medlineplus/phenylketonuria.html.

Phthalates – A group of chemicals used to make plastics more flexible and harder to break, also known as plasticizers. They are used in products, such as vinyl, adhesives, detergents, oils, plastics, and personal-care products.
Ref: National Report on Human Exposure to Environmental Chemicals. 2011. Fact sheet: Phthalates. Centers for Disease Control and Prevention. http://www.cdc.gov/exposurereport/Phthalates_Fact Sheet.html.

Physical activity – Any bodily movement produced by the contraction of skeletal muscle that increases energy expenditure above a basal level. Physical activity generally refers to the subset of activity that enhances health.
Ref: National Center for Chronic Disease Prevention and Health Promotion. 2011. Physical activity for everyone: Glossary of terms. Centers for Disease Control and Prevention. http://www.cdc.gov/physicalactivity/everyone/glossary/index.html.

Age-appropriate physical activity – Physical movement that is suitable for a specific age.

Moderate physical activity – Levels that are at intensities faster than a slow walk, but still allow children to talk easily. It increases your heart rate and breathing rate. You may sweat, but you are still able to carry on a conversation; you can talk, but you probably can't sing.
Ref: Nemours Health and Prevention Services. 2009. *Best practices for physical activity: A guide to help children grow up healthy – For organizations serving children and youth.* Newark, DE: Nemours Health and Prevention Services. http://www.nemours.org/filebox/service/preventive/nhps/paguidelines.pdf.

Structured physical activity – Caregiver/teacher-led, developmentally appropriate, and fun physical movement. Structured activity should include: a) Daily planned physical activity that supports age-appropriate motor skill development (the activity should be engaging and involve all children with minimal or no waiting); and b) Daily, fun physical activity that is vigorous (gets children "breathless" or breathing deeper and faster than during typical activities) for short bouts of time.
Ref: Nemours Health and Prevention Services. 2009. *Best practices for physical activity: A guide to help children grow up healthy – For organizations serving children and youth*. Newark, DE: Nemours Health and Prevention Services. http://www.nemours.org/filebox/service/preventive/nhps/paguidelines.pdf.

Unstructured physical activity – Physical movement that is child-led free play. Unstructured activity should include: a) Activities that respect and encourage children's individual abilities and interests; and b) Caregiver/teacher engagement with children, support for extending play, and gentle prompts and encouragement by caregivers/teachers, when appropriate, to stay physically active.
Ref: Nemours Health and Prevention Services. 2009. *Best practices for physical activity: A guide to help children grow up healthy – For organizations serving children and youth*. Newark, DE: Nemours Health and Prevention Services. http://www.nemours.org/filebox/service/preventive/nhps/paguidelines.pdf.

Vigorous-intensity physical activity – Rhythmic, repetitive physical movement that uses large muscle groups, causing a child to breathe rapidly and only enabling them to speak in short phrases. Typically children's heart rates are substantially increased and they are likely to be sweating.
Ref: Nemours Health and Prevention Services. 2009. *Best practices for physical activity: A guide to help children grow up healthy – For organizations serving children and youth.* Newark, DE: Nemours Health and Prevention Services. http://www.nemours.org/filebox/service/preventive/nhps/paguidelines.pdf.

Physical therapy – The use of physical agents and methods (such as massage, therapeutic exercises, hydrotherapy, electrotherapy) to assist a child with physical or mental disabilities to optimize their individual physical development or to restore their normal body function after illness or injury.

Pica – A pattern of eating non-food materials (e.g., dirt or paper).
Ref: Medline Plus. 2008. Pica. Medical Encyclopedia. http://www.nlm.nih.gov/medlineplus/ency/article/001538.htm.

Picaridin – An EPA registered synthetic ingredient formulated for use in insect repellents.
Ref: Centers for Disease Control and Prevention. 2010. Insect repellent use and safety. http://www.cdc.gov/ncidod/dvbid/westnile/qa/insect_repellent.htm.

Picocuries – A measure of concentration of radiation per liter of air.

Plagiocephaly – Refers to a head that is abnormally shaped from a variety of causes.
Ref: Eunice Kennedy Shriver National Institute of Child Health and Human Development. 2007. Positional plagiocephaly. National Institutes of Health. http://www.nichd.nih.gov/health/topics/positional_plagiocephaly.cfm.

Pneumonia – An acute or chronic disease marked by inflammation of the lungs and caused by viruses, bacteria, or other microorganisms and sometimes by physical and chemical irritants.

Poison Center – Service that provides poison expertise treatment advice by phone. All poison centers can be reached by calling the same telephone number: 1-800-222-1222. Poison centers are staffed by pharmacists, physicians, nurses, and poison information providers who are toxicology specialists.
Ref: American Association of Poison Control Centers. About AAPCC. http://www.aapcc.org/dnn/About/tabid/74/Default.aspx.

Polybrominated diphenyl ether (PBDE) – Flame-retardant chemicals that are added to plastics and foam products to make them difficult to burn.
Ref: Agency for Toxic Substances and Disease Registry. 2004. ToxFAQs for Polybrominated diphenyl ethers (PBDEs). http://www.atsdr.cdc.gov/toxfaqs/tf.asp?id=900&tid=183/.

Polymer panels – A glass-like panel that is made of polymers and which serves to protect or add design elements to a living/play area.

Pooling – A practice in larger child care settings where children of various ages are brought together as they arrive at the beginning of the day or depart at the end of the day to consolidate the number of staff needed to meet child:staff ratios.

Postural drainage – Body positioning resulting in the gradual flow of mucous secretions from the edges of both lungs into the airway so secretions can be removed from the lungs by coughing.

Potable – Suitable for drinking.

Prenatal – Existing or occurring before birth (as in prenatal medical care).

Preschooler – A child from achievement of self-care routines (such as toilet learning/training) and the age of entry into a regular school; usually three to five years of age (thirty-six to fifty-nine months of age).

Prescription medications – Medications that can only be prescribed by a licensed practitioner (such as a physician or nurse practitioner).

Primary care provider – A person who by education, training, certification, or licensure is qualified to and is engaged in providing health care. A primary care provider coordinates the care of a child with the child's specialist and therapists.
Ref: Donoghue, E. A., C. A. Kraft, eds. 2010. *Managing chronic health needs in child care and schools: A quick reference guide.* Elk Grove Village, IL: American Academy of Pediatrics.

Professional development – A continuum of learning and support opportunities designed to prepare individuals for work with and on behalf of young children and their families, as well as opportunities that provide ongoing experiences to enhance this work. These opportunities lead to improvements in the knowledge, skills, practices, and dispositions of early childhood professionals. Professional development programs encompass both education and training programs: Education programs help learners to "...have a deep foundation of factual knowledge, understand facts and ideas in the context of a conceptual framework, and organize knowledge in ways that facilitate retrieval and application." Education programs are broad based: They include learning experiences specific to a primary area of inquiry (e.g., child development, early childhood education, or related fields including elementary education and early childhood special education), as well as subjects of general knowledge (e.g., mathematics, history, grammar). Education programs typically lead to an associate's, baccalaureate, or graduate degree or other credit-based certification. These programs provide the foundations for a lifetime of professional practice, expanded upon through experience and ongoing professional development. Education programs also may include continuing education programs that lead to the award of continuing education units (CEUs), but not college credits. Training programs are specific to an area of inquiry and set of skills related to an area of inquiry (e.g., a workshop series on positive discipline for preschoolers). Completion of training participation can lead to assessment for award of the Child Development Associate (CDA) Credential or another type of credential, CEUs, clock hours, or certification.
Ref: National Research Council. 1999. *How people learn: Bridging research and practice*, 12. Eds. M. S. Donovan, J. D. Bransford, J. W. Pellegrino. Washington, DC: National Academy Press.

Projectile – A fired, thrown, or otherwise propelled object.

Prone – Lying face-down.
Ref: Merriam-Webster. 2009. Prone. Medline Plus Medical Dictionary. http://www.merriam-webster.com/dictionary/prone/.

Prosthetic devices – An artificial body replacement adapted to reproduce the form and, as much as possible, the function of the missing part.

Protective barrier – Type of containment or deflector system that surrounds and obstructs primarily vehicle passage into a play area, such as bollards and posts. Barriers must pass impact tests for the highest speed limit allowed and posted on the street, road or parking lot adjacent to the outdoor play area.
Ref: ASTM International (ASTM). 2009. F2049-09b: Standard safety performance specification for fences/barriers for public, commercial, and multi-family residential use outdoor play areas. West Conshohocken, PA: ASTM.

Pseudomonas aeruginosa – A type of organism that is commonly a contaminant of skin sores but that occasionally causes infection in other parts of the body and is usually hospital-acquired.

Psychosocial – Involving aspects of social and psychological behavior (as in a child's psychosocial development).

Purulent – Containing pus, a thick white or yellow fluid.

Purulent conjunctivitis – Also known as "Pink eye," a white or yellow eye discharge, often with matted eyelids after sleep, and including eye pain or redness of the eyelids or skin surrounding the eye. This type of conjunctivitis is more often caused by a bacterial infection, which may require antibiotic treatment.

PVC (polyvinyl chloride) – Chemical, made up of many chains of vinyl chloride, used to make a variety of plastic products including pipes, wire and cable coatings, and packaging materials. PVC is made up. Vinyl chloride is a known carcinogen.
Ref: Agency for Toxic Substances and Disease Registry. 2006. Public health statement for vinyl chloride. http://www.atsdr.cdc.gov/phs/phs.asp?id=280&tid=51/.

Quality rating and improvement system (QRIS) – A systemic approach to assess, improve, and communicate the level of quality in early and school-age care and education programs. Similar to rating systems for restaurants and hotels, QRIS award quality ratings to early and school-age care and education programs that meet a set of defined program standards.
Ref: National Child Care Information and Technical Assistance Center. About QRIS. http://nccic.acf.hhs.gov/qrisresourceguide/index.cfm?do=qrisabout#1/.

Radon – A radioactive gaseous element formed by the disintegration of radium that occurs naturally in the soil. Radon is considered to be a health hazard that may lead to lung cancer.

Reflux – An abnormal backward flow of stomach contents into the esophagus.

Registration – Permission from a state that is required to operate a child care facility. Some states use this term to describe their regulatory process instead of the word licensing.
Ref: National Child Care Information and Technical Assistance Center, National Association for Regulatory Administration. 2010. The 2008 child care licensing study. http://naralicensing.org/display common.cfm?an=1&subarticlenbr=205.

Rescue breathing – The process of breathing air into the lungs of a person who has stopped breathing. This process is also called artificial respiration.

Respiratory syncytial virus (RSV) – A virus that causes colds, bronchitis, and pneumonia.

Respiratory tract – The nose, ears, sinuses, throat, and lungs.

Return demonstration – An individual demonstrating what (procedure, technique, etc.) they just learned.

Rheumatic fever – A severe infectious disease often occurring after a strep infection. Rheumatic fever is characterized by fever and painful inflammation of the joints and may result in permanent damage to the valves of the heart.

Rhinorrhea – Excessive mucous secretion from the nose.
Ref: Merriam-Webster. 2009. Rhinorrhea. Medline Plus Medical Dictionary. http://www2.merriam-webster.com/cgi-bin/mwmednlm?book=Medical&va=rhinorrhea.

Rhinovirus – A virus that causes the common cold.

Rifampin – An antibiotic often prescribed for those exposed to an infection caused by *Haemophilus influenzae* type b (Hib) or *Neisseria meningitidis* (meningococcus), or given to treat an infection caused by tuberculosis.

Ringworm – A fungal infection that may affect the body, feet or scalp.
Ref: Aronson, S. S., T. R. Shope, eds. 2009. *Managing infectious diseases in child care and schools: A quick reference guide*. 2nd ed. Elk Grove Village, IL: American Academy of Pediatrics.

Roseola – A viral infection causing rash in infants and children that primarily occurs between six and twenty-four months of age.
Ref: Aronson, S. S., T. R. Shope, eds. 2009. *Managing infectious diseases in child care and schools: A quick reference guide*. 2nd ed. Elk Grove Village, IL: American Academy of Pediatrics.

Rotavirus – A virus that causes diarrhea and vomiting.
Ref: Aronson, S. S., T. R. Shope, eds. 2009. *Managing infectious diseases in child care and schools: A quick reference guide.* 2nd ed. Elk Grove Village, IL: American Academy of Pediatrics.

Rubella – A mild viral illness usually lasting three days, with symptoms of red rash, lowgrade fever, swollen glands, and sometimes achy joints also known as German measles, three-day measles, or light measles.

Safety vacuum release system (SVRS) – A system or device capable of providing vacuum release at a suction outlet (as in a swimming pool) caused by a high vacuum occurrence due to a suction outlet blockage. SVRS devices must allow for the vacuum release with or without the suction outlet cover(s) in place, and shall operate in such a way as to not defeat or disengage other layers of protection installed to protect against suction entrapment.
Ref: North Carolina Department of Environment and Natural Resources. 2005. Top 20 frequently asked questions about SVRS and anti-entrapment drain covers. http://www.deh.enr.state.nc.us/ehs/quality/svrs_faq05.doc.

Salmonella – A type of bacteria that causes food poisoning (salmonellosis) with symptoms of vomiting, diarrhea, and abdominal pain.

Salmonella paratyphi – The bacterium responsible for paratyphoid fever. This Salmonella serotype has three forms: A, B, and C.
Ref: Centers for Disease Control and Prevention. 2008. National typhoid and paratyphoid fever surveillance. http://www.cdc.gov/nationalsurveillance/typhoid_surveillance.html.

Salmonella typhi – The bacterium responsible for causing the life-threatening illness typhoid fever.

Salmonellosis – A diarrheal infection caused by *Salmonella* bacteria.

Sanitize – See Appendix J: Selecting an Appropriate Sanitizer or Disinfectant.

Scabies – An infestation of the skin by small insects called mites.
Ref: Aronson, S. S., T. R. Shope, eds. 2009. *Managing infectious diseases in child care and schools: A quick reference guide*. 2nd ed. Elk Grove Village, IL: American Academy of Pediatrics.

Scarlet fever – A fine red rash that makes the skin feel like sandpaper caused by a streptococcal infection.
Ref: Aronson, S. S., T. R. Shope, eds. 2009. *Managing infectious diseases in child care and schools: A quick reference guide*. 2nd ed. Elk Grove Village, IL: American Academy of Pediatrics.

School-age child – For the purposes of early care and education settings, a child at the entry into regular school, including kindergarten through sixth grade.

School-age child care facility – A facility offering activities to school-age children before and after school, during vacations, and non-school days set aside for such activities as caregivers'/teachers' in-service programs.

Screen time – Time spent watching TV, videotapes, or DVDs; playing video or computer games; and surfing the internet.
Ref: Guide to Community Preventive Services. 2010. Obesity prevention: Behavioral interventions to reduce screen time. http://www.thecommunityguide.org/obesity/behavioral.html.

Screening – Examination of a population group or individual to detect the existence of a particular disease (such as diabetes or tuberculosis). See also Developmental screening.

Secondary infection – When a person is infected by an organism that had originated from the illness of another person. The first person infected has the primary infection, and any persons infected from the originally infected person is said to have contracted a secondary infection.

Secretion – Wet material, such as saliva, that is produced by a cell or a gland and that has a specific purpose in the body.

Sedentary activity – Non-moving activity like reading, playing a board game, or drawing.
Ref: Nemours Health and Prevention Services. 2009. *Best practices for physical activity: A guide to help children grow up healthy – For organizations serving children and youth*. Newark, DE: Nemours Health and Prevention Services. http://www.nemours.org/filebox/service/preventive/nhps/paguidelines.pdf.

Seizure – A sudden attack or convulsion due to involuntary, uncontrolled burst of electrical activity in the brain that can result in a wide variety of clinical manifestations, including muscle twitches, staring, tongue biting, loss of consciousness, and total body shaking.

Sensory table – A piece of equipment consisting of a liner set inside of a frame; water and sand are popular fillers, but almost anything can be used.
Ref: Hunter, D. 2008. What happens when a child plays at the sensory table? *Young Children* 63(6): 77-79.

Sepsis – An infection that involves the presence of pathogenic organisms or their toxins in the blood or body tissues.

Serotype – A group of intimately related microorganisms distinguished by a common set of antigens. For example, Salmonella has many serotypes including typhimurium and enteritidis.
Ref: Merriam-Webster. 2009. Serotype. Medline Plus Medical Dictionary. http://www2.merriam-webster.com/cgi-bin/mwmednlm?book=Medical&va=serotype/.

Serum – The clear liquid that separates in the clotting of blood.

Sexual orientation – An emotional or affectional attraction to another person. This includes heterosexuality (attraction to the opposite sex), homosexuality (attraction to the same sex), and bisexuality (attraction to either sex).
Ref: American Psychological Association. Sexual orientation and homosexuality. http://www.apa.org/helpcenter/sexual-orientation.aspx.

Shelter-in-place – The process of staying where one is located and taking shelter, rather than trying to evacuate.

Ref: National Association of Child Care Resource and Referral Agencies, Save the Children. 2010. Protecting children in care during emergencies. http://www.naccrra.org/publications/naccrra-publications/publications/8960503_Disaster Report-SAVE_MECH.pdf.

Shiga toxin-producing *E. coli* (STEC) – Bacterial intestinal tract infection that causes diarrhea.

Shigella – A type of bacterium that causes bacillary dysentery or shigellosis, a diarrheal infection.

Shigellosis – A diarrheal infection caused by the *Shigella* bacterium.

SIDS – See Sudden Infant Death Syndrome (SIDS)

Small family child care home – See Family child care

Special facility for children who are ill – See Facility for children who are mildly ill

SSRI (selective serotonin reuptake inhibitors) – A type of medication used to treat depression, anxiety disorders, and some personality disorders.
Ref: National Institute of Mental Health. 2010. What medications are used to treat anxiety disorders? http://www.nimh.nih.gov/health/publications/mental-health-medications/what-medications-are-used-to-treat-anxiety-disorders.shtml.

Stackable cribs – Cribs that are built in a manner that there are two or three cribs above each other that do not touch the ground floor.

Staff – All personnel employed at the facility, including directors, caregivers/teachers, and personnel who do not provide direct care to the children (such as cooks, drivers, and housekeeping personnel).

Standard precautions – Use of barriers to handle potential exposure to blood, including blood-containing body fluids and tissue discharges, and to handle other potentially infectious fluids and the process to clean and disinfect contaminated surfaces.

Standing orders – Orders written in advance by a health care provider that describe the procedure to be followed in defined circumstances.

Staphylococcus – A common bacterium found on the skin that may cause skin infections or boils.

Streptococcal pharyngitis (strep throat) – A disease caused by a *Streptococcus* bacterium.
Ref: Aronson, S. S., T. R. Shope, eds. 2009. *Managing infectious diseases in child care and schools: A quick reference guide*. 2nd ed. Elk Grove Village, IL: American Academy of Pediatrics.

Streptococcus – A common bacterium that can cause sore throat, upper respiratory illnesses, pneumonia, skin rashes, skin infections, arthritis, heart disease (rheumatic fever), and kidney disease (glomerulonephritis).

Structured physical activity – See Physical activity

Substitute staff – Caregivers/teachers hired for a temporary time frame (one day or for an extended period of time), who work under direct supervision of a trained, permanent caregiver/teacher.

Suction – The removal of respiratory secretions or mucous of a child to aid in breathing.

Sudden Infant Death Syndrome (SIDS) – The sudden death of an infant under one year of age, which remains unexplained after a thorough case investigation, including performance of a complete autopsy, examination of the death scene, and review of the clinical history.
Ref: American Academy of Pediatrics, Task Force on Sudden Infant Death Syndrome. 2009. The changing concept of sudden infant death syndrome: Diagnostic coding shifts, controversies regarding the sleeping environment, and new variables to consider in reducing risk. *Pediatrics* 123:188.

Supine – Lying on the back or with the face upward.
Ref: Merriam-Webster. 2009. Supine. Medline Plus Medical Dictionary. http://www2.merriam-webster.com/cgi-bin/mwmednlm?book=Medical&va=supine/.

Swaddling – The act of wrapping an infant tightly in a blanket.
Ref: Healthy Children. 2009. Responding to your baby's cries. American Academy of Pediatrics. http://www.healthychildren.org/English/ages-stages/baby/crying-colic/Pages/Responding-to-Your-Babys-Cries.aspx.

Systemic – Pertaining to a whole body rather than to one of its parts.

TB – See **Tuberculosis**

Tdap – Abbreviation for the immunization against tetanus, diphtheria, and pertussis.

Thermal injury – Bodily injury due to burns.

Thrush – A yeast infection predominately produced by the *Candida albicans* organisms causing mouth infections in young infants.
Ref: Aronson, S. S., T. R. Shope, eds. 2009. *Managing infectious diseases in child care and schools: A quick reference guide*. 2nd ed. Elk Grove Village, IL: American Academy of Pediatrics.

Toddler – A child between ambulation to accomplishment of self-care routines such as use of the toilet, usually thirteen through thirty-five months of age.

Touch supervision – Within an arm's reach or able to touch the child at all times. This concept has derived from the supervision of children during water play.
Ref: American Academy of Pediatrics. 2004. Policy statement: Swimming programs for infants and toddlers. *Pediatrics* 114:1126.

Toxoplasmosis – A parasitic disease usually causing no symptoms. When symptoms do occur, swollen glands, fatigue, malaise, muscle pain, fluctuating low fever, rash, headache, and sore throat are reported most commonly. Toxoplasmosis can infect and damage an unborn child while producing mild or no symptoms in the mother.

Transmission – The passing of an infectious organism or germ from person to person.

Tremolite – A mineral that can occur in fibrous form (an asbestos).
Ref: Agency for Toxic Substances and Disease Registry. 2001. Toxicological profile for asbestos. http://www.atsdr.cdc.gov/toxprofiles/tp61-c10.pdf.

Tributyltin oxide – A volatile organic compound, used as a wood preservative.
Ref: American Chemical Society. 2008. Tributyltin oxide. http://portal.acs.org/portal/acs/corg/content?_nfpb=true&_pageLabel=PP_ARTICLEMAIN&node_id=841&content_id=WPCP_008064&use_sec=true&sec_url_var=region1&__uuid=0e0ad17e-1ead-4697-9c59-0d591d56bdd4/.

Tricolosan – A chemical with antibacterial properties; used in consumer products such as detergents, soaps, skin cleansers, deodorants, lotions, creams, toothpastes, and dishwashing liquids.
Ref: Centers for Disease Control and Prevention. 2009. Triclosan. http://www.cdc.gov/exposurereport/pdf/Triclosan_FactSheet.pdf.

Tricyclic antidepressants – Any of a group of antidepressant drugs (as imipramine, amitriptyline, desipramine, and nortriptyline).

Ref: Merriam-Webster. 2009. Tricyclic antidepressant. Medline Plus Medical Dictionary. http://www.merriam-webster.com/dictionary/tricyclic antidepressants/.

Tuberculosis (TB) – A disease caused by an infection with the bacteriaMycobacterium tuberculosis that usually involves the lungs but could affect other parts of the body.

Tummy time – The time an infant spends on his stomach (tummy) throughout the day. Tummy time is only for when the infant is awake, alert and being watched.
Ref: Healthy Children. 2010. Back to sleep, tummy to play. American Academy of Pediatrics. http://www.healthychildren.org/English/ages-stages/baby/sleep/pages/Back-to-Sleep-Tummy-to-Play.aspx.

Ulcerative colitis – A disease that causes inflammation and sores, called ulcers, in the lining of the rectum and colon.
Ref: National Institute of Diabetes and Digestive and Kidney Diseases. 2006. Ulcerative colitis. http://digestive.niddk.nih.gov/ddiseases/pubs/colitis/.

Under-immunized – A person who has not received the recommended number or types of vaccines for his/her age according to the current national and local immunization schedules.

Unitary surface material – A cushioned surface material (such as rubber mats or a combination of rubberlike materials held in place by a binder) for placement under and around playground equipment that forms an uninterupted shock absorbing surface.

Universal precautions – See Standard precautions

Vacuum breaker – A device put on a pipe containing liquid (such as drinking water) to prevent the liquid from being sucked backward within the pipe.

Varicella-zoster – An illness with rash and fever caused by the varicella-zoster virus, also known as chickenpox.
Ref: Aronson, S. S., T. R. Shope, eds. 2009. *Managing infectious diseases in child care and schools: A quick reference guide*. 2nd ed. Elk Grove Village, IL: American Academy of Pediatrics.

Vector borne diseases – A disease in which the pathogenic microorganism is transmitted from an infected individual to another individual by an arthropod (e.g., insect) or other agent, sometimes with other animals serving as intermediary hosts.
Ref: Center for International Earth Science Information Network. CIESIN thematic guides: Changes in the incidence of vector-borne diseases attributable to climate change. Columbia University. http://www.ciesin.columbia.edu/TG/HH/veclev2.html.

Vegan – Individual who does not eat meat, poultry, fish, eggs, or dairy products; the individual only eats plant foods.
Ref: Healthy Children. 2010. Vegetarian diets for children. American Academy of Pediatrics. http://www.healthychildren.org/English/ages-stages/gradeschool/nutrition/pages/Vegetartian-Diet-for-Children.aspx.

Vegetarian – An individual who does not eat meat, poultry, or fish. Variations of vegetarians include: Lacto-ovo-vegetarians who consume eggs, dairy products, and plant foods and lacto-vegetarians who eat dairy products and plant foods but not eggs.
Ref: Healthy Children. 2010. Vegetarian diets for children. American Academy of Pediatrics. http://www.healthychildren.org/English/ages-stages/gradeschool/nutrition/pages/Vegetartian-Diet-for-Children.aspx.

Ventilation – Method of controlling the environment with air flow.
Ref: Occupational Safety and Health Administration. Ventilation. U.S. Department of Labor. http://www.osha.gov/SLTC/ventilation/index.html.

Venlafaxine – A medication in a class of medications called selective serotonin and norepinephrine reuptake inhibitors (SNRIs).
Ref: Medline Plus. 2009. Venlafaxine. Drugs and Supplements. http://www.nlm.nih.gov/medlineplus/druginfo/meds/a694020.html.

Viandas – Root vegetables common in some diets.
Ref: Block, G., P. Wakimoto, C. Jensen, S. Mandel, R. R. Green. 2006. Validation of a food frequency questionnaire for Hispanics. *Preventing Chronic Disease* 3(3): 1-10. http://www.cdc.gov/pcd/issues/2006/jul/pdf/05_0219.pdf.

Vigorous-intensity physical activity – See Physical Activity

Virus – A microscopic organism, smaller than a bacterium, that may cause disease. Viruses can grow or reproduce only in living cells.

Volatile organic compound (VOC) – Emitted gases from certain solids or liquids. VOCs include a variety of chemicals. Many types of household products contain VOCs, including paints, paint strippers, adhesives, cleaners, pesticides, building materials, and office equipment.
Ref: The National Women's Health Information Center. 2009. The environment and women's health: Frequently asked questions. http://womenshealth.gov/faq/environment-womens-health.cfm#hh.

Volunteer – An individual who is not paid and gives their time to work at an early care and education program. See Standard 1.3.2.3 for qualifications.

Water play activities – Activities that involve the use of water such as swimming, wading, sprinklers, and water play tables.
Ref: Milnes, S. Web-based learning units. Wonderful water. Better Kid Care, Penn State University. http://betterkidcare.psu.edu/angel units/onehour/waterplay/waterlesson.html.

West Nile virus (WNV) – An infectious disease due to a virus spread by infected mosquitos.
Ref: Aronson, S. S., T. R. Shope, eds. 2009. *Managing infectious diseases in child care and schools: A quick reference guide.* 2nd ed. Elk Grove Village, IL: American Academy of Pediatrics.

A

B

*Corrected page number in second printing, August 2011

*Corrected page number in second printing, August 2011

*Corrected page number in second printing, August 2011

*Corrected page number in second printing, August 2011

D

*Corrected page number in second printing, August 2011
***Addition to Index in second printing, August 2011

*Corrected page number in second printing, August 2011
***Addition to Index in second printing, August 2011

G

H

*Corrected page number in second printing, August 2011
**Corrected to "staff" from "stall" in second printing, August 2011

*Corrected page number in second printing, August 2011

*Corrected page number in second printing, August 2011

J

K

L

*Corrected page number in second printing, August 2011

M

*Corrected page number in second printing, August 2011

P

Q

R

*Corrected page number in second printing, August 2011

S

*Corrected page number in second printing, August 2011

*Corrected page number in second printing, August 2011
**Corrected to "of" from "by" in second printing, August 2011
***Addition to Index in second printing, August 2011

T

*Corrected page number in second printing, August 2011
**Corrected to "surface" from "swimming" in second printing, August 2011

U

V

W

*Corrected page number in second printing, August 2011

Z